ADOLESCENT DEPRESSION

A Johns Hopkins Press Health Book

Francis Mark
MONDIMORE, MD

Patrick
KELLY, MD

ADOLESCENT DEPRESSION

2nd
Edition

A Guide for Parents

Johns Hopkins University Press
Baltimore

Note to the reader: This book is not meant to substitute for medical care of people with depression or other mental disorders, and treatment should not be based solely on its contents. Instead, treatment must be developed in a dialogue between the individual and his or her physician. Our book has been written to help with that dialogue.

Drug dosage: The author and publisher have made reasonable efforts to determine that the selection of drugs discussed in this text conform to the practices of the general medical community. The medications described do not necessarily have specific approval by the U.S. Food and Drug Administration for use in the diseases for which they are recommended. In view of ongoing research, changes in governmental regulation, and the constant flow of information relating to drug therapy and drug reactions, the reader is urged to check the package insert of each drug for any change in indications and dosage and for warnings and precautions. This is particularly important when the recommended agent is a new and/or infrequently used drug.

© 2002 Francis Mark Mondimore
© 2015 Johns Hopkins University Press
All rights reserved. Published 2015
Printed in the United States of America on acid-free paper
9 8 7 6 5 4 3 2 1

Johns Hopkins University Press
2715 North Charles Street
Baltimore, Maryland 21218-4363
www.press.jhu.edu

Library of Congress Cataloging-in-Publication Data
Mondimore, Francis Mark, 1953–
    Adolescent depression : a guide for parents / Francis Mark Mondimore, MD, and Patrick Kelly, MD. — Second edition.
    pages cm. — (A Johns Hopkins press health book)
    Includes bibliographical references and index.
    ISBN 978-1-4214-1789-9 (hardcover : alk. paper) — ISBN 978-1-4214-1790-5 (pbk. : alk. paper) — ISBN 978-1-4214-1791-2 (electronic) — ISBN 1-4214-1789-8 (hardcover : alk. paper) — ISBN 1-4214-1790-1 (pbk. : alk. paper) — ISBN 1-4214-1791-X (electronic) 1. Depression in adolescence—Popular works. I. Kelly, Patrick, 1978– II. Title.
    RJ506.D4M66 2015
    616.85′2700835—dc23   2015002501

A catalog record for this book is available from the British Library.

Figures 3-1, 3-2, 3-3, 5-1, 5-2, 5-3, 7-1, 8-1, and 15-1 by Jacqueline Schaffer.

Special discounts are available for bulk purchases of this book. For more information, please contact Special Sales at 410-516-6936 or specialsales@press.jhu.edu.

Johns Hopkins University Press uses environmentally friendly book materials, including recycled text paper that is composed of at least 30 percent post-consumer waste, whenever possible.

The authors dedicate this book to their parents,

Frank and Winifred Mondimore,

and Pat Kelly, Sr., and Vicki Kelly

CONTENTS

PREFACE

Francis Mondimore's essential publication of the first edition of *Adolescent Depression* fundamentally changed the conversation among adolescents, parents, and providers when it comes to this condition. He brought to light a different (and correct) view of depression as a biological illness that needs to be taken as seriously as diabetes or any other medical condition, altering forever the way in which parents see their children.

But, as with all things, work in the study and treatment of adolescent depression has progressed, and we thought that you, the reader, could benefit from being brought up to date on the latest information. In the thirteen years that have elapsed since the book's initial publication, many changes, large and small, have affected the field of psychiatry. Every chapter in this new edition has been updated to reflect the most current evidence base in terms of diagnosis, treatment, and advice for both parents and children. We cover and explain new treatments, both medication and psychotherapy. In an extensive discussion of bipolar affective disorder in young persons, we attempt to examine rationally how and why this diagnosis, once perceived as extremely rare, has suddenly become so common. We also introduce discussions of new topics, such as the interface between autism and depression. One of the biggest changes in the field of psychiatry, a new version of our basic system of diagnosing patients, has recently rocked the psychiatric field and is an essential change for parents and adolescents to understand so they can have an educated discussion with their physician.

We go through the changes relative to young persons and how this new way of looking at psychiatric conditions may change your child's treatment, diagnosis—or both.

Nonetheless, the central message of this text remains the same. For a long time, mental health professionals thought that serious depression was an illness only adults were likely to develop. The general belief among psychologists and psychiatrists was that children might get a little sad or upset about some disappointment or frustration, but that they weren't emotionally mature enough to experience true depression. Gloominess and "angst" were thought to be almost universal among adolescents, but only temporary —just a developmental stage that they would emerge from unscathed.

Research done in the 1990s demolished these myths. We now realize that young people do indeed get seriously depressed. In fact, as is becoming clear, depressive illnesses and bipolar disorders that start in adolescence may be more serious and more difficult to treat than adult-onset mood disorders. A 2013 study sponsored by the Centers for Disease Control and Prevention estimated that 4 percent of young people between the ages of 3 and 17 years had been diagnosed with a depressive illness, with adolescents more likely than their younger counterparts to be diagnosed (up to 13 percent).[1] It's been estimated that nearly one in five persons will go through a period of serious depression during their lifetime, and research increasingly indicates that many of these people will have had their first encounter with depression as teenagers.

Some parents still struggle with the idea of their child being treated for a psychiatric illness, seeing a therapist, or taking medication for a problem that they may think—and hope—might be "just a phase." We hope to persuade you in this book that serious depression in adolescents is an illness— an illness that can be effectively treated.

Clinical studies have shown that depression is underdiagnosed in young people and undertreated as well. A study in 2000 found that only 20 percent of seriously depressed adolescents in a community sample received any treatment for their problem. The same study found high rates of relapse in these young people, and even more disturbing was the finding that, by their twenty-fourth birthday, many of them had developed other psychiatric problems in addition to depression, most commonly alcoholism and drug abuse.[2]

We now know that depression comes in many forms and is often the symptom of a collection of emotional illnesses that psychiatrists call mood disorders. Some adolescents with a mood disorder are troubled by "down" and sad feelings—the feelings people usually think of when they hear the word *depression*. But other adolescents with a mood disorder have predominantly irritable moods with angry outbursts, temper tantrums, and destructive rages, problems that seem to bear little relationship to what most people think of as depression. Can the same illness really look so different from one young person to the next? Why? These are some of the questions we hope to answer in this book.

This is not a "how to talk to your teenager" book. Adolescent mood disorders are complex, poorly understood, and potentially dangerous illnesses, and parents want the facts about these illnesses. What are the danger signals of serious depression in teenagers? How are mood disorders diagnosed? What are the implications of the different diagnoses? How does depression relate to other problems, like drug abuse, attention-deficit/hyperactivity disorder (ADHD), and eating disorders? What are the available treatments? How can parents of an adolescent with a mood disorder help their child get the best treatment possible? What else can parents do? You'll find answers to all these questions in this book.

We have organized the book by dividing it into four parts. Part I, Symptoms, Syndromes, and Diagnosis, focuses on recognizing serious depression in adolescents and on understanding why mood disorders are real illnesses. It reviews some of the unique issues of emotional development during adolescence that may explain why mood disorders express themselves differently in young people than in adults. We also try to explain something about the diagnostic process in psychiatry and the classification of mood disorders.

Part II, Treatment, reviews the different medications and other medical treatments used to treat depression, as well as the types of psychotherapy and counseling that have been shown to be useful, how these very different treatments relate to each other, and why a combination of both medication and therapy is the most useful approach to treating depression.

Part III, Variations, Causes, and Connections, discusses other problems that often complicate the picture in depressed adolescents, such as ADHD and eating disorders and the dangerous and frightening issues of suicidal behavior and "cutting." A chapter on the inheritance of mood disorders and evidence for the genetic basis of these illnesses rounds out this part of the book.

Part IV, Getting Better and Staying Well, contains the real-world, practical information you need to maximize the effectiveness of treatment and minimize the chances of relapse and complications. Finding a good treatment team, dealing with insurance issues, and handling such emergencies as dangerous behaviors and hospitalization are some of the issues covered here. We specifically seek to open the "black box" of mental health treatment and diagnosis in chapter 16, wherein we describe the various, seemingly innumerable types of mental health professionals and what their particular roles in your child's treatment should be. We also expose our own means of reaching a diagnosis, and give general guidelines (and warnings) to parents about what to look for when seeing a psychiatrist.

WE HOPE THAT AFTER READING THIS BOOK YOU WILL better understand the symptoms, the treatments, the complications, and what we know about the causes of mood disorders in adolescents. More important, we hope you will feel better equipped and more confident about helping your depressed adolescent get the most out of treatment, on the road to recovery, and on the path to becoming a happy and healthy adult.

ACKNOWLEDGMENTS

Patrick Kelly

My first and most gracious acknowledgment goes to Francis Mondimore, without whom this book would not have been possible. This is both for the obvious reason, but also, and more important, for his mentorship. He taught me how to write, how to think, and how to be a good psychiatrist (or at least try, by modeling myself after such a great one).

I'd also like to thank our editor, Jacqueline Wehmueller, whose encouragement and advocacy are critical to any success that this book might have.

And thanks to Michael Lindsay, without whose unwavering support this book would be an unrealized dream.

Above all, I'd like to thank you, the readers of this book. Psychiatrists get to close up their office and go home at night. Any person or family member who has struggled with depression knows that it is a twenty-four-hour-a-day, seven-day-a-week struggle against the darkness, and that continued striving toward success, such as by educating yourself through this work, is sometimes the bravest and most difficult thing you can do. Thank you.

Francis Mark Mondimore

I'd like to thank those who have helped me in the writing of this book. First, many, many thanks to Sallie Mink, RN, of DRADA (Depression and Related Affective Disorders Association) at Johns Hopkins, who suggested the project to me in the first place and who was a constant source of support and encouragement.

Thanks to all my colleagues in the Affective Disorders Section of the Department of Psychiatry and Behavioral Sciences at Johns Hopkins, especially Anthony Drobnick, MD, for feedback, encouragement, and support.

Thanks to Jacqueline Schaffer for her handsome illustrations, and special thanks to all the wonderful staff of Johns Hopkins University Press, most especially my editor, Jacqueline Wehmueller. I have been fortunate indeed to work with such a dedicated and talented group of people.

And thanks, once again, to Jay Allen Rubin, my biggest fan and frankest critic, for always being there.

ADOLESCENT DEPRESSION

Introduction

For many years, psychiatrists and psychologists proposed that serious depression was rare, even impossible, in children and adolescents. We now know this is not true. In fact, you'll see the words *adolescent depression* in magazine articles and newspaper stories practically every day.

Often the term appears in a context that is frightening for parents worried that their child may be depressed: a story about adolescent drug abuse or suicide. Parents can become so frightened at the thought of these destructive and violent problems affecting their family that they can't decide what to do next. Sometimes the thought "my child would *never* do something like *that*" tempts parents to minimize the severity of the symptoms of this treatable illness, perhaps allowing them to talk themselves out of seeking psychiatric evaluation for their teenager. On the other hand, it's possible to panic, perhaps rushing off to an emergency room in the middle of the night after finding some gloomy poetry that a teenager has left lying around. What should parents do if they think their adolescent might have a problem with serious depression? If an adolescent has been diagnosed with serious depression, what are the implications? How best to help?

We would be lying to you if we said that adolescent depression was something psychiatrists understand completely. But there is a lot we *do* know about depression in young people. Admittedly, quite a lot was initially based on what we knew about adults. Using this knowledge as a springboard, psychiatry found some significant differences in the form the de-

pressive illness can take in younger persons who are still undergoing phe-
nomenal amounts of biological growth and development, not to mention
the psychological tasks of defining themselves.

That word *illness* is key. What is unequivocally clear is that serious depression is the symptom of an illness—actually a group of illnesses, called
mood disorders. The symptoms of depression should be approached in the
same way we would approach *any* symptoms that might indicate a serious
illness: taking the potential problem seriously, getting the adolescent to an
evaluation by the proper professional expert as soon as possible, and par-
ticipating in treatment by monitoring symptoms and treatment response,
being supportive and encouraging, and following through on any other recommendations from the treatment team.

The horror stories you read in newspapers are often the result of *not* following this approach—a serious depression that has gone unrecognized or,
worse, that was suspected but not treated, for a variety of reasons: fear of a
"mental illness" diagnosis, misinformation about psychiatric medications
based on rumors and inaccuracies, or the erroneous idea that mood disorders are not "real" diseases. Parents of a child with diabetes don't generally
worry over "what the neighbors will think" about their child's diagnosis
and treatment. Parents of a child with leukemia don't usually blame themselves for their child's illness or wonder "what did we do wrong?" Serious
depression *is* a serious medical illness and should be approached no differently from any other illness.

When physicians see an adolescent who may be suffering from depression (we'll discuss later why a physician, preferably a psychiatrist trained
in the treatment of children and adolescents, needs to be one of the first
professionals involved), their approach will be the usual medical approach
to symptoms and illnesses: getting all the facts about the symptoms, performing an examination of the patient, perhaps doing some lab tests, and
making a diagnosis. That symptoms are mostly emotional rather than
physical—sadness, loss of interest in things, rather than abdominal pains
or fever—doesn't change anything about needing a medical approach to
what may turn out to be a medical problem. The examination involves talking and listening to the patient rather than using a stethoscope or blood
pressure cuff, but psychiatrists have years of training that enable them, by

just this method, to draw out mental experiences from patients and pick up subtle changes in psychological functioning that are the signs of illness.

Like physical illnesses, mood disorders have characteristic patterns of symptoms and a characteristic "natural history," that is, a predictable way in which the illness usually runs its course. To make predictions about a medical problem, a diagnosis must first be made. The most important prediction a diagnosis allows is a prediction of what treatment will be effective at restoring the patient to health.

In psychiatric illnesses, as in no other group of medical problems, people get distracted by "why" questions and forget to focus on "what" questions. For the surgeon treating a person with a broken leg, *why* the patient's leg is broken (a car accident? skiing mishap?) is of relatively little interest. The *what* question (What's wrong with this patient? His leg is broken *here* and *here*) is the focus of attention. The answers to these kinds of questions determine the treatment plan. Psychiatry is not that much different: treatment is determined by answering the question "What kind of depression does this person suffer from?" Major depressive disorder? The depression of bipolar disorder? The minor, temporary depression we call an adjustment disorder? The answer must be determined before other questions become relevant: Is he depressed because he broke up with his girlfriend? Because he didn't get into the college that was his first choice? These kinds of questions are related to the search for diagnosis, but they usually become really relevant only *after* a diagnosis has been made.

This way of thinking about people and their emotions doesn't come naturally to us. We have all experienced being sad after a loss or apprehensive in the face of uncertainty, so we expect that all bad emotional feelings come about in this way. We have become accustomed to expecting to find reasons for unpleasant emotions in a person's life and experience. But this kind of analysis can lead us dangerously astray in the case of serious depression: looking for "reasons" can distract from the diagnosis, and thus delay the treatment, of a serious illness.

A more familiar example will illustrate. Perhaps your child, like many children, went through a period of having "tummy aches" on school mornings if she was nervous about school or simply didn't want to go. But the question that popped into your mind that first morning was probably not

"Why doesn't my child want to go to school?" but rather "What's wrong with my child? What illness might explain these pains?" It's probably a safe bet that you took your child's temperature, put her to bed and watched her closely, and perhaps called or even took her to the pediatrician to make sure it wasn't an illness, such as food poisoning or appendicitis, that needed medical attention. You would wonder about the judgment of any parent who didn't take these steps, wouldn't you? Even a visit to the emergency room wouldn't be an overreaction if the child seemed to be in extreme distress. Only after medical problems had been ruled out, when it was clear that the child wasn't ill, would it have been appropriate to start looking for psychological explanations: reasons that the child might not want to go to school.

The book begins, then, by describing the symptoms of these illnesses: mood disorders. Understanding how psychiatrists approach a problem with adolescent depression, make a diagnosis, and decide on a treatment plan is an important first step for the parent who wants to know how to help.

Since the first version of this work was published in 2002, the field of psychiatry, particularly that branch focusing on younger patients, has experienced many changes. These changes have affected every aspect of this book—including even the meaning of the title. "Adolescent" is now a more ambiguous term and encompasses a larger group. The new generation of millennials, as opposed to Generation X-ers, are experiencing something of a prolonged adolescence. Traditionally, the field of "child" psychiatry focused on patients until they turned 18, at which point they were considered adults. Although this is still true in many legal situations (including some relating to their care, which we deal with later in the book), an entirely new focus on "transitional aged youth," those between approximately 16 and 24, has emerged. These young persons are in many ways more similar to their younger neighbors in age than to their older ones—many are still in school, still struggling to define their individual identity, unmarried and without children, sometimes still depending on (or even living with) their parents. They differ from the prior generation in other ways as well, including an increased suspiciousness of psychiatry and psychiatric treatment, yet an increased willingness to share all aspects of their lives (including psychiatric diagnoses), sometimes with negative social ramifications. Later on in the book, we discuss how adolescents can sometimes misuse social media to spread messages that inadvertently harm themselves or others, including bullying and sharing dark, sometimes graphic, stories of their own struggles. The face of adolescence has shifted, providing an increased challenge to these young persons and to their parents.

The term in the other half of the title, "Depression," has also experienced some changes in what it encompasses and signifies. Since 2002, depression has been increasingly recognized (in many cases, thanks to this book) in younger and younger children. This has been a boon to patients because their symptoms are getting treated, and the stigma surrounding the condition is lessening. Other trends have cropped up, however, that may have been less helpful. Primary pediatricians began to get increasingly involved in psychiatric treatment, and up to around 2005, there was a large increase in antidepressant prescriptions. There seemed to be such a swing of the pendulum that providers saw a particular type of these medications—SSRIs, or selective serotonin reuptake inhibitors—as a sort of cure-all for any low mood, with little to no attention paid to the psychological overlays of real-world problems that were either the causes of or the result of the depression.

In 2005, the situation changed, when the FDA put a black box warning (the most severe warning possible) on these medications based on the results of a study (later debunked) that seemed to indicate that these medications may double the rates of suicide in adolescents. As we now know, the factor most likely to predispose an adolescent to suicide is untreated depression, but the pendulum had swung again. Now no pediatricians would prescribe these critical medications; even general psychiatrists were fearful. Even today, many providers feel uncomfortable prescribing medications to address depression, leaving many people untreated. This is why it is crucial for patients and parents to acquire an in-depth understanding of these medications—including when the medications should and, sometimes more important, should not be used—and to have an educated and enlightened discussion with their psychiatrist before beginning on any path of treatment.

Although we focus in this book on the changes in the psychiatric field, the foundations of our science are still rooted in the same guiding principles. We urge readers not to do that which is most tempting—to skip ahead to the "treatment" section of this text. Treatment must be guided by diagnosis. Medicating a low mood that is not the result of the illness of depression is like trying to treat seasonal allergies with an antibiotic (a drug useful only for addressing bacterial infections)—no effect at all. Similarly, ignoring a serious depression through the misunderstanding that the "blues" will go away on their own can have the same result as withholding antibiotics from a serious bacterial infection—dire consequences indeed. Before jumping ahead to pick your child's medication, first spend some time learning what exactly may be behind her symptoms and which symptoms are important to pay attention to. We want to take you down the same path we as psychiatrists would take in diagnosing a patient and developing a treatment plan. This book is organized to do exactly that. Many complain that psychiatry and psychiatric treatment is at best a mystery, at worst a guessing game. We hope to open this subject up and show you precisely how a good psychiatrist will come to a conclusion about what has been afflicting you or your child and how to best help in recovery.

Part I

SYMPTOMS, SYNDROMES & DIAGNOSIS

WHAT IS DEPRESSION? Doesn't everybody feel down now and then, especially teenagers? How can we tell when depression is serious? These are some of the questions we answer in this first part of the book.

We begin with a chapter on what depression is, how to recognize it, and more important, how it differs from the normal "downs" everyone experiences. This chapter also has an introduction to some of the theories of what causes depression, including a discussion of how we have learned that biological changes in the brain are at the root of serious depressive illness.

In chapter 2, we take a closer look at the psychology of adolescence and explain why depression often takes different forms in adolescents than in adults—so different that it may be hard to recognize.

Chapter 3 gets into the nitty-gritty of the diagnostic process in psychiatry, with an introduction to how psychiatrists think about depression and mood disorders, then an outline and description of the different types of depression that are seen in adolescents.

The part ends with a more detailed look at the diagnostic scheme for mood disorders that is currently used by the American Psychiatric Association: the *Diagnostic and Statistical Manual of Mental Disorders* (the *DSM*). As of this writing, the *DSM* has recently undergone its first revision in over a decade, one that changes the fundamental way it views patients. We discuss how adolescents are seen in both versions. Most important, we explain why it's critical not to view the *DSM* as the "bible of psychiatry," as it has often been called, but rather to see it as an imperfect work in progress that is a helpful guide to, but not the ultimate authority on, understanding treating actual patients in the real world.

Depression

Some Definitions

The word *depression* comes from Latin roots that mean "pressed down." Many of the common words we use to describe the feelings of depression describe, in one way or another, a downward direction or position. People talk about feeling "down in the dumps" or "low" or simply "down." The many synonyms for depression that begin with the same two letters, like "*des*pondent" and "*de*jected," share the Latin-derived prefix *de-*, which signifies a downward direction (as in "*de*scend").

Other words for depression cast it as the *opposite* of something: we say we are "unhappy" or "discontented," emphasizing the opposite of the good feelings of happiness or contentment. Still other words for depression conjure up the *absence* of something: the depressed are said to be "gloomy," a word that denotes an absence of light; or "dispirited," an absence of that vital spark of life we call spirit; or "desolate," the absence of just about everything. All these words capture something of the feeling of depression.

But if you listen to people who have suffered from serious depressive illnesses talk about their experiences (more on why we psychiatrists see this as an illness in a bit), you soon learn that depression is not a moving down or away from something and not really a lack of something; rather, it is a something that comes over its sufferers and imposes itself on them. William James, the great nineteenth-century American psychologist-turned-philosopher, who suffered from depression, said that, far from an absence of something, depression is "positive and active anguish...wholly unknown to healthy life."[1] William Styron, the Pulitzer Prize–winning author of the novel *Sophie's Choice*, wrote in his memoir of severe depressive illness, *Darkness Visible*, of feeling "a poisonous fogbank roll in upon my mind."[2] The prolific author J. K. Rowling introduced us to the Dementors in her Harry Potter novel series. "Dementors are among the foulest creatures that walk this earth...they drain peace, hope, and happiness out of the air around them. Get too near a Dementor and every good feeling, every happy memory will be sucked out of you... You'll be left with nothing but the worst experiences of your life."[3] They were one of the most feared specters in Harry's world and perfectly personified the effects of a depressive episode—which the author is public about having experienced in her life. In a separate interview, she described her bout with depression as the "absence of being able to envisage that you will ever be cheerful again. The absence of hope. That very deadened feeling, which is so very different from feeling sad."[4]

From the ancient Greeks comes the word *melancholy*, derived from their words for "black bile," the bodily fluid whose excess they believed caused the state of misery we now call depression. They conceptualized depression as caused by a disturbance of bodily functioning, an out-of-balance state of the four vital bodily fluids called "humors" (the other three were water, blood, and yellow bile). After several thousand years of attempts at other explanations, this idea should strike us today as an astonishingly modern one, an idea that some have now returned to with such phrases as "chemical imbalance" to describe where depression comes from.

But to define depression accurately, we need to define another word, *mood*, because any definition of depression must include the idea of *low mood*. Our mood includes our happiness or sadness, our state of optimism or pessimism, our feelings of contentedness or dissatisfaction with our situation, even physical feelings such as how fatigued or robust we feel. Mood is like our emotional temperature, a set of feelings that expresses our sense of emotional comfort or discomfort.

When people are in a good mood, they are confident and optimistic, relaxed and friendly, patient, interested, content. The word *happy* captures part of it, but good mood includes a lot more. The mental picture most people have of the boisterous adolescent is a good illustration of what *good mood* means. Many teenagers feel confident and energetic and have a sense of physical well-being; they sleep soundly and eat heartily. It's easy for them to be sociable and affectionate; the future looks bright, and the moment is ripe for starting new projects.

In a low mood, an opposite set of feelings takes over. People tend to turn inward and may seem preoccupied or distracted by their thoughts. The word *sad* captures some of the experience, but low mood is a bit more complicated. There may be a sense of emptiness and loss. People with low mood find it difficult to think about the future and, when they do, find it hard not to be pessimistic or even intimidated by it. Teenagers may be impatient and irritable, losing their temper more easily and then feeling guilty about having done so. They have difficulty being affectionate or sociable, so they avoid others and prefer to be alone. Energy is low, motivation ebbs away, and interest is dulled. Self-doubt takes over; they become preoccupied, worrying even more than usual about how other people see them. As you will see later in this part of the book, depression is sometimes complicated and difficult to spot, especially in adolescents. But the core feature of depression, its defining characteristic, is the cluster of symptoms we call *low mood*.

NORMAL AND ABNORMAL MOODS

Some of life's stresses and the normal human reactions to them are such everyday experiences that common terms have been coined for the associated mood changes—and most people recognize these mood changes as quite normal. Moving to a new community where we don't know anyone often leads to a sense of dislocation and loneliness that we know as *homesickness*, an unpleasant experience that may last for days or even weeks, a mood that everyone has probably experienced at one time or another. When someone close to us dies, we experience a profound sense of sadness and loss that can become temporarily incapacitating—the deep sorrow that we call *bereavement* or mourning.

At the time of various milestones of personal achievement, we experience changes of mood in the other direction. On the occasion of a graduation or winning a championship game or a coveted scholarship, a teenager can be filled with joy and pride and a sense of limitless optimism, feelings that can be nearly overwhelming. We wouldn't call any of these moods "abnormal," even though they can be extreme.

Like many other things we can measure in human beings—body temperature, blood pressure, hormone levels, for example—a person's mood state normally varies within a certain range. People, especially adolescents, are not in the same mood state for long; it is quite normal for everyone to have ups and downs of mood. So, low mood is sometimes *normal*. But there are other times when it is not, when it is the symptom of a *mood disorder*.

THE *SYMPTOM* OF DEPRESSION

Just like physical pain, then, periods of low mood are universal human experiences. People grieve when a loved one dies, are disappointed when an eagerly anticipated trip must be canceled, are heartbroken when a romance ends unexpectedly. In these cases, feelings of depression seem normal. No one would think of low mood in such circumstances as a symptom of anything pathological.

It's not difficult to think of situations when even physical pain can be regarded as almost normal. If the initial lawn mowing in the spring is the first bout of vigorous physical exercise after months of wintry inactivity, waking up the next morning with stiff and sore muscles is no surprise. Spend too much time out in the sun without proper protection, and a painful sunburn results. But no one thinks of after-exercise soreness as a muscle disease or would call the pain from a sunburn an abnormal reaction. Some healing needs to take place in both cases, but neither makes one worry that something in the body isn't working as it should.

But if you woke up one morning after mowing the lawn with achy muscles and joints *as well as* a fever, headache, and scratchy throat and cough, you wouldn't blame these symptoms on unaccustomed exercise. The other symptoms that accompany the sore muscles, especially the fever, indicate that something else is going on—in this case, probably a nasty virus. The *collection* of symptoms points toward a viral infection, even though one of the symptoms—the muscle aches—might be expected after too much physical exertion. A *clinical syndrome* includes a collection of symptoms and clinical findings that point toward a particular illness or group of illnesses.

When depressed mood is accompanied by certain other symptoms (table 1-1), such as disordered sleep and appetite, and includes severe irritability or a severe loss of energy and interest in usual activities, one should suspect that the individual might be suffering from a depressive *illness*—even if there are reasons that would explain one of the symptoms: low mood. Psychiatrists begin to consider the diagnosis of a mood disorder when they find that the patient has the *syndrome* of depression.

THE *SYNDROME* OF DEPRESSION

The core *symptom* of depression, low mood, can show up in many different situations, some of which can be called normal, such as feelings of bereavement during a period of mourning. The *syndrome* of depression indicates the presence of a serious medical problem that requires treatment. A case history will illustrate.

Table 1-1 Symptoms of Depression

Mood Symptoms
  Depressed mood
  Pervasive, constricted quality of mood
  Irritability
  Loss of ability to experience pleasure (anhedonia)
  Guilty feelings
  Loss of interest in usual activities
  Social withdrawal
  Suicidal thoughts
Cognitive (Thinking) Symptoms
  Poor concentration
  Poor memory
  Indecision
  Slowed thinking
  Loss of motivation
Bodily Symptoms
  Sleep disturbance
    Insomnia
    Hypersomnia
  Appetite disturbance
    Weight loss
    Weight gain
  Fatigue
  Headaches
  Constipation
  Worsening of painful conditions

▼ Susan had been thinking for weeks about how to bring it up to her husband. "Tom, I think we made a mistake taking Charlie out of Springfield."

"What do you mean?" said her husband, putting down the newspaper he'd been reading. "Edgemont is the best prep school in Columbia; how could it be a mistake? What makes you think that?"

Susan had closed her book and laid it on her lap. She looked down at its cover, then up at her husband sitting across the den, and said, "I think Charlie's unhappy at Edgemont. He misses his friends at Springfield."

Tom's face, which had frowned with concern briefly, relaxed at this. He picked up the newspaper from his lap and started to scan the columns again. "Is that all you're worried about? He'll get over it, Sue. He had to change schools twice during junior high because of our transfers, and he handled it without any problems." Then Tom lowered the paper again. "Does he talk about missing his friends?"

"Well, I asked him how school was going the other day, and he told me he wasn't sure. He said he felt like he wasn't fitting in, that he's felt disconnected since school started."

"That's not so unusual for a kid starting at a new school at this age. Teenagers are so sensitive about that kind of thing."

"Charlie also said he's worried he might not be as smart as the kids at Edgemont. Tom, that's not like Charlie at all. He's a smart boy, and he's always known it. He's always been so confident about himself."

"Well, I still think it's some kind of adolescent phase. This is only November; give the kid a chance to settle in. Besides, it's not like he was against transferring into Edgemont."

Tom had gotten an important promotion within his company the previous spring—with a hefty salary increase. Tom and Susan could now afford to send their son to a prestigious private school and had asked Charlie what he thought about transferring. "Wow, that would be super!" Charlie had said enthusiastically. "Springfield is a good school and all, but Edgemont Prep! Have you seen their computer labs?"

Tom continued, "Charlie talked all summer about how much he wanted to join some of the computer clubs at Edgemont."

"Well, that's just it. He hasn't."

Tom's face became more serious. "He hasn't?"

"No. He seems to have lost interest in computers altogether."

"Are you sure?"

"Do you remember that computer graphics thing he ordered last month for his PC? So his computer games would work better? It finally came last week, and I put it on his desk in his room." Susan looked down at her closed book again. "I was putting clean clothes in his bureau this morning, and I found it in the bottom drawer."

"Well, maybe it was the wrong piece; maybe it was incompatible or something."

"He hadn't even opened the package. He'd just stuffed it in a drawer."

"Wow, that's not like Charlie at all."

"Another thing," Susan continued. "He goes right to his room when he comes home from school and sleeps. I can't get him to come to dinner at all. I'm sure he's lost weight."

"Well, that's not so unusual, is it? Kids sleep more at this age, don't they?" Tom asked.

"I don't know—not this much, I don't think," said Susan. "Last Sunday, he was in bed most of the day and all night. That can't be normal."

"He has been extra quiet the past few weeks. Let me talk to him and see what I can find out."

"Please do, Tom. I'm worried."   ▲

Let's review the facts of this "case" for a moment. The most significant fact is that Charlie's mother has noticed that Charlie is just not himself. Though you won't find this listed in diagnostic manuals, it's significant and typical of mood disorders. The individual seems to undergo a change in so many aspects of emotional life that those around him, even if they can't quite list details, notice that he is simply different. Sometimes parents have trouble pinning it down, but often, if they think about it, they realize that the activities, enthusiasms, and energy they've come to take for granted in their teenager seem to have drained out of him. Sometimes parents will be tempted to doubt these subtle intuitions that something is wrong and, like Tom in this vignette, ascribe what they notice to "a phase" their teenager is going through. This is usually a mistake. Susan has noticed that her son's energy level, motivation, and interest level have changed. Her intuition that this isn't normal is quite correct and must not be simply dismissed in the face of a contrary opinion, even if that opinion comes from the son himself.

This is a critical point, particularly when it comes to young people. Adolescents are still discovering who they are and how they feel. They may not have the language to describe their feelings, or even be in touch enough with their emotional state to detect such a variation. The official term for this state is *alexithymia*, meaning a lack of awareness regarding one's internal emotional thermometer. Even the *Diagnostic and Statistical Manual of Mental Disorders (DSM)* recognizes this problem, particularly in this age group. Although we don't typically stick to the letter of the *DSM* criteria unless we are embarking on a scientific study, for the reasons we give throughout this book, these criteria do allow the official, full-fledged diagnosis of depression in children and adolescents even if they deny having a low mood, as long as those around them take notice of the low mood. In fact, this conflict between how adolescents identify feeling and how others perceive them can lead to struggles. When adolescents feel down or low, they can perceive others pointing this out as criticism rather than an observation. They can become defensive, even angry—emotions that, of course, could be amplified if they are in fact depressed. In most cases, attempting to "prove" to them that they are depressed devolves quickly into a power struggle and an argument, so this approach usually isn't that helpful. Agreeing to disagree, and keeping one's eye on the adolescent—prepared to respond should the situation not improve—is usually a better course of action.

But what specifically can point to a low mood, even if those experiencing it don't recognize it themselves? Let's again look at the facts of the case above. Psychiatrists use the word *anhedonia* to designate a loss in one's ability to enjoy things. It is one of the defining features of the depressive syndrome and worth discussing in more detail. Derived from the Greek word for "pleasure," *anhedonia* can be defined as loss of the ability to experience pleasure. One of Charlie's favorite things seems to be his computer—which makes his stuffing a new, unopened piece of hardware into a drawer an indicator of something very wrong. When depressed, adolescents will lose interest in sports, friends and socializing, extracurricular activities, or favorite classes or subjects. They have much more difficulty deriving any pleasure from listening to music, going to a movie, or engaging in the sports or hobbies they usually enjoy. This is an important feature and, at times, can be somewhat deceiving. A depressed adolescent may be able to have something of a mildly pleasurable experience, but the stimulus required to get her that brief moment of sunshine is far higher than what would usually make her happy.

For example, one of us has treated a patient whose parents thought she was not depressed. "She had fun on her birthday. We took her to her favorite place, Disneyland, with all her friends, and she seemed to enjoy herself; she was just a little shyer than usual." This girl was eventually diagnosed with depression. Her old self, her well self, would have been delighted to go to Disneyland. She would have had trouble sleeping due to her excitement, talked constantly in the car on the way there, and run from her parents toward the characters to embrace them. Her last trip, while she was depressed, did bring on a few smiles, and she did seem to enjoy the new ride, but she was far more subdued than would be expected. And this is the difference: depression causes a change in our behavior, in who we are and what we like to do. It is not so black and white as to mean that a depressed person can never, under any circumstances, derive any pleasure from anything. Rather, it means that the amount of pleasure derived from a given task is much lower than usual. Another patient of ours was so depressed that the only thing she found pleasurable was eating doughnuts, though she was simultaneously afraid to gain weight. So she would take an entire box of doughnuts and lick the frosting off them—her only pleasurable experience in an otherwise miserable existence.

Great writers, artists, and musicians who suffered from depression have left us poignant and vivid descriptions of this unresponsiveness to pleasure. In his novel *The Sorrows of Young Werther*, Johann Wolfgang von Goethe has his main character express a loss of responsiveness to the joys and beauty of nature: "Nature lies before me as immobile as on a little lacquered painting, and all this beauty cannot pump one drop of happiness from my heart to my brain."[5] People with depression describe food losing its taste, colors draining away from sunrises and landscapes, flowers losing their textures and perfumes—everything becoming bland, dull, and lifeless. For some, the bright and beautiful things in the world become a source of anguish rather than pleasure. The nineteenth-century Austrian composer Hugo Wolf described a terrible sense of sorrowful isolation during his depressions, a feeling of separation from the world of ordinary pleasures—all the more painful when it occurred in springtime: "What I suffer from . . . I am quite unable to describe. This wonderful spring with its secret life and movement troubles me unspeakably. These eternal blue skies, lasting for weeks, this continuous sprouting and budding in nature, these coaxing breezes impregnated with spring sunlight and fragrance of flowers . . . make me frantic. Everywhere this bewildering urge for life, fruitfulness, creation—and only I . . . may not take part in this festival of resurrection, at any rate not except as a spectator with grief and envy."[6]

Now imagine what it is like when these terrible feelings come over young persons who are just learning to make sense of their feelings, adolescents who are still trying to understand their emotional reactions to the world. Young adolescents, especially, will have difficulty identifying and describing their internal emotional states, and the word *depression* often doesn't mean much to them. This may be one of the reasons that low mood in adolescents sometimes is associated with prominent irritability. Frightened and frustrated by their depressive feelings, young people sometimes lash out at anyone and anything around them. In some adolescents, the irritability can even be the most prominent aspect of their change of mood. This is such a common phenomenon that it is even recognized in the *DSM*. To qualify to enter even the most strict research study, an adolescent can have a purely irritable mood instead of a self-expressed "depressed" mood and still meet full criteria.

Another differentiating factor between a "normal" low mood and the depressive syndrome is that individuals with a mood disorder lose the normal *reactivity* of their mood states. When persons who do not suffer from a mood disorder go through a period of low mood, such as after a romantic disappointment, the loss of a job, or a period of homesickness, they retain the normal *reactivity* of mood, that is, the normal changeability of mood in relation to what is going on around them.

Anyone who has attended a funeral and then returned to the home of the bereaved afterward has probably observed—and perhaps experienced—this normal reactivity of mood. Mourners who might be grief stricken during the funeral service or at the graveside can often relax, reminisce about good times they had with the person who has died, and enjoy catching up with friends and relatives perhaps not seen for a long time. The reactivity of mood is also retained in the lonely or homesick person who goes to the movies, can lose himself in a good film, and forget about his longing for more familiar surroundings. If the depressed mood is a "normal" one, we are able to dispel the feelings of bereavement, isolation, or disappointment—even if it's only for a few hours.

The depressed mood of the syndrome of depression, on the other hand, is frequently *constricted*. Years ago, AM radio stations used to give away free radios, gifts that came with only one catch: they couldn't be tuned to any of the sponsoring station's competitors. These radios were built to receive only the signal of the station that gave them away. The mood state of the person suffering from a depressive disorder is like one of those radios, "set" to receive only one mood signal: depression. The mood of the syndrome of depression is a relentless, pervasive gloom that continues from one day to the next, week after week. As William Styron said of his own depression, "The weather of depression is unmodulated, its light a brownout."[7]

We've just discussed the under-reactive, constricted mood of a true depressive syndrome. It is worth pointing out that, in some cases, the mood state actually appears to be hyper-reactive. An adolescent will suddenly seem touchy and irritable, will explode at the slightest provocation, and will continue a fight against all attempts at amelioration. Though not the most common pattern, we must emphasize that what is lost in a depressive syndrome is the "normalness" of mood reactivity—for most people it diminishes, though for some it seems to be on a hair trigger. However, it is always focused on the negative, sad, or angry aspects of a person's life.

Perhaps the most continuous characteristic of the depressive syndrome is a preoccupation with negative thoughts: depressed individuals often find their thinking dominated by thoughts of inadequacy or loss, regret, and even hopelessness. In depressed adolescents, worries about not "measuring up" in some way that seems out of character for them are not uncommon. Charlie's worry that he's not smart enough to compete in his new school would be a typical kind of negative thought, especially indicative of depression since, as his mother says, he's never been troubled by such a worry. Guilty ruminations are especially characteristic of the syndrome of depression, and psychiatrists often make a special point to ask about guilty feelings when evaluating a person for depression. Unrelenting ruminations on themes of guilt, shame, and regret are common in the depressed states of mood disorders, and they are uncommon in "normal" low mood states. An adolescent who talks about being responsible for his difficulties in some way, who describes himself as "lazy" or "worthless," may be seriously depressed. Individuals experiencing the normal depressed mood that comes after a personal loss usually attribute their bad feelings to the fact that a loss has occurred—only in unusual circumstances will they think they are to blame for the problem and be preoccupied by guilty feelings or feelings of shame. The individual with a depressive syndrome, on the other hand, frequently feels to blame for his troubles, and sometimes for other people's troubles as well. The presence of guilty preoccupations is very significant for making a diagnosis of the syndrome of depression.

ASSOCIATED SYMPTOMS OF DEPRESSION

So far we've concentrated on the mood changes seen in the depressive syndrome. But there are other symptoms as well, changes beyond the change in mood.

Severe depression almost always causes a change in sleeping pattern. Depressed persons frequently suffer from insomnia, but also from its opposite, sleeping too much (*hypersomnia* is the technical term). A peculiar rhythmic pattern of sleep disturbance and mood changes through the day sometimes seen in depressed persons is called *diurnal variation of mood* (*diurnal* is a word used in biology to refer to a twenty-four-hour cycle). Persons with this pattern fall asleep at the usual time and without much difficulty but wake up very early in the morning after only a few hours of sleep. Lying awake hours before sunrise, they experience their lowest mood of the day during this early morning period, and minor problems and regrets seem magnified and overwhelming. They notice a gradual lifting of their mood as sunrise approaches, and when the morning light comes, they can often rouse themselves and start their daily activities despite feeling worn out from fretting for those troublesome hours. As the day goes on, their mood continues to improve little by little until, by day's end, they feel nearly back to their normal self. They typically go to bed and can often fall asleep easily, but several hours later, they awaken depressed, and the cycle repeats itself.

Sleep changes in adolescents can be difficult to identify. Most adolescents go through a period of going to bed later and later, usually in order to stay awake doing fun activities, with subsequent awakening later and later in the day (the technical term is *sleep phase advance*, and it has indeed been shown through research that some adolescents, and adults, have a biological clock that prefers this state). So, how is one to differentiate between the normal changes in sleep pattern that occur as children become more social and focused on fun and those that indicate a depressive episode? Although many adolescents stay awake to enjoy themselves, depressed adolescents do so because it is the only time of the day when they feel good. As fits the diurnal variation discussed above, most persons with depression can only really feel halfway good toward the end of the day, and they want to stay up late to enjoy this period. Nondepressed adolescents will eventually fall asleep, and their body will want to make up for the late hour when they retired by causing them to sleep later. (It is not unusual for an adolescent to sleep past noon if not awakened by an alarm or another person.) Those with the depressive form of insomnia, however, will frequently awaken on their own after only a few hours of sleep and be unable to return to rest despite extreme fatigue.

In depression, as for many adolescents, getting up in the morning is a chore and can result in a transient irritability and grumpiness. For the majority of young persons, however, this quickly dissipates once they arrive at school. In depression, adolescents are persistently irritable or sullen, have trouble attending to class, and may even fall asleep (as opposed to socializing with friends).

But what of hypersomnia? It is true that some people do not experience this early morning awakening when depressed but instead want to sleep seemingly all the time. This holds true for adolescents as well and can be a key defining characteristic of those going through a depression. As we've said, many adolescents enjoy their free evening time and take advantage of it by staying awake. Those with depression will frequently return from school or other activities and either take prolonged and frequent naps or stay up to complete homework but retire unusually early—at times before their parents. In both cases, what is most critical to notice is a *change* from a regular routine. And remember, as with low mood, sleep disturbance is but a single symptom that must be evaluated in conjunction with other symptoms to diagnose the syndrome of depression.

Appetite is usually disturbed in depressed individuals. As with sleep problems, changes occur in both directions: eating too much or too little. Individuals can lose or gain a significant amount of weight during periods of depression. (We discuss the deliberate self-starvation and compulsive eating of *eating disorders* in chapter 13; these behaviors seem to be complex syndromes deserving their own dedicated discussion.)

Of the other bodily symptoms that occur in depression, a sense of fatigue with prominent low energy and listlessness is one of the most striking. Headaches, constipation, and a feeling of heaviness in the chest are common, as are other, more difficult-to-describe uncomfortable physical sensations. Whether these symptoms are caused by depression itself or arise from the lack of restful sleep, lack of exercise, and poor eating habits that depression brings is not clear. Depression seems to lower the pain threshold: depressed individuals seem more sensitive to pain and are more distressed by it.

Even young children can identify a physical pain and are able to describe a headache or a stomachache, but they may not be able to identify and name a painful psychological state. The young adolescent who may not quite understand the concept of low mood may instead complain of headaches that make her want to spend time in bed. In young adolescents who are depressed, uncomfortable physical symptoms may result in frequent physical complaints that overshadow complaints of low mood.

Depression changes thinking as well as mood. Depressed persons can experience slowing and inefficiency in their thinking and often complain of memory and concentration problems. Charlie's complaint that he's not as smart as the other students in his new school might be understood better in this way. It's possible that he is indeed not performing as well as some of the other students in his classes, but his concentration is probably adversely affected by his depression. When concentration is impaired, memory can seem to be affected as well: when we can't concentrate, our ability to register and later retrieve information is also impaired. Falling grades at school are very common in adolescent depression, and though certainly due in part to the energy and motivation problems depression causes, they are probably also caused by what psychiatrists call *cognitive* symptoms. From the Latin *cognoscere,* meaning "to know," this term refers to problems in concentration, thinking, and memory. We know, for example, that in depressed elderly persons, these sorts of thinking problems can be so severe that depression can be misdiagnosed as Alzheimer's disease. In adolescents, on the other hand, these problems may be misconstrued as ADHD (attention-deficit/hyperactivity disorder). We have seen many adolescents whose parents brought them in for an evaluation for "new-onset ADHD" when in fact the adolescent is in the throes of a depressive episode. This type of distinction is why it is absolutely critical to seek help from a qualified psychiatrist when seeking an accurate diagnosis. Analyzing individual symptoms without looking at the larger pattern can easily lead one down the incorrect path. We spend more time discussing the overlap between depression and other psychiatric disorders, like ADHD, later in this book.

MOOD DISORDERS: REAL ILLNESSES

Because everyone has gone through periods of low mood at one time or another, many people think they understand depression. Even the associated symptoms of the depressive syndrome sometimes accompany normal low mood states briefly or in a much milder form: a bit of trouble falling asleep for a night or two or a temporary loss of appetite are not that unusual after a serious disappointment or loss.

These facts can make it tempting to think that serious depressive disorders must follow the same "rules" as ordinary low mood states. They don't. Serious depressions don't get better on their own after a few days. Seriously depressed adolescents can't "shake off" their mood states or get their minds off their troubles by concentrating on school or sports or friends. They can't "get over" whatever preoccupations with loss or failure their depressive illness inflicts on them. They can't "get ahold" of themselves or "shape up," "move on," "lighten up," do something about their situation, pull themselves up by their bootstraps—or any of the things people can often do to get past a period of low mood. Adolescents with mood disorders are in the grip of their illness, and their symptoms stay with them day after day, week after week, relentlessly. It's thought that this is due to real changes of functioning in certain brain "centers" or "circuits."

It is tempting, however, to fall back on our own experiences with low mood as well as our experiences with people in general and to attribute the seriously depressed adolescent's inability to "get over" his depression symptoms to being unmotivated, lazy, stubborn, or simply not trying hard enough. This misunderstanding of what serious depression really is can lead to major problems. At worst, it can lead to the conclusion that there is nothing wrong with the teenager that time, encouragement, or stricter discipline won't solve. It might lead to the conclusion that the seriously depressed adolescent is simply "troubled" and that a few counseling sessions or a few weeks of talking to a therapist will take care of the problem. Although counseling and therapy are certainly important aspects of treating all types of depression, medical intervention, *treatment with medication,* is the mainstay of treatment of serious depressive disorder.

How do we know this?

THE CHEMISTRY OF MOOD

One of the greatest revolutions in medicine occurred during the seventeenth and eighteenth centuries, when physicians began to realize that the workings of the human body followed the rules of science. Indeed, the word *science* came to be used in its modern sense during this time and replaced the older term *natural philosophy.* Today, we take for granted that the heart is a pump and that we can understand a lot about the way it works if we understand how pumps work. After the Frenchman Jean Léonard Marie Poiseuille elucidated the laws of physics that determine the flow rate, pressure, and other properties of liquids flowing through glass tubes, it quickly became apparent that the flow of blood through arteries and veins follows the same principles. Philosophical speculations on the heart as the source of love, loyalty, and other poetic qualities and feelings disappeared and were replaced by cold hard mathematical rules and principles.

It took several hundred more years for us to realize it, but as is now quite clear, the functioning of the brain follows scientific principles as well and depends on processes that follow the rules of biochemistry (the chemistry of living things). We also know that the brain is the organ of emotions and thinking, so it follows that, at some level, thinking and emotions depend on these biological and chemical processes. It also follows that when those processes go awry, abnormalities of thinking and emotions result.

If you think about it for a moment, you'll realize that it really isn't such a new idea. People have used various chemicals to change thinking, emotions, and behavior for thousands of years. Almost as soon as we figured out how to raise crops, we discovered how to ferment some of them and began using ethyl alcohol (the alcohol in alcoholic beverages) to change the way we feel. We found substances that dull the perception of pain (aspirin from the bark of willows, morphine from poppies), substances that boost mood and energy level (caffeine from coffee beans, cocaine from coca leaves), and even substances that induce abnormal mental experiences such as hallucinations (*Psilocybe* mushrooms and the peyote cactus, among others). Ancient peoples attributed these effects to spirits or demons or gods, but during the early part of the twentieth century, biochemists isolated the active ingredients from these natural materials, and several decades later, neuroscientists discovered specific mechanisms of action for some of them (such as the discovery of receptors in the brain to which morphine binds). Our understanding of these mechanisms increased, and today, the number of naturally occurring psychoactive substances (those having an effect on the activities of the brain and nervous system) has now been far surpassed by the number of manufactured ones. We take it for granted now that chemicals, either naturally occurring or synthetic, can alter the biochemical functioning of the brain and thus alter thinking and emotions.

During the middle decades of the twentieth century, researchers discovered that several pharmaceuticals had specific effects on mood. Reserpine is a pharmaceutical extracted from the root of an Indian shrub, *Rauvolfia serpentina*. Ancient Hindu writings mention the use of the plant for medicinal purposes, but not until the 1950s was it discovered to have a potent effect on blood pressure, becoming the first effective agent to treat hypertension (high blood pressure). As was also noted, some patients who took the medication to control their blood pressure developed serious depression. Low mood gradually developed over a period of weeks and soon was accompanied by all the other manifestations of the depressive syndrome—several patients taking this drug committed suicide.

In 1951, several doctors prescribing iproniazid, a pharmaceutical used to treat tuberculosis, noticed an interesting side effect in some of their TB patients: it helped with depression. Patients with low mood, sleep and appetite disturbances, and other symptoms of serious depression had a remission of these symptoms after taking iproniazid for several weeks. Physicians at the time were puzzled by this development, as iproniazid was known to cause sometimes significant and uncomfortable side effects; however, despite the symptoms of the patients' illness and the effects of the treatment, their mood actually improved. The first *antidepressant* medication had been accidentally discovered.

In part II of the book, in the discussions of treatments, you will see that *all* the original medications used to treat mood disorders were discovered more or less accidentally. But accidental or not, the discovery of pharmaceuticals that can cause the depressive syndrome and of others that can make it better unequivocally points to the existence of a *biochemistry of mood*. A mood disorder, then, must be what occurs if something goes wrong with this chemistry.

In this chapter, we've started to give you a picture of adolescent depression, with an emphasis on the most common symptoms and an overview of some approaches to understanding it. In the next chapter, we fill in some details of this complicated picture with some facts derived from research on what is still a poorly understood illness.

Normal Adolescence and Depression in Adolescence

I t is not too far off the mark to say that our understanding of serious depressive illnesses in young people is several decades behind our understanding of depressive illnesses in adults. Fortunately, the field is catching up fast. But experts still disagree on many of the most basic facts about depression in adolescence. How frequently does serious depression occur in young people? What exactly are the symptoms? What is the best treatment approach? What are the risk factors for depression in young people? Are there protective factors? How likely is it that depression will continue to be a problem into adulthood for any given individual? Are there common complications of the illness? We go into each of these questions in turn and try to give the best, most up-to-date information regarding the answers as we understand them. But the number one question most people have for us is this: "Is *my* child depressed?" To answer this most perplexing query, it is essential to first give more information on the symptoms of depression, then to cover the changes even nondepressed adolescents go through in this life stage of nearly constant change and development.

MORE ON SYMPTOMS

There was no such thing as a field of child psychiatry before the 1930s, when Adolf Meyer, then the director of psychiatry at the Johns Hopkins Hospital, recognized a need for specialized treatment of children and adolescents. This effort was primarily driven by members of the pediatrics department, who believed themselves somewhat neglected in regard to psychosocial supports for what were obviously suffering children and families. Leo Kanner was recruited to chair the first division of child and adolescent psychiatry in the world. Kanner used his experience to gather information for his book *Child Psychiatry*, published in 1935.[1] He was ahead of his time in his assertions that children could indeed suffer from severe psychiatric abnormalities, an idea that was unfortunately ridiculed and derided by the very people who initially funded his studies—the pediatricians. They despised the idea of pathologizing what they considered the "normal," or reactive, transient depressive symptoms that they believed were a perfectly ordinary part of growing up.

In an article entitled "The Menace of Psychiatry," the famous Chicago pediatrician Joseph Brennemann wrote, "There is a menace in psychologizing the school child, psychiatrizing his behavior and over organizing his habits and his play."[2] Many took his argument to be that children cannot suffer as adults can, furthering an antipsychiatry movement within pediatrics. In fact, Dr. Brennemann clarified later that his ire was directed at the "charlatans" of psychiatry, who claim that every child is suffering from a severe psychiatric illness in need of frequent, extensive (and expensive) treatment that only they are capable of carrying out. He did believe that children can suffer from the same mood disorders as adults, but that careful time and attention must be paid to diagnosing and treating these more significant conditions so that they are neither missed nor overdiagnosed. In that, many psychiatrists would agree. But Brennemann was too late—his message was (mis)heard loud and clear by the pediatric community. Leo Kanner wrote that there "is a tendency among pediatrics to ridicule and resent any psychiatric offerings" in terms of diagnosis and treatment.[3] This unfortunate divide is only recently being mended, primarily by the increasing preponderance of research that has proved that adolescents (and children as well) show the same symptoms of depression as do adults and can develop the full depressive syndrome. In 1987, a study was conducted of 296 children and adolescents between the ages of 6 and 18 years who had been referred to a clinic specializing in child and adolescent depression and were carefully examined for depressive symptoms. A statistical analysis of the pattern of symptoms found that "the similarities across the school age in the [symptoms] of major depressive disorder far outweigh the few differences."[4] The clusters of symptoms included mood symptoms, negative thinking, anxiety symptoms, and appetite problems, and they paralleled the adult symptom pattern in both the children and the adolescents examined. A more recent study, focused on older adolescents (ages 14 to 18), also found that depressed teenagers had symptoms typical of adult depression (table 2-1).

This research also indicates that despite the similarities across age groups, some subtle patterns of symptom differences show up as one looks closely at different ages. Younger adolescents, just like small children, seem to have more in the way of anxiety symptoms: fearfulness and nervousness. They show clinging behaviors, unexplained fears, and physical symptoms of anxiety such as stomachaches and stress headaches. Older adolescents suffer more from loss of interest and pleasure, and they have more in the way of morbid thinking: thoughts of death and suicide. Conversely, they may be more likely to be irritable and angry than either younger children or adults. This special form of depression, present though less common in other age groups, has the danger of being mistaken for other psychiatric diseases (such as bipolar affective disorder, discussed in chapter 3) and can place the adolescent at great risk of misdiagnosis and ineffective treatment.

Another set of symptoms now recognized to occur in some severely depressed adolescents are what are called *psychotic symptoms*. *Psychosis* is an unfortunately vague term that is nevertheless frequently used in psychol-

Table 2-1   Symptoms of Adolescent Depression

Symptom	Percentage of Adolescents Reporting
Depressed mood	97.7
Sleep disturbance	88.6
Thinking difficulties	81.8
Weight/appetite disturbance	79.5
Anhedonia	77.3
Worthlessness/guilt	70.5
Loss of energy	68.2
Thoughts of death/suicide	54.5

Source: Peter Lewinsohn, Paul Rohde, and John Seeley, "Major Depressive Disorder in Older Adolescents: Prevalence, Risk Factors and Clinical Implications," *Clinical Psychological Review* 18, no. 7 (1998): 765–94.

ogy to describe various symptoms of losing touch with reality, specifically, hallucinations and delusions. Hallucinations are sensory perceptions without actual sensory stimuli: hearing voices when no one is present, or seeing things that no one else can see. Delusions are false beliefs that preoccupy the person with such conviction that he cannot be persuaded otherwise. He may be convinced that he has a terrible incurable illness such as cancer or AIDS or believe that his family has lost all its money, and that he will soon be homeless or institutionalized. In depressive illnesses, the delusional beliefs usually have depressing themes such as these, and the person may believe he has committed some terrible sin or crime and fear severe punishment. The hallucinations seen in psychotic depression are depressing as well: the individual may hear voices calling him bad names or condemning him, telling him he is worthless or a failure. The visual hallucinations are usually frightening and grotesque, of devils or monsters. Delusions or hallucinations in adolescent depression seem to be uncommon, but when present, they signal an especially severe illness.

It is important, however, to distinguish the intersection of what we would call a hallucination with the imaginary world of a child. A true hallucination is, as listed above, a *true* sensory perception without a stimulus. This means that the child actually hears, through his ears, another voice. The child can point to where it is coming from, and in severe cases may try to find the speaker located in his wall. An *imagined* sensory perception, or a *misinterpreted* sensory perception, is another matter entirely and is not necessarily indicative of any malign process at all. We realize that these distinctions are subtle and difficult to tell apart. Who has not known children with imaginary friends they insist are real? Do parents rush to the hospital, fearing their child is psychotic, or instead engage and possibly humor their beloved youngster by setting an extra place at the table? And who themselves has not had the experience of believing they heard their name called only to realize it was either another word entirely or (more eerily but not any more unusual) that no one was there at all? Does this indicate the sort of break with reality with which we usually associate hallucinations? Certainly not, if we experience it ourselves, but if a friend were to tell us about all the invisible people calling her name, would we not begin to worry a bit? Answering these sorts of questions—what is a hallucination and what is not?—is exactly what psychiatrists spend their lives doing and why they must work so hard and spend so much time to reach an accurate diagnosis.

We talk about how to find a skilled psychiatrist, and why it is so important to do so, later in the book. As we go along, however, try not to become overwhelmed as we present these sorts of subtle differences that we as psychiatrists must pay such close attention to. We are not attempting to write a textbook or to teach readers how to become psychiatrists. We do feel it is essential, however, to open the curtain on the world of those who daily diagnose and treat adolescents with depression and to give as clear and as accurate a picture as possible of what this illness looks like, without cutting any corners or softening any of the difficult ambiguities we regularly must face.

MORE ON ADOLESCENCE

The first person to formulate a psychological theory of adolescence was the American psychologist and educator G. Stanley Hall, who believed that emotional turmoil and crisis were always characteristic of this developmental period, something to be endured rather than understood. Writing at the beginning of the twentieth century, Hall proposed that the entire history of the human race had become part of each individual's genetic endowment and that the psychological development of each individual retold the story of human history. Borrowing a German phrase used to describe the sweeping romantic sagas of Schiller and Goethe, Hall characterized adolescence as a period of Sturm und Drang, "storm and stress," a phrase that was used to characterize adolescence for decades afterward. Hall saw adolescence as a recapitulation of the conflicts of preindustrial civilization: a time of crusades and revolutions, great chivalry and great cruelties, self-sacrifice and brutal domination, fervent loyalty and unscrupulous treachery. Adolescents passed through a time of rapidly changing moods and emotions, unbridled optimism giving way to despair, melancholy alternating with youthful exuberance, before a mature, rational adult emerged from the chaos. Even after the genetic and historical components of Hall's ideas had been discredited, his concept of inevitable emotional storminess during adolescence persisted, becoming incorporated into psychological theories that followed and even into popular thinking about adolescence.

It turns out that the "storms" most adolescents go through are fairly minor and short lived—perhaps better thought of as passing cloudbursts. Surveys of teens and their parents through the 1960s and 1970s indicated that adolescents generally tend to have positive self-concepts and place high value on the approval of their parents. A modern study, from 2011, evaluating more than 300,000 high school students, found similar results.[5] It seems, then, that though some bickering between teens and their parents about such everyday issues as what clothing they wear and what time to be in at night is common, serious conflict is not actually the norm. Sir Michael Rutter, a British child psychiatrist who has extensively researched and written about adolescent issues for several decades, puts it this way: "It is evident that normal adolescence is *not* characterized by storm, stress and disturbance. Most young people go through their teenage years without significant emotional or behavioral problems. It is true . . . that there are challenges to be met, adaptations to be made, and stresses to be coped with. However, these do not all arise at the same time and most adolescents deal with these issues without undue disturbance."[6]

A theory of adolescence that has better withstood the test of time is that of the great American psychologist Erik Erikson, who invented the term *identity crisis* in the 1960s to characterize the uncertainty, self-questioning, and existential confusion he believed was inevitable during adolescents' search for their place in the world. Erikson's concept of the identity crisis of adolescence remains one of the best formulations of these issues. Although the word *crisis* conjures up a meaning of danger and even possible catastrophe, Erikson's use of the word is more like that of the Chinese, encompassing a meaning of opportunity as well. "Turning point" might capture the idea better. According to Erikson, the main issue that confronts and preoccupies adolescents is a search for their identity as a person.

Erikson's theory has roots in psychoanalysis but emphasizes the interplay between the individual and society. You may be familiar with the "Eight Stages of Man," which he devised as the outline of his theory (table 2-2). Each of Erikson's stages represents a developmental task that confronts individuals at a particular age as they encounter ever-widening and complex social situations, expectations, and responsibilities. Erikson proposed that each stage has the possibility of a positive or a negative outcome. If individuals are able to manage a positive outcome at any particular step,

Table 2-2 The Life Cycle Stages Proposed by Erik Erikson

Stage	Age	Psychosocial Crisis
I	Infancy	Trust versus mistrust
II	Toddlerhood	Autonomy versus shame and doubt
III	Preschool age	Initiative versus guilt
IV	School age	Industry versus inferiority
V	Adolescence	Ego identity versus role confusion
VI	Young adulthood	Intimacy versus isolation
VII	Middle age	Generativity versus self-absorption
VIII	Old age	Integrity versus despair

they move on to the next with enhanced psychological coping and developmental tools. If the crisis is not well managed, the negative attribute will interfere with the next step in development, and psychological problems are more likely.

Erikson postulated that adolescence is the first time a person begins to ask, in a serious way, "Who am I?" Also pressing for attention are the related questions: "Where did I come from?" "What do I want to become?"

Bodily changes—physical growth, hormonal changes, the onset of menstruation in girls, and voice changes in boys—force the adolescent to come to terms with a new body image. Experimentations with the use of cosmetics in girls, with facial hair and body building in boys, and with clothing and hairstyles their parents don't approve of in both sexes (not to mention piercings and tattoos) are adolescents' efforts to discover their bodies and attempts at self-invention and self-definition.

During this time, greater psychological development allows adolescents to interact in more sophisticated ways with others, and they become much more preoccupied with what others think of them, often comparing these perceptions with how they feel about themselves. This may explain why teens seem determined to be centers of attention but simultaneously complain of feeling as if they are constantly being scrutinized and are "on stage." They crave feedback but at the same time are worried about what they might hear about themselves. As adolescents seek roles and models outside the home, the peer group becomes increasingly important as a reference point and sounding board. Idolization of athletes, musicians, and movie stars is part of this search for self-definition and of developing a vocational identity, the beginnings of thinking about a career.

Sexuality is another aspect of personal identity that adolescents begin to explore, and exploration of the physical aspects of sexuality is only part of the process. Adolescents first begin to feel attraction to specific people, which can be a source of strength and bonding with nonromantic friends, as they discuss their crushes and "likes," or a source of distress, teasing, and torment if those attractions are different from the norm within one's peer group. Adolescents live in an interesting era now, when individual expression is tolerated to an extent never before seen, particularly in America. Adolescents are exploring whole new definitions of sexual and gender expression and feeling supported and cared for while doing so. It is not the place of this book to judge these expressions, merely to point out how disruptive new feelings and new hormones can be to the development of the adolescent mind.

The sexuality most commonly explored through adolescence is more about relationships, about learning to emotionally pair with another and see oneself through that person's eyes, than it is about any simple physical act. Crushes and infatuations with unobtainable partners occur, with inevitable disappointment. The teenager may establish a sense of identity through couple-hood: "Who am I? I'm her boyfriend." The personal feedback of the youthful love affair helps the adolescent reflect on, redefine, and revise his image of himself. As Erikson explained it, "That is why many a youth would rather converse, and settle matters of mutual identification, than embrace."[7]

The adolescent's move toward autonomy and away from parental authority and control also means giving up some measure of parental protection and nurturance, often before secure and comfortable emotional self-reliance is possible. A stage of substituting dependence on a peer group for dependence on parents is not unusual, explaining the intense devotion among friends, cliques, and teams so often seen at this age. Extreme peer group conformity in choice of clothing styles, behavioral norms, and even the heroes and idols of the group provides acceptance and solidarity. Selection of foods and entertainment and use of language and slang expressions are in strict conformity to the peer group. Disdain, intolerance, and even cruelty toward those who act differently are common. This is a time when adolescents can become vulnerable to pathological group allegiances as well: gangs, religious cults, militaristic organizations—all groups that exploit the adolescent's tendency to view the world in terms of black and white. This is even more worrisome today with the boom of the Internet and social media, in that teens can join groups from radically different geographic regions—physical proximity is no longer enough to limit the activities of young persons. Many examples of these phenomena exist, but a particularly striking one is of online groups espousing the ideals of eating disorders, not as life-threatening psychiatric illnesses in need of treatment, but as lifestyle choices equally deserving of respect as vegetarian eating or regular triathlon training, and in the same class of healthy living. These "pro-ana" (pro-anorexia) and "pro-mia" (pro-bulimia) sites describe how much self-control and discipline these lifestyles require, placing their practitioners in a special class of person who is able to achieve "success." Eating disorders are discussed in far greater detail in chapter 13, but we use this example to show the power of social media in connecting people around the globe, at times around ideas that promote negative behavior rather than positive.

For many teenagers, the mental work accomplished in this stage of development results in succeeding in the beginning stages of determining their own identity and learning to trust themselves, balanced with a willingness to take in feedback from others and re-evaluate their values and goals in order to continue growing. The possible negative outcome of this stage, *identity diffusion*, results in an individual who is constantly bedeviled by self-doubt and either morbidly preoccupied with the opinions of others or defiantly indifferent to them. Some adolescents attempt to escape feelings of alienation and anxiety by using alcohol and drugs. In Erikson's most comprehensive consideration of adolescence, *Identity, Youth, and Crisis,* he summed up the dilemma of identity confusion by quoting Biff, a character in Arthur Miller's play *Death of a Salesman:* "I just can't take hold, Mom, I can't take hold of some kind of life."[8]

Like any developmental theory, Erikson's proposals about adolescence should not be taken as a blueprint for every individual. Most important to remember is that psychological development during adolescence is a process, not an event; it proceeds in fits and starts over a period of years (and of course, our search for the answer to the question "who am I?" is never really over at any age). Later theorists expanded and elaborated Erikson's ideas, emphasizing that the process is usually disorganized and erratic and that adolescents inevitably go through at least some period of partial identity diffusion with its accompanying feelings of alienation.

The concept of *developmental foreclosure* has been proposed by American psychologist James Marcia to describe the process whereby the adolescent identifies and commits to some aspect of self-definition by incorporating the goals and values of others without the personal searching and self-examination inherent in true identity exploration.[9] The youth espouses the political or religious views of parents or significant others, sometimes fervently, but without an open exploration and consideration of alternatives. If, for some reason, some aspect of this "foreclosed" identity no longer fits, a temporary crisis can ensue until the adolescent readjusts or perhaps even reinvents this aspect of her identity. An adolescent who has unquestioningly accepted the teachings of the church she was raised in may be forced to question her allegiance to the denomination if she finds her developing political or social ideology at odds with its dogma. A period of questioning, searching, and perhaps stress and confrontation ensues before one or the other jarring element of identity is adjusted.

Inevitably, all this testing, exploring, questioning, and adjusting is psychologically stressful. The adolescent suffers disappointments in relationships, disillusionment with cherished ideas or values, frustration that the answer to "who am I?" keeps changing, anxiety that the answer to "what do I want to become?" isn't as clear as it seemed during childhood. It should not be surprising, then, that anxiety and low mood are common in adolescence.

Michael Rutter and his colleagues studied thousands of children and adolescents on England's Isle of Wight in an attempt to measure the frequency of psychological symptoms and illnesses in the population. They found that more than two-fifths of the 14- to 15-year-old boys and girls they interviewed reported substantial feelings of misery or depression. As Rutter concluded, "It seems that feelings of misery and depression are particularly common during adolescence and are more frequent during this age period than during either earlier childhood or adult life."[10] Many other studies have come up with similar findings.

What can we make of all this "misery" in adolescents? We know from similar studies (discussed below) that only a fraction of these adolescents have severe depression or mood disorders. Rather than depression, it may be more accurate to say that adolescents are prone to periods of *demoralization*.

In his classic book about psychotherapy, *Persuasion and Healing,* Johns Hopkins psychiatrist Jerome Frank states, "A person becomes demoralized when he finds that he cannot meet the demands placed on him and cannot extricate himself from his environment." Demoralized persons are "conscious of having failed to meet their own expectations or those of others, or of being unable to change the situation or themselves."[11] Where could we read a better description of adolescents' dilemma? Repeatedly finding themselves in strange new situations loaded down with expectations from parents, peers, and themselves, and often feeling powerless to affect the outcome, adolescents face big questions.

"In order to function," Frank states, "everyone must impose an order and regularity on the welter of experiences impinging upon him. To do this, he develops out of his personal experiences a set of...assumptions about himself and the nature of the world in which he lives, enabling him to predict the behavior of others and the outcome of his own actions."[12] This set of assumptions is called one's *assumptive world.* When something happens that disrupts a person's assumptive world, the environment suddenly seems unpredictable and a little scary. The individual may react with anxiety, feelings of loss of control and of being trapped, powerless, and, yes, miserable and depressed for a time—the state of affairs that Frank calls demoralization.

In the process of identity development, adolescents' assumptive world is constantly being upset and jostled by new experiences that can throw it into doubt. They spend weeks getting up the courage to ask out someone they think is just right for them only to be turned down ("Maybe I'm not as good-looking/popular as I thought"). They fail an exam ("I'm not as smart as I thought"), or don't make the team ("not as athletic..."), or lose the audition ("not as talented..."). Even positive accomplishments like getting good grades can raise questions about negative identities ("I must be a nerd"). Adolescents often assume that what happens to them indicates something about what kind of person they are. They react strongly to disappointments and setbacks, because they wonder what such events indicate about who they are and what their future will be like. A slight setback that adults would react to with only minor disappointment often causes adolescents to feel much more upset and disappointed and to question themselves in profound ways.

Reading through this, you might wonder why more adolescents don't need treatment for symptoms of demoralization. But as Rutter puts it, these challenges, adaptations, and stresses "do not all arise at the same time"; that is, only under rare and unusual circumstances is the adolescent faced with so many crises simultaneously that they overwhelm psychological resources to cope.

Jerome Frank developed his concept of psychological demoralization in the course of doing research on the effectiveness of psychotherapy. He studied persons with demoralization symptoms such as "depression" (low mood) and anxiety so severe that they sought professional psychological treatment. As Frank discovered, the crucial elements that make psychotherapy effective for these individuals are surprisingly simple: patients must have faith that the therapist cares about them and knows how to help them. Frank's theory was later validated through research into what psychiatrists call *resilience* in young people—that is, their ability to suffer through adverse events in life and come out the other side relatively unscathed. Scientists looked at all sorts of factors in life that could be supportive—other people, religiousness, wealth, social standing, and so on. What they found was elegant and moving in its simplicity. It turns out that the most critical factor in increasing resilience in children is that they have just one person, a single individual, they feel deeply bonded to and can go to in times of crisis. This single individual can make the difference in a person being defeated by life events or growing from them and becoming stronger. Fortunately, most teens have any number of persons in their lives who meet these requirements; they are surrounded by concerned, supportive, and experienced persons, such as parents, teachers, coaches, clergy, even older friends—the list could go on and on—who can help them through periods of uncertainty and discouragement.

All adolescents go through periods of discouragement, suffer from occasional feelings of not fitting in, and are bothered by uncertainty about the future. We must be careful not to "medicalize" this growth process (as Anna Freud is guilty of doing, exemplified by her comment that "to be normal during the adolescent period is by itself abnormal"[13]), and we must remember that a majority of the teenagers in the studies by Rutter and others did *not* report undue depression or "misery."

WHEN IS DEPRESSION "SERIOUS"?

At this point, you may be a little confused. We told you earlier that depression is a serious illness but just spent several pages telling you that adolescent complaints of being "miserable" are not uncommon and do not represent *clinical* depressions—that is, they do not usually warrant medical treatment. The way to understand this better is to recall the discussion in chapter 1 about depression the *symptom* and depression the *syndrome*. In this chapter, we've put an even finer distinction on the issue and have talked about the difference between *depression* and *demoralization*. But how are these related? Can one cause the other? Blend into the other? Where does intense demoralization end and the depressive syndrome begin?

At this point in time, the answers to these questions are not fully known. We know it is not uncommon for adolescents to pass through periods of "miserableness" quite unscathed. But we know that some of this miserableness is a prelude to, or an aspect of, a mood disorder. We also know that adults with mood disorders can have an episode of serious depression triggered by psychological stress and demoralization.

The big mistake that people make in deciding whether to seek treatment for a person with depression is to think that if he seems to have "real" reasons to be depressed, he won't need treatment because he'll "get over it" as soon as he deals with those reasons. A related error is thinking that this individual needs counseling or therapy but not medical treatment. This is not too different from the middle-aged man with chest pains trying to persuade himself that "it's only heartburn" rather than going to the nearest emergency room. When an individual has the signs and symptoms of the syndrome of depression, it's time to get professional help, not to try figuring out whether he has "reasons" to be depressed.

Because we have several ways of understanding depression, one perspective based on biology and the disease model, and a second perspective based on psychology and understanding how people react to events in their lives, it's tempting to think we should be able to categorize depressions in the same way: "biological" and "psychological." We've already led you into this way of thinking a bit, with the discussion of *depression* differentiated from *demoralization*. If only an understanding of people were so easy!

This categorizing of depressions works fairly well in some clear-cut cases at the extremes of the categories. No one would say that a teenage football player who sulks and broods for a day or two after his team misses a chance to be in the state playoffs is suffering from a biologically based mood disorder derived from some misfiring of his physical brain. Similarly, no one would say that Charlie from chapter 1 is simply discouraged, suffering from "normal" teenage angst. This boy is clearly ill.

But there is a large area between these extremes, where differentiation between biological and psychological depressions is not only impossible but also probably meaningless. Another great student of human behavior, Alfred Kinsey, the pioneering researcher on sexuality, said, "The world is not divided into sheep and goats ... Nature rarely deals with discrete categories. Only the human mind invents categories and tries to force facts into separated pigeonholes."[14] Our mental lives involve a complex interplay between biology and psychology that is poorly understood and probably cannot be teased apart. One set of forces affects the other, and there are probably complex feedback loops and an intertwining of influences and processes that make attempts to do so futile.

Michael Rutter, in talking about causes of psychological problems, makes the point that this entanglement of causation is also apparent in physical illnesses as well: we know that a germ called the tubercle bacillus causes tuberculosis. But we also know that genetic factors play a role in resistance to infection and to some extent determine who gets infected. We know, too, that nutritional status is important, that malnourished individuals are much more vulnerable to TB, making it in some ways an illness of poverty. To say that poverty causes tuberculosis isn't quite correct, but to say that tuberculosis is caused by a germ and leave it at that omits a lot of factors that need to be identified in order to treat the illness. Talking too much about what is "biological" and what is "psychological" in depression is simply a waste of time. Serious depression is both.

Not too long ago, psychiatrists and psychologists (more on the differences between these two professions in a bit) made the mistake of relying too much on theories to guide their treatment of depressed patients and not enough on research data and experience. We spent too much time trying to understand depressed persons rather than diagnosing and treating mood disorders. We now know that serious depressive syndromes must be treated medically and that psychotherapy alone will usually not make the patient better. But we also know that people with depressive illnesses are usually demoralized and need support, encouragement, education, and guidance. Adolescents with serious depression should not be denied either kind of treatment just because the details of their symptoms seem to suggest that either depression or demoralization predominates.

So, back to the original question posed earlier: What constitutes *serious* depression? Although you really need a medical or psychology degree and years of clinical training to be able to answer this question for any given individual, you can get some sense of what serious depression is like by rereading chapter 1 for the details of the depressive syndrome. Also, there are some red flags that should always make parents worry that their teen might be seriously depressed:

— *Persistent change in mood*: gloominess, sadness, grouchiness, or irritability that persists over several weeks, on more days than not, such that the teenager seems consistently different from her usual self
— *Loss of interest and enjoyment* in most of the activities that the adolescent usually spends time doing
— *Persistent changes in sleep habits and appetite*: complaints of insomnia, sleeping too much, loss of appetite or increased appetite that results in a weight change of ten pounds or so, persistent complaints of tiredness or low energy, looking tired or haggard all the time
— *Change in self-attitude*, that is, a change in the way the adolescent feels about himself: feeling worthless or useless; self-critical statements about not being as good as other kids; feeling that he is lazy, stupid, ugly, a failure, or good-for-nothing
— *Falling grades*, loss of concentration, complaints that schoolwork is suddenly more difficult
— *Preoccupation with death or illness, especially thoughts of suicide*

The next step in understanding adolescent depression is to learn about the different disorders that exhibit the depressive syndrome. Several decades of research have led to our current classification of the various mood disorders. The depressive syndrome shows up in all of them, but the severity and pattern of the depressive symptoms, their course over time, and some associated symptoms indicate that they are probably different illnesses. Research has also shown that the treatments of these various disorders sometimes need to be very different.

In the next chapter, we discuss the mood disorders of adolescence.

The Mood Disorders of Adolescence

When the mental health community started thinking about serious depression as an illness and began to do research on the symptoms of depression, the course of the illness, and its response to various treatments, they found that serious depression shows up in different forms. These forms differ in severity and types of symptoms and in the timing of symptom development. This research has resulted in our current classification system of mood disorders.

PSYCHIATRIC DIAGNOSIS

Diagnosis is just as important in treating emotional problems as it is in treating physical illnesses. Diagnostic classification has two purposes in medicine: (1) to make predictions about the course of an illness and (2) to aid the clinician in selecting the treatment most likely to be effective. In the practice of psychiatry, since the physical basis for most psychiatric illnesses has yet to be discovered, classification systems are largely derived from studying groups of patients with different combinations of symptoms and seeing whether the groups vary in the course of their illness or in their response to medications.

As different types of medications have become available to treat mood disorders, the classification system of mood disorders has continued to evolve. In this chapter, we describe various subtypes of mood disorders. These are the subtypes that currently seem to make sense to clinicians, because they serve one of the two purposes of diagnosis mentioned above: (1) they allow for a better prediction of the course of the illness, and (2) they allow for a rapid selection of effective therapy—saving the patient time that would be wasted trying an ineffective medication. In 2013, the American Psychiatric Association released a new version of their diagnostic manual, the *Diagnostic and Statistical Manual of Mental Disorders*. This fifth edition, often called the *DSM-5*, contains significant changes in the world of adolescent mood disorders for just the reasons mentioned above. It turned out that an increasingly common diagnosis in young persons, bipolar affective disorder, predicted neither the illness course nor the treatment response, as it did in adults. In fact, longitudinal studies of these children diagnosed as having bipolar affective disorder showed that a re-evaluation of their symptoms once they reached adulthood much more closely matched the syndrome of depression, or that of an isolated anxiety. How can such a seeming error be made? How can a child "have" one syndrome at one point in her life and another one later on?

The proliferation of the diagnosis of bipolarity in children helps us illustrate this critical point. No one, neither adolescents nor adults, can be diagnosed in such a way that the diagnostician is absolutely certain that this is and will be the person's underlying syndrome for the rest of his life. Humans, especially adolescents, are evolving and changing creatures, constantly in flux. In medicine, some (though surprisingly few) illnesses remain permanently with individuals in exactly the same way throughout their lives—and these are mainly genetic disorders. In most cases and especially in psychiatry, people need continual re-evaluation to ensure that their condition has not evolved into something else, and that the diagnosis was correct in the first place. In the world of child psychiatry, we know that certain individuals seem to have multiple diagnoses piled on top of them, which can prove confusing to children and parents alike. Much of our time is spent explaining how a child can "have" ADHD at 5, an anxiety disorder at 7, major depression at 12, and then bipolar disorder at 15.

In reality, all of our diagnoses in psychiatry are clinically based—we do not (yet) have the detailed definitive testing, such as a blood test or brain scan, as do so many other fields of medicine. We must think carefully and rationally about what is happening in a person's life at this moment, compared to what has happened before—with no knowledge of what is yet to come. People change, and so with time we are able to see new and more subtle facets of their underlying selves to clarify what we think may be going on in their psyche, including any psychiatric illnesses they may have. It is not so much that an adolescent "used to have" one condition and now "has" a totally different one replacing the first as it is likely that the developmental changes a child goes through are paralleled by changes in the pattern of symptoms, which now more closely matches the description of one syndrome than another.

Take, for example, the symptom of an inability to pay attention. In one snapshot, a child may appear happy and engaged in fun activities but struggle in class and with homework. This child may be given the diagnosis of ADHD. Later in life, as his brain develops and social pressures increase, he may again experience this symptom of difficulty concentrating, but it may be accompanied by frustrations, low mood, a feeling of failure, anxieties about ever succeeding, trouble sleeping, a lower appetite, a withdrawal from friends and fun activities—you get the picture, which now appears to much more closely approximate the depressive episodes we have described.

In this chapter we discuss the various faces of mood disorders in adolescence. Remember that even if someone's symptoms closely match those listed here, this does not mean that this person has a given diagnosis or, more dangerously, has been misdiagnosed. It may merely mean that the person's most recent appearance closely matches a particular description. This is a trap that even experienced clinicians can fall into. Many adolescents have been diagnosed with bipolar affective disorder based on current *symptoms* when they have the *syndrome* of depression with perhaps a greater expression of irritability in that given moment than would be expected. The most recent version of the *DSM*, fifth edition, attempts to clarify these sorts of errors by further emphasizing the long-term pattern of symptoms rather than a simple cross-section. We discuss all of this more as we go through each form of mood disorder in greater detail.

At least once a month, it seems, we see a patient who requests to be "tested for clinical depression," the implication being that a blood test of some type will be able to detect the "chemical imbalance" that underlies serious mood problems. It's not an unreasonable request. Unfortunately, it's not a request that can be satisfied—not just yet. We don't have a blood test or an x-ray or a biopsy that can make the diagnosis of a mood disorder (or, for that matter, that can be used to confirm the diagnosis of most problems that psychiatrists treat).

This is because the biological and chemical basis of mood disorders remains a nearly complete mystery—no one knows what to test for. Despite literally hundreds of years of examining the bodily fluids and brain tissues of individuals with mood disorders, first with the naked eye, then with microscopes, then with x-rays and scanning devices, and more recently with incredibly sophisticated biochemical probes, no one has been able to find any abnormalities that can be accurately and reliably measured in people with this illness and used to aid in the diagnosis of these disorders. Though scientists have certainly tried! In the 1980s, something called the dexamethasone suppression test was employed in patients with low mood to try to differentiate between demoralization and depression. In theory, people who are depressed for a long time begin to produce higher and higher levels of cortisol, a stress hormone. Their bodies become less sensitive to the effects of this stress response and produce more and more. In most persons, if something that looks like cortisol (in this case, a steroid called dexamethasone) is introduced to the body, it senses this increase and relaxes its own production, lowering the cortisol level. The exhausted bodies of depressed persons seem blunted to this response and, perhaps wanting more and more cortisol, don't respond the same way. It seemed to be a good test in theory and was in clinical use for a number of years, but under rigorous study it didn't turn out to be a clinically useful test—the "sensitivity" (a statistical term used to describe the percentage of time the test is right when it comes out positive vs. the percentage of time it's wrong) was 50 percent, so it was wrong half the time.[1]

Today, the work on the genetics of mood disorders holds the promise that genetic markers for the illness may be discovered in the not-too-distant future—suggesting that a blood test might be possible to identify at least some cases of the illness. Although some individuals with mood disorders have been identified as having subtle brain-scan abnormalities—again suggesting a possible diagnostic tool—the clinical applications of these findings are still far off. Modern psychiatrists are left with the same diagnostic tools available to nineteenth-century psychiatrists: their eyes and ears.

We psychiatrists listen to patients and their family members describe symptoms. What has changed? What doesn't feel right? When did it start? Do the symptoms come and go or stay all the time? We observe the patient for the signs of mood disorders described in chapter 1 by performing a *mental status examination*, the psychiatrist's equivalent of the physical examination. This consists of observing speech patterns and behavior, questioning about mood and thinking processes, and evaluating other aspects of mental functioning, such as concentration and memory. In adolescents, information about these aspects of life from other sources (generally parents, sometimes others, such as teachers) can be as important or at times even more important pieces of the puzzle. After this process of history taking and examination, a picture of the person, of her symptoms and the course of her troubles, emerges. We identify a particular diagnostic category that seems a good fit with the clinical information, and once this is done, we can make predictions about the future course of the symptoms and, perhaps more important, select a treatment that has a good chance of relieving them.

MAJOR DEPRESSIVE DISORDER

Major depressive disorder is the name given to the mood disorder characterized by the development of the full-blown depressive syndrome. Research indicates that major depressive disorder is the most common mood disorder of adolescents and young adults.[2]

The illness usually has a fairly definite beginning, and over a period of weeks, the various symptoms of depression gradually come over the adolescent one by one until the full syndrome is present (table 3-1). The symptoms can last for months, with studies indicating that seven to nine months is typical—an entire school year for an adolescent.[3] The symptoms can vary tremendously in severity from fairly mild symptoms that affect the teen's level of functioning only moderately to severe cases in which social, school, and home life are all significantly affected.

In chapter 1 we met the parents of Charlie, who was showing the typical symptoms and course of illness of major depression. Charlie's symptoms included low mood, withdrawal, low energy, sleep and appetite problems, loss of interest in his usual pursuits, feeling bad about himself—symptoms that came on gradually over a period of weeks and basically drained the spark out of this previously energetic, confident boy.

Sometimes, however, major depression can look rather different, espe-

Table 3-1   Symptoms of Major Depression

Mood Symptoms
    Depressed mood
    Dysphoric mood
    Irritability
    Loss of ability to feel pleasure (anhedonia)
    Loss of interest in usual activities
    Social withdrawal
    Feelings of guilt or worthlessness
Cognitive (Thinking) Symptoms
    Poor concentration
    Poor memory
    Indecision
    Slowed thinking
    Thoughts of death, suicidal thinking
Bodily Symptoms
    Sleep disturbance
        Insomnia
        Hypersomnia
    Appetite disturbance
        Weight loss
        Weight gain
    Fatigue
    Headaches
Symptoms of Psychosis
    Delusional thinking
    Hallucinations

cially when the mood change is to irritable rather than low. In these adolescents, the irritable, miserable mood (psychiatrists often use the term *dysphoria*) is so disruptive to the adolescent's social world, especially the family, that other symptoms of major depression are obscured. Another case study will illustrate this.

▼   Heather's mother tried not to worry when her bright and usually bubbly 15-year-old daughter seemed to spend more Saturday afternoons listening to music in her room and fewer with her friends at the mall. But when Heather dropped out of the choral society, Maggie knew something was wrong.

"It's no fun anymore" was Heather's explanation for dropping out of the student choir only a month before the spring concert. "It's really boring; that stuff is for nerds anyway," she said, with a shrug of her shoulders, when her mom asked about it.

This explanation didn't quite sit right with Maggie, but she could guess what the real reason might be. Heather had auditioned to be a soloist in the concert and had been very disappointed that she wasn't chosen to sing any of the solo pieces. The choir director had told her that she wasn't quite ready for solo work yet but urged her to audition again for the fall concert. The director had also started telling the girls who were having trouble with their parts to stand next to Heather on the risers. "Heather has a strong voice and great intonation; she'll help carry you until you get the part down better," she would tell them in front of Heather and the whole group.

Heather had at first seemed to get over her disappointment, but as the weeks went by, it seemed singing was a chore rather than a source of joy and pride. "She didn't mean what she said about my having a good voice," Heather said angrily when Maggie reminded her of her music teacher's encouraging words. "She said that to humiliate me in front of *everyone*." So saying, Heather burst into tears and ran up to her room.

"Heather's just going through a stage," Maggie's sister reassured her one afternoon when they met at the grocery store. "Don't you remember when my Matt dropped off the swimming team with hardly an explanation and started writing poetry at all hours of the night? Kids' interests change all over the place at this age. They're finding themselves, that's all."

"I don't know," Maggie replied warily. "Heather's interests haven't changed. She seems to have lost interest in *everything*. She got lower grades in two subjects on her last report card, and besides she's so . . . oh, I don't know, so *mean* all of a sudden."

"Mean?" her sister asked.

"Well, she's so sarcastic about everything. She has Beth in tears several times a week."

"Big sisters criticize little sisters all the time at this age. It makes them feel grown up."

"I don't know, Fran. Heather and Beth always got along so well. They've never been mean to each other."

"Heather's never been a teenager, either," Fran soothed, patting Maggie's hand on the grocery cart. "And believe me, it gets worse when they're juniors; but you'll get through it somehow. Everyone does!"

Things did get worse. And much worse than Fran had predicted. There were screaming matches between Heather and her mother and father, Phillip, several times a week. Heather's grades continued to drop, and she took to spending most of her time in her room listening to music. Several times, Maggie had awakened in the middle of the night still hearing the music playing softly in Heather's room. She'd gone in to turn it off only to find her daughter still awake, sometimes in tears, but unable to say why she was crying.

Heather started coming in later than her curfew on weekends and often had alcohol on her breath.

Maggie and Phillip got a phone call from one of Heather's teachers warning that summer school might be a good idea if Heather wasn't able to turn her grades around. "I'm worried about Heather, and I think you should be too. Some of the answers on her tests make me think she's not concentrating in class like she should. She doesn't seem to be able to grasp the concepts this semester." But Heather flew into a rage when Maggie and Phillip told her about the call from her teacher. "And I will *not* go to summer school! Don't even think about it! I'll kill myself first!" she hissed ominously through clenched teeth.

Maggie felt alone and bewildered in dealing with her changed daughter. Fran shook her head sympathetically and suggested Maggie and Phillip go to "Tough Love" meetings. Phillip started staying later at the office to avoid the tension at home, and one night had only half-jokingly threatened to leave home "until she's 21 and a normal person again—I'll send you a check every month but you can call me when this part is *over*." Even 12-year-old Beth seemed to be out of the house most nights, needing to "study" with classmates. "I work better with someone else there," she explained sheepishly. "And it's hard to concentrate at home."

And there was no talking to Heather about much of anything. Maggie had made up her mind several times to make an appointment for Heather to see a therapist, but then things would go better for a day or two and she'd hope that the worst was over. And when things seemed to be getting worse, Maggie would become terrified at how Heather might react to the idea of seeing a mental health professional, and she would put the idea off "until she's in a better mood."

Late one evening, the phone rang. Maggie picked up the receiver expecting to hear Heather with her latest excuse for being out later than she should be. Instead, Maggie heard a woman's voice, a woman who seemed to be calling from some crowded place with phones ringing and some kind of beeping sound in the background.

"Mrs. McAllister? This is Ruth calling from the emergency department at St. Luke's Hospital." Maggie felt something in the middle of her chest drop to the soles of her feet. "We have Heather here and—"

"Oh my God, is she all right?"

"Yes, Mrs. McAllister, she's not hurt. There was a car accident, but Heather was not injured. She's fine physically, but—"

"Oh, thank God. We'll come right over to bring her home. Should we—"

"Well, ah . . . yes, you need to come over, but the doctor wants to talk to you about admitting Heather to the hospital."

"I don't understand. I thought you said she wasn't injured."

"No, she wasn't, but the psychiatrist thinks that she needs—"

"Psychiatrist? But what—"

"Heather drove off in her friend's car and ran off the road out by St. Mary's cemetery. The police found her passed out in the driver's seat with alcohol on her breath."

"Oh, God" was all Maggie could say.

"She was pretty alert by the time she got here, but the psychiatrist thinks she's very depressed. She wants to admit Heather at least overnight and see her in the morning, to see if she's still feeling suicidal."

"Depressed? Suicidal? But she's never—"

"Heather had two bottles of over-the-counter pills in her pocket, and we think she was planning to take an overdose. These particular pills probably wouldn't have caused anything serious, but anytime someone tries to hurt themselves we need to—"

Maggie wasn't listening anymore. Depressed? But depressed people are sad and gloomy, Maggie thought, not like this. Why did they think Heather was depressed? She didn't have anything to be depressed about. Could not getting the solo part in the spring concert have caused all this? No, that made no sense at all.

"We'll come right away," she said, and hung up the phone. ▲

Because Heather's problems seem at first glance so different from Charlie's, it doesn't seem possible that they have the same illness: major depression. But when we review Heather's symptoms, they're not really so different.

First, of course, there is the mood change. Heather is mostly irritable and dysphoric rather than suffering what we typically call a low mood. But the mood change is dramatic and pervasive, with her all the time, every day, week after week. Next, she's lost interest in school, in going with her friends to the mall, and she complains that singing is no fun anymore; she's developed a loss of pleasure in things, which you might remember is called *anhedonia*. Heather is in her room alone much of the time and isn't sleeping at night. She's having crying spells frequently. Her teacher has noticed poor concentration, and her grades are dropping.

Heather feels bad about herself and doesn't think she's a good singer after all; she even thinks that the music teacher's compliments were some kind of sarcastic ploy meant to make fun of her. This misinterpretation of the reality of the situation is, in fact, the kind of idea that can become increasingly preoccupying and gradually turn into a *delusion*, a psychotic symptom in which a person has a preoccupying false belief.*

Noting Heather's use of alcohol is also critical in diagnosing her depression. Although substance use and abuse can certainly be stand-alone problems in adolescents or in adults, sometimes substance-abuse problems get started and are sustained by a mood disorder and can be understood as secondary to it. The start of alcohol misuse (and anything that approaches regular use is *misuse* in adolescents) accompanied by the other symptoms are a strong indicator of the seriousness of Heather's problems. And, lastly, the serious attempt to harm herself carries a lot of weight and puts her collection of symptoms squarely into the category of major depression.

---

*Remember that in depressive disorders, the content of delusional beliefs is depressing in some way. In *A Mind That Found Itself*, written in the nineteenth century, author Clifford Beers describes his battle with a mental illness that was almost certainly a mood disorder. In one scene, he describes how, on a train ride to the psychiatric hospital, he noticed people standing on the station platforms reading the newspaper as the train passed through. Beers relates how convinced he was at the time that they were reading about him, about his long history of mental illness, and about what a failure he had been. These themes of shame and failure are typical of a mood disorder.

Because of her mostly irritable rather than depressed mood state, and because of her outwardly directed disruptive behaviors, especially toward her family, a superficial appraisal of Heather's situation might suggest that her problem is being *bad* rather than *sad*. But remember that diagnosing the syndrome of depression requires looking at many aspects of emotional life and behavior in addition to mood, and when this kind of survey is done with Heather, we come up with quite a list: a pervasive mood change, withdrawal from friends and family, low energy, poor concentration, sleep problems, loss of interest in usual pursuits, feeling bad about herself (to the point that she thinks life just isn't worth it and she tries to harm herself)—virtually the same list as Charlie's. Heather's diagnosis is the same as well: major depression.

No one is quite sure why this irritable mood is more common in adolescents than in adults. Irritability can certainly be a part of the picture in adults, but it is rarely the most prominent aspect of the mood syndrome as it can be in adolescents. Research shows that irritability as an expression of severe depression is most striking during adolescence. Though the syndrome of major depression is far rarer in prepubescent children, the symptoms these young ones experience more closely resemble depression in adults, with low mood and energy level. Thus, the mood change that takes place in severe depression before and after adolescence can be different from that seen during adolescence. Why?

It is tempting to speculate that the struggle for independence and separation from family that preoccupies most adolescents somehow makes them more "prickly" and reactive in their interactions with parents and authority figures. Perhaps depression exaggerates the tendency toward defiance that is part of every teenager's drive to find and assert his independence. This theory would state, then, that psychological issues particular to adolescence shape the depressive feelings and result in the prominent irritability. But this is pure speculation, and this very important question remains unanswered.

Onset of depression following a loss or disappointment of some type is not uncommon. In Heather's case, the disappointment was a rather minor one, and this is *not* typical. More commonly, the loss is a significant one, such as the death of someone close, parental divorce, or the breakup of a serious relationship. The exposure to the suicide of someone close has been strongly linked to the development of major depression in adults. One might want to conclude from these sorts of data that loss and stressful events can cause major depression, but this conclusion would not be quite correct, for several reasons. First, some adolescents who get depressed do not seem to have a significant stressful event preceding the development of their depression. Second, many teens who suffer a significant loss do not go on to develop severe depression. A 1995 study compared the occurrences of stressful life events in teenagers with and without major depression. It found no statistically significant difference in the total number of stressful events in the two groups.[4] That said, this is still an active field of research within psychiatry, because it seems like stressful life events should be associated with depression. And they are, but that doesn't mean they *cause* the depression. A 2010 study seemed to show a high correlation between stressful life events and depression but failed to show that these events caused the depression. In fact, this and other studies indicate that the road can go both ways, in that those who experience major depressive episodes are more likely to experience stressful life events because of their condition (failing grades, the end of romance, and similar events).[5] One expert on the relationship between depression and stressful events put it this way: "Undesirable events are . . . neither necessary nor sufficient to explain the onset of an episode of depression."[6] It's possible that rather than "causing" depression, stress and especially loss trigger the development of a depression in an adolescent who is vulnerable in some way, perhaps because of genetic factors (more on genetics in chapter 15).

How common is major depression in adolescents? Some of the most recent studies have found that 8 to 10 percent of adolescents will enter a major depressive episode in any given year.[7] This is about the same rate that adults report (7 percent), which has been interpreted to mean that adult major depressive disorder is an illness that starts in adolescence.[8] Girls and women seem about twice as likely to experience major depression than boys and men once they enter into puberty (before that stage, both genders seem to be about equally predisposed).[9]

You may have noticed that we have used two similar-sounding terms: major depressive *episode* and major depressive *disorder*. Is there a difference? The answer to this question takes us into a discussion of the course that mood disorders take. We talk about "episodes" of mood disorders because they are illnesses that usually come and go throughout a person's lifetime. A person with major depressive disorder has an illness that takes the form of periods during which he has all the symptoms that make up the depressive syndrome: these periods are the major depressive episodes. Put another way, major depressive *disorder* is a psychiatric illness characterized by recurrent major depressive *episodes.*

Research has shown that in children and adolescents, a major depressive episode lasts, on average, approximately seven to nine months.[10] But a percentage of these young people have episodes that last longer; a small percentage will still have symptoms one to two years after the beginning of their illness, and in up to 10 percent, symptoms can last even beyond this if untreated.

Another striking fact about adolescent depression is its tendency to recur. In one study of adolescents with major depression, over a period of five years researchers checked in with 196 adolescent patients who'd had an episode of major depression. This study found that 47 percent of the adolescents experienced another episode of depression within the five-year period.[11] Other research suggests that for adolescents who have had major depression, up to 70 percent will go through another period of major depression within the next five years.[12] The patients in these studies are usually from clinics and hospitals, so the results tend to show what the more severe forms of the illness can be like. Also, the researchers often do not take treatment into account. In some of these studies, the teens were getting only psychotherapy, some were taking medication as well, and some were getting little or no treatment. (That many teens with serious depression, even after getting a diagnosis by a professional, either never get into treatment or stop treatment after a short period is a finding in study after study of this type.)

These numbers are sobering. Major depressive disorder in adolescents can cause lengthy periods of symptoms, and once an adolescent has had an episode, the risk for recurrence is high.

DYSTHYMIC DISORDER

Like many words used in the field of medicine, *dysthymia* comes from Greek roots. The prefix *dys-* is from a word that means "bad" or "difficult," and the root *thymia* comes from the Greek word for "mind." In psychiatry, the meaning of this root word has altered a bit and usually refers to "mood." Dysthymia, then, is an illness characterized by "bad mood." How is it different from major depressive disorder?

Persons with dysthymic disorder suffer from a smoldering low-grade depressive syndrome that persists over a period of many months, sometimes for years. It is an illness that can remain undetected and thus untreated for a very long time. These individuals sometimes see a psychiatrist for the first time as adults, when they finally come to realize that the bad feelings they have constantly struggled against are *not* normal. When asked how long they have felt depressed, many of these patients say, "As long as I can remember." Because the symptoms can develop insidiously and smolder on without precipitating a crisis, dysthymic individuals can lose track of the onset of their depressed feelings and eventually seem to forget what "normal" feels like. One of us once treated a young man, whom we will call Max Phelps, with precisely these problems.

▼   Max was the most serious-looking 13-year-old I had seen in a long time. His khakis, white shirt, and blue-striped tie added to this impression, making him look almost like a little college professor rather than a young teenager.

"Max really didn't want to come today, doctor," his mother was saying. "But he said he would as long as he didn't have to miss school to come to the appointment."

"Why was that, Max?" I asked. "Kids don't often mind missing an hour or two of school, even if it is a trip to the doctor's office."

"I don't want to have to explain to people," he answered. "Other kids are too nosy about stuff. I didn't want to have to deal with a lot of questions."

Mrs. Phelps filled in Max's story. She had noticed her youngest son becoming more and more miserable over a period of many months. "He mopes around the house or sits and watches television. His grades have slipped again this year and—"

"No, they haven't," Max said with a bit of irritation showing in his voice.

"Yes, they have, Max," his mom said. "You went from a 3 to a 2 in English in December." Mrs. Phelps looked up at me. "Now I know that's not a bad grade by any means. But it's the pattern we're worried about. He has dropped a grade point in at least one subject every semester for the past two years. Maybe it's not exactly a drastic drop, but his performance has been drifting downward for months." She looked over at her son. "Don't you agree, Max?"

"I guess so," he said, looking down.

"Have you noticed any sleep problems or eating problems?" I asked.

"No, not particularly," Mrs. Phelps replied.

"Max?" I asked.

"Huh?" he said.

"Max, honey, talk to the doctor," his mom said soothingly. She looked up at me. "He doesn't seem to be paying attention half of the time. Do you think this might be why his grades are dropping?"

"I don't know why you have to say that over and over again," Max said. "It really makes me angry."

It turned out that anger was becoming more and more of a problem as well. Max was persistently defiant at home, often about little things. "Max made his bed every day almost from the time he started kindergarten. I don't think he's made it for a year. Now, I know a lot of boys his age don't, but it just doesn't seem right for Max. He's always been so eager to help around the house."

"How is Max getting along with his friends?" I asked.

"OK," Max responded.

I looked over at Max's mom. "Yes?" I asked.

"Well, it's hard for me to tell," she said. "He spends plenty of time with his friends, but he seems to worry a lot that nobody likes him."

"Mom!" Max said a little sharply.

"Max, honey, I'm just telling the doctor what you've told me so he can help you to feel better."

Max peered down at his shoes with a stony look.

"He just seems so miserable all the time," Max's mom said. "I see his friends run up the street yelling and laughing, and then Max comes along after them almost shuffling his feet, like it's almost too much effort. He wasn't this way before." Mrs. Phelps looked over at her son wistfully. "I remember him on his tenth birthday, so full of fun and energy. But something's changed; something has been creeping up on him for a long time now. It's happened so slowly that I didn't realize it for a long time."

The "something" was depression, and the pattern was dysthymic disorder. "You did just the right thing to bring Max in," I said. "I think we can make this 'thing' go away." ▲

We like the word *smoldering* to describe dysthymic disorder. And just as a gust of wind can fan a smoldering fire into flame, stress can inflame the illness and cause symptoms of irritability to flare up. Because the symptoms aren't usually as dramatic as those of major depressive disorder, they may be easier to miss, but dysthymia can be just as dangerous.

Dysthymia, like depression, seems less common in the very young, but is certainly not unheard of—studies have shown that children as young as 5 years old can be affected. These young people have a gloomy, pessimistic, down mood and are often preoccupied with feeling unloved and left out. They feel bad about themselves and worry that they don't measure up in various ways.

In a study that attempted to contrast and compare the symptoms of dysthymic disorder and major depressive disorder, the dysthymic children were younger, had fewer guilty feelings, had less sleep or appetite disturbance, and didn't suffer from the severe loss of pleasure that is characteristic of major depression. Their mood symptoms (depressed and irritable mood) and feelings of being unloved and without good friends were about the same (table 3-2).

One of the most significant findings of this study is that early-onset dysthymic disorder seems to be an indicator for problems with other, often more severe mood symptoms later in life. As with an episode of major depression, a diagnosis of dysthymic disorder is a predictor of increased risk for more problems with depression in the future. In the study, a group of children was observed over a period of up to twelve years, and during that time, 80 percent of the children with dysthymia had another episode of a mood disorder. More than two-thirds of the fifty-five children with early-onset dysthymic disorder went on to have an episode of the more severe collection of symptoms of major depression. Most of the time, these children's symptoms worsened into major depression with no completely well time in between, a phenomenon that has been called *double depression.* In double depression, the more severe symptoms of major depression become superimposed on symptoms of dysthymia. In this group, the second and third years after the beginning of dysthymic symptoms were the period of highest risk.[13]

These findings have been interpreted to indicate that dysthymic disorder might be best thought of as a subtype or a precursor of other mood

Table 3-2 Depressive Symptoms in Children with Dysthymic Disorder and Major Depressive Disorder

Symptom	Percentage of Children Reporting the Symptom	
	Dysthymic Disorder	Major Depressive Disorder
Depressed or sad mood	91.7	80.0
Feeling unloved	55.6	48.9
Feeling friendless	41.7	40.0
Irritability	55.6	71.1
Anger	63.9	62.2
Anhedonia	5.6	71.1
Guilty feelings	13.9	31.1
Social withdrawal	8.3	53.3
Impaired concentration	41.7	67.4
Thoughts of wanting to die	16.7	42.2
Reduced sleep	22.2	62.2
Reduced appetite	5.6	46.7
Fatigue	22.2	64.4
Disobedience	58.3	43.2

Source: Maria Kovacs, Hagop Akiskal, Constantine Gatsonis, and Phoebe Parrone, "Childhood-Onset Dysthymic Disorder," *Archives of General Psychiatry* 51 (1994): 365–74.

disorders and may not really be a separate mood disorder after all. These findings also give new meaning to the idea that dysthymia is a "smoldering" type of depression, because in many of these young patients, the symptoms flare up into full-blown major depression.

How common is dysthymic disorder? From studies of large groups of children and adolescents, researchers have estimated lifetime rates for dysthymia of between 0.1 and 8 percent in young people.[14]

PREMENSTRUAL DYSPHORIC DISORDER

There is another, more subtle, form of depression that deserves special discussion. Recall that we earlier discussed how most girls and women are at twice the risk of developing depression than their male peers. This increased risk starts when the woman begins puberty and reverses after menopause. Although the field of psychiatry does not exactly know yet what causes depression, there is no doubt that our hormones play a large role in determining and regulating our mood. This is true for men as well, as can be seen most clearly in older men, as the level of testosterone begins to decline and depression risk increases. But it is also apparent in women who have a regular, cyclical variation of hormones as their bodies prepare for procreation. Premenstrual dysphoric disorder (PMDD) has only recently become an officially recognized entity with the advent of the *DSM*, fifth edition—prior to this, it was discussed in the literature but not officially recognized. (Women with these symptoms had to be given the diagnosis of depression not otherwise specified [NOS], a rather unsatisfying and seemingly contradictory diagnosis.)

Many adolescents report some symptoms, both physical and emotional, within about one week before their menstruation. What we are discussing here is something quite different from these anticipated symptoms. Just as most people have experienced low mood in the past but have not gone through a major depressive episode, the normal premenstrual syndrome and that of PMDD are entirely separate entities. In PMDD, the woman experiences all and exactly the same symptoms as a person with major depressive disorder. What separates PMDD from major depression is not symptoms but timing. A woman in the throes of PMDD suffers only during the week before menstruation (a hormonally tumultuous time known as the *luteal phase* of the menstrual cycle). Outside that time, the woman may be unaffected by depression of any sort, or may suffer from a dysthymia or major depression that seems to significantly worsen during this time. The condition can be serious to the point of impairment in some patients, so that they cannot function at school or work; they may entertain suicidal thoughts. Some have reported experiencing the most severe depressive symptoms, including hallucinations, when at their worst.

We have said all along that the diagnosis of major depression is made not only by the severity of symptoms but also on the symptoms' tenacity, their pervasiveness. The diagnosis of PMDD can be particularly difficult because the symptoms are not consistent—someone incapacitated by her depression can appear to be perfectly fine the next week. What can be examined, however, is a long-term pattern in which an adolescent consistently experiences the same symptoms in the same time frame before her menses. And it can be a critical diagnosis to make, as it nearly always requires biological treatment (that is, medications) rather than psychotherapy. Treatment of depression and its related entities is something we talk more about later, but for now it is important to note that the treatment for PMDD is somewhat different than that for routine major depression, so the distinction between the two can mean the difference between continual suffering and recovery.

PMDD is rare. Although almost 80 percent of women experience some premenstrual symptoms, and approximately 20 percent have symptoms that "interfere with life," only about 1.3 percent experience true PMDD.[15] This disorder is even less common than the other depressive disorders we have been discussing. Rare as PMDD is, we make it a point to routinely ask every female patient we evaluate about any relationship between her depression and her menstruation, because it makes a significant difference when determining what sort of treatment we would undertake.

BIPOLAR DISORDER

Bipolar disorder, or more formally bipolar affective disorder, in children and adolescents is a topic of some debate, even among the most revered experts in the field. The subject has become so extensively argued that it could be the subject of an entire book unto itself. Within these pages, we give an overview of what bipolar disorder is, what it is not, and how it relates to depression. This will necessitate a somewhat lengthy discussion in the midst of a book that is supposed to be devoted solely to adolescent depression, but given the wild increase in diagnosis of bipolar disorder (and a close cousin, mood disorder NOS) in adolescents, we feel it deserves a good amount of thoughtful conversation.

First, according to the *DSM* and the field of psychiatry, what exactly is bipolar affective disorder? The description can be discerned from a careful examination of the name itself: *bi-* (meaning two), *polar* (therefore having two poles), *affective* (relating to mood) disorder. The following case study illustrates these "two poles" of mood as they play out in the life of a teenager whom we will call Kelly.

▼ Finally, finally, thought Anne, the treatment was working! Her daughter Kelly had always been a bit of a bookworm, sure, but so was the rest of the family. Because of Kelly's introverted nature, it had taken Anne some time to recognize that her daughter had started to become depressed. It shouldn't have been that big of a surprise, really, since depression ran in her husband's family, but at first it was hard to believe it had happened to their child. Still, seeing the psychiatrist was the best thing they had ever done. Since starting treatment, her daughter had come back to herself. She found a renewed love of books, her small but close group of friends had gotten back together, and her schoolwork had recovered.

Ever since she turned 16, though, Kelly had started to come out of her shell in a way that no one had expected. She was hanging out with more friends, and Anne's shy, introverted daughter had actually gone out for the school play! In fact, some of the things she was doing were firsts for the whole family. Anne and her husband were quiet people, as was their younger son, Allen, so Kelly joining the cheerleading squad was new to all of them. Anne wasn't all that surprised that Allen was a bit jealous, but some of the things he was saying about Kelly were getting out of control, that she's "so energetic it's like she's on crack." The truth was that both Anne and her husband were really excited to have such a well-rounded child and thought that maybe the psychiatrist had "cured" her.

As Anne was lost in her thoughts, the door slammed open, and Kelly bounded into the room.

"Hi, Mom! How was your day? Mine was great! I got a role in the play, and cheerleading practice was just the best! I can't believe I never got into it before. You know I think I'm the best in the whole squad; I'm teaching other people how to do what I do! Maybe next I'll start that home ec class—I just love cooking lately, and I'm really great at it! I was watching a cooking show the other day, and they were making pizza. That's something we haven't had for a while. Why don't we go out for pizza tonight? My favorite is pepperoni, but I've gotta watch those pounds . . ."

Anne started to lose focus. Her daughter did tend to ramble on lately, but you had to forgive her—she had so many new, exciting things to talk about. It was a little surprising that Kelly was so interested in home ec. Truth be told, she was pretty useless in the kitchen, although she seemed to be working hard at learning to cook. Last week, Anne woke to the sound of pots and pans banging around at three in the morning and found her daughter baking up a storm.

"Are you even listening?!" yelled Kelly.

Anne broke out of her reverie and felt a little shocked. While she had been thinking, Kelly had walked right up to her and was yelling in her face.

"I said I'm going to a party and asked like a billion times for the car keys!"

Now that was strange. Kelly knew she wasn't allowed to go out at night when she had a test the next day.

"Sweetie, you know you have that English—" Anne picked up her purse almost without thinking about it, right as Kelly ripped it out of her hands, so hard Anne lurched forward.

"You can't stop me!" yelled Kelly again, as she took out the car keys, threw the purse to the floor, and ran out the front door.

Anne knew that kids could be moody, but this was ridiculous. Anne reached for the phone and dialed. Her husband picked up after two rings.

"Steven, it's me. Kelly ran out of the house again. No, she grabbed the ones to your car. I still keep mine in the dresser after last time. Look, I know you hate these interruptions. Just please come home. Yes, you told me this is exactly how it started with your brother. That's why I'm worried!" ▲

Some people with severe depressions have other types of abnormal mood states in addition to their depressions, periods that are in many ways quite the opposite. During these episodes, they experience increased physical energy and psychological agitation. Instead of being slowed down and lethargic, they feel sped up and energized. Their thoughts can race so much that their speech can't keep up; they jump from topic to topic, and they don't make sense. Their mood state can be giddy and high, or extremely irritable. But whether the abnormal mood state is pleasantly high or irritable, these individuals are abnormally energized, restless, and activated. These are some of the symptoms of *mania* (table 3-3).

People with bipolar disorder can also have a strange mix of the activation and agitation of mania combined with the negative thinking and mood of depression, a separate mood state called a *mixed affective state*, or simply a *mixed state*. Mixed states are very dangerous, because depressing thought patterns are combined with excess energy, restlessness, and an inner sense of pressure and tension. This negative energy puts these individuals at high risk for hurting themselves with suicidal behaviors.

Originally, the name for the illness characterized by periods of depression and periods of manic symptoms was *manic-depression* (or *manic-depressive illness*, or *disorder*). More recently, the term *bipolar disorder* has come to be used almost universally.

Table 3-3   Symptoms of Mania

Mood Symptoms
   Elated, euphoric mood
   Irritable mood
   Grandiosity
Cognitive (Thinking) Symptoms
   Feelings of heightened concentration
   Accelerated thinking ("racing thoughts")
Bodily Symptoms
   Increased energy level
   Decreased need for sleep
   Erratic appetite
   Increased sexual feelings
Symptoms of Psychosis
   Grandiose delusions
   Hallucinations

Bipolar symptoms can be dramatic and extremely dangerous, but they can be rather subtle as well. Individuals may not have the frenzied, disorganized extreme mood state of mania but may instead have *hypomania* (*hypo-* is the Greek prefix meaning "below"), a less severe "high" in which they are overconfident, tend to be reckless and lose inhibitions, and have a giddy over-optimism that causes them to take unaccustomed risks and to exercise poor judgment.

Many parents might think this sounds precisely like most of the teenagers they have met—a little indestructible, a little overconfident, and somewhat reckless. Remember how we distinguished true depression from more transient and understandable sadness? In mania and hypomania, these characteristics constitute a *change* from someone's normal temperament and way of behaving and feeling. Additionally, they are not usually the result of something that has occurred in the person's life. Every teenager who has a first date may be a little giddy, but for teenagers suffering from mania (yes, it sounds strange to say that someone is "suffering" from excessive happiness, but the same word is used—we get to why later), their high mood descends on them from out of the blue, usually with little or no correlation to what's happening in their lives. Some people cycle through different moods almost daily, feeling gloomy then giddy then irritable for brief periods with hardly any moments of normal mood. This is why we say that someone *suffers* with mania, because that the elevated mood cannot last indefinitely. According to most experts, there is no unipolar manic psychiatric illness, unlike depression, which can be unipolar. We both have experience with patients afflicted with bipolar affective disorder who secretly (or not so secretly) want their manias to last forever and sometimes despise medications for "taking away the highs." But what goes up must, in fact, come down, and people experiencing mania do inevitably enter a depression. It is this wild swing of emotion that brings about the suffering—as, at times, do the activities in which a manic person engages. Persons in a manic state tend to lose all sense of consequence to their actions. They will shoplift, speed, cheat on their loved ones, and so on. Once the mania lifts, only then do they experience the repercussions of their actions and have to face them head on, often while falling into a depressed state, which amplifies their negative feelings tremendously.

CONTROVERSIES SURROUNDING BIPOLAR AFFECTIVE DISORDER IN CHILDREN

The bipolar affective illness and all its variations are well described in adults, but much less so in children. Psychiatry is only beginning to understand how these illnesses show up in younger people. This may seem confusing, because the prevalence of bipolar affective illness in children seems to be exploding. How can there be an exponential increase in the diagnosis of an illness, the symptoms of which even the most revered experts disagree on? This was the challenge facing the committee writing the new version of the *DSM*, the *DSM-5*, and it came up with quite a creative answer to this perplexing question.

From a historical perspective, bipolar disorder was traditionally thought to be extremely rare in young people—even though research data on adults indicated that the first symptoms of bipolar disorder usually appeared before the age of 20. Perhaps because of a reluctance to diagnose children with an illness known to be a lifelong problem, and perhaps because of a hesitation to prescribe for children the powerful medications used to treat its symptoms, bipolar disorder in young children received little attention from researchers until quite recently. At the time of publication of the *DSM-IV* (1994) and the *DSM-IV-TR* ("text revision," 2000), the prevalence of children and adolescents diagnosed with bipolar affective disorder was small. Then, suddenly, something changed. From 1997 to 2003, the number of persons younger than 18 diagnosed with this condition increased forty-fold, from about 0.025 percent of children to about 1 to 2 percent—the same proportion as seen in adults.[16,17] What had been a seemingly rare and mysterious condition had become rather commonplace. When we say that a psychiatric illness is "rare," we mean that the population with a particular illness is small relative to the general, unaffected population. Imagine a room filled with one hundred adolescents—a school lunchroom, for example. In this scenario, in 2004, one of those children would be diagnosed with bipolar affective disorder. This may not seem like all that much, but now imagine a room filled with four thousand young people—a moderately sized liberal arts college, for example. In 1997, only one of those young persons would have been diagnosed with bipolar affective disorder. Quite a difference! And the numbers continue to rise.

There is another, more nebulous diagnosis in the *DSM* called "mood disorder not otherwise specified." It is similar to depression NOS, though even more vague. It is ideally meant to capture all those people who we believe have a mood disorder (something in the depressive or bipolar scales) but who do not meet strict criteria for any specific disorder. Its use, however, has unfortunately grown to describe those adolescents with any sort of extreme emotional state, however transient—among children aged 1 to 17 years old, "mood disorder" was the single most common diagnosis and reason for hospitalization in 2011, edging out even medical diagnoses like asthma and injury.[18]

This extreme increase caught the attention of some of the most renowned experts in the world of psychiatry and invited a number of questions. What was happening? Were children becoming more ill? Was bipolar affective illness occurring earlier and earlier in a person's life? Had the whole of human history missed out on the early development of such a serious condition in the young? Or was it psychiatry's fault—had we lost our way and were misdiagnosing huge swaths of the population? Unfortunately, the last answer seems to be the correct one.

How could this have happened? Essentially, psychiatrists had begun to broaden their definition of what the bipolar syndrome looked like in young people. Some psychiatrists even thought they could predict it.

Recall that mania and hypomania can be characterized by elevated energy, impulsivity, and a giddy or happy mood, *or by those same symptoms combined with irritability*. Some experts felt that the "childhood presentation" of bipolar affective disorder could be different from that of adults, in that it is more frequently characterized by an irritable mood than an elated one (as it is in depression). They reasoned that the combination of wild temper tantrums, disinhibited behavior (such as destroying property), and irritability may be the "bipolar" of childhood.

In bipolar affective disorder of all types, there is a phenomenon known as *kindling*. The name comes from the idea of kindling a fire—what starts off as a small flame can grow to be a large bonfire, given sufficient time. Research has shown that bipolar affective disorder seems to get worse the longer it remains untreated and the more episodes of mania or depression the person has. The episodes become more frequent, more severe, and more difficult to treat. Traditionally, researchers had always been most concerned about the initial "flame"—the first episode of mania. But in the early 2000s, some investigators tried to reach even further back, to find the spark behind the flame.

DISRUPTIVE MOOD DYSREGULATION DISORDER

Though poorly characterized in the literature, there seemed to be a group of children who were angrier and more irritable than their peers. They weren't really depressed, in that they didn't have the other symptoms we typically think of (social isolation, sleep pattern changes, low mood, suicidal thoughts, and so on). In fact, some of their symptoms were a little closer to mania: the children were more likely to act before thinking rather than thinking before acting (called *disinhibition*), seemed to have a restless quality, were aggressive, seemed to need less sleep (as opposed to being unable to sleep but being tired the next day), and so on. These children didn't seem to have discrete "episodes" like adults—in a way, they were like a pilot light yet to turn into a full flame, a little kernel of bipolar affective disorder just waiting to pop. Could this be the precursor to adult bipolar affective disorder? Is this what it looked like in childhood? Early evidence seemed to suggest that, yes, children with this collection of symptoms had family histories of bipolar affective disorder, and yes, some of the same medications seemed to help. The word got out, and psychiatrists expanded their practice to include more and more children with this diagnosis.

Others at the pinnacle of the field disagreed with this theory. As evidence mounted, the explanation that these children had bipolar affective disorder seemed thinner and thinner. One study examined a large cohort of adults with true bipolar affective disorder. Few if any of them had had this constellation of symptoms as children, no more than the nonpsychiatrically ill population, and about 20 percent had had their first true manic episode as an adolescent (none as children). Another study followed a group of children diagnosed with bipolar disorder longitudinally and found that they were far more likely to develop true major depressive or anxiety disorders as adults (with no episodes of mania or hypomania). These experts were concerned by the trend of expanding the bipolar phenotype to include what they saw as normal childhood reactions to life stressors. They took the stance that pediatric bipolar affective disorder should be treated no differently than adult bipolar affective disorder, that a child must meet exactly the same criteria as adults, and that a child who was irritable and throwing tantrums was simply that and was at no higher chance of developing bipolar disorder (and needing medications) than any other child. Irritability, by itself, can be a symptom in several psychiatric conditions and life circumstances—everything from a major depressive episode to simply having a bad day.

Regardless of this undecided debate, many in the field began diagnosing children who experienced an episode of irritability as having mood disorder NOS or bipolar affective disorder. Essentially, psychiatrists had changed their practice from using a quite rigid definition of bipolar disorder to using a looser one that encompassed wider and wider groups of children. Child psychiatrists made this change not out of malice or laziness, but because they had no other way to characterize this population. Unfortunately for the young person, this diagnostic change had dire consequences. As we've said, this diagnosis was the number one reason for hospitalization among this age group, so many children were admitted to a psychiatric hospital. Many others were started on medications to "control their bipolar affective disorder." Although medications can be helpful and at times necessary, they can have side effects, so many of these children may have been exposed to unnecessary uncomfortable physical changes (such as weight gain and fatigue).

Sitting down together, the *DSM-5* committee on mood disorders faced a conundrum. No one would argue that bipolar affective disorder is unheard of in adolescents. There were young persons out in the world who needed to be accurately diagnosed and treated for their sake and the sake of their families. At the same time, this committee had to figure out some way to tease apart more accurately who actually had the *syndrome* of bipolar affective disorder and who may have been having some similar *symptoms* of mania (such as irritability) for another reason. This much larger group of children could not simply be thrown out of the *DSM*. In *DSM-5*, the committee explains its trial between the Scylla of underdiagnosis and the Charybdis of overdiagnosis:

> During the latter decades of the 20th century, this contention by researchers that severe, non-episodic irritability is a manifestation of pediatric mania coincided with an upsurge in the rates at which clinicians assigned the diagnosis of bipolar disorder to their pediatric patients. This sharp increase in rates appears to be attributable to clinicians combining at least two clinical presentations into a single category. That is, both classic, episodic presentations of mania and non-episodic presentations of severe irritability have been labeled as bipolar disorder in children. In DSM-5, the term bipolar disorder is explicitly reserved for episodic presentations of bipolar symptoms. DSM-IV did not include a diagnosis designed to capture youths whose hallmark symptoms consisted of very severe, non-episodic irritability, whereas DSM-5 . . . provides a distinct category for such presentations.[19]

How, indeed, does the *DSM-5* accomplish this goal? Here is their solution in their own words:

> Unlike in DSM-IV, this chapter "Depressive Disorders" has been separated from the previous chapter "Bipolar and Related Disorders" . . . In order to address concerns about the potential for the overdiagnosis of and treatment for bipolar disorder in children, a new diagnosis, disruptive mood dysregulation disorder, referring to the presentation of children with persistent irritability and frequent episodes of extreme behavioral dyscontrol, is added to the depressive disorders . . . Its placement in this chapter reflects the finding that children with this symptom pattern typically develop unipolar depressive disorders or anxiety disorders, rather than bipolar disorders, as they mature into adolescence

and adulthood ... The core feature of disruptive mood dysregulation disorder is chronic, severe persistent irritability. This severe irritability has two prominent clinical manifestations, the first of which is frequent temper outbursts ... The second manifestation of severe irritability consists of chronic, persistently irritable or angry mood that is present between the severe temper outbursts.[20]

Disruptive mood dysregulation disorder (DMDD), then, was their solution. They firmly separated this cohort of children into those with a true cyclical, independent syndrome with both manic episodes and depressive episodes and those best described as irritable with temper tantrums out of proportion to, but in response to, life circumstances.

It should be noted that this book is being written mere months after the creation of the *DSM-5*. Change takes time, and many psychiatrists have yet to adopt the practice of using the diagnosis of disruptive mood dysregulation disorder. This lag occurs for several reasons—medical billing has yet to figure out where this diagnosis fits in the reimbursement scheme; hospitals and universities have not yet altered their documentation to incorporate it; there is a significant dearth of research on its prevalence and availability; and, quite simply, old habits die hard. (By the way, a dearth of research always makes practitioners nervous. We like to think we practice based on evidence—in fact, lack of research was what kept premenstrual dysphoric disorder from being officially recognized in the main body of the *DSM* for twenty years.) We believe that the changes made in the *DSM* concerning pediatric bipolar disorder are positive ones that can spare children and their families from unnecessary treatments and hospitalizations while still providing help to those who need it. That said, no one, not even psychiatrists, has a crystal ball, and so we have little idea as to how this diagnosis will be clinically used and how it will evolve over time. Future research may show that disruptive mood dysregulation disorder does not exist as an entity and instead is merely a descriptive term for those children who have trouble controlling their anger. The evidence behind DMDD is in its infancy; but the evidence for bipolar affective disorder, in its traditional form, is decades long, so we can speak about that, at least, with some confidence. For the remainder of this chapter, we discuss only those adolescents meeting criteria for the bipolar disorder spectrum as defined in the

DSM-5. Along this spectrum, psychiatrists agree that there are three major subtypes of bipolar disorder: *bipolar I*, *bipolar II*, and *cyclothymia*.

BIPOLAR I

Bipolar I is the designation for the classic variety of bipolar disorder characterized by full-blown manic attacks and deep, paralyzing depressions. A schematic representation of the moods of bipolar I is shown in figure 3-1.

The pattern of abnormal mood episodes seems to vary widely, and the pattern of the illness is almost as individual as the person who has the illness. Symptoms of bipolar I usually begin in the late teens or early twenties, so the diagnosis is important to consider in young people with any type of mood disorder. Like the other mood disorders, bipolar I is what physicians refer to as a *relapsing and remitting illness*—during the course of the illness, its symptoms come and go of their own accord and may disappear, without any treatment at all, for months or even years at a time. Clinical studies on the course of bipolar disorder performed in the years before effective treatments for this disorder were available document and illustrate the pattern of bipolar disorder symptoms that existed when the illness was not treated—what physicians call the *natural history* of the illness.

In a 1942 study, researchers looked at the records of sixty-six patients with "manic-depressive psychosis," some of whom had been under observation for up to twenty-six years. These patients went through what we

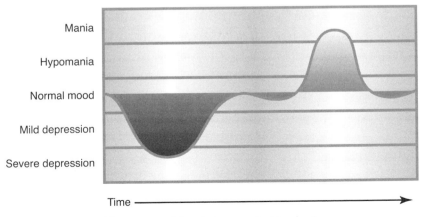

Figure 3-1 Mood changes in bipolar I

now call episodes of the illness, periods of severe depression or mania that lasted for several months (though sometimes much longer) and then went away on their own, with the patient's emotional state returning to normal. Although a few patients seemed to have had only one episode of illness in the period of the study, about one-third had two to three episodes; one-third, four to six episodes; and one-third, more than seven. A few had twenty or more episodes (table 3-4). Unfortunately, when a person is diagnosed with bipolar I disorder, there is no way to know whether the individual will have another two or three episodes during his lifetime or more than twenty.

Bipolar I is the classic manic-depressive illness, with fully developed manic episodes and episodes of severe depression. It is also characterized by long periods of "hibernation," when the symptoms temporarily disappear. The number of episodes varies enormously, but individuals who have only one or two episodes seem to be the exception rather than the rule. Before the availability of effective treatments, the average length of each episode, if untreated, was about six months (in the 1942 study discussed above, the average duration was about six and a half months), but episodes that lasted years and years were not at all uncommon (table 3-5).

Bipolar I disorder seems to be uncommon in teenagers. In 1995, an important study on mood disorders in high school students was published in the *Journal of the American Academy of Child and Adolescent Psychiatry*.[21] To find out how common the various subtypes of mood disorders were in high school students, these researchers interviewed 1,709 boys and girls between the ages of 14 and 17 who attended a high school in western Oregon.

Table 3-4 Episodes of Illness in Sixty-Six Adult Patients with Bipolar Disorder

	Number of Episodes	Percentage of Patients
	1	8
	2–3	29
	4–6	26
	More than 7	37

Source: Data from Thomas A. C. Rennie, "Prognosis in Manic-Depressive Psychosis," *American Journal of Psychiatry* 98 (1942): 801–14, quoted in Frederick Goodwin and Kay Redfield Jamison, *Manic-Depressive Illness* (New York: Oxford University Press, 1990), 133.
Note: This study was done before the availability of any effective treatment for bipolar disorder.

Table 3-5   Features of Bipolar I Disorder

Mood
  Fully developed manic episodes
  Fully developed depressive episodes
Other Features
  Untreated episodes lasting an average of six months

The students were interviewed twice, about a year apart. Only two cases of bipolar I were identified; that is, two students had a history of a full-blown mania, the main diagnostic criterion for bipolar I. Bipolar affective disorder type I is extremely rare in younger children and should prompt a second opinion evaluation by an expert in the field.

BIPOLAR II

Bipolar II is characterized by fully developed depressive episodes and episodes of *hypo*mania. Figure 3-2 shows a schematic representation of the moods of bipolar II.

When lithium became available in the United States in the 1970s, and researchers were trying to find better diagnostic criteria for bipolar disorder, several noticed a large group of patients who didn't have a history of fully developed manic episodes, but who seemed to have a bipolar disorder nonetheless. These people had severe depressions, but their "highs" never developed into mania. Were they "manic-depressives" who were still early in the course of their illness and simply hadn't had time to have a fully de-

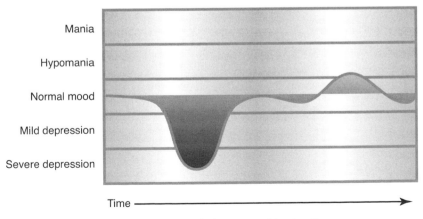

Figure 3-2   Mood changes in bipolar II

veloped manic episode? Several studies attempting to answer this question concluded that these patients did *not* usually go on to have fully developed mania. In one study, less than 5 percent of the patients with recurrent depressions and hypomania eventually became manic.[22] Several studies also showed that many patients with this type of disorder had relatives with a bipolar mood disorder also characterized by major depressions and hypomanias.[23] Although people with bipolar II sometimes have family members who have bipolar I or depressive disorders (without either mania or hypomania), the disorder frequently seems to show up in an identical form in affected families: family members of a person with bipolar II who have mood disorders also tend to have the bipolar II symptom pattern.[24] People with bipolar II disorder also seem to be at higher risk for alcoholism.[25] (See table 3-6 for a list of features characterizing bipolar II.)

Compared with people who have bipolar I disorder, those with bipolar II seem to have more problems with depression—in fact, the depression is sometimes so prominent that many receive a diagnosis of depressive disorder and don't get treatment for bipolar disorder at all. In a study from the National Institutes of Health published in 1995, 559 adult patients diagnosed with a *depressive* disorder were observed over time, some for up to eleven years. Almost 9 percent of them developed symptoms of bipolar II.[26] The first hypomanic episode could usually be documented within several months of the onset of severe depression, but sometimes it took up to nine years for the correct diagnosis to become clear. Some of these 559 "depression" patients also developed a manic episode; that is, they actually had bipolar I, but this was far less common (only 3.9 percent). This study also found that patients with bipolar II disorder had longer depressive episodes (about a year) than those with bipolar I (about six months).

The study of Oregon high school students described above found eleven adolescents (about 0.6 percent) who had had a major depressive episode and had also gone through a period of elevated or irritable mood and other symptoms of hypomania, the pattern of bipolar II.[27] As you might have already figured out, this is about five times the number of students with bipolar I disorder. This finding is consistent with several studies in adults indicating that bipolar II may be more common than bipolar I.

Recall that this study took place prior to the explosion of bipolar affective diagnoses in children. It was undertaken at a time when researchers

Table 3-6 Features of Bipolar II Disorder

Mood
  Fully developed depressive episodes
  Hypomanic episodes
Other Features
  Increased sleep and appetite during depressions
  Depression, sometimes more chronic than with bipolar I
  Family history of bipolar II
  Later age at first hospitalization
  Fewer hospitalizations
  Possible increased risk for alcoholism

still had a more "pure" view of what bipolar affective disorder had to be in children and young adults. Though we do not have access to the actual tools used to describe these young people in their hypomanic states, the states are described as episodes and include distinct periods of elated mood as well as distinct periods of irritable mood that are presumably different from the adolescents' normal mood. Therefore, the results likely encompass those who with some certainty would fit into the bipolar II category. A more recent study may be slightly more suspicious for lumping those with depressed irritability in with the bipolar population.

CYCLOTHYMIC DISORDER

Cyclothymic disorder, or cyclothymia, is characterized by frequent short periods (days to weeks) of mild depressive symptoms and hypomania separated by periods (which also tend to be days to weeks) of fairly normal mood. By definition, the person does not have either fully developed major depressive episodes or manic episodes. A schematic representation of the moods of cyclothymia is presented in figure 3-3.

Individuals with cyclothymic disorder have frequent ups and downs of mood with only comparatively few periods of "normal" mood. Cyclothymic disorder also begins early in life—in the late teens or early twenties. Although many persons with this disorder never develop more severe mood symptoms, a significant number of them eventually have a fully developed depression or manic episode; that is, they develop bipolar disorder. In one study, about 6 percent of patients with the cyclothymic pattern eventually had a manic episode, putting them into the bipolar I category, but a higher

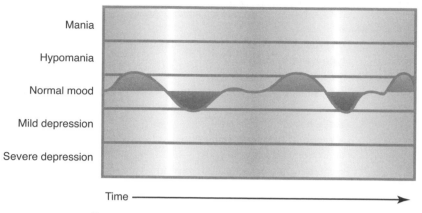

Figure 3-3 Mood changes in cyclothymia

number (25 percent) developed severe depression—they turned out to have bipolar II.[28] Perhaps half of people with the cyclothymic pattern never develop symptoms of "full-blown" bipolar disorder—a finding that makes cyclothymia a true diagnosis in its own right (table 3-7).

Family history studies suggest some relationship between cyclothymia and other bipolar disorders. People with cyclothymia often have relatives with bipolar disorder but rarely have relatives suffering from depressions only. Treatment experiences seem to confirm this relationship—the mood swings of cyclothymic disorder often respond to many of the same treatment approaches as the bipolar disorders do. Cyclothymia was at one time thought to be a personality type, not an illness. Research indicates that this is not true.

In the Oregon study, 5 of the 1,709 students surveyed were diagnosed with cyclothymic disorder. These students had suffered from ups and downs of mood with periods of significant depression but had never experienced the full syndrome of a major depressive episode.[29]

BIPOLAR "SPECTRUM" DISORDERS

If you look at the end of the section on bipolar disorders in the American Psychiatric Association's *Diagnostic and Statistical Manual*, you will see a category titled "Bipolar Disorder Not Otherwise Specified" (also called simply "bipolar NOS"). This odd category exists because the developers of the *DSM* recognized that some patients seem to have a kind of bi-

Table 3-7   Features of Cyclothymic Disorder

Mood
    Frequent alternation between mild depression and mild hypomania
    Short, irregular cycles (days)
    Only short periods of normal mood
Other Features
    Pattern appears in late teens, early twenties
    Frequently mistaken for problems with "personality"
    Sometimes develops into bipolar I or bipolar II disorder

polar disorder but don't really fit the usual picture for bipolar I or II or for cyclothymia.

Psychiatrists have long recognized the existence of many forms of bipolar disorder. For many years, clinicians have described various types of "soft" bipolar disorder, mostly in patients who came to be treated for depression and whose illness seemed related to bipolar disorder.[30] Terms such as *pseudo-unipolar depression* and *bipolar III* have been coined to describe various types of severe depressions that have some features of bipolar disorder but do not fall into traditional categories for bipolar diagnoses. Research into these less defined categories of bipolar disorder are ongoing, but none are officially recognized in the *DSM*.

As more and more treatments for bipolar disorder become available and as more research on the mood disorders is done, we are finding that many patients who suffer from mostly depressive symptoms can benefit from treatment with medications for bipolar disorders and may, in fact, have a type of bipolar disorder. Although we haven't yet figured out how to classify and accurately diagnose these problems, it is becoming clear that they are related in some way to bipolar disorders and that many depressed patients who don't seem to have classic "manic-depressive illness" benefit from medications used to treat those disorders. In the treatment section of this book, we begin to hint at the reasons this may be, but the utter truth is that we simply don't know. From a research standpoint, we do know that people have individual responses to medications: one person's symptoms of depression may respond better to, say, Zoloft (sertraline), while another person with exactly the same symptoms will respond better to Prozac (fluoxetine). The simple fact is that the field of psychiatry has not yet evolved to the point where we can say why this is so (though genetic studies are coming closer to answering the question), any more than we can answer why some individuals with seemingly unipolar depression do much better when a medication for bipolar affective disorder is added to their regimen. This is why having a good psychiatrist who is continually evaluating and reassessing your child's treatment is essential.

MORE ON DIAGNOSIS

As you've probably noticed from the discussion thus far, the boundaries between the various depressive disorders of adolescence are not very clear. Studies indicate that children and adolescents with dysthymia can eventually develop major depressive episodes. Does it make sense to change such a child's diagnosis to major depressive disorder? Did one illness turn into another? Did the child have major depressive disorder all along? If so, why give the problem two different names?

It is useful to remember that modern psychiatry's tendency to split different mood problems into separate diagnostic categories depending on symptom pattern and duration is comparatively new. In fact, the category of mood disorders as a subgroup of psychiatric disorders is only about two hundred years old. Before that, such words as *insanity* and *madness* were used loosely to refer to almost any kind of severe psychiatric problems, even for illnesses we now recognize as medical illnesses that can cause psychiatric symptoms, such as central nervous system syphilis and Alzheimer's disease. The term *melancholia* was used to refer to illnesses we would call severe depression, but this was thought of as a type of "madness" too.

At the beginning of the twentieth century, the great German psychiatrist Emil Kraepelin wrote a new edition of his influential textbook of psychiatry and coined the term *manic-depressive insanity* to encompass *all* the relapsing psychiatric disorders characterized by abnormal mood states. What we now call major depressive disorder, dysthymia, and the various types of bipolar disorder would have been considered forms of manic-depression. Dr. Kraepelin believed that each of these illnesses was a variation of one illness: "In the course of years I have become more and more convinced that all [mood disorders] only represent manifestations of a *single morbid [disease] process*."[31] Kraepelin proposed that seemingly different mood disorders share the same fundamental causes and therefore can never be accurately separated into distinct categories. To modern ears, this makes a certain sort of intuitive sense. What seems to be affected in all the conditions described above is the regularity and integrity of someone's mood state, hinting that a single area of the brain or a single mechanism is affected. Though this may be true, it is similar to saying (and please forgive the analogy), "All cancers represent manifestations of a single morbid process." This is, in a sense, true—in cancer, cells lose the ability to control their own growth and begin to invade surrounding areas. But there are hugely significant differences in the various causes of this change, how it occurs, in which cells, how quickly they grow, how they are treated, and so on. We would argue that mood disorders are similar: they can certainly be grouped roughly together, but in their subtle distinctions, they prove themselves to be different beasts indeed. The *DSM-5* committee seems to be taking a similar view, by separating depressive disorders from bipolar disorders in the fifth edition.

For parents wondering what treatment is best for their depressed child, this discussion might seem a rather useless debate about theoretical matters, the psychiatric equivalent of medieval theologians debating the number of angels that can dance on the head of a pin. But if you remember what we said previously about the importance of diagnosis in predicting the future course of an illness and in helping select treatment, it becomes clearer that this "theoretical debate" has significant practical implications. Research on treatments is meaningful only if the researchers agree on the diagnosis of the individual being treated.

For a time after the first antidepressant medications became available, in the early 1960s, these medications were thought to treat just about any kind of depression. People who suffered from mild, moderate, or severe depressions, with or without the associated symptoms of the depressive syndrome, were often prescribed a "mood elevator," as these pharmaceuticals were sometimes called. The belief then was that antidepressants treated the symptom of depression no matter what the cause, just as aspirin will bring down a feverish person's temperature whether the fever is caused by the flu, pneumonia, or malaria.

Soon it became apparent that antidepressants were of tremendous benefit to some people who complained of depression but seemed to have no effect on others, and that the medications could cause some depressed individuals to develop a manic episode (those who, as we now realize, had a bipolar disorder). By studying the characteristics of patients for whom these medications did or did not work, it became possible to predict with better accuracy which patients antidepressants would help.

Now we have several dozen different antidepressants available, another half dozen or so mood-stabilizing medications, plus several other classes of medications that seem to be helpful in some mood disorder patients. Unfortunately, we are still not very good at predicting precisely which medication will work best for which patient. One of the first steps in getting better at this is improving our diagnostic categories.

Another problem in trying to make a diagnosis in a young person is that mood disorders are, by their nature, relapsing and remitting disorders: symptoms develop, go on for a time, and then may go away on their own, without any treatment. As you have seen, our diagnostic categories are based on how the symptoms fluctuate over time. In a young person who is suffering from depressive symptoms for the first time, an accurate diagnosis may be impossible simply because the course of the illness hasn't had time to play out.

Despite these problems with diagnosis, there are a few facts most psychiatrists agree on. The division of mood disorders into two broad categories based on whether the individual has only depressive symptoms or has depressive as well as manic or mixed symptoms seems to be an important distinction. The terms *unipolar depression* and *bipolar depression* (or *disorder*) describe these two types of depression problems. The bipolar disorders have several subcategories as well, as we've described above. We have already seen that depressive disorders are further subdivided into *major depressive disorder* and *dysthymic disorder.* The foundation for medical treatment of unipolar depressions tends to be antidepressant medications, and treatment for bipolar disorders is usually mood-stabilizing medications. But either type—or both types—of medication may be used in some patients with either type of disorder, because such combinations have been shown to be necessary and effective for some patients.

Some interpret this as proving that Dr. Kraepelin was right after all, that all the mood disorders stem from a "single morbid process." Others insist that we just haven't figured out the right system of categories and diagnostic methods.

So, what is the bottom line here? Psychiatric diagnosis is imprecise and difficult, and the making of a diagnosis must often be tentative. The diagnosis is helpful in predicting the probable course of the illness over time but less helpful in selecting a particular medication.

THE IMPORTANCE OF TREATMENT

Although mental health professionals may disagree about the classification of depressive disorders of adolescence, there is little disagreement about the importance of treatment. Three facts underscore the importance of getting treatment started quickly and making sure the person stays in treatment: (1) depression causes adolescents to suffer significant impairment in many areas of functioning; (2) serious depression is associated with other psychiatric problems, especially substance abuse; and (3) serious depression is a relapsing illness, and adolescent depression can lead to depression in adulthood.

One of the most important reasons for aggressive treatment of depressive disorders in adolescence is the tremendous toll these illnesses take on the functioning and development of teenagers if untreated. As you have seen in this chapter, the symptoms of these disorders can go on for many months, even years, if not treated.

The consequences are far more than repeating classes or being held back a year in school (though these consequences can be significant enough, particularly for adolescents with depleted internal resiliency thanks to depression). These illnesses can essentially shut down the developmental process during a period of very important emotional growth and change. In chapter 2, we reviewed the developmental "tasks" of adolescence, essentially the struggle for differentiation from parents and establishment of a personal identity. Adolescence is a time when important groundwork is laid for mature social functioning and for educational and career development. The adolescent begins to learn to navigate independently in the world and to develop interpersonal skills such as negotiation and compromise. These require a strengthening of self-confidence and healthy independence, exactly the things the adolescent is deprived of by depression. A year of developmental "shutdown" can require several years of "catch-up" to overcome.

In a study that compared the school performance of sixty-two depressed adolescents (average age about 15 years) with thirty-eight adolescents who had no psychiatric illness, the depressed adolescents showed a variety of impairments.[32] In addition to lowered school achievement, these young people were more likely to have behavioral problems in school, they complained that they didn't like their teachers, and their parents received more teacher complaints about them—all illustrating how this illness poisons school life and relationships for the affected adolescent.

There is also evidence that a period of depression has long-lasting effects on adolescents even after they recover from an episode of the illness. The researchers who conducted the Oregon study discussed earlier found that depressed adolescents were "scarred" by the experience of depression in long-lasting ways.[33] They compared a group of students who had never been depressed with a group who had developed and recovered from a major depressive episode. When the adolescents were studied several months after the depressed students had recovered, problems with excess worrying and social withdrawal were found to be more common in the once depressed than in the never depressed group. The formerly depressed students also had less emotional independence and tended to need more emotional support and approval from others. And cigarette smoking was more common among the formerly depressed students. Perhaps the most instructive finding of this study was that only about a quarter of the adolescents who had gone through a depression had received treatment of any kind for their mood problems.

How long does it take to catch up? In 2013, researchers looked at more than one thousand Canadian adolescents (ages 16 to 17) using the national health registry.[34] After two years, those adolescents who had had a depressive episode were more impaired in the realms of educational achievement, employment, social supports, and self-reported health and self-efficacy. At the end of ten years, to some extent the depressed adolescents caught up with their peers in most areas (marital status, employment, financial status). In only two areas were the formerly depressed adolescents behind, but they are two critical areas indeed: level of social support and perceived self-efficacy and health. At least into these individuals' late twenties, the social ramifications of this illness are still evident. It should be noted that this study did not examine those who had been in treatment and those who had not. If more of these teens had gotten treatment and thus been depressed for a shorter time, would depression's "scars" have been milder and perhaps less frequently observed?

Another reason for aggressive treatment of depressive disorders in adolescents is the tendency for depressed adolescents to have other mental health problems, especially behavioral problems. In a study of sixty-seven adolescents with major depression, nearly one in six had behavioral problems severe enough to warrant the diagnostic label "conduct disorder."[35] Young people receiving this diagnosis have serious behavioral problems, such as aggressiveness (bullying others and fighting), destroying property, stealing, truancy, and running away from home. Another study found that these types of severe conduct problems sometimes develop as a complication of the depression and persist even after the depressive symptoms go into remission.[36]

Perhaps the most serious problem associated with depressive disorders is substance abuse. The vignette about Heather illustrates just how dangerous a combination this is. Depressed adolescents, especially girls, are at higher risk than depressed adults for substance abuse, especially as they progress into early adulthood,[37] and the combination of problems puts adolescents at a much higher risk of suicidal behaviors than does either problem alone.

Lastly, the finding that adolescent depressive episodes predict problems with serious depression in adulthood further emphasizes the need for early identification and treatment. Another study looked at the outcome of adolescent major depressive disorder in early adulthood by interviewing young adults who had participated in a study of adolescent major depression about seven years earlier. The results were striking: more than two-thirds of the depressed adolescents had suffered at least one recurrence of major depression. Even more striking was the effect of recurrent depressions on the functional level of the young person. Individuals who had suffered multiple major depressive episodes in the previous years completed less schooling, reported less satisfaction with their lives and more impairment in relationships with friends, and scored lower on a functional rating scale. Also, more had become parents. The individuals who had not suffered a recurrence did not differ from a never depressed control group on any of these measures.[38] These findings show just how important it is to prevent recurrences of depression in adolescents.

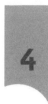

Mood Disorders

A *Summary of Diagnostic Categories in the* DSM

Parents who read a diagnosis in their child's medical records or insurance statements often have questions about the diagnostic categories used by mental health professionals and have concerns about the implications of various diagnostic terms. Psychiatry is one of the few medical specialties that have a more or less official list of disorders and diagnoses. In this chapter, we take a closer look at the latest version of this list, the fifth edition of the *Diagnostic and Statistical Manual of Mental Disorders* (the *DSM-5*), developed and published by the American Psychiatric Association. We present here a brief overview of the *DSM* and explain some of the diagnostic terminology for depressive and other mood disorders.

WHAT IS THE *DSM*?

The roots of the *DSM-5* go at least as far back as the United States Census of 1840, which included the category of "idiocy/insanity" in its classification system of American citizens. By 1880, there were seven categories into which persons with mental illness could be placed: mania, melancholia, monomania, paresis, dementia, dipsomania, and epilepsy.[1] In 1917, the American Medico-Psychological Association (the forerunner of the American Psychiatric Association) developed a statistical manual for use in mental hospitals that included various categories of diagnoses. As time went on, other organizations interested in the statistics of mental illness (such as the Veterans Administration and the United States Army) developed their own statistical manuals. The World Health Organization, after the Second World War, included a long section on mental disorders in the sixth edition of its *International Classification of Disease* (the *ICD 6*).

In 1952, the American Psychiatric Association published the *Diagnostic and Statistical Manual: Mental Disorders*, the *DSM-I*. This work differed from previous statistical manuals because it contained a glossary that described the symptoms of the different disorders. Thus, in addition to containing an official list of categories of mental illness, the *DSM-I* provided guidance to the clinician in making psychiatric diagnoses. By the time the third edition of the manual appeared in 1980 (the *DSM-III*), each category of psychiatric disorders had a list of *diagnostic criteria*—symptoms and other characteristics of each disorder that were thought to define it and to set it apart from other psychiatric disorders. This was a large leap forward in psychiatric diagnoses, as all psychiatrists began to speak the same language. Now, when a patient goes to a new doctor and her medical records indicate a diagnosis of, say, "panic disorder" or "anorexia nervosa," the new doctor knows (if previous psychiatrists did their job well, of course) that the patient has had certain symptoms and not others and that the symptoms have troubled her for a certain period.

The *DSM-III* allowed psychiatric research to flourish. Previously, it was difficult to do a study on a group of "depressed" patients, because (as we've shown) this one word could encompass persons experiencing dozens of varying *syndromes*, all of whom shared the *symptom* of low mood. Use of the *DSM* in research means that when you read in a study of some particular psychiatric disorder in a professional journal that "the patients met the *DSM* diagnostic criteria" for that disorder, you can be sure that all the patients in the study had a certain well-defined collection of symptoms and other characteristics in common and that the researchers are not mixing psychiatric "apples and oranges." The *DSM-III* allowed researchers to create a long list of criteria that patients had to meet in order to be included in a study (for example, they must have five symptoms of depression, not merely low mood; must have them for a specific length of time; and so on). The *DSM-III* suffered from the same problems as later versions, in that the checklist of depressive symptoms captured a nonuniform population—one person could have the syndrome of major depressive disorder, while another had just lost a loved one—but still, this advance led to a proliferation of research around these conditions. Sometimes, the research supported the classifications delineated in the *DSM-III*, and other times it suggested that some symptoms needed to be included, or thrown out, of various descriptions. All of this came together fourteen years later to create the *DSM-IV*, which was the pinnacle of psychiatric diagnosis until recently. Now, almost ten years after that edition's release, researchers and clinicians have again come together to update the *DSM*, resulting in the *DSM-5*. Some of these updates were again based on research proving, or disproving, existing classifications. Others were updates to expunge seemingly outdated notions, or to clarify the practice of psychiatry more than the research (recall our discussion of mood disorders and dividing them into two separate chapters in the *DSM*).

A word of warning about the *DSM* is needed here. Because the manual contains a list of psychiatric diagnoses followed by succinct and clearly written criteria for making those diagnoses, it has the unfortunate effect of making psychiatric diagnosis look easy. It is tempting for individuals who do not have any psychiatric training to see the manual as a series of symptom checklists that can be easily applied to make the diagnosis of mental illness. This is not the case, for a number of reasons.

First of all, only with an enormous amount of training and experience can one gain an appreciation for the wide range of *normal* emotions and behaviors and have a sense of what falls outside this normal range. Significant clinical experience and judgment are needed to decide what constitutes an "irritable mood" or an "increase in energy" that is *clinically* significant. The *DSM* is full of diagnostic criteria that use qualifiers—"*clinically* significant," "*marked* impairment," "*excessive* involvement in..."—all requiring judgment based on experience. Even some counseling and therapy professionals, if they have not trained in a setting where they have had the opportunity to see very sick patients, may not really have an appreciation for what constitutes *severe*—simply because they have never seen and worked with severely depressed patients. Nonprofessionals, of course, usually have even less experience with the range of normal and abnormal moods. Without the experience of seeing and treating many patients with depressive illnesses, it is impossible to accurately separate normal from abnormal mental experiences or clinically significant mood changes from those that are within the range of normal. In psychiatry as perhaps in no other field, the dictum "a little knowledge is a dangerous thing" holds true.

Second, many *medical* conditions can mimic abnormal mood states. Dozens of pharmaceuticals can cause depressed or euphoric states in some persons, and drugs of abuse can cause all kinds of mood changes and psychoses in almost anyone. Almost all the *DSM* diagnoses contain "exclusion criteria" for medical conditions, such as "the symptoms are not due to . . . a general medical condition." Only a clinician trained in the diagnosis and treatment of physical illness will be able to pick up these sorts of problems.

Third, just as the range of normal experience and behavior is enormous, so is the range and complexity of abnormal mental experiences and behaviors—they cannot be contained in any one book and certainly not all described in a few dozen diagnostic categories.

Last, and perhaps most important, the *DSM* is designed to see the patient in one "plane," rather than three dimensionally. It does not discuss the origin of a syndrome so much as its current symptoms. We discussed earlier how a young person can be diagnosed as ADHD at 5, anxiety at 8, depression at 10, bipolar at 16—to anyone familiar with the *DSM*, it is fairly clear how this can happen. An anxious child, constantly alert to threats in his environment, can certainly have trouble regulating his attention at a young age, as could a traumatized child. Though they may "meet criteria" according to the *DSM* for the diagnosis of ADHD, in reality these symptoms could be the result of their anxiety or trauma. Only through a thorough evaluation, followed by serial examinations and a process of truly getting to know the child and his experiences, can a clinician make such a determination. Filling out a checklist certainly does not suffice and, for inexperienced clinicians, can be the origin of misdiagnosis.

For these reasons, we are not going to list the *DSM* diagnostic criteria for the disorders described in this chapter. We don't want to tempt nonclinicians to engage in self-diagnosis or diagnosis of family members. The *DSM* is easily available in libraries—but it should be considered a reference book for clinicians, not a textbook of psychiatry.

A MULTIAXIAL DIAGNOSTIC SYSTEM

You, the reader, are engaging in this discussion at an interesting time. The multiaxial diagnosis was included in the *DSM* at version III and has been the mainstay of psychiatric assessment for more than thirty years. It can be tremendously useful in dividing up and more clearly thinking about different "types" of diagnoses in separate categories (more on that in a moment). Despite its usefulness, it had the unfortunate effect of setting psychiatry somewhat apart from the rest of the medical fields, because psychiatry is the only specialty that uses its own particular method of discussing diagnoses. As such, the *DSM-5* no longer requires the use of the multiaxial system, though it is still in use by most psychiatrists at the time of this writing. We have already discussed that change takes time, and though the *DSM-5* has only been available for a short while, we expect that the multiaxial system will not go anywhere soon. It is possible, as time marches forward, that fewer and fewer clinicians will choose to employ the multiaxial system in diagnosing their patients, so it is helpful for you to be familiar with, though not attached to, this methodology.

A multiaxial *DSM* diagnosis always lists five types of diagnoses and other pieces of clinical information on patients in five separate categories, each of which is called an *axis*.

Axis I	Clinical disorders
Axis II	Personality and intelligence
Axis III	General medical conditions
Axis IV	Psychosocial and environmental problems
Axis V	Assessment of level of functioning

The reason for this complexity is that, to put it plainly, people are complex creatures, and an understanding of their mental life requires looking at them from several different angles.

On *axis I* is listed the psychiatric illness or condition that is being treated or studied. This is where a mood disorder diagnosis would go, as would diagnoses such as attention-deficit/hyperactivity disorder or panic disorder or alcohol abuse. Because symptoms of a psychiatric illness might be expressed differently depending on a person's personality and intellectual ability, these two factors are also recorded for every patient—on *axis II*. A diagnosis of a personality disorder would be listed here. A person with "avoidant personality disorder," for example, is socially inhibited, hypersensitive to negative comments or reactions from others, and constantly fearful of criticism and rejection. These individuals are so sensitized to criticism that they see it everywhere and avoid making friends or even going to social activities. They withdraw from life and function below their true capabilities because of these fears and preoccupations. This pattern of thinking, relating, and behaving is called a personality disorder because it seems ingrained in the individual's personality from an early age rather than the expression of an illness imposed on him at some point in life. Similarly, personality disorders do not cycle like mood disorders. Rather than being episodic, these conditions are ingrained in every aspect of the person's interactions with the world and are consistent aspects of his being.

Personality disorder diagnoses are not made very often in adolescents, for several reasons. The most important one is that in young persons, personality style is still under development. Personality traits that are present in childhood often do not persist into adult life. Another reason is that prolonged periods of depression can negatively affect adolescents' ways of thinking about themselves and their relationships. You've already seen how depression can adversely affect how young persons relate to others and color their view of themselves and their world. It's not difficult, then, to see how a chronically depressed young person can seem to have the personality style and show the behaviors of avoidant personality disorder briefly described above and thus seem to meet the criteria for this diagnosis. But to make a diagnosis of a personality disorder would be to miss the most important problem: depression. Technically, a diagnosis of personality disorder can be made in someone under the age of 18 if the personality traits have been present and causing problems for at least one year. Nevertheless, for the reasons we've mentioned, most psychiatrists are reluctant (or at least they should be) to make a personality disorder diagnosis in an adolescent, especially an adolescent who is or has been depressed.

Axis III is the place to list any medical problem the individual may have. Examples would be high blood pressure, asthma, kidney failure, or migraine headaches. The axis III diagnosis is sometimes very important in treating a patient with a mood disorder because mood symptoms can be caused or affected by medical conditions, such as thyroid problems or medications being taken for a medical problem. Medication that an adolescent might be taking for asthma, for example, can cause nervousness and anxiety.

On *axis IV* are listed problems in and stresses from the environment that may contribute to the patient's difficulties—parental divorce, serious illness in the adolescent or another family member, a move to a new community, chronic poverty, living in an unsafe neighborhood. These factors can also affect how individuals cope with illness as well as their response to treatment. Axis IV information is especially important in the mood disorders, since environmental stressors can be an important precipitating factor for an episode of illness.

On *axis V*, the clinician records an assessment of the patient's functional level, using a 1 to 100 rating scale called the Global Assessment of Functioning (GAF) Scale. This assessment is a judgment of how impaired (or unimpaired) a patient is by symptoms in everyday life. On this scale, a score of 80 or above indicates basically normal everyday functioning, below 50 indicates serious impairment such as recurrent unemployment due to psychiatric illness, and below 20 indicates a level of impairment that suggests the need for psychiatric hospitalization. This axis is more useful to researchers and statisticians than to clinicians, but it rounds out a picture of the patient, capturing strengths as opposed to afflictions.

MOOD DISORDER CATEGORIES IN THE *DSM*

We've already discussed the two main depressive disorder categories: major depressive disorder and dysthymic disorder. *Major depressive disorder* is the most frequently diagnosed depressive disorder of adolescence. It is characterized by one or more major depressive episodes and periods of recovery between episodes. *Dysthymic disorder* is the smoldering disorder in which symptoms persist for months at a time. According to the *DSM*, symptoms must persist for at least one year in children and adolescents. (Adults must show symptoms for two years.)

In the *DSM*, serious depressive illnesses that don't quite fit the diagnostic criteria for either of these disorders are called "depressive disorder not otherwise specified" (depressive disorder NOS). This is something of a "wastebasket" category and a good example of why the *DSM* should not be considered a psychiatric "bible" when it comes to understanding and treating patients. An adolescent who has had symptoms of dysthymic disorder for 364 days would technically need to be diagnosed with depressive disorder NOS until, on the 365th day, the diagnosis could be changed to dysthymic disorder—obviously not a meaningful distinction for an individual patient. People with severe depression who don't have enough symptoms on a *DSM* checklist also technically need to be put into this category. The *DSM* should be seen as a guide to diagnosis and treatment, not a textbook. It would be wise to repeat our favorite quote from Alfred Kinsey here: "The world is not divided into sheep and goats . . . Nature rarely deals with discrete categories. Only the human mind invents categories and tries to force facts into separated pigeonholes."[2] We've already discussed some of the difficulties in separating depressive disorders in young persons into discrete categories and some of the problems with symptom overlap. (Compare table 4-1 to tables 4-2 and 4-3 to see how the mood disorder checklists have changed from the fourth edition to the fifth.)

The *DSM* also provides several other descriptive terms, called *specifiers*, that can be added to the main diagnosis to better describe the current episode of mood problems. The clinician can call the episode *mild, moderate,* or *severe.* If the patient has not had any episodes in two months, the disorder can be designated *in remission (in full remission* if there have been no symptoms for two months, *in partial remission* if only a few symptoms exist or the remission has been for less than two months). In the DSM-IV, if the patient has all the symptoms of major depression continuously for a period of at least two years, major depression is said to be *chronic.*

The specifier *with melancholic features* can be added when the patient's depressive episode is dominated by loss of ability to experience pleasure (anhedonia) and by guilty feelings, loss of appetite, and the classic daily fluctuation of mood (early morning awakening, with the mood lifting slightly as the day progresses)—in short, the "textbook" depressive syndrome so eloquently described by William Styron in *Darkness Visible.*

Another clinical syndrome (more common in pure depressive disorders than in the depressive phase of a bipolar disorder) has been called *atypical depression.* People with this syndrome retain reactivity in their mood (for example, their mood brightens when good things happen). In fact, they seem to have a "hyper-reactive" mood and an especially difficult time with rejection in interpersonal relationships—even when not in an episode of depression. They also tend to have changes in appetite and sleep of the less common pattern: eating and sleeping too much.

The specifier *with psychotic features* can be added if the patient has hallucinations or delusional beliefs during the illness, such as those described in

Table 4-1   Mood Disorders in the *DSM-IV*

Major Depressive Disorder
    Full syndrome of severe depression
        Severity specifiers
            —mild, moderate, severe (with or without psychotic features)
            —in partial or full remission
        Special syndrome specifiers
            —with melancholic, catatonic, or atypical features
            —with postpartum onset
        Longitudinal course specifiers
            —with or without full inter-episode recovery
            —with seasonal pattern
            —chronic
Dysthymic Disorder
    Smoldering, low-grade, long-standing depression
        —early onset (before age 21)
        —late onset (after age 21)
        —with atypical features
Depressive Disorder NOS
Bipolar Disorder I
    Mania and severe depression
Bipolar Disorder II
    Severe depression and hypomania
        Specifiers for bipolar disorders:
            Severity specifiers
            —mild, moderate, severe (with or without psychotic features)
            —in partial or full remission
            Special syndrome specifiers
            —with melancholic, catatonic, or atypical features
            —with postpartum onset
            Longitudinal course specifiers
            —with or without full inter-episode recovery
            —with seasonal pattern
            —with rapid cycling
Bipolar Disorder NOS
    "Soft" bipolar and bipolar spectrum disorders
Cyclothymic Disorder
    Depressive symptoms and hypomanias
Substance-Induced Mood Disorder
    Mood Disorder Due to a General Medical Condition

Table 4-2   Depressive Disorders in the *DSM-5*

Major Depressive Disorder
    Full syndrome of severe depression
        Severity specifiers
            —mild, moderate, severe
            —with mood congruent or incongruent psychotic features
            —in partial, in full remission or unspecified
        Special syndrome specifiers
            —with melancholic, catatonic, or atypical features
            —with anxious distress
        Longitudinal course specifiers
            —with or without full inter-episode recovery
            —with seasonal pattern
            —with peripartum onset
Dysthymic Disorder/Persistent Depressive Disorder
    Smoldering, low-grade depression
        Severity specifiers
            —mild, moderate, severe
            —in partial, in full remission or unspecified
        Special syndrome specifiers
            —with melancholic, catatonic, or atypical features
            —with anxious distress
        Longitudinal course specifiers
            —with pure dysthymic syndrome
            —with intermittent major depressive episodes
            —with peripartum onset
        Timing modifiers
            —early onset (before 21)
            —late onset (after 21)
Premenstrual Dysphoric Disorder
    A time-limited major depressive episode surrounding menses
Disruptive Mood Dysregulation Disorder
    Chronic irritability thought to be related to a low-level depression
Substance/Medication Induced Depressive Disorder
Depressive Disorder Due to Another Medical Condition
    Unspecified Depressive Disorder

Table 4-3   Bipolar and Related Disorders in the *DSM-5*

Bipolar Disorder I
  Mania and severe depression
Bipolar Disorder II
  Severe depression and hypomania
    Specifiers for bipolar disorders:
      Severity specifiers
        —mild, moderate, severe
        —with mood congruent or incongruent psychotic features
        —in partial or full remission
      Special syndrome specifiers
        —with melancholic, catatonic, atypical or mixed features
        —with anxious distress
      Longitudinal course specifiers
        —with peripartum onset
        —with seasonal pattern
        —with rapid cycling
Bipolar Disorder NOS
  "Soft" bipolar and bipolar spectrum disorders
Cyclothymic Disorder
  Depressive symptoms and hypomanias
Unspecified Bipolar and Related Disorder
  "Soft" bipolar and bipolar spectrum disorders
Substance/Medication Induced Bipolar and Related Disorder
  Bipolar and Related Disorder Due to Another Medical Condition

---

chapter 2. The specifier *with catatonic features* is added if the patient shows symptoms of catatonia, a rare syndrome in which the individual lies (or sometime sits or stands) motionless for long periods staring into space and has other unusual physical mannerisms, such as rigid posturing, grimacing, or meaninglessly repeating whatever is said to him. Both of these problems are unusual in adolescent depressions.

Another set of specifiers describes the course of the illness over time, called *longitudinal course specifiers*. Mood disorders may be *with* or *without full inter-episode recovery*, depending on whether the individual is completely free of symptoms between episodes or not.

Some people have a mood disorder in which they have repeated depressive episodes occurring regularly in the winter and sometimes hypomanic or manic symptoms in the summer. This illness has been called *seasonal af-*

fective disorder. In DSM-IV, the specifier *with seasonal pattern* is added to the diagnosis of major depressive or bipolar disorder.

Lastly, patients with a bipolar disorder who have had at least four episodes in twelve months have a disorder *with rapid cycling.*

When drug intoxication or medical problems mimic depressive episodes, the DSM diagnoses *substance/medication-induced depressive disorder* or *depressive disorder due to another medical condition* are used. When the mood problem is due to a medical condition, the medical condition and type of mood change are specified in the diagnosis (as in, for example, "mood disorder due to hyperthyroidism, with manic features"). When the problem is due to substance abuse, the type of mood change and whether the symptoms came on during intoxication or withdrawal are specified. (Examples would be "alcohol-induced mood disorder with depressive features, onset during withdrawal" and "cocaine-induced mood disorder with manic features, onset during intoxication.")

CONTROVERSIES IN THE USE OF THE *DSM*

There have been enormous controversies surrounding the use of the DSM in the diagnosis of psychiatric problems in children and adolescents. Although these controversies don't touch very directly on the use of DSM diagnoses for mood disorders, a brief discussion is still warranted. The misuse of psychiatric diagnosis is, and should be, an important concern for parents.

The problems with the DSM arise with the various diagnoses that get applied to children and adolescents with behavioral problems: problems involving high activity levels, defiant behaviors, and disruptive and destructive behaviors. The main criticism usually leveled at the DSM is that it "medicalizes" problems in children that are really no more than normal behavioral and developmental variations of one type or another. The parents of a child who is more energetic and less attentive than his classmates get a letter from the teacher recommending that the child be evaluated for attention deficit disorder. When does "inattention" become attention deficit disorder? How does anyone decide what constitutes a "disorder"?

In earlier chapters, we made the point that most of the problems psychiatrists are called on to treat do not have any known physical basis—no abnormalities on brain scans or blood tests (what are called *biological markers* for psychiatric illness). This means that the diagnostic criteria are basically things that the person experiences or does: thoughts, feelings, and behaviors. A problem arises when what are identified as "symptoms" are experiences or behaviors that are not outside the realm of normal except in degree.

There is little disagreement that hearing voices when no one is speaking is not normal. And the frenzied disorganization of mania can't be mistaken for normal high spirits. But what about a childhood diagnosis such as *conduct disorder*, for which the symptoms are behaviors like fighting, setting fires, disobedience, and running away? How does one decide when "bad behavior" becomes "*really* bad behavior," and therefore becomes conduct disorder? Even more slippery is *oppositional defiant disorder*, for which the diagnostic criteria include things like "often loses temper," "often argues with adults," "is often angry and resentful," and "is often touchy or easily annoyed by others." An adolescent who has had these characteristics for six months, to the point where they cause "clinically significant impairment" in her school or family life, would meet the *DSM* criteria for this diagnosis. Now, from what you already know about depression, you can see that a depressed adolescent may be all of these things. Does Heather in the vignette in chapter 3 have both major depressive disorder *and* oppositional defiant disorder? Although, technically, she does not, because the *DSM* diagnosis of oppositional defiant disorder cannot be made when the symptoms occur during an episode of depression, you can see how complicated and difficult the issue of psychiatric diagnosis can sometimes be. For every voice calling for the early identification and treatment of psychiatric problems in young people, there seems to be another one warning that overdiagnosing and, worse, overmedicating young people is the real problem, and a more sinister one at that.

How are these controversies important for the parent of a depressed adolescent? First, they reinforce what we have been saying about the *DSM* being only a guide to psychiatric diagnosis—and a decidedly imperfect one. Second, they should make parents cautious and questioning about the diagnosis of a behavioral disorder in their child if they notice signs of depression. Using the *DSM* criteria for behavioral disorders as a checklist to assess difficult behaviors and assign diagnoses such as conduct disorder and oppositional defiant disorder, while missing a depression or other causes of these clusters of behaviors, happens all too frequently—especially when the *DSM* is in the hands of persons without much training in the assessment of psychiatric illnesses. Third, and perhaps most important, parents should be skeptical of some people's insistence on the opposite view: that the behavioral symptoms of serious depressive illnesses are no more than "bad behavior" and, worse, that punishment rather than treatment is necessary to teach adolescents about the "consequences" of their bad behaviors.

Unlike some other *DSM* categories, depressive disorders in adolescence have a clear demarcation from normal behaviors and need medical treatment. That treatment is the subject of the next part of the book.

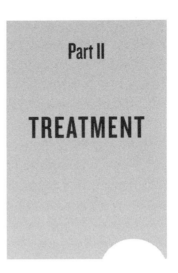

Part II

TREATMENT

I N THESE CHAPTERS, we discuss the available treatments for adolescent depression. We now have a wide range of options, from pharmaceutical and other medical treatments to specific types of psychotherapy that have proved especially helpful in treating depression.

Chapter 5 introduces some of the special considerations that must be given to the use of medications in the adolescent age range. After all, some adolescents are physically more like children, whereas others are close to adults. Are medications given in different dosages to adolescents? Are the medications known to be effective in treating adult depression also effective in adolescents? These are some of the questions answered here. We also present a brief introduction to what we know about the chemical workings of the brain and how the medications used to treat depression work.

In chapters 6 through 8, we talk more specifically about medical treatment, reviewing the various pharmaceuticals used to treat these illnesses. In chapter 8, we include some less frequently used medications, some alternative treatments for depression, and electroconvulsive therapy—still a valuable resource for the treatment of mood disorders. This chapter ends with a discussion of several promising experimental treatments for severe depression. Finally, chapter 9 covers the role of counseling and psychotherapy in treating adolescents with depression.

Medication Issues in Adolescence

5

W
e know that the medications used to treat adult disorders don't always work in quite the same way in children and adolescents. Unfortunately, textbooks, research articles, and prescribing guidelines from pharmaceutical manufacturers often provide only limited guidance about the use of medications to treat psychiatric problems in children and adolescents. One reason for this is that far fewer good research studies have been conducted on the use of psychiatric medications in these younger patients than on their use in adults. Pharmaceutical research is more difficult to do in young people, for a variety of reasons. Parents who would willingly volunteer to be in a drug study are often much less willing to volunteer their children for research, making it difficult to recruit research subjects. Issues of informed consent to be a research subject are much more complicated when minors are involved, making researchers reluctant to tackle the issue. Not only are these studies more challenging to do, but the financial returns for pharmaceutical companies are often far lower: children and adolescents usually represent a smaller "market" for medications than do adults.

These factors have added up to a lack of information about the use of psychiatric medications in children and adolescents compared with that available for prescribing to adults. The prescription of psychiatric medication to young people is often what is referred to as "off-label" prescribing, a term we explain below.

PHARMACEUTICALS AND THE FDA

The United States Food and Drug Administration (FDA) is responsible for determining that a pharmaceutical is safe for use in humans and that it is effective for the illness or symptoms for which the manufacturer claims it is effective. The FDA's process of determining the safety of pharmaceuticals is quite thorough, perhaps the most thorough and rigorous in the world. It is credited with preventing an epidemic in the United States of birth defects caused by thalidomide, which occurred in other countries during the 1960s. Thalidomide was widely used in Europe but had not been approved for sale in the United States when it was discovered to cause severe deforming birth defects in children whose mothers had taken it during pregnancy.

A pharmaceutical company performs, sponsors, and encourages research on a drug it wants to sell and then presents the research results to the FDA in support of its request to sell the drug and market it to physicians. Once the drug is approved, the product can be sold in the United States, and the FDA regulates how the drug is "labeled" for use. This "labeling" is the information on the product insert distributed with the drug to physicians and patients. Only the indications for a medication that have been evaluated by the FDA may be listed on the label. For example, antibiotic manufacturers are allowed to list only those illnesses for which the antibiotic has been proved effective by the FDA. Now, doctors may know from research studies and experience that a certain medication works for other illnesses and may legally prescribe it as they see fit. The FDA does not regulate how physicians can prescribe a given pharmaceutical. Doctors can legally prescribe an approved drug for *any* purpose they want to, based on their knowledge of the medical research literature and using their medical judgment—even if the FDA has not reviewed the effectiveness of the drug for that particular use. When a doctor prescribes a pharmaceutical for an illness or symptom that is not covered in the drug's labeling, this is called *off-label* prescribing.

There are several reasons that physicians quite frequently prescribe pharmaceuticals for off-label indications. Once a drug has been approved for sale, manufacturers are often very conservative about requesting the FDA to approve a new use for the drug (called the drug's *indication*), even if clinical research shows the new use is an effective one. For example, research had shown quite clearly that antidepressant medications were effective in the treatment of panic attacks for many years before the FDA labeled any antidepressants for treating panic disorder; many antidepressants are still not labeled for this use but are widely and safely prescribed for panic attacks. Research had shown that the antiepilepsy medication divalproex was a safe and effective treatment for manic symptoms for many years before its manufacturer, Abbott Laboratories, requested that its brand of divalproex, Depakote, be approved to treat mania. Off-label prescription of a pharmaceutical for a particular condition often precedes FDA-approved prescribing for that condition by years, even decades. As of this writing, the antidepressant sertraline (Zoloft) is labeled for the treatment of obsessive-compulsive disorder in children 6 to 17 years old but not for the treatment of depression, even though more prescriptions are probably written to treat depression than obsessive-compulsive disorder in this age range.

At other times, the off-label use of medications is driven more by marketing than by medical knowledge. It is obviously in the pharmaceutical company's financial interest to sell as much of its product as possible. To this end, drugs were once "marketed off label" for all sorts of uses that had not been evaluated by the FDA. For many years, the medication Neurontin was used off label as a treatment for bipolar affective disorder, even though later evidence would show that it had no effect on the condition. More recently, Johnson and Johnson has agreed to a $2.2 billion settlement for charges that it was actively pushing the use of medications off label. The manufacturer was accused of creating a misleading marketing campaign targeting aggression in elderly patients, implying that the medication (risperidone, or Risperdal) had been proved safe and effective, when in fact it had not been specifically studied in this population at all and, once it was, was shown to be potentially harmful. Furthermore, they were accused of giving payments and kickbacks to elder care facilities and to physicians for using and promoting the use of the medication in this manner. The federal government was particularly interested in this case as virtually all the medication was being paid for by Medicare, which means in essence that the taxpayers were funding this potentially inappropriate prescribing.

In an effort to minimize extraneous uses of medications, the FDA now strictly regulates how a drug is advertised and marketed to physicians by representatives of pharmaceutical companies. Physicians can still prescribe any medication as they choose, but under the newer legislation, a pharmaceutical company's sales representatives are not permitted to discuss off-label uses of their company's products when they make marketing visits to physicians, nor are they allowed to discuss off-label uses in any of their marketing materials. Some locations have gone a step further. In many major medical centers, pharmaceutical representatives are not even allowed on the grounds except under strictly regulated circumstances, to prevent biased prescribing by the centers' physicians.

As you read this discussion, we worry that you may take our message to be that "pharmaceutical companies are evil, and the FDA is there to prevent their opportunistic parasitism on the ill." This is simply not true. Although they are businesses, they also donate millions of dollars' worth of medications per year to those in need, contribute to charities, and participate in untold billions of dollars in research to help us understand illnesses better. Of course they would prefer that physicians prescribe only the medications that they manufacture, but they also understand that not every medicine works for every patient. In our personal interactions with pharmaceutical representatives, we have never found them to be unnecessarily pushy; nor have they been insulted or affronted when we discuss the use of another company's medications instead. It is true, however, that the FDA takes its job very seriously and wants to ensure that all medications taken by patients are safe, effective, and given for their best interest. This has led the FDA to be exceedingly cautious before approving a new medicine, some may feel overly so.

What are the reasons for the inconsistencies and delays in getting a medication FDA approved? There are several. Perhaps the most important is that once a medication has been approved for one indication, a pharmaceutical manufacturer may decide that it's not particularly advantageous to request a new indication, especially if the new indication is for a less common condition. The expense of going through an FDA approval process may not be offset by the increase in sales that marketing the drug for the new indication would bring about—especially since doctors are able to prescribe the medication off label anyway. This means that the labeling of any pharmaceutical is usually an incomplete guide to the use of a medication and illustrates why a physician must have a familiarity with the clinical research literature to make prescribing decisions. The popular *Physicians'*

Desk Reference (the PDR) is *not* a good source of information about medications and prescribing for this very reason: the *PDR* is only a compilation of the FDA labeling for medications. If physicians limited themselves to only FDA-approved uses of pharmaceuticals, many patients would go untreated for conditions for which proven remedies are available.

Just as a pharmaceutical company may decide it's not financially advantageous to ask the FDA to label a drug for a new indication, the company may decide there are no financial incentives to ask the FDA to label a drug for prescription to children and adolescents. If you glance through the *PDR*, you'll notice that for many medications, it makes no mention of uses in children and adolescents and gives only the recommended doses in adults. Many psychiatric medications fall into this category. The FDA is addressing this vacuum, and policy revisions are in the works with new requirements to address the use of medications in young people when approval is sought for new pharmaceuticals.

DOSE ADJUSTMENTS AND OTHER DIFFERENCES FOR YOUNG PEOPLE

The dosing of medications is more complicated for young people than for adults. On the one hand, because children are physically smaller than adults, pediatric doses of medication are often smaller than adult doses. But then again, a healthy 16-year-old who is mature for his age may be physically bigger than many adults and require a dose of medication in the adult range, perhaps even at the top of the adult range. Sometimes a dosing guide is available that calls for a calculation of the appropriate dose of a medication based on body weight—but physical size differences between children and adults are only a part of the story. Many medications are absorbed into fat tissue, and at various ages young people and adults have different proportions of fatty tissue. This factor can be especially important in adolescents, because the distribution of fat tissue can change dramatically during puberty over a short time, especially in girls, requiring more frequent dosage adjustments than in adults.

Young people sometimes absorb medications from the gastrointestinal tract into their bloodstream more rapidly than do adults. This means that after a dose of medication, the level of medication in the blood rises more rapidly and to a higher peak level in adolescents than in adults. This can cause more sleepiness or other side effects immediately after taking the medication. Splitting the dose of medication into several doses throughout the day may help with this problem, but doing so means there are twice or even three times as many opportunities to forget to take a dose.

Young people and adults also eliminate medications differently. The amount of medication active in the body is determined by a balance between how much is going in and how much is going out: the main organ in charge of the "going out" part is the liver, which chemically breaks down most medications into inactive forms, which are then usually eliminated through the kidneys into the urine. In children, the liver is larger in proportion to overall body size than it is in adults. This means that children may eliminate a medication more quickly and may therefore need a surprisingly higher dose than would be expected from their physical stature.

All these differences decrease, of course, as a young person grows from child to adolescent to young adult. But remember that the timing of these physical changes can vary quite a bit from one individual to another. One particular 15-year-old might need to take a pediatric dose of a medication, while another might require an adult dose, because of these differences in physical maturity.

In addition to dosing differences, there may be important efficacy differences between young people and adults. That is, just because a medication is effective in adults for a particular problem doesn't mean it will be equally effective for what seems to be a similar problem in a child or adolescent. The most striking example of this is the difference in efficacy of certain antidepressants. The class of antidepressants called tricyclic antidepressants has been used with great effectiveness to treat depressive disorders in adults for many years, and it was assumed that tricyclics must be effective in childhood depression as well. But in several clinical studies done in the 1980s, tricyclics appeared no more effective than placebo (a sugar pill) in treating childhood depression. (Other types of studies do show some efficacy; we discuss this controversy in the next chapter.) It may be that the different symptoms often seen in younger depression patients are a reflection of variations in the chemical basis of their depression, or perhaps a difference between the developing nervous system and the mature brain makes younger patients respond to some medications differently.

All these issues mean that the dosing rules and guidelines for prescribing most psychiatric medications for young people are still developing. A glance through the *PDR* is *not* a good way to get information about medications. A discussion with the prescribing physician about the reasoning for picking a particular dose of medication *is*.

HOW PSYCHIATRIC MEDICATIONS WORK

A number of years ago, psychiatrist and neuroscientist Nancy Andreason wrote the book *The Broken Brain*, about new discoveries in biological psychiatry.[1] The title makes the point that psychiatric illnesses such as major depressive disorder, bipolar disorder, and schizophrenia are caused by biological and chemical malfunctions of the brain, not repressed memories or traumatic childhoods. Although we still don't know exactly what these malfunctions are, we are getting close to understanding some of the biological mechanisms that might be involved in the symptoms of mood disorders.

To understand the treatment of mood disorders with medications, you should know a little bit about how the brain works. Patients and parents frequently ask, "What does this medication *do*?" The answer to this question turns out to be complicated, so in this chapter, we're going to give a brief overview of the functioning of the human nervous system, just enough to help you understand a little bit about how psychiatric medications work.

Many people imagine that the human brain is a kind of wonderful computer. Although this is a vast oversimplification of the true capabilities of the brain, it's a good place to start in trying to understand how this fantastic organ of the mind works.

Like the computer that we used to write these words, a human brain receives input, processes the information it receives, and then delivers output. Like a computer, it stores information and often uses this stored information to help process the input it receives. The brain receives its input from the sense organs—the eyes, ears, taste buds, touch receptors, and so forth—and delivers output in the form of behavior.

The simplest example of this input-processing-output circuit in our nervous system is the spinal reflex. This circuit is so simple and so automatic in its operation that it richly deserves its label, *reflex*, meaning a simple behavior that requires no "thinking" to be effectively carried out. If you inadvertently touch the hot surface of a stove or a candle flame, a nerve ending detects the resulting tissue damage and fires a message along a nerve fiber (a sensory nerve) that ends in the spinal cord. Here, the first nerve communicates with another nerve, which dispatches a message down again through another fiber (a motor nerve) to activate the arm muscles to pull the finger back from the source of heat (figure 5-1). If you've ever actually had this experience, you may have noticed that your hand pulled away before you even felt the pain. This is because the brain, where consciousness resides, is not yet involved. (The message that is eventually sent up to the brain from the level of the spinal cord responding to the pain signal is more or less an "FYI" message that will be stored in the memory system. Hopefully, this painful memory will lessen the chances of the same thing happening again.)

Let's look at a more complicated example of the input-processing-output circuit—one that is more than a reflex. Say you're walking down the street and pass a florist shop with a sign in the window that reads, "Don't forget, next Sunday is Mother's Day!" You realize with a start that you *have* forgotten, so you go into the shop, pull out your credit card, and order some flowers. This is not really so different a process from the spinal reflex: input (seeing the sign), processing (I forgot!), and output (ordering the flowers). There are a lot more steps (and some very complex ones) this time around: seeing the sign, using the language functions of the brain to draw meaning from all those little shapes we call letters, drawing on memories of what is expected of you on Mother's Day, an emotional tone generated by your feelings for your mother that affects the process—just to name a few. A complex interaction of many, many nervous system functions is going on, some fairly simple (the posture reflexes that let you walk into the shop without falling are nearly as simple as the spinal reflex example above) and others more complex (the arithmetic functions that allow you to answer the question, "How big an arrangement can I buy without going over my credit limit?"). The processes are so complex, in fact, that no computer built today is capable of anything approaching as complex a processing task as this.

You may know that a computer computes by means of many thousands of microscopic switches embedded in its processing chip. The pattern of "on" and "off" in the switches is what stores information, and the flow of input signal through these switches is the processing. The human brain contains about eleven billion nerve cells, or neurons, but as powerful as a computer with eleven billion switches might be, our brain is much more

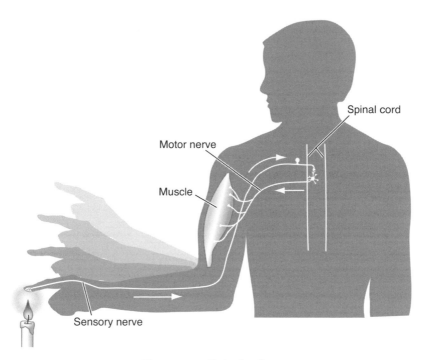

Figure 5-1   Spinal reflex

impressive than that. The neuron is not simply a switch that is either "on" or "off"; rather, it is an impressive microprocessor in its own right. Each neuron receives input from many other neurons, processes this information, and sends output to many others. The brain is not simply a biological computer with billions of switches. It is more like a network of billions of computers, each capable of being individually programmed. Every neuron in the brain may receive input and transmit signals to up to fifty thousand other neurons. This makes the number of *all* the possible connections between neurons in the human brain incomprehensibly huge, a hyper-astronomical number on the order of the number of molecules in the universe. (Even if we could figure out how to build such a computer, there'd be no place on the planet big enough to put it.) This almost unimaginable complexity explains why the capabilities of even the most powerful computers are puny compared with those of the human brain.

Like computers, the human nervous system uses electrical signals to do much of its work, as well as chemical signals called *neurotransmitters*.

Let's go back for a moment to the spinal reflex to examine how these signals do their jobs. Remember that in this reflex, a pain signal from the finger travels up a nerve fiber into the spinal cord. As you might guess, this is an electrical signal, a change in the electrical charge of the nerve fiber that travels as a pulse along the length of the fiber until it reaches a *cell body* that resides in the spinal cord. This cell body is one of the eleven billion tiny computers we mentioned earlier (except that it's in the spinal cord, not in the brain). When a sufficient number of pain signals arrive at the cell body, this microscopic CPU starts communicating with the motor nerve responsible for pulling away the finger, and when the motor neuron computes that it's necessary, this neuron fires its own pulse of electrical energy down the motor nerve to the muscles. The signals by which the neurons communicate with each other are the chemical ones we mentioned above: molecules called neurotransmitters. Most of the medications used in psychiatry work by affecting neurotransmitters in one way or another.

One neuron sends a chemical signal to another at a site called the *synapse*, an area where the two neurons nearly touch, separated only by an ultramicroscopic space called the *synaptic cleft*. The first neuron (the *presynaptic neuron*) releases packets of neurotransmitters that flow across the narrow synaptic cleft and link up with targets called *receptors* on the next cell (the *postsynaptic neuron*); the neurotransmitter molecules fit into their receptors like keys fit into locks. There needs to be some mechanism for this signaling system to be turned off and reset, of course. After neurotransmitter molecules in one pulse link up with receptors across the synapse, they must somehow be removed in preparation for the next pulse. This happens in a variety of ways in different cells, but one of the most important mechanisms is *reuptake* into the cell that released them. A reuptake pump on the presynaptic neuron removes neurotransmitter molecules from the synapse and takes them into the interior of the cell, where they are repackaged for re-release (figure 5-2).

There is a constant level of neurotransmitter release across the synapse, a steady tone of chemical signal that pulses up at times. The neurons are not just "switches" that can be set only to "on" or "off" but rather tiny information-processing units that are constantly communicating with other neurons to which they are functionally linked.

Now let's return to mood disorders. What is "broken" in these illnesses? As you will see, much of what we know about the biological and chemical

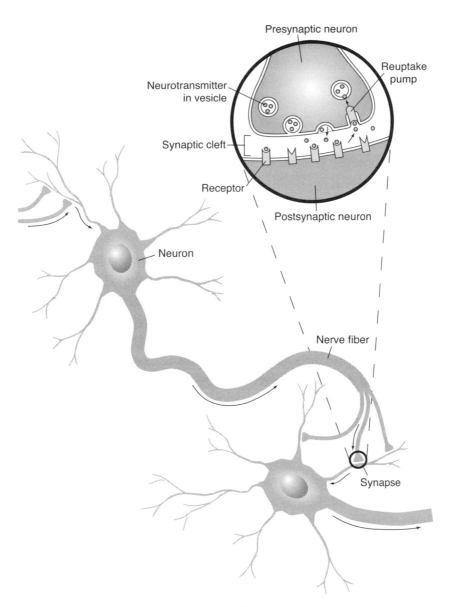

Figure 5-2 Synapse

basis of mood disorders was discovered *after* an effective medication had been accidentally discovered. In a backwards kind of investigative process, by figuring out where in the brain these medications are active and what they do to brain chemistry (usually by observing the effects of these pharmaceuticals on brain preparations in test tubes), we have found clues about the location and function of the "broken" mechanisms in mood disorders.

In chapter 1, we mentioned that the first pharmaceutical to have antidepressant effects, iproniazid, was discovered accidentally when doctors noticed that depressed tuberculosis patients taking the drug for their lung disease had improvement in their mood symptoms. In 1957, another breakthrough in the treatment of mood disorders occurred when Roland Kuhn, a Swiss psychiatrist, discovered that a compound originally developed as an antihistamine also had remarkable therapeutic effects on depressed patients. He reported his results in a Swiss medical journal, in a paper titled "The Treatment of Depressive States with G 22355 (Imipramine Hydrochloride)."[2] Unlike iproniazid, imipramine is still used as an antidepressant medication.

For many years, brain scientists had only vague ideas about the answer to the question, "What does imipramine *do*?" When some of them started to look at the effect of this pharmaceutical on brain chemistry, they discovered that imipramine was a powerful inhibitor of the reuptake of a group of neurotransmitters called *neurogenic amines,* or *neuroamines,* the most important of these being *norepinephrine.*

Remember that neurons turn off their chemical signals (turn *down* is probably more accurate) by scooping up neurotransmitter molecules from the synapse and repackaging them. Just as partially closing the drain in a bathtub while the water is running will cause the tub to begin to fill with water, blocking the reuptake of neurotransmitter molecules has the net effect of *increasing* neurotransmitters in the synapse. This observation, that antidepressants increase the number of neurotransmitters in the synapse by blocking their reuptake, led to the *amine hypothesis* of mood disorders. This hypothesis basically stated that an abnormally low level of norepinephrine caused depression and that, in bipolar disorder, too high a level caused mania.

Further work soon indicated that this explanation was too simplistic. As more antidepressant medications were discovered, it was found that some effective ones seemed to have little effect on the norepinephrine system. Fluoxetine (Prozac) is one of a family of pharmaceuticals that are powerful inhibitors of the reuptake of another neurotransmitter, called *serotonin*, but they have little direct effect on norepinephrine. Some antidepressants also seem to affect other neurotransmitters too, especially one called *dopamine*. As a result of these discoveries, the amine hypothesis was revised, and the proposal was put forward that mood is regulated by a complex interplay of several chemical circuits in the brain. It is now thought that the interplay of activity among all these systems is disrupted in depression and in mania (and actually, it was later discovered that imipramine may be so effective because it has activity in all these chemicals, not just norepinephrine).

Another argument against a simplistic theory involving too much or too little norepinephrine is an observation about the time course of the antidepressant-induced chemical changes in the brain. Antidepressant-induced changes in neurotransmitter levels at the synapse occur almost immediately after the drug is taken—in a matter of hours. But, as is well known, several weeks are required for these agents to start alleviating the symptoms of depression. If the problem were simply too little neurotransmitter in the synapses of certain brain circuits, why would it take several weeks after the drug raised transmitter levels at the synapse for the symptoms of depression to get better? It has been suggested that the neurons respond to these higher levels of neurotransmitters by changing their receptor molecules, either making them more sensitive to the neurotransmitter or putting more of them on the surface of the postsynaptic cell. The idea is that antidepressants work by triggering an "up-regulation" of receptor sensitivity in the neuron. This hypothesis continues to be popular among neuroscientists interested in the chemistry of mood disorders.

This idea fits nicely with some of the work done on the chemical mapping of the brain. Several nuclei of cells (*nucleus* here means a group of neurons) deep in the brain that use norepinephrine as their neurotransmitter project a vast network of fibers that terminate on sheets of cells contained on the convoluted surface of the brain, the cerebral cortex. The cerebral cortex, thought to be responsible for many of our most complex "higher" brain functions, is rich in cells with receptors for norepinephrine. This system seems to be ideally organized to affect the tone of functioning of the entire cerebral cortex—making it a good candidate for the target system of antidepressants. There are serotonin pathways that originate deep in the brain and project widely across the cortex too, as well as pathways that use other neurotransmitters. The balance of activity among these different systems and their interaction with each other are probably very important in the regulation of mood. These neurotransmitter systems are most likely the sites where antidepressant medications do their work.

Because of the uniquely therapeutic effects of *lithium* in bipolar disorder and its important antidepressant effects, a lot of effort has gone into trying to figure out the site of lithium's activity in the brain and its effect on brain chemistry. Lithium doesn't seem to affect neuroamine levels the way antidepressants do, and it doesn't interact with neuroamine receptors or reuptake pumps. In fact, it doesn't have any of the types of direct effects on cells that the antidepressants have (though there is an additional neurotransmitter, glutamate, over which lithium seems to have some pull). Only in the last few years has the probable site of lithium action been found, and it's not at the synapse at all. Lithium (and perhaps the newer mood stabilizers as well) seems to work at a different cellular level: *inside* the neuron.

Although the precise fit between a neurotransmitter and its receptor molecule has often been compared to the precise fit of a key into a lock, it has become apparent that the receptor is much more than just a lock. Starting in the 1970s, scientists were able to elucidate the structure of cellular receptors and discover the details of these complex and elegant mechanisms. Receptors on the surface of the cell are coupled with structures called G *proteins,* which extend through the cell membrane (the outer covering of the cell) and link up with a complex array of other proteins and enzymes within the cell that help regulate various cellular functions (figure 5-3). The G proteins act as transducers, converting data from outside the cell (this data being the presence or absence of neurotransmitters bound to the receptor molecules) into functional changes inside the cell. They don't do this directly but by a complex cascade of chemical events that probably also includes turning genes inside the cell on and off.

There is evidence that lithium has direct effects on G proteins, but scientists have recently started to focus on several other groups of molecules that work inside the cell as *second messengers.* The neurotransmitters, molecules that bring messages from other cells to the neuron, are considered the *first* messengers. The *second* messengers are molecules *inside* the cell

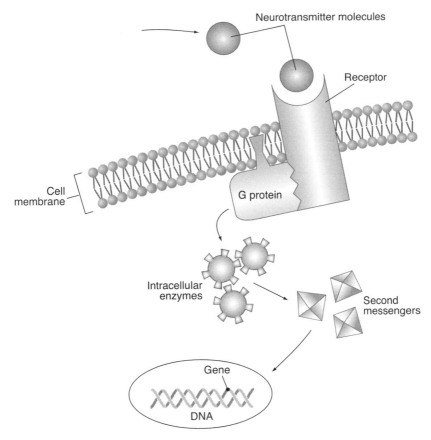

Figure 5-3   Receptors and G proteins

that are activated by G proteins to travel within the neuron to activate various cellular switches in the cell membrane and in the cell nucleus, the main control center of the neuron. Several lines of evidence support the alternative idea that lithium acts by inhibiting enzymes responsible for the manufacture of several second messenger molecules.

One might think of the G protein–second messenger system as a communications and activity-monitoring system for the neuron, constantly assessing the level of neurotransmitter activity and, perhaps by turning genes on and off, constantly altering and adjusting the functioning of the neuron in response to this activity. This process might be a necessary part of maintaining mood within a normal range, and it might control mood by somehow "tuning" the responsiveness of our mood state to experiences and environment. Perhaps mood disorders are the result of a broken G protein–second messenger system in neurons of the norepinephrine and serotonin circuits that regulate mood: the system's sensitivity gets incorrectly tuned too high or too low, and abnormal changes of mood result. (This might explain why the highs and lows of bipolar disorder are *both* effectively treated by lithium. Perhaps the lithium ion fits into and stabilizes the shape of one of the component molecules of this system or in some other way helps the system to work better and to do its job more effectively, thus stabilizing mood.)

This idea may also explain why antidepressants take several weeks to work. One important concept to appreciate is that science is continually discovering more and more actions of the supposedly "selective" serotonin reuptake inhibitors and their counterparts. It turns out that the serotonin receptors are themselves connected to the G protein system and therefore may affect the neuron in a similar way to lithium. Antidepressants may artificially raise neurotransmitter levels in the synapse to very high levels, high enough so that even a "broken" G protein–second messenger system can respond, turning on genes that start making receptor molecules or other cell components necessary to retune the neuron, a process that takes several weeks.

Antidepressants have even more functions. One of their strongest feats is an ability to protect the brain from damage. Some studies have suggested that depression is associated with an area of the brain called the *hippocampus*. In depressed patients, this area seems to be smaller than in those who are not depressed. For a long time, it was thought that the neurons in the brain do not recover in the same way as other neurons do. If, say, one were to have a stroke and some of the neurons died, those neurons would never be replaced. The brain may eventually rewire itself to avoid the broken area, but that area itself would never recover. Researchers were understandably surprised to discover that when depressed patients were treated with antidepressants, the hippocampus seemed to grow. This seemingly astounding feat may be due to the antidepressants' ability to stimulate a particular chemical in the brain that promotes development of brain synapses, called brain-derived neurotrophic factor (BDNF).

It may be a while before we understand how all the molecular and cellular pieces of this complicated story fit together, but the work to unravel the basic cause (or causes) of mood disorders is proceeding rapidly. Adolescent patients and their parents frequently complain that they feel they are guinea pigs when it comes to picking medications to treat mood disorders, because there's no way to know which medication or combination of medications will work best for a particular person. When we understand exactly what is "broken" in these illnesses, the job of treating them will become much easier and also much more systematic.

Antidepressant Medications

A ntidepressant medications have been used for several decades in treating children and adolescents, and the odds are that the first medication to be recommended for your child will be an antidepressant. These highly effective medications are safer than ever, and more and different antidepressants are being introduced every year.

Talking about this group of medications illustrates how the name of a class of medications often doesn't do them justice in describing their true range of efficacy. Medications listed as "antidepressants" have been found to be effective treatments for a whole variety of problems besides depression. In fact, more antidepressant prescriptions may be written to treat problems other than depression than to treat the illnesses for which these medications are named. Tricyclic antidepressants are effective in the treatment of panic attacks, obsessive-compulsive symptoms, and attention-deficit/hyperactivity disorder. Imipramine is effective in treating enuresis (bed wetting).

TRICYCLIC ANTIDEPRESSANTS

Although tricyclics are now prescribed less frequently than other, newer antidepressants, we start with this group because they were the first antidepressant medications developed and because they still provide the standard by which all promising new pharmaceuticals for treating depression in adults are usually judged. As with most psychiatric medications, however, their use in adolescents for the treatment of depression has been mainly based on their proven effectiveness in adults. They are now being used less and less frequently in younger patients because of studies that have thrown significant doubt on the assumption that they are just as effective in children and adolescents. In fact, adolescents who are prescribed these medications tend to be those who have not responded to the more common, newer types of antidepressants. Psychiatrists call these patients *treatment resistant*, or *treatment refractory*. This is by no means intended to imply some sort of fault on the part of the patient—rather, it simply indicates that this individual has a type of depression that for whatever reason does not seem to respond chemically to antidepressants as it should (assuming, of course, that the individual has been thoroughly and correctly diagnosed and treated). In many cases, the switch to a tricyclic is done because these chemicals tend to be involved with more neurotransmitters than the selective antidepressants (the *selective* serotonin reuptake inhibitors, or SSRIs). Table 6-1 shows a list of tricyclic antidepressants. These pharmaceuticals are called *tricyclics* because of the three rings in their chemical structure (figure 6-1).

Although some of these medications have an effect on serotonin systems in the brain, the primary effect of the tricyclics seems to be an inhibition of reuptake of the neurotransmitter norepinephrine by neurons. As we discuss in chapter 5, reuptake of neurotransmitters into the neuron after they have been released into the synaptic cleft and done their work (signaling the next cell) is the means by which the synapse is "reset." Norepinephrine is usually quickly removed from the synapse and pumped back into the cell

Table 6-1   Tricyclic Antidepressants

Generic Name	Brand Name
Amitriptyline	Elavil
Amoxapine	Asendin
Clomipramine	Anafranil
Desipramine	Norpramin
Doxepin	Sinequan
Imipramine	Tofranil
Maprotiline	Ludiomil
Nortriptyline	Pamelor
Protriptyline	Vivactil

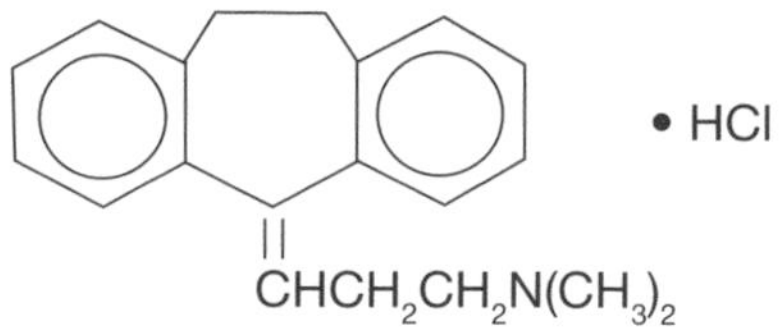

• HCl

CHCH$_2$CH$_2$N(CH$_3$)$_2$

AMITRIPTYLINE

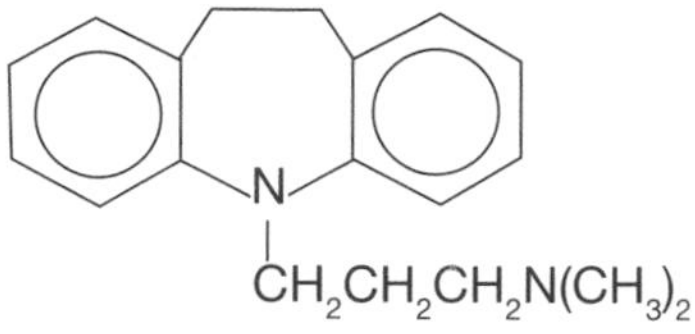

CH$_2$CH$_2$CH$_2$N(CH$_3$)$_2$

IMIPRAMINE

Figure 6-1   Chemical structure of two tricyclic molecules, showing their characteristic three-ringed structure

that released it, to turn off and reset the system. By blocking the removal of norepinephrine, tricyclics seem to prolong or intensify norepinephrine's message to the postsynaptic cell.

This effect of tricyclics on norepinephrine in neurons was one of the first chemical effects of a medication active in the brain to be measured in the laboratory. The observation that tricyclics *increased* the amount of norepinephrine in the synapse, along with the discovery that certain other medications used to treat high blood pressure *reduced* norepinephrine—and were observed to cause depression in some patients—led to the early amine hypothesis of mood disorders: the theory that depression was caused by too little norepinephrine (and mania presumably by too much). However, further testing indicated that tricyclics increased amines in the synapse within hours of a person's taking them, whereas the therapeutic effects of antidepressants were known to take several weeks. This led to a search for alternatives to the amine hypothesis.

Following the discovery that tricyclics cause a change in the number and sensitivity of norepinephrine receptors on the postsynaptic neuron, it was suggested that this "down-regulation" of the norepinephrine system by tricyclics was the therapeutic effect of these medications for which researchers had been looking. But other, newer antidepressants don't have this down-regulating effect on norepinephrine.

The fundamental biochemical effect of antidepressants that is actually responsible for their benefits still remains a mystery, though science is getting closer and closer to the answer by looking deeper into the cell itself. It is thought that the change in neuroamine signaling at the synapse caused by antidepressants may set off a cascade of events involving second messenger systems that eventually result in the improvement of the symptoms of depression, likely by altering the genetic expression of the neuron. Unfortunately, how these medications work remains largely unknown.

Although studies show that these medications are far less effective for children than for adults, the principal reason that tricyclics are now infrequently prescribed as antidepressant medications is their many side effects. As with all medications, some patients take these medications easily and without unpleasant side effects, but many have to put up with a few problems to get the benefits. Fortunately, all the side effects are dose related, and most are temporary.

As we mentioned in chapter 5, Roland Kuhn found imipramine, the first tricyclic, among a group of compounds that had some antihistamine effects.[1] It's not surprising, then, that these medications affect some people in the same way antihistamines do, causing mild sleepiness and sometimes what some of our patients have called a "weird" or "spacey" feeling for the first day or two after starting to take them. Tricyclics block another neurotransmitter, called *acetylcholine*, that is used in a part of the nervous system that regulates many automatic functions of the body, such as digestion. The resulting *anticholinergic* side effects include a slowing down of the gastrointestinal tract, causing constipation and dry mouth. This system also controls focusing of the lens of the eye and emptying of the urinary bladder, and tricyclics can cause blurry vision and urination difficulties, although usually only in high doses. Tricyclics also cause weight gain in many patients.

There have been several reports of sudden death in children taking desipramine, one of the tricyclic antidepressant medications, and a more recent sudden death in a child taking imipramine.[2] This appears to be an extremely rare event: fewer than a half dozen such cases have ever been reported. The cause has been presumed to be a sudden heart-rhythm problem, so your doctor should always ask about a family history of abnormal heartbeats (called arrhythmias) or any other sudden, unexplained cardiac death. Additionally, many published guidelines recommend that, before starting to take a tricyclic antidepressant, children and adolescents have an electrocardiogram to make sure there is no undiagnosed heart problem.

Overdoses of tricyclics are very dangerous and are responsible for many of the completed suicides by overdose by people with mood disorders. For adults, the lethal overdose is up to twenty times the normal dose, but children are more sensitive to the toxic effects of these medications, and just a handful of tablets can be fatal in a small child. For this reason, these medications must be scrupulously safeguarded in households with small children.

Accurate blood tests are available to measure tricyclic antidepressant levels in the bloodstream. The level at which these medications have their maximum efficacy, as well as ranges that are associated with side effects and toxicity, has been determined by clinical trials. These blood tests are useful in adjusting the dosage of medication, especially if a usually adequate dose doesn't seem to be helping.

Children and adolescents eliminate these medications more quickly than do adults, perhaps because the size of the liver, the organ responsible for breaking down these medications, is proportionately larger in children than in adults. For this reason, monitoring of blood levels is especially important in adolescents to be sure they are getting the proper dose.

We've referred several times now to studies that have questioned the efficacy of these medications in treating depression in young people. There has been a discrepancy in results between what are referred to as *open* studies and *double-blind* studies of tricyclic medications in young people.

In an open study, the medication under investigation is given to a group of patients with the disorder for which the medication is thought to be effective, and the investigators simply assess how many patients get better and how many do not. Open studies have shown that between 60 and 80 percent of children have a therapeutic response to tricyclics, and significant recovery rates have been found in adolescents as well.[3]

There are two problems with open studies that can trick researchers into thinking a medication is effective when it really isn't. The biggest factor is the *placebo effect*. This is the beneficial effect that comes from taking a medication that is prescribed by a trusted source who is convinced of the effectiveness of the medication and who thus convinces the patient that the medication will help. When a person in a white coat writes a prescription or one in a white uniform gives you a pill, a powerful set of psychological factors is put into action that can make you feel significantly better. In an earlier chapter, we discussed the beneficial effect on demoralization of encouragement from a trusted source. It's easy to see, then, how the placebo effect can be especially powerful with antidepressant medications. The other factor that can mislead researchers in an open study is their own desire to get positive results: no matter how objective the researcher tries to be, there will always be a tendency, perhaps only an unconscious one, to accentuate the positive in measuring improvement in patients. Both these factors can lead to a finding in clinical trials of a medication benefit where there really isn't any.

Double-blind studies eliminate these misleading factors and are the most powerful type of medication trial possible—so much so that this type of study is now pretty much required for all new medications. In a double-blind placebo-controlled study, subjects who are similar in age, diagnosis, severity of illness, and so forth and who agree to be in the study are divided into two groups. One group (the *experimental* group) gets the medication that is being tested, and the other group (the *control* group) gets an identical-looking but inactive tablet, the placebo. The study participants do not know whether they are taking the new medication or the placebo, and neither do the clinicians who are examining them for improvement—hence the term *double*-blind. Only after the trial is over is the group membership of the participants revealed, and the results of the two groups are then compared. Improvement is measured objectively by using checklists of symptoms and various severity rating scales that have been verified as reliable and valid. (In some studies, instead of a placebo, the control group receives a standard medication for the disorder being studied. This allows researchers to study the use of new medications for serious illnesses for which it would be unethical to give patients a dummy pill and not have them receive available treatment for their condition. This type of study would be double-blind, but not placebo-controlled.)

Several double-blind placebo-controlled studies of tricyclic antidepressants in children and adolescents have shown no advantage of the drug over placebo.[4] Critics of these studies have argued that many of the subjects in the studies were only mildly depressed and were perhaps demoralized rather than suffering from a mood disorder, and thus were quite likely to have a placebo response. Some of the studies were of very small groups of patients and thus might not pick up the response for statistical reasons. Other studies have been criticized for not following up on the patients long enough to detect significant improvement and for using measures of improvement that were not sensitive enough.[5]

In cases such as this, when the evidence seems contradictory, scientists will sometimes undertake a vast review of all available research on a particular topic to compare it. This can be done in a couple of ways. In a *meta-analysis,* researchers collect all published (and sometimes unpublished) results of various trials. They then use statistical methods to analyze the studies so that they are comparing apples to apples. This allows them to see which studies had positive results and which had negative results and to look deeper to any possible errors or mistakes that may have skewed the results one way or another. Sometimes the summary of these results is enough to help researchers answer their question of why different studies about the same subject come up with different results. If they wish to take their analysis a step further, they can use this information as part of a *systematic review.* In a systematic review, researchers seek to answer bigger questions, such as "Which patients should we treat with tricyclic antidepressants?" by interpreting and applying the results of the meta-analysis. The review requires a more careful approach in looking at each trial and trying to determine what if any biases might have been present and how they would have affected the results.

In 2013, the Cochrane Collaboration, widely regarded as possibly the best and most thorough research body in existence, completed these procedures to review the treatment of children and adolescents with tricyclic antidepressants. By looking at all available randomized controlled trials to date, Cochrane researchers found no difference between adolescents taking tricyclic medications and those taking placebo in terms of their depression remitting. Despite not fully improving, children taking tricyclics experienced a slight decrease in the severity of some depressive symptoms, based on a particular self-report scale they were given (about 3 percentage points, taking a child from a depression severity of 90 to one of 87—not much of a difference). These children also experienced significantly more side effects (as would be expected). This particular analysis even evaluated whether tricyclic antidepressants may be a good backup option after treatment with an SSRI did not work, and even then these children had no greater response than those given a placebo medication.[6]

It seems reasonable to conclude that tricyclic antidepressants are not as effective in young people as they are in adults—though perhaps unreasonable to conclude that they are completely ineffective. We still have no good way of analyzing a given person's brain chemistry to tell exactly which would be the best medication for her. It is certainly the case that some adults have been depressed for the majority of their lives, and only when they try a particular medication (say, one SSRI versus another) does their depression seem to lift. The research can say that, on a population scale, tricyclic medications don't seem effective for children and adolescents, but the studies can't say that for Shaun sitting in the psychiatrist's office, there is no possibility that a tricyclic might be helpful. Because of this, many psychiatrists have moved tricyclics way down the list of options but haven't crossed them off entirely.

This difference in efficacy between adults and children has yet to be explained. Perhaps there are differences in the biology of depression in younger people; perhaps the chemical pathways that these drugs affect are less developed in the immature brain and thus less responsive to these medications. What is clear, however, is that tricyclic antidepressants must be prescribed with caution in young people and should not be the first choice among antidepressant medications, especially since, as you will see in the next section, safer medications with more clearly proven effectiveness are now available.

SELECTIVE SEROTONIN REUPTAKE INHIBITORS

A new pharmaceutical that had none of the tricyclics' side effects and was not toxic in overdose caused something of a sensation when it was introduced in 1988. That pharmaceutical was fluoxetine (Prozac), and "sensation" sums up the response to this medication quite well. A Prozac capsule showed up on the covers of *Newsweek* and *New York* magazines, the drug was featured in many other magazine and newspaper articles, and for a time it seemed that nearly everyone was either taking Prozac or reading the book *Listening to Prozac* (or *Talking Back to Prozac* or *Prozac Nation*). Prozac was touted by some as a miracle drug that was going to change the world. Many physicians were prescribing Prozac for everything from deep depression to simple mundane sadness, because it was seen as so safe that a mindset of "it can't hurt" started to develop.

The inevitable backlash to this enthusiasm took about another year to fully develop, but once it did, psychiatrists couldn't *pay* their patients to take Prozac. Full-page ads in *USA Today* denouncing the drug appeared for weeks, and various talk show hosts found people who gladly came on national television to swear that Prozac had made their lives miserable. In children, this mindset became especially fixed in October 2004, when the FDA placed a *black box* warning, the sternest warning available to this body, against prescribing selective serotonin reuptake inhibitor (SSRI) medications in adolescents due to a concern about "increased suicidality." This warning was based on the results of a study that seemed to indicate that SSRIs may *double* the rates of suicide in adolescents. Unfortunately, these results were a fairly superficial view of the evidence. First of all, the absolute numbers were miniscule—in the two thousand children in the study, two in the control group expressed suicidal thoughts, whereas four did in the experimental group. More important, these were thoughts only—no suicide attempts or events occurred during the study at all. Finally, subsequent studies have been unable to replicate these results.

Despite these facts, the black box warning remained foremost in the minds (and fears) of doctors as well as parents. For many years, pediatricians and many psychiatrists would not even think of medicating depressed adolescents for fear of "causing" suicidality. In reality, untreated depression is the most important risk factor for suicide, not treatment with an SSRI, so many young people with depression were in a precarious state.

Now, public (and professional) opinion is swinging back toward the middle as more of the facts emerge. Prozac and similar pharmaceuticals that have since been introduced (table 6-2) are extremely safe and have a record of side effects vastly superior to that of tricyclic antidepressants. The most encouraging fact in the treatment of serious depression in young people is that, unlike the tricyclics, this group of medications has shown unequivocal benefits in double-blind placebo-controlled studies in children and adolescents.

Table 6-2   Selective Serotonin Reuptake Inhibitors (SSRIs)

Generic Name	Brand Name
Citalopram	Celexa
Escitalopram	Lexapro
Fluoxetine	Prozac
Fluvoxamine	Luvox
Paroxetine	Paxil
Sertraline	Zoloft

These new antidepressants also differ from tricyclics in that they have little direct effect on norepinephrine in the brain; instead, they block the reuptake of another neurotransmitter into neurons, another amine compound called *serotonin*. The potent and specific blockade of serotonin reuptake by these agents gives this class its name: *selective serotonin reuptake inhibitor*. As with the tricyclics, the effect on serotonin in the synapse seems to occur at the receptors, and there is some evidence that serotonin is actually the more important neurotransmitter in the treatment of depression. Scientists are discovering, however, that despite their name, these medications have more effects on the brain than had initially been appreciated, such as potentially protecting neurons from damage and reducing inflammation in the brain. The development of these new agents, which help with depression but seem to work differently than the tricyclics, has provided more clues to the underlying biology of mood disorders.

Unlike most other psychiatric medications, most of the SSRIs have FDA-approved dosing guidelines for children and adolescents. In many cases, this approval was given several years after the drugs were labeled for use in adults, again proving the point that off-label prescribing is not unusual for psychiatric medications in young people.

The main side effect of the SSRIs is gastrointestinal discomfort. Many patients experience nausea for the first couple of days after starting to take one of the SSRIs, and a few have diarrhea or constipation. We call this a side effect, but it's actually not. In fact, the majority of the serotonin in our bodies, almost 90 percent, is used as a signaling mechanism not in our brains, but in our digestive tract. Scientists are only recently appreciating the complex neurological structure required to maintain our digestive processes, finding an entire neuronal network similar in complexity to our spinal cord residing in and around our gut. So, it is easy to see why medications that affect serotonin signaling would have an effect on this region as well. The gut is remarkably good at maintaining its equilibrium, so once it becomes used to these medications, the gastrointestinal effects are quickly gone (typically within a few days).

These medications (especially fluoxetine) are also somewhat stimulating in some patients, and though this is just what some depressed people need, others feel unpleasantly nervous or "wired" on these medications. In children, this can present as agitation or irritability, which might make prescribing SSRIs for adolescents seem contradictory. We've already said that depression can cause irritability in some adolescents, so why would we give them a medication that could potentially make it worse? The answer is that the irritability of depression and the irritability of SSRI treatment are entirely different. In these medications, this side effect is transient and passes quickly—within a day or two—and is mild. Also, these side effects occur in a small portion of the population taking these medicines. Most important is that once the sufferer of even the most severe side effects is over this brief hump, the benefits of the medication take hold, and the irritability overall lessens substantially.

Unusually, a person may suffer the converse of the side effects described above, such as feeling sleepier than usual, or having slightly less energy. Many patients report that SSRIs seem to curb their appetite a bit, and they also notice some weight loss, especially early on in taking an SSRI. This is, of course, a potential concern in young people who are still growing. Someone who is going to have these side effects usually notices them immediately; none of them sneak up on a person who has been taking an SSRI for weeks or months.

In adults, SSRIs have been reported to cause an unpleasant blunting of emotions; patients complain of being apathetic and indifferent to events, of being unable to get excited or enthusiastic about anything.[7,8] This appears to be a problem only at high doses and does not often trouble patients taking the usual antidepressant dose.

Another side effect that has been described is a change in sexual functioning, specifically a noticeable decrease in sexual interest (loss of libido) or difficulty in reaching or inability to reach orgasm. The frequency of these problems was at first difficult to gauge, because these sorts of side effects were often not asked about during clinical trials. But as more people have been treated with SSRIs since they were introduced in the early 1990s, it has become apparent that this is a significant problem affecting at least one-third of patients. We don't want to get into a discussion of the complicated issue of adolescent sexuality here, but for a young and insecure individual, sexual side effects may be very important. We have had cases of young persons, usually boys, who stop their medications and refuse to restart them but will not tell us why. Through gentle questioning, it eventually became apparent that sexual side effects were behind their sudden departure from treatment. In many cases, the concern was not an inability to perform with a partner but merely how a decrease in sexual desire made them feel separate and different from their peers, further isolating an already depressed individual. Various strategies are available for dealing with these problems when they occur, so it is critical for clinicians to ask about these features with every adolescent started on medications, particularly when an abrupt, unexplained disinterest in further treatment develops. Weekend "vacations" from the medication have been reported to be helpful, as well as the addition of other medications that seem to block these effects, but sometimes a switch to another antidepressant in another class is the only solution (though often an effective one).

Some side effects of SSRI medications may not be noticed outside exceptional circumstances. Some people who stop their medications abruptly (if they, say, forget to bring their pills on a vacation) feel almost as though they have the flu for a day or two—they feel slightly feverish, slowed down, and achy. These symptoms are not dangerous, and they pass fairly quickly, but they can be uncomfortable.

Like most psychiatric medications, SSRIs are metabolized in the liver, and the details of this process have been studied more carefully for this class of medications than for most other psychiatric drugs. Many SSRIs cause a partial blockade of the cellular machinery responsible for breaking down many other medications in the liver, so they can increase the time it takes for the body to get rid of medications. This means that levels of those medications in the body will rise. For example, if an adolescent who is taking theophylline (Theo-Dur and others) for asthma starts taking fluvoxamine (Luvox) for depression, her level of theophylline can rise to toxic levels because the antidepressant slows down theophylline metabolism. For this reason, *all* physicians caring for a patient need to know about any change of medications; they need to pay close attention to drug interactions with SSRIs—and for that matter, with all medications.

OTHER, NEW, ANTIDEPRESSANTS

Since the early 1990s, a whole series of new antidepressants have come on the market that are neither tricyclics nor SSRIs (table 6-3). Most of these pharmaceuticals don't share many common features, so there isn't a good class name for them; you'll sometimes see many of these new agents listed as "atypical" or "second generation" antidepressants. They have a variety of effects on norepinephrine, serotonin, and even other neurotransmitters; some have more than one effect on these systems, so they are thought to provide different ways of manipulating the chemical systems in the brain that are concerned with mood. Their side-effect profiles vary widely: some are more like tricyclics, others more like SSRIs.

SEROTONIN-NOREPINEPHRINE REUPTAKE INHIBITORS

As the 1990s progressed, psychiatrists began to notice a population of patients who had depression that did not respond to the SSRI medications but who were amenable to treatment with the tricyclic antidepressants. By this time, tricyclics were considered a second-line medication, primarily because of the significant side effects and potential lethality in overdose, not to mention the need to get blood drawn for levels periodically. Psychiatrists, and pharmaceutical companies, tried to develop a chemical that had the benefits of the tricyclics but the side-effect profile of the SSRIs. Although the general consensus was that the primary brain chemical responsible for depression was serotonin, this was clearly (as we have discussed) not the full picture. The biggest difference between these two chemicals seemed to lie somewhere in their ability to also target norepinephrine. In 1994, Wyeth introduced the chemical venlafaxine (Effexor), touting it as the perfect antidepressant. This *serotonin-norepinephrine reuptake inhibitor* (SNRI) was active on both serotonin and norepinephrine, like a tricyclic, but had a mild side-effect profile and was nonlethal, like an SSRI.

As it turned out, this description was not strictly true. First of all, at low doses, venlafaxine isn't very active in norepinephrine at all—only at

Table 6-3   New Antidepressants

Generic Name	Brand Name
Serotonin-Norepinephrine Reuptake Inhibitors (SNRI)	
Venlafaxine	Effexor
Desvenlafaxine	Pristiq
Duloxetine	Cymbalta
Dopamine-Norepinephrine Reuptake Inhibitors (DNRI)	
Bupropion	Wellbutrin

higher doses does this benefit become apparent. Furthermore, most patients will tell you that the side effects are indeed more significant than an SSRI, even severe for some. That said, the SNRI was immensely helpful to those patients who did not respond to an SSRI, proving that it did indeed have a place in the pharmacological lexicon of psychiatry. Since its inception, venlafaxine has been placed into an extended release formulation so that it needs to be taken only once a day (as opposed to three times a day). Additionally, other medications in the same class (duloxetine [Cymbalta] and desvenlafaxine [Pristiq]) have been created with more or less the same intent.

In terms of side effects, adding norepinephrine to the equation did add some unanticipated consequences. Norepinephrine is used in the body in a way similar to adrenaline. Patients with too much of this chemical can see a small though significant rise in their heart rate or blood pressure. Also, abrupt withdrawal from these medications can cause a somewhat unusual subjective feeling, almost like small electrical jolts in the muscles, which, though not painful, can be uncomfortable.

Although evidence now shows that SNRIs can be effective for children and adolescents (particularly older adolescents), they have still not been approved by the FDA for these indications and so are typically reserved by psychiatrists for patients who do not do as well on initial treatment with an SSRI.[9] There is some evidence that they may also be helpful for children with attention deficit disorder[10] or chronic pain,[11] so some psychiatrists may use them as a first-line agent for children with these types of problems in addition to depression.

By now, you are probably seeing a pattern in antidepressant medications. Since we do not yet know how exactly these medications do what they do, how they help alleviate depression, researchers are trying to think of every combination possible in helping patients who are suffering with this condition. We have talked about serotonin and serotonin plus norepinephrine, and now we will discuss norepinephrine plus dopamine. Many of you will be familiar with dopamine as the "pleasure chemical" or the "reward chemical" —it is so potent that in particularly susceptible people, it reinforces gambling or drug use to the exclusion of other interests in life. For some, depression constitutes primarily a loss of pleasure in life, so what better way to try to eliminate depression than by stimulating an increase in dopamine? It turns out that dopamine is rather short lived in the brain, so pure dopaminergic drugs don't work the way we would like. But when combined with norepinephrine, dopamine does seem to be helpful. Commonly marketed today as bupropion (Wellbutrin), *dopamine-norepinephrine reuptake inhibitors* (DNRIs) are somewhat different from the antidepressants we've discussed so far.

Bupropion is a widely prescribed antidepressant, popular not so much for what it does do as what it doesn't. Its side effects seem to be quite different from the tricyclics, SSRIs, and SNRIs. It is almost never associated with weight gain and for many leads to a slight weight loss, typically by lowering the appetite. It has few if any sexual side effects, and stopping the medication abruptly does not lead to the same flulike symptoms. Bupropion does have one side effect that can be quite serious, though. In some persons, it has been shown to lower the seizure threshold to the point that epileptic seizures develop. This is a very rare side effect but is notable in people who are already prone to seizures or who have other conditions that may predispose them to this condition (eating disorders, for example, can cause imbalances in the nutritional status of a person, making them more likely to seize).

As an antidepressant, bupropion seems to be about as effective as the other medications. It seems particularly helpful for those depressive symptoms characterized by fatigue, low energy, and sleeping and even eating too much—what was called *atypical* depression at one point. It also helps persons with seasonal affective disorder—a milder depression that seems to come on in the winter, thought to be due to the effect of reduced sunlight. Like the SNRIs, DNRIs have some action in the norepinephrine family of neurotransmitters, so they have been used for people who have both depression and attention deficit disorder. Finally, the dopamine activity seems to blunt the highs and lows of addiction, so DNRIs have been used to help those interested in quitting smoking (when marketed as Zyban). Because bupropion seems to work by a somewhat different mechanism than the SSRIs, it is commonly added to these medications for those patients who don't have full remission of their depression.

Although many SNRIs and DNRIs are used frequently in children and adolescents, they are not approved by the FDA for this purpose and so are, with few exceptions, reserved for young patients who do not respond adequately to one of the first-line medications, typically an SSRI. There are other alternate antidepressants out there, and more are being developed as this is written, so it is important for parents to have open, direct, and potentially lengthy conversations with psychiatrists about why they chose a certain medication, what they are hoping to accomplish with its use, what side effects are possible or can be expected, and how long they expect it to take before the patient and parents see a benefit. More information, in this case, is always a good thing.

MONOAMINE OXIDASE INHIBITORS

You've already heard about iproniazid, the drug developed to treat tuberculosis that caused mood elevation in some patients who took it for their lung disease. In addition to its effect on the tubercle bacillus, iproniazid causes inactivation of an enzyme in the body that metabolizes amine compounds in the nervous system. This enzyme, called *monoamine oxidase,* is responsible for gobbling up molecules of norepinephrine, serotonin, and several other neurotransmitters. Inactivating monoamine oxidase has the effect of increasing the amounts of these compounds in the nervous system, and this effect, in some as yet poorly understood way, may be the mechanism by which these medications alleviate the symptoms of depression. This effect on the enzyme gives this class of pharmaceuticals their name: *monoamine oxidase inhibitors,* or MAOIs (table 6-4).

Monoamine oxidase is also present in the lining of the intestine and in the liver; a number of naturally occurring substances in foods are close

Table 6-4 Monoamine Oxidase Inhibitors (MAOIs)

Generic Name	Brand Name
Phenelzine	Nardil
Selegiline	Eldepryl, Emsam
Tranylcypromine	Parnate

enough chemically to norepinephrine to need deactivation before they are absorbed into the bloodstream. The importance of this becomes clear when we tell you that another name for norepinephrine is nor*adrenaline*. Tyramine, an amino acid that has adrenaline-like effects on blood pressure and heart rate, is present in high enough concentrations in some foods to cause dangerous cardiovascular problems in persons taking MAOIs (table 6-5). A number of pharmaceuticals, including the ingredients of many over-the-counter remedies, also have adrenaline-like effects. Persons taking MAOIs therefore need to observe certain dietary restrictions and, even more important, need to *scrupulously* read the labels of any over-the-counter medication they are considering—or better yet, consult their pharmacist before taking any pharmaceutical bought over the counter.

Medications of this type also interact with other drugs that are prescribed or commonly used in emergency rooms for various problems. Anyone taking an MAOI must be sure to inform all his treating physicians that he is using this medication. He should also consider wearing an alerting bracelet, so that if he is brought unconscious to an emergency room after an accident or a sudden illness, the ER personnel will be aware that he's taking an MAOI.

Other side effects accompany MAOIs too. These medications can be stimulating and cause nervousness, insomnia, and excess perspiration. Dizzy spells, especially when suddenly getting up from lying down, can occur. MAOIs block a blood pressure reflex that usually maintains blood pressure when we stand up, and the sudden drop in blood pressure on standing (called *orthostatic hypotension*) causes light-headedness. Weight gain, water retention, and sexual dysfunction may also occur.

As you might predict from the foregoing discussion, MAOIs are seldom used in the United States unless other antidepressants have failed to be effective, and they are even more rarely used in adolescents. Indeed, taking a medication that would mean not eating pepperoni pizzas seems too much to ask of a teenager. Nevertheless, MAOIs are sometimes uniquely effective

Table 6-5   Foods to Avoid while Taking MAOIs

Fava or broad beans
Aged cheese (cream and cottage cheese permitted)
Beef liver or chicken liver
Orange pulp
Pickled or smoked fish, poultry, or other meats
Sauerkraut
Packaged soups
Fermented bean curd (tofu)
Yeast and protein dietary supplements
Summer (dry) sausage (e.g., pepperoni)
Soy sauce
Sour cream
Draft beer and many wines

Note: This list is not exhaustive, and some items included here are low enough in tyramine that some physicians allow one or two servings per day. Patients, and parents, should get a complete list and discuss the specifics of the diet with a knowledgeable physician, pharmacist, or nutritionist before starting to take an MAOI.

treatments for depression. Almost every psychiatrist we've ever spoken with has had the experience of effectively treating a particular patient with an MAOI after no other antidepressant had helped.

In an attempt to avoid these unpleasant side effects, one company had the idea to bypass the digestive system altogether. It found a way to deliver one type of MAOI, called selegiline (Emsam), through a person's skin. Users place a patch, similar to a nicotine patch, on their body and wear it throughout the day. A small, even dose of selegiline is delivered directly to the bloodstream. In this way, the tyramine in food can still be deactivated. Even the manufacturer admits, however, that you can maintain a normal diet only at the lowest dose of the medication, which is unlikely to be effective for the majority of people; above this dose, you must still maintain a strict tyramine-free diet, difficult for most people and nearly impossible for an adolescent.

ANTIDEPRESSANT THERAPY: SOME GENERAL CONSIDERATIONS

In 2012, the Cochrane Collaboration completed another meta-analysis investigating the use of "newer" antidepressants (the SSRIs and their variations listed above) for the treatment of depression in children and adolescents. They found them to be effective, particularly in adolescents (over 12 years old) rather than children. The majority of the studies used fluoxetine, since it is the only FDA-approved medication for depression and therefore, for multiple reasons, far easier to study than unapproved medications. The study found, however, that "there was no evidence that one particular type of newer generation antidepressant had a larger effect than the others."[12] The safety and effectiveness of the SSRIs are perhaps the most clearly supported by research, but which SSRI (or, in rare cases, other medicine) should be chosen as the first-line drug? What dose should be used? How long does one wait before deciding that a medication isn't working? What then?

When studies have compared antidepressant medications in large groups of (adult) patients for the treatment of depression, no single pharmaceutical has ever been proved to work better or faster than any other. There is no "best" antidepressant. If there were, we wouldn't find several dozen different ones on the market in the United States. Neither is there a "strongest" antidepressant medication. The usual dose of one may be higher, in milligrams, than that of another, but this has nothing to do with effectiveness.

We've already mentioned the evidence for superior efficacy of SSRIs over tricyclics in adolescents, but we have no evidence that one SSRI is superior to another. Considerable evidence suggests that some adult patients who get better with tricyclic medications do not improve on taking SSRIs, and vice versa. The same could well be true for adolescents: there may be a small group of adolescents for whom tricyclic medications are *more* effective than SSRIs, but the proportion of these patients to other patients responsive only to SSRIs is so small that statistical analysis doesn't "see" them in the studies done so far.

Because of this lack of proven superiority of any particular agent, subtle differences in side effects are often used to make a choice among antidepressant medications. An antidepressant that is mildly sedating might be a good choice if insomnia or anxiety is a prominent symptom of depression in a particular patient. A medication that tends to be somewhat stimulating might be a choice if the patient is lethargic and having problems with energy level. One that stimulates appetite might be a major problem for one adolescent but just what is needed for another. Physicians' experience with a particular medication may make it a first among equals in their prescribing for patients. Indeed, a medication that a particular doctor has had a lot of experience with in prescribing for patients probably *is* a better medicine than a similar one that is prescribed less often—for this doctor's patients at least.

We've already discussed some of the problems in deciding on a dose for adolescents. Fortunately, more data are becoming available all the time to help with this. Most of the SSRIs are already labeled for use in young patients (though usually for reasons other than depression, such as panic disorder or obsessive-compulsive disorder). Remember, too, that doses of all medications in older adolescents are usually not so different from those used in adults, and probably little alteration in treatment will be needed from that used for adults. No radical biological shift occurs on an adolescent's eighteenth birthday that makes him suddenly an adult physiologically. Treatment decisions for some 17- and 16-year-olds may be the same as those for adults.

One of the most frustrating aspects of antidepressant therapy is the lag time between starting medication and improvement in symptoms. Most studies of depressed patients first starting to take an antidepressant medication report some improvement of symptoms within two weeks. But it often takes longer for improvement to be noticed. The sequence of events brought about in the brain by antidepressant treatment most likely involves a re-engineering of neurons on some level, probably through turning on genes in these cells. This process takes time. It's not unreasonable to wait four to six weeks before giving up on a medication. Even when a medication is beginning to help, it may take a long time for its *full* benefit to become apparent.

Studies of depressed adults indicate that depressive symptoms continue to improve for up to three months after starting to take antidepressant medications. Unfortunately, this lag time is not usually the same for the side effects as for the efficacy. Most of the bothersome effects of these medications (sedation, appetite changes, sexual side effects) seem to occur through some other, more direct route than genetic manipulation and often appear within days of starting a medication. We often hear parents and patients complain that a medicine "made them worse" than they were before, which can of course seem true if the only effect you are feeling from a medication is a little nausea in the midst of a depression. The best and only counsel we can give is that these side effects do, fortunately, resolve quickly. Patience is the most important virtue when treating depression with a medication, though one that is frequently difficult to find when in the midst of deep suffering.

What options are available if a medication doesn't seem to be helping? Raising the dose is often the first choice. A switch to an antidepressant in a different class is another. At some point, adding another medication is often tried. Some patients respond to combinations of antidepressants or a combination of an antidepressant and another type of medication, such as a mood-stabilizing medication. Use of the maximum dosage has been studied, both in adults and in adolescents. The Treatment of Adolescents with Depression Study (TADS) found that after maximizing the dose of antidepressant, about 60 percent of patients improved significantly.

Within the last few years, a study concerning the Treatment of SSRI Resistant Depression in Adolescents (TORDIA) looked at patients who did not seem to respond well to the first antidepressant tried. The results of this study are still being evaluated, though the initial results seem to show that changing to another SSRI resulted in a further 60 percent of those patients getting better (so, along with the 60 percent who responded to the first medicine, about 15 percent of adolescents in the study still had depressive symptoms). This number was the same as when adolescents were switched to another type of antidepressant (in this study, the SNRI venlafaxine). So, many psychiatrists will first try one or two SSRI medications, then, if there isn't an adequate response, move on to alternate antidepressants. If the child still doesn't seem to be getting better, adding another type of medication, like a mood stabilizer (what we call *augmenting* the antidepressant), can be hugely helpful.

We have no way to know beforehand which patient will respond to which antidepressant. And we have no way to know which, if any, side effects a particular person will develop. Unfortunately, some trial and error is required in the process of finding the medication or combination of medications that works best with the fewest side effects. The clues to how a person will respond to a medication seem to reside within the genetic code of the individual. One of the greatest clues we have lies in the response to medication of a close family member. If we are seeing a patient with, say, an older brother who also had depression but had an excellent response to fluoxetine (Prozac) with no side effects, that would be the first medicine we would reach for, as it is likely that the patient will respond in the same way. In chapter 15, we talk in more detail about how an individual's genes interact with medications, a relatively new field of science known as *pharmacogenomics*. Several commercially available genetic tests aim to take some of the guesswork out of prescribing psychiatric medications by providing the prescriber with information about which medications are more likely to be effective or to cause side effects in a particular patient. Although prescribing antidepressant medications can accurately be described as an art rather than a science, this is changing quickly.

Mood-Stabilizing Medications

T rue mood stabilizers are medications that have both antimanic and antidepressant effects. They are usually the foundation for the treatment of people with bipolar disorders, and they are used for other problems as well. Mood stabilizers, especially lithium, are often used in combination with antidepressant medications to treat depression that is unresponsive to an antidepressant alone. At the end of this chapter, we discuss how physicians go about making the decision to treat an individual with a mood stabilizer.

LITHIUM

In the second century AD, the Greek physician Soranus of Ephesus recommended that physicians treating patients suffering from mania should prescribe "natural waters, such as [from] alkaline springs."[1] Roman physicians recommended that their patients "take the waters" at various springs for a whole variety of physical and mental ailments. The little town of Spa in eastern Belgium, Bath in England, Wiesbaden in Germany, and dozens of other towns in Italy and Greece that were the sites of natural springs became centers for healing. As the science of analytical chemistry developed, curious chemists and physicians evaluated these various springs and found that the waters of many were rich in lithium.

In the middle of the nineteenth century, lithium compounds were tried as treatments for gout and kidney stones. Unfortunately, the approach was unsuccessful and was soon abandoned. Nevertheless, this work led to formulation of pharmaceutical preparations of lithium compounds and to information on the range of safe doses for lithium preparations in humans.

In the 1940s, lithium came to medical attention again when lithium chloride was introduced as a substitute for table salt (sodium chloride) for people with medical problems, such as heart disease and high blood pressure, that required them to be on a low-sodium diet. But when heart patients were given saltshakers full of lithium salts to sprinkle on their food, the results were catastrophic for some. Because lithium is toxic in surprisingly low concentrations, substituting lithium chloride for sodium chloride turned out to be a disaster. There were many reports of severe lithium poisoning and even several deaths. The use of lithium as a salt substitute ended, and the episode had the effect of giving lithium a bad reputation among physicians.

So it was very much a chance occurrence that led to the discovery of lithium's beneficial effects on mood disorders in 1948. John F. J. Cade, MD, senior medical officer in the Mental Hygiene Department of Victoria, Australia, was working in his laboratory on trying to determine whether some toxin might be present in the urine of individuals with manic-depressive illness. Cade was especially interested in urea and uric acid, by-products of protein metabolism found in urine, and was testing the toxicity of these compounds by injecting small amounts of them into guinea pigs.

One of the technical problems with his work was that uric acid is rather insoluble in water, making it difficult to prepare injectable solutions of higher concentrations. Looking for a soluble urate salt to use instead of uric acid, Cade consulted prior research and discovered that uric acid was easiest to dissolve in water when it was combined with lithium as lithium urate. He injected small amounts of lithium urate into the guinea pigs and noticed that uric acid seemed to be much less toxic in this form. This suggested to Cade that the lithium component of the compound might have some sort of protective effect against urate toxicity. To determine what the effect of the lithium ion might be, he injected lithium carbonate (the carbonate ion is a harmless substance, found, for example, as sodium carbonate in baking soda)* and discovered that "after a latent period of about two hours the animals, although fully conscious, became extremely lethargic and unresponsive to stimuli for one to two hours before once again becoming normally active."[2]

As Cade admitted in his original paper, "It may seem a long distance from lethargy in guinea pigs to excitement in psychotics,"[3] but doctors of the time were desperate for new treatment possibilities. So Cade decided to administer lithium preparations to several patients who were chronically agitated. The effect on individuals with mania was dramatic:

CASE I—W.B., a male aged fifty-one years, who had been in a state of chronic manic excitement for five years, restless, dirty, destructive, mischievous and interfering, had long been regarded as the most troublesome patient in the ward. His response was highly gratifying. From the start of treatment on March 29, 1948, with lithium citrate he steadily settled down and in three weeks was enjoying the unaccustomed surrounding of the convalescent ward. As he had been ill so long and confined to a "chronic ward," he found normal surroundings and liberty of movement strange at first. He remained perfectly well and left the hospital on indefinite leave with instructions to take a dose of lithium carbonate, five grains, twice a day. He was soon back working at his old job.

CASE VIII—W.M., a man of fifty years, was suffering from an attack of recurrent mania, the first of which he had had at the age of twenty. The present attack had lasted two months and showed no signs of abating. He was garrulous, euphoric, restless and unkempt when he started taking lithium. Two days later he was reported to be quieter. By the ninth day he was definitely settling down and the following day commenced work in the garden. By the end of two weeks he was practically normal—quiet, tidy, rational, with insight into his previous condition.[4]

At this point, Dr. Cade had treated ten manic patients with lithium, and all ten had shown the same dramatic improvement. One would think the news of Cade's discovery would have spread like wildfire. It did not. In fact,

---

* Many chemicals, including medications, consist of two parts called *ions*, one of which is positively charged (such as lithium or sodium) and the other negatively charged (such as chloride or carbonate). When the two parts exist together as a *compound,* the charges cancel each other out, and the system is stable.

not until several decades later did the United States Food and Drug Administration approve lithium for the treatment of bipolar disorder. Part of the reason for this delay was the state of world psychiatry following the end of the Second World War. Much of European psychiatry, especially German psychiatry, was in ruins, literally and figuratively. In the United States and England, psychoanalytic theories had replaced the traditional medical practices of evaluation, diagnosis, and treatment with the prescription of "the talking cure" for all emotional problems. Accurate psychiatric diagnosis simply didn't exist. Ronald Fieve, the American psychiatrist who would champion the use of lithium in the United States in the 1970s and who was instrumental in getting American psychiatrists to prescribe it for their patients, observed that during the late 1940s and the 1950s in New York, he "rarely met with the diagnosis of manic-depression . . . It had virtually disappeared. Most cases of excitable, talkative, and elated behavior were being diagnosed as schizophrenia."[5]

But a Danish psychiatrist, Morgans Schou, realized that Cade's discovery was a real breakthrough (noting in a 1954 paper that "it is rather astonishing that [Cade's] observation has failed to arouse greater general interest among psychiatrists").[6] Schou quickly became convinced of the effectiveness of lithium in treating acute mania, and he was one of the first clinical researchers to become convinced of another therapeutic effect of the drug: its ability to prevent further episodes of illness (lithium's preventive, or *prophylactic,* effect). Schou had a more difficult time convincing his colleagues around the world that lithium could prevent recurrences of bipolar disorder and that patients should take it even after their acute symptoms had subsided. In 1967, Schou and his colleague Paul Christian Baalstrup reported on eighty-eight patients who had taken lithium for several years and had experienced a dramatic reduction in the frequency and duration of their mood episodes. Several patients who had been sick for several weeks out of every year experienced a complete remission of their illness that lasted for more than five years: their illness had essentially stopped (figure 7-1).[7]

As Schou and his colleagues treated more and more patients with lithium, their findings that lithium favorably altered the course of bipolar illness became so clear that they had ethical qualms about doing a more rigorous placebo-controlled study—one in which patients with bipolar disorder

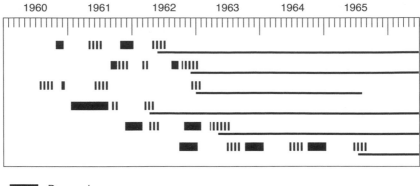

Figure 7-1 This graph illustrates data from six patients in Baalstrup and Schou's early study of the protective effect of lithium against the relapse of bipolar symptoms. Each line represents the symptom course of one patient. In all these patients, when lithium was started, episodes of depression and mania stopped completely. *Source*: Data from Paul Baalstrup and Morgans Schou, "Lithium as a Prophylactic Agent: Its Effect against Recurrent Depressions and Manic-Depressive Psychosis," *Archives of General Psychiatry* 16, no. 2 (1967): 162–72.

would be divided into two groups, some to receive lithium and the others a placebo. Several British psychiatrists scolded the Danes for reporting their results without a placebo-controlled study, so Baalstrup and Schou did a lithium discontinuation study in which they selected patients who had been stable while taking lithium for at least a year, divided them into two roughly equal groups, and in one group substituted a placebo for the lithium. The results were dramatic: of the thirty-nine participants whose lithium was replaced with the placebo, twenty-one relapsed within five months; *none* of the forty-five participants still taking lithium had a relapse.

It took a few more years to show that lithium is an effective antidepressant as well, but by the early 1980s, clinical studies had clearly shown that lithium is also an effective treatment for depressive syndrome.[8] Also clearly proven is that adding lithium to antidepressant medication can benefit people who have had an incomplete response to an antidepressant. This use, often referred to as antidepressant *augmentation*, can effectively turn a poor or incomplete therapeutic effect into a complete one.[9] Its antidepressant properties are thought to come from a completely different mechanism than most traditional antidepressants, which may be one reason it is so effective.

THERAPEUTIC PROFILE

Lithium is a naturally occurring element found in mineral springs, seawater, and certain ores. Like its close cousin, sodium, it is never found in its pure form in nature; it is always combined with other ions as a salt of one type or another. Lithium is mined on an industrial scale for use in the manufacture of ceramics and batteries. Therapeutic lithium preparations usually contain lithium carbonate. (See the therapeutic profile in table 7-1.)

Because it is an element, lithium is not metabolized within the body, and because lithium ions are so similar to sodium ions, the body handles lithium in much the same way it handles sodium. Lithium is rapidly absorbed through the gastrointestinal tract, enters the bloodstream, and is eliminated from the body by being filtered out by the kidneys.

Descriptions of the effects of a pharmaceutical in the body always include a vital statistic called its *half-life*. This is a measure of how quickly the body gets rid of a medication. Specifically, it is the time required for half the amount of the drug to be eliminated or metabolized by the body. Put another way, it is the time the body takes to reduce the level of the medication by half. The half-life of lithium in children and adolescents is about the same as in adults: approximately eighteen hours.[10] Another useful number, which can be derived from the half-life statistic for any medication, is the time required for the level of medication to build up to a constant level in the body—the time required for the amount taken in to equal the amount

Table 7-1 Therapeutic Profile of Lithium

Medication class:	Mood stabilizer
Brand names:	Eskalith, Eskalith CR, Lithobid, Lithonate, Lithotabs
Generic names:	Lithium carbonate, lithium citrate (liquid preparation)
Half-life:	14 to 30 hours
Metabolism:	None
Need for birth control:	Probably mandatory (see text)
Other considerations:	Blood levels extremely important

eliminated: the equilibrium point. By a series of mathematical steps that we don't need to detail here, it can be shown that the equilibrium point is the same for all medications: five half-lives. This means that since the half-life of lithium is roughly one day, it takes about five days for lithium, when first taken, to reach a steady level in the bloodstream. It also means that if the lithium dose is changed, it takes about five days for the blood level to stabilize at a new level.

Because of the toxic effects and even deaths that were reported when heart patients sprinkled lithium salt freely on their food, there was a significant delay in the acceptance of lithium as a therapeutic agent. Lithium is a powerful pharmaceutical, one that must be treated with respect. It has a very low *therapeutic index*, meaning that the difference between the therapeutic dose and a toxic dose is small.* Fortunately, lithium can be measured in the bloodstream accurately and fairly cheaply, and the dosage adjusted accordingly.

Monitoring of lithium levels in the blood is important not only to prevent toxicity but also because clinical studies have clearly demonstrated that, for most individuals, lithium needs to be present in the bloodstream at a certain level to be effective.[†] Clinical studies indicate that the therapeutic range for maximum efficacy is the same in adolescents and adults. But just what that level should be has been a matter of some debate.

An important study from the Massachusetts General Hospital found that a level of between 0.8 and 1.0 meq/L (milliequivalent per liter, a chemical measure of concentration) was most effective. In this double-blind study, adults with bipolar disorder were divided into two groups: a "standard dose" group, whose lithium levels were kept between 0.8 and 1.0 meq/L, and a "low dose" group, whose levels were maintained between 0.4 and 0.6 meq/L. The result was that the relapse rate in the "low dose" group was more than double that in the "standard dose" group (table 7-2).

There is more to these data than may initially meet the eye, however.

---

* To be more precise, the therapeutic index is the ratio of the largest dose producing no toxic symptoms to the smallest dose routinely producing the desired therapeutic effects.

† We speak of a "therapeutic level" in discussing the effective range of lithium in the bloodstream for treatment, not a "normal level." Lithium is a trace element in the body, normally present in undetectable concentrations.

Table 7-2 Comparison of Higher and Lower Lithium Levels in Relapse Rates of Bipolar Disorder

Treatment Group	Any Relapse	Depressed	Mixed/ Manic	Hypo- manic	Withdrew from Study
Standard dose range (0.8–1.0 meq/L)	6 (12%)	3 (6%)	3 (6%)	0	24 (51%)
Low dose range (0.4-0.6 meq/L)	21 (44%)	1 (2%)	17 (35%)	3 (6%)	11 (23%)

Source: Data from Alan Gelenberg, John Kane, Martin Keller, Phillip Lavori, Jerrold Rosenbaum, Karyl Cole, and Janet Lavelle, "Comparison of Standard and Low Levels of Lithium for Maintenance Treatment of Bipolar Disorder," *New England Journal of Medicine* 321, no. 22 (1989): 1489–93.
Note: Percentages are rounded.

Many more patients from the "standard dose" group than from the "low dose" group dropped out of the study because of side effects. The take-home message seems to be that levels closer to 1.0 meq/L are more protective, but that many people have trouble taking such a high dose because of side effects. Many psychiatrists compromise and try to maintain their patients at levels between these two. Dr. Schou, whom many consider the father of lithium therapy, has recommended levels of 0.5 to 0.8 meq/L for the treatment of bipolar disorder in adults.[11] Some people, however, clearly have good control of their symptoms with even lower levels, elderly persons, for example. Lithium levels thus need to be individualized for individual patients, and as Dr. Schou also points out, "Changes in lithium levels as small as 0.1 to 0.2 [meq/L], upward or downward, may substantially improve patients' quality of life during maintenance treatment."[12]

The lithium level rises in the bloodstream after every dose, peaks in about two hours, and then begins to fall again. If a patient takes his lithium two or three times a day, there will be several peaks and valleys. Because the level is rising and falling throughout the day, in checking lithium level it is important that the blood be drawn at a time when the result can be correctly interpreted. The convention that has been adopted is to use a twelve-hour level, making it convenient to draw blood in the mornings. For most people, this means getting to the lab twelve hours after their bedtime dose (for example, at 11 a.m. if the bedtime dose was at 11 the night before), without having taken their usual morning dose.

Lithium is approved for use in treating bipolar disorder in adolescents over the age of 12. Given what we've said about the variability of physical maturity in adolescents, you may wonder why the FDA doesn't label lithium and other drugs as approved for people of a certain height or weight rather than a certain age. The short answer is that this is simply how the FDA decided to do things. Remember that pharmaceutical labeling is a *guide* to prescribing medications, not *rules* for prescribing them.

Clinical research indicates that lithium is as effective for treating bipolar disorder in adolescents as it is in adults.[13] The research on using lithium as an augmentation of antidepressant treatment is more limited for adolescents than for adults, but the results are encouraging. In open trials of lithium as an augmentation of tricyclic antidepressants, about half the adolescents who had not had an adequate response to a tricyclic alone got better when lithium was added. This is about the same response usually seen in adults.[14] There have been case reports of lithium also helping the newer antidepressants to work better.[15] One of the most convincing reasons to consider lithium in certain populations is that it seems to reduce suicide. This has been shown time and again, most recently in a large meta-analysis of more than 6,000 adolescents.[16] No one understands exactly why, but in some way lithium reduces both suicidal thinking and suicide itself. The effect seems to be seen even in patients who continue to have other symptoms of depression that lithium did not reduce.

SIDE EFFECTS

Individuals vary widely in their sensitivity to side effects of lithium (and of all medications, for that matter). Some people have none; others have several. Fortunately, almost all of lithium's side effects can be eliminated or managed (table 7-3).

Many of the side effects are *dose related*: the higher the lithium dose, the more severe the side effect. One management strategy, then, is simply to lower the lithium dose. The advantages of higher levels are clear, as noted above, but most physicians will aim to maintain patients at the lowest possible dose that controls their symptoms.

Because of its similarity to sodium, lithium has some of the same effects that an increased sodium (table salt) intake would have: increased thirst, increased urination, and water retention. These side effects are often tem-

Table 7-3 Treatable Side Effects of Lithium

Side Effect	Remedy
Nausea, diarrhea	Take immediately after meals; switch to a controlled-release preparation
Weight gain	Diet and exercise
Tremor	Cut out caffeine-containing beverages; take beta-blocker medications
Flare-up of preexisting dermatological condition	Dermatological preparations
Hypothyroidism	Thyroid medications

porary and subside as the body adjusts to the medication. If they do not, the judicious use of medications that promote urination and excretion of excess body water (diuretics) can help. DO NOT ALLOW YOUR CHILD TO TAKE DIURETICS WITHOUT CONSULTING A PHYSICIAN! Some diuretics have the effect of raising lithium levels and can cause severe lithium toxicity. The regular lithium dose must usually be lowered and blood levels of lithium must be scrupulously monitored if a patient takes diuretics regularly. There have been reports of persistent and severe increased urination (*diabetes insipidus*, which has nothing to do with *diabetes mellitus*, the common "sugar diabetes") that progresses over time. A few cases of impaired kidney functioning have also been reported. Both these problems are rare and slow to develop. Nevertheless, in addition to monitoring lithium levels, blood tests that measure kidney functioning are routinely ordered for patients taking lithium.

Lithium is irritating to the gastrointestinal tract and can cause nausea or diarrhea; taking it on a full stomach can ease these problems considerably. A fine shaking in the hands (tremor) can occur at higher lithium levels; medications used to treat tremors, called beta-blockers, are frequently prescribed and can be very helpful. Weight gain can be an annoying side effect and unfortunately has an equally annoying remedy: diet and exercise.

Between 5 and 35 percent of people treated with lithium develop depression of thyroid gland functioning (hypothyroidism).[17] A test of thyroid functioning is the third in the battery of blood tests routinely ordered for persons taking lithium.

Lithium can cause flare-ups of preexisting skin conditions, but only rarely causes the new onset of dermatological problems. Individuals with acne, psoriasis, or other dermatological problems may need closer follow-up from their dermatologist.

Because those who start taking lithium for a mood disorder as an adolescent will often continue doing so into adulthood, it's important to note that lithium has been associated with birth defects. By the time a woman misses her period after conceiving, development of many of the embryo's major organs is already well under way. Stopping a medication after a woman *knows* she is pregnant may be too late to prevent a birth defect. Women of childbearing age have usually been advised to practice birth control while taking lithium if there is any chance of becoming pregnant. Some more recent data suggest that children born to women taking lithium have only a slightly increased chance of birth defects. The decision of how to go about lithium treatment during pregnancy is something of a debate, but often the risks of a recurrence of mental illness far outweigh the risks to the developing child, and many practitioners today recommend that patients stable on their medications should continue to take them throughout pregnancy.[18] That said, it is an individual decision, and women taking lithium who want to get pregnant should have a discussion with their psychiatrist and obstetrician about the risks of taking lithium and of stopping it. Lithium is secreted in breast milk, so women taking lithium should not breast-feed.

Another of lithium's side effects that troubles a significant number of people is a noticeable dulling of mental functioning. Patients complain that their ability to memorize and learn is affected and that they have a difficult-to-describe sense of mental sluggishness. A particular complaint is word-finding difficulties. For years, clinicians downplayed these complaints as coming from people who simply weren't used to being "normal," individuals who just missed the mental hyperalertness of hypomania. This view seemed to be supported by research using psychological tests on persons taking lithium for the treatment of bipolar disorder, research that has been basically inconclusive. But when nonpatient volunteers were administered lithium and similarly tested, a small but definite drop in their performance was found,[19] proving that this lithium-induced mental sluggishness is a real problem for some people. This side effect should be checked into for adolescents who seem to be having difficulties in school, even though their mood problem is under better control. This is a dose-related side effect and is another reason to strive for the lowest possible maintenance dose of lithium that still controls mood symptoms adequately.

VALPROATE (DEPAKOTE)

The development of valproate (brand names include Depakote and Depakene) for the treatment of mood disorders is another convoluted study in serendipity. Valproic acid is a carbon-containing compound similar to several others found in animal fats and vegetable oils: a fatty acid. It was first synthesized in 1882 and used as an organic solvent (a liquid in which other substances dissolve) for many years, for various purposes. Many decades ago, pharmacists used it as a solvent for bismuth salts, which were used to treat stomach and skin disorders.

In the early 1960s, scientists looking for treatments for epilepsy were working with a group of new pharmaceutical compounds that appeared promising but were difficult to dissolve. They discovered that valproic acid was an effective solvent for the compounds they were testing, and they started using it to dissolve their test drugs for animal experimentation. As they tested their various new pharmaceuticals, the results they obtained seemed confusing—until someone realized that it didn't matter *which* of the new pharmaceuticals was used. As long as *any* of them was dissolved in valproic acid, the drug was found to be effective in stopping epileptic seizure activity. It soon became obvious that the valproic acid was stopping the seizures, not what was dissolved in it. By 1978, valproate was approved by the FDA for use in treating adult epilepsy,[20] and it is now approved for and widely used in the pediatric population as well.

In the 1960s, there were some reports that valproate might be helpful in mood disorders, and throughout the late 1960s and early 1970s, a French psychiatrist named Pierre A. Lambert published a series of papers about using it to treat bipolar disorders. After the discovery that another antiepilepsy medication, carbamazepine, was effective in treating mania, interest in the possibilities of valproate as a mood stabilizer grew. In the mid-1980s, several studies on the use of valproate in treating bipolar disorder were published by American psychiatrists, and ten years later, valproate had become firmly established as an effective antimanic medication and a mood stabilizer in adults; it is now FDA approved for use in bipolar disorder (in adults only, for now). Less research has been done on adolescents, but the available data indicate that valproate is effective for adolescents with bipolar disorder.[21] Because one of valproate's first uses was for seizure disorders in children and adolescents, there is a large amount of information on dosing, safety, and side effects in young people.

Valproate's therapeutic action in bipolar disorder (or in epilepsy, for that matter) is still largely unknown. We do know that it improves neuronal transmission in the brain that is mediated by the neurotransmitter *gamma-aminobutyric acid* (GABA). GABA seems to have an inhibitory or modulating effect on many brain circuits, and valproate's effect may be through its ability to regulate the amount of GABA in the brain. Valproate is also increasingly recognized as a chemical that alters the gene expression of neurons, protecting them in the brain and making them overall less excitable (and therefore less likely to produce seizures and, potentially, the wide mood swings of bipolar affective disorder).

THERAPEUTIC PROFILE

Valproate is known to be an effective treatment for acute mania. It also appears to be effective in preventing the recurrence, and reducing the severity, of episodes of bipolar disorder. Its effectiveness in treating acute depressive episodes of bipolar disorder has been less impressive, so it may be less likely to help as an antidepressant augmentation agent than lithium in the long run, though a head-to-head study of these medications for this purpose has not yet been completed. (See the therapeutic profile in table 7-4.)

In reading about this medication, you'll notice the many names it goes by: valproate, valproic acid, divalproex sodium, not to mention the brand names, Depakote and Depakene. Valproate is the name of the negative ion. When associated with a hydrogen ion, the result is valproic acid; in combination with a sodium ion, it becomes sodium valproate. Depakote, a preparation manufactured by Abbott Laboratories, consists of a stable combination of sodium valproate and valproic acid called divalproex sodium. (Depakene is Abbott's brand name for their valproic acid preparation.)

Valproate seems to be more effective than lithium for certain subgroups of patients: those with rapid cycling (four or more mood episodes per year) and those with mixed mania, that is, a mixture of manic hyperactivity and pressured thinking and depressed or unpleasant mood.[22] Valproate is also

Table 7-4   Therapeutic Profile of Valproate

Medication class:	Mood stabilizer (anticonvulsant)
Brand names:	Depakote, Depakene
Generic names:	Divalproex sodium, valproic acid
Half-life:	6 to 16 hours
Metabolism:	Affected by other antiepilepsy drugs
Elimination:	By liver and kidneys
Need for birth control:	Probably mandatory
Other considerations:	Blood levels helpful to adjust dose; blood tests for liver inflammation needed

much less toxic than lithium. One big disadvantage of valproate is that it does not seem to be as helpful as lithium in treating acute depression. Nor is it very effective in preventing recurrences of depression.[23] This suggests that valproate may be a better choice for individuals with rapid cycling or with mixed mania, but that those with classic euphoric mania and major depression may have better control of their symptoms with lithium.[24] As with antidepressants, however, overall conclusions about how a medication affects a *group* of patients is at best a guess of how it will affect a *particular* patient. Treatment of yourself or your child can often be a process of repeated trials to find the right medication or combination of medications.

Like lithium, valproate can be measured in the bloodstream; unfortunately, it is more difficult to measure and requires a more expensive test. Blood levels above 45 mcg/mL (micrograms per milliliter) have been shown to be necessary for the therapeutic effect to occur, and side effects become more problematic at levels greater than 125 mcg/mL.[25] Several studies have shown that valproate is helpful in cyclothymia, bipolar II, and "soft" bipolar disorders, and that lower doses and lower blood levels are required than in the treatment of bipolar I.[26] As with lithium, in measuring valproate levels, blood should be drawn twelve hours after the last dose of medication.

Valproate has also been used to treat more general behavioral problems in children and adolescents, specifically impulse problems, aggressiveness, and severe temper tantrums, though evidence for this use is still somewhat controversial, and it has not been approved by the FDA for any of the above.[27] Valproate has significant antianxiety effects and is sometimes prescribed for this reason, especially in Europe.

Valproate has a milder side-effect profile than lithium and is not nearly as toxic in overdose. Side effects that are common as an individual starts taking the medication include stomach upset and some sleepiness. These problems usually go away quickly. Increased appetite and weight gain can occur. Mild tremor also occurs and can be treated with beta-blocker medication. A few patients report hair loss, usually temporary, which resolves even more quickly with vitamin preparations containing the minerals zinc and selenium.[28] Most dandruff shampoos contain selenium, and these help combat this type of hair loss too.

Cases of severe liver problems have been reported in patients taking valproate. These occurred almost exclusively in young children (under age 2) taking the drug for control of epilepsy, most of whom had other medical problems and were taking several different medications. A 1989 review article stated that no fatalities from liver problems caused by valproate had ever been reported for individuals over the age of 10 who were taking only valproate.[29] Just to be on the safe side, however, a blood test that can detect liver inflammation is done for those taking valproate for the first time and is repeated at appropriate intervals while they are taking this medication. Because valproate also, though rarely, causes a drop in blood cell count, a complete blood count is usually done as well. These are very rare problems. Even when they do occur, they develop slowly and usually during the first six months of therapy and thus can be picked up with routine blood tests. Nevertheless, individuals taking valproate should be on the lookout for signs of liver or blood count problems: unusual bleeding and bruising, jaundice (yellowing of the eyes and skin), fever, and water retention.

Valproate has been associated with birth defects, so women in the child-bearing years should practice birth control while taking valproate if there is any possibility of becoming pregnant. There is also controversy about the frequency with which valproate causes multiple ovarian cysts (polycystic ovaries) in women who have taken it for many years. A study demonstrated that up to one in ten young women treated with valproate develop this condition.[30] This is an important consideration in prescribing this medication to adolescent girls.

CARBAMAZEPINE (TEGRETOL)

After the introduction of carbamazepine (brand names include Tegretol and Epitol) for the control of epilepsy in the 1960s, several reports appeared indicating that, when taking this medication, people with epilepsy who also had mood problems not only had good control of their seizures but had improvement in their psychiatric symptoms as well. It was a small step to test carbamazepine in patients with mood problems who did not suffer from epilepsy. Much of the earlier work on the use of carbamazepine in treating bipolar disorder was done by Japanese clinicians looking for an alternative to lithium, which was not approved for use in Japan until years after it was available in the United States. In 1980, a study appeared in the *American Journal of Psychiatry* titled "Carbamazepine in Manic-Depressive Illness: A New Treatment."[31] Although carbamazepine has been used to treat epilepsy in children and adolescents for many years, it is currently not labeled by the FDA for the treatment of psychiatric disorders in children or adolescents (or adults, for that matter). Although it seems that carbamazepine may be helpful for children and adolescents with bipolar affective disorder,[32] the effect is smaller than that of either lithium or valproic acid, and it has never been investigated for use in depression.

THERAPEUTIC PROFILE

Carbamazepine is one of those medications that don't seem to have any particular advantage in most studies on groups of psychiatric patients, but it works well—in fact, works when other medications do not—in some individuals. In one well-designed double-blind study, manic patients who took carbamazepine actually seemed to do worse than those taking lithium.[33] But most psychiatrists have had a patient like "Ms. B.," whose case history was reported in a paper from the National Institute of Mental Health in 1983:

CASE 2. MS. B., a 53-year-old woman, had a history of treatment resistant, rapid cycling manic-depressive illness that required continuous state hospitalization from 1956 to her admission to NIMH in 1978. She had been non-responsive to [antipsychotic medications, tricyclic antidepressants] and lithium . . . After institution of carbamazepine, both mood phases improved dramatically and she was able to be discharged...During a subsequent hospitalization her severe mania again did not respond to [antipsychotic medications] and she was not able to leave the hospital until she was treated with carbamazepine.[34]

The authors of this study noted, "Additional improvement appeared to occur when [antipsychotic medications] were used in conjunction with carbamazepine or when lithium and carbamazepine were used in combination." This has become carbamazepine's niche: a second-line mood-stabilizing agent for patients who do not respond to other agents, often used in combination with other agents. (See the therapeutic profile in table 7-5.)

A series of case reports published in 1999 supports carbamazepine's effectiveness in the treatment of bipolar disorder in adolescents. The cases included a 17-year-old girl and a 14-year-old boy who had classic bipolar symptoms with severe depressions and manias. Both had only a partial response to lithium and significant side effects with it. Because of these problems, these children had stopped taking the medication several times and had suffered relapses. Both had excellent remissions of their symptoms on taking carbamazepine, and because they didn't have side-effect problems, they were willing to take it continuously and therefore stayed well.[35]

Like the other mood-stabilizing medications, carbamazepine can be measured in the bloodstream, and the blood levels are used to adjust the dose. Unfortunately, not much work has been done on blood levels of this medication in patients with bipolar disorder, so the therapeutic range used for the treatment of epilepsy is usually the target that psychiatrists aim for in their patients.

Table 7-5   Therapeutic Profile of Carbamazepine

Medication class:	Mood stabilizer (anticonvulsant)
Brand names:	Epitol, Tegretol
Generic name:	Carbamazepine
Half-life:	18 to 55 hours (shortens after time)
Metabolism:	Complex: affects and is affected by other drugs
Elimination:	By liver and kidneys
Need for birth control:	Probably mandatory
Other considerations:	Blood levels helpful to adjust dose; blood tests for liver inflammation and blood abnormalities needed

Carbamazepine is metabolized in the liver, and like some other drugs, it causes the levels of liver enzymes that metabolize it to increase. This means that the longer a person takes carbamazepine, the better the liver becomes at getting rid of it. So after a few weeks, the blood levels of the drug may go down, and the dose may need to be increased. This increase in liver enzymes can also affect other medications that the patient might be taking, including certain tranquilizers, certain antidepressants, other epilepsy medications, and some hormones, including birth-control preparations. It is essential to inform all physicians involved in a person's care that she has started taking carbamazepine, so that dosage adjustments can be made.

SIDE EFFECTS

Carbamazepine can produce the sort of general side effects caused by many medications affecting the brain: sleepiness, light-headedness, and some initial nausea. These problems tend to be short lived and dose related.

As with valproate, there have been rare cases of liver problems, so blood tests for liver inflammation are routinely done. There have also been rare reports of dangerous changes in blood cell counts, so blood counts are also done, especially in the first several weeks of therapy. Some cases of a rare but dangerous skin reaction called Stevens-Johnson syndrome have occurred. Although all these problems are uncommon, patients should be on the watch for the development of a rash, jaundice, water retention, bleeding or bruising, or signs of infection.

LAMOTRIGINE (LAMICTAL)

Lamotrigine (brand name Lamictal) is another antiseizure medication that appears to have therapeutic effects for people with mood disorders. Studies began to appear in the 1980s showing that it was a useful add-on therapy for people with epilepsy who were already taking other antiseizure medications. During the early investigations of this use, researchers noted that patients who took lamotrigine for seizure control reported an improvement in their mood and sense of well-being—even if it hadn't helped much with their seizures. Lamotrigine has several effects on the brain that might explain its efficacy in bipolar disorder. It appears to inhibit release of the neurotransmitter *glutamate*, an amino acid that causes stimulation of various neural circuits. Lamotrigine is also thought to affect at least one of the same second messenger systems that lithium affects, the *inositol triphosphate system*.[36] It is approved as a mood stabilizer for bipolar affective disorder in adults, though not in children.

THERAPEUTIC PROFILE

The most exciting aspect of lamotrigine's profile is its apparent effectiveness in depression, including both bipolar and unipolar depression (table 7-6).[37] One of the first reports on its use in the treatment of bipolar disorder described a patient who had suffered from rapid-cycling bipolar I disorder since he was 14.[38] In the year before starting to take lamotrigine, he had been either depressed or manic continuously with no period of normal mood. When the research team first saw him, he was severely depressed and had not responded to lithium, carbamazepine, or an antidepressant. On taking lamotrigine, his depression symptoms gradually improved, and eleven months later, he hadn't had a recurrence of either depressive or manic symptoms. There are other reports of lamotrigine being helpful in cases of extremely treatment-resistant major depressive disorder in adults.[39]

Other studies indicate that lamotrigine works well with other mood stabilizers in treatment-resistant patients and can sometimes turn a partial medication response into a more complete one.[40] Lamotrigine is a welcome addition to the present array of mood stabilizers—especially in light of its apparent antidepressant effects.

Lamotrigine has a half-life of about twenty-four hours, and the body's ability to metabolize it is affected by taking carbamazepine and valproate. Blood levels are not routinely ordered for lamotrigine because of its low toxicity and because therapeutic effects have not been correlated with a particular blood-level range.

SIDE EFFECTS

Aside from some initial nausea or gastrointestinal upset and the sort of side effects that many medications affecting the brain can cause— sleepiness, light-headedness or dizziness, and headache—lamotrigine has a good side-effect profile. The most serious side effects reported are severe types of skin rashes, Stevens-Johnson syndrome and toxic epidermal necrosis (TED). This last severe rash has the effect of a whole-body third-

Table 7-6   Therapeutic Profile of Lamotrigine

Medication class:	Mood stabilizer (anticonvulsant)
Brand name:	Lamictal
Generic name:	Lamotrigine
Half-life:	15 to 24 hours
Metabolism:	Complex: affected by other drugs
Elimination:	By liver and kidneys
Need for birth control:	Recommended
Other considerations:	Rarely causes severe skin rashes, but has a generally good side-effect profile

degree burn and has been fatal in some cases. The likelihood of this problem developing has been greatly reduced by the practice of starting the medication at a very low dose and raising the dose quite gradually. Although this means it takes a lot longer (several weeks) to get to a therapeutic dose, the technique has greatly reduced the number of serious rashes. Also, the rash problem seems to be more frequently seen in individuals who have had other dermatological reactions to medications. Unfortunately, TED has been reported more often in young people than in adults, so lamotrigine is not recommended by the manufacturer for children under the age of 16. Patients should examine their skin carefully, especially during the first several weeks of therapy, and stop the medication and get in touch with their doctor at any sign of skin rash. Despite this frankly scary though uncommon side effect, lamotrigine can be an excellent option for adolescents who have not responded to other medications.

OTHER MOOD STABILIZERS

Several other agents seemed to show promise for the treatment of bipolar disorder. The evidence for these agents is still in the early stages of development, although unfortunately, it doesn't appear to be as encouraging as the evidence for the medications described above. For the most part, the promise of these medications is based on a few case reports of a therapeutic effect in adults; in some cases, they are medications in the same class as other pharmaceuticals already shown to be helpful.

Gabapentin (brand name Neurontin) is yet another antiseizure medication that initially seemed to be a mood stabilizer as well. As with the others, reports of beneficial effects on mood disorder symptoms in people being treated for epilepsy came first, and a few indicators of effect in bipolar disorder followed. A large study of gabapentin found no difference from placebo in effect on patients with bipolar affective disorder.[41] That said, as is so often the case, for the rare patient who seems to respond to nothing else, it can be a virtual miracle cure. One case report concerned a man with bipolar disorder who refused to take lithium and who had liver disease and low blood counts caused by alcoholism.[42] Because he wouldn't take lithium, and his medical problems made the use of valproate or carbamazepine risky, gabapentin was tried. He had a "dramatic" decrease in manic symptoms, his sleep pattern returned to normal, and best of all, he reported no side effects. Gabapentin is not metabolized in the liver and so does not affect the blood levels of other medications; it doesn't need blood-level monitoring and has a good side-effect profile.

Oxcarbazepine (brand name Trileptal) is an antiepilepsy drug similar to carbamazepine. Several encouraging studies from Germany were published in the 1980s describing its use in treating bipolar disorder in adults, but the drug was not approved for use in the United States until January 2000. The case of a 6-year-old girl with severe bipolar disorder who was successfully treated with oxcarbazepine appeared in the *Journal of the American Academy of Child and Adolescent Psychiatry* in 2001. This little girl had mood symptoms with severe aggression and violent behaviors that included breaking windows and knocking doors off their hinges. She had not benefited from lithium but had "full mood stabilization" after six weeks of taking oxcarbazepine. After three months, her mother reported that she was "fabulous," and her teacher said she was a "little angel."[43] This one case report contrasts with larger studies, which don't seem to show that it is helpful for children or adolescents as a population. Oxcarbazepine has fewer side effects than carbamazepine and has not been associated with the dangerous skin rashes and blood count problems occurring with that drug.

Other antiepilepsy drugs that have attracted the interest of clinical researchers on bipolar disorder are *topiramate* (Topamax) and *tiagabine* (Gabatril). Neither of these has shown any appreciable effect on mania or depression, unfortunately.

Research clearly indicates that lithium, valproate, carbamazepine, and lamotrigine are effective for the treatment of bipolar disorder in adults. The studies on younger patients are more limited, but the results have been encouraging. Adding mood-stabilizing medications, primarily lithium, to an antidepressant medication for adult patients who have treatment-resistant depression is also clearly helpful and can turn a partial remission of symptoms into a complete one. Again, there is less research on this use in adolescents, but what is available supports the view that this is an effective strategy. Thus, mood-stabilizing medications seem to have a place in the management of both bipolar disorders and depressive disorders.

These medications have also been used to treat behavioral problems that have some overlap with the symptoms of mood disorders. It's important that we have a quick sidebar about what exactly a "diagnosis" means in psychiatry, so that it's crystal clear what these medications are treating and how they are supposed to help. Some diagnoses in the *DSM* and in psychiatry refer to conditions that are caused by inborn biological causes over which the person has no control. These diagnoses speak to the *etiology*, the origin, of the condition. Major depression is one such diagnosis, as is bipolar affective disorder.

Other diagnoses are merely descriptive terms used to identify a cluster of behaviors. They don't speak to where the condition comes from or what causes it; instead, they simply are a checklist of different symptoms or characteristics, usually behaviors, that tend to go together. In children, two such diagnoses are *oppositional defiant disorder* and *conduct disorder*. Putting "disorder" at the end of their names may lead some to believe that these diagnoses describe conditions that descend on the poor sufferer without any hope of avoidance. In fact, *conduct disorder* is a diagnosis given to children and adolescents who are aggressive, destructive, and disobedient, and who break the rules and often the law with behaviors such as stealing. There is no description of why they do this, and possibly no underlying neurological cause to begin with; instead, there's a pattern of behavior, of things the person willfully does, that are collected under a single term.

Consequently, when a medication is given to a patient to "treat" one of these disorders, it is not the same as giving an antidepressant to correct the chemical imbalance of depression. Rather, medications used for these conditions usually help the patient with her behaviors in a more roundabout fashion. We have spoken about how the initial trials of lithium in animals showed it to have a sedating, calming effect. In patients with bipolar affective disorder, lithium can reduce impulsivity (or at times creativity) and create a sort of sleepy, lackadaisical mood. In an irritable, angry, disobedient adolescent, this same sort of change may be seen as "treating" her "condition," though in fact it is more likely taking away some of the energy she uses to fuel her negative behaviors.

Now, it is not necessarily the case that an adolescent has either a biological mood disorder or a behavioral conduct disorder. More frequently than not, the two go together. An adolescent develops low mood, irritability, anger, and social isolation, and deals with these feelings by lashing out and having little concern for the consequences. He may begin to develop a behavioral disorder as the result of a mood disorder, or the two may develop independently.

With this caveat in mind, it is worth mentioning that several studies have looked at the effectiveness of mood-stabilizing medications for these behavioral problems; some of the studies have demonstrated beneficial effects, though others have not. Lithium has been shown to help with aggressiveness in children and adolescents in some studies, as has valproic acid.

Based on these sorts of studies on the effects of mood-stabilizing medications on behavioral problems, some child psychiatrists will prescribe a mood stabilizer to a patient whose mood syndrome is complicated by aggressive, irritable, impulsive behaviors, even if the classic bipolar symptoms don't seem to be present. We are not necessarily against this practice, if it is helpful to the child, but we remind patients and parents that the medications are not the path to curing a behavioral disorder. They are useful merely for managing the symptoms while the patient undergoes more targeted treatment, usually psychotherapy, to change behavior patterns and become more positive.

WHY, AND HOW, TO USE MOOD STABILIZERS IN DEPRESSION

Combinations of medications in the treatment of severe mood disorders are becoming the rule rather than the exception. Almost by definition, early-onset mood disorders are severe mood disorders, and when the adolescent has a family history of bipolar disorder, it might be reasonable to add a mood stabilizer to his medication. How should the psychiatrist choose among the different mood stabilizers for a particular patient? It has been suggested that younger children seem to tolerate lithium better than older adolescents, because they are not as troubled by the weight gain and dermatological problems (remember that lithium can worsen acne). That said, children are usually less tolerant of the accompanying blood draws, and parents have to be careful that their child doesn't get dehydrated, as dehydration can increase the blood lithium level. For older adolescents who may have trouble with lithium side effects, valproate may be more appropriate, especially since these teenagers often have more problems with aggressiveness, which valproate has been shown to help.[44]

Even more so than with the antidepressants, the decision to add a mood stabilizer to an adolescent patient's medications and making a choice among the available mood-stabilizing medications is more art than science. The published clinical studies on the use of these drugs for children and adolescents nearly always end with a sentence or two bemoaning the lack of research that proves the pattern of efficacy of these medications in young patients with mood disorders.

All of this makes it crucial that parents understand the target symptoms for which a mood stabilizer is being used, so they can help monitor their child for improvement, or lack of improvement, of these symptoms.

Other Medications and Treatments

Although antidepressant and mood-stabilizing medications are the primary treatment of depression and bipolar disorders, a variety of other medications are often used as adjunctive treatments. Sometimes these medications are used temporarily to relieve severe symptoms of irritability or anxiety, and sometimes they are an ongoing part of the patient's treatment. Only some of the following medications are approved by the U.S. Food and Drug Administration for the treatment of mood disorders in young persons, so their use is still somewhat controversial. Despite this, one class (the atypical antipsychotics) are some of the most frequently prescribed psychiatric medications in this age group and therefore need to be discussed.

As this is written, multiple government regulatory agencies are evaluating how these medications are used. If you recall our discussion in chapter 6 of SSRI medications and how they were being given out like candy for every instance of apparent sadness, you will understand the climate of a few years ago in which some of these medications, considered relatively benign in the short term, were used to treat every type of anger or aggression. An increased understanding of the long-term effects of these chemicals on the developing body is now beginning to curb this practice.

ANTIPSYCHOTIC MEDICATIONS

A difficulty that immediately arises in discussing antipsychotic medications is their unfortunate name. *Psychotic* is an imprecise term at best, and these medications have many more uses than simply treating psychotic symptoms. This group of medications has also been called the *major tranquilizers,* a label that perhaps more accurately describes the usefulness of these pharmaceuticals in treating mood disorders. They can provide substantial and fast relief of the restlessness and mental anguish of severe depression and calm the agitation of mania. We discussed mood stabilizers in the previous chapter. In a large study, antipsychotics were found to be startlingly more effective than any mood stabilizer in acute mania in adolescents,[1] though we have also discussed how some practitioners may misdiagnose "mania." Some may confuse the *symptom* of agitation for the *syndrome* of mania, when in fact the agitation could be due to any number of different causes.

Before we get into the details of antipsychotic medications, a brief explanation about the word *psychosis* is in order. Psychosis can be thought of as a mental state or disorder in which a person's ability to comprehend the environment and react to it appropriately is severely impaired. The layperson's definition of *psychotic* might be "out of touch with reality." The person who is hearing voices (hallucinations) or who has bizarre idiosyncratic beliefs (delusions) is psychotic. The word also has a connotation of a severe disorganization of thinking and behavior, usually with restlessness and agitation. The manic syndrome is a good example of a state of psychosis, and in chapter 4, we talked about "psychotic features" in depression.

In the 1930s, pharmaceutical compounds called *phenothiazines* were synthesized in Europe and were found to have antihistamine and sedative properties. One in particular, chlorpromazine, was found to be useful in surgical anesthesia because it deepened anesthetic sedation more safely than other available agents. In the early 1950s, two French psychiatrists carried out several clinical trials using chlorpromazine to treat highly agitated patients suffering from schizophrenia and mania. They noticed that in addition to its quieting and sleep-promoting effects, chlorpromazine made the hallucinations and bizarre delusional beliefs of many individuals with schizophrenia practically disappear. It also decreased the severity of the disorganization of thinking and agitated behavior seen in patients with acute mania. Chlorpromazine, in other words, had a *specific* effect on the cluster of symptoms usually referred to as "psychotic" symptoms, and thus the name for this group of drugs came about: *antipsychotic medications.* Occasionally, they are still referred to as *neuroleptic* medications (or *neuroleptics*), from *neuroleptique*, the French word coined from Greek roots that means, roughly, "affecting the nervous system." The term *major tranquilizers* was coined to distinguish these medications from *minor tranquilizers*, medications used for sleep problems and anxiety. But because these agents are much more than just "tranquilizers," this term has fallen out of favor too. The far-ranging effects of this group are more than simply "antipsychotic," but until a better term comes along, *antipsychotic medications* is what we're stuck with.

The main chemical effect of all the pharmaceuticals in this class is a blockade of dopamine receptors in the brain. In people with schizophrenia, neural circuits that use dopamine as their neurotransmitter may be dysfunctional in some way, and this may cause the bizarre hallucinations and disorders of thinking typical of that illness. Antipsychotics may work by affecting these systems in some as yet unknown way. Whether these medications alleviate the psychotic symptoms that sometimes complicate bipolar disorder in a similar fashion is also not yet known.

After the development of the original group of antipsychotic medications (table 8-1), the phenothiazines, in the 1960s and 1970s several other potent dopamine-blocking medications were developed. The side-effect profile of these newer medications was marginally better than that of the phenothiazines, but they did not represent much of an advance therapeutically.

More recently, several new antipsychotic medications have been introduced that not only have substantially fewer and less severe side effects but also are more effective for many patients (table 8-2). These agents are called *atypical* or *second generation* antipsychotic medications because although they block dopamine receptors (though not as potently as their predecessors), they differ from the typical antipsychotic medications in that they are also active at serotonin receptors. As you might guess, this effect is thought to explain why these medications might be more helpful in mood disorders. Among these medications, aripiprazole (Abilify), que-

Table 8-1 Traditional Antipsychotic Medications

Generic Name	Brand Name
Chlorpromazine	Thorazine
Fluphenazine	Prolixin
Haloperidol	Haldol
Loxapine	Loxitane
Molindone	Moban
Perphenazine	Trilafon
Thioridazine	Mellaril
Thiothixene	Navane
Trifluoperazine	Stelazine

tiapine (Seroquel), olanzapine (Zyprexa), and risperidone (Risperdal) are approved for treatment of mania in bipolar affective disorder type I.

THERAPEUTIC PROFILE

Antipsychotic medications are effective in reducing the symptoms of delusions or hallucinations that accompany a true psychotic episode. In their role as major tranquilizers, they are strongly sedating and can quickly calm an agitated patient, though unlike the benzodiazepines, they are nonaddicting. Antipsychotics are given primarily for this purpose in such intense environments as the emergency room, and they are rapidly effective and safe. There is good evidence, particularly in adults, that they can be used long term to augment antidepressant effects (particularly the second generation antipsychotics, which seem to affect the serotonin system), as well as reduce the agitation and irritability that tend to accompany the more adolescent forms of depression. Manic patients can find quick relief

Table 8-2 New Antipsychotic Medications

Generic Name	Brand Name
Clozapine	Clozaril
Olanzapine	Zyprexa
Quetiapine	Seroquel
Risperidone	Risperdal
Ziprasidone	Geodon
Aripiprazole	Abilify
Asenapine	Saphris
Lurasidone	Latuda

of their euphoric or irritable states, and these medications can be a helpful augmentation to mood stabilizers for long-term maintenance of a stable mood. Similarly, in a young person with severe symptoms of irritability or aggressiveness, antipsychotic medications may be prescribed temporarily to reduce these symptoms until other medications have time to become effective.

SIDE EFFECTS

The original antipsychotic medications have significant effects on muscle tone and movement, side effects caused by the dopamine blockade these agents cause. The newer agents do not cause these side-effect problems nearly as often, so they are now used much more frequently. In textbook discussions of these medications, you will see these problems referred to as *extrapyramidal symptoms,* or simply EPS. Dopamine is the main neurotransmitter in a complex circuit of brain areas called the *extrapyramidal system,* which coordinates movement. The term *extrapyramidal* contrasts this system with another brain system, called the *pyramidal* system because its main fibers are carried in triangular-shaped bundles into the spinal cord (the *spinal pyramids,* or *pyramidal tract*). The pyramidal system controls the quick, accurate execution of fine muscle movement, and the extrapyramidal system makes sure that the rest of the body moves as needed for the smooth and graceful execution of these movements. Antipsychotic medications, by blocking the dopamine receptors in these extrapyramidal centers, can cause movements to become stiff and slow. *Acute dystonic reactions* are muscular spasms that usually involve the tongue and facial and neck muscles; these spasms are more common in young male patients. People taking antipsychotic medications can also develop an uncomfortable restlessness called *akathisia,* felt mostly in the legs. A person with akathisia often feels the need to walk or pace and can appear agitated though he is in fact merely uncomfortable.

Fortunately, all these side effects are treatable, either by lowering the dose of medication or by adding one of several medications that are also used to treat Parkinson's disease. Although the side effects are uncomfortable, they are not dangerous and usually respond quickly to treatment.

People who took older antipsychotic medications over many years sometimes developed a side effect called *tardive dyskinesia* (TD). This consists of repetitive involuntary movements, usually of the facial muscles: chewing, blinking, or lip-pursing movements. There is no good treatment for TD other than discontinuing the medication. Because TD seemed to persist in some individuals even after they stopped taking the medication, it used to be thought that these problems were permanent. As it turns out, some TD symptoms *do* go away with time.

The great advantage of the newer antipsychotic medications is that most patients who take them have none of these extrapyramidal movement problems. For years, many believed that these medications were hands down safer for children (in some cases, this evidence may have been due to a manipulation of data by pharmaceutical companies, as we discuss below). However, there are several different side effects to consider, and experts are constantly debating which profile is more detrimental to the developing young body.

Although the possibility of movement disorders is significantly lower with atypical antipsychotics, the atypical antipsychotics seem to have a fundamental and unavoidable effect on the way the body metabolizes and uses food. A cluster of conditions, together labeled the *metabolic syndrome*, may develop. In this syndrome, the body's cells become much less sensitive to the insulin we all use to signal that it is time to convert the free sugars floating in our bloodstream into energy. In extreme cases, diabetes develops and requires treatment with additional medications. The way the body uses fats also changes. People begin putting on weight, sometimes in surprising amounts, rather quickly. This is partially an effect of increased appetite but also seems related to a change in how the body stores excess energy. Cholesterol, triglycerides, and lipids all increase. Children develop the cholesterol profiles of 50-year-olds. Most of the time, stopping the antipsychotic can reverse some, but not all, of these effects. Strict diet and exercise are helpful, though difficult for young persons.

Atypical antipsychotics can also alter the way our bodies produce certain hormones. We all have a certain amount of the hormone *prolactin* secreted by our brains. This hormone has many effects, but one of them (as can be deduced by the name) is to signal to a woman's body that it is time to begin producing milk. Antipsychotics, particularly the second generation class, increase this hormone. In some cases, this can cause breast tissue formation (*gynecomastia*) and milk production (*galactorrhea*), even in males.

In 2013, the results of a large study evaluating a second generation antipsychotic indicated that this effect was transient and quickly returned to near normal, and so was clinically negligible.[2] In fact, the study (paid for by the maker of this antipsychotic) had accidentally incorporated a statistical error; the incidence of milk production in boys was actually double what was originally reported. In most men, this is reversible by stopping the medication, but it can take some time to return to normal, which can be an excruciating experience for a young man trying to find his social place in the world.

There are, fortunately, few potentially lethal side effects of second generation antipsychotics, but one deserves further discussion. The first atypical antipsychotic, clozapine, was synthesized in laboratories in the 1960s but was not marketed in the United States until 1990. One of the reasons clozapine took so long to get on the market is that it causes a dangerous drop in the number of white blood cells (a condition called *agranulocytosis*) in about 1 percent of patients.[3] This problem might have meant the end of the line for clozapine were it not found to be highly effective in treating patients with schizophrenia who derived no benefit from traditional antipsychotic medications. Dramatic case studies of patients with chronic treatment-resistant schizophrenia basically "awakening" from years of unrelenting psychotic symptoms after they started taking clozapine sustained the interest of clinicians and pharmaceutical researchers in this medication. Following the discovery that the risk of agranulocytosis could be substantially reduced if the white blood cell count was monitored weekly, clozapine treatment became available to larger groups of patients.

None of the other atypical antipsychotics causes this problem, so weekly blood tests are not necessary with these medications. Clozapine is usually reserved for patients who have not responded to other types of antipsychotics, so it is rarely used in young persons; but it is not an unreasonable possibility if someone has tried two or three other medications with little response.

CONTROVERSIES

A good number of clinical studies have reported on the safety and efficacy of atypical antipsychotics in the treatment of schizophrenia in young people. This is probably because symptoms of schizophrenia often begin in adolescence, and these medications are the foundation of medical treatment of this illness. Until recently, there existed much less clinical research on the use of these medications in adolescents with mood disorders—even less than on the use of antidepressants and mood stabilizers. A 1999 article in the *Journal of the American Academy of Child and Adolescent Psychiatry* titled "Antipsychotics in Children and Adolescents" does not even mention the use of these medications in young people for the treatment of mood disorders.[4]

In the early 2000s, prescribing patterns changed rapidly. We spoke earlier about how, at around the same time, there was an explosion in the diagnosis of bipolar affective disorder in young people (see chapter 3). Accompanying this increase in diagnosis was a rapid increase in the use of atypical antipsychotic medications in an attempt to rapidly and definitively reduce the symptoms of these youth. We didn't know as much about these medications' side effects at the time, so when comparing something like risperidone (a once-daily pill that required no special precautions or monitoring) to something like lithium (with its blood draws and potential for overdose), the choice seemed clear. Between 1993 and 2002, the number of prescriptions for atypical antipsychotics to young people increased six-fold.[5] About one in ten outpatient psychiatry visits of a child or adolescent resulted in the prescription of an antipsychotic, and over half of all children and adolescents admitted to a psychiatric hospital were discharged on one of these drugs regardless of the diagnosis.[6]

In one disturbing trend, the rates of antipsychotic prescribing to children in foster care was found to be much higher than those for children not in foster care. Although about 10 percent of non-foster-care children were on these medications, over 40 percent of foster care children were taking them. It was also found that a high percentage of these children were on more than one such medication at a time (a practice known as *polypharmacy*, which could expose them to more risks of side effects), and that some children were on significantly higher doses than were allowed by the FDA even for adults. Finally, few if any of these children were being routinely monitored for the metabolic effects described above. There was not the same degree of difference in *diagnoses* between foster care and non-foster-care children, seeming to imply that the medications were no longer tied to their intended use. This was all revealed in a congressional report published by the Government Accountability Office.[7] Although no definitive conclusions were drawn, the patterns seemed to suggest that these medications were used to control behavioral outbursts in a fragile and often underserved population.

Among the child psychiatry community, the combined realization that long-term use of these medicines had increasingly harmful effects and that they were seemingly overprescribed, particularly to the underserved, was not a pleasant one. Active discussions are being held within virtually all major academic centers about how to address these trends. In some cases, states are taking up a call to action as well—Maryland, for example, has introduced a peer review program in which physicians will have to submit proof that the proper blood tests and physical examinations are being performed on all children taking antipsychotic medications. This text is being written in the midst of these shifts, though we are certain that psychiatry will settle on an appropriate way to use these critical medications so that those most in need get the help they deserve, while maintaining judicious use and monitoring in all patients.

BENZODIAZEPINES

The benzodiazepines (table 8-3) are widely prescribed for severe anxiety and insomnia in adults, and are used extensively in hospital settings for young people with situational anxiety and worry. They can help relax a child before an invasive procedure, for example, or ease muscle spasms associated with certain illnesses. These uses are time limited, however, so that a young child is exposed to benzodiazepines for only a matter of weeks. For chronic management of anxiety outside the hospital, these medications are probably best avoided. Benzodiazepines can be abused, and it's possible to become psychologically dependent on and even physically addicted to them. (Withdrawal symptoms in persons taking high doses of these medications can include serious problems, including seizures.) Also, their sedating effects decrease over time, and after several weeks of use, their effectiveness as tranquilizers decreases. For these reasons, benzodiazepines are best thought of as temporary measures.

ST. JOHN'S WORT

Hypericum perforatum, commonly known as St. John's wort, is one of about three hundred *Hypericum* species, shrubby perennial plants with

Table 8-3 Benzodiazepine Medications

Generic Name	Brand Name
Alprazolam	Xanax
Chlordiazepoxide	Librium
Clonazepam	Klonopin
Clorazepate	Tranxene
Diazepam	Valium
Lorazepam	Ativan

bright yellow flowers that grow in most temperate regions of the world. Teas and other extracts of St. John's wort (often simply called hypericum) have been recommended by herbalists for centuries to treat everything from insomnia to the painful viral skin infection called shingles. In the late 1980s, hypericum was investigated as a possible treatment for HIV infection, when researchers discovered that it had activity against retroviruses—activity that, unfortunately, did not translate into clinical usefulness against HIV infection. Most of the scientific work so far on hypericum has been done in Germany, where there is intense interest in herbal medicine, and where herbal preparations are more widely available and perhaps more seriously regarded as valid treatment options for major illnesses. Several studies have compared hypericum extracts with placebo and with a standard antidepressant. The results of the earlier studies were generally encouraging, suggesting that hypericum extracts had an antidepressant effect that is clinically significant in some people. A 1996 article in the *British Medical Journal,* which systematically reviewed twenty-three different studies, including a total of 1,757 patients, found that hypericum extracts "are more effective than placebo for the treatment of mild to moderately severe depressive disorders."[8] The review concluded that people taking hypericum preparations generally reported fewer and less severe side effects than those taking standard antidepressants. Hypericum is approved in Germany, and it makes up 6 percent of all prescriptions written to adolescents for depression.[9]

But much work remains to be done to better understand which groups of patients will benefit from hypericum and which should be treated with better-established agents. Problems with the design of many of the original studies (all done on adults, by the way) have made it difficult to draw conclusions about the relative effectiveness of the two approaches, hypericum versus antidepressant medication. For example, in two studies comparing hypericum with the tricyclic antidepressants imipramine[10] and amitriptyline[11] in people with depression, the prescribed doses of the antidepressants in the studies were low—so low, in fact, that they would be considered ineffective by most psychiatrists.* Another problem is that these studies often lump together people with mild depression and people with more severe depression, making it difficult to know what kind of depression hypericum is helpful for: mild depression, severe depression, or both.

One study that avoided all these problems tested St. John's wort against placebo in two hundred patients who had been rigorously evaluated and diagnosed with major depression. This study concluded that "the results do not support significant antidepressant or antianxiety effects for St. John's wort when compared to placebo in a clinical sample of depressed patients" and that "persons with major depression should not be treated with St. John's wort, given the morbidity and mortality risks of untreated or ineffectively treated major depression."[12] Thus, at present, it is difficult to recommend hypericum preparations for anyone with serious depression.

Some proponents of St. John's wort emphasize that it is a "natural" remedy and therefore inherently safer and better than "synthetic" pharmaceuticals. This argument is flawed on multiple levels. It is important to understand that herbal preparations are *not* inherently safer than or superior to chemically synthesized compounds. Toxic substances such as nicotine and strychnine are found in plants, and some of the deadliest poisons we know of, the amatoxins, occur naturally in the death cap mushroom, *Amanita phalloides*.[13] Another important point: the lower incidence of side effects of herbal preparations can often be attributed to the lower concentration of the active compounds in these preparations, an advantage that is easily duplicated by using low doses of synthetic pharmaceuticals. But natural chemicals do not necessarily have fewer side effects. We have already discussed the use of lithium for the treatment of bipolar affective disorder. Although it is a completely natural substance—in fact, one of the most ba-

---

* These studies compared effectiveness of hypericum preparations with doses of 75 mg of imipramine, a dose most psychiatrists would probably consider barely in the effective range, and 30 mg of amitriptyline, a dose that is definitely subtherapeutic for most patients.

sic in nature, an elemental salt—it can have significant side effects and can even be toxic in overdose.

Nevertheless, discovery of a pharmacologically active plant compound has often formed the basis for development of a much larger number of useful new drugs and led to other exciting discoveries. The chemical isolation of opium from the poppy plant led to the development of dozens of safer and more potent pain medications as well as to the discovery of similar compounds in the brain (called *endorphins*)—now the basis for an entire new branch of neurochemistry. As we learn more about hypericum, it may turn out that a whole new class of safer and more effective antidepressants will emerge, derived from the active compounds found in St. John's wort.

OMEGA-3 FATTY ACIDS AND FISH OIL

There are several nutrients that we must consume in our diet, albeit in small quantities, to remain healthy, compounds that our body cannot manufacture but that are nevertheless necessary for normal cellular functioning. The most familiar of these are, of course, vitamins, compounds manufactured by some plants and animals but not by humans. Their name, from the Latin word *vita*, meaning "life," indicates just how important to health they are. Unless we eat foods that contain the vitamins we need, serious illness results. Scurvy, beriberi, and pellagra are three, now thankfully unfamiliar, illnesses that result from deficiencies of, respectively, vitamin C, vitamin B_1, and niacin. All these illnesses have significant central nervous system symptoms, especially B_1 deficiency, which causes severe central nervous system degeneration.

Another group of necessary nutrients is the *essential fatty acids*, a collection of complex molecules found in some vegetables and other plant sources but in much larger amounts in most fish. Nutritionists have long touted the health benefits of diets rich in seafood, and the lower incidence of breast cancer and heart disease in the Japanese population has been attributed to a diet rich in seafood.

There is growing evidence that essential fatty acids, especially a subgroup called *omega-3 fatty acids* (table 8-4), may be useful in the treatment of mood disorders. The particular compounds thought to have the most health benefits have tongue-twisting names typical of complex organic compounds: eicosapentaenoic acid (EPA) and docosahexaenoic acid (DHA).

Table 8-4 Omega-3 Fatty Acids in Fish

High in Omega-3 Fatty Acids
(more than 1,000 mg per serving)
  Salmon
  Tuna
  Trout
  Mackerel
  Anchovies
  Sardines
  Herring
Moderate in Omega-3 Fatty Acids
(500–900 mg per serving)
  Halibut
  Rockfish
  Swordfish
  Yellowfin tuna
  Whitefish
  Smelt
  Sea bass
Low in Omega-3 Fatty Acids
(less than 500 mg per serving)
  Catfish
  Shellfish: shrimp, crab, lobster
  Cod
  Flounder
  Mahi mahi
  Sea trout
  Perch

Several preliminary studies have indicated that omega-3 fatty acids, taken as fish oil capsules, are beneficial for individuals with mood disorders. One study showed that patients who took fish oil capsules in addition to their usual treatments for bipolar disorder had fewer relapses of mood symptoms over a period of four months than patients who took placebo capsules containing olive oil.[14] All subjects in this study were adults with bipolar I or II disorder, and all were taking a number of other medications during the study. Despite these limitations, the results were exciting because they pointed to a whole new approach to the treatment of mood disorders with a new set of compounds. Other than mild gastrointestinal discomfort and a fishy aftertaste, fish oil capsules have no significant side effects.

Unlike bipolar disorder, studies on adolescent depression seem to have more mixed results. One study showed no difference between omega-3 fatty acid supplements and placebo,[15] while others showed almost unbelievably strong effects,[16] in some cases similar to SSRIs.[17]

The possible mechanism of action of omega-3 fatty acids has been described in studies, which show that these compounds are incorporated into cell membranes in association with molecules that are known to be involved in cell signaling. They seem to be active at some of the same points in cellular signaling mechanisms where lithium and valproate are thought to work. Given that valproate is, after all, a synthetic fatty acid, the idea that natural fatty acids might have benefits in mood disorders shouldn't seem strange at all.

Other circumstantial evidence has also been cited to support the importance of omega-3 fatty acids for good mental health. Archeological and epidemiological studies suggest that modern humans consume much less food rich in fatty acids than did ancient peoples, and that, compared with our ancestors, we may be deficient in these important compounds. This fact, combined with the evidence that the prevalence of depression is increasing and the age of onset of mood disorders is decreasing, has been cited as further evidence of a link between these important compounds and mental health.[18]

In most of the studies referred to above, much higher doses of fish oil were used than are generally recommended by nutritionists, who also suggest eating more fish rather than taking capsules. Whether such a high dose of omega-3 fatty acids was a necessary element in the findings of the study is not known. A study that investigated the benefits of eating more fish high in omega-3 fatty acids for preventing stroke found an incremental benefit: the more fish the research subjects incorporated into their diet, the lower their risk of stroke became.[19]

Omega-3 fatty acid therapy is at this point an unproven treatment for mood disorders, so it should not be substituted for proven treatments. One of the best uses of these compounds seems to be augmenting the efficacy of an antidepressant. In a study comparing omega-3 fatty acids to an SSRI, the combination of both was more effective than either by itself.[20] Another study found that patients with recurrent depression maintained on an SSRI had further improvements in their symptoms and fewer relapses in as few as three weeks when omega-3 fatty acids were added to their regimen.[21] Given the apparently low risk of these compounds, supplementation of standard treatments for mood disorders with fish oil capsules, under the supervision of a physician, may be an option some patients will want to explore.

EXERCISE

In recommending a certain treatment for depression, psychiatrists often compare the potential risks of a treatment with their potential benefits. We have endeavored throughout this text to take you through some of that thought process by clearly identifying what symptoms or disorders a certain treatment may be able to help (for example, an atypical antipsychotic may calm the agitation of mania) and what harm it may cause (that same antipsychotic may negatively affect certain features of metabolic functioning in the body). Weighing these risks and benefits for a particular individual is the only reasonable way to arrive at a treatment regimen. There is one treatment, however, that has recently seen a surge of positive evidence with no significant risks—exercise.

Depression can sap one of energy and of joy. Exercise understandably seems like the opposite of what a depressed person wishes to engage in. Psychiatrists see this view of exercise in nearly every depressed patient admitted to the psychiatric hospital. When suffering from depression, even getting out of bed in the morning seems like a struggle, let alone engaging in more strenuous activities. And yet, returning to the normal activities of living can be one of the most powerful and helpful additions to depression treatment. In psychotherapy, the concept of *behavioral activation* means exactly that—introducing a plan to help a depressed individual return to her life activities, such as going to work or simply completing her morning routine.

It's easy to see why this is helpful from a psychological perspective, but are there other factors at play? We know about many of the positive biological effects that exercise has on the body. Could some positive effects also be happening in the brain, to help regulate mood? Some evidence is building that exercise has a neuroprotective effect on brain tissues similar to the effects of lithium or the SSRIs and, if so, may help in depression recovery. Exercise also induces the release of all sorts of chemicals known to improve mood (in extreme cases, this can be the "runner's high" that some athletes achieve).

Analysis of the effects of exercise on depression, particularly in children, is a relatively recent development but is growing in strength. In 2001, over 2,000 British students were interviewed for depressive symptoms and level of physical activity over the course of two years.[22] It turned out that the chance of developing depression was reduced by about 8 percent for each hour of weekly physical activity. So, it seems that activity may have some preventive function against developing depression. But what about children who are already depressed? A more recent prospective study tries to answer this question. Thirty depressed adolescents not on medication were enrolled in an aerobic exercise program or passive stretching (the control group) for three months.[23] Many thought it would be difficult to encourage the adolescents to participate, but about 80 percent of both groups completed the study. At the end, not only had both groups experienced improvement in their depression (the exercise group about twice as quickly as the stretching group), but these improvements continued to hold true up to one year later, regardless of whether the adolescents continued their program. Both groups also had positive effects in other areas of their lives, including school performance and peer relationships.

In general, exercise should be considered in the treatment for any adolescent depression (for those adolescents who are simply not up to the task, even mild physical activity, such as stretching or going for walks, seems to be helpful). This is not to say that exercise can replace medications or dedicated psychotherapy, particularly for those with severe depression, but rather that it needs to be considered as complementary treatment when discussing the management of this illness in a suffering adolescent.

"MEDICAL" MARIJUANA

Some of the readers of this text will think that this section was placed in this chapter by mistake. Indeed, there will be a much more extensive discussion of marijuana in a later chapter on substance abuse. Others of you, in certain states, will know (or know of) persons who are prescribed marijuana for various psychiatric conditions, including anxiety and attention-deficit/hyperactivity disorder (ADHD). During the writing of this text, one of us moved from Maryland to California and was surprised, to say the least, to have young patients being prescribed this substance for these uses. This practice is controversial at best. There is no evidence to our awareness that marijuana has any ability to help ADHD (and in fact, it can mimic many of the symptoms). Although some patients find it relaxing, chronic marijuana use has consequences to cognitive learning and development that make it a poor choice as an antianxiety medication for use in young persons. And given this drug's potential mood-destabilizing properties in some vulnerable individuals, particularly those with mood disorders, the prescription of marijuana to adolescents is unlikely to help in the long term and can in fact be harmful.

ELECTROCONVULSIVE THERAPY

No survey of the available treatments of serious depression is complete without a discussion of electroconvulsive therapy, or ECT. A highly effective treatment for severe depression and also for both phases of bipolar disorder, ECT often provides dramatic and rapid relief of symptoms when other treatments have failed. Unfortunately, patients and their families resist this treatment because of myths and misconceptions about it. A review article titled "Half a Century of ECT Use in Young People" confirms the effectiveness of this treatment in children and adolescents, and the authors conclude that "serious complications [are] very rare."[24]

Too often, the popular media refer to ECT as "shock treatments," with all the unpleasant connotations of that term: *shock* defined as an unpleasant jolt or blow, or reminding one of the pain of an electric shock, such as the painful spark of static electricity that comes from touching a doorknob after crossing a carpeted room on a dry winter day. Calling ECT "shock treatments" is a bit like referring to modern surgery as "knife treatments"—accurate in a crude sort of way, but doing injustice to what is now a safe and effective treatment that can be literally life saving.

Although the effectiveness of ECT in mood disorders was not a completely accidental discovery, the theory originally proposed to explain its benefit has been shown to have no validity, so the development of modern ECT was a kind of happy accident nonetheless. In the early 1930s, the Hungarian physician Joseph Ladislas von Meduna proposed that there was a mutual antagonism between epilepsy and schizophrenia: patients who suffered from epilepsy did not suffer from schizophrenia, and vice versa. Modern research has shown this is not the case, but von Meduna—convinced of this idea based on his examination of the microscopic appearance of the brain of persons with the two conditions—conducted animal experiments attempting to find a way to artificially produce seizure activity. In 1935, he published a paper reporting a dramatic symptom improvement following artificially induced seizures in several patients with schizophrenia. Von Meduna used injections to produce seizures, but several years later, two Italian psychiatrists reported that seizures could be produced by briefly passing a low-voltage electrical current through the skull by means of electrodes applied to the scalp. Ugo Cerletti and Lucio Bini developed their technique in animals and then tried it on several patients with schizophrenia; they also reported remarkable success.

Although individuals with some forms of schizophrenia often did show improvement in some of their symptoms after these treatments, it quickly became apparent that severely depressed patients showed improvement that was little short of miraculous. With "electroshock" treatments, these patients had complete recovery from their symptoms within a matter of days.

One of the first articles to appear in the professional literature on ECT was a 1942 report on the treatment of two adolescents with ECT by two French psychiatrists. The following year, the same clinicians reported on a series of thirty young people with a variety of conditions who were treated with the new procedure. These physicians concluded that ECT was safe in this age group and was most effective in the treatment of "melancholia." Interest in ECT spread quickly around the globe.

Like many seemingly miraculous treatments, ECT was overprescribed at first and probably administered to many hundreds of persons whom it had little chance of helping. It's important to remember, however, that these were desperate times in psychiatry. With the discovery of antipsychotic medications nearly a decade away, and the discovery of antidepressants nearly two decades away, "little chance" of helping was better than no chance at all. Because ECT is a highly effective treatment for mania, some institutions were inclined to use it for any and all highly agitated patients, and sometimes on merely uncooperative ones. Another negative factor was that in the first decade or so after its development, ECT had serious complications. An epileptic seizure is a violent event: all the muscles of the body contract simultaneously for a few moments, sometimes with such force that broken bones result. Also, breathing stops and heart-rhythm irregularities can occur, which can even be fatal when not appropriately monitored.

The nearly indiscriminate overprescription of a therapy that had serious potential side effects led to a backlash against ECT. In the late 1960s and 1970s, although modern anesthetic techniques were making ECT safer, and more careful research was being done to determine which psychiatric disorders the treatment helped with and which it did not, the damage to ECT's reputation was already done. (The film *One Flew Over the Cuckoo's Nest*, awarded the Oscar for best movie in 1975, which depicted ECT as it would have been administered several decades earlier, certainly didn't help ECT's reputation.) State hospitals drew up regulations sharply curtailing its use, and legislation was in effect briefly in California banning the procedure. The prescription of ECT for young people was even more vigorously opposed and even banned completely in several states for various groups of children and adolescents.

Fortunately for those who can benefit from ECT, the pendulum has swung back to center. Modern ECT is safer than most surgical procedures, side effects are minimal, and indications for its use have been clarified. A 1999 survey of twenty-six individuals who had received ECT before the age of 19 reported that "the vast majority considered ECT a legitimate treatment and, if medically indicated, would have ECT again and would recommend it to others."[25] The American Academy of Child and Adolescent Psychiatry recommends ECT for certain adolescents, and notes that "despite misperceptions among the media, patients and families, and even physicians, ECT is a safe and beneficial procedure, and one with a high response rate."[26]

MODERN ECT

Electroconvulsive therapy has been greatly improved by developments in anesthetic techniques. ECT is usually done in the recovery room of the surgical suite of a hospital, the area where surgical patients are taken for observation immediately following an operation. This location is used because ECT treatment is over in about sixty seconds, and most of the "treatment" time is actually the ten minutes or so it takes for the patient to awaken from anesthesia. Some large psychiatric hospitals have their own treatment suites that are equipped like a recovery room.

Patients are usually hospitalized during a course of ECT, although increasingly, ECT is given as an outpatient procedure, just like same-day surgery. Sometimes a patient starts a course of ECT in the hospital and finishes it as an outpatient.

Electroconvulsive therapy is now done under general anesthesia just as safely as is surgery. Because each treatment lasts only a few minutes, intravenous barbiturate is used instead of the inhaled anesthetics used in most surgery. The crucial anesthetic advance for ECT was the introduction in the 1950s of agents called *muscle relaxants*, or more properly, *neuromuscular blocking agents*. These medications, also given intravenously, temporarily paralyze the patient by blocking nervous center transmission to the muscles. This prevents the violent muscle contractions during seizures that characterized early ECT.

Immediately before the treatment, a patient usually receives an injection of a medication that prevents abnormal heart rhythms, an IV is started, and the patient is put to sleep with a barbiturate and then given the muscle relaxant. The patient is asleep and completely relaxed in less than five minutes. Electrode disks similar to those used to take cardiograms are applied to the scalp. Modern ECT equipment, designed specifically for this purpose, delivers a precisely timed and measured electrical stimulus: usually a half-second to several seconds in duration. In *bilateral* treatments, an electrode is applied over each temple; in *unilateral* treatments, where the object is to stimulate only half the brain, one electrode is placed in the middle of the forehead and the other at the temple. (Unilateral treatment causes less post-ECT confusion and memory problems—side effects discussed below—and is now used almost exclusively. Occasionally, unilateral treatments don't work as well, and some patients must therefore receive bilateral treatments.)

The "seizure" in modern ECT is pretty much an electrical event only, with few or none of the jerking movements that usually characterize seizures. Most ECT machines used today also record an electroencephalogram (a measurement of the electrical activity of the brain) through the same electrodes used to deliver the stimulus, so the physician can see how long the induced "seizure" lasts—usually twenty-five to forty-five seconds.

A few brief muscle contractions might be observed during this time, but the muscle relaxant keeps the patient nearly motionless. There is usually a brief quickening of the heart rate and increase in blood pressure, which also signal that the "seizure" has occurred. The anesthetist applies a facemask breathing device to deliver oxygen to the patient until he wakes up five or ten minutes later and the treatment is over.

The only patients who absolutely can't receive ECT are those with medical conditions so severe that even ten to fifteen minutes of general anesthesia is too dangerous, for example, patients with severe cardiac or lung disease.

Typically, when the decision is made to give a course of ECT, most or even all psychiatric medications are stopped. (Sedative medications often shorten and otherwise interfere with the ECT "seizure," as do the antiepilepsy mood stabilizers. Lithium seems to make patients more prone to episodes of confusion after treatments.)

Patients awakening from anesthesia are a bit groggy, of course, and often are also slightly fuzzyheaded and feel "spacey" for another hour or so. This is probably related to the treatments themselves, not just the anesthesia, and resembles the mild postseizure confusion sometimes experienced by people with true epilepsy. Occasionally, a more severe period of confusion called delirium is seen, especially after bilateral treatments and especially toward the end of a course of treatments. Sedatives can treat this problem quickly, but when it occurs, consideration should be given to stopping the treatments or giving them less often.

The most troublesome possible side effects of ECT relate to its effect on memory; about two-thirds of patients report that ECT affects their memory in some way. The most common memory loss is for events occurring during the several weeks of the ECT treatments. Treatments are typically given three times a week, and a patient usually needs six to twelve treatments for complete recovery, so a course of ECT will last two to four weeks. Patients commonly lose memory for some events that occurred during those weeks. Some also suffer *retrograde amnesia*: memory loss for a period before they started receiving ECT. This is thought to occur because ECT somehow disrupts the process by which shorter-term memories become incorporated into longer-term memory. (If you've ever lost an hour's worth of computer work because you didn't save your work before something untoward locked up your computer, you get the idea. The short-term memories that are still in the brain's memory "buffer" seem to be lost due to ECT.) Patients who have successfully completed a course of ECT may not remember checking in to the hospital, or may not recollect a home visit or trip they took with their family during the treatments. This problem seems to be worst just after receiving ECT. In a study of forty-three patients interviewed about their memory a few weeks after completing ECT, some reported difficulty remembering events from a period of up to two years before their treatment. But when the subjects were tested again seven *months* after their treatment, these more distant memories were almost completely recovered.[27] One explanation for this finding is the known effect that severe depression has on memory. Several studies indicate that complaints of memory problems after ECT correlate better with the severity of patients' depression than with how they do on memory tests.[28] Unilateral ECT appears to sharply reduce the number of memory complaints.[29]

We should be clear about the effects of ECT on memory. Although there is an associated short-term memory loss for the period before or during ECT, many studies have shown that ECT has a *protective* effect on long-term memory. It seems to prevent the development of dementia and other conditions of long-term memory loss when patients who have received ECT reach an older age. This may be due to the remission of their depression to the ECT itself—the reason is not yet clear. What is certainly clear is that there are no negative effects of ECT on memory in the long run.

Data on the effect of ECT on memory in young people are scarcer than for adults, but one study of a group of adolescent patients who received ECT for bipolar disorder found that only 2 percent of them complained of any memory problems.[30] A more rigorous study of the longer-term effects of ECT on thinking and memory in adolescents—ten patients who had received ECT before the age of 19—involved testing learning ability and short-term memory and asking questions about their subjective sense of their memory ability. The testing was done an average of two years following the course of treatment. No differences were found in learning, short-term memory, or complaints about memory between the subjects who had received ECT and a similar group of subjects who had also been depressed but had never received ECT.[31]

The mechanism by which ECT works continues to be profoundly mysterious. During seizure activity, the neurons of the brain fire simultaneously and rhythmically, and there is a massive discharge of many neurotransmitters. We used to compare ECT to cardiac defibrillation: just as applying a current to the heart can "reset" abnormal rhythms in cardiac muscle, perhaps ECT "resets" rhythmic discharges in the brain in some way. But newer work seems to indicate that, as with other treatments for bipolar disorder, the effect occurs at the level of the individual neurons. Animal experimentation indicates that ECT, like lithium, affects G proteins within the neurons. It may be that ECT, like lithium, works on the neuronal "tuning" mechanisms: the G protein–second messenger system discussed in chapter 5.

PRESCRIPTION OF ECT FOR ADOLESCENTS

Electroconvulsive therapy is perhaps the most effective treatment there is for severe depression and severe mania and often works more quickly than medications. Naturally, it should be a treatment consideration whenever a person continues to be severely depressed despite antidepressant medication treatment. It is *rapidly* effective: many patients have dramatic improvements after three or four treatments, that is, after five to seven days. Severely suicidal individuals, or those who have stopped eating and drinking and are in danger of malnutrition and dehydration—any patients for whom profound depression has become an imminently life-threatening illness—are candidates for ECT. For these individuals, the effectiveness of ECT can seem truly miraculous, as this account shows:

> On February 10, 1977, electroconvulsive treatment was administered for the first time to a 16-year-old female who had not eaten, spoken or walked unaided for the past four months... The first treatment produced an unclenching of the fists... The second treatment produced consumption of small amount of fluids... The fifth was productive of eating and talking normally... She was allowed to go home two days after the [seventh] treatment and for the past three months has been getting along nicely and doing all things previously done in a satisfactory fashion.[32]

Electroconvulsive therapy is also a highly effective treatment for mania. A review in the *American Journal of Psychiatry* of fifty years' experience of the use of ECT for treating mania found that it provided complete symptom remission or marked improvement in 80 percent of the manic patients studied. Many of the patients in these studies had failed to respond to many other available treatments—making this success rate all the more impressive.[33] ECT seems to work more quickly in mania than in depression. One study found that patients with mania recovered after an average of six treatments, about half the usual requirement for the treatment of depression.[34] Severely manic patients whose highly agitated state becomes physically dangerous are obvious candidates for ECT.

Although ECT can quickly interrupt an episode of depression or mania, the effect of the treatment doesn't usually last more than several months. Thus, medication treatment will still be necessary to sustain the benefit of ECT and keep the patient's mood state stable after the treatments are finished. Some experts are now recommending that medication be started before the treatments are finished. Depressed patients with bipolar disorder who receive ECT can become slightly hypomanic. Obviously, it's time to stop the treatments when this occurs. Unlike antidepressants, however, ECT does not seem to increase the cycling of the illness.[35]

A survey of adolescents who had received ECT and of their parents illustrates how difficult and frightening it is for parents to give consent for ECT for their children. Most of the parents volunteered, even before being asked by the researchers, that the decision was very difficult and the prospect of the treatment frightening at the time they were asked to agree to it for their child. The use of electricity and the induction of seizures was the scariest part for them. But once the treatments were over, attitudes about them were positive. All the parents (and the adolescents too) said they thought ECT had been a helpful treatment that should be available to treat severe depression in young people.[36]

Your child's psychiatrist should be up to date on the most recent recommendations regarding use of ECT in children and adolescents. The American Academy of Child and Adolescent Psychiatry recommends the treatment "when there is a lack of response to two or more trials of [medication] or when the severity of symptoms precludes waiting for a response to pharmacological treatment." That said, each of us has had many experiences of patients for whom ECT was not only effective but life saving.

OTHER NEW TREATMENTS

TRANSCRANIAL STIMULATION

Repetitive transcranial magnetic stimulation (TMS, or sometimes rTMS) is a new therapeutic technique similar to ECT that has been shown to be effective in treating mood disorders, with several devices receiving FDA approval for treating adults with depression. TMS is still in the early phase of research with adolescents, but preliminary results are encouraging, particularly when TMS is used as an adjunctive treatment for patients for whom antidepressants help but are not fully effective.[37] The great advantage of TMS over ECT is that TMS is much simpler to administer: no seizure activity is induced by the treatment, and therefore no anesthesia is necessary.

This technique takes advantage of a principle of electromagnetism called *induction* (in which a magnetic field induces an electrical current in a nearby conductor) to deliver an electrical stimulus to the brain without applying electrical energy to the scalp (as in ECT). During TMS treatments, a magnetic coil is held against the scalp, and the magnetic field that develops in the coil causes electrical current to flow through nearby neurons under the skull (figure 8-1). No electricity passes through the skull as in ECT, only magnetic waves. Because the electrical current that is generated in the brain tissue by TMS is so small, a seizure does not occur—which is why no anesthesia is necessary. Pulses of magnetic energy are delivered over a period of about twenty minutes while the patient simply sits in a chair. The patient is awake and alert through the whole procedure. Other than some soreness from muscle stimulation, there appear to be no side effects of any kind.[38]

Transcranial magnetic stimulation has been used for a number of years to do brain mapping. Mapping of the motor areas of the brain involves stimulating a brain area and measuring for electrical activity in muscles controlled by that area. Stimulating sensory areas of the brain can cause a person to feel tingling in the part of the body that sends sensory messages to that brain area. Sophisticated TMS techniques are also being used to study language functions, as well as the organization of complex movements.

It is possible to give a placebo TMS treatment, allowing valid research on the efficacy of TMS in depression. When the TMS coil is applied to the

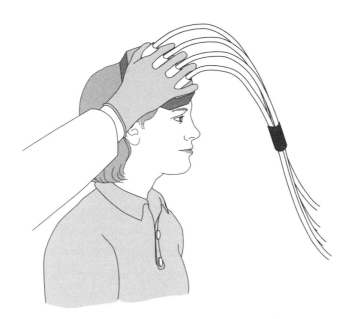

Figure 8-1 Transcranial magnetic stimulation

scalp at a slightly different angle from that used to give treatments, it does not cause electrical current to flow through the brain tissue and thus will not have the usual TMS effect. Because the muscles are still stimulated, the slight muscle soreness associated with the treatment still occurs, and research subjects have no way of knowing whether they are getting a sham treatment or the real thing. This makes the all-important double-blind placebo-controlled studies fairly easy to do.

Several studies indicate that the brain areas known as the left prefrontal lobes are less active than normal in depression. This finding has led researchers to try TMS treatments on depressed patients by stimulating the left prefrontal lobes. Early results have been very promising. In one of the first studies on TMS in the treatment of depression, twelve patients received twenty TMS stimulations of two seconds each over a period of twenty minutes every weekday for two weeks.[39] Either before or after the two weeks of therapy, the subjects were given two weeks of sham treatments (the placebo), during which the TMS coil was held at an angle that would not cause brain tissue stimulation. The patients were tested for depressive symptoms by trained investigators using a standardized questionnaire. Neither the subject nor the investigator giving the mood questionnaire knew whether the patient was receiving real or sham TMS (making the study double blind). The study found statistically significant mood improvement after TMS treatments but not after the sham treatments. Several patients continued TMS after the completion of the study and experienced even further clinical improvement in their depressive symptoms. Another study found similar results in a group that included some individuals with bipolar disorder.[40] In several studies, patients with drug-resistant depression showed improvement after TMS.[41]

Transcranial magnetic stimulation is in its infancy. All indications are that it will be safe, but its efficacy remains untested in the young. The strength of the magnetic stimulation that is most beneficial, the exact placement of the coil, the number of treatments, and the duration of therapy are all under investigation at various centers around the world. Will TMS, like ECT, be effective in bipolar depression as well as in unipolar depression? How about in mania? These and many other questions remain to be answered. Perhaps the biggest unanswered question is, How does TMS work? It has always been thought that the seizure is the necessary therapeutic factor in ECT. Does TMS work in a different way? Or is it some kind of "gentler" ECT that works by a similar mechanism but without causing a seizure? (If the TMS coil is made to generate a strong enough magnetic field, a seizure can indeed be triggered with this technique, perhaps supporting the latter explanation.) As with so much of the science of psychiatry, these questions remain unanswered. What is known, however, is that this safe, effective treatment is more and more available and may find a home in helping treatment-resistant adolescent depression when medications don't seem to be enough.

VAGAL NERVE STIMULATION

Vagal nerve stimulation (VNS), another experimental approach for severe treatment-resistant depression, is also currently under investigation. Because it is sometimes discussed in the media, a brief description is in order. The vagal nerve (or *vagus*) is a long nerve that emerges from the base of the human brain and travels down the neck and into the chest and abdomen; it regulates several vital bodily functions, such as digestion and heart rate. Its connections in the brain are through important centers thought to be involved in emotional regulation, specifically mood regulation. VNS is done by means of a pacemaker-like device that must be surgically implanted to deliver the tiny electrical signals that stimulate the vagus.

Animal studies done as early as the 1930s demonstrated that electrical stimulation of the vagal nerve produced changes in the electrical activity of the brain. In the 1980s, it was demonstrated that VNS could control epileptic seizures in dogs. By the 1990s, VNS had become available for the treatment of intractable epilepsy in humans, first in Europe and then in the United States. And by the end of 2000, about six thousand patients worldwide had received VNS, almost all of them for the treatment of epilepsy. As with antiepilepsy medications that later turned out to be effective mood stabilizers, VNS was noted to have beneficial effects on mood in several of the patients who received it to treat their seizures. Several epilepsy patients had substantial antidepressant effects from VNS, even though the treatment didn't improve their seizure control.

In one of the first studies of VNS treatment in depression, thirty adults received VNS for severe, treatment-resistant depression; some of these patients had taken up to five different medications and received ECT, with little benefit. About half of the patients benefited from VNS.[42] This is still an experimental treatment, and as of this writing, there are no reports of its use in young people for depression, though it has been used extensively to combat seizures in all ages and has been fairly safe. Given the invasive nature of placing the device, VNS is not likely to find a place in treating depression in a younger age group for some time, if ever.

Counseling and Psychotherapy

Medical treatments such as pharmaceuticals often form the foundation of the treatment of serious mood disorders, but counseling and psychotherapy are important, perhaps indispensable, additional therapeutic interventions for these illnesses. Parents are often interested to know the answers to two very different questions about the treatment of depression with counseling and psychotherapy: first, whether this form of treatment is *necessary,* and second, whether it is *sufficient.* Put another way, these questions become "If medications are going to make the depression better, why bother with psychotherapy?" and "Is it possible that psychotherapy alone will successfully treat depression and make medication treatment unnecessary?" We hope to persuade you that the "medication *versus* therapy" perspective is not a good way to think about the treatment of depression.

THE "BIOLOGY-PSYCHOLOGY" SPLIT IN PSYCHIATRY

In the early twentieth century, after the discovery of the biological causes of mental illnesses such as general paresis (central nervous system syphilis) and cretinism (mental retardation due to thyroid deficiency), psychiatric illnesses were divided into two categories: *organic* and *functional.* Organic psychiatric illnesses were "real" illnesses, caused by germs, or abnormal hormone levels, or something else that could be seen under a microscope or measured in a blood test. In functional illnesses, on the other hand, it was assumed that nothing was wrong with brain functioning, at least not in a physical sense. Patients with severe depression, manic-depressive illness, and even schizophrenia were having some kind of abnormal reaction to life events.

The question then became, Why do some people have these abnormal kinds of reactions while others do not? It was at this point that the attempt to understand and treat these illnesses turned away from medicine and toward psychology. Sigmund Freud spent his lifetime treating and trying to understand people who were unhappy in their relationships, disappointed in themselves for choices they had made, perhaps confused and anxious about life decisions they were facing. Freud and his followers developed a large and sophisticated system of understanding human behavior based on understanding childhood development. They developed the "talking treatment" for psychiatric problems: psychotherapy. This basically consisted of helping patients understand themselves better: let go of grudges, resentments, and fears triggered by traumatic experiences and learn better, more mature coping mechanisms. This approach has come to be called *dynamic* psychology or psychiatry and is based on the belief that mental life is best understood as a dynamic interplay between emotions and intellect, present circumstances and unconscious memories of past experiences, and many other psychological factors.

Although this approach was extremely successful in helping people with a wide variety of problems and symptoms, practitioners of dynamic psychotherapy soon discovered that it didn't make much of an impact on the symptoms of persons with major psychiatric illnesses such as schizophrenia or bipolar disorder. The explanation given was that these individuals were too disturbed or too immature or that their families were too dysfunctional for patients to benefit from therapy. Then a revolution occurred: imipramine, lithium, chlorpromazine, and other effective medications for "functional" illnesses were developed. Persons with depressive disorders, bipolar disorders, and schizophrenia, along with their families, started leaving the therapists who often seemed to be blaming them for their illnesses for a new kind of doctor: the biological psychiatrist, the pharmacotherapist, someone who would treat them for a "real" illness.

For a time there was a kind of schism in American psychiatry between those who believed that dynamic psychology best explained mental illnesses and those who believed that biology was the key that would unlock the mysteries of psychiatric disorders.

In the mid-1970s, this biological psychiatry–dynamic psychiatry split was in full swing. Many departments of psychiatry in university medical centers proudly identified themselves as either "biological" or "psychodynamic" in their approach. Usually each camp denigrated the other: psychodynamic psychiatry was "touchy-feely" soft science based more on nineteenth-century literary theory than medicine; biological psychiatrists were "pill pushers" who didn't even talk to their patients and had no appreciation for the human experience.

But a few departments of psychiatry taught their students and resident physicians that mental experiences were not just a series of chemical reactions or simply a collection of dynamically interrelated thoughts and feelings, but both. People with mood disorders are still people, still subject to disappointments and loss and relationship problems and blows to their self-esteem. To see their moods as just the expression of so many chemicals to be fine-tuned with more chemicals was to do them a great disservice. This schism has now healed for the most part, and even the most ardent biological psychiatrists understand that a psychodynamic understanding of the patient is *always* important.

Although there is certainly a place for dynamic psychotherapy in modern psychiatry—*including* traditional Freudian psychoanalysis and the psychoanalytic couch—the variety of available psychological treatments has broadened tremendously in the past twenty-five years or so. Sophisticated techniques have been developed that work for particular kinds of problems. Some involve individual sessions with a therapist, others a group setting. Some are focused on a particular problem, such as family problems; some are symptom-focused, such as on depression or panic attacks; some are designed to last only a few sessions, while others are more open ended. Some are not therapy in the traditional sense at all but are support groups made up of individuals who offer guidance and support to each other and don't even include a "therapist." Research is also being done to determine which psychological treatments work best for which problems. The prescription of a certain kind of counseling or therapy for a particular kind of problem is often backed up by as much research as the prescription of a particular medication.

IS PSYCHOTHERAPY ALONE SUFFICIENT?

A number of reasonably well-designed clinical studies show that some forms of psychotherapy are by themselves effective treatments for many cases of adolescent depression. It's difficult, however, to decide from these studies which cases of adolescent depression can be successfully treated with psychotherapy alone. It seems clear from this work that psychotherapy alone is *not* effective for the treatment of *severe* depression.

Some studies showing that psychotherapy is successful in treating adolescents with depression have recruited their research subjects from schools by means of screening questionnaires that identified students with symptoms of depression. Often, comparisons are made between a group of adolescents who receive treatment and a group who are put on a waiting list, that is, those receiving no treatment at all. Given that it would be unethical to identify individuals with a serious medical problem and then not get them into treatment quickly, we can assume that the adolescents in many of these studies were, by and large, not severely depressed.

Some studies have actually excluded severely depressed adolescents right up front. A 1996 study titled "A Controlled Trial of Brief Cognitive-Behavioral Intervention in Adolescent Patients with Depressive Disorders" (*cognitive-behavioral* therapy is a specific type of psychotherapy that we discuss later in this chapter) found that psychotherapy had a "clear advantage" in a group of depressed adolescents.[1] In this study, research subjects were chosen from individuals applying to an outpatient clinic specializing in adolescent depression. Although this would suggest that a group of more seriously depressed young people was being studied, a closer reading of this paper reveals that any adolescent "taking or likely to require antidepressant medications" was excluded from the study. Almost always, studies of children and adolescents exclude severe symptoms (psychosis, suicidality), which are usually associated with more severe depressive episodes.

Rather than focusing entirely on which patients psychotherapy can help, several studies of the treatment of adolescent depression with psychotherapy have tried to figure out why this treatment *doesn't* help some patients. One such study attempted to compare the efficacy of several different types of therapy in 12- to 18-year-olds with major depression.[2] It found that therapy was not very helpful for 21 percent of the adolescents who had been recruited into the study. These subjects had chronic depressive symptoms during 80 percent of the time the study was conducted—over a period of about two years. (This study had already eliminated more difficult to treat and severely ill patients by excluding adolescents with bipolar disorder, substance abuse, and other complicating factors.) The researchers reported that the subjects who did not respond to psychotherapy treatment had been assessed at the beginning of the study as being more severely depressed.

A study titled "Which Depressed Patients Respond to Cognitive-Behavioral Treatment?" also found that the nonresponders were the subjects who were more depressed at the beginning of the study.[3] This study also measured "impairment" in the subjects at the beginning of the treatment and found that adolescents who were having more trouble functioning in school and at home were less likely to benefit from psychotherapy. Perhaps the most interesting finding was that no particular pattern of individual symptoms predicted which subjects would benefit—that is, there weren't any "red flag" symptoms that seemed to predict that psychotherapy wouldn't work, symptoms such as suicidal thinking or significant weight loss. Subjects who had more symptoms and were functioning poorly didn't do as well with psychotherapy as did subjects with fewer symptoms who were functioning more normally. (This study had already excluded adolescents who were taking antidepressant medications.)

These studies would seem to indicate that psychotherapy alone can be sufficient to treat adolescents with less severe depression—but just what *less severe* is has not been defined very well. Clinical judgment and experience are still the requirements for successfully prescribing treatments for depression, whether medication or psychotherapy.

An important last note to add is that psychotherapy alone is *never* sufficient to adequately treat bipolar disorder. Adolescents with bipolar disorder are uniformly excluded from such studies, and a large clinical literature on adults with bipolar disorders indicates that medication must always be their primary treatment.

IS PSYCHOTHERAPY ALWAYS NECESSARY?

The related question of whether psychotherapy is always required for treating depressed adolescents is also an important one to try to answer. If medication is the more effective treatment for severe depression, why bother with time-consuming and expensive psychotherapy treatment? The TADS trial, which we spoke about in discussing SSRI treatments, looked at this question.[4] One of the major findings in the study was that regardless of the origin of the depression (whether a biological major depressive disorder or a more moderate low mood due to life circumstances), psychotherapy was helpful. This was true both for the group taking medications and for the group taking a placebo. The combination of medications and psychotherapy was the most effective intervention in the study, possibly suggesting that psychotherapy should always be considered in the treatment of depression.

One of the problems with doing this kind of research, and in making any specific recommendations, is that the term *psychotherapy* can cover a lot of territory. It might be helpful to stop for a moment and explore exactly what *psychotherapy* means. Dr. Jerome Frank, who spent his career researching the techniques and effectiveness of psychotherapy, defines it as any technique that attempts "to heal through persuasion" and characterizes the process as one of "employing measures to restore self-confidence and help [the patient] find more effective ways of mastering his problems." Frank emphasizes that psychotherapy works insofar as it can "clarify . . . symptoms and problems, inspire hopes, provide [the patient] with experiences of success or mastery, and stir him emotionally."[5]

Psychotherapy, then, is not just giving advice and encouragement (though these are certainly important constituents of the process); it also helps people to make sense of their negative feelings, understand the source of these feelings, and make the changes necessary to relieve them. Part education and part inspiration, psychotherapy tries to help the patient step outside herself and see her situation objectively, in order to identify changes in thinking and behavior that will make things better for her. Frank's research indicates that a crucial ingredient is the ability of the therapist to persuade the patient that things *can* get better.

MATCHING THE PSYCHOTHERAPY TO THE PATIENT

Different therapists use different theories to help their patients make sense of their situations. Freud and his followers emphasized a person's early childhood experiences as the most important issues, and other theories after Freud have focused on communication, changing thinking patterns, or family dynamics. The healing power of psychotherapy depends on the patient's being able to make use of new ways of thinking about his situation. This means that the type of therapy needs to be matched to the patient's problems and to his way of looking at them. This is important because each family of psychotherapy takes a different view regarding most aspects of how to make this improvement happen and places different demands on the patient, the therapist, and the systems surrounding both. We'd like to briefly discuss each broad type of therapy so that you and your family can have some concept of which type might be helpful to your situation and understand what you can expect when beginning a psychotherapeutic journey.

COGNITIVE-BEHAVIORAL THERAPY

In the 1960s, Dr. Aaron Beck and his colleagues developed a theory of depression, and a psychotherapeutic treatment, called *cognitive therapy.*[6] This type of psychotherapy has been researched more thoroughly than most others and has a proven track record in helping with symptoms of depression; in some studies, it has been found to work as well as, or even better than, antidepressant medication for some patients.[7]

The theory of cognitive therapy maintains that people who are chronically or frequently depressed have developed a distorted view of themselves and of the world and have adopted certain patterns of thinking and reacting that perpetuate their problems. This emphasis on thinking, or *cognition,* lends the theory and the therapy their name. Research has shown that depressed adolescents tend to (1) think negatively about themselves, (2) interpret their experiences in a negative way, and (3) have a pessimistic view of the future. Cognitive theory calls this the *cognitive triad.*[8]

The theory further proposes that all this negative thinking causes a person to develop a repertoire of mental habits called *schemas,* or *negative automatic thoughts,* that spring into action and reinforce the negative thinking.

▼ John was a 17-year-old high school junior whose application to enroll in a summer creative-writing seminar at the local university had just been turned down. He came to his therapy session and brought along a lengthy critique of the short story he had included with his application, a critique handwritten by the seminar's director, a well-known local author.

"You see, I should have known better than to apply for this seminar. Phillip Preston, no less, gives me the bad news. Now I'm never going to be a writer."

"Why do you say that?" I asked.

"If someone like Preston thinks I can't write, I might as well give up. That's the last time I bother trying something I'm not cut out for."

"Did he say he thought you couldn't write?"

"Well, no, of course not."

"I see; this famous author and writing teacher doesn't tell his students what he thinks?"

"Well, no. That's not true. In fact, he's got a reputation for coming right out with his opinions to his students. He's supposed to be really tough but honest."

"But he treats you differently from everyone else?"

John began to get a little annoyed. "Well, I wouldn't think so, but how should I know? I've never met the guy."

"What do you make of the fact that Professor Preston wrote to you himself?"

"Well, I did think it was unusual. My friend Ann just got a form letter with her rejection."

"Could it mean he was impressed with some aspects of your writing and wanted to encourage you?"

"He said the story was, quote-unquote, 'promising,'" John said a little sarcastically. "But I figured he was just being nice to a dumb kid."

"So, Professor Preston doesn't mean what he says?"

"But his comments were really negative," John went on glumly. "He went through the whole story, the plot line, the characters, everything, and shot them down one by one."

I continued to reinterpret John's negative take on everything: "He must have spent several hours with your story if he gave you back such a carefully detailed critique. Don't you think?"

"Yeah, I guess he wouldn't have taken all that time and trouble if he thought it was completely worthless. He told me to apply again next year, but—"

"But he was just being nice?"

John was quiet and seemed to be thinking hard.

I went on, "Didn't you tell me that juniors aren't usually accepted into this seminar?"

"Right," John said. "Mrs. Robinson had told me not to get my hopes up, that she'd never had a junior get accepted."

"So, this wasn't really such a surprise for either of you."

"Well, actually she seemed surprised. 'I thought you would be my first junior to get accepted,' she said when I told her."

"But, she didn't mean it? Just being nice?"

John frowned.

"What did your Mrs. Robinson say when you showed her Preston's note."

"Well, I didn't show it to her. She told me to come by her office to discuss some of my other stories and applying next year, but I haven't yet."

"Because?"

John stopped talking and just the smallest hint of a smile appeared at the corners of his mouth. I went on, "Because Mrs. Robinson is being encouraging to you just to be nice?"

John nodded sheepishly. Then he asked, "Are you saying there's a pattern here?"

"What do you think?" I asked.

"You guys," he said, definitely smiling now. "You always answer a question with another question. Do they teach you that in therapist school?"

I couldn't resist: "What do *you* think?" ▲

John is down on his talents and assumes everybody else is, too. In situations that can be interpreted in many different ways, both positive and negative, he tends to go for the negative rather than seek alternative, positive explanations. When something positive happens or is said to him, he ignores it or explains it away somehow (called *negative attributions*). This, in turn, causes him to do things that reinforce his negative thinking (like missing out on the support and encouragement his teacher obviously wants to give him when he comes to her office), and the vicious cycle repeats itself.

Cognitive-behavioral therapy (CBT) is an active form of therapy. Patients are asked to monitor and record their thinking and behavior patterns. There is an emphasis on diary keeping, and "homework" is often assigned. The therapist challenges the cognitive distortions and helps patients identify automatic negative thoughts and reinterpret events more positively. There is an emphasis on the here and now, not on the past, and patients are taught to modify behaviors and ways of thinking about themselves and what happens to them (a process called *cognitive restructuring*). Many patients and families like this type of therapy because it tends to help more quickly than other types, and how it works is transparent and clearly explained. Also, it establishes concrete, structured ways to help in various situations, including emergencies.

Cognitive-behavioral therapy is the best-studied type of psychotherapy for the treatment of depression in young people, and it has been proved effective in the treatment of less severe depression.

INTERPERSONAL PSYCHOTHERAPY

Interpersonal psychotherapy (IPT) is based on the premise that depression is best understood in the context of personal connections, and that regardless of its underlying causes, depression is always inextricably intertwined with the adolescent's interpersonal relationships. IPT does not assume that relationship problems *cause* depression, but it is thought that addressing relationship problems can alleviate depressive symptoms, regardless of the individual psychological or even biological contributions to depression. Originally developed to treat depression in adults, this type of therapy has been adapted for adolescents to focus better on the relationship issues common in this age group. IPT helps the adolescent deal with problematic or unsatisfying relationships and attempts to restructure relationships to make them more fulfilling.

Like cognitive-behavioral therapy, IPT is an active type of psychotherapy and focuses on the here and now, principally on enhancing communication in the adolescent's important relationships: with parents and peers and in dating relationships. IPT tries to help the adolescent learn a more open communication style and become better at listening to others. The therapist tries to help the adolescent become aware of his need to develop adultlike expectations of himself and an increased understanding of his parents' point of view. IPT works to clarify role expectations and to address role disputes and transitions. By enhancing relationships and problem-solving skills, IPT helps strengthen the adolescent's peer and family relationships, providing an enhanced support system that he can turn to when negative things happen. It is thought that this helps the adolescent become more resilient and less likely to become depressed in the future. According to some literature, this type of therapy may be particularly suited to adolescents embedded in a cultural system that values strong family and social ties.[9]

In a study of 12- to 18-year-olds treated for depression with IPT for twelve weeks, patients reported a significant decrease in depressive symptoms and an improvement in their overall social functioning and functioning with friends and in dating relationships. They also reported improvement in their ability to think of alternative solutions to problems, to try them out, and then to use them to address difficulties.[10]

FAMILY THERAPY

There are many definitions of family therapy, but all types involve face-to-face work with multiple family members to focus on the interactions and dynamics of family relationships. This differs from interpersonal psychotherapy in a number of ways. First of all, the adolescent is no longer the single identified patient. Rather, the family as a unit is the "patient," and the goal is to help the family as a whole by working with each of its individual members equally. As such, all identified persons in the family are expected to attend the therapy sessions and work equally hard at making and sustaining positive change. In effective family therapy, this can mean a drastic increase in progress, because many people are working hard to improve the relationships, not just one. It can be a useful frame for an adolescent who is reluctant to enter therapy for fear that she will be identified as the "broken" one in need of "fixing." The family therapy approach may also be helpful when other clear sources of stress (between parents, or between siblings) are clearly affecting the adolescent. And, of course, parents who have their own history of depression may find this type of therapy particularly attractive, as it allows a more open discussion, and a deeper bonding, between themselves and their children over this common experience in a safe way.

The goal of family therapy for depressed adolescents is to decrease depressive symptoms and improve the adolescent's level of functioning by identifying and changing problems in the interactions within the family that may be responsible for initiating or exacerbating depression. As with interpersonal psychotherapy, there is less concern with the cause or causes of the depression than with current negative relationships among family members.

A depressed adolescent typically isolates herself from family members, and the irritability and disruptive behaviors that are often part of the picture of adolescent depression can poison family life. Situational stressors can cause a depressed adolescent to withdraw from family life and to rebuff parental expressions of concern that her depressive behaviors elicit. This rejection of parents' attempts to comfort and be helpful frustrates parents in turn, and they can then become angry and critical. This makes the adolescent more angry, guilty, and depressed. A vicious cycle of blame and hostility can start that becomes self-sustaining and difficult to interrupt.

Family therapy tries to help the family reestablish constructive relationships by decreasing adolescent isolation and parental criticism and bolstering family cohesion. The therapist attempts to stimulate reattachment within the family by increasing trust and desire for parental love and support in the adolescent and by helping parents reestablish themselves in their roles as empathetic caregivers.

Often the therapist will attempt to reframe depression-related behavioral problems as symptomatic problems in family relationships rather than problems that emanate only from the depressed adolescent. This may involve understanding depressive behaviors as actually fulfilling a positive function within the family. (Mom and Dad are having problems in their relationship; Johnny is acting up because he thinks a crisis will bring the family closer together.) This often has the effect of absolving blame and shifting the family's focus from "whose fault is this?" to "how do we work together to make things better?"

Family therapists encourage all family members to get their feelings out in the open in constructive ways and to improve interpersonal communications. The therapist helps the family negotiate practical family issues such as curfew, chores, and dating, balancing the need for parental authority with the adolescent's need for increasing autonomy.

Because family therapy is so wide ranging and individualized to each family situation, it has been difficult to research its effectiveness. Many studies have indicated, however, that family stresses and tensions predict relapse of depressive illnesses in adolescents. This suggests that family therapy is important when these kinds of tensions exist within the adolescent's family. Recent evidence seems to suggest that this approach can reduce depressive symptoms, even suicidal ideation, in depressed adolescents as effectively as many other therapies described in this chapter.

INSIGHT-ORIENTED PSYCHOTHERAPY

Insight-oriented psychotherapy (or *dynamic psychotherapy*) consists of individual meetings with a therapist, usually over an extended period (months or even years), in which the person in treatment discusses her past and present experiences and feelings with a goal of better self-understanding, acceptance, and personal growth. Disappointments and accomplishments, affections and enmities, fears, inspirations, passions, and worries—all are, as psychotherapists are fond of saying, "grist for the mill" of therapy. Patient and therapist will, of course, talk about such symptoms as sadness and anxiety as well, but insight-oriented psychotherapy tries to understand symptoms as signals that indicate underlying conflicts rather than as the focus of treatment in and of themselves. This more traditional type of psychotherapy emphasizes exploration of the *meaning* of symptoms and the development of self-awareness and maturity.

This type of therapy is different from most of those listed above as the therapist aims to be "nondirective." That is, psychodynamic psychotherapists never tell a patient to do anything—no homework, no assignments. Many times, therapists will even resist interpreting particular interactions, as the goal is to help patients reach their own understanding of situations without therapists muddying the waters by inserting their own opinions. The thinking behind the therapy itself, that deeper understanding on the part of the patient will naturally lead to change in behavior and attitudes, is one of the reasons that it takes such a long time, but this form of therapy is described by patients as incredibly powerful and empowering, as patients reach most of the insights seemingly on their own (though the careful, subtle guidance employed by the therapist is precisely what makes this one of the most difficult therapies to master). More mature adolescents who have good communication skills, who are capable of the introspection and self-reflection that this type of treatment requires, and who are motivated to understand themselves better are more likely to benefit from insight-oriented therapy. It also tends to be more effective for patients who can maintain a relationship, who are comfortable discussing emotions, and who are not inclined to have continual crises.

Dealing with psychological traumas and setbacks—past and present—that cause understandable feelings of sadness or anger or anxiety is a focus of insight-oriented psychotherapy, as are thinking patterns, self-attitudes, and interpersonal styles that disrupt a person's ability to be happy in relationships, effective in school or work, carefree in play, and confident about making decisions about the future. The complexity and subtlety of this kind of therapy is why psychotherapists often study and train in their profession for almost as many years as physicians do in theirs and why people are sometimes in therapy for months, even years, at a time. It is also why this kind of psychotherapy is such an intense, powerful experience and the therapeutic relationship between patient and therapist so unique.

Insight-oriented psychotherapy is often referred to as "open ended" and can continue as long as the patient continues to feel that she is benefiting from it. The goals of treatment are individual and can be quite far ranging. For these reasons, efficacy research on this type of treatment has been nearly impossible to do. That said, recent studies have attempted to compare insight-oriented psychotherapy to more modern techniques, such as cognitive-behavioral therapy. The results have been mixed. Some studies show the insight-oriented approach to be superior, some inferior, though most show it to be equivalent to CBT for the treatment of depression. It really is a matter of you and your child discussing treatment options with your child's psychiatrist and matching the type of therapy with your child's particular strengths and interests.

GROUP PSYCHOTHERAPY

Group therapy can be particularly helpful for adolescents, because they are often much more willing to talk about their feelings and difficulties to peers than to adults. Feedback and observations may have a much more powerful effect on an adolescent if coming from peers rather than from an adult therapist. In a group, young people can model and practice social skills and benefit from companionship and mutual support of others their age.

The therapist usually encourages group members to problem solve for each other and give feedback and support to one another. Group members are helped to better recognize feelings in themselves and in others, are coached on social problem solving, and are taught how to negotiate to resolve conflicts.

Group therapy is usually an adjunctive treatment to another type of psychotherapy rather than the sole treatment for depression, often to address a particular problem such as poor social skills. Substance-abuse treatment is frequently done in a group setting, where modeling of behaviors and roleplaying exercises are helpful for the adolescent to begin developing a substance-free coping and lifestyle. Group therapy helps teenagers see that others their own age have similar problems (sometimes *worse* problems) and helps them experience firsthand how peers successfully or unsuccessfully go about dealing with difficulties and setbacks. Some of the most robust evidence, ironically, relates to helping those adolescents with social anxiety—those least likely to want to participate in groups! Practicing interactions with other young persons in a nonthreatening environment tends to make these individuals more comfortable in other settings as well. Consequently, this treatment may also be good for depressed adolescents who seem to be especially asocial.

DIALECTICAL BEHAVIORAL THERAPY

In 1987, Marsha Linehan, a professor and practicing psychologist at the University of Washington, published a paper in which she outlined an adaptation of the principles of cognitive-behavioral therapy for individuals with particular problems.[11] A certain subgroup of patients, many with diagnosed mood disorders, had a difficult collection of characteristics. They seemed more irritable than sad, though they certainly had both facets; they frequently sought out, then rejected, help and authority; they sometimes had suicidal thoughts, and some responded to these thoughts with risky behaviors; they could be socially isolated; they frequently did not want to go to therapy or treatment, and had difficulty staying in therapy once started, as they rejected the idea that anything was "wrong" with them. To the attentive reader, this seems strikingly similar to our earlier descriptions of the depressed adolescent. Therefore, although this type of therapy was initially created to treat a related though separate entity (called borderline personality disorder), it will be discussed here as it can frequently be helpful in major depression in young people.

Dr. Linehan believed that cognitive-behavioral therapy had many strengths as a modality. It was concrete and easy to follow, focused on positive change, and was rapidly effective. What she did not like, however, was that some patients seemed to find it rather punitive and invalidating. For some depressed persons who are already more likely to perceive their situations and surroundings as negative, going to a therapist weekly who (kindly, but distinctly) tells you a litany of everything you are doing wrong and what you need to change can leave them feeling invalidated. Dr. Linehan noticed in her research that the rate of persons who started but prematurely terminated therapy was relatively high for CBT, and she thought she might understand why. She set out to rebalance CBT to be both validating and focused on improvement. By validating the intense struggles of the depressed person to do even the most basic of activities, while providing the skills to take on more and more challenges, a therapist can help a patient feel understood and motivated to take on the challenge of the cognitive-behavioral technique. These dialectical dilemmas are at the core of dialectical behavioral therapy (DBT) and its principles. (In a dialectic, two opposing viewpoints are resolved into a higher truth in which both are accurate—for example, "I'm doing the best I can *and* I have to change and do better.")

Like CBT, the DBT treatment itself focuses on challenging cognitions and helping the person learn skills to improve himself and his situation. It also incorporates additional domains beyond CBT, including mindfulness and distress tolerance, all aimed at helping a person accept his current circumstances without reacting emotionally. All of us have probably said things we later regretted in the heat of the moment, usually in an argument. A person struck with an irritable temperament due to depression may be even more likely to do so, setting him up for further rejection from his loved ones, deepening his sense of sadness and loneliness. DBT teaches specific concrete skills to use in just such a situation, linking the base emotional state of "I'm really mad right now and he has no right to say that to me" to the intellectual understanding of "In the greater context, I know he cares for me and I don't want to hurt this relationship." Combining the emotional and intellectual understanding of a situation results in what Linehan calls the "Wise Mind," or wise understanding, from which the correct actions may follow.

As we've discussed, DBT was initially created to treat another condition entirely. However, studies in adolescents have shown that DBT can be helpful for some of the core symptoms of depression as well, including low mood, irritability, impulsivity, and difficult interpersonal relationships. Although DBT is certainly not for every patient, it may yet find a home in treating depressed adolescents, particularly those with prominent irritability.

ACCEPTANCE AND COMMITMENT THERAPY

Acceptance and commitment therapy (ACT) is a relatively new type of treatment in the field of behavioral psychology. Although it superficially seems similar to cognitive-behavioral therapy, or other behavioral therapies, in the types of exercises it asks the patient to do, it is quite different. Almost all of the above treatments aim in some way to reduce the uncomfortable feelings and experiences accompanying depression. In CBT, this is accomplished by challenging background thoughts and behaviors, thereby controlling them; DBT takes this a step further by mitigating even the therapeutic experience itself, tempering it with understanding and acceptance. Interpersonal psychotherapy, family therapy, and group therapy all look to improve an adolescent's relationships, in one way or another, in order to improve uncomfortable interactions that worsen the depression. Insight-oriented psychotherapy seeks to resolve discomfort of which the person may not even be aware, so-called unconscious conflicts, leading the person to change. ACT is different in that its goal is specifically *not* to resolve this discomfort, but rather to allow the person to function *despite* it.

ACT bases its principles on reducing something called experiential avoidance. Many people experience uncomfortable events throughout the day. Sometimes, this is a phone call that we know we have to make even though we don't want to. Or it may be our anxiety at public speaking, or going to a party. Our natural response is usually to try to avoid these experiences. The more discomfort, the greater the avoidance. In the long run, though, avoidance actually makes us *more* uncomfortable, not less. All of the above therapies, through one method or another, aim to reduce this discomfort, allowing us to reduce the avoidance. An extreme example is in the context of CBT, in which patients are asked to undertake uncomfortable ventures. A person afraid of flying, for example, will be taken through a stepwise series of exercises aimed at lowering this fear. First, she will be asked to look at pictures of planes. Then, the therapist may take her for lunch at the airport. Next, she may (at least in the pre-TSA days) be taken onto a grounded plane and asked to sit in a seat—all the while practicing relaxation exercises until she feels more comfortable and learning to control her catastrophic thoughts ("We're going to crash!") by confronting them. Finally, she may take a short flight. ACT is different. Although the end result, flying on a plane, may be the same, the goal of the therapy would be for the patient to *accept* that flying is scary and that she will be uncomfortable, but to *commit* to getting on the flight anyway. This will reduce her avoidance of many things (the flight, her own fear), making it seem less scary and more tolerable in the long run, improving the chances of future trips.

ACT therapists do not attempt to challenge negative or scary thoughts. Rather, they encourage the patient to notice them, realize that they are just thoughts, and return to being present in the moment. This approach teaches patients to get in touch with their core self, the entity observing the thinking, and realize that their selves and their thoughts are separate things. It also emphasizes that thoughts are just that, thoughts, not facts. Rather than practicing distraction or relaxation in the face of fear, the ACT practitioner notices the thoughts and the fear and, instead of running from them, attends to them as they are in the present moment. ACT is much more meditative and present focused than the other therapies, and some adolescents find these qualities more appealing. The ACT approach does not try to "fix" the depression or negative experience, but rather encourages the person to accept it and move on, another appealing factor to some who already resent the idea that they are "broken."

In adults, ACT has shown to be effective in lowering depression scores and in improving functioning, particularly when depression is combined with other negative experiences, such as chronic pain.[12] There is increasing evidence that it can be useful in adolescent depression.[13] Although ACT is new to the field, it represents a fairly radical departure from prior approaches and may be a consideration, although few practitioners specialize in children and adolescents.

CHOOSING A THERAPY AND A THERAPIST

Some therapists are clear about the type of treatment they use. You would be able to tell by glancing at their website that they are a "CBT therapist" or a "family therapist." More frequently, however, it will take a phone call or an initial meeting to determine what specific modality a therapist employs. Many therapists are experienced in multiple treatments and will be able to adjust their therapeutic style based on their assessment of what will work best with a particular patient. A really good therapist will be able to shift back and forth as the therapy progresses, perhaps being more encouraging and directive when the adolescent is still very depressed and more passive, making the adolescent work harder, as he gets better.

Sometimes, it's not difficult to decide which psychotherapeutic technique has a good chance of being helpful for a depressed adolescent. The depressed person who tends to be self-blaming and too hard on himself and whose depression is not complicated by disruptive behaviors or substance abuse might be a good candidate for a cognitive-behavioral approach. If the adolescent relates easily to adults and usually completes the kinds of homework assignments that this treatment orientation uses, so much the better. If the depressed adolescent's irritability and disruptive behaviors have resulted in such a toxic family atmosphere that family members can hardly speak to each other without arguing, family therapy would seem like a good place to begin. Sometimes during the course of treatment, complex issues are identified that call for the more in-depth approach that insight-oriented therapy provides. An adolescent who identifies a history of sexual trauma, for example, may need longer-term psychotherapy to deal with the complex issues that such a history raises, even after the depressive symptoms have abated.

Rather than seeking out a therapist with a particular theoretical orientation or type of training, focus on finding a therapist who is experienced in the treatment of adolescents and who is good at what she does. Usually, the treating psychiatrist will be familiar with good therapists in the community, as will pediatricians, school counselors, and clergy.

In addition to getting treatment for depression symptoms, the depressed adolescent usually needs treatment for the *consequences* of having been depressed. If a hospitalization has been necessary, the return to school may be quite difficult. The young person will need to cope with the curiosity and possibly the cruelty of classmates and acquaintances, and will need help and support in formulating answers to their questions and responses to their teasing. Studies have indicated that peers often perceive the depressed adolescent as shyer and less popular than other children as well as more apt to be teased by peers. Depressed adolescents may have been outcasts and felt isolated for a while before getting treatment and will usually need help integrating back into their social situation, a situation that may have been uncomfortable for a long time.

Sometimes depressed adolescents have developed a dysfunctional peer group that they need to break away from. The youth may have developed relationships with younger, more immature children because of his poorer social skills, or with peers who are substance abusers or who engage in delinquent behaviors. The adolescent recovering from depression will need considerable therapeutic support to be able to leave these dysfunctional but nevertheless comfortable relationships and to develop relationships with healthier and more functional peers.

Adolescents also need to make peace with having a psychiatric illness and probably with taking medications, and they need help incorporating these experiences into their self-identity and coping with the stigmatization of psychiatric treatment. For all these reasons, psychotherapy is always an important component of the treatment of depression. Even if an adolescent has an excellent response to medications, she will need help dealing with these sorts of issues. All these goals can be addressed by any of the above discussed types of psychotherapy, though each will go about it in different ways.

THE PSYCHIATRIST-PSYCHOTHERAPIST: AN EXTINCT SPECIES?

You have probably noticed that throughout this chapter, we usually refer to the psychiatrist and the psychotherapist as two different individuals. Unfortunately, this has become more or less the rule rather than the exception in American psychiatry. It would, of course, be preferable for all sorts of reasons for the person prescribing medication and the person doing psychotherapy to be the same individual. But for a variety of complicated reasons, most adolescents with mood disorders will see a psychiatrist for medication management and a nonphysician therapist (often a social worker or psychologist) for therapy. (We discuss the various types of mental health professionals and their unique expertise in chapter 16.) Some of the reasons for this are the changes in medication management of mood disorders that have come about with the development of new medications: so many different pharmaceuticals are now used in psychiatry that staying skilled in their use has become increasingly time consuming. Perhaps even more significant, though, is that as more effective medications become available for more psychiatric problems, increasing numbers of people want to (and need to) see a psychiatrist for their treatment. There simply aren't enough psychiatrists to do medication management and therapy too, especially in busy clinics. Because medical school and psychiatric training take longer and cost more than the training required to become a psychotherapist, psychiatrists are usually more expensive than other professionals. This is particularly true for psychiatrists who have received additional training to become board certified in child and adolescent psychiatry, a field currently experiencing a national shortage. When the administrator of a busy clinic or an HMO is looking to staff a mental health program, *split treatment* (psychiatric treatment split between a psychiatrist for medication management and a nonphysician therapist for psychotherapy or counseling) means more cost-effective treatment for patients.

The superior cost-effectiveness of split treatment allows so many more patients to receive psychiatric treatment so much more cheaply that it's difficult to envision a return to the days when psychiatrists did therapy and prescribed medications. Fortunately, there are excellent training programs for clinical social workers, psychologists, and counseling professionals that are producing superb psychotherapists. And as we have seen in this chapter, psychotherapy is becoming more specialized too. It has become nearly impossible to be both an expert therapist and an expert psychopharmacologist. For all of these reasons, two professionals rather than one will usually share the medication management and the therapy of the adolescent with a mood disorder.

Part III

VARIATIONS, CAUSES & CONNECTIONS

IN THIS GROUP OF CHAPTERS, we explore several related conditions and problems that frequently complicate the picture of adolescent depression. Chapter 10 addresses the complicated relationship between mood disorders and attention-deficit/hyperactivity disorder. ADHD is a common childhood diagnosis in adolescents who suffer from mood disorders. The links between these two problems are real but also complex and controversial. We explain what ADHD is (and isn't) and introduce some of the controversies surrounding its diagnosis and treatment.

Chapter 11 discusses the diagnosis of autism and how it relates to mood disorders. Since the first edition of this book, there has been a large increase in the number of children and adolescents diagnosed with autism or one of its variants (including Asperger's syndrome). Many children with these conditions at times express similar symptoms to the symptoms seen in a mood disorder, and some will have both autism and an underlying mood disorder as well. Helping persons afflicted with both of these conditions can be difficult for physicians and parents alike, and we discuss some possible approaches here.

In chapter 12, we review alcoholism and substance abuse, looking at how these problems, for most people who suffer from them, are almost inextricably interwoven with mood disorders. This topic may well be the most important of the "connections" covered in this part of the book, because the problem of substance abuse is so common and because it is the most dangerous. Numerous studies show that the combination of a mood disorder and substance abuse is perilous. Individuals with both problems are at far greater risk of harming themselves with suicidal behavior.

Next comes a review of the symptoms, classification, and treatment of eating disorders. These mysterious illnesses are seen predominantly, though not exclusively, in young women, most of whom also suffer from a mood disorder. Anorexia nervosa is one of the deadliest of all psychiatric conditions, and its successful management requires vigorous and sustained treatment of both the disordered eating behaviors and the mood disorder that so frequently fuels and sustains them.

In chapter 14, we discuss "cutting," a complication of depression that is occurring with increasing frequency and seems in many ways surprisingly similar to substance abuse and some eating disorder symptoms. It is also frequently a manifestation of a mood disorder, but as with substance abuse and eating disorders, it requires specialized treatment in its own right. This chapter also takes up the topic of suicidal behavior among adolescents.

The last chapter in this part turns away from more clinical matters and toward a more scientific one, to a topic often of intense interest to adolescents with mood disorders and their families: the genetics of mood disorders.

Attention-Deficit/Hyperactivity Disorder

No book on psychiatric problems in adolescents would be complete without a discussion of attention-deficit/hyperactivity disorder (ADHD). Depending on whom you talk to, ADHD is either an undiagnosed epidemic, with thousands of young people going untreated, or an overblown fraud that has resulted in the needless prescribing of potentially addictive pharmaceuticals to a significant percentage of children and adolescents. As is usually the case with any issue that involves human behavior, the truth is more complicated, and neither of these extreme views seems to be quite correct. In this chapter, we discuss the diagnosis and treatment of ADHD and give you some idea of how this controversy has come about. We also discuss the relationship between ADHD and mood disorders.

WHAT IS ADHD?

To understand attention-deficit/hyperactivity disorder, it's useful to examine more closely what is meant by *attention*. Psychologists have conceptualized *attention* as requiring the following separate steps and processes:

1. Becoming aware of new information in the environment (the *stimulus*)
2. Beginning to process the detected information, and filtering out competing stimuli

3. Shifting attention when appropriate to the task at hand, while resisting the shifting of attention to nonessential stimuli
4. Organizing a response to the incoming information

It is important to note that the normal attention process involves focusing on some information in the environment and actively screening out other information. If you are making a presentation to a new client at her office and hear the siren of an emergency vehicle outside, you may pay attention to the siren for a moment, but you'll then shift your attention back to the business meeting. Chances are, if another vehicle sounding its siren goes by, you won't even be consciously aware of it. In some ways, this screening out of stimuli is the more important aspect of attention.

The other important concept to understand regarding ADHD is that of *executive function*. This set of brain functions, possibly unique to humans, involves self-control and behavioral regulation, suppression of impulses, and planning and sequencing of behaviors. The executive control center of the brain allows us to think about our situation and about what might happen in the future and to plan how we can influence what happens to us for the better. Executive functions mature as a child grows into an adult. These functions seem to be carried out in the frontal lobes of the cerebral cortex, the most advanced area of the human brain. We know that this area of the brain continues developing during adolescence, which seems to provide evidence that this area is where these mature types of brain functions are carried out. In addition to problems with attention, persons with ADHD have problems with executive function. This explains their impulsivity, or inability to plan well or to delay gratification, and their tendency to overreact emotionally to stresses with angry outbursts.

A diagnosis of ADHD is considered when a child, adolescent, or adult has problems with level of attention or executive functioning that seem inconsistent with his age and expected level of maturity. The problem with making this diagnosis comes in deciding what is appropriate at any given age.

The first description of children for whom we would today make a diagnosis of ADHD was given in 1902 by British psychiatrist George Still, in a paper titled "Some Abnormal Psychical Conditions in Childhood."[1] Still described forty-three children with serious behavioral problems: aggressiveness, temper outbursts, defiance, and severe attention problems.

Many of the children had epilepsy, intellectual disabilities (formerly classified under the umbrella of "mental retardation"), or other evidence of brain damage of some kind. He suggested that these children had a "defect in moral control," meaning that they could not regulate their behavior normally. From the 1930s through the 1950s, psychiatrists emphasized the relationship between these problems and brain injuries of various types, whether actual brain trauma from accidents or damage from childhood brain infections such as what sometimes results from measles. At the same time, psychiatrists recognized that the behavioral and attention problems of these children resembled those of individuals who had suffered damage to their frontal lobes. The term *minimal brain damage* was coined to identify these cases. By the 1960s, it was recognized that many of the children and adolescents with these symptoms had no history of brain injury, so the term was changed to *minimal brain dysfunction* (MBD). More recently, the term ADHD has been used, to acknowledge that this problem may or may not be due to "brain dysfunction," and that the cause of the symptoms of ADHD is unknown.

For several decades now, the number of children and adolescents (and adults) whose problems are grouped under the ADHD umbrella has been growing significantly. Whereas the individuals given the predecessor diagnoses of ADHD were severely disturbed, often intellectually disabled, and brain-damaged children, today, adults with college degrees are being prescribed stimulant medication for ADHD because of concentration problems at work. Between 1990 and 1993, the quantity of the stimulant medication methylphenidate (Ritalin) manufactured in the United States nearly tripled, from about eighteen hundred to more than five thousand kilograms annually.[2] Are pediatricians and psychiatrists getting better at recognizing subtle cases of ADHD? Or are these medications being overprescribed? The jury remains out on this issue.

The difficulty in diagnosing this disorder is that the behaviors assessed occur along a continuum and are not abnormal in themselves: a level of attention and executive control that seems abnormal for a person of one age might be perfectly normal in someone younger. If, in the example of the business meeting given above, you interrupted your presentation by rushing over to the window every time an emergency vehicle went by, this would clearly not be age-appropriate behavior. But if a 4-year-old were to do so, no one would be surprised or would consider the child's behavior abnormal. Children are more easily bored than adults and are more easily distracted by interesting and unusual stimuli in their environment. They become more able to focus as they get older.

Age is not the only variable that affects attention and executive functioning. Just as there is a range of body height and weight that is considered normal, brain functions vary among individuals within a range that can be considered normal. At all ages, people vary in their ability to concentrate and attend. When we use more common terms such as *patience* or *maturity* to describe some of the elements of executive function, it becomes obvious that people also vary in these qualities within a wide range of "normal."

So how does one decide how impulsive is too impulsive? Or how active is hyperactive? What amount of "fidgetiness" is normal for a 7-year-old boy? And how does one objectively measure it? The psychiatrist needs to answer these kinds of questions when considering a diagnosis of ADHD.

Simply giving an individual a trial of stimulant medication to see whether it helps cannot be used as a diagnostic tool, because stimulant medications will improve behavior in healthy children as well. Stimulants *always* help with attention and concentration. This is why they are so prone to be abused.

Although the diagnosis of ADHD is difficult to make for some children, others have such severe problems with attention and executive functions that their behavior is clearly outside the range of normal functioning. There is no doubt that these children have a disorder and need help. What is the clinical picture in these children?

The two faces of the ADHD coin are that of inattention (attention deficit) and that of hyperactivity. People with this condition tend to have difficulty regulating their attention. Many people believe that ADHD describes an inability to pay attention to any single thing for a prolonged time. This isn't true. As we've said above, ADHD is an inability to direct one's attention to the task at hand regardless of outside stimuli. We have parents who come to us feeling that their child cannot possibly have ADHD. "He can play video games for hours! He's just lazy and doesn't want to do his homework." In truth, no single picture could be more indicative of ADHD than such a child. Video games are designed to constantly grab one's attention, with bright colors, loud noises, and constant action. Children with ADHD almost get pulled into the game and are able to stop scanning their environment for other stimuli. Parents will call their child's name over and over again without getting a response, not because the child is being willful, but rather because the child's entire attentional focus has been sucked into the flashing, blinking screen. Trying to attend to a less interesting task like homework is almost physically impossible for those with significant ADHD, and any other random stimulus (the family pet walking by, the phone ringing) will derail their current train of thought, so they have to start over.

The other face of ADHD is that of the hyperactive child seemingly driven by a motor. These children truly cannot sit still for any period. They seem to have more energy than any one person should. They impulsively do things without thinking about them. In psychiatric parlance, these two types of ADHD are called, respectively, the *inattentive* type and the *hyperactive/impulsive* type. Most children with ADHD have aspects of both types, but some have primarily the inattentive type. As these children tend to be more quiet and distractible, they are often overlooked by teachers. After all, they are not causing any problems but are rather passively sitting in their chair, thinking about something else. This subtype tends to affect girls more than boys and is usually diagnosed later on, usually around the third or fourth grade, when "learning to read" becomes "reading to learn." At this point, children need to use skills acquired in the first and second grades to comprehend increasingly complicated material. These skills were never laid down in children with inattentive ADHD, and their grades begin to suffer significantly.

What are the consequences of ADHD? In younger children, these problems may lead to poor grades, classroom disruptions, placement in special classes, and disciplinary suspension or even expulsion from school. Peers perceive a child with ADHD as irritating and immature (*executive functioning* is, after all, another term for what we often call *maturity*). Other children may exclude a child with ADHD from their activities, so his social skills can suffer. Peers learn quickly that it is easy to tease children who have ADHD and to set them up to get into trouble with adults. ADHD is not a benign disorder by any means, and aggressive treatment is necessary to prevent the sorts of problems these children encounter over time.

Attention-deficit/hyperactivity disorder persists into adolescence in about three-quarters of the children diagnosed with the condition. Because many of these adolescents have not acquired the basics of learning, it interferes with school performance, self-esteem, and family relationships and predisposes teenagers to high-risk behaviors. Adolescents with ADHD have worse driving habits, more accidents, and more traffic tickets. They have first intercourse at an earlier age, more sexual partners, less use of birth control, more sexually transmitted diseases, and more teen pregnancies than their peers without ADHD (all of which are likely related to increased impulsivity and a reduced sense of the consequences of their actions, or, again, immaturity).[3]

TREATMENT ISSUES

There are two main types of treatment for ADHD (as for almost any psychiatric condition): psychotherapy and medication. The "psychotherapy" for ADHD is actually more weighted toward the surrounding environment than toward the child herself. It includes parent management training (a sort of cognitive-behavioral training for parents in how to effectively manage a child with ADHD), and can also include school accommodations, such as a "decreased stimulation" environment, a high teacher-to-student ratio, and tutoring. More advanced children and adolescents can also be enrolled in study skills training. In terms of medication, the mainstay of treatment is and always has been stimulant medications, of which there are two types, *amphetamines* (table 10-1) and *methylphenidates* (table 10-2). The safety and efficacy of stimulant medications for the treatment of children and adolescents with ADHD is one of the most studied areas in the field of psychiatry. In contrast to the small amount of research on the efficacy of most other psychiatric medications in children, more than 150 randomized controlled studies have been conducted on the use of stimulant medications in children and adolescents.

These studies indicate that stimulant medications improve attention and concentration and decrease impulsive behaviors such as fidgetiness and interrupting in the classroom, and that these effects are sustained over time. Stimulant medications are unlike most of the other medications we've discussed in that they take effect almost immediately. Whereas depressed individuals must wait two to four weeks for their antidepressants to become effective, a stimulant may improve ADHD within hours.

There is much less evidence that stimulant medications help with the

Table 10-1   Stimulant Medications—Amphetamine Class

Generic Name	Brand Name
Amphetamine/dextroamphetamine	Adderall
Dextroamphetamine	Dexedrine
Lisdexamphetamine	Vyvanse

Table 10-2   Stimulant Medications—Methylphenidate Class

Generic Name	Brand Name
Methylphenidate	Ritalin, Methylin
Methylphenidate	Daytrana (topical patch)
Methylphenidate–Extended Release	Concerta

behavioral "fall-out" of ADHD. Research data indicating that medication makes a difference for problems with academic performance, peer relationships, and social skills are scarce. For these reasons, it is important to realize that medication for ADHD is only part of a comprehensive treatment plan that should include interventions in the school (such as smaller class size, increased supervision, and sometimes specialized programs to enhance social skills). Counseling and psychotherapy and sometimes family education and therapy are also extremely important to address the many types of problems afflicting children who have ADHD.

So what treatment do you pick for your child? The largest landmark study of the treatment of ADHD to date is the Multimodal Treatment Study of Children with ADHD (MTA).[4] Researchers followed almost six hundred children with ADHD who received medication, behavioral treatment, both, or no intervention (a placebo control). The children were followed for fourteen months to see how they responded. In the end, the combination of medications and therapy was the most effective. These children also ended up on lower total doses of medications than the medication-only group. Medications alone were helpful, though not as much (and at mostly higher doses). Behavioral treatment alone was no more helpful than the placebo treatment, statistically speaking. This seems to indicate that most children with ADHD should be involved in both therapy and medication management, though in a pinch, medications can help those with pure ADHD who have no sign of a mood disorder.

MOOD DISORDERS AND ADHD

Psychiatrists use the term *comorbidity* to describe two separate conditions or illnesses that frequently occur together in the same person. There is a high degree of comorbidity between ADHD and mood disorders—in some studies, as high as 75 percent.[5]

The diagnosis of both ADHD and mood disorders is difficult in young people, and the relationships between the two diagnoses are, at this point, still poorly understood. Many of the symptoms are similar (an inability to pay attention, impulsivity, irritability, disruptive behavior). The symptoms of ADHD and mood disorder can be differentiated in many youths, but some adolescents seem to have both disorders simultaneously. In one study of children already diagnosed with ADHD, 21 percent were also found to meet the diagnostic criteria for bipolar disorder by age 15. That is, they seemed to have both disorders. The children with ADHD who eventually developed bipolar symptoms had more severe symptoms and more disturbed behaviors. However, an even larger percentage of the children diagnosed with ADHD met the criteria for a diagnosis of major depression: 29 percent had major depression by age 11, and by age 15, 45 percent—nearly half—had been diagnosed with major depressive disorder.[6]

How do we understand the children whose ADHD seems to develop into a mood disorder? Did they really have ADHD symptoms in the first place, or do early-onset mood disorders mimic ADHD in their early stages? Are ADHD and early-onset mood disorder two separate illnesses that share similar symptom pictures but have different causes? Why? And what do we make of the extremely high comorbidity between ADHD and mood disorder? The answers to these questions are not yet known, and the nature of the connection between ADHD and pediatric mood disorders is unclear.

It has been suggested that the link may be genetic. In studies that look at the family members of children with ADHD, the families are found to have high rates of mood disorders. Children of parents with mood disorders have high rates of ADHD. The researchers studying the group of young people with ADHD described above investigated the prevalence of mood disorder in the family members of these children. They found that relatives of children with ADHD and bipolar disorder were five times more likely to have bipolar disorder than were family members of children with only ADHD. They also found high rates of major depression among relatives of the children with ADHD and bipolar disorder. The researchers speculate that ADHD with bipolar symptoms is a particular subtype of ADHD.[7] Or perhaps these are two separate illnesses that happen to co-occur frequently because the genes that cause them are close to one another on the chromosome and are thus usually inherited together (more on chromosomes in chapter 15). The only certainty about this mysterious connection is that much research in the area remains to be done.

The practical issues raised by comorbidity have to do with treatment. Specifically, if an adolescent has a combination of ADHD and a mood disorder, *both* will need to be treated. This makes treatment particularly difficult, as stimulant medications have been shown to worsen both the symptoms and the overall course of bipolar disorder (in adults, at least).

The combination of ADHD and bipolar disorder seems to be especially difficult to treat, and combinations of medications are often necessary. In a study of adolescents being treated for a manic episode with lithium, researchers compared treatment responses in adolescents with and without a history of childhood-onset ADHD. The adolescents with the ADHD history took significantly longer to get better during lithium treatment than did those with no history of ADHD symptoms. This appears to be further evidence that the combination of ADHD and bipolar disorder may be a subtype of illness and that it is especially challenging to treat.[8]

We know that stimulant medication can precipitate mania in patients with bipolar disorder. We know that early-onset depressions not uncommonly predict the development of mania and bipolar disorder later in adolescence. Therefore, the use of stimulant medications in depressed children must be approached with extreme caution. Many clinicians recommend avoiding stimulant medications completely in young persons with bipolar disorders.

OTHER MEDICATIONS

Although tricyclic antidepressant medications have not proved very helpful in the treatment of young people with depression, their efficacy in the treatment of ADHD is clearly proven. The newer antidepressant bupropion (Wellbutrin) has also been shown to be helpful. The problem here is the same as with stimulant medications: the possibility of precipitating mania in a predisposed adolescent.

Clonidine (Catapres, Kapvay) and guanfacine (Tenex, Intuniv), medications used to treat high blood pressure in adults, have proved helpful in ADHD. Whereas stimulant medications help with both inattention and impulsivity/hyperactivity, clonidine and guanfacine seem to be effective in reducing impulsivity/hyperactivity, though may not be as robust in treating inattention. These medications work primarily by lowering the excitement level throughout the nervous system. The human nervous system has two ways in which it can influence the body. The *sympathetic* nervous system tends to heighten awareness and excitement. It is one of the many systems responsible for the "fight or flight" response. The *parasympathetic* nervous system is primarily responsible for maintaining a calm state while the body is at rest. It is able to lower pulse, blood pressure, and breathing rate and induces a state of relaxation. These two systems are constantly in flux to maintain the body in the appropriate state for the situation. Clonidine and guanfacine seem to act by lowering the sympathetic system's ability to affect the body, effectively helping a hyperactive, impulsive individual feel more calm. As they have no stimulant effect at all, they can be useful in patients with comorbid ADHD and mood disorders. However, because they aren't all that helpful regarding pure inattention, they are rarely used in isolation and are often combined with other medications.

Recall that the most commonly prescribed antidepressants work by affecting serotonin, norepinephrine, and/or dopamine—three major chemical transmitters in the brain. The main classes are selective serotonin reuptake inhibitors (SSRIs, like Paxil and Prozac), the serotonin-norepinephrine reuptake inhibitors (SNRIs, like Effexor and Cymbalta), and dopamine-norepinephrine reuptake inhibitors (DNRIs, like Wellbutrin). In 2002, one pharmaceutical company began testing a pure norepinephrine reuptake inhibitor (NRI) for the treatment of depression. Although it seemed ineffective in treating depression, the researchers found that it was helpful in maintaining attention. Further investigations led the FDA to approve this medication, atomoxetine (Strattera), for the treatment of ADHD. It has some advantages over other treatments for this condition. Atomoxetine is not a stimulant, so the risk of it worsening a mood disorder is low. It is also not a controlled substance according to the FDA, as stimulants are, so adults with certain jobs (such as the military) are able to use it. Atomoxetine has some disadvantages too. Although it seems helpful for inattention, it has almost no effect on hyperactivity. It is more like an antidepressant than a stimulant in that it can take weeks to work. For persons who cannot take stimulants for one reason or another, however, atomoxetine has certainly carved out a niche for itself in the treatment of ADHD.

TREATMENT FOR YOUR CHILD

With all the complications delineated above, how is a parent to even begin understanding the complex treatment of a child or adolescent with a mood disorder and ADHD? How can these conditions even be told apart? As with all psychiatric illnesses, the first step is to find a qualified psychiatrist (ideally a child and adolescent psychiatrist) experienced in treating this combination of conditions. This doctor will be able to help determine which symptoms belong to which condition and develop a treatment plan unique to your child's situation. As we've said, many children need both some form of psychotherapy and medication. In cases of mild to moderate symptoms of depression and ADHD, some medications (an SNRI or a DNRI) may be able to treat both. Most persons with ADHD and a mood disorder, however, require more than one medicine to help them become the happiest, most stable, most functional people they can be. Finding the right combination can be something of a journey and is not really an endpoint so much as a continuing discussion, as both mood disorders and ADHD tend to change as the person grows and changes. That said, many highly successful people have both ADHD and a mood disorder, and the secret to their success is starting and staying in effective treatment.

Autism, Asperger's, and Related Disorders

We've just spent some time discussing the interaction of mood disorders and another condition, ADHD. We demonstrated how the conditions can share some symptoms and may be confused for each other. Sometimes ADHD and mood disorders can be comorbid; that is, two conditions exist in the same patient simultaneously, creating unique challenges in treatment. Other conditions that can add complexity to mood disorders in adolescents are autism spectrum disorders (ASD).

Autism spectrum disorders are increasingly common. The cause of this rising prevalence is a topic of debate, even among experts. Some believe that environmental factors are making this condition more common in children. Increased screen time (video games, TV, and so on) has been suggested as a possible cause, as have food additives, wheat or lactose allergies, proximity to electrical wires (which emit subtle magnetic fields), paint additives, chemicals used in carpet and furniture manufacturing, detergents, pollution, certain infections, older paternal age, and others. One popular notion, that vaccines led to increased rates of autism, was later debunked as a scam perpetrated by competing vaccine manufacturers using falsified data. There are, however, certain genetic illnesses associated with autism, such as fragile X syndrome (so named because in people who have this syndrome, one arm of the X chromosome appears under a microscope to be thin and easily breakable).

Other experts believe that there is no real increase in the percentage of children with autism. Rather, they think pediatricians, psychiatrists, and other clinicians are paying more attention to this condition and recognizing it more and more frequently in young persons who have vague and poorly understood social difficulties. Regardless of which side of the debate you are on (and at this point, whether ASD is increasing is still a debate, with facts backing up both sides of the argument), more and more children are being diagnosed with this condition. Young persons with autism, just like all young persons, may be prone to depression and mood disorders. In this chapter, we do not try to give a complete discussion of autism, which is an incredibly complex condition. Rather, our goal here is to help parents, adolescents, and professionals better understand how a mood disorder might appear and be managed in children who, to an extent, already have some of the symptoms of depression and are by definition less able to describe their internal emotional state.

AUTISM: A HISTORY

As with so many psychiatric conditions, the history of autism is fraught with disbelief, lack of acceptance by the scientific community, misdiagnosis, and poor treatment. The term itself, *autism,* was first used by a German psychiatrist, Paul Eugene Bleuler. He was, unfortunately for the future of this disorder, also the first to describe the schizophrenic diagnoses, illnesses dealing primarily with psychosis. When Bleuler saw people who had schizophrenia who were more internally involved than externally engaged, who had retreated into themselves to the exclusion of the world around them, he labeled them autistic. The word *autism* is from the Greek word *autos*, meaning "self," with the suffix *-ismos*, which refers to a state of being. He coined the term around 1910. We now know that Bleuler was describing a particular cluster of *symptoms* without proper appreciation for fully describing the underlying *syndrome.* The term *autism* was used to characterize adults who had clear patterns of psychosis characteristic of schizophrenia as well as symptoms of internal preoccupation and internalization. When children were seen to have some of the same symptoms, even in the absence of any signs of psychosis, they were presumed to be suffering from some sort of infantile schizophrenia and were treated as such.

The first introduction of autism as a cluster of symptoms that might represent an independent condition came in the 1930s from two independent sources. The first was from Hans Asperger (for whom Asperger's syndrome was later named). An Austrian psychiatrist, Asperger used the term *autism* to describe children who showed "a lack of empathy, little ability to form friendships, one-sided conversations, intense absorption in a special interest, and clumsy movements."[1] He published a paper detailing four such cases in 1944. At about the same time, Leo Kanner, an American psychiatrist practicing at Johns Hopkins Hospital (and now widely regarded as the father of modern child psychiatry), acting independently, published a case series about eleven young persons characterized by "lacking affective contact with others; being fascinated with objects; having a desire for sameness; and being non-communicative in regard to language before 30 months of age."[2] Kanner suggested the now-defunct theory that this condition was produced by a combination of a biological predisposition and parents "lacking in genuine warmth." (We now know that parenting styles have nothing to do with the generation of autism, though parents and family members play a critical role in treatment.)

In fact, Asperger's and Kanner's descriptions seemed to diverge later in their careers. Whereas Kanner patients tended to be low functioning and have great difficulty getting on in life, some of Asperger's patients were quite successful. He described them as "little professors" (a term still used today) for their ability to pontificate wildly about their narrow focus of interest. The children Asperger described tended to be more eloquent and have more intact language than the children Kanner studied. Later in life, one of Asperger's patients became a fairly famous astrophysicist, one who went on to correct an error in Isaac Newton's original physics, an error he had noted as a child. Another of Asperger's patients was Elfriede Jelinek, an Austrian writer and Nobel laureate.

As America entered the 1950s and 1960s, a time when psychoanalytic theory held sway and most conditions were thought to be caused by life experience and internal conflicts, the idea that autistic children were the result of cold parenting was increasingly popular. The famous "refrigerator mother" theory of autism (and of schizophrenia—the two conditions were not yet fully separated) was made famous by Bruno Bettelheim in Chicago.

This theory lost influence as the science of psychiatry became more robust. Of siblings raised in the same household by the same parents, one child would have autism and another would not. Also, it was noted that children of parents who had mental illness were more likely to have autism than children whose parents did not, even if the children of parents who had mental illness were not raised by them. Finally, if two siblings were separated at birth and raised in different households and one developed autism, the other was significantly more likely to have autism than the general population. The biological side of this condition began to take hold as the causal factor, eventually eclipsing parenting styles entirely, though this took some time, until about the 1980s.

With the publication of the *DSM-III*, also in the 1980s, autism was firmly differentiated from schizophrenia, being classified as a developmental disorder rather than a mental illness. Developmental disorders are, almost by definition, biological and do not occur because of life experiences or psychological conflicts. As the century progressed, the late 1990s and early 2000s saw an increase in both the recognition and the prevalence of autism, estimated to affect 1 in 250 children (now thought to be a low estimate, but at the time a striking number).

It was at this time that other causes for autism, biological but not necessarily genetic, were explored. In 1998, a famous British medical journal, the *Lancet*, published a paper showing a link between the measles, mumps, and rubella (MMR) vaccine and an increased rate of autism in children. The author of the study, Dr. Andrew Wakefield, published a case series of twelve young people who purportedly developed symptoms of autism shortly after being vaccinated with the combined vaccine. His stance was that children should be vaccinated by three separate vaccines, and that something in either the manufacture of this combined product or the interaction of the strains themselves was to blame. This stance was problematic because the vaccine was not available as individual strains, only as the combined product.

It was later revealed that Dr. Wakefield had significant motivation to publish his (now recognized as) fraudulent paper. First, he had received more than £400,000 from lawyers involved in unrelated class action lawsuits against the vaccine manufacturer, seeking to widen their class action population and build evidence against this company. Second, Wakefield had obtained patents to manufacture his own vaccines (not surprisingly, the three separate viral strains as individual shots), which he planned to sell. The paper was finally retracted from the *Lancet*, with editorials in this journal and others citing it as "containing manipulated evidence," "fraudulent," and "the most damaging medical hoax of the last 100 years."[3]

The idea that autism is caused by external environmental influences is still a popular one. Although many of these ideas do not have firm scientific evidence, that does not make them incorrect. The human body is incomprehensibly complex, the human mind more so, and we are in all likelihood simply too scientifically naive to find definitive answers to these questions. Today, autism is seen as even more prevalent—as many as one in sixty-eight children are diagnosed with an autism spectrum disorder, with boys experiencing the condition at five times the rate of girls.

SYMPTOMS OF AUTISM

The symptoms of autism are classically divided into three main domains of function. According to the *DSM*, for the diagnosis of autism, the child must experience a failure to meet milestones in these domains before the age of 3. In about 20 percent of cases, a child who was presumably developing normally will regress, losing milestones. If this happens after age 3, however, something else is likely at play.

The first domain, and usually the most obvious to parents, is social interaction. Children who have autism simply do not bond with their parents in typical ways. These children are disinterested in their mother's and father's voices. Although they may seek out their parents to have their needs met (to be fed, for example), they couldn't care less about the human interaction that is typically such an integral part of the experience. Children who have autism fail to make consistent eye contact and do not respond to their parent's smiling face. When crying and upset, they neither seek out nor respond to parental attempts at caring and comfort. As they age, they do not play *with* other children so much as they play *beside* them. (Called *parallel play*, this is normal in younger children but tends to stop by about age 4, when typically developing children play with each other.) When children with autism do play with others, they typically use people as tools to their own ends, so that other children find them bossy and demanding. In conversation they do not so much speak *with* other people as *at* them, delivering mini-lectures on topics of interest. They frequently miss the subtle signals that their companion would like to move on to another topic or another person, and stay with the topic incessantly, refusing to cease the monologue. Children with autism rarely have friends but, unlike painfully shy children who also tend to stay alone, they have no desire for them. This pattern persists through the rest of their lives. To a greater or lesser extent, they seem to have no need of other people, aside from a certain intellectual appreciation. (We once had a patient tell us that he was engaged to be married simply because that is what people seemed to expect of him, and yes, it would probably be helpful to have someone split the responsibilities of keeping up a home.)

The second domain, the one usually most evident to the rest of the world, is language. To be diagnosed with autism, again according to the *DSM*, children must have a delay in the development of the spoken word. Some children with autism never develop the power of speech. Those who do frequently repeat what they hear, sometimes repetitively, but cannot process and internalize language in the usual way, to use it to communicate with others. Being able to repeat a favorite movie, word for word, is the kind of ability often seen as a sign of early brilliance in young children. But if they are merely repeating without internalizing the meaning of these words, this may in fact be a sign of autism. This tendency for children to repeat verbatim what they hear from others, called *echolalia*, was one of the first autistic symptoms identified by Kanner. As children with autism age, they are unable to play with language, to understand the subtleties of meaning that allow for puns, jokes, and sarcasm. This makes them the object of much teasing by their peers in school, though unusually, they don't seem to mind much (because they do not understand that they are being teased). A few people with autism, on the other hand, became fascinated by how the intonation of a word could change its entire meaning and went on to become authors, intellectually researching but never truly understanding the expressiveness of language.

The third area of function is that of fixed, repetitive interests and behaviors. Children with autism find one, usually narrow, area of focus and stick to it relentlessly. An autistic child interested in dinosaurs can out-lecture a professional paleontologist. In play, children with autism tend to be unimaginative and concrete. For example, they will not act out scenes or play with a dollhouse but might merely move the toy doll's arm up and down repetitively. They often become focused on part of a toy rather than on the whole object (repetitively spinning the wheel of a car instead of pretending to drive it, for example). Many insist on sameness and routine, playing the same game over and over again. They will insist that parents replay the same movie, or scene from a movie, endlessly. Any disruption in routine or sameness (rearranging furniture, or taking a different route to school) can result in an emotional explosion. In many children with autism, this repetitive nature also comes out in body movements, such as wringing or flapping their hands.

Some individuals on the autism spectrum turn their fixed interest into successful careers, such as the patient of Asperger who became a renowned astrophysicist. For others, the single-minded focus proves more problematic, as they avoid necessary activities to pay full attention to their particular focus, becoming upset, even enraged, when removed from it.

There are other, more subtle, signs of autism that are not part of the official diagnostic parameters in the *DSM*. Many children with autism appear to have the symptoms of ADHD, such as difficulty maintaining attention for a long period, or conversely, difficulty breaking attention from interesting objects. They may appear impulsive and have difficulty sitting still. They are frequently forgetful and cannot follow complex instructions. These shared symptoms were so common, in fact, that according to the *DSM-IV*, it was not possible to diagnose ADHD in a child with autism, because all the symptoms of ADHD were inherent in the autism diagnosis. This has changed in the *DSM-5*, because ADHD symptoms can be an important and treatable aspect of autism, and ADHD requires a diagnosis to justify treatment with the correct medications.

Many children with autism have wild and extreme temper tantrums and are poorly able to self-soothe when upset, or to accept soothing from others. Most if not all have sensory eccentricities. Broadly speaking, sensory experts divide sensory issues into *sensory seeking* or *sensory avoidant* categories, though this is usually a gross oversimplification, because many children have aspects of both. Some children will insist on eating only white foods, for example, or on eating strange and exotic foods for the textural differences. Many children with autism cannot stand the tags on the backs of T-shirts, almost as if they are painful. They may run screaming from the sound of the toilet flushing, or throw open the door to better hear an ambulance siren. Some cannot stand to be swaddled or held; for others, it seems to be the only thing that will help them calm down. Many children who are more sensory seeking use behaviors their parents see as harmful to help them regain a calm state, such as scratching themselves or banging their heads against a wall.

AUTISM VERSUS ASPERGER'S SYNDROME: THE SPECTRUM OF AUTISM

Many changes have occurred to the diagnosis of autism in the last decade. Some of the biggest were in how experts view the illness itself and how it is categorized in the *DSM*. The *DSM-IV* categorized autism as one of five disorders under the umbrella of pervasive developmental disorders (PDDs). We have discussed how mood disorders tend to appear as episodic illnesses—at times present, and at other times in remission—and how treatment with medications can make the illness entirely (or mostly) inactive. The pervasive developmental disorders are different. They are, as their name describes, *pervasive*, meaning that they are not limited to a single area of the person's functioning, such as mood or ability to pay attention. The symptoms seen in autism affect socialization, communication, and range of interests—areas that are likely to affect a person's entire sphere of life. Furthermore, PDDs are *developmental*. These disorders interfere with a child's development and are apparent early in life. This also contrasts with mood disorders, which are usually seen later, such as in adolescence, after a normal period of development.

One of the pervasive developmental disorders, Rett syndrome, has known genetic causes, and another, childhood disintegrative disorder, is controversial as to whether it exists at all. A third PDD category is "pervasive developmental disorder not otherwise specified" (PDD NOS). PDD NOS is, like mood disorder NOS, a nonspecific entity meant to capture children and adults who seem to have some features of a PDD but who do not fit cleanly into one category or another. Autism and Asperger's disorder are the remaining specific diagnoses of the five under the PDD umbrella in the *DSM-IV*. What is the difference between autism and Asperger's disorder?

The answer can be seen in the contrast between the research of Kanner and that of Asperger. Whereas Kanner worked with a group of young children who exhibited language delay (or absence), intellectual disability, and low function, Asperger had a somewhat different cohort of patients. We have already described how one revised the face of modern physics and another won a Nobel Prize. This subset of patients capture what later became known as, fittingly, Asperger's disorder. Among children, the most striking difference between autism and Asperger's is that the second group has no formal language delay (though their internalization and understanding of language still suffers in the understanding of pragmatics). People who have Asperger's disorder tend to have a normal or slightly above average IQ. Some have what are known as *splinter skills*. Anyone who has seen the movie *Rain Man* is familiar with this phenomenon. Although these persons are limited in many other ways, some of them excel in a single, narrow form of functioning. From memorizing the phone book to correcting classic theorems of Newton, splinter skills are more classically a feature of Asperger's disorder. Children who have Asperger's tend to be higher functioning than those who have autism. Though socially awkward, children with Asperger's disorder survive and sometimes excel in school. They have restricted interests, but they are often able to turn this restriction into a strength rather than a weakness. They usually exhibit a lack of social awareness or need for interaction similar to people with autism, and many people with Asperger's have sensory sensitivities and experience emotional explosiveness when routines are altered.

We've spent some time describing and delineating the different types of pervasive developmental disorders. Now we will share a secret—experts in PDDs know that the formal name of the diagnosis really doesn't matter much. Many psychiatrists have treated patients who fit every criterion for Asperger's disorder but must receive the diagnosis of autism because of a very small language delay. This is true in reverse as well—a severely "autistic" child whose symptoms were not diagnosed before the age of 3 cannot ever receive a diagnosis of autism and instead must be categorized as PDD NOS. The *DSM*, as we've said, is a research guide that has expanded to clinical circles, but it is frankly not all that useful when trying to determine the syndrome underlying a particular collection of symptoms. This was recognized by the *DSM-5* committee, and they did away with all these various categorizations and now label Asperger's syndrome, autism, and related conditions under autism spectrum disorder (ASD).

This decision was, as could be expected, controversial. Many people diagnosed with Asperger's disorder did not want to be lumped with every other form of autism, and some experts felt that it was a giant step backward in our treatment of this condition. As such, the committee instead added modifiers. So take for example a young man who in the past received the diagnosis of Asperger's disorder. Under the *DSM-5*, depending on his symptoms, this young man will be diagnosed with "autism spectrum disorder, without accompanying intellectual impairment, without accompanying language impairment, mild severity." Other modifiers include "associated with a known medical or genetic cause" and "associated with another neurodevelopmental, mental, or behavioral disorder"—which brings us to our next topic.

AUTISM AND MOOD DISORDERS

How does autism, regardless of its origin, interact with mood disorders? We've discussed the symptoms of autism: lack of interest in socialization and possibly social withdrawal; a minimal outward expression of emotionality; sleep problems; outward emotional instability, such as crying spells for seemingly no reason; finicky appetites and preferences; lack of interest in pursuits outside of a restricted interest; seeming inability to focus; and emotional reactivity and temper tantrums, which may appear as irritability. Imagine you are a psychiatrist sitting in your office. Now, imagine parents describing these symptoms in their child. You can imagine how easy it would be to think that this person might be depressed. And then, upon interviewing the child, you realize that his affect is constricted due to disinterest, not sadness. Although he may not be paying attention to you, the interviewer, he is engrossed in spinning the wheel of a toy truck or lining up his crayons in rainbow color order. He is animated while performing these tasks, though he rarely answers your questions. When he does speak, it is usually to repeat what you or his parents have said.

This boy is not depressed, he is autistic. It is uncommon, though not unheard of, to confuse the two. What is more difficult is determining if a young person already diagnosed with a pervasive developmental disorder becomes depressed. Almost by definition, children who have autism have difficulty understanding and describing their emotional world. They do not understand feelings and emotions in others and therefore have little reference point for themselves. Extensive questioning is likely to result in little meaningful information on internal symptoms. What makes this problem even more pressing is that autistic children are more likely, not less, to experience depression than the general population. According to studies, up to 24 percent of children and, surprisingly, over 50 percent of adults with autism spectrum disorders have experienced a major depressive episode.[4] Rates of depression increase along with IQ, placing those children with so-called high-functioning autism or Asperger's disorder at greater risk.[5]

There are debates on how to best approach diagnosing depression and mood disorders in this group of individuals. Many psychologists and other mental health professionals use tools to help with diagnoses in all their patients. These usually take the form of self-reports, handouts that parents and children fill out that are then "scored" by the provider. As we discuss in chapter 16, although psychological tests can be helpful, the best way to get a clear diagnosis is through a clinical interview with a trained professional experienced with the relevant population. We advise parents to be wary of providers who rely more on such reports than on face-to-face time, or who see these tools as definitive diagnostic markers (which they certainly are not). Some studies show that these tools are even less helpful when used in an autistic population, making diagnosis of a mood disorder even more troublesome.

Recall that autism is a pervasive developmental disorder. For the most part, the symptoms a child has are fairly consistent and stable. Mood disorders, on the other hand, are cyclical. The average length of a major depressive episode (untreated) is a little over seven months. When someone becomes depressed, her mood and behavior change. In adolescents, this frequently takes the form of irritability. When looking for depression in children with ASD, we look for a relatively sudden change in their behavior and mannerisms. For example, children with autism may be particularly interested in and attached to inanimate objects. A piece of string, for example, was one of our patient's constant companions. If they lose interest in this essential component of their life, we become concerned. If their emotional outbursts increase, or last longer, we begin to consider depression. In persons who can poorly describe their internal emotional experience, their external actions, and more specifically a change in their behavior patterns, signal times of distress.

APPROACHES TO TREATMENT OF THE CHILD WHO HAS AUTISM

The mainstay of treatment for autism is psychotherapeutic behavior modification. For the most part, medications are not effective in treating autism. Pharmacology can be helpful for individual symptoms, but addressing the core syndrome, the autism itself, is at this point an unknown territory. Various studies are constantly ongoing, but as of yet, there is no hard evidence that we can treat autism as we can mood disorders. There is evidence for treatments with oxytocin, the so-called love hormone, but its use is still preliminary and limited to research studies.

Even symptomatic treatments are difficult at best. Many children with autism spectrum disorders are highly ritual and routine based. If their routine changes (if they must sit in a different seat at school, for example, or if their favorite pencil is missing from their backpack), they can become almost unaccountably enraged. This feature is similar to some children with severe anxiety or obsessive-compulsive disorder, so enterprising psychiatrists began prescribing SSRI medications to try to address this anxiety. Disappointingly, a Cochrane review of nine studies found "no evidence of effect of SSRIs in children with autism spectrum disorders."[6] It seems, then, that as with so many other things, trying to work backwards from a particular symptom to the cause was ineffective. Even though these children had symptoms similar to the symptoms of anxious children, the syndrome was entirely different and not helped by the SSRI.

For children who seem to have depression and autism spectrum disorders, though, SSRIs do seem to be helpful. This is because the medicine is doing what it was designed to do: address the depression, not the symptoms of autism. In fact, from a medication standpoint, the treatment of depression does not look all that different whether the child has autism or not. We do know that children with autism are more sensitive to medication side effects, so we may start at a lower dose, but the choice of medication is not likely to be all that different. If on the other hand, the adolescent seems to have symptoms of bipolar disorder, we may make a different choice, and here we are about to contradict ourselves. In chapter 8 we spent some time discussing why antipsychotic medications are not a good first choice for mood stabilization in young people, and now we are about to describe why they may be our first choice for mood stabilization in children who have autism.

We do have some treatments that seem effective, and that are approved by the FDA, for treating a particularly troubling aspect of the autistic syndrome: aggression. When children with autism spectrum disorders become irritated, they frequently lash out, not appreciating the results of their actions. We once treated a patient whose method of getting his mother's attention was to run over and bite her arm (not because he wanted attention for attention's sake, but just because he needed something, like the phone from her purse, that only she could provide). He did not appreciate that this hurt his mother, put her at risk for infection, and so on. He had merely at some point realized that biting his mother interrupted her from whatever activity she was engaged in and forced her attention to him. Two medicines are currently approved for aggression in children with autism, both atypical antipsychotics: Risperdal (risperidone) and Abilify (aripiprazole). In children with autism, these medications are effective in reducing this type of aggression as well as the emotional outbursts that children have when frustrated. When children with autism spectrum disorders become uncomfortable, they are far more likely to act out aggressively than children who do not have autism. So, children in the midst of a mood disorder can quickly become violent—again, not with the specific intent of breaking objects or hurting people, but more out of simply not recognizing the consequences of their actions. A medication that addresses both problems (the mood disorder and the consequent aggression) would then be ideal, and these antipsychotics seem to fit this niche.

One aspect of treatment that is critical but frequently ignored is that of the parent. Multiple studies have shown that parents of children with pervasive developmental disorders have higher degrees of feeling sad, overwhelmed, and isolated than parents whose children do not have such a disorder.[7] Caring for a child with an autism spectrum disorder is a daunting task, and any treatment approach needs to take you, the parent, into consideration. Fortunately, there are many resources available for helping families, as we cover in the resources section at the back of the book. These include help groups, online communities, and practical resources such as school advocates and respite care for autistic youth. Remember what they tell you on the airline—put your own oxygen mask on first, before helping those around you. The same goes for parenting—you need to be sure to take care of yourself and your needs to be able to address your child's.

Alcohol and Drug Abuse

I n the last third of the twentieth century, young Americans achieved extraordinary levels of illicit drug use, either by historic comparisons in this country or by international comparisons with other countries.[1] As terrible as this assessment is for the health of American youth, the truth is that it has even more troubling implications for adolescents with serious depression and other mood disorders. We know from studies of adults that the combination of substance abuse and mood disorders is especially deadly: persons who have mood disorders and who also abuse alcohol or drugs have a greatly increased risk of completed suicide. Severe depression complicated by alcoholism or drug abuse has been found to be one of the most frequent diagnostic pictures in study after study on the psychiatric diagnoses of suicide victims. In a 1993 study, clinicians reviewed the medical records and interviewed the relatives of almost fourteen hundred adults who had died by suicide, in an attempt to make psychiatric diagnoses of the suicide victims. This study, which found that most of the suicide victims had suffered from a mood disorder, also found that *nearly half* (48 percent) had suffered from alcoholism or drug abuse.[2]

ADOLESCENT SUBSTANCE ABUSE

Surveys indicate that among adolescents, the number who try alcohol or drugs (substance *use*) is much higher than the number who use these substances regularly, which in turn is higher than the number who develop serious dependence and addiction problems. There are two important progressions that adolescents may move along as they develop substance-use problems. The first involves how often and how seriously they use, and the other involves which particular drugs they use.

The *stages of use* of adolescent drug use and abuse illustrate how the abused substance becomes a bigger and bigger part of the adolescent's mental life:

1. Curiosity (or pre-abuse) stage
   Does not use: opportunity for prevention
2. Experimentation stage
   Accepts alcohol or drugs from others
   May try drugs for fun and peer acceptance
   Does not usually show behavioral changes
3. Drug-seeking stage
   Seeks out a steadier supply of abused substance (either own supply or a peer group with easy access to substances)
   Needs more drugs to achieve the same feeling (tolerance)
   Uses more drugs, and more often, than planned
   Uses drugs more regularly to get high and to escape reality
4. Drug-preoccupation stage
   Has a significant loss of control over drug use
   Has less regard for the consequences of drug use
   Develops legal and relationship problems
5. Addiction
   Finds drugs necessary to feel *normal*
   Uses drugs daily, or even several times daily

As you will see later in the chapter, several factors determine how far along this continuum, and how quickly, an adolescent will progress. We'll jump the gun a little and tell you that depressed adolescents progress farther and faster than nondepressed adolescents.

The other type of progression is according to *substance type*, reflecting the use of increasingly "hard" drugs with increasingly severe health and legal consequences:

1. Drugs legal for adults
   Tobacco
   Alcohol
   Marijuana (in some states, under certain circumstances)
2. Less addictive illegal drugs
   Marijuana (in states where it is still illegal)
   Stimulants (ecstasy, methamphetamines, and "club drugs")
3. More addictive drugs
   Cocaine
   Narcotics

There is no doubt that tobacco and alcohol are indeed "gateway" drugs that often precede the use of illicit and increasingly dangerous substances. A glance at the results of various surveys of adolescent drug use verifies the alarming progression some adolescents make along this continuum: one review of the subject noted that adolescent cigarette smokers were 16 times more likely to use alcohol and 11.4 times more likely to use illegal drugs than nonsmoking peers. Adolescents who used alcohol were 7.5 times more likely to use marijuana and 50 times more likely to experiment with cocaine than nondrinkers. Adolescents who smoked marijuana regularly were 104 times more likely to use cocaine.[3] The farther the adolescent moves along this continuum, the farther she is likely to go. It becomes apparent that even cigarette smoking puts some young people at the beginning of a rapid trajectory of drug use that can end in physical addiction to extremely dangerous substances.

Social factors such as patterns of use among peers and the availability of particular drugs in a particular community will affect a youth's entry into and movement through this continuum. Age factors are also relevant: "huffing," the inhalation of glue and paint fumes, for example, tends to be more of a problem in younger adolescents. It is important not to regard *legal* substances as necessarily of low risk: more people die each year of tobacco-related illnesses than of any other substance-related illness. Alcohol-related illnesses and tobacco-related deaths far outnumber those due to any illegal drug. Nevertheless, increasing social impairment, legal consequences such as arrest and incarceration, and increasingly severe medical problems usually go hand in hand with the use of the "hard" drugs.

Adolescent drug abuse is a complex issue. A survey of all the substances that can be abused and the ramifications of their use for adolescents with mood disorders would require its own book. Therefore, in the following sections we cover only a few substances likely to be abused, in their order of prevalence in adolescents: (1) alcohol, because it is the most widely abused substance, except for tobacco; (2) marijuana, because it is the most widely abused *illegal* substance and can now in some areas be obtained legally; and (3) MDMA, or "ecstasy," because its rate of use by adolescents is extensive and because it has an undeserved reputation of being a "safe" high. In addition, we will discuss another substance with an alarming recent increase in use and abuse by young people: the ever-expanding category of substances collectively known as methamphetamines.

ALCOHOL ABUSE

Many medical definitions of alcoholism have been proposed over the years, and none of them involves the popular notions of what defines alcoholism: such behaviors as drinking alone or drinking before noon. Several decades of public education seem to have made most people aware that only a minority of persons with alcohol problems wind up as bleary-eyed panhandlers on downtown streets and that an alcoholic might well be able to hold down a job, pay taxes, and mow the lawn every Saturday morning. Fewer people realize, however, that an alcoholic can be someone who goes to high school and manages to maintain passing grades. As a groundbreaking article for pediatricians states, "Teenagers can and do become alcoholics."[4]

The National Council on Alcoholism and Drug Dependencies includes several factors in its definition of alcoholism: *impaired control over drinking, preoccupation with alcohol use, continued drinking in spite of adverse consequences*, and *denial*. This definition can just as easily be applied to any kind of substance abuse.

All definitions of problem drinking include a person's *loss of control* over drinking, perhaps the most important part of the definition. A teenager who drinks when alcohol is available even though he had made the decision not to is showing a loss of control over drinking. So is a young alcoholic who goes to a party intending to have one or two beers and ends up having seven or eight.

Preoccupation with alcohol means spending more and more time thinking about alcohol, about where and how to get it and how to drink without getting caught. Having availability of alcohol in mind when deciding which friends to hang out with and which parties to go to is a part of this preoccupation. Soon, alcohol is not just a part of social activities but rather the axis around which everything else revolves.

The alcoholic adolescent *continues to drink despite adverse consequences*, as alcohol begins to replace everything else as the most important thing in life and becomes the center of his world. No price is too high to pay to use it. Parental disapproval and punishment, falling grades, loss of friendships or privileges, even legal problems will not deter the alcoholic from his pursuit of alcohol.

Another important aspect of any definition of alcohol abuse (or any drug abuse) is alcoholics' *denial* of the seriousness of their problem with alcohol. The word *denial*, when used as a psychological term, means more than just a refutation or saying no. Rather, it is one of the many psychological *defense mechanisms* we all use to manage psychological conflicts and anxiety. Sigmund Freud originated the concept of defense mechanisms, and his daughter, the child therapist Anna Freud, elaborated on his ideas about them. Sigmund Freud believed that a part of the mind he called the *ego* is constantly trying to balance conflicting demands that impinge on it from within and without each individual. He called the ego's attempts to manage these conflicts *defense mechanisms* (or, more properly, *ego defense mechanisms*). Denial, formulated as an immature way to manage psychological conflict, works by simply rejecting the very existence of one "side" of the conflict. The alcoholic who wants desperately to continue drinking and does not want to think of himself as a problem drinker (and thus have to *stop* drinking) deals with these opposing sets of desires by telling himself and everyone else that he does *not* have a drinking problem. It's important to emphasize that someone in denial truly *believes* that the thing he is denying is really *not true*. The alcoholic in denial *believes* that he does *not* have a drinking problem. When the teenage alcoholic says, "I can stop anytime I want to" or "I don't drink any more than my friends do," he is not simply making excuses for continuing with a behavior he knows is a problem. Rather, the problem drinker truly believes the things he tells others about his drinking.

Although alcohol is physically addicting, and the withdrawal symptoms of abrupt cessation of heavy alcohol use are potentially fatal, a person can certainly have a drinking problem and not be *physically* addicted. Because adolescents do not have the degree of access to alcohol that adults do, true physical addiction to alcohol is less common in this age range. An important signal of physical addiction is a need to drink daily to prevent feeling "nervous" or "shaky." Persons with severe alcohol addiction also experience blackouts, episodes of memory loss that occur after a bout of heavy drinking. Blackouts may range from not remembering everything that happened at a party where the teenager became intoxicated to not remembering going to the party at all.

A person with a mood disorder is more prone to drinking than a person without a mood disorder. Individuals who have mood disorders can experience a brief reprieve from their depression in the mild euphoria induced by alcohol. Unfortunately, this experience sets them up for more problems in the future. Alcohol is in fact a depressant and can precipitate and maintain depressive episodes over the long term. In fact, some practitioners will not start an antidepressant on a person who is actively drinking because as many as one-third of those with depression who stop drinking will have a spontaneous remission of their low mood, because their depression was a pure psychological and biological consequence of their alcohol use.

MARIJUANA ABUSE

For the quarter century or so that the National Institute on Drug Abuse has been surveying drug abuse among young people in the United States, marijuana has been the most widely used illicit drug. In 2000, 89 percent of high school seniors reported that they thought they could get marijuana either "very easily" or "fairly easily." More than 75 percent of tenth-grade students and nearly 50 percent of eighth-graders reported the same thing. Obtaining marijuana has become even easier given the medical uses of marijuana for adults in certain states and the recent legal recreational use in others.

For many years, it was commonly believed that no one became physically addicted to marijuana and that it was therefore a comparatively "safe" drug to get high on. This is because cannabinoids, the active components of marijuana, are absorbed into the fat tissues during use and are slowly released when marijuana use stops, making for a sort of tapering off that often prevents withdrawal symptoms. Studies have demonstrated, however, that chronic marijuana users develop all the signs and symptoms of physical addiction. The main criteria for addiction are the development of *tolerance* to the effects of the drug and *withdrawal symptoms* when the drug use stops. In a study in which volunteers were given the same measured doses of cannabinoids daily for four weeks, the volunteers reported that the marijuana seemed to become "weaker" and that their high was becoming progressively less intense, demonstrating their development of tolerance to the drug. A number of these volunteers became irritable and hostile and developed sleep problems after the drug was stopped.[5] Other studies have confirmed that persons who use marijuana regularly and then stop completely can develop anxiety and panic, depressed mood, irritability, loss of appetite, insomnia, and physical symptoms such as changes in heart rate and blood pressure, sweating, and diarrhea.

Because these effects develop several days after stopping the drug, users can convince themselves that they are only using the drug to "self-medicate" preexisting anxiety or depressive symptoms. A regular marijuana user might say she uses it to "calm her nerves," when in fact the use is to ward off the development of withdrawal symptoms.

Marijuana abusers have the same problems with loss of control as do alcoholics, becoming increasingly preoccupied with the drug and continuing to use it despite adverse consequences. A study at the University of Colorado surveyed more than two hundred adolescents who had been admitted to a substance-abuse facility because of problems with alcohol and other drugs. This is definitely a skewed population, but nevertheless, the researchers had no trouble demonstrating the full-blown marijuana dependence syndrome: 97 percent of these adolescents had continued to use after realizing marijuana caused problems for them, and 85 percent reported that it interfered with home and school life or that they had been high in a situation where it was dangerous, such as while driving. Smaller but still significant numbers reported that they had given up other activities to get or to use marijuana and that they spent a great deal of their time getting, using, or getting over the effects of cannabis. Two-thirds of these youths reported withdrawal symptoms, and a quarter said they had used it before entering treatment in order to stop having withdrawal symptoms.[6]

There's little doubt that for these young people, marijuana was a powerful and addicting drug whose grip on them had become unbreakable. As with alcohol, some individuals appear to use marijuana "socially" and maintain control over their use, but many do not. We examine the factors that seem to help predict these differences a little later. Clearly, however, marijuana's reputation as a benign drug is undeserved.

We are fortunate authors to have colleagues willing to advise us on our writing. One such person, residing in a state in which marijuana is legal for medical purposes, believed the above discussion to be "old fashioned" and "not up to date with the current literature," to be "condemning marijuana and deriding its potential medical uses." To be perfectly clear, we are not here to weigh in on the debate as to whether marijuana is useful in medical settings or safe for recreational use. There are many drugs that have important medical or social uses, but whose inappropriate use is devastating to some individuals. Alcohol, for example, is perfectly legal for persons of a certain age. A class of medications called benzodiazepines (Valium, Xanax) work very much like alcohol and are used medically for a multitude of conditions. Pain-killing narcotics, which we discuss later, are used every day in hospitals across the country for lifesaving purposes. There is no contradiction in our minds between saying that a substance may have rational medical and even recreational use, and simultaneously saying that certain persons can develop an addiction to these same substances that harms their lives and their futures. We like to clearly point out that certain persons, especially those with a preexisting mood disorder, may be at more risk of developing addiction and need more help to break it once it has developed. Similarly, overuse of any of these substances (marijuana included) can replicate many of the symptoms of a biological mood disorder and be problematic in itself. Add to these facts the research findings showing that serious damage to the developing brains of adolescents can be caused by alcohol and marijuana and it becomes clear that the use of these substances is extremely risky for some individuals, especially if they are of a certain age.

Separate from marijuana, and pre-dating much of its legalization for medical purposes, a new crop of substances started to be seen in the United States. These were the "synthetic marijuanas," and they went by names such as spice and salvia. Unlike marijuana, these substances were being legally sold to anyone who asked for them in certain stores. People using these substances argued that they were legal and therefore must be safer than true marijuana. This argument is fundamentally flawed because of the nature of how substances gain legal or illegal status. In fact, both spice and salvia are significantly more potent than most naturally occurring marijuana. Nonmedical substances (those that do not have to go through the FDA) are "innocent until proven guilty"—that is, they are legal until they are made illegal. In essence, chemists took the cannabinoids, the active ingredients in marijuana, and chemically altered them just enough for them to be outside the definition of marijuana according to the law (thus producing a legal substance), then sold them on the street. The advent of synthetic marijuana use has been particularly problematic for the psychiatric communities, as these substances seem to be uniquely proficient at causing psychotic episodes in their users that can last for as long as the substance is in the body (which, since they are fat soluble, can be weeks). Legal status aside, we strongly encourage avoidance of all such substances, particularly in persons who may already have a preexisting psychiatric illness, which includes mood disorders.

AMPHETAMINES (CRYSTAL METH, ECSTASY, AND "CLUB DRUGS")

Amphetamines include a group of compounds (of which methamphetamine is the most abused) that are potent stimulants of the central nervous system. "Speed," "crystal meth," "ice," and "bath salts" are street names for these pharmaceuticals. They make the user feel alert, energetic, and often elated. The user experiences increased initiative, motivation, and self-confidence; enhanced concentration; and often an increase in activities and productiveness without a need for sleep. Because both physical and mental performance are enhanced, these drugs are prone to be abused by athletes, students cramming for exams, long-distance drivers, and others who desire to artificially boost their alertness and performance. The effects are brief, however, and users often experience depression and fatigue after only a few hours of amphetamine use, which may require several days of recuperation. Longer-term use or binges of heavy use over several days usually cause a crash into more severe depression, with low mood, fatigue and listlessness, and loss of interest and pleasure in activities—the gamut of symptoms of a depressive illness. Changes in appetite also occur, as well as vivid, unpleasant dreams and other sleep disturbances that can take weeks to subside completely.

The parent compound, amphetamine, is one of the stimulant medications used to treat ADHD. Diversion of these drugs from legitimate use is a source of some of the amphetamines used illicitly, but they are easily manufactured in basement laboratories from ephedrine, a related compound found in over-the-counter cold and allergy preparations, along with other fairly easily obtained chemical ingredients.

For a time in the late 1990s, a group of amphetamine derivatives started to eclipse the parent compounds in popularity, especially among young people. These substances are sometimes collectively referred to as "club drugs," or "designer drugs," and of them "ecstasy" is the most popular. The annual survey of adolescent drug use conducted by the National Institute on Drug Abuse noted a marked increase in the use of ecstasy in the late 1990s. Ecstasy is the compound MDMA (an abbreviation of its chemical name, 3, 4-methylenedioxy-methamphetamine), and a related compound is MDA (3, 4-methylenedioxy-amphetamine). Although both are illegal now, these drugs were first synthesized in the 1910s by pharmaceutical companies as possible appetite suppressants. No therapeutic use for the compounds was ever discovered, and there was little interest in them until the 1970s, when MDA (called the "love drug" for a time) began to be illegally manufactured and widely abused, prompting the Federal Drug Enforcement Administration to declare MDA and MDMA illegal substances. Underground laboratories worked to make more powerful variations of these compounds, and in the process they produced compounds that were not covered under laws against the selling, distribution, and possession of illegal substances (hence the term *designer* drugs). By 2000, nearly two hundred of these drugs had been synthesized.[7] A pill that is called "ecstasy" may, in fact, be any one of these compounds.

Although MDMA is chemically derived from amphetamine, the molecule has structural similarities to mescaline and is often classified, like LSD, as a hallucinogen. Unlike LSD, MDMA does not usually cause hallucinations, but as with other drugs in this group, users report feeling that their emotions are deeper and more meaningful and that they achieve profound self-understanding and develop new perspectives and insights about themselves and their relationships. Intense sexual arousal is often noted as well (the reason, perhaps, why MDA was called the "love drug"). The amphetamine-like euphoria and confidence the drug produces makes these experiences all the more intense and powerful. When abused, the adverse psychological effects are, as might be expected, a combination of those reported to occur with amphetamines and hallucinogens: psychotic episodes, panic, and depression.

An individual's decision to use a particular drug is determined by a balance between the perceived benefits and the perceived risks of using the drug. (This is more the case prior to the development of dependence, after which cravings take on a life of their own, and decision making is impaired.) If the perceived benefits (such as the quality of the "high" and the other pleasurable effects the drug induces) outweigh the perceived risks (adverse physical and psychological reactions; the legal consequences of drug possession or distribution), the user will decide to use. The National Institute on Drug Abuse's annual survey of patterns of drug abuse among adolescents has noted that the abuse of new drugs spreads very quickly, because it takes only a few rumors and testimonials about the "benefits" to generate interest and willingness to experiment. It usually takes much longer for evidence of serious adverse effects to accumulate and even longer for this news to be disseminated. For an illustration of this pattern, one has only to think of the decade or so during which cocaine was touted as a harmless "party drug" and widely considered nonaddictive. MDMA and its derivatives were in this "grace period" as the twenty-first century began, unfortunately abetted by uncritical media (as the spread of misinformation about cocaine was abetted). "Experiencing Ecstasy," an article published in January 2001 in the Sunday *New York Times*, reads in places like an enthusiastic endorsement of the drug and mentions little of the rapidly accumulating evidence on the dangers of MDMA.[8] Increasingly seen in the psychiatric and toxicological literature are reports of several sudden deaths in users, psychotic episodes, prolonged depressions, memory impairment, and thinking problems.

It seems that MDMA exerts its effects by potently altering the levels of serotonin in the brain. You might remember from chapter 6 that one of the groups of antidepressant medications has the effect of *boosting* serotonin levels in the brain. Serotonin seems to play a significant role in mood regulation, acting as a modulator for various brain circuits. MDMA (as well as other substances that cause a high) seems to set off a kind of serotonin "storm" that results in intense pleasurable experiences. The aftermath of this storm is an "exhaustion" of the cells that produce serotonin and, consequently, a depletion of serotonin levels in the brain. This probably accounts for the symptoms of depression that follow MDMA use. A much more worrisome aftermath of MDMA use is suggested by experimental studies in rats and monkeys. The results demonstrate that MDMA actually destroys serotonin-producing neurons in the brain. The implication of this for human users is certainly not clear yet, but we know that there is a gradual loss of neurons as individuals age, a loss that is not usually significant because of the brain's excess capacity. It has also been shown that chronic MDMA users have lower levels of serotonin than nonusers (though it cannot be definitively proved that this is due to loss of neurons). On formal cognitive testing, chronic users have significant impairment in certain types of memory and in higher cognitive functions, like executive function (see the discussion of executive function and ADHD in chapter 10).[9] If users of MDMA have depleted their "excess" serotonin neurons, killing them off by taking MDMA over a period, there is the possibility that psychiatric problems will emerge as these individuals age and progressively worsen as time goes on. Unlike mood problems brought on by alcohol use, these problems are likely to be permanent.[10]

The most recent iterations of designer drugs include "bath salts." These substances are a group of synthesized amphetamine-like compounds in the form of large crystals that superficially resemble the harmless soap-like bathing crystals, from which they derive their name. Initially developed and sold in Europe in the mid to late 2000s, they first came to the attention of the U.S. market in 2010. As with the synthetic marijuana mentioned above, these were legal compounds in the United States and so were sold over the counter in such innocuous places as gas stations and cigarette stores. In a further attempt to delay investigation of their contents, most if not all such products have clear labeling on their exteriors that they are "NOT FOR HUMAN CONSUMPTION." This warning is flippantly ignored by the person using the substance.

Around this time, poison control centers began to see an increase in patients with what seemed to be the symptoms of amphetamine intoxication (paranoia, excitability, high heart rates, panic-like symptoms, and in extreme cases, hallucinations or even heart attacks), but their toxicology tests were negative for the typical culprits, including cocaine and amphetamines. Eventually, these centers discovered the rampant use of these bath salts and since that time have put out major warnings against their use. Bath salt use was so problematic, in fact, that the United States Navy produced a warning/educational video distributed to its active service members, entitled "Bath salts: It's not a fad...It's a nightmare!" In this video, a male recruit in his early twenties opens a package containing bath salts that he has ordered from another country. After ingesting them, he attacks his friends and his girlfriend because of his disturbing hallucinations. This admittedly graphic video has as of this writing almost one million views and has developed rapid popularity among news outlets.[11] Given extreme effects of bath salts, they have successfully been made illegal in the United Kingdom and Canada and are currently illegal in forty-one states, with legislation pending in the remaining nine. Fortunately, the message that bath salts are dangerous seems to be getting through. Between 2012 and 2013, the number of teens reporting that bath salts "involve significant risk to the user" increased by 25 percent.

MOOD DISORDERS AND SUBSTANCE ABUSE

Research indicates that adolescent drug *use* appears to be more closely related to a teen's social and peer factors, whereas substance *abuse* seems to be more closely related to biological and psychological factors. This is evident from looking at the numbers of adolescents who fall into "drug *use*" versus "drug *abuse*" categories in research surveys. The National Institute on Drug Abuse's annual survey of adolescent drug use for the year 2013 indicated that about 70 percent of high school seniors had drunk alcohol and 50 percent had used an illicit drug sometime in their lives (the most common illicit drug used was by far marijuana, which was used by about 45 percent of adolescents, followed by prescription pain killers at 21 percent). Data from other surveys suggest, however, that the number of adolescents with a substance-*abuse* problem, though large enough to be of grave concern, is significantly smaller, around 10 percent.[12] In these studies, the biological and psychological factors associated with adolescent substance abuse are a family history of substance abuse (probably indicating a genetic predisposition) and a psychiatric diagnosis in the adolescent, the most common being ADHD and other behavioral problems and mood disorders. Studies also indicate that depressed adolescents are much more likely to progress from substance *use* to substance *abuse.*

Does having a mood disorder make adolescents more likely to use and abuse drugs and alcohol? Can alcoholism or drug abuse trigger the development of a mood disorder in someone who is genetically vulnerable? Do mood disorders and substance-abuse disorders have a common biochemical or genetic cause? There is some evidence to support an answer of yes to all three of these questions. Substance-abuse problems have been reported to precede the development of mood problems, to occur simultaneously, and to follow them.

Several studies support the idea that depression puts young people at risk for the development of substance abuse. In one study, 76 percent of adolescents with substance-abuse problems who had been referred to a psychiatric clinic had depression problems, and in most of these youths, the psychological problems had *preceded* the substance-abuse problems, sometimes for up to a year.[13] This supports what has been called a "self-medicating" link between substance abuse and depression: the adolescent finds that alcohol or drugs numb the psychic pain of depression, at least temporarily. After a time, however, the substance abuse takes on a life of its own because of the powerful addictive potential of these chemicals. At this point, the depression and substance abuse feed on each other. The adolescent drinks or uses drugs to get temporary relief from his feelings of depression, but since one of the after-effects of this high is a crash into worse depression, he uses again, and crashes again—and on and on the cycle spins, ever faster and more out of control.

Some studies have shown the development of alcohol and drug abuse preceding the development of mood disorders. The idea has been put forth that substance abuse somehow leads to depressive disorders. It's clear that alcohol and drug abuse adversely affect mood in the short run, especially stimulating drugs such as cocaine, amphetamines, and ecstasy. Perhaps ongoing use of drugs and alcohol can lead to more long-term problems with mood as well.

All abused substances appear to work by stimulating "reward" centers in the human brain. You have probably heard descriptions of experiments in which laboratory animals will push a lever that delivers an electrical stimulus to certain brain regions rather than push another one that delivers food to their cage, and they will continue to do so until they're practically dead from hunger. When a similar lever device is used to deliver an intravenous dose of alcohol or another drug, the substances the laboratory animals will willingly and persistently self-administer in this way are almost exactly the same ones that humans use to get intoxicated: narcotics, cocaine, and certain stimulants and tranquilizers. And these are the same substances that humans abuse and become addicted to. Some drugs, including ecstasy and cocaine, affect these brain centers quickly and powerfully; others, such as marijuana, work more slowly, but they all work in the same way: by disrupting the normal operations of the brain's "feel good" circuitry. Perhaps repeated episodes of drug use disrupt this circuitry in more profound and long-lasting ways and a mood disorder is the result. (Remember that animal studies have demonstrated that MDMA kills serotonin neurons in the brain.)

Finally, it may be that similar biological and psychological factors underlie the development of *both* mood disorders and substance-abuse disorders and that both types of problems are better thought of as two sides of the same coin.

TREATMENT ISSUES

Numerous clinical studies have shown a strong connection between adolescent substance use and adolescent mood disorders. One study followed up on a group of about seven hundred young people for approximately nine years to examine the relationship between substance use and depression. Not surprisingly, it found that depressed adolescents were more likely to use drugs and alcohol. It also found a roughly linear correlation between depression and drug use: the rate of depression problems went up in proportion to the severity of substance use. Put another way, the more severe the substance-use problem, the more likely the adolescent was to be suffering from a depressive disorder.[14]

But what about the question of whether one type of disorder *causes* the other? This question has important ramifications for treating these problems in individuals. If the self-medication hypothesis is true and depressed adolescents use alcohol and drugs in an attempt to "treat" their depressed feelings, this would suggest that successful treatment of the mood disorder should make the substance-abuse problem simply go away on its own. If the substance abuse is causing the mood disorder, then remaining abstinent from the abused substances should make the mood disorder go away. Research studies support both scenarios, which probably means that both can occur.

We think most psychiatrists who treat mood disorders have seen these two scenarios in patients, and most would agree that when a mood disorder and a substance-abuse problem occur together, they are best thought of as two problems that *both* need aggressive treatment. Either of these problems can precede and seem to trigger the other, which then takes on a life of its own and therefore requires treatment of its own as well. In our experience, patients who do not get treatment for both problems will not recover from either.

The first goal of treatment for substance abuse is to interrupt the drinking or drug use. Admission to a psychiatric hospital or other treatment facility is sometimes necessary to remove adolescents from an environment where they can still obtain and use alcohol or drugs. Family involvement is critical for treatment to be successful, by improving communication among family members and helping parents to provide guidance and set limits with the adolescent. In psychiatry there is a phenomenon called *codependence.* This is a somewhat loaded term that carries many, sometimes incorrect or exaggerated, social meanings. When psychiatrists use the term, they are usually trying to describe a simple pattern of behavior. In this pattern, one party in a relationship (in our scenario, an adolescent addicted to drugs) behaves in a dysfunctional way (misses school, for example, or commits crimes). The other person (usually the parent) inadvertently starts to support the behavior by shielding his child from the consequences of her behaviors. This usually happens with the best of intentions, that of protecting his child. What quickly transpires, however, is that the addict is increasingly insulated from the consequences of her actions, and the parent is increasingly called on to provide his protection, even if this means compromising his values. Usually this pattern becomes particularly problematic when the addict is asked to give up her addiction. Psychiatrists are constantly confronted by parents and children who want to get clean but find the process difficult and prematurely terminate the attempt. The father will sign his daughter out of rehab because it is uncomfortable or causes her suffering (even knowing that this temporary suffering is in her best interest). The mother will invite her son home from juvenile hall, knowing full well that he is likely to steal money again for drugs. This can be one of the most challenging aspects of addiction for a family to face, and it is why we always recommend that parents and loved ones pursue their own support during the treatment of the addict. This can take the form of support groups (such as Al-Anon) or even entering mental health treatment to work through their own feelings and distress. It is not usually appropriate for the same psychiatrist to treat both the child and the parent, because the psychiatrist must always have the best interest of the single identified patient in mind, which can be complicated when treating multiple members of the same family. It is becoming more and more common for psychiatry and therapy to be provided by different individuals, and in such a scenario, it may be valid for a family therapist to treat both the child and the adult, or for each to have an individual therapist as well as an individual psychiatrist.

Studies of adult alcoholics and cocaine abusers have shown that regular use of intoxicating substances alters brain functioning. Specifically, functioning is disrupted in the prefrontal cortex, an area of the brain thought to be involved in the executive functions such as self-control, delay of gratification, and inhibition of impulses (as we discuss in chapter 10). Studies of brain metabolism show that only after many *months* of sobriety do these brain areas function normally again.[15] During this time, the recovering substance abuser is still at grave risk of relapse. The treatment of substance-abuse problems must therefore be a long-term commitment. A brief "detox" admission to a hospital or several weeks of intensive outpatient treatment is not sufficient to have a long-lasting effect on substance abuse in an adolescent who has progressed beyond the experimentation stage of alcohol or drug use.

Although alcohol and drug use may stop for several months after intensive treatment, many studies have shown that abstinence does not last if the youth doesn't get maintenance treatment of some kind. According to one study of the treatment of adolescent drug abuse based on the twelve-step program of Alcoholics Anonymous, just as many adolescents who had completed a short-term treatment program relapsed by the twelve-month mark as those who hadn't even completed the program.[16] Often the adolescent needs help in developing an alcohol-free and drug-free lifestyle and in making some necessary major changes in his peer group and recreational activities, changes that the adolescent can make only with time, counseling, and support.

Some young people can move from a hospitalization or detoxification program of several days'—or weeks'—duration to outpatient care. This is often possible if the adolescent's functioning level and school and family life were not too severely affected by drug use. If drinking and drug use have reduced the adolescent's life to shambles, however, longer-term residential treatment will be necessary.

Adolescents who have dropped out of or been suspended from school, or who have developed run-away and other disruptive behaviors that make returning to live with the family tense and difficult, will probably need the structured rehabilitation of a residential or "halfway house" setting. These young people require the professional supervision and guidance, structure, and support provided in these settings to make the changes in behavioral patterns necessary to maintain their sobriety. Should this eventuality occur, it is the perfect opportunity for a parent to enter into her own treatment. Even though seeing her child destroy his life through an addiction is terribly traumatic, few things are as painful for a parent as having her child taken away from her for such a long period, especially knowing that he will likely be in psychological distress during the treatment. To brave through the experience, parents might find professional help invaluable in supporting their correct, though difficult, choices.

Adolescents who abuse alcohol and drugs to any substantial degree essentially stop the process of psychological maturation. Their emotional development is arrested at the point where they started using substances heavily. An 18-year-old who has been smoking marijuana regularly for two or three years may have the emotional maturity of a 15-year-old and will lack the more mature coping, problem-solving, and communication skills expected for her chronological age. When this adolescent gets clean, parents may be disappointed that their child seems to be immature for her age. The adolescent may find it difficult to feel comfortable with same-age peers. For all these reasons, counseling and psychotherapy, including family therapy, are often necessary and extremely beneficial for all involved. We discuss more about how to cope better with substance-abuse issues in the family in chapter 17.

Eating Disorders

E ating disorders make up a group of psychiatric syndromes that share the common element of a distortion of normal eating behaviors. Individuals with an eating disorder may eat too little or too much, but they all share a preoccupation with food, calories, and weight that comes to be all-engrossing and pathological, often with dangerous, sometimes even deadly, consequences. Ninety-five percent of persons with eating disorders develop them between the ages of 12 and 25, and 90 percent are women. Therefore, according to statistics, eating disorders are predominantly disorders of adolescent girls, and most of these individuals have mood disorders as well.

▼ Jennifer had blacked out for only a moment, it seemed, but she was still glassy-eyed and quiet when the ambulance arrived. The phys ed teacher had whisked horrified students out of the gym and called the school nurse, Mrs. Coleman, who found Jennifer's pulse to be alarmingly low and was having trouble taking her blood pressure. When Mrs. Coleman hiked up the sleeve of the girl's sweatshirt to take her blood pressure, she was taken aback by how skinny Jennifer's arm was.

"Has this girl been sick?" she asked.

"Not that I know of," replied the teacher. "At least not anything serious, I don't think. She's missed a few days here and there, but that's all."

They heard the sirens wailing up the school driveway. Good, thought Mrs. Coleman, they're here.

She looked down at Jennifer again. "Why are you wearing these heavy sweats in June?" she asked. Perhaps the girl had become overheated and fainted.

"I'm always cold," replied Jennifer listlessly.

The gymnasium doors clanged open, and three paramedics in sharply pressed blues briskly walked in. Mrs. Coleman and the teacher stood back, and Jennifer was on the gurney in seconds. One of the paramedics pumped up the blood pressure cuff that was still on the girl's arm and listened intently with her stethoscope. "Sixty-five over forty," she gasped. Another paramedic had already pricked Jennifer's finger and squeezed a drop of blood into what looked like a handheld calculator. He read the number that glowed on its little screen. "Her blood glucose is only thirty-seven, Kate." Kate looked down at Jennifer. "Are you diabetic, honey? Do you take insulin?" Jennifer shook her head weakly.

"What did you have for breakfast today, sweetie?"

"A vitamin pill."

"We're going to start an IV on you, Jennifer." In a moment, Jennifer, the gurney, and the three paramedics were moving toward the door. "Tell her parents we're taking her to Memorial. We'll need them to sign for treatment." The gymnasium doors clanged shut. As the echoes of the door's banging died away, the siren's wail started up and then faded.

Mrs. Coleman turned to the teacher. "Has this student seemed tired to you lately? Has she had trouble keeping up with the others in this class?"

"No. Jennifer's always full of energy. But this isn't really a class; it's an aerobics group for junior girls with weight problems. Participation is voluntary."

"Weight problems?" Mrs. Coleman said. "Carol, that girl does *not* have a weight problem."

"I started the group last month, and Jennifer was the first to sign up. I didn't think she looked overweight, but it's hard to tell with those baggy clothes she always wears."

Mrs. Coleman looked thoughtful for a moment, and then asked, "Do you ask these girls how much weight they want to lose when they sign up?"

"They fill out a form with their current weight and their goal weight. I remember that Jennifer left those questions blank. I just thought she was embarrassed—"

Mrs. Coleman wasn't listening anymore. She realized that this girl probably *did* have a weight problem, but not the kind of problem an aerobics class would help with. When she spoke with Jennifer's mother on the phone, she asked about the girl's eating habits.

"They're terrible. I know she's too skinny. But she won't eat with us anymore. I almost think it's better that way because every meal turned into a screaming match. We can't even talk about it around here. Her father gets so mad about it that I worry about his blood pressure getting out of control again."

"Mrs. Andrews," the nurse said slowly, "I think Jennifer might have an eating disorder." ▲

By the time pop singer Karen Carpenter died of anorexia nervosa in 1983—an event that brought eating disorders to the consciousness of most Americans for the first time—physicians had been aware of this mysterious group of psychiatric illnesses for more than two centuries. Dr. R. Morton wrote in a 1694 treatise on "consumptions" (an old word for any illness characterized by a physical wasting away) of "a nervous atrophy . . . a wasting of the body without any remarkable fever, cough, or shortness of breath" that he attributed to a "distemper'd state of the brain." In 1874, the English physician William Withey Gull coined the term *anorexia nervosa* to describe "a morbid mental state" that resulted in extreme weight loss. Gull realized that the weight loss was not due to a bodily illness like tuberculosis or an intestinal disease but was instead the result of "simple starvation."

But it was the French alienist (*alienist* is a nineteenth-century term for a psychiatrist) Charles Lasègue who first captured the essential elements of this form of the illness: a "refusal of food" that becomes "the sole object of preoccupation and conversation" such that "the circle within which revolve the ideas and sentiments of the patient becomes more narrowed." Lasègue described the disconnect between the patient's appearance and her perception of her appearance as well as her distorted assessment of her nutritional needs: "The patient, when told that she cannot live upon an amount of food that would not support a young infant, replies that it furnishes sufficient nourishment for her, adding that she is neither changed nor thinner." Lasègue also recognized the upheaval the syndrome causes in families and the frustration and powerlessness of the parents of these patients. He noted that the family "has but two methods at its service which it always exhausts—entreaties and menaces."[1]

In the 1980s, it was increasingly recognized that self-starvation is not the only serious abnormal eating syndrome. Also described were individuals, often of normal weight, who binged on huge amounts of food in a matter of hours or even minutes and then caused themselves to vomit what they had eaten. The terms *binge-purge syndrome* and *bulimia nervosa* (or simply *bulimia*) were coined to describe this condition.

More recently, descriptions have appeared in the psychiatric literature of overweight patients who binge but do not induce vomiting or use other means to compensate for their increased calorie intake, and the diagnosis *binge-eating disorder* was officially adopted in the *DSM-5*.

It has been suggested that perhaps the biggest group of persons with abnormal eating behaviors does not fit neatly into any one of these classifications; these individuals have elements of several eating disorders or shift from one clinical picture to another over time. Abnormal eating syndromes cover a wide range of problems, from those posing only minor risks to health to those that are life threatening.

As with adolescent substance abuse, the topic of eating disorders is enormous and complex. What follows, then, is a brief overview of the main symptoms of the disorders, just to introduce them and to make it easier to understand the interplay between these syndromes and the mood disorders.

ANOREXIA NERVOSA

The most dramatic and severe of the eating disorders is anorexia nervosa. People with this disorder believe they are overweight, even obese, and restrict their food intake to lose weight. They lose their objectivity about calories, weight, and appearance, and they continue to think they are overweight despite the emaciated appearance of their bodies. Their drive to lose weight takes on a life of its own, and despite their steadily decreasing weight, they continue trying to lose even more. The syndrome is, in a sense, incorrectly named, because the word *anorexia,* a medical term for "loss of appetite," does *not* characterize these individuals (except perhaps in the advanced stages of starvation, when their brain functions are abnormal in many different ways). People with anorexia do not lose their appetite but rather *fight* their hunger, and after a time, the struggle against their appetite becomes an end in itself, the focus of all their energies.

Often, the individual starts out with a desire to lose what might indeed be extra pounds, but then she cannot identify or be satisfied with a healthy goal weight. She may identify an initial goal weight of, say, 110 pounds, but after reaching this initial goal decides to get down to 105. At 105 pounds, the new goal becomes 100, then 95, and eventually the only goal is to weigh less than the day before—with no end in sight. She becomes convinced that if she starts to gain weight, she will lose control of her eating and her ability to maintain her weight and will become enormously obese. In other cases, the person realizes she is thin but nevertheless worries that some part of her body, such as her abdomen or buttocks, is "fat." Either way, eating comes to be viewed as a vice; taking needed nourishment is "giving in."

As others notice the girl's increasing thinness with alarm, eating and meals become more and more tense. As Lasègue observed in the families of his patients, "the delicacies of the table are multiplied in the hope of stimulating the appetite; but the more the solicitude increases, the more the appetite diminishes. The patient disdainfully tastes the new [foods] and after having thus shown her willingness, holds herself absolved from obligation to do more."

Individuals suffering from anorexia not only fast but also exercise excessively to lose weight. They may use laxatives and diuretics (fluid pills) to decrease calories and weight. To avoid the stares and comments of others, they dress in baggy clothing that conceals their emaciation.

Eventually, the physical consequences of starvation begin to take their toll. Menstruation stops, heart rate slows, and hands and feet become cold as the body attempts to conserve calories. Skin becomes dry, the hair may fall out, and the person complains of fatigue and is noted to be listless and lethargic. Dizzy spells and fainting occur. Eventually, sodium and potassium imbalances affect cellular functions, heart-rhythm abnormalities develop, and the girl can die from cardiac arrest.

The treatment of anorexia nervosa focuses first on refeeding the patient in order to reverse the distortions in thinking that are due to starvation.

Then, a lengthy retraining process must occur during which the patient relearns normal eating patterns and changes her feelings about herself, her weight, and her relationship with food and calories. In many cases, this eventually proves impossible to accomplish outside a carefully controlled setting. Just as many substance abusers must enter rehab to terminate their unhealthy relationship with drugs, so do many people who have anorexia require admission to a psychiatric hospital to interrupt their unhealthy relationship with food.

BULIMIA NERVOSA

The hallmark of bulimia nervosa is binge eating, during which the individual eats an enormous amount of food, often sweet high-calorie foods, over a period of an hour or so. She may eat an entire gallon of ice cream at one sitting, dozens of doughnuts, pizzas by the carton, candy by the pound, usually stopping only when physically incapable of taking in any more food. A binge is a private affair undertaken secretly and alone; the food consumption is frenzied, joyless, and obsessive, and the bulimic feels out of control, almost "out of body," while it is happening.

When she cannot force another bite, the bulimic is overcome with disgust and shame at what she has done and seeks a way to rid herself of the calorie load. The vast majority of people with bulimia do this by forcing themselves to vomit. This provides them relief from the physical discomfort brought on by the binge and also reduces their fear of gaining weight from such an enormous intake of calories. In the early stages of the disorder, individuals with bulimia usually stimulate their gag reflex by putting a finger or spoon down the throat, but later in the course of the disorder, they often become adept at vomiting at will. Those who do not manage this may actually develop a callus on the first knuckle of their finger from the repeated abrasions caused by their teeth during self-stimulation to induce vomiting. Individuals with bulimia also misuse laxatives and diuretics to get rid of calories and water weight.

The binge is often an unplanned and impulsive response to some uncomfortable emotional state. Like those with anorexia nervosa, these girls and young women are abnormally preoccupied with their weight and body image and, outside their binges, are often strictly controlling their diet and avoiding high-calorie foods.

Individuals with bulimia nervosa are usually impulsive in other areas of their lives, and they often have a history of substance abuse, self-mutilation, and suicide attempts. Many people with anorexia also have bulimic behaviors, and approximately 40 percent of them have a more prolonged bulimic phase in the course of their illness or recovery.[2]

Most individuals with bulimia are of normal weight or are slightly overweight. Physical complications of bulimia nervosa are mostly related to the purging behaviors discussed above, including vomiting. These purging practices are dangerous. They can cause severe dehydration or imbalances in the body's natural electrolytes that can lead to cardiac arrhythmias or seizures. The stomach acid repeatedly forced up the throat can cause blistering and, over the long term, cancer.

Binge-eating disorder describes the behaviors of people who binge but do not purge, use laxatives, or engage in other behaviors to get rid of the extra calories. Their binges have exactly the same qualities as those of a bulimic—they can be impulsive or, conversely, highly ritualized. The person feels physically unable to stop and can eat well over her daily allotment of calories in one sitting. We once treated a patient who would consume three family-sized buckets of fried chicken in a single episode—he would begin crying halfway through but was still unable to stop the bingeing episode. As might be expected, many people with binge-eating disorder are overweight.

The treatment of bulimia nervosa includes helping patients identify the precipitating factors of a binge, addressing their distorted body image and abnormal attitudes toward food, and teaching them healthy eating habits and coping patterns other than binge eating during periods of emotional distress. As with anorexia, persons with bulimia have a great fear of food and can be highly resistant to entering treatment. Though many are of normal body weight (as opposed to people with anorexia), they fear that giving up their abnormal behaviors (primarily the purging) will result in their ballooning up to an enormous weight. Forcing a patient to refrain from vomiting after even a normal-sized meal can result in a seemingly calm, rational patient flying into a violent rage. As may be expected, treatment of bulimia is similarly difficult to treatment of anorexia and may require an inpatient psychiatric stay.

UNDERSTANDING EATING DISORDERS

Like substance-abuse problems, eating disorders are best understood as complex self-reinforcing *behaviors* that entrap vulnerable individuals. The challenge to understanding eating disorders in this way is that of understanding how self-starvation and bingeing and purging can possibly be self-reinforcing, that is, why patients, on some level at least, are *attracted* to these behaviors in the same way substance abusers are attracted to alcohol and drug use. It helps to first identify the vulnerabilities that are the setup for these behaviors.

Social and cultural factors are very important. Eating disorders are seen almost exclusively in industrialized countries where food shortage is not significant. Western culture's glorification of thinness in females is also a significant factor. One need only glance through any magazine marketed to teenagers to see the idealized feminine physique: willowy thin supermodels or buxom but toned and wiry beach beauties—often photographed and touched up in such a way as to make them look even thinner than they are in real life. Surveys show that up to 70 percent of young women in Northern Europe and the United States feel they are overweight even when they are thin or normal in weight. Most girls simply do not have the genetic endowment needed to look like the women they constantly see depicted in magazines, on billboards, and in films and television programs. Adolescent boys feel some of the same pressures, but the emphasis is on being muscular rather than thin. This is one of the reasons eating disorders are thought to be so much rarer in males (and perhaps why steroid abuse is almost exclusively a problem of young men).

There is also something of a class consciousness attached to thinness, exemplified by the old saying that "a woman can never be too rich or too thin." In contrast to cultures in which food is scarce and plumpness is valued, where food is plentiful, slimness and the avoidance of obesity are valued and associated with wealth. Being overweight is associated with laziness, poor self-control, and self-indulgence; thinness is associated with good health and self-discipline. Young people constantly see and hear that thin is good and fat is bad, and they incorporate these ideals into their view of what sort of body type is attractive and desirable.

While some young people are relatively unaffected by this barrage of messages about weight and appearance, those with serious self-esteem problems can take these messages to heart in a very serious way. Adolescence is a time of difficult transitions and worries about identity and fitting in. Fears about sexual maturation crop up for younger adolescents, and older ones may equate entering adulthood with being abandoned and isolated. The adolescent fears losing control of her life in several important ways and may feel ineffective and helpless to influence the outcome of these developmental processes. At this point, some adolescents become preoccupied with food and weight control to distract themselves from these frightening issues.

When they restrict their food intake and experience weight loss, these young women experience a surge of competence, self-confidence, and control. Complimentary and congratulatory comments from others on successfully losing weight further reinforce weight loss as an admirable goal. Fasting and food preoccupation become a "safe place" where the girl feels in control and knows that her efforts will pay off in predictable and measurable ways. The girl with anorexia begins to take pride in her ability to adhere to stricter, narrower, and more abnormal diets and to restrict further and further. Thinness, fasting, and exercise come to be seen as virtues and eating as a vice. The adolescent becomes intoxicated by her success at losing weight and by reaching ever more ambitious weight-loss goals.

Experiments to study the psychological effects of starvation, in which healthy volunteers have gone on extremely restricted diets, have shown that constantly hungry people begin to think about food constantly, talk about food constantly, and even have dreams about food. As her food intake decreases, the girl with anorexia experiences ever stronger, and now physiologically induced, food cravings. She finds that she must work even harder to keep the weight off. She develops increasingly irrational fears about what would happen if she were to begin to eat normally, imagining that her body would balloon to immensely obese proportions if she were to stop restricting. More fasting leads to more craving and hunger, which leads to more food preoccupation, more fear of losing control—and this leads to more fasting. A vicious circle has developed: the young woman with anorexia has become intensely fearful of eating, and fasting is the only way she knows of to deal with her anxiety. There is no escape.

Eventually, malnutrition begins to affect brain functioning. At this point, the individual becomes physically incapable of making good decisions about eating or realizing how dangerous a situation she is in. This is why, at very low weights, hospitalization is necessary to accomplish refeeding.

Individuals with bulimia follow a comparable course. They are affected by the same sociocultural factors regarding thinness and also start out worried about their weight. They often go on diets that are unreasonable and overly strict, and their initial binges are the result of impulsive and out-of-control eating to quickly alleviate their hunger pangs. Alternatively, the binge may have developed as a means of dealing with depression, loneliness, and anxiety. In either case, binge eating becomes the coping mechanism and simultaneously the cause of shame, guilt, and disgust. The bulimic starts purging to rid herself of the physical discomfort and calories that result from the binge, but this behavior (and perhaps the weight gain that results from it as well) causes more shame and guilt, precipitating more binge eating, and another vicious cycle begins.

In the treatment of eating disorders, normal eating behaviors and healthy attitudes toward food and body need to be retaught to the patient. She must also learn new ways of coping with uncomfortable feelings and address self-image and self-esteem issues. For many of these individuals, there is also an underlying mood disorder that fuels the maladaptive coping mechanisms and that requires treatment in its own right.

MOOD DISORDERS AND EATING DISORDERS

Many people with eating disorders have mood disorders as well, usually depression. One clinical study of American high school girls with eating disorders found that more than 80 percent of them suffered from a depressive disorder, mostly major depressive disorder.[3] Another study found that dysthymic disorder was more closely associated with eating disorders than major depression.[4] But whatever the details, the pattern is clear: the combination of an eating disorder and a mood disorder occurs too often to be explained away as simply coincidental. The cause or causes for this correlation are hotly debated. There is some evidence that genetic factors are at play. A study of twin girls with anorexia nervosa found evidence that genetic risk factors are important for the development of the eating disorder and "substantially contribute to the observed comorbidity between anorexia nervosa and major depression."[5] Perhaps personality traits such as obsessiveness or a tendency to be shy and introverted have a genetic basis, and perhaps these traits interact with social cues to set up the adolescent female for anorectic behaviors. We know that a person's degree of impulsivity has some genetic basis and that a tendency to be impulsive is frequently seen in individuals with bulimia.

The bad feelings that arise from a mood disorder may precipitate eating disorder behaviors and sustain them over time. An Italian study of patients with bulimia found that many of them had a *prodrome*, or preliminary phase, to their eating disorder characterized by low self-esteem, depressed mood, loss of interest and pleasure in activities, and irritability—all symptoms of depression.[6]

The relationship between eating disorders and mood disorders is likely one of complex interactions that differ from one individual to another. The optimal treatment of the combination is quite clear, however: when they occur together, *both* problems require treatment. As with the combination of substance abuse and mood disorders, treating one problem does not usually make the other go away.

Several double-blind placebo-controlled studies have shown that patients with bulimia can reduce the frequency of their binges when they are prescribed antidepressant medications as part of an overall treatment plan that includes psychotherapy and therapy aimed at the eating disorder behaviors.[7] Studies on antidepressant treatment of patients with anorexia nervosa at first appeared to be less impressive, but more recent studies suggest a reason to be optimistic. It seems that antidepressants have little effect when the patient with anorexia is still significantly underweight, perhaps explaining the results of studies on still-malnourished hospitalized patients that have not shown antidepressants to be of much benefit. When fluoxetine (Prozac) was given to patients who had been discharged from the hospital at normal weight, however, the medication had a significantly beneficial effect on relapse rates. Perhaps biochemical abnormalities in the brains of malnourished, underweight patients prevent antidepressant medications from working properly, and only when weight has returned to normal can medication be effective.[8]

The treatment of severe eating disorders is complex and requires a team of experts. Severely malnourished patients are best served in psychiatric hospitals that have a special eating disorders unit and a treatment team that is experienced in the therapy of such disorders. In addition to treating the abnormal eating behaviors, all the treatment options for addressing the mood disorder that usually accompanies an eating disorder are required. A psychiatrist with experience in treating eating disorders, mood disorders, and children and adolescents is optimal, though it may be difficult to find someone with this level of expertise, as the only specialty of the three eligible for separate certification by a governing board is that of child and adolescent psychiatry. Additional members of the treatment team should include experienced psychotherapists, family therapists, and nutritionists, all of whom are necessary to treat these complex and very dangerous illnesses.

"Cutting" and Other Self-Harming Behaviors

W e have described in the last two chapters two types of self-harming behaviors that frequently complicate mood disorders: substance abuse and eating disorders. As Drs. Paul McHugh and Phillip Slavney point out in their book *The Perspectives of Psychiatry,* a disorder is something people *have* whereas a behavior is something people *do.*[1] This distinction is important when developing a treatment plan for a psychiatric problem. Treating a disorder is often easier than stopping a behavior. In this chapter, we talk about a group of behaviors often seen in people with mood disorders, behaviors in which individuals intentionally injure themselves. "Cutting" behaviors and other forms of self-mutilation, as well as the ultimate self-harming behavior, suicide, fit into this category.

SELF-MUTILATION

This account from Jill (14 years old) appeared in the *New York Times:*

I was in the bathroom going completely crazy, just bawling my eyes out, and I think my mom was wallpapering—there was a wallpaper cutter there. I had so much anxiety, I couldn't concentrate on anything until I somehow let that out, and not being able to let it out in words, I took the razor and started cutting my leg and I got excited about seeing my blood. It felt good to see the blood coming out, like that was my other pain leaving me too. It felt right and it felt good for me to let it out that way.[2]

Self-mutilation is deliberate *nonsuicidal self-injury* (NSSI), usually by cutting or burning the body. By definition, it is self-injury that does not involve the desire to end one's life; the self-injury is, rather, an end in itself. This behavior inspires horror and disgust and seems utterly irrational to others, but it is increasingly common. Even suicide is, in a sense, easier to understand as possibly arising out of a desire to end suffering or out of a profound hopelessness and despair. The intentional self-infliction of pain and disfigurement, on the other hand, is incomprehensible, at least at first glance. Unfortunately, self-mutilation is not rare, and it has been estimated that "cutters" and other individuals who repeatedly harm themselves number in the millions—this behavior occurs in about a thousand persons per hundred thousand population per year.[3] Among young persons being treated for other psychiatric conditions, the prevalence can be as high as one in five.[4] Like substance abuse and eating disorders, self-inflicted injury is a complex behavior with no single "cause." Rather, it is best understood by examining the variety of factors that are involved in its development. Self-mutilation occurs in vulnerable individuals, is precipitated by emotional distress of various types, and is then sustained by additional and usually different factors.

In this section, we discuss what has been called *repetitive*, or *episodic*, *self-mutilation*. Elsewhere in this book, we describe other forms of self-harm, such as the repetitive head-banging occurring in severely developmentally disabled persons and the self-mutilation in response to hallucinations or delusional ideas in individuals with psychotic illnesses. Repetitive self-mutilation, on the other hand, occurs in nonpsychotic individuals who cannot resist impulses to harm themselves physically.

Again, it's important to stress that this is not suicidal behavior, that is, individuals are not acting out of a desire to end their life. Rather, they report that the behavior gives them rapid, though short-lived, relief from a variety of uncomfortable emotional states such as depression, anxiety, and anger. They describe how, while they are engaging in the self-harming behavior, they go into a trancelike state (called *dissociation*) and do not experience pain from their actions. Usually the individuals feel guilty and ashamed afterward and attempt to conceal what they have done. This pattern shares many behavioral elements with eating disorders, especially bulimic behaviors, and in fact, many patients with repetitive self-mutilation behaviors have eating disorders too.

Secondary effects of the behaviors help sustain them. As with eating disorders, it's quite a challenge to understand how self-mutilation can make a person feel *better* in any way and what feelings draw people to hurt themselves again and again. As with eating binges, episodes of self-mutilation seem to start out with a building sense of inner tension or distress that gradually increases to a point where it is unendurable. Patients report that injuring themselves provides an instant relief of this unbearable tension. They compare the relief they experience to lancing a boil, popping the lid off a pressure cooker, or bursting a balloon. The injury focuses frustration and emotional pain in the harmful act, and some patients report a sense of regaining control of their mental state by their self-injury. This sense of relief may last for hours, and the person often goes into a deep sleep afterward. Sometimes the act is highly ritualized, including a careful laying out of the cutting instruments and the materials to bandage the wound afterward.

The range of self-injuring behaviors is broad. Some individuals make only superficial skin scratches with their fingernails or pick at skin blemishes. At the other end of the continuum are those who collect razor blades, surgical gauze, and antiseptics and make careful incisions, which they then cleanse and bandage. Burning with lit cigarettes or heated metal objects is another common method of self-harm. For some people, self-mutilation seems to be a brief, time-limited behavioral syndrome, playing out over weeks or months. Only a minority of persons who repeatedly injure themselves go on to develop a sort of addiction to the behavior that can go on for years. Many of these individuals have mood disorders, but we still don't know how many mood disorder patients repetitively self-injure themselves or how many self-injuring individuals have a mood disorder. As with eating disorders, the individuals who self-mutilate appear to be predominantly female. The most important personality vulnerability factor seems to be impulsiveness. One study of women with self-mutilating behaviors found that about half of them had a history of or later developed an eating disorder, and about one-fifth had a history of alcohol or drug abuse, compulsive stealing, or shoplifting.[5]

The ability of the self-mutilating behavior to shock and horrify others, especially family members, is another proposed explanation for how such behaviors develop. Rendering family members (and therapists) gasping and helpless, as these behaviors do, can be a potent and dramatic way to act out anger and replace fear and depression with feelings of power and control.

The number of persons with this problem is growing, and it's fairly clear that young females are especially at risk. Articles and books in the lay press that describe and discuss "cutters" have appeared with increasing frequency.[6] The practice of self-mutilation has been glorified through the vast availability of information on the Internet. Sites like YouTube and Instagram carry sometimes graphic depictions of self-injury.[7] The same kinds of social factors that influence the development of eating disorders may be at work to increase the numbers of young women who are drawn to "cutting" behaviors. In 1992, *People* magazine published excerpts from a biography of Princess Diana that revealed not only her eating disorder behaviors but her repeated episodes of cutting herself as well. Film idol (and teenage heartthrob) Johnny Depp displayed scars on his forearm and told *Details* magazine in 1993 that he cut himself with a knife to mark special times in his life.[8] Just as the glorification of thinness and the societal pervasiveness of dieting lead increasing numbers to attempt to lose weight and trap a few of them into eating disorder behaviors, the glamorizing and romanticizing of self-injury in the famous may be leading more and more to try cutting. The increasing prevalence and acceptance of such body modification behaviors as tattooing, piercing, and scarification (producing tissue injury to develop decorative scars) among young people may also be a factor, reducing the barriers to trying cutting by making painful and visible assaults on the body more acceptable.

The treatment of self-mutilation resembles that of eating disorders: the individual must be persuaded to give up a behavior that, however perverse, is powerfully addictive. Treating underlying depression is, of course, always necessary. Therapy to identify other sources of uncomfortable emotional states and to help the individual learn alternative ways of coping with them is extremely important. Treating repetitive self-mutilation is complex and requires intensive, long-term multidisciplinary therapy, preferably by specialists in the treatment of these problems.

A specific technique for treating patients who engage in repetitive self-mutilation is a form of cognitive therapy called *dialectical behavioral therapy* (DBT). We discussed DBT in chapter 9 as a form of therapy that may be helpful for many young people with depression. DBT focuses on emotional regulation and distress tolerance, on learning to cope with negative feelings without acting irresponsibly to end them. DBT has now been validated to help with many different forms of negative experiences, but it was specifically created to help patients with chronic suicidal or nonsuicidal self-injury, particularly those with borderline personality disorder.[9] Dr. Marsha Linehan, the founder of this technique, later admitted that she was a former cutter herself and that this influenced her development of DBT: "I developed a therapy that provides the things I needed for so many years and never got."[10] DBT focuses on helping the patient identify and interrupt the thinking and emotional processes that lead up to an episode of self-mutilation (or other poorly adaptive behaviors, such as aggression) and consists of weekly individual psychotherapy and group therapy sessions. There is a strong emphasis on learning how to tolerate distressing emotional states, on learning to better regulate emotions, and especially on changing behavior patterns to eliminate self-harm. For adolescents who have repetitive problems with self-mutilation, seeking out a therapist who is trained and experienced in DBT is an essential part of the treatment process. DBT has also been shown to help in multiple domains beyond self-injury, including generally tolerating distress and reducing emotional reactivity. As you can imagine, in many ways it is tailor-made for the tribulations of adolescence. In fact, a modified form of DBT specifically for adolescents includes their parents in the treatment, which can greatly reduce strife in this relationship. This form of DBT externalizes the dialectical debate. Whereas classic DBT focuses on the internal mental processes of a single person, DBT for adolescents works on bringing together the sometimes opposing viewpoints of parent and child.

In the introduction to an issue of a psychiatric research periodical devoted to the topic of self-mutilation, the scientific editor, a well-known psychiatrist, stated, "The typical clinician treating a patient who self-mutilates is often left feeling a combination of helpless, horrified, guilty, furious, betrayed, disgusted and sad."[11] As in treating other destructive but addictive behaviors, the intense and specialized treatment required for self-injury behaviors is often difficult and time consuming; recovery can be frustratingly slow. Fortunately, more and more research on the causes and correlates of this syndrome is being done, and the number of therapists who are skilled in its treatment is increasing.

ADOLESCENT SUICIDE

In the chapters in this part of the book, we have been discussing complex behaviors that often complicate mood disorders but that are shaped and precipitated by many factors and influences—behaviors that do not have any simple cause. Suicidal behavior also falls into this category.

We discuss the danger signals of an impending suicide and talk about suicide prevention later in this book (chapter 18). Here, we want to discuss adolescent suicide a bit more abstractly and address some misconceptions about suicide in this age group.

The rates of suicide among adolescents rose steadily in the United States during the second half of the twentieth century. In 1956, the completed suicide rate among 15- to 19-year-olds was just over 2 per 100,000 individuals per year, a number that turned out to be the lowest of the century. By the mid-1980s, this number had increased nearly five-fold, to about 11 per 100,000 per year. Most strikingly, boys almost entirely accounted for this dramatic increase in the number of adolescent suicides, with the suicide rate for males in this age range approaching 20 per 100,000 per year in 1988. The rate has declined slightly since then, likely due to increased education and a larger awareness of adolescent depression itself. The adolescent suicide rate hit a low of 10 per 100,000 in 2000, though since then it has crept back up slightly to 12 per 100,000 in 2013. During this time, suicide rates for young women stayed about the same, so this fluctuation is again almost entirely due to increased rates among young men.[12]

The number of adolescents who make *suicide attempts* is far larger than the number who actually kill themselves. For every adolescent who commits suicide, more than a hundred others have made an attempt. Most of these attempts do not result in any injuries, and many are medically inconsequential, such as taking a handful of aspirin tablets or making superficial scratches on the wrists. Studies have indicated that only about 2 to 3 percent of adolescents who have made a suicide attempt seek medical treatment.

Studies also show that twice as many adolescent girls than adolescent boys make a suicide attempt, but more than five times more boys than girls actually kill themselves. Boys who attempt suicide do so by more lethal means. In fact, of all suicide attempts resulting in death, half involve a gun and a quarter involve suffocation (which includes hanging). These two methods are those most commonly attempted by boys. It has been suggested that those who *attempt* suicide and those who "succeed" in killing themselves are two different (though overlapping) groups. But a review of the research studies on individuals who make suicide attempts and on those who die from completed suicide reveals that, aside from the differences in sex ratio, the characteristics of the two groups don't appear so terribly different clinically. Also, most adolescents who actually kill themselves have previously made a suicide attempt. It appears that both groups usually suffer from psychiatric problems, most commonly mood disorders.

For many years, mental health experts held on to what might be called the "Romeo and Juliet" theory of adolescent suicide, the idea that adolescence is a time of stress and that any individual exposed to an intolerable amount of psychological stress is at risk for suicide. The theory was a natural outgrowth of the early Sturm und Drang ideas about adolescence that we discussed in chapter 2: that all adolescents are volatile, impulsive, and raging with emotions, and those who attempt suicide are, like Romeo and Juliet, simply more volatile and impulsive and under greater environmental stress. This is clearly not the case. The majority of adolescent suicide victims suffered from a mood disorder. Environmental stressors seem to play some role in the behavior, but the underlying psychiatric illness appears to be the most important factor. For this reason, suicide prevention programs aimed at adolescents are beginning to shift away from "stress management" models to programs that educate adolescents and their families on how to recognize mood disorder symptoms and on the importance of treatment.

One model for understanding and preventing adolescent suicide, increasingly accepted in psychiatry, is that developed by David Shaffer and his colleagues at Columbia University in New York (figure 14-1). This multifactorial model proposes that suicidal thinking originates in an adolescent because of an underlying psychiatric disorder, but it smolders under the surface until more active consideration of suicide is precipitated by some stressful event; at that point, actual suicidal behavior is either facilitated or inhibited by a combination of mostly external factors.

Numerous studies have found that almost all adolescents who commit suicide suffer from depression, forming the basis for the proposed first step of this model: development of an underlying psychiatric disorder. Studies of adolescent suicides indicate that the most common underlying disorders are mood disorders. In boys, a combination of a mood disorder and a substance-abuse problem is especially dangerous. In a study of 6,483 adolescents aged 13 to 18, 12 percent had considered suicide, and 4 percent had attempted. Twenty-four percent of those who had attempted suicide abused alcohol, and 35 percent abused other drugs. Seventy-five percent of those who had attempted suicide also suffered from a mood disorder. More than 50 percent of this last group had shown signs of the disorder that were severe enough for them to already be in mental health treatment prior to their suicide attempt.[13]

The suicide attempt is precipitated in these vulnerable individuals by what Shaffer calls a *stress event,* an event such as being in trouble with the police or at school, the breakup of a relationship, or simply a recent distressing or humiliating experience. Often the stress event can be understood in relation to the underlying disorder: the stress event leads to an acute emotional crisis, with the development of extreme anxiety, dread, and hopelessness; a sense of inner tension and agitation builds, and the adolescent feels compelled to "do something."

At this point, external factors either facilitate or inhibit suicidal behavior. A strong religious belief about the sinfulness of suicide would be an inhibitory factor, whereas living in a culture where suicide is seen as an acceptable solution to problems (as was formerly the case in Japan) would be facilitating. The availability of a supportive, trusted influence such as a family member, a close friend, or a therapist to help soothe and decompress the situation would be an inhibitory factor. Studies suggest that feelings of connectedness to family are protective against suicide. Being or feeling isolated and unable to reach out for comfort or support, on the other hand, appears to facilitate suicidal behavior. This factor has been cited as important in understanding the much higher rate of suicidal behavior among adolescents who experience questions and conflicts over same-sex romantic at-

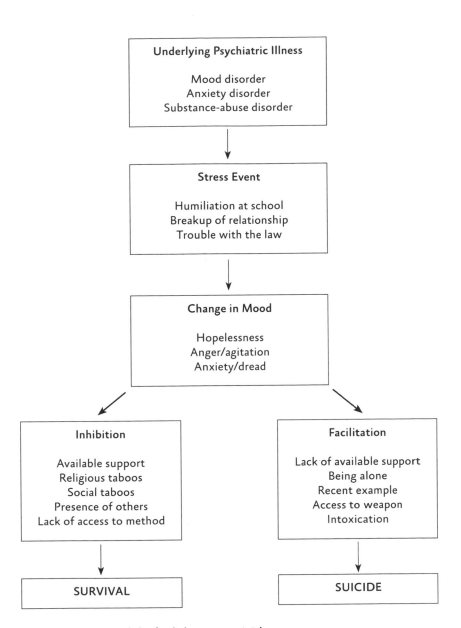

Figure 13-1 A model of adolescent suicide
Source: Described in David Shaffer and Leslie Craft, "Methods of Adolescent Suicide Prevention," *Journal of Clinical Psychiatry* 60, suppl. 2 (1999): 70–74.

traction and who feel unable to discuss this issue with family, friends, or the other usual sources of support.[14]

Another facilitating factor is the recent suicide of someone known to the adolescent or even someone simply living in the same community, serving as a model for suicidal behavior. The issue of *suicide contagion* has received attention: adolescent suicides often occur in clusters, and the suicide of one adolescent may lead to a series of suicide attempts by others. In February 1990, a physician notified the Centers for Disease Control (CDC; now the Centers for Disease Control and Prevention), the federal agency that investigates epidemics and the spread of illnesses, that two adolescent boys had committed suicide in Santa Fe County, New Mexico, within four days of each other. The New Mexico Department of Health investigated and found that the number of persons under the age of 20 who had been evaluated for a suicide attempt or suicidal thinking had *tripled* that month, a finding interpreted as strongly suggesting that one suicide can lead others to make an attempt. The study also found that the rate of suicide attempts had been consistently lower during June, July, and August for the preceding three years, giving support to the idea that school problems can be a precipitating factor for suicidal behavior.[15] A more recent Canadian study found even higher numbers, that adolescents were four and a half times as likely to attempt suicide after a schoolmate had done the same.[16]

Media coverage of an adolescent suicide that seeks to comfort a community may have the unwanted effect of promoting the clustering of suicides. Portrayals of a poignant family and community tragedy, with emotional descriptions of grieving friends and family and of moving eulogies given at well-attended funerals, have the effect of presenting suicide in a positive way and making it more acceptable. In 1994, the CDC issued media guidelines for reporting on suicide and listed several aspects of media coverage that may promote suicide contagion, including presenting simplistic explanations for suicide or presenting suicide as an understandable way of coping with personal problems ("John had recently broken up with his girlfriend"). Focusing on the victim's accomplishments and positive characteristics is also discouraged, as it may make suicide more attractive to vulnerable adolescents who feel that those around them do not appreciate them.

Other suicide facilitators include opportunity and access factors, such as being alone at home and the availability of a highly lethal suicide method, such as access to a gun. It is quite clear that the presence of a firearm in the home greatly increases the risk of suicide. One study showed that the presence of *any* firearm increased adolescent suicide risk, and whether the weapon was a handgun or a long gun, kept loaded or unloaded, locked up or not, made no difference.[17]

Perhaps the ultimate facilitating factor is intoxication of some type. Not only does a substance-abuse diagnosis greatly increase the risk of suicide, but most persons who kill themselves have alcohol in their bloodstream when they do so.

Public health efforts at suicide prevention in adolescents are increasingly focusing on the start of the process that leads to suicide: identifying the psychiatric disorder and getting the adolescent into treatment. Although hotlines and crisis services have been popular efforts, there is little research evidence to suggest they have much effect on suicide rates in a community. Efforts to educate high school students and parents about the self-identification of depression and referral for treatment also show no clear effect. Actually screening students for symptoms of depression and suicidal thinking and making further evaluation and treatment available to students who screen positive for symptoms may be the most effective means of reducing suicide rates in the community. According to a study by the CDC in 2009, 16 percent of all children in grades nine through twelve have seriously considered suicide, and almost 10 percent report attempting suicide within the past year.[18]

Suicide is still the third leading cause of death for those aged 15 to 24 years old. That said, recent data indicate that reduction in adolescent suicide coincided with the introduction of more effective SSRI antidepressant medications, and some have suggested that improved treatment of serious depression in adolescents may be an important factor in this welcome trend. Many factors are at work, however, and much research into the causes of and solutions to suicidal thoughts and behaviors remains to be done before the startling epidemic of adolescent suicide over the last fifty years or so can be truly under control.

The Genetics of Mood Disorders

A s has long been recognized, mood disorders cluster within families. Dr. Emil Kraepelin, who more or less invented the modern concept of mood disorders, wrote in his landmark textbook of psychiatry about one family in which "of the ten children of the same parents who were both probably manic-depressive by predisposition, no fewer than seven fell ill the same way; of the five descendants of the second generation, four have already fallen ill."[1]

For many years, research on the genetics of mood disorders was hampered by foggy diagnostic criteria and a lack of laboratory methods to identify genes. But this is changing. Not only have psychiatrists become more skilled in the diagnosis of mood disorders, but the biochemical methods available to locate and identify genes on the human chromosomes have become tremendously more sophisticated. These developments will, sooner or later, lead to a better understanding of the genetic mechanisms of mood disorders, which will in turn lead to better diagnosis and treatment of these illnesses.

GENES, CHROMOSOMES, AND DNA

A brief discussion of the principles of *genetics*, the scientific study of the inheritance of biological attributes, is necessary before turning to a discussion of the heredity of mood disorders.

The patterns and rules of inheritance in living things were first described by Gregor Mendel, an Austrian monk who, over many years, performed elegantly planned and executed experiments with plants, mostly garden peas, in his monastery garden. Prior to Mendel's work in the latter half of the nineteenth century, it was thought that the traits of one parent were simply blended with those of the other parent in their offspring, who thus had traits that were intermediate between those of the two parents. Mendel discovered that this was not always or even usually true. He found, for example, that crossing a pea plant that produced tall plants with a pea plant that produced short ones (which he did by transferring pollen from one plant to the other) did not give rise to seeds that produced medium plants—that is, an intermediate form. Instead, Mendel discovered that *all* the seeds formed from this cross gave rise to tall plants (figure 15-1A). When he then crossed the offspring plants and planted the next generation of seed, exactly *three-quarters* of them produced tall plants and *one-quarter* produced short plants (figure 15-1B). There were no intermediate forms and no blending of traits. The offspring received either a "tall" inheritance or a "short" one—there were no "in-betweens." Mendel concluded that each parent contributed something that determined plant size, and these "somethings" were distributed to the next generation, determining plant size in that generation. These "somethings" are now called *genes*, the units of inheritance.

We now understand that genes are sets of instructions for building proteins. All plants and animals are constructed (in part) and operate by means of proteins. Myosin (muscle protein), hemoglobin (the oxygen-carrying protein of red blood cells), and collagen (the structural protein of skin and cartilage) are just a few examples. Even the nonprotein structural materials of the body, such as the calcium salts in our bones, depend on proteins. Proteins called enzymes direct the manufacture of bone from calcium salts by expediting certain chemical reactions. Many hormones are proteins (insulin, for example), and those that are not (such as testosterone and cortisol) are manufactured by protein enzymes. In earlier chapters, we discussed some members of the protein family that are of enormous interest to those studying mood disorders: G proteins and the receptors for neurotransmitters. All proteins are built according to specifications contained in genes.

For many years, it was believed that genes were proteins also, that genetic information was somehow encoded in protein molecules. But by the

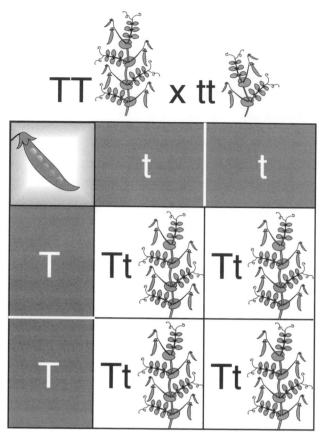

Figure 15-1 *Above*: Mendel's cross between a tall (*TT*) and a short (*tt*) pea plant. Each offspring (seed) receives two tallness genes, one from each parent plant. The seeds from this cross grew all tall plants because all received the *tall* gene (*T*), which dominates over the *short* gene (*t*). *Next page*: When the next generation of plants is crossed, one-fourth of them receive no *tall* gene (*T*) and therefore grow short plants.

mid-1940s, experiments with bacteria had proved that a far simpler family of biochemical compounds, called *nucleic acids,* contained the genetic information. In 1953, James Watson and Francis Crick published a paper in the British scientific journal *Nature* describing the structure of the most important of these compounds, deoxyribonucleic acid (DNA). With this discovery, the modern age of genetics had begun.

DNA molecules are long spiral chains, their links consisting of four simpler compounds called nucleotides. The four types of DNA nucleotides,

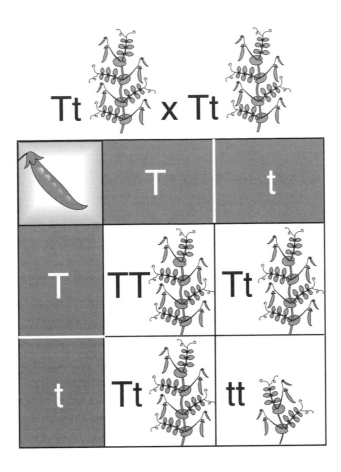

containing adenine, cytosine, guanine, and thymine (usually abbreviated as A, C, G, and T), are the elements of an elegantly simple code used to write out instructions for the manufacture of proteins. Just as you can write out a Morse code version of *Hamlet* using only dots and dashes, you can write out instructions for building hemoglobin, myosin, collagen, or any other protein using A's, C's, G's, and T's. That's what DNA does. You can think of the physical structure of a gene as the section of a DNA molecule that codes for one protein.

When the DNA molecule is doing its work in the cell, it is unraveled and stretched out and surrounded by a whole retinue of ultramicroscopic attendants busily reading the coded instructions and making proteins. When it's time for the cell to divide, another set of attendants carefully coil the DNA molecule into a compact cylinder and surround it with protective proteins to form the threadlike structures you probably looked at under the microscope in high school biology: the chromosomes.

GENETIC DISEASES

Sometimes the pathways from a certain gene to a certain protein to a certain trait or disease are easy to follow (although, in medicine, as we'll see, the understanding of these paths has usually been approached from the other direction: disease to protein to gene). Sickle-cell anemia is one disease for which the pathway from gene to disease is easy to follow. If you looked at the blood of a person with sickle-cell anemia under the microscope, instead of seeing the normal saucer-shaped red blood cells, you'd see abnormal crescent-shaped (sickle-shaped) cells. When scientists had the biochemical methods to look at the components of blood cells, they discovered that people with sickle-cell anemia had an abnormally shaped hemoglobin molecule, which tended to form abnormal chains within the cell, stretching the normally disk-shaped cells into the characteristic sickle shape seen under the microscope.

Because hemoglobin is easily purified, it was one of the first proteins whose structure was completely described (a feat that earned Cambridge University biochemist Max Ferdinand Perutz the Nobel Prize in 1962). Sickle-cell hemoglobin (hemoglobin S) was found to differ from normal hemoglobin by only a few atoms, the equivalent of a single substitution of one nucleotide for another in the gene of the DNA molecule. Because of a number of biochemical factors that made the hemoglobin gene especially accessible and easy to work with, scientists could pinpoint its location early on in the search for genes that caused human diseases. We now know that at one particular spot on the DNA molecule of persons who have sickle-cell anemia, there is an A instead of a T in the set of instructions. An abnormal hemoglobin molecule results from the reading of these incorrect instructions. The abnormal hemoglobin causes the abnormally shaped red blood cells, which block blood vessels and result in the symptoms of the disease. The pathway from abnormal gene to abnormal protein to abnormal cells to symptoms was completely described.

Genes have been identified and located for several other human diseases whose inheritance patterns indicate that they are single-gene illnesses. In some cases, this has been possible even though the identity or function of the protein that the abnormal gene codes for is unknown. Huntington's disease (or Huntington's chorea), the degenerative brain disease that afflicted folk-singer Woody Guthrie and his family, is one example. We know that the affected gene, the HTT gene, produces a protein called *huntingtin*, but we don't know what precisely the function of this protein is in the brain.

Scientists searching for "disease genes" now often use *linkage studies* to locate and identify genes. These studies take advantage of the fact that genes located close to one another on the same chromosome tend to stay together when the chromosomes undergo the process that apportions them into egg or sperm cells. In linkage studies, geneticists use gene maps that show the location of marker genes. First, DNA tests are performed on a blood sample of persons with the condition being investigated as well as on unaffected family members. Scientists then perform sophisticated mathematical analyses of the presence or absence of marker genes in affected and unaffected subjects to find an association between the condition and marker genes. If an association is found, the known location of the markers pinpoints the location of the gene for the condition. This method has been highly successful in locating the genes for several other single-gene diseases, including cystic fibrosis and Duchenne muscular dystrophy.

Studies have indicated that depressive disorders and bipolar mood disorders are probably related genetically at least some of the time. Serious depression is two to ten times more likely to occur among relatives of persons with bipolar disorder than in families of persons who don't have the illness. When we examine the family tree of persons with major depressive disorder, however, the data are not quite as clear; more persons with bipolar disorder than would be expected are found in some studies but not in others. This has been interpreted as indicating that when major depressive disorder shows up in families with bipolar disorder, the depressive illness is genetically similar to bipolar disorder, but that depressive illness in the absence of bipolar disorder in the family has more varied causes and may or may not share the same genes as bipolar disorder.

When several genes might be involved in an illness, the problem of gene identification becomes tremendously more complicated. And if the illness takes several forms or is difficult to diagnose, the task becomes monumental. Unfortunately, all of this applies to mood disorders. Most scientists looking for genetic causes of mood disorders agree that these are not one-gene illnesses like sickle-cell anemia or Huntington's disease. Mood disorders are caused, in all probability, by several different genes, perhaps as many as a dozen or so. The illnesses take many different forms and are sometimes difficult to diagnose.

In the late 1980s, several reports appeared that purported to link a mood disorder, specifically bipolar disorder, to specific regions of chromosomes. The most significant report was of an Amish family that seemed to carry a gene for bipolar disorder on one end of chromosome 11 (human cells have twenty-two pairs of chromosomes, numbered 1 through 22, and a pair of sex chromosomes). In this study, the researchers thought they had overcome at least one of the usual hurdles to finding a "bipolar gene." This particular family pedigree seemed to indicate Mendelian (that is, single-gene) inheritance at work. Even if several possible genes could cause bipolar disorder, this particular family seemed to pass on the disorder through only one gene. Mathematical analysis of previously identified DNA markers pointed to chromosome 11, and the statistical significance of the findings appeared solid. Zeroing in on a mood disorder gene seemed within reach.

These results were called into question within months, however, when another team of scientists took a look at the mathematical analysis. But it was the issue of diagnosis that ultimately scuttled this ambitious study. Several of the individuals who had been classified as unaffected when the data were originally collected developed symptoms of bipolar disorder later on. When the new numbers were crunched, the results fell apart completely.[2]

Linkage studies have pointed to several different locations on different chromosomes as possible sites for "mood disorder genes," but results are still preliminary. The most promising candidates currently are genes involved in creating a certain type of channel in the neuron. When a neuron gets a signal to release neurotransmitters (for example, serotonin or norepinephrine), the mechanism by which this occurs is quite complicated. It's not as simple as the electrical impulse directly shooting forth the chemicals. In fact, the impulse causes channels in the neuron to open and allow the entrance of calcium ions. As the concentration of calcium in the neuron increases, other chemical changes occur, leading to the release of neurotransmitters. In certain genome-wide studies, a particular gene, CACNA1C, has been closely associated with the development of bipolar disorder. Functionally, this makes sense—lithium, one of the oldest and best-studied medications used to control this condition, lowers the influx of calcium, essentially making the neurons less excitable. Although it would be silly to think that this one gene is responsible for all of bipolar disorder (in studies, most persons with the genetic mutation do not develop bipolar disorder), it is certainly reasonable to say that scientists may very well have found a strong risk factor for developing the condition.

Looking for genes involved in major depressive disorder has been even more challenging, because this disorder can be more difficult to diagnose. A 2014 review article examining "the nine published genome-wide association studies" for major depressive disorder found, in the authors' words, no significant genetic associations, a conclusion echoed in many of the papers and reviews of the field.[3] Studies of *childhood-onset* major depressive disorder, however, have demonstrated that this form of the illness is especially likely to run in families, suggesting that studies of the childhood-onset illness will prove the most useful for studying genes for major depression.

People who develop mood disorder symptoms most likely have inherited *several* genes that predispose them to these illnesses. There is even some thought that these are relatively common genes that many people carry without ever developing a mood disorder. Perhaps a certain number of genetic "hits" are necessary to make a person vulnerable to developing mood disorder symptoms, and perhaps certain environmental conditions are needed as well. Furthermore, genetics don't seem to tell the entire story of bipolar disorder.

Monozygotic twins are those sets of siblings who have exactly the same genetic information. Almost immediately after the mother's egg is fertilized (forming the *zygote*), it splits in half, forming two zygotes from the original one (*mono-*). Two separate eggs that happened to be fertilized at the same time result in *dizygotic twins*, that is, twins originally from two (*di-*) zygotes. Even in monozygotic twins, if one twin develops bipolar disorder, the second twin has only about a 70 percent chance of developing the condition—leaving 30 percent up to other factors, likely the environment. These findings and factors make the search for mood disorder genes all the more daunting.

WHAT WE KNOW

Until we identify specific genes and discover what proteins these genes code for, we can talk about the inheritance of mood disorders in only a general way. What we can say is that the children of persons with mood disorders have an increased risk of developing a mood disorder. Assigning a number to that risk is tough, owing to some of the same problems that have made the search for mood disorder genes so difficult, especially problems of diagnosis. But the risk appears to be several times that of the general population, around 10 percent, for those with a family history of the disease.

The risks in bipolar disorder can be quantified more precisely. The chance that a child whose parent has bipolar disorder will also develop bipolar disorder parallels the numbers above for mood disorders in general: the risk is about 10 percent, several times the risk for the general population. However, children of persons with bipolar disorder are also at a higher risk for unipolar (depression only) illness, and when you add this risk in, the percentages go up into the high twenties. This means that the children of persons with bipolar disorder have about a one in four chance of developing some kind of mood disorder and about a one in ten chance of developing bipolar disorder.[4]

Persons with mood disorders need to be alert to signs and symptoms of mood disorders in their children and get them into treatment if these signs appear. Although we may be uncertain about the details of the inheritance of these illnesses, we are not at all uncertain about the importance of early diagnosis and treatment.

THE SEARCH CONTINUES

Several factors make scientists optimistic about eventually discovering genes for mood disorders. In 1999, scientists of the Human Genome Project and Celera Genomics announced the "first draft" of the full sequence of human chromosomal DNA. Specifically, the pattern of A's, C's, G's, and T's in human DNA had been worked out. Based on this work, scientists can now perform multiple types of chemical analyses on an individual DNA strand to look for small or previously unknown mutations. Researchers can now look for single nucleotide polymorphisms (called SNPs, pronounced "snips"), changes in a single genetic base pair, across the entire genome.

But the number of identified genetic markers used in the linkage studies that *will* determine gene locations continues to rise. These markers, like signposts along the length of the chromosome, designate particular locations in the DNA molecule: the more genetic signposts there are, the easier it will be to find a particular gene. More precise diagnoses will also help, as will the study of larger family pedigrees and the development of technological advances—both biochemical methods and more powerful computers and software to do the mathematical analyses.

Even when genes are identified and tests developed that can look for these genes in individuals, predictions about who will develop symptoms will probably still be imprecise. Several genes are likely involved and genetics is unlikely to be the whole story. Environmental factors are probably operating to determine who will and will not be affected: psychological and perhaps physical stresses and traumas may be important. Some evidence suggests that viruses play a role in the development of some psychiatric disorders. So even when a gene or genes are identified and can be tested for, finding that a person has a mood disorder gene will probably mean that she has a much higher chance of developing symptoms than someone who does not have the gene, but that developing them is not a certainty—the risk is not 100 percent. This will raise many difficult questions about who should and should not be tested and who is entitled to know the test results (siblings? spouse? employers? insurance companies?).[5]

But finding the genes responsible for mood disorders may lead to new treatment approaches that will benefit everyone with these illnesses. Gene identification, and identification of the function of these genes or their gene products, will undoubtedly shed light on the biochemical basis of mood disorders. It may then be possible to design medications or other treatments based on knowledge about the causes of symptoms at the cellular or biochemical level—rather than stumbling on treatments by accident, as has been the case so far. This science is called *pharmacogenomics*. It is already widely used in the treatment of cancer and certain other conditions and is just beginning to be examined for use in psychiatry. Genetics research is one of the most challenging but also the most promising areas of investigation of mood disorders and could truly revolutionize the treatment of these illnesses.

Part IV

GETTING BETTER & STAYING WELL

K EEP IN MIND THAT DEPRESSION and other mood disorders of adolescence are not "cured" by any of the treatments discussed in part II of this book. We are getting better and better at treating these problems, but talk of cures is still years, perhaps even decades, in the future. In the meantime, however, many things can be done to promote good mental health. Millions of individuals who have been diagnosed with mood disorders are living happy, healthy, and productive lives. Unfortunately, many are not. These chapters are intended to help you and your adolescent maximize the chances of staying in the first category and out of the second.

But if you're looking for a simple list of do's and don'ts, we're afraid you will be disappointed. Instead, in chapter 16, we lay out some general principles that underlie the sorts of advice and recommendations usually given to patients in the doctor's office or clinic. We hope that after reading this chapter, you'll have a better understanding of why some of the do's and don'ts that you hear from the doctor and therapist are so important. We also address what the terms "doctor" and "therapist" actually mean and describe in detail the various types of mental health professionals so that you can make more informed decisions when seeking treatment for yourself or your child.

Adolescent depression doesn't just affect the teenager. Inevitably, family members are affected in countless ways, both directly and indirectly, and chapter 17 addresses this aspect of the illness. We go over what family members can do—and just as important, what family members cannot and should not try to do—to help their loved one who has a mood disorder.

In chapter 18, we've collected together some principles for dealing with emergencies and highlighted the types of emergency situations that, in our experience, patients and their families often fail to prepare for. It's so tempting to put off thinking about and planning for things that we hope won't happen; we emphasize in this chapter how important it is not to give in to this temptation and how easy it is to be prepared for emergencies.

Finally, we provide a short chapter that looks into the future and explores some of the exciting possibilities that may help us to better understand mood disorders. With this knowledge, it should be possible to improve the diagnosis and treatment of these illnesses, and perhaps one day, we might be able to cure them.

Strategies for Successful Treatment

This chapter presents some principles of good treatment for mood disorders in adolescents. In depression and bipolar disorder, perhaps as in no other kind of medical problem, treatment must be carefully tailored to each patient's needs. In part III of this book, we discussed how complex treatment can be when a person has complicating problems such as substance abuse or an eating disorder along with a depressive disorder. But even when these complications are not in the picture, the best treatment approach to adolescent depression is often a matter of much dispute. Experts frequently disagree on what should be considered standard treatments for these illnesses, which often makes treating patients more of an art than a science.

The prescription of medications for the treatment of adolescents with mood disorders is frequently off label (see chapter 5), and new medications are being touted all the time as useful for treating mood disorders years before they are approved, or even evaluated, by the FDA. How should parents make decisions about medication, about choosing a therapist, about hospitalizing their child? How can parents know whether their child is receiving the best possible treatment?

Because these illnesses are so complex and poorly understood, and because the treatment for each individual must be so, well, individualized, we cannot say which medication should always be tried first or tell you at what point a different or an additional pharmaceutical should be tried. We can lay out some principles that underlie successful treatment and that will usually, though perhaps only slowly, put your child on the road to recovery.

DIAGNOSIS, DIAGNOSIS, DIAGNOSIS

You've probably heard the old saw that the three most important factors in the real estate business are location, location, location. A similar saying would be well heeded by all mental health professionals: the three most important factors in the development of a treatment plan in medicine are diagnosis, diagnosis, diagnosis.

Occasionally, we speak to a parent who is interested in getting a consultation about her adolescent's problems and who tells us something like, "Our son has been diagnosed with major depressive disorder, ADHD, obsessive-compulsive disorder, generalized anxiety, separation anxiety, and a learning disorder, and his therapist is wondering if he's not developing a personality disorder, too. We want to be sure he's getting the proper treatment for all his diagnoses so that doesn't happen." Not infrequently, the adolescent is on a different medication for *each* of his "diagnoses" and is experiencing so many side effects that any kind of normal functioning is impossible.

This problem of accumulating diagnoses in psychiatry seems to us to be a direct result of the checklist method of the *DSM*, which lists different symptoms of various disorders and asks for several from this column and a few from that one to meet diagnostic criteria. It's easy to go through these various diagnostic checklists and, before you know it, compile a collection of "diagnoses" on the patient's chart. But this is not what the diagnostic process is all about. Rather, the job of the diagnostician is to put together *all* the information about symptoms, family history, medical history, and the findings on examining the patient in order to formulate a coherent diagnostic impression that pulls together the entire story—in *one* diagnosis if possible.

The overlap of the symptoms of bipolar disorder and ADHD is a good example of how this kind of diagnostic confusion can develop. Some of the symptoms of ADHD, such as impulsivity, impatience, disorganized thinking, and poor concentration, are also seen in adolescents with bipolar disorder. These are distressing symptoms that deserve attention, but more important, they deserve the right kind of attention. If they are an expression of the mood changes of bipolar disorder, then medication for ADHD won't help. (In fact, the medications used to treat ADHD, stimulants and antidepressants, may make things worse.) Adolescents with depression are especially vulnerable to irritable mood states that lead to behavioral problems, which might suggest an additional diagnosis of conduct disorder, oppositional defiant disorder, or again, bipolar disorder. We want to persuade you that giving these young people additional *diagnoses* often doesn't clarify their situation; it just confuses the picture. This is a central tenet that is critical to, but often forgotten in, the diagnostic process. If a child is diagnosed at age 7 with ADHD, but later on it is discovered that he had the symptom of inattention only because of a developing depression, some clinicians will diagnose him with ADHD and depression, rather than re-evaluating the picture in light of new evidence and removing prior diagnoses.

In the field of medicine, such errors of continuation without critical examination are called "chart viruses." These include statements, recorded in the diagnostic record, that may or may not continue to be true. In hospitals, these diagnoses lay indolent and spread throughout the hospital record, only becoming virulent when they seem most applicable. For example, a person asked while in the hospital how her headaches are doing, even though she hasn't had a headache for twenty years, may be experiencing the results of a chart virus. These chart viruses can infect the field of psychiatry as well—not through bad intentions, but rather through the reluctance to doubt previous clinicians' diagnostic acumen without becoming familiar with a case in depth.

When we see a patient, particularly a young one, who seems to have too many diagnoses, we wonder how much information gathering and critical thinking went into the diagnostic process. The same applies when there seem to be too many medications. Does the patient really have several different disorders that need treatment with different medications—an antidepressant for depression, a tranquilizer for anxiety, a mood stabilizer for "mood swings," and so on? Or have too many medications accumulated to treat various symptoms of one underlying disorder?

Making a diagnosis is the process of attempting to identify the one process that can explain all the patient's symptoms. There is a scientific principle called *Occam's razor,* named after the medieval theologian-philosopher who developed it, William of Occam (or Ockham). This principle states that the simplest explanation for a phenomenon is always preferable to a more complex one and is more likely to be correct. Obviously, a patient may have two or three or four different disorders that require different treatment approaches. But if all the symptoms can be understood as expressions of *one* disorder, treating that one will likely alleviate all the symptoms. Even when there are clearly several problems, formulating the relationship between them often makes the treatment plan priorities clear. For example, an adolescent may have a depressive disorder that is "fueling" eating disorder behaviors and precipitating alcohol abuse. These three problems all need attention, but unless the depression that is driving the behavioral problems is aggressively treated, treatment aimed solely at behavioral problems will not be very effective. We have seen many young people go through extensive (and expensive) substance-abuse rehabilitation programs only to relapse as soon as they leave the program, because a mood disorder underlying the substance-abuse problem was never identified and properly treated.

Such mistaken thinking can run the other way as well. An adolescent with recurrent substance-abuse issues and problems with stealing, who sometimes feels morose when the result of his actions run into him (for example, failing a test from partying the night before), may appear depressed at that time. This does not mean that he has a major depressive disorder and that a simple medication will cure all his problems. At the risk of sounding redundant, taking the time and energy to determine the true diagnosis and to develop a well-rounded and thought-out treatment plan is critical to success.

Another diagnostic pitfall is putting too much emphasis on psychological testing and rating scales. We occasionally see parents who have been told their child has a particular psychiatric diagnosis solely on the basis of psychological testing (meaning paper-and-pencil testing) or even of a score on some rating scale administered by someone. Frequently, parents think this is the definitive diagnostic procedure.

Sometimes parents insist that psychological testing be administered to their child as part of the assessment. Rating scales and psychological testing are helpful tools for the diagnostic process, but they are not sufficient in themselves to make a psychiatric diagnosis and are rarely the final answer to the diagnostic process. Many people think that a psychological test is like an x-ray: by means of trick questions and other mysterious methods, a psychological test will reveal what's "really" there, just as an x-ray can reveal a break in a bone that is otherwise undetectable. This is nonsense. In fact, the opposite may be true. One of us once treated a very bright child who, unfortunately, leaned toward the lazy side. He quickly found a particular quirk of many psychological tests, that those who do more poorly are asked fewer questions. He found that by intentionally flubbing examinations, the testing would be over sooner. The subpar results of his testing clearly did not match up with his clinical picture according to the psychiatrist, and so the test was quickly declared invalid for this child—in this instance, the acumen of the physician was far more important than any testing. Most psychological tests simply compare the way an individual answers standardized test questions with the way groups of others have answered the same questions, then assume that the individual being tested resembles the group whose answer patterns are closest to his answers. Psychological tests are useful for helping to identify personality styles quickly, but they don't do a good job of making diagnoses of psychiatric disorders. A depression rating scale might show that someone is depressed, and might even be able to say whether he is mildly or severely depressed, but it won't do a good job of determining whether he is suffering from major depressive disorder, bipolar depression, dysthymic disorder, or more minor temporary depression. And when a person is depressed, psychological tests aren't even that good at what they usually do best—revealing personality style—as the depression will alter the profile of answers. If the individual being tested isn't very honest in completing questions, the results will be practically meaningless.

This is not to say that psychological testing is never useful. It is accurate and precise in grading people on the mental abilities that we call intelligence. The same goes for tests of memory, some types of problem-solving abilities, and other types of mental functioning (again, this is true only as long as the person is answering honestly and putting forth her best effort). Paper-and-pencil tests are also helpful in screening large groups of people for the possibility that they might have some psychiatric disorder, identifying those who need a more in-depth evaluation for a particular problem (in psychiatry, these kinds of tests are globally known as *screeners*, because they screen for potential problems and hint at further evaluation but make no attempt at actual diagnosis). Various rating scales are useful in assessing changes in the severity of a disorder's symptoms over time. An individual who is suffering from depression might fill out a depression rating scale at each visit to the doctor or therapist, who can then make a more accurate assessment of progress, or lack of it, by following how the scores change over time.

The decision to give an adolescent an antidepressant cannot be made on the basis of a depression questionnaire. The diagnosis of attention-deficit/hyperactivity disorder cannot be made on the basis of a score on a screening test for ADHD. A battery of psychological tests is rarely necessary for the accurate diagnosis of mood disorders; a thorough psychiatric assessment is sufficient (and, as we make clear in the next section, necessary). Like any other laboratory test, a psychological test can answer a specific question that comes up during a psychiatric assessment (How intelligent is this person? How introverted is this person compared with most people?). But putting an individual through a battery of tests to "see what shows up" is not good practice.

One last warning about the diagnostic process. In a popular book for parents about mood disorders in young people, we read something to the effect that parents should be wary of a doctor who "takes too long to make a diagnosis." We are going to tell you the exact opposite: beware of a doctor or therapist who seems too eager to make a diagnosis, especially multiple diagnoses, too quickly. Adolescent mood disorders are often complex, subtle, and difficult to diagnose, especially if the adolescent has come to treatment reluctantly or has trouble describing how she feels. If there are complicating factors like substance abuse or behavioral problems, it may take several visits over a period of weeks or even months to get the best sense of how the various problems relate to each other and what the best treatment approach should be. Quick, confident diagnoses may feel satisfying—like an answer to the question "What is wrong with my child?"—but frequently lead to sloppy, ineffective treatments.

CHOOSING THE TREATMENT TEAM

We hope we have convinced you by now that adolescent-onset depressive disorders are serious illnesses that require serious treatment by specialists. The foregoing section should make it clear that the diagnostic process is vital in starting treatment on the right track. For that reason, a full evaluation by a board-certified psychiatrist experienced with adolescent mood disorders, or even better, by one specifically board certified in child and adolescent psychiatry, should be part of the treatment process as early as possible. There are places for many different types of professionals in the treatment of depression, but the point of entry should be with an individual who has the most training and experience in the treatment of psychiatric illnesses: a psychiatrist. Sometimes this is impossible, as busy psychiatric clinics will insist on initial appointments with a therapist, but the psychiatrist should still be involved as soon as possible.

Psychiatrists have attended medical school, where they have learned about the structure and biological functioning of the human body (anatomy and physiology); the biological chemistry of the body and the principles of treatment with medication (pharmacology and therapeutics); the methods for examining bodily and mental functioning by physical examination, mental status examination, laboratory tests, and medical imaging (x-rays, MRI scans [magnetic resonance imaging], and other methods); as well as the principles of treating medical and surgical diseases. After medical school, psychiatrists train in the specialty of psychiatry for four or more years, applying what they have learned in medical school about diagnosis and treatment of disease to the evaluation and treatment of psychiatric problems of all types. They also learn a set of therapeutic skills that are somewhat different from those of their colleagues in other medical specialties: the principles of psychotherapy. By studying the works of behavioral scientists—Freud, Erikson, and others—psychiatrists learn about the theories of psychology, and by counseling and doing therapy with patients, they learn the practice of psychotherapy. At the conclusion of their training, most psychiatrists apply for certification by the American Board of Psychiatry and Neurology. They undergo two full days of examination, including written tests and a review of cases on video. These exams are created by experienced psychiatrists who have themselves passed the tests. The examiners have a vested interest in making the tests challenging, for by certifying the performance of the test takers, they are welcoming them to the public as representatives of their own profession. Applicants who pass these rigorous examinations are said to be *board certified* in general psychiatry. This board certification is somewhat equivalent to obtaining a black belt in martial arts. Though it seems like the final point of mastery to the uninitiated, it is really only the beginning of the psychiatrist's practice and opens the door for further specialization. An old saying is this: "The path to black belt is about the creation of technique. The path beyond black belt is about learning to implement technique effectively."

Part of the requirements for general psychiatry training is that, at some point, trainees must spend two months working with children and adolescents. The form this work takes, however, can be highly variable. In the training program at Johns Hopkins Medical School, senior trainees work on child inpatient units for that time, receiving a good overview of the most intense forms of treatment. At other programs, however, first-year trainees (called interns) may only have to observe a clinical session once a week, leading to a thin experience. Alternatively, they may work in a college counseling center or somewhere similar, which certainly doesn't help them later when their patient is a 12-year-old. For psychiatrists interested in treating younger patients, a separate training follows their general psychiatry residency. Called a *fellowship*, it entails two additional years of working exclusively with children and adolescents. Psychiatrists who enter this realm of work train with a variety of experts in the diagnosis and management of conditions in young people, and in various settings. After completion of this work, the trainees are eligible for board certification in child and adolescent psychiatry, an additional full day of testing and examination.

One thing that many people don't know is that no authority requires psychiatrists to receive board certification for treating young people (and there are psychiatrists who decide simply that they'd like to add younger people to their patient list, without having any sort of experience in the matter). In fact, any licensed physician could in theory open a psychiatry practice with no experience at all. Therefore, it is up to you, as an educated consumer, to ask any potential providers about their training and board certification. You can also go to the American Board of Psychiatry and Neurology website (abpn.org) and look up the current status of any physician you are considering seeing.

Psychiatrist clearly signifies a specific type of training. The term *psychotherapist* more appropriately describes what someone does, rather than how the person was trained. The term describes anyone who does counseling and psychotherapy, regardless of professional education and training experiences. This can include psychiatrists as well as a number of other professionals. At times this number can seem daunting, and more professionals are becoming involved all the time. Just as physicians typically place letters after their names, such as MD (for medical doctor) or DO (for doctor of osteopathy), most if not all psychotherapists will have some letters after their names that tell you something about their educational and professional background.

A *psychologist* has a doctoral degree in the science of human behavior: psychology. Psychologists usually place PhD (doctor of philosophy) or PsyD (doctor of psychology) after their names. The field of psychology covers the whole range of mental life and functioning: language development, how visual images are represented in the brain, the neural basis of learning, crowd behaviors, and the accurate measurement of intelligence— these are only a few of the areas within this immense and fascinating field. Psychologists may focus on understanding normal human—or animal— behaviors through research (experimental psychology); on the dynamics of groups of individuals (organizational psychology); or on the treatment of psychological problems (clinical psychology). *Clinical psychology* is the subspecialty of the field involved in the treatment of emotional problems. Clinical psychologists usually have a four-year college or university degree plus several more years of education toward their final degree. Clinical psychologists have focused on theories of human behavior as they relate to the development of psychological problems, have learned various methods of psychological assessment (such as giving and scoring intelligence tests, personality assessments, and other tests of mental functioning), and have learned about psychological disorders and psychological treatments: counseling and psychotherapy. Doctoral-level psychologists must go on to complete a year of postgraduate training (called an *internship* or sometimes a *residency*), in which they gain practical experience in assessing patients and doing therapy. There is no national accrediting body for clinical psychologists, but most states require psychologists to be licensed in order to see patients. Typical licensure requirements include passing a written and sometimes an oral examination and having completed a degree and an internship in a program approved by the American Psychological Association.

After psychologists achieve their doctorate degree, they may go by the title "doctor," but this is not the same as being a medical doctor—most psychologists have no training in the practice of medicine. Although some states have given psychologists permission to prescribe certain psychoactive medications, we shudder to think of anyone taking a prescription written by a professional who has no training in how it might affect her physical body, or interact with other medications she may be taking. Many mental health professionals see the medications we prescribe as benign; they underappreciate how significant the effects of medications can be. A colleague of ours was asked if it might be possible to put together a training on the effects of medications for prescribing psychologists, so that they might begin to appreciate the medications' more general effects on their patients. He replied "There already is one. It is four years long and called medical school." We firmly agree.

Many, perhaps even most, psychotherapists have a degree in social work, a field that emphasizes the interactions of individuals with their various social groups: their family, community, and culture. A *clinical social worker* specializes in helping individuals, couples, or families with emotional or relationship problems by means of counseling and psychotherapy. Most clinical social workers have a master of social work degree (MSW), though some have a doctoral-level degree (DSW or PhD). Many social workers instead list their licensure after their names. An LGSW is a licensed graduate social worker. After additional training and supervision, a social worker may apply for licensure as a licensed certified social worker, or LCSW. After yet more training and experience, licensed certified social workers may apply for an added modification so that they are recognized as an LCSW-C (in which the last C stands for "clinical," the subspecialty of social work focused on direct mental health treatment of patients, much like clinical psychology). Social workers may apply for membership in the Academy of Certified Social Workers of the National Association of Social Workers after submitting professional references and passing a written examination if they have a master's degree in social work from an approved program and two years of supervised social work experience. The letters ACSW in a social worker's title indicate this membership. A more advanced certification is the diplomate in clinical social work, requiring additional years of experience and a more advanced examination. These social workers use the designation DCSW to indicate this certification. The American Board of Examiners in Clinical Social Work is another organization that issues a certification in advanced practice to social workers who have a master's degree in clinical social work from an approved college or university program, have practiced in the field for five years and seen clients under supervision for a certain number of hours, and have had colleagues and supervisors attest to their competency. Clinical social workers with this certification add the designation BCD after their name.

Some psychiatrists decide to limit their practice to psychotherapy and become primarily psychotherapists, though this is becoming increasingly rare. Individuals with degrees in nursing may also work as psychotherapists. Often they have taken advanced training in therapy to do so. Their names typically end in RN (registered nurse, an associate degree), BSN (bachelor of science in nursing, a college degree), or MSN (master of science in nursing). All these providers must practice under a licensed physician. Nurse practitioners (NPs) and doctors of nursing practice (DNP) are in many states able to practice independently. These professionals, in contrast to psychologists, have training in the physical body and in the medications they prescribe.

Some psychotherapists have a degree in counseling and have trained specifically in this field. *Counseling* differs from psychotherapy in its emphasis on giving advice and guidance rather than treating disorders. School counselors often have this kind of training background. A more advanced degree in counseling allows counselors to put LCPC (licensed clinical professional counselor) after their names. Alternatively, a counselor with a college degree may choose instead to get licensure as a marriage and family therapist (MFT). These therapists, as their title indicates, typically focus more on couples and family therapy than on individual therapy, so they are not as likely to work individually with children. Though there is certainly a lot of overlap between counseling and psychotherapy, counseling can be thought of as helping psychologically healthy individuals to improve and enhance their functioning and coping skills, and psychotherapy as treating individuals with psychological problems, helping them return to normal functioning. Clergy may get training in pastoral counseling and even pursue advanced training in psychotherapy. Pastoral counselors usually emphasize spiritual growth, of course, and the religious and ethical principles of their particular faith will guide their work with clients. The National

Board of Certified Counselors offers various certifications in counseling to individuals with diverse educational backgrounds.

Of all these professionals, the one with the most training and experience in the treatment of persons with illnesses is the psychiatrist. It's difficult to think of a reason that parents who suspect serious depression in their child shouldn't *begin* the evaluation with a psychiatric consultation, but this isn't always possible. Many busy mental health clinics practice an alternative structure in which a patient meets with a therapist or counselor first, before seeing the psychiatrist later. Typically this is because of the relatively small number of psychiatrists and is not ideal. This shortage of psychiatrists is a problem especially in child and adolescent psychiatric clinics. As of 2013, there were only about eight thousand board-certified child and adolescent psychiatrists in the country, about one for every ten thousand children. This severe deficiency of child and adolescent psychiatrists is a well-recognized phenomenon. We are obviously aware that not everyone will be able to find a board-certified child and adolescent psychiatrist in his area, but if possible, it really is the best option. If you are faced with a situation in which a child and adolescent psychiatrist is unavailable, be certain to question the psychiatrists you consider for your child about their training and experience with this age group. Far from being insulted, any qualified psychiatrist will be delighted to inform you, and impressed that you care enough and know enough to ask.

As with choosing any other physician, choosing a psychiatrist must usually start with a review of your medical insurance plan. Psychiatry is considered a specialty referral, and depending on your coverage, some phone calls and investigation will be necessary and will save a lot of headaches later. If your family is enrolled in a health maintenance organization (HMO), your child will be able to see only a psychiatrist approved by the plan and usually only with the referral of your child's primary care physician. If your family is covered by a preferred provider organization (PPO), the primary care referral may or may not be necessary, and you may be able to go outside the organization's list of approved doctors for psychiatric care at a lower reimbursement rate (you will be required to pay for a higher percentage of the fee).

HMOs and PPOs frequently outsource their mental health services. This usually involves contracting with a particular mental health practice or other provider group. Sometimes this group provides all treatment services; sometimes it provides certain services and manages others, contacting other providers and approving treatment with them upon receipt of written treatment plans. (Chapter 18 goes into more detail on these insurance issues.)

More and more psychiatrists, especially child psychiatrists, are opting not to participate in insurance plans because of all the paperwork and other kinds of extra work involved in dealing with managed care organizations. These practitioners require their fees be paid in full at the time of each visit; patients must then submit receipts to their insurance plan and deal with the reimbursement issues themselves. Unfortunately for individuals needing care, the best practitioners often fall into this category, making for some difficult financial decisions. Many psychiatrists will operate on a sliding scale, so it is always worth calling to inquire.

Once you know what your options are from an insurance standpoint, you can narrow your decision making. Pediatricians usually have a consultative relationship with a psychiatrist, or with a psychiatric practice, to whom they are confident referring their patients. This is perhaps the best referral source. If you live in a community where there is a university with a medical school, the medical school will have a department of psychiatry and usually a practice affiliated with the faculty. These clinics can often be the best resources available, but because of their value, they typically fill up quickly.

Some psychiatrists choose to provide a full range of services, including psychotherapy. Many do not, so it may be necessary to assemble a treatment team including both a psychiatrist and a separate psychotherapist. Choosing a psychotherapist will involve a similar process. It may be easier, in fact, because psychiatrists almost invariably have working relationships with several psychotherapists to whom they refer their patients. Because the fees of nonphysicians are usually lower than psychiatrists' fees, paying a psychotherapist out-of-pocket may be a bit more feasible. But remember that psychotherapy sessions are often weekly for many months, so the total outlay may be substantial. Given the devastating effects of untreated depression on the lives of adolescents, however, this is clearly a good investment.

Another factor to keep in mind when going through this selection process is that the management of mood disorders is a long-term proposition. One of the most important requirements for successful treatment is a *long-term* relationship with the treatment professionals. We cannot emphasize this point strongly enough. One of your goals in selecting a professional is to find someone who will be providing care for *years* to come.

Do not be afraid to get a second opinion about treatment. When your child doesn't seem to be benefiting from treatment, getting another clinician to take a fresh look at the diagnosis and treatment plan can be very helpful. The treating physician will not, or at least *should* not, object to a request for a second opinion. In fact, a physician often welcomes the opportunity to get some help and advice in managing a difficult case. Many university medical centers provide consultation services and often have mood disorder experts on the staff. The consultant will be able to help most if he can review as many treatment records as possible, so some advance work on your part, collecting records in preparation for a consultation, is well worth the effort. The consultant's report usually has a "have you thought of . . ." tone and will often raise questions rather than answer them, but this approach is usually the most helpful for the clinician who already knows the patient well and who will thus be able to incorporate new ideas into the treatment plan.

Beware, however, of the temptation to get too many opinions in a tough case. It is *not* useful to radically alter a treatment approach every month or so based on yet another consultant's recommendation; a parade of experts can result in more confusion than clarity.

The treatment of mood disorders must often adjust to the clinical situation: medications are started and stopped, added and taken away; therapy may need to be more intense and frequent at times, but the patient may be able to take a "vacation" when things are going well. Especially for adolescents, who often have trouble expressing their feelings and who sometimes are just plain oppositional, having a psychiatrist and a psychotherapist who know them well is a tremendous asset in their treatment.

Keep a treatment record for your child. This can be in chart form, as in figure 16-1, or it can simply be a diary. Record what medications your child has taken, including dates of starting and stopping, doses of medications, and blood levels (if they have been ordered). List any side effects or problems your child has had with the medications and also the treatment response.

This sort of list is extremely useful in many different situations: if there is a change in doctors, if you request a second opinion, or if treatment seems to have stalled for some reason and a detailed review of all treatments and responses is needed to see what hasn't yet been tried. Many parents assume that the physician is keeping a detailed history of each patient's prescriptions. The reality is that they probably are not. The information is available, but it may be embedded deeply within the individual progress notes and treatment records. Keeping your own succinct "cheat sheet" can be one of the most important contributions you make toward your child's improvement.

ELIMINATING PATHOLOGICAL INFLUENCES: MOOD HYGIENE

The word *pathological* is derived from the Greek word for "disease," and by *pathological influences,* we mean factors in the patient's environment that make illness symptoms worse or more difficult to treat. Just as an adolescent with diabetes must make lifestyle changes (including dietary changes, such as what to eat and the timing of meals) as a part of controlling blood sugar, so an adolescent with a mood disorder must make lifestyle changes to have the best control of mood symptoms. Sometimes this means a minor adjustment, sometimes a major overhaul, but this is *not* an optional part of the recovery process.

What is meant by *mood hygiene*? Simply put, it refers to practices and habits that promote good control of mood symptoms in persons with mood disorders. *Hygiene* is a word that we probably don't use as much as we should in medicine—and we certainly don't use it as much as we used to. Hygeia was the Greek goddess of health, the daughter (or in some versions of the story, the wife) of Aesculapius, the god of medicine (figure 16-2).

Hygiene, or *hygienics,* is the science of the establishment and maintenance of health (as opposed to the treatment of disease) and concerns itself with conditions and practices that are conducive to health. The hygienic conditions and practices we think of today are usually related to cleanliness, but the word has a much broader meaning. Johns Hopkins University's School of Hygiene and Public Health (founded in 1916; now the Bloomberg School of Public Health), University of London's School of Hygiene and Tropical Diseases (1924), and other such institutions were founded to study methods for the prevention of disease and for promoting and improving the

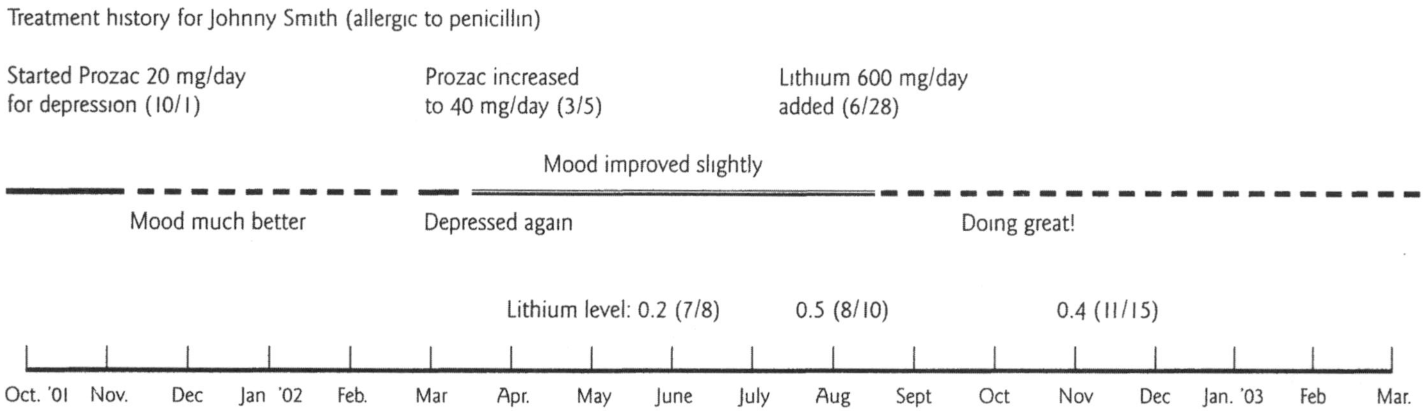

Treatment history for Johnny Smith (allergic to penicillin)

Started Prozac 20 mg/day
for depression (10/1)

Prozac increased
to 40 mg/day (3/5)

Lithium 600 mg/day
added (6/28)

Mood improved slightly

Mood much better

Depressed again

Doing great!

Lithium level: 0.2 (7/8)   0.5 (8/10)   0.4 (11/15)

| Oct. '01 | Nov. | Dec | Jan '02 | Feb. | Mar | Apr. | May | June | July | Aug | Sept | Oct | Nov | Dec | Jan. '03 | Feb | Mar. |

Figure 16-1 A sample treatment record. This sort of chart is extremely helpful in recording medication response, especially when a mood disorder is difficult to treat and multiple medications have been tried.

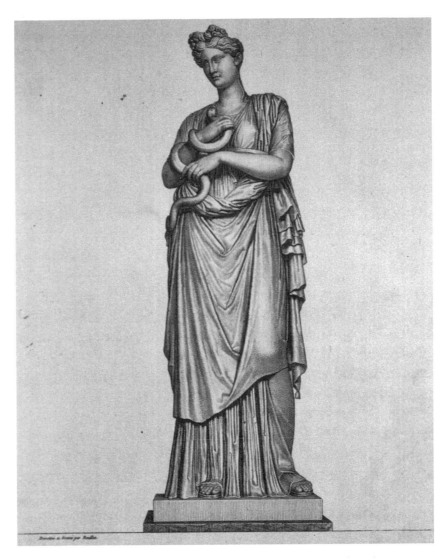

Figure 16-2 Hygeia. *Source*: Courtesy of the National Library of Medicine.

health of whole communities. Pre-dating these was the Mental Hygiene Association, founded in 1909 by former asylum inmate Clifford Beers (who probably had bipolar disorder) and now called the Mental Health Association; its purpose is to promote emotional health and well-being and to advocate for better and more available treatment for psychiatric illnesses.

Several areas of research on mood disorders, especially bipolar disorder, show just how important preventive measures can be for improving symptom control in these illnesses. Things like stress management and lifestyle regularity make a big difference.

One of the most astute students of the study of mood disorders, German psychiatrist Emil Kraepelin, noticed in his patients with mood disorders that early in the course of illness, their mood episodes often came on after a stressful event in their lives. In the final edition of his textbook of psychiatry (which was almost ten times longer than his first edition), published early in the twentieth century, Kraepelin noted: "In especial, the attacks begin not infrequently after the illness or death of near relatives . . . Among other circumstances there are occasionally mentioned quarrels with neighbors or relatives, disputes with lovers . . . excitement about infidelity, financial difficulties . . . We must regard all alleged injuries as possible sparks for the discharge of individual attacks."

Kraepelin was quick to point out that these events were triggers, not causes, and that "the real cause of the malady must be sought in permanent internal changes which . . . are innate." Kraepelin noticed, however, that later in the course of the illness, attacks occurred "wholly without external influences," and he proposed that at this later stage, "external influence[s] . . . must not be regarded as a necessary presupposition for the appearance of an attack."[1]

Research has shown that severe depressive episodes in many young persons are preceded by the death of someone close to them or by some other loss or difficulty. One study found a significant association between adolescent depression and repeated episodes of loss or significant separation during childhood. The most interesting finding of the study was the lack of an association between depression and only one episode of serious loss. *Multiple* events were necessary to trigger depression.[2] Studies on adults with bipolar disorder have shown that the initial and early mood disorder episodes are often related to psychological stresses, but that after several episodes, the illness can take on a life of its own, and episodes are more likely to arise spontaneously.

These sorts of findings are quoted to support the idea of a *kindling* phenomenon in mood disorders: a match held to a pile of wood may start a small flame that quickly dies out; but if the process is repeated often enough, a fire is kindled, and no more matches are needed. In a similar way, repeated episodes of psychological stresses, especially loss, set off a chain of events in vulnerable individuals (perhaps individuals who have inherited a genetic vulnerability to mood disorders) and an episode of depression results.

An interesting parallel in animals can be demonstrated by repeatedly giving animals small doses of stimulants, such as cocaine. Over time, animals become *more* rather than less sensitive to the stimulant, and repeatedly giving the same small dose causes *increasing* amounts of behavioral stimulation in the animal. A close examination of the brain cells of these animals, with and without the prolonged stimulant treatment, reveals that a certain gene that was not previously active has been turned on by the repeated stimulant exposure. This same gene can be made to turn on by stressing the animals (by depriving them of water, for example). This work with animals, showing that electrical and chemical stimulation as well as stress can bring about long-term changes in behavior (possibly through alterations in gene function), is thought by many experts to be highly relevant to the study of mood disorders.[3] The observation that anticonvulsant medications, which have "anti-kindling" effects, are highly effective in treating bipolar disorder is one piece of evidence cited in support of this line of thinking.

Several direct observations on patients indicate that kindling may occur in individuals with mood disorders. First, patients sometimes have more environmentally triggered mood episodes early in the course of their illness and more spontaneously occurring episodes later. Second, they sometimes have an acceleration in their illness as they age, with episodes occurring more and more frequently as time goes on. And third, mood episodes make patients more sensitive to stress than they might otherwise be and more likely to relapse. In a study of fifty-two adult patients with bipolar disorder followed up for two years, those who relapsed during the time of the study were much more likely to have experienced some stressful event. In this group of patients, those with a greater number of prior mood episodes were *more* sensitive to these stresses: they were more likely to relapse under stress, and they relapsed more quickly.[4] The worsening of depressive illnesses as individuals age has been demonstrated in many studies.

Given the observations that (1) psychological stress can make a person with bipolar disorder more vulnerable to having a mood episode, and that (2) as the person has more and more episodes, the symptoms can be triggered by smaller and smaller amounts of stress and adversity, then (1) *preventing* relapses of depressive episodes is extremely important, and

(2) individuals with mood disorders need to work hard to minimize situations of emotional stress in their lives.

PREVENTING RELAPSE WITH MEDICATION

After the development of antidepressant medications made the medical treatment of severe depression widely available in the 1960s, the question quickly arose of how long antidepressant medications should be prescribed. Although we do not have enough information yet to answer this question definitively, the information we do have supports long-term treatment.

Studies in adults clearly indicate that an antidepressant medication that has been effective for an individual with a serious depression should be continued for at least twelve months. We tell patients and parents of patients that anyone who has had a serious depression that has responded to treatment with an antidepressant medication shouldn't even consider discontinuing the medication for at least a year. For some individuals, this becomes difficult. Taking a daily pill, which may have minor but annoying side effects, to prevent a depression they do not feel, seems less and less important. For other individuals, however, it is a blessing. They recognize that they had been more depressed and more severely depressed than they had ever realized while in the grip of their illness. These are the individuals who had never really known what a normal mood was like before starting on medication. Not infrequently, these patients come to their appointment at the twelve-month mark ready to plead with us to let them *continue* taking antidepressant medication. They never need to plead. We are only too happy to let individuals who have been helped by antidepressant medication take it for as long as they wish. We are convinced by our personal experiences of treating many patients with mood disorders that every relapse of depression increases the chances of the illness becoming more difficult to treat. Research data clearly indicate that early-onset depression is a more severe illness. Some guidelines for the treatment of adults with depression recommend that individuals with the onset of severe depression before the age of 20 take medication indefinitely because of the higher probability of relapses.[5] Instead of asking, "Why should I continue taking antidepressant medication?" people who have had serious depression should probably ask, "Why *shouldn't* I continue taking antidepressant medication?" Individuals who have a family history of either bipolar disorder or recurrent major depressive disorder are especially well advised to take this long view.

For individuals with bipolar disorder, the evidence for the necessity of long-term treatment with medication is much more compelling. True bipolar disorder is clearly a relapsing illness that must be treated continuously and indefinitely to prevent the development of episodes. This piece of evidence re-affirms how essential it is to reach—and get—a correct diagnosis. Many irritable adolescents receive a misdiagnosis of bipolar disorder, which sets them on a path of taking medications for years of their lives that they may not have needed in the first place.

ADDRESSING SUBSTANCE ABUSE

The surest recipe for treatment failure in mood disorders is the continued use of intoxicating substances. For many reasons, adolescents with mood disorders must not drink alcohol and must certainly not use marijuana or other drugs.

The first is that alcohol and many drugs have direct toxic effects on the brain. In the chapter on substance abuse, we mentioned that drugs such as ecstasy have been shown to kill neurons. We know that chronic alcoholics develop memory problems and the wide-ranging decline in all mental abilities that psychiatrists call dementia. These damaging effects are more significant in the developing brain (neurons and their interconnections are still growing and developing in an adolescent's brain). Substance abuse in young people is thought to interfere with the brain's developmental process and may disrupt brain development in permanent ways that, currently, we can only guess at.

By altering the chemical functioning of the brain, substance abuse has effects on mood as well. Persons who abuse alcohol and individuals who are crashing from binges of cocaine or amphetamines can go through profound depressive episodes that seem to be directly related to the chemical effect of the intoxicating substances. It's thought that the high of getting intoxicated from alcohol or anything else results from a massive stimulation of the pleasure centers of the brain. These centers become exhausted and depleted of their chemical messengers because of this massive overstimulation, and this depletion is what is thought to result in the depressive crash and other mood changes that occur after intoxication. Thus, for individuals undergoing treatment for mood disorders, getting intoxicated interferes with the therapeutic process to relieve depression or to stabilize mood. A simple way of thinking about this is that getting intoxicated depletes the chemicals that antidepressants are trying to boost. We tell patients that drinking or getting high when under treatment for depression is like punching holes in a bucket that you are trying to fill with water—continued substance abuse makes treatment for a mood disorder pretty pointless.

We believe that abuse of marijuana is the most harmful in this regard, because it is the most insidious. Because marijuana is slowly absorbed into the fat cells of the body and slowly released between episodes of "getting high," crashes into depression and obvious withdrawal symptoms are less apparent. It's as if the usual time line for these phenomena gets so stretched out as to become almost undetectable. We've seen many persons with depression in all age ranges who refused to stop using marijuana because they were convinced that marijuana had no effect on their mood, or that it even helped their depression—and whose depressions never quite went into remission.

A striking lesson in how marijuana use can be a powerful obstacle to treatment of depression comes through in the story of a young adult one of us was treating for severe depression. We'll call him Joe.

▼ Joe's severe depressions only partially responded to aggressive treatment with medications. A combination of quite a few medications was the only approach that kept him out of the hospital, and he was nearly nonfunctional in his family life and was unable to work. Joe insisted that marijuana was the only thing that helped him feel better for a few hours, and he absolutely refused to give it up.

One day, I stepped into the clinic's waiting area to ask Joe to come back to the interviewing room for his medication appointment, but I didn't see him among the patients waiting for their appointments. There was a young man with a neck brace who looked familiar, but it seemed that Joe must have stepped out to the restroom. When I turned to the receptionist and asked if she knew where Joe had gone, the young man with the neck brace stood up. It was Joe, looking so bright-eyed, relaxed, and energetic that he was unrecognizable.

It turned out that Joe had been in a swimming accident that had injured him badly enough to put him in a rehabilitation hospital for nearly three months—long enough for the marijuana to get out of his system completely. His depression steadily improved over this period, and by the time he got out, most of his medications had been discontinued, and he was taking only a single antidepressant. We had both learned an important lesson about the connection between depression and substance abuse the hard way (though it had certainly been a lot harder on Joe). ▲

Substance abuse is, in a way, a means of coping with adversity by retreating into getting high. As we explained in chapter 12, substance abuse also has the effect of crowding out other activities like school and family life. Another activity it crowds out is emotional maturation. Learning how not to get caught takes the place of learning how to trust and be trusted. Learning how to find and secure a steady supply of alcohol or drugs takes the place of learning how to make and keep healthy relationships with peers. Planning for the next high takes the place of planning for the next five years. Every mental health professional who has worked with adolescents can tell you that young people who are substance abusers seem to stop maturing emotionally at the age they started using. A 19-year-old who is able to stop using alcohol or drugs may have the emotional development of a 13-year-old, if that's when he started using. Catching up from this "maturity deficit" can take several years and a lot of therapy.

The most difficult issue parents face when their child is abusing substances is knowing how much intervention on behalf of the adolescent is helpful and how much is *enabling*. The concept of enabling a substance abuser has developed out of the treatment literature on alcohol abuse and refers to helpful actions on the part of family members that turn out to sustain rather than stop the substance abuse. The classic example is the wife of an alcoholic who calls her husband's boss to report that her husband is "sick" and won't be in to work, when he is actually hung over from his latest alcoholic binge. Rather than helping her husband, she is actually enabling him to escape the consequences of his alcoholism—consequences that could force him to face his problem and decide to get treatment. Parents must decide how much interceding on their child's behalf with school authorities, other family members, and even the police is helpful and how much is enabling their child to remain a substance abuser. Because adolescents have a difficult time appreciating the long-term consequences of their actions, this is an even tougher problem. At what point is "tough love" too tough? There are no easy answers. In his powerful account of his daughter's struggle with alcoholism, Senator George McGovern writes, "The trouble with waiting for people to 'hit bottom' is that they may do so only after they have destroyed their lives or the lives of others."[6] (More on this dilemma in the next chapter.)

ADOPTING A LIFESTYLE THAT PROMOTES MENTAL HEALTH

Just as physical stress is to be avoided by persons with certain physical problems, psychological stresses need to be identified and addressed by individuals who suffer from mood disorders. Although most of us have little control of when and how stress and conflict come into our lives, we sometimes have *some* control, and we can learn how to better manage the stress and conflict we can't avoid—and here we will put in another plug for counseling and therapy. Serious, *vigorous* attention to any ongoing sources of significant stress is critical in the management of mood disorders. It's no accident that family therapy is so often recommended as an adjunct treatment in adolescent mood disorders. Numerous clinical studies show that ongoing family conflict is a major risk factor for relapse of depressive disorders in adolescents.[7] Relationship difficulties, too much advanced coursework at school, an overly ambitious schedule of extracurricular activities—all these things can make for too many demands, too much stress, and can be risk factors for relapse of the mood disorder.

Adolescence is a time of developing lifestyle habits that will last a lifetime. Putting things off until the last moment invariably raises stress levels. Eliminating procrastination as a way of dealing with things goes a long way toward eliminating a lot of stresses. A growing body of research supports the notion that external regulators like regular sleep and activity schedules help with mood stability. *Establishing and sticking to a personal schedule* is essential. Establishing regular times for going to bed and getting up in the morning—seven days a week, if possible—is highly recommended. Adolescents need more sleep than adults, not less. For many 12 to 18 year olds, nine to ten hours every night is optimal (though rarely possible). Research on sleep shows that many other lifestyle factors contribute to or detract from good sleep. Adolescents might consider cutting caffeinated beverages out of their diet completely, or at least making a habit of not drinking caffeine-containing soft drinks or coffee or tea after noon. Heavy meals late in the day should be avoided. Regular exercise has been shown to benefit sleep and has many other benefits besides, on blood pressure, for example. These factors are even more important for adolescents with mood disorders because of possible medication side effects on appetite and energy level. Several medications increase appetite and can be mildly sedating at first. Attention paid to healthy diet and exercise habits will go a long way toward improving energy level and avoiding unwanted weight gain. Consultation with a nutritionist can be helpful, and developing an exercise program through the physical education department at school is often an option.

It is impossible in these few paragraphs to distill this process of taking stock of personal conflicts and stresses and to detail the kind of individual attention it takes to deal with them. There's no list of helpful hints or do's and don'ts that we can give you here. Rather, we are recommending *serious examination* and *fundamental change*. This change may involve something as minor as cutting back on participation on a team or as major as changing schools. Adolescents face many important decisions: decisions about selecting a high school and a college, after-school jobs and career paths, and for older adolescents, moving away from home and sometimes even getting married. These decisions need to be considered even more thoughtfully and carefully for those with a mood disorder. Counseling and psychotherapy are an invaluable help in sorting through options and making these decisions.

The Role of the Family

hen a child is miserable, parents want to make things better. Small children aren't very hard to cheer up. They will delight in a little toy surprise, a trip to a fast-food restaurant, helping mom or dad in the kitchen or with washing the car. But when an adolescent is seriously depressed, no amount of cheering up can help. Worse, when the symptoms of depression take the form of oppositional behavior and irritability, parents may discover that their child has become a hostile stranger who seems intent on tearing the family apart. Parents may be frightened and angered to discover that their son or daughter is drinking, using drugs, or engaging in other dangerous behavior. It's easy to be so paralyzed by fear and anger that ordinary decisions become overwhelming.

As in any illness, the role of the family includes support, understanding, and encouragement of the person who is ill, and the role of the parent includes nurturing, protecting, and supervising. The first step in being able to provide this kind of support is understanding some important facts about the illness. It's also vital to get the help and support *you* need to be there and be strong for your child.

RECOGNIZING SYMPTOMS

Never forget that someone with a mood disorder does not have control of his mood state. People who do not suffer from a mood disorder sometimes expect the person who does to be able to exert the same control over his emotions and behavior that they themselves are capable of. When we sense that we are letting our emotions get the better of us and we want to exert some control over them, we tell ourselves things like "snap out of it," "get a hold of yourself," or "pull yourself together." We are taught that self-control is a sign of maturity and self-discipline. We are indoctrinated to think of people who don't control their emotions well as being immature, lazy, self-indulgent, or foolish. But you can only exert self-control if the control mechanisms are working properly, and in someone with a mood disorder, they are not.

People with mood disorders cannot "snap out of it," as much as they would like to (and understand that they *desperately* want to do so). Telling a depressed adolescent something like "pull yourself together" is simply cruel; in fact, it may reinforce the feelings of worthlessness, guilt, and failure already present as symptoms of the illness.

The first challenge facing family members is to change the way they look at behaviors that might be symptoms of the illness—behaviors like not wanting to get out of bed, being irritable and short tempered, or being "hyper" and reckless or overly critical and pessimistic. Our first reaction to these sorts of behaviors and attitudes is to see them as laziness or meanness or immaturity and to be critical of them. In a person with a mood disorder, this almost always makes things worse: criticism reinforces the depressed adolescent's feelings of worthlessness and failure, and it alienates and angers the hypomanic or manic individual.

Keep in mind, however, that these behaviors are symptoms primarily when individuals are in the midst of an episode of a mood disorder. Our response to some of these same behaviors in adolescents who are not experiencing an episode should not necessarily be the same as when they are. We have both treated patients who are perfectly well (what we would term *euthymic*) but claim to suddenly develop a deep depression if and only if they are asked to participate in things they would rather not do; they then return to euthymia after the stressor is relieved. One of us even treated a patient who eventually admitted that there was an upside to being depressed. As she put it, "My boyfriend is only nice to me when I'm depressed," meaning that he took care of her and did not expect her to act or function independently. Just as an accurate diagnosis is essential in putting together an effective medical and psychiatric treatment plan, it is also critical in creating a "family" treatment plan that helps you best address behaviors that may—or may not—be symptoms of an underlying illness.

This is a hard, but critical, lesson to learn: don't always take behaviors and statements at face value. Learn to ask yourself, before you react, "Could this be a symptom?" Little children frequently say "I hate you" when they are angry at their parents, but parents know that this is just the anger of the moment talking and that these are not their child's true feelings. Irritable, depressed adolescents will say "I hate you" too, but this is the illness talking, an illness that has hijacked their emotions. The depressed adolescent might also say, "It's hopeless. I don't want your help." Again, this is the *illness* and not your child rejecting your concern.

GETTING INVOLVED IN TREATMENT

Frequently, parents don't know what role to take in their child's treatment, and sometimes the seemingly contradictory messages given by therapists and psychiatrists can be confusing. Be interested in your child's life, but not nosy. Be assertive and set limits, but do not be overly controlling. Be sensitive to changes in your child's behavior, but don't jump to conclusions. Inform the therapist of all you observe about your child, but don't expect the same in return. Respect your child's privacy, unless you're afraid for her safety! In many ways, negotiating the role of the parent in treatment is similar to negotiating the role of the spouse in a relationship, and it requires the same amount of careful consideration, and possibly continual adjustment. Although we go through some general guidelines here (and into some specifics especially around the delicate nature of confidentiality), your role as parent is best understood through a continued discussion with both your child and your child's therapist.

Different therapeutic modalities will require different levels of involvement. In discussing medication effects, parents and child will be expected to report on everything and anything they've observed that may be helpful or a side effect. Cognitive-behavioral therapy is similar in that parents can participate in the treatment, both in the office and at home, when their children are trying to use the skills they've learned. In psychodynamic treatment, on the other hand, parents may learn to expect a closed door with very little, if any, information at all. Different phases of treatment will also require different levels of involvement. During standard outpatient therapy during a relatively stable time, parents may be able to take a small step back. Should an emergency develop or a hospitalization be required, however, parents sometimes have to take time off from work due to the necessary level of involvement.

Every individual's health care information is protected from unauthorized access by a law entitled HIPAA (the Health Insurance Portability and Accountability Act of 1996). In short, this law makes the identifiable health information of each individual his or her own property. There are exceptions to this, of course. For the purposes of this discussion, the health information of children is the property of their parents or legal guardians. Certain states have made exceptions to this rule in regards to reproductive and psychological health, but generally, parents have the legal obligation and the right to consent to or deny psychiatric treatment and medications for their children under the age of 18. The details of said treatment, however, are a little murkier. Parents have a right to ask questions and get answers about their child's treatment, particularly medications. The intimate details of individual therapy sessions, however, are expected to be confidential between the therapist and patient, provided that there is no risk to the child's health or safety. If, for example, a patient stated that she was planning on committing suicide, the clinician would legally have no choice but to tell the parents. However, should the parents ask, "Is Sally still dating Tommy? She won't tell me," the clinician will usually decline to answer or, in the best-case scenario, encourage that sort of a discussion with all parties in the room. Most clinicians lay out these delicate ground rules about privacy issues at the beginning of treatment.

On the other hand, after age 18, the patient is the only person who has the right to his own treatment information and records, a change that can feel both abrupt and shocking to parents. Psychiatrists experienced at dealing with these matters will always make parents aware of this change well before the child's adulthood (years before, preferably) and will attempt to negotiate the terms of this adulthood with the child. Unfortunately, this change can come at exactly the time when parents are most curious about the activities of their children, who may even have moved to college or elsewhere. The therapist cannot answer simple questions from parents, such as "Did Mark come to his appointment today?" Doing so would be considered a breach of ethics, unless the patient has explicitly signed a legal document giving the clinician permission to discuss his treatment with his parents.

Fortunately, many therapists are savvy enough to directly involve parents in the treatment of their children. Many clinicians will see parent and child together, at least initially. As the child ages, more and more time is spent with him alone, although the parent is usually brought in toward either the beginning or the end of the session for more information and discussion. Some clinicians will also give parents their own time to discuss their child's life; however, even these individual sessions must follow the confidentiality rules described above. Remember, your child is the patient. He should be given all (well, most) of the same rights you would expect from your own treatment provider. Just as you would probably not appreciate your therapist telling your child all about your own session, so would your child appreciate some degree of confidentiality in his. Your own individual meetings with his therapist should not be seen as your chance to "see into his mind," or to find out all the little details about his life that he wants to keep private. Quite the opposite! These are chances to discuss any changes you have observed and how you should best handle them.

Even though you are expected to respect your child's privacy in therapy, you are also expected to participate in the treatment as far as it affects your relationship with your child and your interactions. Your child's treatment isn't exactly like seeing another type of physician. You should not expect to drop them off at the door and pick them up in an hour. Also, don't ask the therapist or psychiatrist to confront your adolescent about behaviors you've observed if you can't be there to back up your observations. We find that separate conversations with the patient and the parents about these sorts of issues often become "yes, he did—no, I didn't" sessions that are simply not helpful for anyone. Going along with your child to doctor's appointments and sharing your observations and concerns during the visit *in your child's presence* eliminates miscommunication and ensures that everyone—therapist, parents, and patient—is operating with the same set of information. This can at times be uncomfortable, but that is exactly what therapy is for—making room for difficult discussions and issues so that they can be resolved productively.

Above all, parents should resist the impulse to bring the therapist to "their side." Conversations in which parents plead, "You can't tell her I know about this, but..." or "Don't tell her but..." can make ongoing therapeutic work difficult, to say the least. In general, children are very sensitive to perceived slights, and any feelings that their therapist and their parents are conspiring against them can ruin any further work that might have been done.

Parents sometimes err on the side of not being involved enough in their child's treatment, however, for fear of being a "tattle-tale"; they assume the clinician will notice the same things they've noticed about changes in moods or behaviors. One of the most valuable ways in which a family member can help in treatment is to provide a clear, undistorted view of the situation to the clinical team treating the adolescent. In our experience, family members are frequently the first to pick up on subtle changes in behaviors and attitudes that signal the beginnings of a relapse. We don't know how many times we have seen a patient in the clinic or even in the emergency room who has reassured us that she was feeling fine, whose behavior and mood seemed normal, whom we sent on her way, making a note in the chart that she was doing well, only to receive a panicked phone call from a parent or other relative a few hours later. "Didn't she tell you that she's lost ten pounds?" "... hasn't slept in three nights?" "... got suspended from school?" Contrary to popular belief, psychiatrists cannot read minds! Communicate your concerns openly, sincerely, and supportively—almost anything that might otherwise seem intrusive can be forgiven. Your goal is to have your child trust you when she feels most vulnerable and fragile. She is already dealing with feelings of deep shame, failure, and loss of control related to having a psychiatric illness. Be supportive, and yes, be constructively critical when criticism is warranted, but above all, be open, honest, and sincere.

Don't ask the psychiatrist or therapist to make parental decisions, and don't abdicate parental authority to the treatment team. The professionals are there to make recommendations and suggestions but not to make family decisions. Saying something like "you can't go to Tampa on spring break because the doctor said you can't" gives the adolescent the message that the parent has ceded authority to the professionals or, even worse, is incompetent to make decisions. It may cut off debate and argument in the short run but will inevitably backfire, actually encouraging defiant behavior. Remember that one of the goals of family therapy is to clarify roles and *your* parental authority. Adolescents need to know and to feel that their parents are in charge in the home. Your psychiatrist will back this up. When our patients ask us if something is OK to do, we always say that they will have to discuss it with their parents. In psychiatry, there's a phenomenon called *splitting*. It's something that every parent will be familiar with. The most common situation is that a child will ask one parent for something (say, staying out past curfew) and, if she doesn't get the answer she wants, ask the other parent. A more wily adolescent may start playing one side against the other or using other tools to manipulate the situation. "Mom said I could stay out late as long as you don't need the car," or "Dad's so strict! It drives me crazy. He won't even let me stay a half hour later! Can you believe that? Of course you can. You're cool, not like dad." For parents, our advice is always to be on the same page.

The exact same thing can happen in treatment. Parents will ask us if it's OK, from a mood disorders standpoint, to change their child's curfew, or to go on a trip. In the absence of a true psychiatric emergency, our reply is almost always, "What do *you* think?"

SAFETY ISSUES

Never forget that mood disorders can occasionally precipitate truly dangerous behavior. The dark specter of suicidal violence haunts those with serious depression, and rageful irritability can lead to frightening assaultive behavior. Violence is often a difficult subject to deal with, because the idea is deeply embedded in us from an early age that violence is primitive and uncivilized, a kind of failure or breakdown in character. Of course we recognize that the person in the grip of psychiatric illness is not violent because of some personal failing, and perhaps because of this, people sometimes hesitate to admit the need for a proper response to a situation that is getting out of control—when there is some threat of violence from the adolescent, toward himself or others.

Although family members cannot and should not be expected to take the place of psychiatric professionals in evaluating suicide risk, it is important to have some familiarity with the issue. As we've mentioned, young people who are starting to have suicidal thoughts are often intensely ashamed of them. They often hint about "feeling desperate," about not being able to "go on," but may not verbalize actual self-destructive thoughts. It's important not to ignore these statements but to clarify them. Don't be afraid to ask, "Are you having thoughts of hurting yourself?" People are usually relieved to be able to talk about these feelings and get them out in the open where they can be dealt with. But they may need permission and support to do so.

Remember that the period of recovery from a depressive episode can be a time of especially high risk for suicidal behavior. People who have been immobilized by depression sometimes develop a higher risk for hurting themselves as they begin to get better and their energy level and ability to act improve. Also, patients having mixed symptoms—depressed mood and agitated, restless, hyperactive behavior—may be at higher risk of self-harm. In fact, there is some evidence that mixed, or dysphoric, mania is the most dangerous mood state in this regard.[1]

Another factor that increases the risk of suicide is substance abuse, especially alcohol abuse. Alcohol not only worsens mood, it lowers inhibitions. People do things when drunk that they wouldn't do otherwise. Increased use of alcohol increases the risk of suicidal behaviors and is definitely a very worrisome development that needs to be confronted and dealt with.

The development of serious suicidal risk calls for action. Have an emergency plan and be prepared to use it. Involve your child and, if possible, the therapist or psychiatrist in developing this plan so that everyone is on the same page and there are no surprises. Don't hesitate to invoke involuntary commitment procedures if you are really worried and your child is not cooperating with the need for evaluation.

A less frequent but nevertheless real risk of violence is the violence toward others that can occur in mood disorders. Friends and family members should not hesitate to call for police help if they feel threatened. "What will the neighbors think?" should not be a concern when anyone's safety is at risk. If the situation is becoming dangerous, don't call the psychiatrist's office or the local emergency room—dial 911. Police officers are accustomed to dealing with psychiatrically ill individuals. They know safe physical restraint techniques, and they will be familiar with psychiatric emergency services in the community. In our experience, police officers will have the same goals you do in the situation: transporting your child quickly and safely to the appropriate health care facility so that he can receive proper treatment.

ARRANGING HOSPITALIZATION AND INVOLUNTARY TREATMENT

Every community has laws and procedures to safeguard individuals who are unable to care for themselves. Laws allowing the removal of children from the care of parents who are abusing them are the most obvious example. Another set of laws allows the treatment of individuals for psychiatric illnesses against their will in certain circumstances. One of the most difficult things parents might be called on to do for their child with a mood disorder is to sign for hospitalization over the child's protest or to initiate involuntary treatment or commitment.

The laws governing the admission of minors to psychiatric facilities and the involuntary commitment laws for adults are usually state laws, so they vary from one state to another; in addition to these state-by-state variations, local procedures can differ from community to community. This means that we can't provide a step-by-step procedure here, only general principles—but in our experience, it's not the procedures that confuse people but the general principles, so we think a brief discussion of this matter is worthwhile.

There are generally two types of admissions to the hospital: voluntary and involuntary. In nonemergency situations, parents must *consent* to the hospitalization. This gives them the legal right to voluntarily admit their child to the hospital. Part of the consent is also the right to refuse to consent—that is, to decline an admission. In some states, minors of a certain age are given the right to consent to or to refuse their own psychiatric treatment independent of their parents' wishes. Other states do not consider the wishes of the minor, relying solely on the parents' judgment. A third option exercised in some areas is to ask the minor to *assent* to this decision. This means that the minor agrees with her parents' decision to have her admitted. Minors cannot admit themselves if the parents do not first consent. Similarly, minors can refuse to assent (that is, they can *dissent*), in which case a judicial process of some kind is typically initiated to protect the rights of the minor. This process is similar to that for minors admitted involuntarily to the hospital. It is to prevent a parent from dealing with a troublesome child by simply signing her into a psychiatric hospital. Thus, the admission of a minor to a psychiatric hospital, though sometimes technically a "voluntary" procedure, might involve a judicial hearing similar to those held in the case of involuntary commitments (sometimes this is true even if the adolescent is willing to be in the hospital).

Law and legal procedures governing the provision of psychiatric treatment (or any kind of medical treatment, for that matter) against a person's stated wishes are based on the knowledge that, first, an individual whose judgment is immature and unformed cannot make sound decisions about medical treatment, and second, an adult whose judgment is clouded by the symptoms of an illness often does not make the same decisions about treatment that he would make if his judgment were not impaired. The delirious motor vehicle accident victim who has suffered massive blood loss may moan, "I want to go home," as he loses consciousness on the stretcher, but the ER team will ignore such a statement and proceed to do what they have to do to save the person's life. It is presumed that if the person were alert and thinking clearly and understood the implications of "going home," he would not make such a request. No one would ask a screaming toddler for written permission for a needed blood test. Similar principles underlie psychiatric commitment law: treatment is given to persons against their will if immature or clouded judgment prevents them from making good decisions about their treatment. Minors fall into this category. Depressed older adolescents may feel so hopeless that they think treatment has no chance of helping. Thinking processes in mania can be so disorganized and scattered that seeking out and cooperating with treatment is not possible. In either case, there are mechanisms to get needed treatment for persons whose immaturity or psychiatric symptoms blind them to the need for it.

Fortunately, these laws also have safeguards built in to prevent confinement in a psychiatric hospital for the wrong reasons. Decades ago, it was easy to invoke commitment law, often requiring only the signature of a relative or family physician to hospitalize a person for weeks or months, even years. People were hospitalized for all kinds of bogus reasons, and serious abuses of individual rights occurred. Laws became much stricter in the 1960s and 1970s to prevent these abuses. The main change was the addition of *dangerousness* as a commitment criterion. Unless an individual's behavior is truly dangerous to self (usually meaning suicidal behavior) or others, the person cannot be committed for involuntary psychiatric treatment. In the case of minors, the need for and appropriateness of the level of treatment are the sorts of criteria used.

Requests or petitions for psychiatric hospitalization do not necessarily mean that the person who is alleged to be psychiatrically ill will be hospitalized. Parents cannot simply sign a child into a facility; only a doctor can admit someone to a hospital. A parent's request for admission or involuntary commitment usually allows the young person to be transported to an emergency room, where a physician will make a decision about hospitalization. The child may be released if she does not meet legal criteria for admission or commitment.

Involuntary commitment is a serious legal procedure in which an individual is confined against his will and temporarily loses some rights of self-determination. For this reason, the law and the courts take involuntary psychiatric treatment very seriously, and many safeguards against abuses are built into the procedures. The person requesting an involuntary commitment must usually appear at the local courthouse or police station to give information and, in some jurisdictions, must make a sworn statement before a judge or magistrate. Parents will be asked for specific and detailed information about their child's behaviors. This is often frustrating for those trying to get help for their loved one. They may feel that being asked a lot of questions is uncaring, or that someone is questioning their judgment or their motives. It's important to remember that in the days when individuals could be confined to psychiatric hospitals simply because a relative or a doctor "thought it was best" for them, significant abuses of civil rights resulted. With serious attention on the part of the issuing magistrate or judge to documenting the facts and a close questioning of the need for psychiatric admission for minors and involuntary treatment of adults, we know the system is working.

Some form of judicial review (a *commitment hearing*) occurs at some point in the process (usually a few days after hospitalization), at which a judge or hearing officer determines that the admission procedure was done properly and legally. Although this is a legal proceeding, it is not a big courtroom scene. Usually a conference room in the hospital is used, only a few people are present, and the proceedings are kept confidential (not a matter of public record). The patient is allowed legal representation—in fact, an attorney will be appointed if the patient does not have one. As noted above, in some jurisdictions, even when both parents and child agree to hospitalization, a similar hearing occurs to safeguard the rights of the minor.

Involuntary commitment for psychiatric treatment does not usually affect people's other legal rights. This is changing, though, and certain states now forbid the possession of firearms to anyone who has had an involuntary hospitalization (sometimes for a limited time, such as five years, and sometimes for life). This change may have rather serious implications for anyone interested in a police or military career and is worth investigating. Other rights, such as wills or other legal instruments the committed person has executed, are not invalidated, and patients do not become legally "incompetent" in other areas. Hospitalization and treatment are the only issues that are addressed in commitment hearings.

We are aware that the topic we're discussing here is frightening. It might seem that a person's liberty and the right of self-determination can be taken away all too easily. At the risk of sounding glib, however, we want to reassure readers that involuntary commitment of an individual is *not* a quick and easy procedure. On the contrary, in our experience, most people are surprised at how difficult it is to invoke these laws, how many safeguards are built into the procedures, and how seriously the strict interpretation of the laws is taken by everyone involved. These laws have been carefully written in the interest of helping, not simply confining, people with severe psychiatric illnesses. In our experience, they are effective at doing just that.

GETTING THE SUPPORT *YOU* NEED

It is important that family members recognize their own need for support, encouragement, and understanding in dealing with adolescent mood disorders. Mental health professionals go home every day and leave behind their work of dealing with psychiatric illnesses, an option that most parents and other family members do not have. Dealing with a seriously depressed adolescent day after day and living with a frequently irritable, cranky teenager can be frustrating and exhausting. The changes and unpredictability of the moods of someone with a mood disorder intrude into home life and can be the source of severe stress in family relationships, straining them to the breaking point.

Perhaps the most difficult challenge is that posed by an adolescent with a mood disorder who is consistently resistant to getting treatment. The most astonishing learning experience for medical students and interns is encountering their first patient who repeatedly refuses to continue with a treatment that will keep him well and that is often the only way to avoid hospitalization. As a resident, one of us had the experience of reading the chart of an adult patient with bipolar disorder who had been admitted to the hospital dozens of times after stopping lithium, and wondering why on earth a person would make such a foolish decision again and again. In perspective, three capsules of lithium a day seemed a small inconvenience compared with spending what added up to several years of this patient's life in a psychiatric hospital. We have since learned that making peace with having this illness and staying in treatment are much more difficult than healthy people realize. Sticking with treatment is especially rough for individuals who must start taking medications at an age when none of their peers have to bother with such things—when the only people they know who take medication are "old people" and "sick people." It's very difficult for a young, physically healthy person who's feeling well to take medication every day. The idea of the medication controlling one's moods and mental processes is also daunting.

But the harder lesson for parents is learning that no one can *force* an individual, even one's own child, to take responsibility for treatment. Unless the individual makes the commitment to do so, no amount of love and support, sympathy and understanding, cajoling or even threatening can make someone take this step. Even parents who understand this at some level may feel guilty, inadequate, and angry at times when dealing with this situation. These are normal feelings. Parents should not be ashamed of these feelings of frustration and anger but should get help with them instead.

But even when the adolescent does take responsibility and is trying to stay well, relapses can occur. Family members might wonder what *they* did wrong. *Did I put too much pressure on her? Could I have been more supportive? Should I have been tougher and set firmer limits? Why didn't I notice the symptoms coming on sooner and get her to the doctor?* A hundred questions, a thousand "if only's." Another round of guilt, frustration, and anger.

On the other side of this issue is another question: How much understanding and support for the adolescent with a mood disorder might be *too* much? What is protective and what is overprotective? Should you call your child's coach with excuses for why she isn't at practice? Should you pay off credit card debts from hypomanic spending sprees caused by dropping out of treatment? When an irritable outburst ruins a family occasion, should the teenager be grounded for her behavior? We've already discussed the concept of enabling a substance abuser to continue abusing by shielding him from the consequences of his problem. The same dynamic can operate even when substance abuse is not at issue. What actions constitute helping a sick person, and what actions are helping a person to be sick?

These are thorny questions and complex issues. To say that they have no easy answers sounds pat and rather feeble, but it is frustratingly true. Punishing the teen for symptoms like irritability and low energy and motivation isn't fair, but not holding the teenager accountable for *any* of her actions isn't helping her either. Clearly, putting the adolescent too much in charge of her treatment is not right, but letting her have no say in treatment decisions isn't right either. Parents need a forum to process their decisions and strategies; by walking through their successes and failures with experienced peers or a professional, they can learn from others. You will need and deserve a lot of support and encouragement for the tough work of helping with these illnesses—just for hanging in there, every day, day after day.

For all these reasons, it's vital that family members seek out support groups and organizations and consider getting counseling or therapy for themselves to deal with the stresses caused by these illnesses. Like many chronic illnesses, mood disorders afflict one but affect many in the family. It's important that *all* those affected get the help, support, and encouragement they need. At the end of this book we have included names and contact information for some reputable organizations that can provide further information and support. Some of these are for parents by parents, and others are led by mental health professionals. Of course, the best way to ensure that you are getting precisely the individualized support you need may be to find your own therapist. This is not the same as seeing your child's therapist regularly, or even taking your child to family therapy. This is about you, sitting alone with your therapist, talking about your concerns. It may seem like an extreme step to consider, but we can say from experience that all parents we have ever engaged with who have taken this step have later told us that it was possibly the single greatest turning point in their family's recovery from their child's mood disorder.

Planning for Emergencies

T he decisions we are forced to make in a crisis situation are frequently not the decisions we would make under other, calmer circumstances. When an emergency arises for which we are unprepared, we are usually forced to make up our response as we go along. One of the best ways to prepare for an emergency is to have a crisis plan ready to go.

In speaking to many readers of the first edition of this book, we learned that some skipped this chapter because "My son was depressed but never suicidal," or "Well, we didn't think we'd need a plan and wanted to get through the book." We caution readers that the best strategy regarding an emergency plan is that "it is better to have one and not need it, then to need one and not have it." Although some people may find even the specter of an emergency stressful and the planning process anywhere from overly laborious to anxiety provoking, take home this message—at the very least, bring up the topic with your child's therapist or psychiatrist. They have put together many, many safety plans in their time and can give you a better and more individualized opinion of what may be best for your family. What follows are some general guidelines that we always consider when having these discussions with families.

Because so many highly effective treatments are available for a mood disorder, we sometimes forget that these disorders are potentially fatal illnesses. And in dealing with a disease that has the potential to become life threatening, the last thing you want is an improvised response to an emergency situation. One of us once faced just such a situation.

▼   The frustration in the nurse's voice was apparent as she spoke into the emergency room phone.

"I hear you, Mrs. Winters," Susan said, "but the magistrate won't approve a petition for involuntary treatment because you think she needs treatment. I need more information before we can—"

Suddenly, Susan put down the phone. "I can't believe it. She hung up on me!" She looked down at her note pad and then turned to me. "Does the name Anne Winters mean anything to you? That was her mom. She wanted someone to come out to their house and bring Anne into the emergency room. She said the girl might be suicidal."

"The name doesn't ring any bells with me," I replied. "Let's try the computer to see if she's ever had any treatment here before; maybe we've got some records. Then we can try calling Mrs. Winters back." As Susan stepped over to the emergency room's computer terminal, I glanced at my watch. It was almost noon, and I had a lunchtime lecture to give. "Susan, I have to go and give my lecture to the medical students. If we have a chart on Anne, can you order it from medical records? I'll be back a little after one, and we can see what we're dealing with and get back with Mrs. Winters."

It was just minutes past one when my beeper went off, with a message to call the emergency room.

"Frank, this is Susan. Mrs. Winters and her daughter are here in the ER. Well, that's not exactly true. Mrs. Winters is here, but Anne won't get out of the car. Do you think you can come down?"

I hadn't done any parking-lot therapy for a while, and as I walked past the "Authorized Personnel Only Please" sign that marked the door to the emergency room, I wondered what I would find. Susan was waiting for me. "I went out and persuaded the girl to come in. They're in room five. Anne has secretly been making cuts on her wrist for several days, so I think she'll need to be admitted. I'll call and see if we have any beds on the adolescent unit."

"How old is the girl? Has she been here before? Were you able to get some records?" I asked.

"She's sixteen, and she was seen about two years ago in the emergency room. We should have the record soon, but the computer information shows that the discharge diagnosis from the ER was major depressive disorder."

"Well, that's some help. Let me go see them."

As soon as I opened the door to the interview room, I could see that (as usual) Susan had sized up the situation pretty accurately. Anne was a tall girl dressed in baggy denim pants that looked to be at least four sizes too big, held up by bright yellow suspenders. She had on a gray sweatshirt with sleeves so long that her hands were invisible. A few brownish smears on one of the sleeves must have been what clued Susan in to asking the girl about hurting herself. She was slumped in a chair in the corner of the room, staring at the floor. Mrs. Winters was smartly dressed in a business suit, which made me think she had been at work before all this started. She didn't wait for me to ask a question to get started.

"The principal called me from school this morning and said Anne had told one of her friends she wanted to die. She's been staying with her father and me since spring break last week and is supposed to be going back to her mother and stepfather this evening. I could tell something was wrong with Anne, but her father's been gone on business for the past several days and I thought we'd talk to her together when he got back. This is a total shock to me. The school counselor suggested I call the doctor Anne was seeing, but when I did, I found out she's retired from practice. Then Anne tells me she hasn't taken her antidepressant for a month—I didn't even know she was on medication!"

Anne answered my questions with only angry glares, so I took Mrs. Winters to another office and let Susan try to sort out what had happened at school with the girl. It took a while to get Mrs. Winters calmed down, and even longer to get the whole story.

Anne's father had shared joint custody of the girl with his ex-wife since they had divorced about three years previously. He had married the present Mrs. Winters a year later. This Mrs. Winters knew nothing about Anne's mood disorder. She had gotten Anne to agree to come to the ER only by threatening to call the police, and she'd been worried the girl would jump out of the car the whole way downtown.

A phone call to Anne's father revealed that the girl had begun psychiatric treatment following the ER visit two years previously. She had started psychotherapy and some medication and after a few months had recovered well from her symptoms. She was no longer in therapy but was supposed to be seeing the psychiatrist every month. I recognized the name of the psychiatrist as a colleague who had retired about three months earlier. I knew for a fact that she had sent letters announcing her retirement several months before she quit her practice group.

It turned out that when Anne ran out of medication, Mr. Winters had persuaded her pediatrician to continue it "until we can make other arrangements." That had been months ago, and Anne still didn't have a psychiatrist.

I heard a knock on the door. Susan peeked in. "Doctor, can I see you for a moment?" "Excuse me," I said and stepped outside. Susan was holding the PPO and HMO list that was posted on the ER bulletin board. "Mr. Winters's medical insurance changed in April, and the new plan doesn't pay here. If Anne needs to be admitted, she'll have to go to Harris Memorial."

As Susan filled in more details of Anne's history and suicidal thinking, it became clear that the girl would indeed need to be in the hospital. "Great," I grumbled. "Her step-mom had a terrible time getting her here. I don't think we should let Mrs. Winters transport the girl. Can you have the secretary call patient transportation, and I'll call—"

Susan's frown stopped me. "Our transportation won't take patients to a hospital outside our system," she said. "We'll need to call an ambulance."

"That will cost them several hundred dollars," I said. "We can't use our people for a three-mile ride?" Susan gave me her best "I don't make the rules, I just follow them" look and said nothing. I took a deep breath and prepared to go in to tell the Winters that it would probably be several more hours before Anne could be admitted to a hospital.   ▲

People usually enjoy making plans—vacation plans, wedding plans, retirement plans. Planning for a psychiatric emergency is much less enjoyable, but if you have a family member with a mood disorder, it is, unfortunately, much more important. Unlike with vacation plans, you won't be disappointed if you don't need to use your emergency plans. But if you do need them, odds are you'll be very glad you made them.

It seems that Mr. Winters was operating under the assumption that his daughter's mood disorder was an easily treated problem that didn't require a specialist. As we've emphasized already, adolescent-onset mood disorders can be difficult to treat, and vigilance to signs of relapse is vital. Mr. Winters made a big mistake switching Anne's care to a busy pediatrician so soon after she had received her diagnosis and started treatment. It also seems that no one was monitoring her medications to be certain that she had a good supply and was taking them regularly, which is unfortunately common. Although many parents want to give their children autonomy over their medications, this is typically easier said than done. It is common for parents to reach the end of the month, time for a new refill, and find the bottle half full with medicine. Clearly, something went wrong. This would be a matter to discuss further with the adolescent or, if it is more appropriate, with his psychiatrist so a more detailed plan can be put in place (for example, taking a pill every night right before brushing one's teeth, and keeping the medicine next to the toothbrush, or setting a reminder on a cell phone). Similarly, many adolescents cannot, or will not, take responsibility for filling their own prescriptions, particularly at a local pharmacy, where they may be recognized by friends. All of these details can be discussed and worked out with the adolescent, preferably in the presence of the psychiatrist.

In the example above, Mr. Winters and his new wife had obviously not had a discussion about Anne's mood disorder and what the step-mom should do if symptoms flared up. Mrs. Winters didn't know what to do or whom to call when Anne refused to come to the ER. Last but not least, the Winters were unfamiliar with their medical insurance plan requirements, so Anne wound up being taken to a hospital where their insurance would not approve hospitalization.

How long would it have taken to avoid all these mistakes? An hour or two? Maybe three? Obviously, this would have been time well spent.

KNOW WHOM TO CALL FOR HELP

Every young person with a mood disorder should be under the care of a child psychiatrist who is familiar with the patient's symptoms and course of illness. This means getting established with a new physician when your family moves to a new community or when any other event (such as the retirement of your child's psychiatrist) leaves your child "uncovered." Changes in insurance plans sometimes force a change in psychiatrist too. Don't put off making an appointment to get your child established as a patient in a new community or with a new practice. Because of increasingly long wait times, it can sometimes take a month or more to get in the office to see someone. It is always better to make an appointment and then cancel if something comes up than to wait for a crisis to prompt an urgent visit. Also, because it can sometimes take months for records to be transferred from one office to another, ask the old office for a copy of your child's records or a letter of introduction that you can take to the new doctor at the first appointment. At the very least, such a letter should include your child's diagnosis and medication or medications.

Be sure to inform your pediatrician or family doctor about your child's treatment for a mood disorder, including diagnosis and any medications your child is taking. Keep a list of these medications on you as well to give to medical staff in case your child is taken to an emergency room or admitted to a hospital for *any* reason.

In choosing a new psychiatrist, there are many practical realities to consider. In addition to asking about the factors we've already mentioned (board certification, experience with adolescent age patients, and so on), don't hesitate to ask how the practice is covered after office hours. Also ask how easy it is to get a routine office appointment. Are appointment times set aside so that patients can get an appointment in a day or two for emergencies? Every psychiatrist or mental health clinic should have some means of seeing patients within twenty-four hours in cases of true emergency. Be sure you know how to contact the psychiatrist or the office at any time of the day or night and what arrangements are in place to handle emergencies. Does the psychiatrist see her own emergency patients, or does everyone in the practice rotate emergency on-call duty? The on-call system, though not ideal, is the standard in many communities, meaning your child may well see a doctor other than his regular one if there is an acute emergency. Are you prepared for such an arrangement, so that your child will be under the care of a psychiatrist who comes highly recommended? Less commonly, some psychiatrists make it clear that they do not have after-hours coverage and that any crisis is expected to be dealt with in the emergency room. If this is the protocol for your psychiatrist, ask which emergency room she recommends, whether the hospital has child psychiatrists available, and what other services are available there.

Which hospital or hospitals does the psychiatrist or the practice have a relationship with? Is it the hospital you prefer? The hospital where your insurance covers inpatient psychiatric treatment? Some psychiatrists do not do inpatient work at all; that is, they do not secure admitting privileges to a hospital but refer patients who need hospitalization to colleagues who do. This is especially true of child psychiatrists. This means a loss in continuity of care and sometimes lost time while a new psychiatrist gets to know the patient. Ask about whether the psychiatrist cares for her patients in the hospital and, if not, to whom she refers her hospitalized patients.

If the answers to these questions are not satisfactory, consider your options. Many psychiatrists are well aware of their own limitations and are more than happy to have a frank discussion about other providers who may be a better fit for your family's needs. Alternatively, ask your family doctor, family members, and friends for recommendations. Call the local chapter of Mental Health America, the Depression and Bipolar Support Alliance, or another advocacy group for a referral. (These groups are listed in the resources, following chapter 19.) Sometimes, your options are limited by medical insurance coverage—which brings us to another important aspect of being prepared.

INSURANCE ISSUES

Be familiar with the details of your medical insurance coverage of psychiatric illness. Unfortunately, most plans do not treat psychiatric illnesses in the same way they treat nonpsychiatric illnesses. For example, for psychiatric illnesses, plans frequently have different and stricter limits on hospitalization coverage, number of outpatient appointments they will pay for, and the percentage or amounts that patients must pay out-of-pocket for certain services (*copayments*). These practices have been minimized to a degree by the 1996 Mental Health Parity Act, the Mental Health Parity and Addiction Equity Act of 2008, and the Patient Protection and Affordable Care Act of 2010. Nonetheless, many people who are working to obtain mental health care for the first time are shocked by the red tape involved, so it pays to contact your insurance provider now to find out the exact details of your coverage.

This does not have to be a confrontational exchange. Many insurance companies have dedicated care coordinators who are invested in maintaining the health and well-being of their company's beneficiaries (thereby financially avoiding the more expensive emergency and hospitalization expenses). Care coordinators can explain exactly what is and is not covered and even how to find providers in your area. Some will contact provider offices on your behalf.

Some of the questions to ask include whether there is a "cap" on psychiatric services. This might be a limit on days of hospitalization or on number of outpatient appointments per year, or it might be a dollar-amount limit to coverage. If your insurance company denies coverage for a hospitalization or for several days of hospitalization, what procedures must you follow to appeal the decision?

Hospital stays of all types are getting shorter, and psychiatric hospitalization is no exception. Hospitalization is reserved almost exclusively for life-threatening emergencies now, and patients are discharged as soon as possible. As a rule, patients are no longer hospitalized on a psychiatric unit or in a psychiatric hospital for weeks or months (an exception might be the inpatient treatment of a very malnourished patient with an eating disorder, and even these stays are becoming briefer). Does the psychiatrist have access to a *partial hospitalization* program? (Sometimes also referred to as a *day hospital.*) This alternative to traditional hospital treatment provides hospital-like monitoring and treatment during the day (or sometimes for only part of the day) but allows patients to return home in the evening and spend the night there. It is a useful treatment option for mood disorders because it offers a way to provide daily monitoring of mood symptoms and treatment response without the disruption to personal and family life that staying in a hospital causes. This can also be a useful transitional step between an acute inpatient hospitalization and returning to the outpatient world. Some insurers cover a partial hospitalization (even insist on it), but others do not. Know where your insurance company and your psychiatrist stand on partial hospitalization.

Everyone these days seems to be talking about *managed care.* If you are a member of an HMO, you are part of the managed care picture. (In a *health maintenance organization,* members pay a monthly fee to receive their medical care from the organization.) But even if you are not in an HMO, aspects of managed care practice probably affect you in one way or another, no matter what kind of insurance you have.

Managed care means that the organization that is financially responsible for your child's medical care (your medical insurance company or HMO, for example) supervises or manages how much medical care your child receives. This is accomplished in a variety of ways, some that may be visible to you, some not. The main purpose of this management is to minimize the use of more expensive types of medical care, usually meaning hospitalization and treatment by specialists. In an HMO, the patient may have to be referred by a primary physician to any specialists (including a psychiatrist) in order to be covered. Lab tests may be covered only if the primary physician approves of them (this can make getting the blood tests needed to monitor therapy with lithium and some other psychiatric drugs inconvenient).

A newer alternative to the HMO is the ACO, or accountable care organization. Unlike the HMO, the ACO is held accountable (hence the name) for both the quality of care it provides to patients and their overall health. This mitigates somewhat the greatest criticism of the HMO, which some felt was designed solely to save money no matter how it affected the health of its members.

Before a person can be admitted to a psychiatric hospital, the physician often needs to get approval for hospitalization from the individual's insurance company, a process called *pre-admission review*. This consists of phoning an insurance company representative (usually a nurse or social worker) and giving the details of the clinical situation that justify a hospital stay. If this reviewer does not think a hospitalization is justified by the facts the physician relates, a doctor-to-doctor review is usually arranged. This pre-admission review can be a lengthy process, involving multiple phone calls to and from insurance company representatives and clinical staff. After the patient is admitted to a hospital, the treating doctor may be called every few days by someone from the insurance company asking why the patient still needs to be in the hospital, a function called *utilization review*. If this reviewer (usually a nurse) thinks your child should be discharged, your child's doctor (and you) will be told that coverage will be denied after a certain date and that you will be financially responsible for any additional inpatient treatment. (A variety of appeals procedures usually kick in at this point if your child's doctor disagrees.) Once limited to inpatient treatment, managed care now monitors outpatient treatment as well, and psychiatrists are being asked to fill out forms specifying a treatment plan and requesting a certain number of office visits. All these hassles are the reasons many psychiatrists who can afford to do so do not participate in insurance plans.

If the insurance plan includes coverage for pharmacy charges, you may not have a choice of brands of medication but will have to take whatever equivalent generic pharmaceutical the pharmacy stocks. Some HMOs have expanded on this theme and limit coverage to certain medications belonging to a broadly defined class, not permitting their doctors even to prescribe others. (For a while, some insurers would not pay for SSRI antidepressants and would insist that tricyclic antidepressants be tried first. Although this is no longer true, many insurers will require a trial of a generic medication before a brand-named one.)

There was a time when medical treatment was controlled by doctors and patients. That time has passed. Managed care methods save millions upon millions of health care dollars. Some people argue that this means more people have access to better medical care because the system is more efficient and effective. Others argue that *managed care* is an oxymoron. But whichever is the case, managed care methods are common in all types of insurance coverage now. Your type of medical insurance will almost certainly determine which hospital your child can be admitted to and may determine which doctor your child can see. Your insurance company will probably supervise the length of any hospitalizations, and limit the number of office visits, and even control which medications can be prescribed. All this means that you should closely scrutinize all aspects of insurance coverage for psychiatric illness—your existing policy and any new policies that you may have to choose from because of job changes. Don't put yourself in the position of getting an emergency room surprise.

Be sure to keep all the information you have gathered in one easily accessible document or folder. Make a list of important phone numbers and other key information you will need at a glance during an emergency. Some of the items you should include are shown in figure 18-1.

MORE ON SAFETY

The most dangerous emergency situation for adolescents with mood disorders, and one that frequently leads to hospitalization, is the development of suicidal thoughts and behaviors. As the parent of a depressed child, *never* lose sight of the fact that mood disorders are potentially fatal diseases.

No firearms should be kept in the home of an individual who has been se-

Psychiatrist			
Name:	Business phone:	After–hours phone:	
Therapist			
Name:	Business phone:	After–hours phone:	
Pharmacy		**Approved Hospital(s)**	
Name:	Phone:	Name:	ER Phone:
Primary Care M.D.			
Name:	Business phone:	After–hours phone:	
Insurance Info.			
Policyholder:	Policy number:	Group number:	Pre–admission contact:

Figure 18-1 Medical information chart. Complete a chart or list with this information and keep it up to date.

riously depressed. For an illness whose symptoms can include suicidal depression and heightened irritability with loss of inhibitions, there is never, *ever* any justification whatsoever for having a gun of any type in the home.

Some parents disagree with this stance. Whether they are in the military or law enforcement, or are simply avid sportsmen who prefer hunting, they will argue that firearms are a perfectly reasonable tool when treated with care and safety (locked in a safe, with the ammunition stored separately, and so on). We are not taking a philosophical stance on the right to bear arms here, but a practical one that is based on many years of scientific research on cold, hard facts. Every study that has ever looked at firearms and suicide risk shows unequivocally that the presence of guns in the home increases the risk of completed suicide.[1] As we discussed in chapter 14, research shows that whether a firearm is a handgun or a long gun, loaded or unloaded, locked away or not is immaterial in the risk of completed suicide. As psychiatrists, and as parents, our job is to minimize that risk as much as possible, which means removing guns from the home.

The appearance of self-destructive thoughts and impulses is frightening both to the adolescent and to those around her. The tremendous stigma and disgrace that have been associated with suicide for centuries still make people reluctant to discuss these thoughts when they occur. This stigma along with notions like "only crazy people kill themselves" complicate what is really a straightforward clinical issue: suicidal thinking is a serious symptom of mood disorders; this symptom must be evaluated quickly by a professional and must be managed swiftly and effectively. Individuals can be intensely ashamed of suicidal thoughts and feel that the development of self-destructive impulses is a kind of failure. It is not a failing in any way, of course, but a symptom of an illness. It is important to see the development of suicidal feelings in a depressed adolescent as a very dangerous symptom of serious illness, just like the onset of chest pains in someone with heart disease. When these symptoms occur, it's not time to wonder what they mean, *it's time to call for help*. And just as with the development of chest pains in a heart patient, the development of suicidal feelings in a person with a mood disorder is often a reason for hospitalization.

Psychiatric hospitalization can be experienced as a terrible failure, but the clinical perspective tells us otherwise. Although we have gotten much, much better at treating mood disorders, our treatment methods are by no means perfect. Sometimes, despite everyone's best efforts, relapses occur: the patient has serious symptoms, such as suicidal feelings, and requires hospitalization. When this happens, it's not time for self-blame or questions like "What did I do wrong?" Rather, it's time for healing.

One more reminder: serious depression can raise many issues of personal safety. These issues need to be anticipated, discussed, planned for, and promptly addressed if and when they occur. Put together a safety plan, and don't be afraid to use it if the time comes.

Looking Ahead

W e have made enormous progress in the last several decades in the field of psychiatry. The diagnosis of depression, bipolar disorder, and other psychiatric illnesses is much more accurate than it was even when this book was first written a decade ago, and the available treatments for these illnesses are far more effective than even a few years ago. But such advances have come about through trial and error, not because of a better scientific understanding of the causes of these diseases. We still do not understand what is "broken" in the nervous systems of individuals with psychiatric illness.

Thousands of scientists are now working on two great enterprises that will eventually lead to a fuller understanding of these illnesses and to new and more effective treatment approaches. The first of these is the field of neuroscience: the study of the biology and chemistry of the brain and nervous system. At the beginning of the twentieth century, physical and psychiatric examinations of patients with brain disorders followed by microscopic study of their brain tissue after death was the only available method to investigate diseases of the brain. Animal experiments conducted along similar lines complemented these studies, but this work resulted in only the vaguest outline of the organization of brain function. The locations of brain areas important for speech, movement, vision, and so forth, were discovered, but psychiatric illnesses remained so mysterious that ideas that had nothing to do with biology—theories such as psychoanalysis—were the only ones that seemed to offer any hope of understanding these problems.

Throughout the last century, however, breakthrough followed breakthrough, mostly in the field of the chemistry of brain functioning, as neurotransmitters were discovered, more powerful electron microscopes allowed the visualization of synapses and other cellular structures, and sophisticated chemical probes allowed scientists to work out the mechanisms by which neurons grow and communicate with each other. The discovery of G proteins inside the cells was another huge step forward, and new discoveries about the workings of the brain are being made every day.

Now, with new technologies for brain imaging such as PET scans (positron emission tomography) and SPECT (single photon emission computed tomography), scientists for the first time can see the brain at work in living persons. These imaging techniques can show changes in blood flow within the brain, locate areas that are hyperactive or abnormally low in activity, and detect abnormally high or abnormally low levels of brain chemicals such as serotonin and dopamine. Functional MRI imaging can show which areas of the brain are active when a person is performing particular tasks and has been helpful in determining how the brain's function changes, in a visible way, when someone is in the throes of a major depression or mania. A similar technique, diffusion tensor imaging, can show the tracts of the brain, how one neuron is connected to another to convey information. All this information is revealing the importance of the interplay of activity between different brain areas in the regulation of mood and is making it possible to identify the responsible circuitry. These techniques are allowing us to see how the brain of a person with a mood disorder functions differently from that of a person who does not have a mood disorder and, perhaps even more interesting, what changes occur when a person receives treatment and is beginning to feel well again.

We should be clear in our message, however. There are some practitioners who, as of the writing of this text, claim that neural imaging or certain EEG techniques can give a definitive diagnosis of ADHD or of mood disorders. They say that they, and they alone, are qualified to make a true diagnosis and recommend treatment. As of now, there is no evidence that any sort of imaging or objective testing of this type is in any way superior to a good old-fashioned diagnostic evaluation with a knowledgeable, experienced psychiatrist. In fact, almost all scientific studies still use the clinical evaluation as the gold standard against which all other tests (whether they be imaging or pencil-and-paper) are compared. Although we all hope for the day when a functional MRI or an EEG can give us the definitive diagnosis, we are simply not there yet, and we would caution any readers to be wary of practitioners who recommend expensive, out-of-pocket tests with little evidence behind the practice.

The second of these great scientific enterprises is the field of genetics. We've covered some of the developments in chapter 15, but if we left any doubt, the future of medicine and of psychiatry lies in understanding how our DNA influences our mood and our functioning, and using this knowledge to target any deficiencies. Here again, the development of new biochemical methods and molecular probes is what has made this research possible. The Human Genome Project, completed in 2003, gives us the full road map of the human genetic material. This analysis has led to other techniques, such as the ability to find very small mutations in an individual's genetic structure that may explain a particular physical or mental variation. The identification of the genes that are associated with mood disorders is only one of the goals of work in this field. Just as important will be understanding the mechanisms by which genes turn on and off and other mechanisms that regulate the expression and work of the instructions encoded in the DNA molecule.

As the genetic basis of the mood disorders is discovered, we may find that our classification system for these disorders is all wrong and that we need a whole new diagnostic system for psychiatric illnesses that is based on which genes are involved in individual patients. Instead of *major depressive disorder* or *bipolar disorder* II, we may be diagnosing patients with something like *21q22 mood disorder*, a name derived from the location of a gene.

A new field within the larger one of genetics is that of *pharmacogenomics*. Rather than looking for genes that are associated with specific illnesses, this search is for genes that are associated with therapeutic response to particular medications, an approach that promises to take the guesswork out of psychiatric therapeutics. A simple blood test may indicate which medication will work best for a particular patient, ending the lengthy and frustrating trial-and-error approach we now must use in finding the right medication for an individual. The field which has perhaps seen the greatest explosion in practical pharmacogenomics is oncology, the study of cancer. Treatment regimens are now custom tailored, not only to the general type of cancer a person has, but to the individual genetic makeup of the cancerous cells and the genetics of the person herself. In the future, the diagnosis and treatment of a particular patient will likely be determined by analyzing a single drop of blood. The phrase "Prozac is probably the best match for your particular type of depression given your serotonin receptor allele, and is the least likely to cause you side effects given your liver enzyme genetic makeup," will sound less like science fiction and more like the next step in reality.

Another promising approach to understanding genetics is *epigenetics*. Although the old adage that "You can't change your genes" still holds true, it turns out that environmental factors can affect how genes operate and can have important implications for health and disease. In 2014, a team of geneticists at Johns Hopkins University led by Dr. Zachary Kaminski published a research paper showing that stress hormones could flip epigenetic "switches" on a particular gene, resulting in a change of gene activity that predicted suicide and suicidal behaviors in persons with depression. This finding suggests that it may be possible to identify depressed individuals who are at highest risk for suicidal behaviors with a simple blood test. Like pharmacogenomics, the promise of epigenetics is just beginning to be realized in the practice of psychiatry.

The two fields of neuroscience and psychiatric genetics are closing in on the causes and mechanisms of mood disorders from different directions. As these two enterprises advance, they will begin to inform each other— that is, advances in one field will lead to advances in the other. Discovering that a gene for a particular protein is associated with a particular mood disorder will tell neuroscientists that the protein is important in the regulation of mood. The discovery of some new enzyme in neurons that is important in neuronal signaling will tell geneticists to focus on the gene for that enzyme in their linkage studies. Little by little, the whole picture will become clearer and clearer.

Advances in many seemingly unrelated fields hold promise for better understanding of mood disorders, too: advances in computer technology, for example. Just as architects now use computers to visualize buildings before they are built, pharmacologists are using computers to visualize the three-dimensional structures of neurotransmitters, receptors, and pharmaceutical agents to design new drugs. It is hoped that new pharmaceuticals that have a better "fit" with receptors or other targets will work faster, at lower doses, and with fewer side effects. In fact, many atypical antipsychotics (including clozapine) and some SSRIs (including fluoxetine, or Prozac) were developed using precisely these methods. Computers are also being used to model and study brain activity. Remember that the brain is much more than just a sophisticated computer: more like a network of millions and millions of individual computers. Advanced computers using *nonsequential neural architecture* to build *neural networks* (made up of many interconnected but independently computing units) show properties that would not be predicted from known principles of computing. These properties are probably highly relevant to the study of human brain activity and psychiatric illness.

Our understanding of the biology of mood disorders is getting better all the time. With each advance we get closer to better diagnostic methods and to safer and more effective treatments. The number of new medications continues to grow, and many more new pharmaceuticals are in the pipeline. With the more sophisticated use of nonpharmaceutical treatments such as transcranial magnetic stimulation, perhaps we'll be able to use lower doses of medications or help medications to work more quickly.

As we take the step from isolating genes to determining the function of those genes, we'll be able to design treatments more effectively and more rationally. This work also holds out the possibility of gene therapy: repairing the code in the DNA that causes mood disorders. The obstacles to be overcome before we can look for this type of cure can only be called daunting, even monumental. But scientists are closing in on these illnesses little by little, and with enough time and enough hard work, a cure might be possible.

As the mechanisms of illness development become known and the genetic vulnerabilities are identified, another exciting possibility emerges: prevention. Genetic data and a better understanding of what triggers the illness may allow the development of prevention programs aimed at averting illness development in individuals known to be at higher risk for a particular disorder. Some people see a darker side to this sort of prevention.

Imagine that a test is developed to determine the genetic risk of a patient, say, developing schizophrenia later in life. Many people who have schizophrenia require expensive medications for a long time, perhaps their entire lives. Now imagine that this test can be given to a newborn, or even in utero. Parents and patients worry that this information will be available to interested parties such as insurance companies or potential employers, cutting off their child's future. This sort of dystopian consequence to our increasing knowledge has been the topic of many science fiction works. Protection of genetic information is still being worked out by legislative bodies, but promising developments include the Genetic Information Nondiscrimination Act of 2008, which aims to eliminate exactly these sorts of discriminatory practices.

People frequently ask us whether they or their child will have to take medication for the rest of their lives. We always tell them that no one knows the answer to this question because no one knows exactly what the treatment of mood disorders might be in the future. Physicians practicing in the 1930s probably could not have imagined that vaccines would one day almost eliminate diphtheria, polio, measles, and other childhood diseases, common, often crippling, and sometimes fatal illnesses they saw so frequently in their patients but were completely helpless to treat. The astonishing developments in neuroscience and genetics hold just this much promise for those afflicted with mood disorders. There is every reason to be hopeful that a time is not too far off when treatments for depression and other mood disorders will be more effective than we can now imagine. But for now, the best way to manage a serious mood disorder is by using every resource available to you. The current evidence suggests that the longer a person can stay well, the lower the person's chance of relapsing into depression or mania. Continued treatment with your child's psychiatrist and therapist is a critical element to your child achieving his full potential.

RESOURCES

Suggested Reading

Samuel H. Barondes, *Mood Genes: Hunting for the Origins of Mania and Depression* (New York: Oxford University Press, 1999).

> *A clearly written and engrossing account of the tough science involved in the search for the genetic basis of mood disorders. An excellent introduction to the science of genetics.*

Robert Hedaya, *The Antidepressant Survival Guide: The Clinically Proven Program to Enhance the Benefits and Beat the Side Effects of Your Medication* (New York: Three Rivers Press, 2001).

> *An ambitious program for avoiding medication side effects that includes prescriptions for diet, exercise, and other lifestyle changes.*

Kay Redfield Jamison, *An Unquiet Mind: A Memoir of Moods and Madness* (New York: Vintage Books, 1996).

> *A powerful and moving narrative written with grace and wit by an international expert on bipolar disorder who suffers from it herself. A treasure of a book that contains some of the most engrossing and vivid descriptions of the experience of bipolar disorder ever written. A "must read" for anyone touched by bipolar disorder.*

George McGovern, *Terry: My Daughter's Life-and-Death Struggle with Alcoholism* (New York: Villard Books, 1996).

> *Senator McGovern's moving account of his daughter Terry's terrible and ultimately fatal addiction to alcohol cannot be too highly recommended for families dealing with an addicted relative. The senator vividly captures the dilemmas and struggles of a family trying to find the balance between helping their daughter without enabling her illness.*

Francis Mark Mondimore, *Bipolar Disorder: A Guide for Patients and Families*, 3rd ed. (Baltimore: Johns Hopkins University Press, 2014).

> *We admit to being more than a little biased about recommending this one but think it's a great resource for learning about bipolar disorder in all its variations. If you found the book you're holding in your hands helpful and want more information in the same style on bipolar disorder, this is your book.*

Francis Mark Mondimore and Patrick Kelly, *Borderline Personality Disorder: New Reasons for Hope* (Baltimore: Johns Hopkins University Press, 2011)

> *Yet another bit of shameless self-promotion, but a book we hope you will find useful. As we've discussed, adolescents are frequently lost, trying to redefine their identity, sometimes doing so in self-destructive ways. This is exactly how a patient with borderline personality disorder exists in the world. If this sounds familiar to you or your family, this book may help unravel some of the mysteries wrapped up in this complex and convoluted syndrome.*

Rolf Muuss, *Theories of Adolescence*, 6th ed. (New York: McGraw-Hill, 1996).

> *This college textbook provides an excellent overview of adolescent psychology by means of well-written chapters on all the major psychological theories from G. Stanley Hall and Sigmund Freud to Erik Erikson and beyond.*

William Styron, *Darkness Visible: A Memoir of Madness* (New York: Vintage Books, 1990).

> *We recommend this book to medical students as one of the best accounts of the symptoms of depression available. A good book for family members to read to better understand the experience of serious depression.*

Support and Advocacy Organizations

All the following organizations provide information, educational resources, and often referrals to support groups and to clinicians in your community who are skilled in treating mood disorders. Get in touch with them all and become a member! In addition to the direct services they provide to consumers, these groups are active in combating the stigmatization of psychiatric illnesses, in advocating for better medical insurance coverage of psychiatric disorders, and in supporting research.

Depression and Bipolar Support Alliance (DBSA)
 55 E. Jackson Blvd., Suite 490
 Chicago, IL 60604
 800-826-3632
 www.dbsalliance.org

International Foundation for Research and Education on Depression (iFred)
  P.O. Box 17598
  Baltimore, MD 21297-1598
  www.ifred.org

Mental Health America (MHA)
  2000 N. Beauregard Street, 6th floor
  Alexandria, VA 22311
  800-969-NMHA
  www.nmha.org

National Alliance on Mental Illness (NAMI)
  3803 N. Fairfax Drive, Suite 100
  Arlington, VA 22203
  800-950-NAMI
  www.nami.org

Internet Resources

All the support and advocacy groups listed above have websites with links to many, many other useful resources. The astonishing range of resources on the Internet continues to grow, but remember that you'll also find inaccurate information, bias, and just plain nonsense online, and it's important to consider information sources very carefully. Here are a few more excellent resources.

American Academy of Child and Adolescent Psychiatry
  www.aacap.org

 Information on child and adolescent psychiatry, including fact sheets for parents and caregivers.

Internet Mental Health
  www.mentalhealth.com

 An excellent site, with information on many different disorders and their treatments, information on many psychiatric medications, and hundreds of reference articles from popular and professional publications.

Medscape
  www.medscape.com

 This is primarily a news site for medical professionals, but it has a "patient information" section with many useful articles and links to other resources.

The Surgeon General of the United States
   www.surgeongeneral.gov

Read the surgeon general's reports online, including comprehensive reports on child and adolescent mental health issues.

U.S. National Library of Medicine
   www.nlm.nih.gov

This site provides free access to Medline, the most comprehensive medical database in the world. You can access more than eight million references in thirty-eight hundred journals. An incredibly valuable resource.

WebMD Health
   www.webmd.com

A comprehensive and reliable source of health information. Thousands of pages on many different disorders, including depression, bipolar disorder, ADHD, eating disorders, and other illnesses. Includes an extensive online discussion group and regular chats on mental health issues.

NOTES

Preface

1. Ruth Perou et al., "Mental Health Surveillance among Children—United States, 2005–2011." *Centers for Disease Control and Prevention Supplements* 62, no. 2 (2013): 1–35.

2. Peter Lewinsohn, Paul Rohde, John Seeley, Daniel Klein, and Ian Gotlib, "Natural Course of Adolescent Major Depressive Disorder in a Community Sample: Predictors of Recurrence in Young Adults," *American Journal of Psychiatry* 157, no. 10 (2000): 1584–91.

Chapter 1   Depression: Some Definitions

1. William James, *The Varieties of Religious Experience* (New York: Penguin Books, 1982), 147.

2. William Styron, *Darkness Visible: A Memoir of Madness* (New York: Vintage Books, 1990), 58.

3. J. K. Rowling, *Harry Potter and the Prisoner of Azkaban* (New York: Arthur A. Levine Books, 1999), 203.

4. *J. K. Rowling: A Year in the Life*, directed by James Runcie (UK: IWC Media, 2007), film.

5. Johann Wolfgang von Goethe, *The Sorrows of Young Werther*, trans. Elizabeth Mayer and Louise Bogan (New York: Random House, 1971), 114.

6. Hugo Wolf quoted in Kay Redfield Jamison, *Touched with Fire: Manic-Depressive Illness and the Artistic Temperament* (New York: Free Press, 1993), 21.

7. Styron, *Darkness Visible*, 19.

Chapter 2   Normal Adolescence and Depression in Adolescence

1. Leo Kanner, *Child Psychiatry*, 3rd ed. (Springfield, Ill.: Thomas, 1957).

2. Joseph Brennemann, "The Menace of Psychiatry," *American Journal of Diseases of Children* 42, no. 2 (1931): 376–402.

3. As quoted in Sebastian Kraemer, "'The Menace of Psychiatry': Does It Still Ring a Bell?" *Archives of Disease in Childhood* 94, no. 8 (2009): 570–72.

4. N. Ryan et al., "The Clinical Picture of Major Depression in Children and Adolescents," *Archives of General Psychiatry* 44 (1987): 854–61.

5. Jerald G Bachman et al., "Adolescent Self-Esteem: Differences by Race/Ethnicity, Gender, and Age," *Self and Identity* 10, no. 4 (2011): 445–73.

6. Michael Rutter, *Changing Youth in a Changing Society: Patterns of Adolescent Development and Disorder* (Cambridge: Harvard University Press, 1980), 87.

7. Erik Erikson, *Childhood and Society*, 2d ed. (New York: Norton, 1963), 228.

8. Erik Erikson, *Identity, Youth, and Crisis* (New York: Norton, 1968), 131.

9. See James Marcia, "The Empirical Study of Ego Identity," in *Identity and Development: An Interdisciplinary Approach*, ed. Harke Bosma, Tobi Graafsma, and Harold Grotevant (Thousand Oaks, Calif.: Sage, 1994).

10. Rutter, *Changing Youth in a Changing Society*, 39.

11. Jerome D. Frank, *Persuasion and Healing: A Comparative Study of Psychotherapy*, rev. ed. (New York: Schocken Books, 1974), 316.

12. Ibid., 314.

13. Anna Freud quoted in Rolf E. Muuss, *Theories of Adolescence*, 6th ed. (New York: McGraw-Hill, 1996), 368.

14. Alfred Kinsey, Wardell Pomeroy, and Clyde Martin, *Sexual Behavior in the Human Male* (Philadelphia: W. B. Saunders, 1948), 639.

Chapter 3   The Mood Disorders of Adolescence

1. The APA Task Force on Laboratory Tests in Psychiatry, "The Dexamethasone Suppression Test: An Overview of Its Current Status in Psychiatry," *American Journal of Psychiatry* 144, no. 10 (1987): 1253–62.

2. P. Lewinsohn, H. Hops, R. Roberts, J. Seeley, and J. Andrews, "Adolescent Psychopathology I: Prevalence and Incidence of Depression and Other DSM-III-R Disorders in High School Students," *Journal of Abnormal Psychology* 102 (1993): 133–44.

3. Boris Birmaher et al., "Childhood and Adolescent Depression: A Review of the Past 10 Years, Part I," *Journal of the American Academy of Child and Adolescent Psychiatry* 35, no. 11 (1996): 1427–39.

4. Douglas Williamson, Boris Birmaher, Barbara Anderson, Mayadah Al-Shab-bout, and Ryan Neal, "Stressful Life Events in Depressed Adolescents: The Role of Dependant Events during the Depressive Episode," *Journal of the American Academy of Child and Adolescent Psychiatry* 34, no. 5 (1995): 591–98.

5. Kenneth S. Kendler and Charles O. Gardner, "Dependent Stressful Life Events and Prior Depressive Episodes in the Prediction of Major Depression—The Problem of Causal Inference in Psychiatric Epidemiology," *Archives of General Psychiatry* 67, no. 11 (2010): 1120–27.

6. Ian M. Goodyer, "The Influence of Recent Life Events on the Onset and Outcome of Major Depression in Young People," in *Depressive Disorders in Children and Adolescents: Epidemiology, Risk Factors, and Treatment*, ed. Cecilia Ahmoi Essau and Franz Petermann (Northvale, N.J.: Jason Aronson, 1999), 241.

7. Ruth Perou et al., "Mental Health Surveillance among Children—United States, 2005–2011," *Centers for Disease Control and Prevention Supplements* 62, no. 2 (2013): 1–35.

8. Ronald C. Kessler et al., "The Epidemiology of Major Depressive Disorder: Results from the National Comorbidity Survey Replication (NCS-R)," *JAMA* 289, no. 23 (2003): 3095–3105.

9. S. Seedat et al., "Cross-National Associations between Gender and Mental Disorders in the World Health Organization World Mental Health Surveys," *Archives of General Psychiatry* 66, no. 7 (2009): 785–95.

10. Birmaher et al., "Childhood and Adolescent Depression."

11. John Curry et al., "Recovery and Recurrence following Treatment for Adolescent Major Depression," *Archives of General Psychiatry* 68, no. 3 (2011): 263–69.

12. Birmaher et al., "Childhood and Adolescent Depression."

13. Maria Kovacs, Hagop Akiskal, Constantine Gatsonis, and Phoebe Parrone, "Childhood-Onset Dysthymic Disorder," *Archives of General Psychiatry* 51 (1994): 365–74.

14. Birmaher et al., "Childhood and Adolescent Depression."

15. S. Gehlert et al., "The Prevalence of Premenstrual Dysphoric Disorder in a Randomly Selected Group of Urban and Rural Women," *Psychological Medicine* 39, no. 1 (2009): 129–36.

16. C. Moreno et al., "National Trends in the Outpatient Diagnosis and Treatment of Bipolar Disorder in Youth," *Archives of General Psychiatry* 64, no. 9 (2007): 1032–39.

17. A. R. Van Meter, A. L. Moreira, and E. A. Youngstrom, "Meta-Analysis of Epidemiologic Studies of Pediatric Bipolar Disorder," *Journal of Clinical Psychiatry* 72, no. 9 (2011): 1250–56.

18. A. Pfuntner, L. M. Wier, and C. Stocks, *Most Frequent Conditions in U.S. Hospitals, 2011*, Statistical Brief 162, Healthcare Cost and Utilization Project (HCUP) Statistical Briefs (Rockville, Md.: Agency for Healthcare Research and Quality, 2013).

19. DSM-5 Committee, *Diagnostic and Statistical Manual of Mental Disorders,* 5th ed. (Washington, D.C.: American Psychiatric Association, 2013). Accessed online at http://dsm.psychiatryonline.org/doi/full/10.1176/appi.books.9780890425596.dsm04#BCFBGAGG.

20. Ibid.

21. Peter Lewinsohn, Daniel Klein, and John Seeley, "Bipolar Disorders in a Community of Older Adolescents: Prevalence, Phenomenology, Comorbidity and Course," *Journal of the American Academy of Child and Adolescent Psychiatry* 34, no. 4 (1995): 454–63.

22. William Coryell, Nancy Andreason, Jean Endicott, and Martin Keller, "The Significance of Past Mania or Hypomania in the Course and Outcome of Major Depression," *American Journal of Psychiatry* 144 (1987): 309–15.

23. G. Cassano, H. Akiskal, M. Savina, L. Musetti, and G. Perugi, "Proposed Subtypes of Bipolar II and Related Disorders: With Hypomanic Episodes (or Cyclothymia) and with Hyperthymic Temperament," *Journal of Affective Disorders* 26 (1992): 127–40.

24. See Sylvia Simpson et al., "Bipolar II: The Most Common Bipolar Phenotype?" *American Journal of Psychiatry* 150 (1993): 901–3.

25. Frederick K. Goodwin and Kay Redfield Jamison, *Manic-Depressive Illness* (New York: Oxford University Press, 1990), 69.

26. Hagop Akiskal et al., "Switching from 'Unipolar' to Bipolar II: An Eleven-Year Prospective Study of Clinical and Temperamental Predictors in 559 Patients," *Archives of General Psychiatry* 52 (1995): 114–23.

27. Lewinsohn et al., "Bipolar Disorders in a Community of Older Adolescents."

28. Hagop Akiskal, "The Prevalent Clinical Spectrum of Bipolar Disorders: Beyond DSM-IV," *Journal of Clinical Psychopharmacology* 16, suppl. (1996): 4S–14S.

29. Lewinsohn et al., "Bipolar Disorders in a Community of Older Adolescents."

30. Hagop Akiskal and Gopinath Mallya, "Criteria for 'Soft' Bipolar Spectrum: Treatment Implications," *Psychopharmacology Bulletin* 23, no. 1 (1987): 68–73.

31. Emil Kraepelin, *Manic-Depressive Insanity and Paranoia,* trans. R. M. Barclay, ed. G. M. Robertson (Edinburgh: Livingstone, 1921; reprinted New York: Arno Press, 1976), 1 (in reprint edition).

32. Joachim Puig-Antich et al., "The Psychosocial Functioning and Family Environment of Depressed Adolescents," *Journal of the American Academy of Child and Adolescent Psychiatry* 32, no. 2 (1993): 244–53.

33. Paul Rohde, Peter Lewinsohn, and John Seeley, "Are Adolescents Changed by an Episode of Major Depression?" *Journal of the American Academy of Child and Adolescent Psychiatry* 33, no. 9 (1994): 1289–98.

34. Kiyuri Naicker et al., "Social, Demographic, and Health Outcomes in the 10 Years following Adolescent Depression," *Journal of Adolescent Health* 52, no. 5 (2013): 533–38.

35. Mark Sanford et al., "Predicting the One-Year Course of Adolescent Major Depression," *Journal of the American Academy of Child and Adolescent Psychiatry* 34, no. 12 (1995): 1618–28.

36. Maria Kovacs, Stana Paulaudkas, Constantine Gatsonis, and Cheryl Richards, "Depressive Disorders in Childhood III: A Longitudinal Study of Comorbidity and Risk for Conduct Disorders," *Journal of Affective Disorders* 15 (1988): 205–17.

37. Uma Rao, "Relationship between Depression and Substance Abuse Disorders in Adolescent Women during the Transition to Adulthood," *Journal of the American Academy of Child and Adolescent Psychiatry* 39, no. 2 (2000): 215–22.

38. Uma Rao et al., "Unipolar Depression in Adolescents: Clinical Outcome in Adulthood," *Journal of the American Academy of Child and Adolescent Psychiatry* 34, no. 5 (1995): 566–78.

Chapter 4 Mood Disorders: A Summary of Diagnostic Categories in the DSM

1. American Psychiatric Association, *Diagnostic and Statistical Manual of Mental Disorders,* 4th ed. (Washington, D.C.: American Psychiatric Association, 1994), xvii. Note that epilepsy was considered to be a mental illness at the time.

2. Alfred Kinsey, Wardell Pomeroy, and Clyde Martin, *Sexual Behavior in the Human Male* (Philadelphia: Saunders, 1948), 639.

Chapter 5   Medication Issues in Adolescence

1. Nancy C. Andreason, *The Broken Brain: The Biological Revolution in Psychiatry* (New York: Harper and Row, 1985).

2. Roland Kuhn, "The Treatment of Depressive States with G 22355 (Imipramine Hydrochloride)," *American Journal of Psychiatry* 115 (1958): 459–64. This is an English translation of Kuhn's 1957 article.

Chapter 6   Antidepressant Medications

1. Roland Kuhn, "The Treatment of Depressive States with G 22355 (Imipramine Hydrochloride)," *American Journal of Psychiatry* 115 (1958): 459–64.

2. C. K. Varley and J. McClellan, "Case Study: Two Additional Sudden Deaths with Tricyclic Antidepressants," *Journal of the American Academy of Child and Adolescent Psychiatry* 36, no. 3 (1997): 390–94.

3. J. Daly and T. Wilens, "The Use of Tricyclic Antidepressants in Children and Adolescents," *Pediatric Clinics of North America: Child and Adolescent Psychopharmacology* 45, no. 5 (1998): 1123–35.

4. Ibid.

5. C. K. Conners, "Methodology of Antidepressant Drug Trials for Treating Depression in Adolescents," *Journal of Child and Adolescent Psychopharmacology* 2 (1992): 11–22.

6. P. Hazell and M. Mirzaie, "Tricyclic Drugs for Depression in Children and Adolescents," *Cochrane Database of Systematic Reviews* 6 (2013): CD002317.pub2.

7. Rudolf Hoehn-Saric, John Lipsey, and Godfrey Pearlson, "A Fluoxetine-Induced Frontal Lobe Syndrome in an Obsessive-Compulsive Patient," *Journal of Clinical Psychiatry* 52 (1990): 343–45.

8. J. Price, V. Cole, and G. M. Goodwin, "Emotional Side-Effects of Selective Serotonin Reuptake Inhibitors: Qualitative Study," *British Journal of Psychiatry: Journal of Mental Science* 195, no. 3 (2009): 211–17.

9. D. Brent et al., "Switching to Another SSRI or to Venlafaxine with or without Cognitive Behavioral Therapy for Adolescents with SSRI-Resistant Depression: The TORDIA Randomized Controlled Trial," *JAMA* 299, no. 8 (2008): 901–13.

10. R. L. Findling et al., "Venlafaxine in the Treatment of Children and Adolescents with Attention-Deficit/Hyperactivity Disorder," *Journal of Child and Adolescent Psychopharmacology* 17, no. 4 (2007): 433–45.

11. R. L. Barkin and S. Barkin, "The Role of Venlafaxine and Duloxetine in the Treatment of Depression with Decremental Changes in Somatic Symptoms of Pain, Chronic Pain, and the Pharmacokinetics and Clinical Considerations of Duloxetine Pharmacotherapy," *American Journal of Therapeutics* 12, no. 5 (2005): 431–38.

12. S. E. Hetrick et al., "Newer Generation Antidepressants for Depressive Disorders in Children and Adolescents," *Cochrane Database of Systematic Reviews* 11 (2012): CD004851.

Chapter 7   Mood-Stabilizing Medications

1. Anastase Georgotas and Samuel Gershon, "Historical Perspectives and Current Highlights on Lithium Treatment in Manic-Depressive Illness," *Journal of Clinical Psychopharmacology* 1, no. 1 (1981): 27–31.

2. John F. J. Cade, "Lithium Salts in the Treatment of Psychotic Excitement," *Medical Journal of Australia* 36 (1949): 349–52.

3. Ibid., 350.

4. Ibid., 350–51.

5. Ronald R. Fieve, *Moodswing: The Third Revolution in Psychiatry* (New York: Bantam Books, 1975), 3.

6. M. Schou, N. Juel-Nielsen, E. Strömgren, and H. Voldby, "The Treatment of Manic Psychoses by the Administration of Lithium Salts," *Journal of Neurology, Neurosurgery, and Psychiatry* 17 (1954): 250–60.

7. Paul Baalstrup and Morgans Schou, "Lithium as a Prophylactic Agent: Its Effect against Recurrent Depressions and Manic-Depressive Psychosis," *Archives of General Psychiatry* 16, no. 2 (1967): 162–72.

8. E. P. Worrall, J. P. Moody, and M. Peet, "Controlled Studies of the Acute Antidepressant Effects of Lithium," *British Journal of Psychiatry* 135 (1979): 255–62.

9. F. Rouillon and P. Gorwood, "The Use of Lithium to Augment Antidepressant Medication," *Journal of Clinical Psychiatry* 59, suppl. 5 (1998): 32–39.

10. Robert Kowatch and John Bucci, "Mood Stabilizers and Anticonvulsants," *Pediatric Clinics of North America* 45, no. 5 (1998): 1173–86.

11. Morgans Schou, "Forty Years of Lithium Treatment," *Archives of General Psychiatry* 54 (1997): 9–13.

12. Ibid., 11.

13. Neal Ryan, Vinod Bhatara, and James Perel, "Mood Stabilizers in Children and Adolescents," *Journal of the American Academy of Child and Adolescent Psychiatry* 38, no. 5 (1999): 529–36.

14. Ibid.

15. G. Walter, B. Lyndon, and R. Kubb, "Lithium Augmentation of Venlafaxine in Adolescent Major Depression," *Australian and New Zealand Journal of Psychiatry* 32, no. 3 (1998): 457–59.

16. A. Cipriani, K. Hawton, S. Stockton, and J. R. Geddes, "Lithium in the Prevention of Suicide in Mood Disorders: Updated Systematic Review and Meta-Analysis," *BMJ* 346 (2013): f3646.

17. American Psychiatric Association, "Practice Guidelines for the Treatment of Bipolar Disorder," *American Journal of Psychiatry* 151, suppl. (1994): 7.

18. Patricia Roy and Jennifer L. Payne, "Treatment of Bipolar Disorder during and after Pregnancy," in *Bipolar Depression: Molecular Neurobiology, Clinical Diagnosis, and Pharmacotherapy*, ed. Carlos A. Zarate and Husseini K. Manji (Boston: Birkhäuser, 2009), 253–69.

19. Frederick K. Goodwin and Kay Redfield Jamison, *Manic-Depressive Illness* (New York: Oxford University Press, 1990), 707.

20. Charles Bowden and Susan McElroy, "History of the Development of Val-

proate for the Treatment of Bipolar Disorder," *Journal of Clinical Psychiatry* 56, suppl. 3 (1995): 3–5.

21. A. Cipriani et al., "Valproic Acid, Valproate and Divalproex in the Maintenance Treatment of Bipolar Disorder," *Cochrane Database of Systematic Reviews* 10 (2013): CD003196.

22. Charles L. Bowden, "Predictors of Response to Divalproex and Lithium," *Journal of Clinical Psychiatry* 56, suppl. 3 (1995): 25–29.

23. Susan McElroy, Paul Keck, Harrison Pope, and James Hudson, "Valproate in Psychiatric Disorders: Literature Review and Clinical Guidelines," *Journal of Clinical Psychiatry* 50, suppl. 3 (1989): 23–29.

24. American Psychiatric Association, "Practice Guidelines for the Treatment of Bipolar Disorder," 21. See also Alan Swann et al., "Depression during Mania: Treatment Response to Lithium or Divalproex," *Archives of General Psychiatry* 54 (1997): 37–42.

25. American Psychiatric Association, "Practice Guidelines for the Treatment of Bipolar Disorder," 10.

26. Frederick Jacobson, "Low-Dose Valproate: A New Treatment for Cyclothymia, Mild Rapid-Cycling Disorders and Premenstrual Syndrome," *Journal of Clinical Psychiatry* 54, no. 6 (1993): 229–34. See also J. A. Delito, "The Effect of Valproate on Bipolar Spectrum Temperamental Disorders," *Journal of Clinical Psychiatry* 54, no. 8 (1993): 300–304.

27. N. Huband et al., "Antiepileptics for Aggression and Associated Impulsivity," *Cochrane Database of Systematic Reviews* 2 (2010): CD003499.

28. Gary Sachs, "Bipolar Mood Disorder: Practical Strategies for Acute and Maintenance Phase Treatment," *Journal of Clinical Psychopharmacology* 16, no. 2, suppl. 1 (1996): 32S–47S.

29. F. E. Dreifuss, D. H. Langer, K. A. Moline, and J. E. Maxwell, "Valproic Acid Hepatic Fatalities II: US Experience since 1984," *Neurology* 39, no. 2, pt. 1 (1989): 201–7.

30. H. J. Talib and E. M. Alderman, "Gynecologic and Reproductive Health Concerns of Adolescents Using Selected Psychotropic Medications," *Journal of Pediatric and Adolescent Gynecology* 26, no. 1 (2013): 7–15.

31. J. C. Ballenger and R. M. Post, "Carbamazepine in Manic-Depressive Illness: A New Treatment," *American Journal of Psychiatry* 37, no. 7 (1980): 782–90.

32. R. A. Kowatch et al., "Effect Size of Lithium, Divalproex Sodium, and Carbamazepine in Children and Adolescents with Bipolar Disorder," *Journal of the American Academy of Child and Adolescent Psychiatry* 39, no. 6 (2000): 713–20.

33. B. Lerer, M. Moore, E. Meyendorff, S. R. Cho, and S. Gershon, "Carbamazepine versus Lithium in Mania: A Double Blind Study," *Journal of Clinical Psychiatry* 48 (1987): 89–93.

34. Robert Post, Thomas Uhde, James Ballenger, and Kathleen Squillace, "Prophylactic Efficacy of Carbamazepine in Manic-Depressive Illness," *American Journal of Psychiatry* 140 (1983): 1602–4.

35. Joseph Woolston, "Case Study: Carbamazepine Treatment of Juvenile-

Onset Bipolar Disorder," *Journal of the American Academy of Child and Adolescent Psychiatry* 38, no. 3 (1999): 335–38.

36. Jonathan Sporn and Gary Sachs, "The Anticonvulsant Lamotrigine in Treatment Resistant Manic-Depressive Illness," *Journal of Clinical Psychopharmacology* 17 (1997): 185–89.

37. A. Trankner, C. Sander, and P. Schonknecht, "A Critical Review of the Recent Literature and Selected Therapy Guidelines since 2006 on the Use of Lamotrigine in Bipolar Disorder," *Neuropsychiatric Disease and Treatment* 9 (2013): 101–11.

38. Joseph Calabrese, S. Hossein Fatemi, and Mark Woyshville, "Antidepressant Effects of Lamotrigine in Rapid Cycling Bipolar Disorder," *American Journal of Psychiatry* 153, no. 9 (1996): 1236.

39. Thomas Maltese, "Adjunctive Lamotrigine Treatment for Major Depression," *American Journal of Psychiatry* 156, no. 11 (1999): 1833.

40. Sporn and Sachs, "Anticonvulsant Lamotrigine in Treatment Resistant Manic-Depressive Illness."

41. Cipriani et al., "Lithium in the Prevention of Suicide in Mood Disorders."

42. Sean Stanton, Paul Keck, and Susan McElroy, "Treatment of Acute Mania with Gabapentin," *American Journal of Psychiatry* 154, no. 2 (1997): 287.

43. Marshall Teitlebaum, "Oxycarbazepine in Bipolar Disorder," *Journal of the American Academy of Child and Adolescent Psychiatry* 40, no. 9 (2001): 993–94.

44. For a discussion of all these issues, see Magda Campbell and Jeanette Cueva, "Psychopharmacology in Child and Adolescent Psychiatry: A Review of the Past Seven Years, Part II," *Journal of the American Academy of Child and Adolescent Psychiatry* 34, no. 10 (1995): 1262–72; and Ryan, Bhatara, and Perel, "Mood Stabilizers in Children and Adolescents."

Chapter 8   Other Medications and Treatments

1. B. Geller et al., "A Randomized Controlled Trial of Risperidone, Lithium, or Divalproex Sodium for Initial Treatment of Bipolar I Disorder, Manic or Mixed Phase, in Children and Adolescents," *Archives of General Psychiatry* 69, no. 5 (2012): 515–28.

2. Robert L. Findling et al., "Prolactin Levels during Long-Term Risperidone Treatment in Children and Adolescents," *Journal of Clinical Psychiatry* 64, no. 11 (2003): 1362–69.

3. In a study of 11,555 patients treated with clozapine, 73 (or 0.63 percent) developed agranulocytosis (of whom 2 died of the infectious complications of the condition). See Jose Alvir, Jeffrey Lieberman, Allan Safferman, Jeffrey Schwimmer, and John Schaaf, "Clozapine-Induced Agranulocytosis: Incidence and Risk Factors in the United States," *New England Journal of Medicine* 329 (1993): 162–67.

4. Magda Campbell, Judith L. Rapoport, and George M. Simpson, "Antipsychotics in Children and Adolescents," *Journal of the American Academy of Child and Adolescent Psychiatry* 38, no. 5 (1999): 537–45.

5. Mark Olfson et al., "National Trends in the Outpatient Treatment of Children and Adolescents with Antipsychotic Drugs," *Archives of General Psychiatry* 63, no. 6 (2006): 679–85.

6. Ric M. Procyshyn et al., "Prevalence and Patterns of Antipsychotic Use in Youth at the Time of Admission and Discharge from an Inpatient Psychiatric Facility," *Journal of Clinical Psychopharmacology* 34, no. 1 (2014): 17–22.

7. Gregory Kutz, *Foster Children: HHS Guidance Could Help States Improve Oversight of Psychotropic Prescriptions*, Testimony before the Subcommittee on Federal Financial Management, Government Information, Federal Services, and International Security, Committee on Homeland Security and Governmental Affairs, U.S. Senate (Washington, D.C.: United States Government Accountability Office, 2011).

8. K. Linde, G. Ramirez, C. D. Mulrow, A. Pauls, and W. Weidenhammer, "St. John's Wort for Depression—An Overview and Meta-analysis of Randomized Clinical Trials," *British Medical Journal* 3, no. 313 (1996): 253–58.

9. Michael Dörks et al., "Antidepressant Drug Use and Off-Label Prescribing in Children and Adolescents in Germany: Results from a Large Population-Based Cohort Study," *European Child and Adolescent Psychiatry* 22, no. 8 (2013): 511–18.

10. E. U. Vorbach, W. D. Hubner, and K. H. Arnoldt, "Effectiveness and Tolerance of the Hypericum Extract LI 160 in Comparison with Imipramine: Randomized Double-Blind Study with 135 Outpatients," *Journal of Geriatric Psychiatry and Neurology* 7, suppl. 1 (1994): S19–S23.

11. R. Bergman, J. Nuessner, and J. Demling, "Treatment of Mild to Moderate Depression: A Comparison between *Hypericum perforatum* and Amitriptyline," *Neurologie/Psychiatrie* 7 (1993): 235–40, summarized in Peter McWilliams, Mikael Nordfors, and Harold H. Bloomfield, *Hypericum and Depression* (Los Angeles: Prelude Press, 1996).

12. Richard Shelton et al., "Effectiveness of St. John's Wort in Major Depression: A Randomized Controlled Trial," *Journal of the American Medical Association* 285 (2001): 1978–86.

13. For a discussion of the plant origins and potent toxicity of several poisons, see Joel Hardman, Alfred Goodman Gilman, and Lee Limbird, *Goodman and Gilman's The Pharmacological Basis of Medical Therapeutics*, 9th ed. (New York: McGraw-Hill, Health Professions Division, 1996), 178–90 (strychnine and related compounds), 146–49 (amatoxins), and 149–54 (belladonna alkaloids).

14. Andrew Stoll et al., "Omega 3 Fatty Acids in Bipolar Disorder: A Preliminary Double-Blind, Placebo-Controlled Trial," *Archives of General Psychiatry* 56, no. 5 (1999): 407–12.

15. Lauren B. Marangell et al., "A Double-Blind, Placebo-Controlled Study of the Omega-3 Fatty Acid Docosahexaenoic Acid in the Treatment of Major Depression," *American Journal of Psychiatry* 160, no. 5 (2003): 996–98.

16. Hanah Nemets et al., "Omega-3 Treatment of Childhood Depression: A Controlled, Double-Blind Pilot Study," *American Journal of Psychiatry* 163, no. 6 (2006): 1098–1100.

17. Shima Jazayeri et al., "Comparison of Therapeutic Effects of Omega-3 Fatty Acid Eicosapentaenoic Acid and Fluoxetine, Separately and in Combination, in Major Depressive Disorder," *Australian and New Zealand Journal of Psychiatry* 42, no. 3 (2008): 192–98.

18. Michael Alvear, "A True Fish Story," www.salon.com, Sept. 9, 1999.

19. Hiroyasu Iso et al., "Intake of Fish and Omega-3 Fatty Acids and Risk of Stroke in Women," *Journal of the American Medical Association* 285, no. 3 (2001): 304–12.

20. Jazayeri et al., "Comparison of Therapeutic Effects of Omega-3 Fatty Acid Eicosapentaenoic Acid and Fluoxetine, Separately and in Combination, in Major Depressive Disorder."

21. Boris Nemets, Ziva Stahl, and R. H. Belmaker, "Addition of Omega-3 Fatty Acid to Maintenance Medication Treatment for Recurrent Unipolar Depressive Disorder," *American Journal of Psychiatry* 159, no. 3 (2002): 477–79.

22. Catherine Rothon et al., "Physical Activity and Depressive Symptoms in Adolescents: A Prospective Study," *BMC Medicine* 8, no. 1 (2010): 32.

23. Carroll W. Hughes et al., "Depressed Adolescents Treated with Exercise (DATE): A Pilot Randomized Controlled Trial to Test Feasibility and Establish Preliminary Effect Sizes," *Mental Health and Physical Activity* 6, no. 2 (2013): 119–31.

24. Joseph Rey and Garry Walter, "Half a Century of ECT Use in Young People," *American Journal of Psychiatry* 154, no. 5 (1997): 595–602.

25. Garry Walter, Karryn Koster, and Joseph Rey, "Electroconvulsive Therapy in Adolescents: Experience, Knowledge, and Attitudes of Recipients," *Journal of the American Academy of Child and Adolescent Psychiatry* 38, no. 5 (1999): 594–99. For an excellent discussion of the history and current practice of ECT, see Max Fink, *Electroshock: Restoring the Mind* (New York: Oxford University Press, 1999).

26. N. Ghaziuddin, S. P. Kutcher, and P. Knapp, "Summary of the Practice Parameter for the Use of Electroconvulsive Therapy with Adolescents," *Journal of the American Academy of Child and Adolescent Psychiatry* 43, no. 1 (2004): 119–22.

27. Larry Squire, Pamela Slater, and Patricia Miller, "Retrograde Amnesia and Bilateral Electroconvulsive Therapy: Long Term Follow-Up," *Archives of General Psychiatry* 38 (1981): 89–95.

28. C. P. L. Freeman, D. Weeks, and R. E. Kendell, "ECT III: Patients Who Complain," *British Journal of Psychiatry* 137 (1980): 17–25.

29. Larry R. Squire and Pamela C. Slater, "Electroconvulsive Therapy and Complaints of Memory Dysfunction: A Prospective Three-Year Follow-Up Study," *British Journal of Psychiatry* 142 (1983): 1–8.

30. S. Kutcher and H. Robertson, "Electroconvulsive Therapy in Treatment-Resistant Bipolar Youth," *Journal of Child and Adolescent Psychopharmacology* 5 (1995): 167–75.

31. David Cohen et al., "Absence of Cognitive Impairment at Long-Term Follow-up in Adolescents Treated with ECT for Severe Mood Disorder," *American Journal of Psychiatry* 157, no. 3 (2000): 460–62.

32. I. Perkins and K. Tanaka, "The Controversy That Will Not Die Is the Treatment That Can and Does Save Lives: Electroconvulsive Therapy," *Adolescence* 14 (1979): 607–17.

33. Sukeb Mukherjee, Harold Sackeim, and David Schnur, "Electroconvulsive Therapy of Acute Manic Episodes: A Review of 50 Years' Experience," *American Journal of Psychiatry* 151 (1994): 169–76.

34. S. Mukherjee, H. Sackheim, and C. Lee, "Unilateral ECT in the Treatment of Manic Episodes," *Convulsive Therapy* 4 (1988): 74–80.

35. Frederick K. Goodwin and Kay Redfield Jamison, *Manic-Depressive Illness* (New York: Oxford University Press, 1990), 661.

36. Olivier Taieb, David Cohen, Philippe Mezet, and Martine Flament, "Adolescents' Experiences with ECT," *Journal of the American Academy of Child and Adolescent Psychiatry* 39, no. 8 (2000): 934–44.

37. Paul E. Croarkin, Christopher A. Wall, and Jon Lee, "Applications of Transcranial Magnetic Stimulation (TMS) in Child and Adolescent Psychiatry," *International Review of Psychiatry* 23, no. 5 (2011): 445–53.

38. See Mark S. George, Eric Wasserman, and Robert Post, "Transcranial Magnetic Stimulation: A Neuropsychiatric Tool for the 21st Century," *Journal of Neuropsychiatry and Clinical Neurosciences* 8 (1996): 373–82.

39. Mark George et al., "Mood Improvement Following Daily Left Prefrontal Repetitive Transcranial Magnetic Stimulation in Patients with Depression: A Placebo-Controlled Crossover Trial," *American Journal of Psychiatry* 154 (1997): 1752–56.

40. Mark George et al., "A Controlled Trial of Daily Left Prefrontal Cortex TMS for Treating Depression," *Biological Psychiatry* 48 (2000): 962–70.

41. A. Pascual-Leone, B. Rubio, F. Pallardo, and M. D. Catala, "Beneficial Effect of Rapid-Rate Transcranial Magnetic Stimulation of the Left Dorsolateral Pre-frontal Cortex in Drug-Resistant Depression," *Lancet* 348 (1996): 233–37; and Charles Epstein, Gary Figiel, William McDonald, Jody Amazon-Leece, and Linda Figiel, "Rapid Rate Transcranial Magnetic Stimulation in Young and Middle-Aged Refractory Depressed Patients," *Psychiatric Annals* 28 (1998): 36–39.

42. A. John Rush et al., "Vagus Nerve Stimulation (VNS) for Treatment-Resistant Depression: A Multi-Center Study," *Biological Psychiatry* 47, no. 4 (2000): 276–86.

Chapter 9   Counseling and Psychotherapy

1. A. Wood, R. Harrington, and A. Moore, "A Controlled Trial of Brief Cognitive-Behavioral Intervention in Adolescent Patients with Depressive Disorders," *Journal of Child Psychology and Psychiatry* 37 (1996): 737–46.

2. Boris Birmaher et al., "Clinical Outcome after Short-Term Psychotherapy for Adolescents with Major Depressive Disorder," *Archives of General Psychiatry* 57 (2000): 29–36.

3. Dinah Jayson, "Which Depressed Patients Respond to Cognitive-Behavioral Treatment?" *Journal of the American Academy of Child and Adolescent Psychiatry* 37, no. 1 (1998): 35–39.

4. John March et al., "Fluoxetine, Cognitive-Behavioral Therapy, and Their Combination for Adolescents with Depression: Treatment for Adolescents with Depression Study (TADS) Randomized Controlled Trial," *JAMA* 292, no. 7 (2004): 807–20.

5. Jerome Frank, *Persuasion and Healing: A Comparative Study of Psychotherapy*, rev. ed. (New York: Schocken Books, 1974), xvi.

6. The standard work on cognitive-behavioral therapy is Aaron Beck, A. John Rush, Brian Shaw, and Gary Emery, *Cognitive Therapy of Depression* (New York: Guilford Press, 1979).

7. The area of comparison studies of cognitive-behavioral psychotherapy and medication in the treatment of depression can be accurately described as a hornet's nest of controversy. It's not difficult to find a study to support any possible view: superiority of medication over psychotherapy, superiority of psychotherapy over medication, and equal efficacy for both. For a nicely designed and well-executed study that found cognitive therapy to be as helpful as imipramine for 107 patients with major depressive disorder, see Steven Hollon et al., "Cognitive Therapy and Pharmacotherapy for Depression, Singly and in Combination," *Archives of General Psychiatry* 49 (1992): 774–81. For readers who would like to jump into the hornet's nest, we suggest Jacqueline B. Persons, Michael E. Thase, and Paul Crits-Christoph, "The Role of Psychotherapy in the Treatment of Depression," and the four (yes, four) accompanying rebuttal/commentary articles in the same issue of *Archives of General Psychiatry*.

8. Beck et al., *Cognitive Therapy of Depression*, 11.

9. Jeannette Rosselló and Guillermo Bernal, "The Efficacy of Cognitive-Behavioral and Interpersonal Treatments for Depression in Puerto Rican Adolescents," *Journal of Consulting and Clinical Psychology* 67, no. 5 (1999): 734.

10. Laura Mufson, Myra Weissman, Donna Morceau, and Robin Garfinkle, "Efficacy of Interpersonal Psychotherapy for Depressed Adolescents," *Archives of General Psychiatry* 56 (1999): 573–79.

11. Marsha M. Linehan, "Dialectical Behavioral Therapy: A Cognitive Behavioral Approach to Parasuicide," *Journal of Personality Disorders* 1, no. 4 (1987): 328–33.

12. Steven C. Hayes et al., "Acceptance and Commitment Therapy: Model, Processes and Outcomes," *Behaviour Research and Therapy* 44, no. 1 (2006): 1–25.

13. Louise Hayes, Candice P. Boyd, and Jessica Sewell, "Acceptance and Commitment Therapy for the Treatment of Adolescent Depression: A Pilot Study in a Psychiatric Outpatient Setting," *Mindfulness* 2, no. 2 (2011): 86–94.

Chapter 10 Attention-Deficit/Hyperactivity Disorder

1. George Still, "Some Abnormal Psychical Conditions in Childhood," *Lancet* 1 (1902): 1008–12.

2. Laurence Greenhill, Jeffrey Halperin, and Howard Abikoff, "Stimulant Medications," *Journal of the American Academy of Child and Adolescent Psychiatry* 38, no. 5 (1999): 503–12.

3. Arthur Robin, "Attention-Deficit/Hyperactivity Disorder in Adolescents," *Journal of the American Academy of Child and Adolescent Psychiatry* 45, no. 5 (1999): 1027–38.

4. MTA Cooperative Group, "Moderators and Mediators of Treatment Response for Children with Attention-Deficit/Hyperactivity Disorder: The Multimodal Treatment Study of Children with Attention-Deficit/Hyperactivity Disorder," *Archives of General Psychiatry* 56, no. 12 (1999): 1088.

5. Thomas Spencer, Joseph Biederman, and Timothy Wilens, "Attention-Deficit/Hyperactivity Disorder and Co-morbidity," *Pediatric Clinics of North America* 46, no. 5 (1999): 915–27.

6. J. Biederman et al., "Attention-Deficit Hyperactivity Disorder and Juvenile Mania: An Overlooked Comorbidity?" *Journal of the American Academy of Child and Adolescent Psychiatry* 35, no. 8 (1996): 997–1008.

7. Stephen Faraone, Joseph Biederman, Douglas Mennin, Janet Wozniak, and Thomas Spencer, "Attention-Deficit/Hyperactivity Disorder with Bipolar Disorder: A Familial Subtype?" *Journal of the American Academy of Child and Adolescent Psychiatry* 36, no. 10 (1997): 1378–87.

8. M. Strober et al., "Early Childhood Attention-Deficit/Hyperactivity Disorder Predicts Poorer Response to Acute Lithium Therapy in Adolescent Mania," *Journal of Affective Disorders* 51, no. 11 (1998): 145–51.

Chapter 11   Autism, Asperger's, and Related Disorders

1. Hans Asperger, "Die 'Autistischen Psychopathen' im Kindesalter," *European Archives of Psychiatry and Clinical Neuroscience* 117, no. 1 (1944): 76–136.

2. Leo Kanner, "Autistic Disturbances of Affective Contact," *Nervous Child* 2, no. 3 (1943): 217–50.

3. Dennis K. Flaherty, "The Vaccine-Autism Connection: A Public Health Crisis Caused by Unethical Medical Practices and Fraudulent Science," *Annals of Pharmacotherapy* 45, no. 10 (2011): 1302–4.

4. Lindsey Sterling et al., "Validity of the Revised Children's Anxiety and Depression Scale for Youth with Autism Spectrum Disorders," *Autism* (Jan. 2014), doi:10.1177/1362361313510066.

5. Susan Dickerson Mayes et al., "Variables Associated with Anxiety and Depression in Children with Autism," *Journal of Developmental and Physical Disabilities* 23, no. 4 (2011): 325–37.

6. Alexander Kolevzon, Karen A. Mathewson, and Eric Hollander, "Selective Serotonin Reuptake Inhibitors in Autism: A Review of Efficacy and Tolerability," *Journal of Clinical Psychiatry* 67, no. 3 (2006): 407–14.

7. Elisabeth M. Dykens et al., "Reducing Distress in Mothers of Children with Autism and Other Disabilities: A Randomized Trial," *Pediatrics* 134, no. 2 (2014): e454–e463.

Chapter 12   Alcohol and Drug Abuse

1. L. Johnston, P. O'Malley, J. Bachman, *Monitoring the Future: National Results on Adolescent Drug Abuse: Overview of Key Findings* (Bethesda, Md.: National Institute on Drug Abuse, 2001), 6.

2. Markus Henriksson et al., "Mental Disorders and Comorbidity in Suicide," *American Journal of Psychiatry* 150 (1993): 935–40.

3. Marjorie Hogan, "Diagnosis and Treatment of Teen Drug Use," *Medical Clinics of North America* 84, no. 4 (2000): 927–66.

4. Sandra Morrison, Peter Rogers, and Mark Thomas, "Alcohol and Adolescents," *Pediatric Clinics of North America* 42, no. 2 (1995): 371–87.

5. Andrew Johns, "Psychiatric Effects of Cannabis," *British Journal of Psychiatry* 178 (2001): 116–22.

6. Thomas Crowley, Marilyn Macdonald, Elizabeth Whitmore, and Susan Mikulich, "Cannabis Dependence, Withdrawal and Reinforcing Effects among Adolescents with Conduct Symptoms and Substance Abuse Disorders," *Drug and Alcohol Dependence* 50 (1998): 27–37.

7. Asbjørg Chrisopherson, "Amphetamine Designer Drugs—An Overview and Epidemiology," *Toxicology Letters* 112 (2000): 127–31.

8. Matthew Klam, "Experiencing Ecstasy," *New York Times*, Jan. 21, 2001, available at www.nytimes.com/2001/01/21/magazine/experiencing-ecstasy.html.

9. Andrew C. Parrott, "MDMA, Serotonergic Neurotoxicity, and the Diverse Functional Deficits of Recreational 'Ecstasy' Users," *Neuroscience and Biobehavioral Reviews* 37, no. 8 (2013): 1466–84.

10. For an excellent summary of MDMA's short-term and long-term effects on the brain, see Michael John Morgan, "Ecstasy (MDMA): A Review of Its Possible Persistent Psychological Effects," *Psychopharmacology* 152 (2000): 230–48.

11. Valerie Kremer, "Navy Medicine Rolls Out New Campaign to Deter 'Bath Salts' Designer Drug Use," *Navy Medicine*, Dec. 20, 2012, available at www.navy.mil/submit/display.asp?story_id=71211.

12. L. D. Johnston, P. M. O'Malley, R. A. Miech, J. G. Bachman, and J. E. Schulenberg, *Monitoring the Future National Results on Drug Use, 1975–2013: Overview, Key Findings on Adolescent Drug Use* (Ann Arbor: Institute for Social Research, University of Michigan, 2014).

13. Timothy Wilens, Joseph Biederman, Ana Abrantes, and Thomas Spencer, "Clinical Characteristics of Psychiatrically Referred Adolescent Outpatients with Substance Abuse Disorder," *Journal of the American Academy of Child and Adolescent Psychiatry* 36, no. 7 (1997): 941–47.

14. Judith Brook, Patricia Cohen, and David Brook, "Longitudinal Study of Co-occurring Psychiatric Disorders and Substance Use," *Journal of the American Academy of Child and Adolescent Psychiatry* 37, no. 3 (1998): 322–30.

15. Michael Lyvers, "'Loss of Control' in Alcoholism and Drug Addiction: A Neuroscientific Interpretation," *Experimental and Clinical Psychopharmacology* 8, no. 2 (2000): 225–49.

16. Paul Bergman, Maurice Smith, and Norman Hoffman, "Adolescent Treatment, Implications for Assessment, Practice Guidelines and Outcome Management," *Pediatric Clinics of North America* 42, no. 2 (1995): 453–72.

Chapter 13   Eating Disorders

1. The complete texts of all three historical accounts can be found in Arnold Anderson, *Practical Comprehensive Treatment of Anorexia and Bulimia* (Baltimore: Johns Hopkins University Press, 1985), 10–29.

2. Richard Kreipe and Susan Birndorf, "Eating Disorders in Adolescents," *Medical Clinics of North America* 84, no. 4 (2000): 1027–49.

3. Peter Lewinsohn, Ruth Striegel-Moore, and John Seeley, "Epidemiology and Natural Course of Eating Disorders in Young Women from Adolescence to Young Adulthood," *Journal of the American Academy of Child and Adolescent Psychiatry* 39, no. 10 (2000): 1284–92.

4. T. Zaider, J. Johnson, and S. Cockell, "Psychiatric Comorbidity Associated with Eating Disorder Symptomatology among Adolescents in the Community," *International Journal of Eating Disorders* 28, no. 1 (2000): 58–67.

5. Tracey Wade, Cynthia Bulik, Michael Neale, and Kenneth Kendler, "Anorexia Nervosa and Major Depression: Shared Genetic and Environmental Risk Factors," *American Journal of Psychiatry* 157, no. 3 (2000): 469–71.

6. A. Raffi, M. Rondini, S. Grandi, and G. Fava, "Life Events and Prodromal Symptoms in Bulimia Nervosa," *Psychological Medicine* 30, no. 3 (2000): 727–31.

7. David Jimerson, Barbara Wolfe, Andrew Brotman, and Eran Metzger, "Medications in the Treatment of Eating Disorders," *Psychiatric Clinics of North America* 19, no. 4 (1996): 739–54.

8. Walter Kaye, Kelly Gendell, and Michael Strober, "Serotonin Neuronal Function and Selective Serotonin Reuptake Inhibitor Treatment in Anorexia and Bulimia Nervosa," *Biological Psychiatry* 44 (1998): 825–38.

Chapter 14   "Cutting" and Other Self-Harming Behaviors

1. Paul R. McHugh and Phillip R. Slavney, *The Perspectives of Psychiatry*, 2nd ed. (Baltimore: Johns Hopkins University Press, 1999), 151.

2. Jennifer Egan, "The Thin Red Line," *New York Times Magazine*, July 27, 1997.

3. Armando Favazza, "The Coming of Age of Self-Mutilation," *Journal of Nervous and Mental Disease* 186, no. 5 (1998): 259–68.

4. Caron Zlotnick, Jill Mattia, and Mark Zimmerman, "Clinical Correlates of Self-Mutilation in a Sample of General Psychiatric Patients," *Journal of Nervous and Mental Diseases* 187, no. 5 (1999): 296–301.

5. Favazza, "Coming of Age of Self-Mutilation."

6. See Egan, "Thin Red Line"; and Marilee Strong, *A Bright Red Scream: Self-Mutilation and the Language of Pain* (New York: Penguin Books, 1999).

7. Stephen P. Lewis, Nancy L. Heath, Jill M. St. Denis, and Rick Noble, "The Scope of Nonsuicidal Self-Injury on YouTube," *Pediatrics* 127, no. 3 (2011): e552–e557.

8. See Armando Favazza, *Bodies under Siege: Self-Mutilation and Body Modification in Culture and Psychiatry*, 2d ed. (Baltimore: Johns Hopkins University Press, 1996), 241.

9. Marsha Linehan, *Cognitive-Behavioral Therapy of the Borderline Personality Disorder* (New York: Guilford Press, 1993).

10. Benedict Carey, "Expert on Mental Illness Reveals Her Own Fight," *New York Times*, June 23, 2011.

11. Alan Frances, "Introduction to Section on Self-Mutilation," *Journal of Personality Disorders* 1 (1987): 316.

12. All information on youth suicide statistics was obtained from the CDC Injury Statistics Query and Reporting System (WISQARS) website. All data are freely available and accessible at www.cdc.gov/injury/wisqars.

13. Matthew K. Nock et al., "Prevalence, Correlates, and Treatment of Lifetime Suicidal Behavior among Adolescents: Results from the National Comorbidity Survey Replication Adolescent Supplement," *JAMA Psychiatry* 70, no. 3 (2013): 300–310.

14. Iris Borowski, Marjorie Ireland, and Michael Resnick, "Adolescent Suicide Attempts: Risks and Protectors," *Pediatrics* 107, no. 3 (2001): 485–93.

15. Centers for Disease Control, "Effectiveness in Disease and Injury Prevention: Adolescent Suicide and Suicide Attempts—Santa Fe County, New Mexico, January 1985–May 1990," *Morbidity and Mortality Weekly Report* 40, no. 20 (1990): 329–31.

16. Sonja A. Swanson and Ian Colman, "Association between Exposure to Suicide and Suicidality Outcomes in Youth," *Canadian Medical Association Journal* 185, no. 10 (2013): 870–77.

17. D. Brent, J. Perper, C. Allman, G. Moritz, M. Wartella, and J. Zelenak, "The Presence and Accessibility of Firearms in the Homes of Adolescent Suicides: A Case Control Study," *Journal of the American Medical Association* 266, no. 21 (1991): 2989–95.

18. Danice K. Eaton et al., "Youth Risk Behavior Surveillance—United States, 2011," *Morbidity and Mortality Weekly Report: Surveillance Summaries (Washington, DC: 2002)* 61, no. 4 (2012): 1–162.

Chapter 15   The Genetics of Mood Disorders

1. Emil Kraepelin, *Manic-Depressive Insanity and Paranoia*, trans. R. M. Barclay, ed. G. M. Robertson (Edinburgh: Livingstone, 1921; reprinted New York: Arno Press, 1976), 165 (in reprint edition).

2. For a more detailed account, which includes references to the original articles, see Eliot Marshall, "Manic Depression: Highs and Lows on the Research Roller Coaster," *Science* 264 (1994): 1693–95.

3. Jonathan Flint and Kenneth S. Kendler, "The Genetics of Major Depression," *Neuron* 81, no. 3 (2014): 484–503.

4. See Elliot S. Gershon, "Genetics," in *Manic-Depressive Illness*, Frederick K. Goodwin and Kay Redfield Jamison (New York: Oxford University Press, 1990), 373–401.

5. For a very readable overview of some of these issues, see Doris Teichler Zallen, *Does It Run in the Family? A Consumer's Guide to DNA Testing for Genetic Disorders* (New Brunswick, N.J.: Rutgers University Press, 1997).

Chapter 16   Strategies for Successful Treatment

1. Emil Kraepelin, *Manic-Depressive Insanity and Paranoia*, trans. R. M. Barclay, ed. G. M. Robertson (Edinburgh: Livingstone, 1921; reprinted New York: Arno Press, 1976), 179–81 (in reprint edition).

2. Ian M. Goodyer, "The Influence of Recent Life Events on the Onset and Outcome of Major Depression in Young People," in *Depressive Disorders in Children and Adolescents: Epidemiology, Risk Factors, and Treatment*, ed. Cecilia Ahmoi Essau and Franz Petermann (Northvale, N.J.: Jason Aronson, 1999), 241.

3. For a complete discussion of these animal models of the kindling phenomenon, see Robert Post, "Transduction of Psychosocial Stress into the Neurobiology of Recurrent Affective Disorder," *American Journal of Psychiatry* 149 (1992): 999–1010.

4. Constance Hammen and Michael Gitlin, "Stress Reactivity in Bipolar Patients and Its Relation to Prior History of Disorder," *American Journal of Psychiatry* 154 (1997): 856–57.

5. Depression Guideline Panel, *Depression in Primary Care*, vol. 1, *Treatment of Major Depression: Clinical Practice Guidelines* (Rockville, Md.: U.S. Department of Health and Human Services, Public Health Service, Agency for Health Care Policy and Research, 1993).

6. George McGovern, *Terry: My Daughter's Life-and-Death Struggle with Alcoholism* (New York: Villard Books, 1996), 187.

7. See Peter Lewinsohn, Paul Rohde, John Seeley, Daniel Klein, and Ian Gotlib, "Natural Course of Adolescent Major Depressive Disorder in a Community Sample: Predictors of Recurrence in Young Adults," *American Journal of Psychiatry* 157, no. 10 (2000): 1584–91; and Mark Sanford et al., "Predicting the One-Year Course of Adolescent Major Depression," *Journal of the American Academy of Child and Adolescent Psychiatry* 34, no. 12 (1994): 1618–28.

Chapter 17   The Role of the Family

1. Stephen Strakowski, Susan McElroy, Paul Keck, and Scott West, "Suicidality among Patients with Mixed and Manic Bipolar Disorder," *American Journal of Psychiatry* 153 (1996): 674–76.

Chapter 18   Planning for Emergencies

1. See, for example, J. E. Bailey et al., "Risk Factors for Violent Death of Women in the Home," *Archives of Internal Medicine* 157 (1997): 777–82.

INDEX

Abilify (aripiprazole), 166, 167, 238
acceptance and commitment therapy
    (ACT), 208–10
accountable care organization
    (ACO), 340
acetylcholine, 121
Adderall (amphetamine/dextroam-
    phetamine), 221
adolescence: age range of, 4–5; bodily
    changes in, 33; dependence and au-
    tonomy in, 34; pathological group
    allegiances in, 34–35; psychological
    development in, 31–36, 81; sexuality
    in, 34; Sturm und Drang of, 31–32, 275
aggression/violence, 324, 325; in ADHD,
    216; antipsychotics for, 168; in au-
    tism, 237–38; in conduct disorder, 83,
    161; in disruptive mood dysregula-
    tion disorder, 67; mood stabilizers
    for, 153, 162, 163
agranulocytosis, 170
Alcoholics Anonymous, 255
alcohol use/abuse, 24, 35, 50, 52, 74, 213,
    241, 242–44; addiction due to, 244;
    definitions of, 242–43; mood disor-
    ders and, 244, 251–53, 313; prevalence
    of, 251; suicide and, 239, 325; treat-
    ment of, 253–56

alexithymia, 16
alprazolam (Xanax), 173, 246
American Academy of Child and Ado-
    lescent Psychiatry, 182, 187, 353
American Psychiatric Association, 7,
    44, 76, 84, 85
amitriptyline (Elavil), 119, 120, 174, 174n
amoxapine (Asendin), 119
amphetamine/dextroamphetamine
    (Adderall), 221
amphetamines: abuse of, 241, 242,
    247–51, 313; for ADHD, 220–21, 248
Anafranil (clomipramine), 119
anger, 16, 19, 29, 57, 59, 96, 162, 203, 216,
    320, 334; in disruptive mood dys-
    regulation disorder, 70; medications
    for, 164; of parents, 318, 330; psycho-
    therapy for, 205; self-mutilation due
    to, 270, 272; suicidality and, 277
anhedonia, 13, 16, 29, 48, 52, 59, 91. *See
    also* loss of interest or pleasure
anorexia nervosa, 214, 259, 260–62, 265,
    267; mood disorders and, 266–67
anticonvulsants, as mood stabilizers,
    151–60, 311
antidepressants, 5, 25, 79–80, 118–39;
    for ADHD, 223–24, 225; blood levels
    of, 122; bupropion, 132–33; chemical

guilt feelings, 11, 13, 19–20, 29, 48, 91, 203, 319; in bulimia nervosa, 266; in dysthymic disorder, 58, 59; of parents, 330; self-mutilation and, 270, 273

gynecomastia, 169–70

halfway houses, 256

hallucinations, 30, 48, 60, 91, 165; antipsychotics for, 165, 166, 167; diagnosis of, 30–31; in mania, 64; self-mutilation due to, 270; substance-induced, 25, 248, 251

hallucinogens, 248

happiness, 9, 10, 17

headache, 13, 22, 29, 48, 89, 158

health insurance issues: choice of psychiatrist, 304–5, 336; copayments, 338; genetic testing, 289, 350; hospitalization coverage, 335, 336, 337, 338–41; managed care, 304, 339–41; medication coverage, 341

Health Insurance Portability and Accountability Act (HIPAA), 321

health maintenance organization (HMO), 212, 304–5, 335, 339–40, 341

history of child psychiatry, 27–28

hopelessness, 19, 270, 276, 277, 320, 327

hospitalization, 66, 68, 70, 155–56, 293, 326–29, 332–43; antipsychotic use and, 171; benzodiazepine use and, 172; for bipolar II disorder, 75; consent and assent for, 326; for dangerousness, 327, 341; for eating disorders, 262, 263, 266, 267–68; for electroconvulsive therapy, 182–83; indicated by GAF Scale, 90; insurance coverage for, 335, 336, 337, 338–41; involuntary, 325, 326–29, 333; parent involvement during, 321; partial/day, 339; pre-admission review for, 340; questions/preparation for, 337–38; return to school after, 211; for substance abuse, 254, 255, 256; for

suicidality, 51, 327, 333, 335, 341, 343; for treatment noncompliance, 330

"huffing," 241

Human Genome Project, 288, 347

hypomania, 64, 66, 68, 71; in bipolar II, 73–75, 92, 94; in cyclothymic disorder, 75–77, 92, 94; electroconvulsive therapy–induced, 187; family reactions to, 319, 330; lithium for, 150; in seasonal affective disorder, 94

identity crisis, 32

identity development, 35–37

identity diffusion, 35

imipramine, 112, 113, 118, 119, 120, 121, 174, 174n, 193, 366n7

impulsivity: in ADHD, 216, 218, 219, 220, 222, 224, 294; in autism, 232; dialectical behavioral therapy for, 208; in eating disorders, 262, 263, 266, 267; in mania, 66, 162; medications for, 162, 220, 224; self-mutilation and, 271; suicidality and, 275

inhalant abuse, 241

insight-oriented psychotherapy, 193–94, 204–5, 320

interpersonal psychotherapy (IPT), 201–2

Intuniv (guanfacine), 224

involuntary commitment, 325, 326–29, 333

iproniazid, 25, 112, 133

irritability, 11, 12–13, 18, 19, 21, 29, 41, 45, 86; in ADHD, 222; antipsychotics for, 167, 168; in autism, 235, 236; behavioral problems and, 295; in bipolar disorder, 67, 69, 74, 75; dialectical behavior therapy for, 206, 207, 208; in disruptive mood dysregulation disorder, 67, 68, 69–70, 93; in dysthymic disorder, 58, 59; eating disorders and, 267; family effects of, 203, 210, 318, 319, 320, 329, 330–31; in major depressive disorder, 48–53; in mania,

medications (*cont.*)

multiple diagnoses, 294–95; noncompliance with, 334, 336; off-label prescribing of, 101, 102–4, 127, 293; placebo effect of, 122–23; for relapse prevention, 312–13; use of, in children and adolescents, 101, 105

melancholia, 10, 31, 78, 84, 91–94, 181

memory problems, 13, 22, 47, 48; alcohol-induced, 244, 313; electroconvulsive therapy–induced, 183, 184–85; MDMA-induced, 249, 250

memory tests, 297

mental status examination, 46

metabolic syndrome, 169

methamphetamine, 241, 247–50

methylphenidate (Concerta; Daytrana; Methylin; Ritalin), 217, 220, 221

monoamine oxidase inhibitors (MAOIs), 133–35; drug and food interactions with, 134–35

mood, 10; chemistry of, 24–26; constricted, 19; diurnal variation of, 20; dysphoric, 48, 52; elevated/euphoric, 64; good, 10–11; hormonal regulation of, 59–60; low, 5, 6, 10–11, 12, 16, 23, 47, 85; normal and abnormal, 11–12; reactivity of, 18–19

mood disorders, 2, 12, 23–24, 28; ADHD and, 222–23; amine hypothesis of, 112, 113, 120; autism and, 235–36; classification of, 41–81; diagnosis of, 2, 3, 43–47, 78–81; in *DSM*, 90–97; eating disorders and, 266–68; genetics of, 285–89, 347–48; importance of treatment for, 81–83; kindling in, 67, 310–11; neurochemistry of, 112–13; not otherwise specified, 66, 68; risk factors for relapse of, 316; specifiers for, 91–94; substance abuse and, 251–53, 313–16

mood hygiene, 307–9

mood stabilizers, 80, 140–63; carbamazepine, 155–57; gabapentin, 159–60; lamotrigine, 157–59; lithium, 140–51; oxcarbazepine, 160; symptoms treated by, 161–62; tiagabine, 160; topiramate, 160; use in depression, 162–63; valproate, 151–54

mood symptoms, 13, 15–20, 47–53

mourning, 11, 13, 18

Nardil (phenelzine), 134

natural history, 3; of bipolar I, 71

negative thinking, 19, 29, 63, 197, 198–201, 209

Neurontin (gabapentin), 103, 159–60

neuroscience research, 345–47

neurotransmitters, 109–14, 281

norepinephrine, 112–13, 119–20, 130–33, 224

Norpramin (desipramine), 119, 121–22

nortriptyline (Pamelor), 119

nurse counselors, 303

obsessive-compulsive disorder, 103, 118, 137, 237, 294

olanzapine (Zyprexa), 167

omega-3 fatty acids, 175–78

oppositional defiant disorder, 96–97, 161, 295

optimism, 10, 11, 31, 64

overdose of drug, 51; lithium, 171, 175; SSRIs, 125; tricyclic antidepressants, 122, 130; valproate, 154

oxcarbazepine (Trileptal), 160

oxytocin, 237

pain, 13; self-mutilation and, 270–72; sensitivity to, 22

pain medications, 175, 246; abuse of, 241, 251; SNRIs, 131

pain signals, 108, 110

Pamelor (nortriptyline), 119

parasympathetic nervous system, 224

parent management training, 220

parents/family, 291–92, 318–31; of child with autism, 238; and consent for treatment, 187, 321, 326; counseling/therapy for, 202–4, 221, 316, 331; enabling by, 315, 331; fears of, 1, 2; involvement of, in treatment, 2, 320–24; overprotective, 330; role of, in arranging hospitalization and involuntary commitment, 326–29; of substance-abusing adolescent, 254–55, 315, 331; support for, 238, 329–31; symptom recognition by, 1, 318–20

Parnate (tranylcypromine), 134

paroxetine (Paxil), 127, 224

pathological influences, 307

Patient Protection and Affordable Care Act, 338

peer relationships: group conformity and pathological group allegiances, 34–35; social media and, 4–5, 35; substance abuse and, 241

personality disorders, 88–89, 207, 273, 294

pervasive developmental disorders (PDDs), 233–35, 236; caring for parents of children with, 238; not otherwise specified, 233, 234

pessimism, 10, 11, 58, 198, 319

pharmacogenomics, 139, 289, 347–48

phenelzine (Nardil), 134

Physicians' Desk Reference (PDR), 104–5, 107

placebo effect, 122–23

polypharmacy, 171

preferred provider organization (PPO), 304–5, 335

premenstrual dysphoric disorder (PMDD), 59–61, 94

Prestiq (desvenlafaxine), 130

privacy issues, 320, 321, 322

protriptyline (Vivactil), 119

Prozac (fluoxetine), 77, 113, 125–27, 128, 136, 139, 224, 267, 348, 349

psychiatrists, 2, 211–12, 299–300, 303, 304; child and adolescent, 2, 300, 304, 305, 336, 337–38; contacting in

emergencies, 337; hospital privileges of, 337–38; interactions with parents, 320–24; selection of, 304–6, 336–38; training of, 299–300, 304

psychoanalysis, 32, 143, 194, 228, 346

psychological testing, 296–98

psychologists, 301–2

psychotherapists, 210–12, 300–301, 302, 303

psychotherapy, 24, 39, 41, 192–212, 316; acceptance and commitment therapy, 208–10; for ADHD, 220, 221, 225; for autism, 236; biology-psychology split and, 192–94; choosing therapy and therapist, 210–12; cognitive-behavioral therapy, 198–201, 320; definition of, 197; dialectical behavioral therapy, 206–8, 273; effectiveness of, 38, 195–96; family therapy, 202–4, 221, 316, 331; group, 205–6; insight-oriented, 193–94, 204–5, 320; interpersonal, 201–2; matching to patient, 198; necessity of, 197; parental involvement in, 320–21

psychotic symptoms, 29–30, 48, 52, 91–92, 165; antipsychotics for, 165–72

quetiapine (Seroquel), 166–67

relapse prevention, 312–13

religious beliefs, 34, 36, 38, 303; suicide and, 276, 377

reserpine, 25

resilience, 38, 81

risperidone (Risperdal), 103, 167, 171, 238

Ritalin (methylphenidate), 217, 221

sadness, 2, 3, 10, 11

safety issues, 324–25, 341–43

Saphris (asenapine), 167

schizophrenia, 107, 143, 180–81, 193, 350; antipsychotics for, 165–72; vs. autism, 227, 228, 229

weight: depression and, 14, 15, 20–21, 29, 41, 48, 196; eating disorders and, 258, 259, 260–67, 272; media messages about, 264–65; obesity/overweight, 258, 260–61, 263, 264, 265

weight changes, drug-induced, 68, 317; atypical antipsychotics, 169; bupropion, 132; lithium, 149, 163; MAOIs, 134; SSRIs, 128; tricyclic antidepressants, 121; valproate, 154

Wellbutrin (bupropion), 130, 132–33, 224

worthlessness, 19, 29, 30, 41, 48, 319

Xanax (alprazolam), 173, 246

ziprasidone (Geodon), 167

Zoloft (sertraline), 77, 103, 127

Zyban (bupropion), 133

Zyprexa (olanzapine), 167

ALSO BY PETER SPIEGELMAN

Red Cat

Death's Little Helpers

Black Maps

THICK
AS
THIEVES

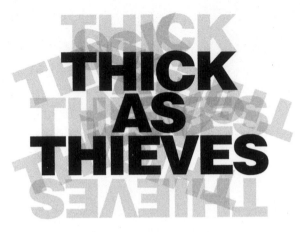

THICK
AS
THIEVES

Peter Spiegelman

ALFRED A. KNOPF   NEW YORK   2011

THIS IS A BORZOI BOOK
PUBLISHED BY ALFRED A. KNOPF

Copyright © 2011 by Peter Spiegelman

All rights reserved. Published in the United States by Alfred A. Knopf,
a division of Random House, Inc., New York, and in Canada by
Random House of Canada Limited, Toronto.

www.aaknopf.com

Knopf, Borzoi Books, and the colophon are registered trademarks of
Random House, Inc.

Library of Congress Cataloging-in-Publication Data
Spiegelman, Peter.
Thick as thieves / by Peter Spiegelman. —1st ed.
p. cm.
ISBN 978-0-307-26317-9 (alk. paper)
I. Title.
PS3619.P543T47 2011
813'.6—dc22   2011017855

Front-of-jacket photograph © NHPA/SuperStock
Jacket design by Evan Gaffney

Manufactured in the United States of America
First Edition

For my parents, Morton and Joyce,
and for my nephew Anthony, who we miss so much

"A plague upon it when thieves cannot be true one to another!"

—Falstaff to Prince Hal,
Henry IV, Part I, act II, scene 2

Acknowledgments

Many thanks are due to many people for their help while I was writing this book: Reed Coleman, for his time and excellent ear; Nina Spiegelman, for her early reading; Denise Marcil and Abner Stein, for their encouragement and enthusiasm; Myron Glucksman, for any number of things; Sonny Mehta, for his support, advice, and supreme patience; and Alice Wang, for—really—more than I can say.

THICK
AS
THIEVES

1

Inside the house now, the three of them stand still in the foyer, in the pale oblong of street light that falls through the transom, and Carr hears voices in the walls. A muted cough from the air ducts, a nervous murmur from the drapes, a creaking sigh from the paneling in the center hall—a muffled chorus, singing only to him. *Home early. Not the maid's night off. Tires in the driveway.* Carr's thighs are lead, and a clamp wraps around his chest. Adrenaline, he knows, but knowing doesn't help. He reminds himself to inhale, to exhale, not too fast. Above his chanting fear he can hear Declan's voice.

"Nothin' like a house in the dark, lad." The brogue that came and went, the rough laughter, the sharper edge of excitement, as if he were talking about a roller coaster. But Carr hates roller coasters, and always has. Inhale, exhale, not too fast.

The odors of the house come to him: lavender, cinnamon, lilac, vanilla, the chemical tang of a disinfectant—like a brothel above a bakery—but Piney Point Village is hardly that kind of Houston neighborhood. He takes another breath and catches a trace of cigars and of dog—an overweight, arthritic Lab that Carr knows is boarded at the vet's all week. Bobby flicks a penlight and follows its beam to a plastic box on the wall.

"No mess," Carr tells him.

"Yeah, yeah, I hear you," Bobby says, irritation and Brooklyn plain in his raspy whisper. He sticks the penlight in his mouth, pops the cover off the box with a thin screwdriver, and pries loose a circuit board from the bracket underneath. He pulls a coil of wire from the wall behind it and picks delicately at the board, teasing up the contacts. Bobby's moves are quick, and there's time to spare when he reaches into his pocket, pulls out something like a matchbook, and snaps it onto one edge of the board. A green LED blinks fast on the matchbook as it talks to the processor in the basement. *Don't worry, be happy.* The blinking is replaced by a steady glow, and Bobby lets the board hang by its wires down along the wall. He hooks the plastic cover on a corner of the bracket and takes the penlight from his mouth.

"Clean enough?" he asks.

Latin Mike answers. "Slick, *cabrón,* like always." Mike is forty, older than Carr, older than any of them, but his rounded San Diego accent makes him sound like a kid.

Carr nods. "Bobby goes downstairs; start by the door to the garage. Mike takes the master. Check your headsets first." Carr touches his own and swings down the mic on its wire arm. "You there, Vee?"

In the darkness Valerie's voice is close, as if her lips are at his ear. "Where else?" she says. Her tone is amber, smoky, a little weary. Carr can almost feel her breath. "All quiet out front. A guy walking a dog at the corner; a drunk in a beemer."

"And in back?" Carr asks.

Dennis answers. "Not even a drunk back here." His voice is young and reedy and tentative, like Dennis himself.

Carr looks at Bobby and Latin Mike. "You guys hear everything?" Bobby barely nods; Mike won't muster even that. Carr looks down. "Clean shoes?"

Latin Mike snorts. "We virgins now, *jefe?*" he says, the *jefe* laden with sarcasm. "We never done this before?" He walks off, into the deeper darkness of the house, and Bobby follows.

Carr takes a long breath and lets it out slowly. He strains to hear them rummaging upstairs and down, but they're silent. No, not virgins. There's a half-moon table in the foyer, black lacquer with a vase of drooping gladiolas on top and a drawer beneath. Carr thumbs his own penlight and opens it.

* * *

Carr has progressed to the office, a mahogany annex to the living room, with many bookshelves but few books. There's a claw-footed desk squatting in the middle, and he's going through the center drawer when Latin Mike's voice crackles in his ear. "Got a box in the master, in the walk-in, behind the suits. Looks like a real piece of shit."

A surge of anger runs through Carr's gut. "Leave it," he says.

"Five minutes max and I'm in this thing."

"I said *leave it*."

"It's low-hanging fruit, *jefe*."

"We're not here for fruit. Now stay off the air unless you find it."

If Mike has an answer Carr doesn't hear it over Bobby's laugh. "You want low fruit, bro, you should see the liquor store goin' on down here. We lift a case of Dom, he'd never miss it."

Carr grits his teeth. There'd been none of this bullshit with Declan. With Deke, once they were inside, it was all business. There was no idle chatter, just that gravelly brogue calling out the numbers, and the clipped, whispered acknowledgments from each of them. Carr knows that Mike and Bobby are fucking with him, trying to get a rise, but he's not going to give them the pleasure. He takes a breath and is about to speak when Valerie cuts through Bobby's chuckles. "You girls want to shut the fuck up while this cruiser passes by?" she whispers.

Mike and Bobby go silent and there's a chunk of ice in Carr's gut. He kills his penlight. Valerie's voice is a low monotone. "Half a block down . . . two houses now . . . goddamn it, he's slowing down. Fuck—is there a backup you guys forgot about? 'Cause he's stopped right in front." Her voice gets softer and the sound of rustling fabric is loud in Carr's ear. He can picture her slouching low behind the wheel.

Bobby starts to talk but Carr cuts him off. "Quiet!" he whispers, and then to Valerie: "We burned or what, Vee?"

"I don't know," she whispers. "I don't . . . wait—he's rolling away. One house down . . . now two. He's at the corner, taking . . . a left."

Something releases in Carr's chest. "Dennis, anything?"

"He just went past. He's hanging a right on Smithdale."

Carr flicks on his light again. Bobby's voice leaps into his ear. "I didn't forget a fuckin' thing, Vee."

"You forgot how to keep quiet," Valerie says, the tension in her voice replaced by anger. "You forgot how to keep your head in the game—you and Mike both."

"Don't drag me into this, *chica*."

"Then shut the fuck up, the both of you, and get back to work."

It's ten minutes later when Bobby calls in. "I got it. On a table at the top of the basement stairs, in a bowl with loose change and gas receipts." Thirty seconds after that, the three of them are in the foyer again.

"Everything buttoned up?" Carr asks.

"Shipshape, *jefe*."

"Bobby?"

"Gotta clean this up," he says, pushing his chin at the box dangling down the wall. He hands Carr the card he's holding and digs in his vest for the screwdriver.

Carr runs his light over the ID card—hard gray plastic, with a picture of an office building on one side and a red nylon lanyard clipped to one end. He turns the card over and looks at the bar codes and mag strip and photo of the bland, balding man in the center. It's a better picture of Jerry Molloy, he thinks, than the portrait above the living room mantel.

2

There are candles burning in green glass spheres, and green paper lanterns hanging, and the air above the patio is tinted the color of an aquarium gone bad. It smells of citronella, and cigarettes, and a hundred clashing colognes. Valerie walks from the bar, a pitcher of Shiner Bock in each hand. She wears a short, flowered dress that clings to her as if it's wet, and her bare arms and legs are gleaming. Her dark blond hair is pinned in a haphazard pile, and her long, limber body is like a burning fuse as she twists through the crowd.

Every eye in the place—male and female—follows her back to the table, though Carr tries to avoid watching. Looking is what she wants, he thinks, and it feels too much like strings being pulled. Still, over the top of his glass, he looks—and so do Bobby, Latin Mike, and Dennis. Because, despite how long they've known her, how many times they've seen her work a room, there is always with Valerie the promise of something they haven't seen before.

Their table is in a far corner, and the four men sit with their backs to the low cinder-block wall that separates the patio from the surrounding hardpan lot. Carr watches the crowd, which is watching them, and he doesn't care for the attention. Valerie slides the pitchers into the center of the table and sits next to Carr. "What's your problem?" she asks.

"You riled up the natives, *chica,*" Mike answers, before Carr can speak.

"Place needs something," Valerie says. "The music sucks." She's smiling and her cheeks are flushed.

"He don't want them noticing us, right, *jefe?*"

Carr leans back and looks up through the rafters and the open roof—at the hovering mosquitoes, the flickering bats, the washed-out stars above. A warm breeze works its fingers beneath his shirt. He's had three beers, and there's a pleasant foaminess somewhere around his forebrain. He knows where Mike is going and he's too tired to follow. He keeps quiet but it doesn't help.

"Like they took us for locals before she crossed the floor?" Bobby says.

Mike gives Bobby a low five. "We blend in, *cabrón;* we natives." Latin Mike looks at Carr and frowns. "They get a bad vibe from us, *jefe.*"

Carr drains his beer glass. "Vibes are one thing; Vee makes us memorable."

"Memorable for sure," Bobby says, and winks at Valerie, who winks back.

Mike snorts. "Face it, *pendejo,* we fit better in Caracas or Recife than we do up here."

Dennis wipes sweat from his face and joins in. "Down there we're just *norteamericanos*—oil workers, contractors, whatever—nobody gives a damn. Just a few more Yankees passing through."

"Speak for yourself, *yanqui,*" Mike says. "But the point is, what the fuck we doing up here? Too much homeland security horseshit—what we need the headaches for? It's not like we have problems finding work."

Carr sighs. "Not this kind of work."

Mike downs half his beer and points a finger at Carr. He's smiling, but with him that's a tactic. "This kind of work is too fucking complicated—too many moving parts."

"You used to worry about the same shit five years ago, if I remember right, but things turned out okay."

"Damn straight I was worried. We had a good thing going, fishing where the fish were stupid—why mess with what works? But Deke was a man with a plan, and there was no arguing with him. Plus, I had faith in the guy."

"And you don't in me."

"No offense, *cabrón,* but you're not Deke."

Carr leans forward. "Sure, Mike, no offense."

"For chrissakes!" Valerie says, and slams her own glass on the tabletop. "Why don't you two get a room if you're going at this bullshit again. This was supposed to be a party." Bobby smirks and Dennis giggles with relief. Under the table Valerie's hand finds Carr's thigh. He doesn't jump, but it's a near thing. Her palm is hot through the fabric of his jeans. Carr nods slowly and reaches for a pitcher. He proffers it across the table.

"Let me top that off," he says, and Mike holds out his glass.

Valerie is right, Carr knows: they've gone around like this a dozen times or more, and there'll be time enough to go around again. But not now. Now, the night before they work again, it's time to drink. It's a lesson he had from Declan, who was ever alert to the peril of idle hands.

"Busy is best for these nippers," he'd told Carr. "Otherwise it's all worry and gossip and chewin' the arses off one another. Keep 'em busy, and when they've done their chores, get 'em pissed." More than tradition, these outings are an antidote to the jitters and jumps and sheer stir-craziness that come to a boil on the eve of every job. But like so much else he's learned from Declan, Carr knows he doesn't do it quite as well. Pirate king, father confessor, jolly Jack Falstaff—Carr is none of these, though he has developed other talents: watchfulness, patience, an attention to detail—the talents of a planner, a technician. Not exactly inspirational, he knows. Not like Declan. Still, one does what one can.

Carr works a smile onto his face and fills glasses until the pitcher is empty. Valerie's hand is gone now, and the music is louder, if unimproved. Valerie is dancing with Mike to something twangy, and Dennis watches them, tapping the tabletop in time to nothing Carr can hear. Bobby is eyeing the local talent. The peaceable kingdom. Carr finishes his beer. He leans back and looks at the wrung-out sky and thinks of limes.

Declan was cutting them the first time they met—a bet with a barman at a marble and frosted glass palace in Las Lomas. Teddy Voigt, Carr's immediate boss at Integral Risk Associates, and the closest thing he'd had to a friend there, had arranged the get-together, not forty-eight hours after Carr had been fired and just forty-eight hours before Carr had to vacate his company-owned apartment—the graceful exit being one of the things Carr had relinquished when he'd hit his most profitable client in the face.

Hunched over the granite bar, Declan was a rhino at a tea party: red-faced, craggy, and ancient next to the silken youth that crowded the

club—more like one of the bodyguards loitering on the sidewalk outside. The paring knife was nearly lost in his fist, but the edge of the blade was a blur and the slices he cut were translucent green petals. Whatever the bet was, Declan won going away, and whatever the prize, Declan declined payment and instead bought the barman a shot of Patrón. Which, Carr came to realize, was essential Declan: good with bartenders, good with knives, good with tactical mercy.

Good at other things too, Carr learned as they bar-hopped across the leafy night, from Las Lomas to an English pub in Polanco to a hipster saloon in Condesa. Good at Gallic bonhomie and fatalistic, self-deprecating humor. Good at oblique but relentless interrogation. Good at large volumes of pricey tequila, chased by even larger volumes of beer. Good, despite how much he'd had to drink, at negotiating the unforgiving chaos of traffic in Mexico City.

Good too at throwing an elbow into a man's windpipe, then breaking his wrist, for slapping a woman to the pavement. That took place in the doorway of their last stop: a workingman's tavern in Santa María la Ribera that was little more than a dim hallway drenched in nicotine and sentimental guitars. The patrons seemed to take the violence in stride, if they noticed it at all, and the smile never left Declan's face. He'd made his pitch to Carr at a table near the kitchen.

Carr comes back to the sound of breaking glass. Dennis and Valerie are on the dance floor but they're not dancing. There's a stunned look on Dennis's face, and a local boy, a wide receiver gone to seed, is laughing and grabbing Valerie around the waist. Latin Mike and Bobby are on their feet, smiling eagerly as three doughy cowboys shoulder through the skittish crowd to help the wide receiver. Valerie looks angry, and looks at Carr, who has visions of broken bottles, flashing lights, the cowboys hauled off in ambulances, his crew simply hauled off.

"Shit," he mutters, and hoists himself off his chair.

In the Ford, on the way back to the hotel, adrenaline has burned off the alcohol and left them with a different kind of buzz. Carr is at the wheel, always three miles over the limit, nice and steady, while Valerie works the radio. Dennis has his face in the rush of humid air from the open window in back, and Bobby and Mike are smoking and joking.

"Fucking Vee," Bobby says, "that guy's gonna be picking his balls outta his nose for a week." He puts a fist forward and Valerie knocks it with her own.

"The way he mauled me, I should've kicked him again."

Mike catches Carr's eye in the mirror. "Three times was enough, *chica*," he says. "Four would make you *memorable*." He and Bobby laugh and Carr shakes his head and pulls into the hotel lot.

Dennis is pale and wobbly getting out of the car; he crosses the parking lot at a jog and disappears into the hotel. Valerie, Bobby, and Mike take their time. Mike lights another cigarette, props his elbows on the Ford's roof, and looks across at Carr.

"Eight o'clock tomorrow," Carr says. Mike and Valerie say nothing. Bobby looks at the low hotel, the rows of windows, mostly black, and the vestigial balconies. He nods absently and heads for the lobby. Carr follows, rubbing the bruises on his forearms and knuckles, not listening to Mike and Valerie, who stand by the car and speak softly.

Carr leaves his room dark and lets his eyes adjust to the yellow haze that seeps through the curtains from the sodium lamps outside. From the window he can see the parking lot and, if he cranes his neck, the car. He can make out Latin Mike's shape, tall, with a plume of cigarette smoke above, and Valerie's silhouette, very close by. Just how close? Carr can't tell from his vantage, and in a while he tells himself he doesn't care. A while after that he stops looking.

The air in his room is like an airplane's: metallic, exhausted, and too cold. Carr switches off the AC, and a ticking silence descends. And then dissolves in the babble of a television from next door. Carr switches on the AC.

His work clothes hang in the closet, and his bag is packed but for his shaving kit and what he's wearing. He strips off his jeans and polo shirt, folds them, packs them away, and looks around the room, rehearsing in his mind the routine for wiping it down: front to back, left to right, floor to head height. Then he brushes his teeth and gets into the shower.

When he comes out, Valerie's key is on the desk. Her shoes are by the nightstand, her dress on the chair, and Valerie herself is in bed, under a sheet, with a hand behind her head and her blond hair fanned across the pillows. Carr can smell her perfume and her sweat, and the cigarette smoke that clings to her like cobwebs. *Just how close?*

Thick as Thieves

"Is he going to behave himself?" Carr asks.

"He'll behave tomorrow."

"And after that?"

Valerie shrugs. "You think you can get to sleep?" she asks.

"No," Carr says, and fastens the chain on the door.

3

The Prairie Galleria, a ten-story structure on Prairie Street, not far from Minute Maid Park, once housed, among other tenants, the Houston offices of a national bank, the Houston outpost of an international consulting firm, and half a dozen energy trading houses. Those businesses are gone now, bought out, broken up, or plain dead, but their bad luck is still etched on the building's blue glass skin, which is stained and cracked in some spots, and missing altogether in others—patched with plywood sheets like rippled, gray scabs.

The current occupants are making the best of the current economy. They're an eclectic bunch, including accountants, lawyers of various stripes—bankruptcy, tax, and divorce the best-represented specialties—a bail bondsman, two dealers in used office equipment, and several real estate liquidators. With the exception of the bail bondsman, none of these firms conduct regular business on Saturdays, so the lobby is quiet when Carr approaches the reception counter at 8:37 a.m.—just two uniformed guards who, Carr knows, work only weekend shifts. The cooling system is cycling low, and the air is thick and smells of someone's breakfast. Carr keeps close to the right-hand wall, out of view of the single security camera. His deck shoes squeak on the marble floor and a line of sweat worms down his ribs. *Inhale, exhale, not too fast.*

Carr hitches up the strap on the nylon briefcase slung over his shoul-

der and pushes the horn-rimmed sunglasses up on his nose. He makes a show of searching the pockets of his sagging blue blazer. The guards have never seen him before, but whatever curiosity they experience is overmatched by heat and apathy, and they barely raise their heads. Carr shifts the Styrofoam coffee cup to his left hand and searches more pockets. The performance settles him down and he nods at the guards and puts a eureka look on his face. He fishes the ID card from his pocket and slides it through the reader on the turnstile that stands between him and the elevator bank. The light on the reader blinks from amber to green and the barrier swings away and Carr walks through. He stops on the other side.

"My guys haven't been in yet, have they?" he asks.

The guards look at each other and back at Carr. "What guys?" the bald one asks.

"IT guys, coming with new computers."

"Nobody's been in."

Carr looks at his watch. "Should be soon. You'll send 'em up?"

The bald guard nods, taps a finger on a keyboard, and squints at the text on the screen. "Yep. That's Molloy, on six?"

"That's me," Carr says, and steps into a waiting elevator. He keeps his head down, away from the camera in the corner, and presses the button for six.

The sixth floor is warmer than the lobby, and quieter, and all Carr can hear after the doors close behind him is the elevator sliding down and the faint push of air from a ceiling vent. Once upon a time, Carr knows, the whole floor belonged to a law firm. It was where they kept their library and conference rooms and archived records, until the markets went south and everything else followed. Then the law firm shut down, the building changed hands, and the new landlords invested in new doors, new wiring, and lots of wallboard, and turned all that teak paneling and Berber carpet into five separate office suites.

Carr looks at the nameplates. To his right, two lawyers and a forensic accountant; straight ahead, behind heavy glass doors and a roll-down metal gate, in the largest suite on the floor, a company called Portrait Capital; and to his left, in the smallest office, Jerry Molloy, tax attorney in semiretirement, currently concluding a one-week visit to his Hill Country home. Carr removes his sunglasses, pulls latex gloves from his briefcase, and turns left.

Molloy's lock is a joke—old and tired—and it surrenders after a few bumps with the power rake. The alarm is even worse—no motion detector, and just a single magnetic contact on the door frame. But Carr doesn't have to fiddle it; he has the code, copied from the slip of paper Valerie discovered taped beneath Molloy's desk blotter two weeks before. Molloy had gone out to lunch—without setting his alarm—and Valerie was ostensibly visiting a divorce lawyer one floor up. It had taken her all of six minutes to find it. A dispirited chirping comes from the smudged plastic box on the wall. Carr taps the keypad and the box goes silent. He locks the office door, wipes a sleeve across his forehead, and looks around.

There isn't much to see. The space is partitioned into two rooms: the one Carr is standing in, with a small window, a small filing cabinet, a small desk for Molloy's part-time secretary, and carpeting the color of car exhaust; and Molloy's office, which is a larger version of the same. Both smell vaguely of old cigar smoke, and neither holds anything of interest to Carr. He takes off his blazer, folds it on Molloy's desk, and rolls up his sleeves. Then he crosses to the far wall and opens a door.

Behind it is a small utility closet, where electrical and telecom lines branch out from the conduits that carry them between floors to provide local service. There are junction boxes on the wall: gray for telecom, beige for electrical, flimsy white plastic for the security system. They're mounted next to the vertical PVC conduits, and bundles of cable snake into and out of them. Carr pulls a penlight and a much handled sheaf of papers from his briefcase and flips pages to the plan of Molloy's office.

The plans tell him that this closet is a recent addition, built when the original office space was subdivided. It shares a wall with another, larger utility closet in the suite next door—a hastily erected wall of gypsum board hung on metal studs. Carr raps on the board and it makes a hollow sound. He pulls a tape measure and a pencil from his bag, checks the plan, and marks a rectangle, two feet wide by three feet high, on the closet wall. Then he takes a headset out.

"You there, Vee?" he says.

"Where else?" she answers. "Everything okay?"

"Fine. Send them in."

Carr looks out the window and watches Bobby and Latin Mike emerge from a rusting blue van parked nose out in the lot across the street. Each has a nylon bag slung on his shoulder, and each is carrying a Dell com-

puter box. Even from six floors up Carr can see the tension in their strides. They wear jeans, dark T-shirts, and sunglasses, but neither really looks the part of IT geek. Bobby comes close—scruffy, freckled, pale, and slightly bloated, as if he lives on fast food—but Mike is a far cry. His heavy shoulders and battered, angry good looks transcend wardrobe and type-cast him as a hardcase, a badass, a thief. Still, Carr knows they'll pass muster with the listless guards in the lobby. They disappear into the Prairie Galleria, and Carr looks again at the van. He tries to make out Valerie behind the wheel but can't.

"Anybody else come in?" he asks.

"The painters and the carpet guys," she answers, "about five minutes ago."

"How many today?"

"Five—same as last week."

The ever-hopeful owners of the Galleria have been painting walls and replacing the carpets in the building's common areas, two floors every Saturday. Carr knows the schedule, and knows they're working down-stairs today, on four and five.

"Nobody else?"

"Not yet."

There's a knock on the door and Carr opens it for Bobby and Mike. Bobby pulls on gloves, looks around, and shakes his head. "What a dump. I had to sit here all day, I'd shoot myself."

"That's why it's good you're not an accountant," Mike says.

"Molloy's a lawyer," Carr says. He points at the closet.

Bobby crouches at the wall, looking at Carr's marks and rechecking the plan. He taps on the wall and shakes his head some more. "Sounds like quarter-inch. Cheap bastards."

Bobby takes a drop cloth from his bag and spreads it beneath Carr's rectangle. Then he removes plastic goggles, a battery-powered reciprocat-ing saw, a set of blades in a plastic box, and a rectangular strip of heavy felt. He's humming softly as he selects a blade, locks it in place, and wraps felt around the saw's motor. Carr doesn't know the tune, but knows that Bobby is nervous. Carr himself is fighting the desire to pace. Bobby squeezes the trigger on the saw and smiles at the dull whirring sound.

"Like a whisper," he says. He wipes sweat off his forehead, sets the blade along a penciled line, and cuts. He's quick and quiet and neat,

and in less than a minute he hands Carr a two-by-three-foot panel of wallboard.

"See—quarter-inch. I could've used my Swiss Army knife." He takes a penlight from his bag and shines it in the hole he's cut. He looks at the metal studs and the back of the wall in the utility closet next door. He taps the wall several times, then takes a Phillips-head screwdriver from his bag and punches a hole in the board. He turns to Latin Mike, who takes the screwdriver from Bobby and hands him the device he's been assembling.

It's an under-door camera, a hand-held video unit with a tiny lens mounted on the end of a thin metal snake. This model has its own light source and an infrared attachment. Bobby powers it up, feeds the snake through the hole, and starts working the controls. Mike leans over his shoulder and peers into the monitor. Carr gives them room and goes to the window.

The sky is yellow and greasy, and though it's hours till noon, the sidewalk already shimmers with heat. Carr's shirt is wet, stuck to his back and ribs, though only some of that is from the temperature. He takes a handkerchief from his pocket and wipes the back of his neck. He looks at the van and thinks of Valerie.

Last night, afterward, they'd been welded together by sweat. The droning of the air conditioner swallowed every other sound, and Valerie's weight on him, and the heat that seeped from her to cover him, and the scent of her skin and of her hair that fell in a honey cascade across his shoulder, swallowed every thought of movement. They were perfectly still and perfectly quiet until she spoke, softly, in his ear.

As he had many times since the first day he'd met her, Carr wondered about Valerie's accent. Like so much else about her it was malleable, indeterminate, like smoke. There were hints of Canada in it sometimes, around the edges of her *r*'s, and at other times a suggestion of farther corners of the Commonwealth—South Africa, or maybe Australia. Other times her speech was flat and neutral, like a newscaster's—straight out of Kansas. It was as supple as the rest of her—stretching, bending, shaping itself like putty to suit the job at hand. Last night, her accent was diluted British, a Surrey childhood not quite undone by decades in the States. He'd heard that one before. He'd heard the sentiment too, though not as often. Twice before, to be exact, twice in the four months they'd been sleeping together.

"We could sleep in. Get room service. Spend the day in bed."

Speaking was an effort for Carr, his words rising up from deep water. "There's no room service here, and we have plans for tomorrow."

"I'm not talking about tomorrow, or about this dump. I'm talking about afterward, someplace with a real bed. Someplace we could take time."

"Time for what?"

"Time out. Time to see what's what—what this is all about."

"Are you asking me to go steady?"

Valerie hadn't laughed or snapped, but simply kissed his ear and gone quiet for a while. "You told me this was it for you," she said eventually. "You said so more than once. So you need to plan for afterward. I'm saying that maybe our plans can line up."

Twice before, and last night was lucky number three. Carr still didn't know what to make of it.

Bobby calls him back. He has the saw in hand again, and Latin Mike is stowing the camera. "It's clean in there—no motion detectors, no infrared, just four walls and a door—your basic utility closet."

Four walls, a door, more junction boxes, and the processing unit of Portrait Capital's security system, which is to Jerry Molloy's alarm as a Porsche is to a vegetable peeler. And that's fitting, as Molloy's office holds only yellowing tax files, while Portrait Capital's safeguards more substantial assets.

4

There are no golden bezants over the door, no neon signs in the window, and no furtive customers lurking out front, but Portrait Capital—Marius Lucovic, founder—is nonetheless a pawn shop, albeit an upmarket one. It doesn't trade in forlorn wedding rings, Grandma's sad china, or handguns of dubious provenance, but the basic deal offered at Portrait— valuables handed over as collateral against a loan—is the same as what's on the table down by the bus station, and the customers are similarly desperate. There are differences, of course: the pawnbrokers at Portrait Capital may be seen by appointment only; they deal exclusively in works of art, authenticated antiques, and pieces of serious jewelry; and the smallest loan that Portrait will consider is for a quarter of a million dollars. Lucovic started the company just after the crash, and business has always been brisk.

Which would, at first glance, seem to explain the motion detectors, pressure sensors, and video cameras, but not quite. While it's true that Portrait Capital often has valuable items on its premises, they're never there for longer than a few hours at a time, and never overnight. Any collateral brought to the office is sent out again by armored courier at the end of the day, to a high-security, climate-controlled warehouse near Ellington Airport. So all the hardware Lucovic installed at the Prairie Galleria is not to defend his high-priced pawn. No, it's to protect the inventory of an entirely different Lucovic enterprise—fencing diamonds.

Diamonds have always been Lucovic's specialty, from his first jewelry store smash-and-grab as a teenager in Zagreb, to his days running conflict stones into Western Europe. Diamond money bought him his ticket to the States, his house in River Oaks, his condos in Vegas and L.A., and the nut to start Portrait Capital. Diamond money is what he launders, month in and month out, through Portrait's several bank accounts, and diamonds are what Carr and Bobby and Latin Mike have come to carry off.

Bobby cuts through the wallboard into Portrait Capital's utility closet—another neat two-by-three-foot section—gets down on all fours, and crawls through. Mike is next, pushing the computer boxes and tool bags, and Carr is last.

This closet is three times the size of Jerry Molloy's, a small room really, and the beams of Bobby's and Mike's utility lanterns cast heavy shadows in the corners. Carr brushes off his pants and joins Mike and Bobby in gazing at the security unit—a large black box, forbiddingly blank but for the name, Ten Argus, in yellow.

Bobby wipes his face on his sleeve and kneels beside the processor. He runs his hand along the bottom edge of the black box, finds a latch, and opens the cover. Inside is an array of densely packed circuit boards, banks of status lights, and three cooling fans. Cables from the sensors installed throughout the office suite feed in through a conduit at the back of the box, along with two dedicated telephone lines and the power supply. Two gray bricks sit at the bottom of the box—backup batteries. Bobby trains his light on it all and stares, as if searching a crowd for a familiar face. He shakes his head.

"It looks different," Bobby says softly. He reaches into a bag and pulls out several sheets of circuit diagrams and starts to hum. He studies the diagrams, while Mike unpacks one of the Dell boxes—Styrofoam, a laptop, a bulky antistatic bag, and cables. Carr gives in to the engine racing in his chest, and paces the little room—four paces by three. He walks to the door, puts his hand on the knob, and imagines what would happen if he opened it and walked across a pressure sensor or stepped into a crossfire of infrared beams. No Klaxons or cruisers, Carr knows—Lucovic doesn't welcome attention, and especially not from the police—but a fast, armed response, the security company guards first, followed closely by Lucovic's own men.

"Okay," Bobby says to no one. He's found what he's looking for in the

thicket of chips, and he folds his diagrams away. Mike powers up the laptop. Bobby opens the antistatic bag and pulls out a large circuit board. He sets the board beside the security system and cables it to the laptop. Carr can see, in the dense mosaic of chips on the board, two large chips with the TEN ARGUS label. Bobby kneels over the laptop and starts typing.

Bobby calls it the Ten Zombie, and he and Dennis built it with specs and components they pinched from a dealer in Sugar Land, whose own offices were scandalously insecure. *Zombie* because, once connected, it will look to the monitoring units on the other end of the dedicated phone line just like the Ten Argus unit installed in the humid little room at Portrait Capital, though in fact it is a hollowed out version of that system, receiving input from no sensors, and reporting only what Bobby instructs it to report. And Bobby has directed it to murmur incessantly that everything is perfectly fine.

Connecting it—swapping the Zombie for the real thing—is the tricky part: the monitor software makes allowances for power surges and line glitches, and that's what Bobby wants the swap to look like, but his window is only seven seconds wide. Latin Mike and Bobby stand by the black box, Mike's hands poised over the phone jacks, Bobby's over the power lines. Carr holds the laptop and the Zombie board, and keeps his eye on his watch. They've practiced this a hundred times or more.

"On three," Bobby says.

They finish with two seconds to spare, not their best time but close. Bobby checks and rechecks the laptop screen, watching the back-and-forth over the phone lines. He gives a thumbs-up and closes the laptop, and Carr gives up an ancient breath. Mike shakes the tension from his arms and shoulders. Their shirts are dark with sweat.

Bobby and Mike pick up the tools and the boxes, and Carr opens the door. The air in the corridor is ten degrees cooler. He blinks in the light, wipes his eyes, and touches his headset.

"We're in," he says.

"Making good time," Valerie answers.

"Things okay down there?"

"It's a fucking swamp," she says.

The office suite is done up in leather and dark wood, someone's notion of staid and bankerly, as gleaned from watching old TV shows. It reminds Carr of a funeral home. Carr leads the way to Lucovic's office,

skirting the reception area where the video cameras stand watch. They pass a floor safe, a glossy, black monster with a handle like a ship's wheel, and the name of a long-defunct bank in gold leaf across the front. It's empty, they know, but Mike gives it an affectionate pat.

Lucovic's office is locked, but not seriously, and once Carr opens it, Mike and Bobby make space. Lucovic's leather chair goes to one side of the room, and his mahogany desk goes to the other, which leaves a wide patch of gray carpet in front of the mahogany credenza that stretches across the back wall. There are bookshelves on top of it and file drawers beneath, and behind one set of drawers—the false ones—is the safe.

It's a Guard-Rite T2100, with steel skin, six thick bolts that anchor it firmly to the floor, and room enough inside to accommodate four bowling balls. Mike spins the combination dial. It's an Ames and Landrieu R720 lock package, and he's drilled ten of them in the past two weeks. Today will make eleven. He opens the other Dell box and unpacks his tools.

Carr watches Mike assemble the drill rig, and Bobby lay out the bits and the borescope. He's pacing again, and Mike doesn't like it.

"You're fucking up my rhythm, *cabrón*. How 'bout you do that someplace else?"

Carr walks his fear and boredom into the hall. He studies the door to Lucovic's office, and the door frame, and the floor, looking for an unseen contact switch, a pressure plate, some other hidden, independent alarm—something Valerie might've missed during her two-week stint emptying trash cans with the cleaning crew. He strains to hear heavy footsteps approaching, even as he tells himself that Valerie doesn't miss those kinds of things.

And then it's Delcan's voice he's hearing again, back in Mexico City, making his pitch at a table by the kitchen. Declan had not hemmed or hawed, but jumped right in.

"I'm a robber, Mr. Carr, a robber plain and simple—cash and highly liquid items only. No art, no stocks, no bonds unless they're the bearer variety, no finished jewels, no cars or boats or fancy stamp collections. Just cash and its closest cousins."

Carr squinted, convinced that Declan was drunk and that this was a joke whose reeling logic eluded him. "A bank robber?" he asked eventually. "Teddy said you were a consultant."

"Not a consultant." Declan laughed. "And I don't touch banks. I don't touch payrolls or cambios either, nor armored cars nor safe deposit boxes—no official money for me. Too much official firepower looking after that stuff, and anyway, who wants to crawl into bed at night with images of sobbing widows in his head, and big-eyed orphans turned out in the cold? Takes the joy from living, don't it? So it's black money only I go for. There's plenty of that lying about, and it leaves you with a nice clean conscience afterward."

Carr peered at Declan through smoke and his own drunken haze, still waiting for the punch line. "So, you rob from the rich and give to . . . ?"

"Myself, Mr. Carr. And it's rich shites I rob from—drug runners, gun-runners, whore runners, human smugglers, kidnappers—the very worst swine. I've lightened the till on all of them."

Carr pulled on his beer, but it didn't help to anchor him. "I can't imagine they're very happy about it," he said finally. "And they've got plenty of firepower of their own, and no hesitation using it."

"That they do." Declan laughed. "But the upside is they don't go whining to the *polizei* either, except maybe to the ones they've got on payroll. And when it comes to security, they tend to go for quantity, not quality, if you know what I mean. Heavy stuff, lots of tech sometimes, but not subtle, and typically with some very large blind spots. And, of course, the boys and me are stealthy bastards—they don't know we exist until we're over the threshold, and then it's in fast, out fast, and clear out of town. We don't leave footprints, and we never—but never—fish the same stream twice."

"Security in obscurity," Carr recited—an old lesson that he knew was only sometimes true. "So what's the downside of your business?"

"What you'd expect: people get cross, they brood over things, they have long memories, and if they catch you they'll kill you all kinds of dead—by which time death will seem like a mercy. But like I said, we're dead sneaky: never been pinched; never come close. We're phantoms, Mr. Carr—black cats tippy-toeing in the black night."

The smoke that swirled around the room seemed to fill Carr's head. "I've got to have a talk with Teddy Voigt. I don't know what he's been telling you about me, but I—"

Declan laughed again. "Teddy said you might be just the ticket."

"The ticket to what?"

"To bigger and better, Mr. Carr—a step up in the league tables."

"I'm not following."

"I'm running a nice enough carnival now. I've got a strongman, a fire-eater, a boy who bites the heads off chickens, and I'm the barker that keeps it all going. Our show does fine, Mr. Carr, a reliable money-spinner, but it's still just a carnival, and I've got bigger plans. I want me a full-blown circus, with three feckin' rings and a fat box office every show. But for that I need a ringmaster: someone to sort out the elephants and monkeys, and stuff the clowns in their wee cars. Someone to make sure the trapeze girl doesn't land in the lion's cage, you see? You understand, Mr. Carr, I need a planner, an organizer. Teddy says that's you."

Carr's mind was stuttering, and organization was the last thing on it. He could muster no more than an adolescent shrug, but Declan had momentum enough for both of them.

"Teddy says you've got an engineer's eye for operations—a talent for breaking big problems into bite-size ones, for finding the shortest paths and the points of failure, and coming up with contingencies and fall-backs. He says—"

"Teddy's talking out of school. He should know better."

The smile widened on Declan's chipped red face, and he ran a hand over his thinning hair. His eyes were cold and probing through the smoke. "He says that you're careful too—that you always pack the belt *and* the suspenders. Caution is a virtuous thing in a planner."

Carr could never put his finger on just when he'd begun to take Declan seriously, to believe that his talk of robbers and ringmasters was more than just drunken digression, or the overture to some elaborate scam. Maybe it was in the long silence that followed Declan's speech, as the smoke and sorrowful music pressed closer, or while Carr sipped at the coffee he'd ordered to replace his unfinished beer. Or maybe, on the heels of another failure, another firing, adrift once again, Carr had been a buyer from the start.

"Maybe you could do with a bit more caution yourself. How do you know I won't go home and call the police?"

"And tell them what? My name? My phone number? You know as well as anyone how disposable those are. And besides, I do my sums, Mr. Carr—I think I know you better than that."

Carr shook his head. "Fucking Teddy."

"Don't go blaming Teddy, either—not too much anyway. Yes, he tells me some things—I expect it for the fee I pay him—but I do my own leg-work besides. So I know about your unfortunate disagreement with your client, and the nice right cross that put an end to your career with Integral Risk. I know about your housing problem, as well. And I know about your brief period of service to your country—very noble that—and how they tossed you out on your arse after all that training. Decided you're not the kind of glad-handing wanker Langley likes for their agent-runners. Imag-inative bunch up there, eh?

"And I know how Teddy recruited you to IR after that, and bounced you around the region a bit, before setting you down in Mexico. And I know that you send a check once a month to your old dad up in Massa-chusetts. Stockbridge, is it? It's not everything about you, I'm sure, but it's enough to give me some comfort you won't be running to the Garda. You're too smart for that, Mr. Carr."

The smile was there, and the furry, conspiratorial chuckle, and there was only the briefest gust of icy air—like walking past an open freezer—when he met Declan's blue gaze. Carr found the implicit threat comfort-ing somehow—a kind of corroboration.

"Many people get killed in your business?" Carr asked finally.

"I won't say no eggs get broken, but we try to avoid it. And truth be told, these aren't altar boys we're dealing with. They're dead-enders—hard boys, or so they fancy themselves—bad insurance risks on the best of days."

"I was wondering more about your own guys."

"When it comes to me and mine, *safety first* is my motto. I'm pleased to say I haven't lost a man yet."

"*Yet.*"

Declan shook his head. "If it's risk you're worried about, I can't change that—it is what it is—but if it's crime that gives you pause, then I'd ask you to think about who it is I'm robbing. They're pricks, every one of 'em—none worse in the world. I'm no Robin Hood, but the fact is I hurt 'em where they live—square in the wallet—which might be more justice than they get from anyone else." Declan smiled again, more broadly this time, impossibly charming, and then he drained his beer. "So what d'ya say, Mr. Carr, you want to run off with the circus?"

Safety first . . . haven't lost a man yet. Carr shakes his head, banishing

the echoes of Declan's voice. No, Carr thinks, you hadn't lost a man until four months ago, when you lost two—shot full of holes and burned to a crisp on the side of the Trans-Andean Highway. And too bad one of those rigid cinders was you.

Then Bobby is shaking him, whispering urgently. "The fuck's the matter with you? You don't hear that?" Bobby points toward the reception area, where the voices are coming from. Carr wipes a hand across his face and listens. They're muffled and indistinct, but he can make out two men, talking and laughing.

"*Chingada!*" Mike's voice is low and harsh. He's standing, clenched, in the door of Lucovic's office, and he's holding a Glock.

"What are you doing with that?" Carr whispers.

"Scratching my ass, *cabrón*—what the fuck you think I'm doing?"

Carr shakes his head. "Stay here, both of you, and put that thing away."

"Time to pack up?" Bobby asks.

"Just stay," Carr says, and he crosses the office suite to a teak-paneled partition that reaches nearly to the ceiling and that on the other side forms the long curving back wall of Portrait Capital's reception area.

The voices are louder here but still muffled, and Carr can tell they're coming from outside the glass doors. Carr lies on the floor and peers through a gap between the corner of the partition and a potted tree. The reception area is still dark, the metal gate is still down, and the glass doors are still closed, but beyond them, in the dimly lit corridor near the elevators, there are two men sitting on the floor. Their T-shirts and baggy white pants are spattered with paint, and they are smoking a joint. The dope smell is cloying and powerful, and it reaches Carr quickly even across the still air. He rolls back around the corner and nearly collides with Bobby, who is holding a little Beretta.

Carr looks at the gun. "For chrissakes—you too?" he whispers.

"Is it the rent-a-cops from the lobby?"

"It's the painters from downstairs, getting high. You want to shoot them?"

Bobby tucks the gun into his back pocket. "So are we fucked or not?"

"I don't know yet," Carr says. He stretches out on the floor again, peeks around the corner for another moment, and then sits up. "Give it a minute. They're down to the roach—let's see if they go back to work when they're done."

"Don't know if Mike's got a minute—he's twitchy as hell."

"He's not alone," Carr says, and he gets low and takes another look. "They're done," he whispers. "The one guy's getting up. He's pocketing the roach. Now the other guy's up. They're . . . fuck these assholes!" Carr turns the corner and stands quickly.

"What's going on?" Bobby asks, but Carr is crossing the office suite at a jog, headed back to the utility closet. Bobby follows. "What's going on?" he asks again.

"They're rattling doorknobs."

"Shit! Did we lock Molloy's door?"

"I don't know," Carr says, and he drops down to crawl through the hole in the closet wall.

"Fucking thieves," Bobby mutters, and he drops too.

They almost make it. Carr is halfway across Molloy's office, headed for his secretary's, and Bobby is just emerging from the utility closet, when there are whispers in the hallway, and the handle on the office door begins to turn. Carr pulls his headset off, jams it in his pocket, and turns his back to the office door. He stands by Molloy's desk and picks up Molloy's telephone. His tone is conversational when he speaks, but his voice is loud—as if the connection is bad.

"Got it, honey—two cases of Lone Star, a case of tonic water, the steaks, the macaroni salad. Anything else?" Bobby freezes in mid-stride, then walks slowly backward until he's up against the wall. His gun is out again and he's sighting along the wall, toward the office door. Carr glares at him and shakes his head minutely.

There's more murmuring in the hall, a suppressed laugh, and the office door begins to open. Bobby works the slide on the Beretta, and Carr slices the air with his fingertips—a gambler refusing a card. Bobby scowls.

"I'll be a while longer," Carr says loudly. "Couple of hours, at least. No, I won't forget the tonic."

The door opens wider and the smell of weed reaches Carr. He's certain he can feel eyes on his back, but his own eyes are locked on Bobby against the wall. And then there's movement in the closet, and Latin Mike is there, lying prone, looking down the barrel of his Glock.

Carr swallows hard. "And the macaroni salad—I won't forget." His voice is shaking and he's trying to catch Mike's eye, but Mike won't see him, won't see anything but the door that's opening wider still. Carr's

lungs lock up, his body tenses, and he takes a half-step to his right, right into Mike's sight line. Bobby draws an audible breath; Mike's Glock doesn't waver.

And then there's laughter in the hallway, a giggled *"Fuck it,"* running footsteps, and the office door falling shut with a decisive click.

The silence afterward is ringing. Carr is conscious only of the pulse in his ears and the sweat running over his ribs. Latin Mike crawls back through the closet wall, and Bobby follows. Carr locks the office door and goes through too, then stands in Lucovic's office while Mike drills the safe.

Two hundred twenty-seven thousand dollars in neatly bundled cash; three million, give or take, in loose polished stones.

5

When the adrenaline washes out, Carr thinks, it's like another country—another planet altogether. On this planet, on this evening, they look like film stars by the swimming pool: Valerie in a slate-blue shift, dark glasses, and a loose French braid; Dennis, Bobby, Mike, and Carr himself all freshly showered, shaved, in crisp shirts and shades of their own. The late-day sun throws sheets of orange light across the pool, the fieldstone deck, the wrought-iron chairs and tables, the sinuous olive trees, and a wide swath of Napa Valley hillside below. The waitress delivers another bottle of Chardonnay, another plate of cheese, and another basket of warm bread to their table. She leaves, and they have the terrace to themselves again.

Latin Mike sips and sighs and stretches in the cooling air. "Nice," he says. "Whose choice?" Carr nods toward Valerie, and Mike smiles. "You can book all my hotels, *chica*." She lifts her wineglass and smiles back.

"Lucky to be here, no, *jefe*?" Mike continues. "Those two stoners could've screwed us up but good."

Carr shakes his head. "The luck was that you didn't start banging away. Otherwise we'd be picking brains off our lapels around now, instead of drinking wine."

"That'd work too," Mike says. "My tastes are simple."

"So instead of nobody knowing anything, we'd have had maybe ten minutes to haul ass before the cops got there. And that works for you?"

Mike shrugs. "Not everybody's so squeamish, *cabrón.*"

Carr takes off his sunglasses. "Not everybody's so stupid, either."

"You saying Deke was stupid, bro? 'Cause he didn't mind a little juice."

"He didn't mind when there wasn't another option."

"Traffic moves fast. There's not always time to figure the options."

"Which is why you're not supposed to figure anything—you're supposed to listen to me. For chrissakes, Mike, we've put months into this gig, and you nearly ended it in the first act."

Valerie mutters something, and Dennis shifts nervously in his chair. Bobby clears his throat. "Which is something we've been wondering about," Bobby says, "ending it in the first act, I mean."

It was hard travel from Houston—dusty, hot, and bumpy—and though he's washed off the grit, Carr can still feel the ride in his shoulders. He looks at Bobby and then at Latin Mike. "We made a deal," he says, "a commitment. We've got big sunk costs in this thing, and so does Boyce. He's not going to like it if we walk away."

Mike clasps his hands behind his head. "*Señor Boyce—el padrino.*"

"Fucking ghost, more like," Bobby says.

Carr rises from the table and walks to the terrace railing. He looks at the darkening vineyards and sighs. He's been down this road before with Mike and Bobby, more than once—do the job, don't do the job; one last run, or not—but with three and a quarter million in swag in a room upstairs, the potholes and blind curves are less theoretical now.

"You've worked for him longer than I have, Mike," Carr says. "You were working for him when I signed on."

"True that, *cabrón,* but I've never met the guy. None of us have had the honor—only Deke and you."

"I didn't ask for it—it's the way Deke set it up. It's the way Boyce wants it."

"But you see how it makes a guy nervous."

"You never had a problem before—no worries about the intel he feeds us, or the logistics; no complaint about the splits or the banking service; no gripes at all that I heard about."

Latin Mike nods slowly, but concedes nothing. "Still, a guy gets older, he starts to like the bird in the hand, right, Bobby?"

Bobby smiles. "Three bucks and a quarter—we used to call that a nice payday."

There's wood smoke in the air, something fragrant, mesquite maybe, mixing with the scents of warm earth, bay laurel, and sage that rise from the hillside. Carr breathes in deeply.

"Back when Declan brought me on, you guys thought half a buck was Christmas morning. Times change; prices rise. Three and a quarter isn't what it used to be, especially after expenses. It's not beach money anymore."

Mike empties his wineglass. "And you're all about retirement, right, *jefe*?"

"I thought we all were. I thought that's what we said the last five times we had this conversation. But if you're saying something different, let's not dick around. Tell me now and I'll tell Boyce when I see him day after tomorrow."

Bobby pops up, as if he's sat on a tack, but he's smiling. "Nobody's saying anything. We're just thinking out loud."

Valerie's laugh is like ice in a glass. "Is that how you split the labor, Bobby—Mike thinks, and you do the out loud part?"

Bobby flips her the bird, but he's laughing too, and so is Dennis, and so—finally—is Mike. Carr is still watching purple shadows spread over the valley when the waitress reappears and says that their table is ready.

It's set with heavy linen, battered silver, and votive candles in thick blue glass. Valerie is at the head, between Bobby and Latin Mike, and Carr sits at the other end, between Dennis and the vacant chair. Valerie's playing hostess tonight, smiling, laughing, keeping glasses filled and conversation weightless. It's a part she plays well: conspiratorial and flattering with Mike; flirtatious and profane with Bobby; and with Dennis simply present to be gazed upon. Carr can relate; he can't look away either.

Candlelight flickers on her arms and throat and softens her elfin features. Her green eyes glow and, as the night wears on, her braid loosens and two honey-colored strands slip down to frame her face. Always in motion, the face, the hands, the voice—lifting, lilting, insinuating. It must be exhausting, Carr thinks—it exhausts him just watching her, but he watches just the same. The room darkens, the crowd thins, wine bottles march steadily past, good soldiers all, and by the time the entrees are cleared Carr is drunk and drifting backward again, to Costa Alegre.

*   *   *

It was off-season in Chamela—white mornings, the narrow pastel streets empty until noon—and Carr was on R & R between jobs, nursing a row of bruised ribs. He was sticking close to his rented casita, swimming, reading, sleeping, and he'd never have seen her if not for Fernando.

Fernando did alarms for Declan when Carr first joined up, and his brother Ernesto did surveillance, but their skills didn't line up with Declan's ambitions and they'd slipped into retirement about a year later—Neto to a sport fishing business on the Riviera Maya, and Nando to invest in Jalisco real estate. Carr had always liked the brothers, their unfussy competence and soft-edged cynicism, and he'd been happy to hear from Nando and accept his invitation to drive up the coast for lunch by a hotel pool.

Nando was thicker, darker, and more jocular than he'd been the last time he and Carr had shared a meal. He was working steadily through a platter of chicken tacos and a long story about some condos he was building in Manzanilla when he paused and pointed with his beer to the far side of the pool. "*Oye, cabrón*—you like a little mystery?"

She wore a green two-piece, and her skin was the color of toast. Her hair wasn't blond then, it was a sun-streaked copper, cut blunt to her shoulders, and there was a tattoo on her lower back, a tangle of blue Sanskrit, that looked as if it had been there a while, but which proved to be window dressing. The freckles were real though, and so were the quick green eyes. And the catch at the back of his throat. And the ache he felt through his arms and fingers.

"*Muy bien, no?*" Nando continued. "At first I think she's a tourist, but then I'm not sure. All week I see guys make their play, and all week she's ice. She shuts them down before they get a word out—even me, if you can believe it. Then these skinny guys check in a couple days ago, from up north, and suddenly she's Miss Congeniality. She lets them buy her drinks, lunch, dinner, whatever, and they're practically slitting each other's throats to get next to her."

"You think she's a working girl?"

"She's working something, *cabrón*. I just can't figure out what."

Nando was flying up to Monterrey that afternoon for his niece's *quinceañera*, and he picked up the check before he left and promised to let Carr buy dinner when he returned. "You keep your eye on her, bro. Maybe you can tell me what the mystery is all about." It took him three days to work it out.

Carr spent a few more hours poolside that afternoon, watching her talk to the skinny men. The next day, he took a room at the hotel and followed her: to the beach with the tall skinny man, into town with the balding one, on the cliff-side hiking trail with the blond one who wore a strand of Buddhist prayer beads around his wrist. Poolside, in the cottony twilight, the men bought her drinks, fidgeted, laughed too long, and looked away from one another and scowled.

The day after that, Carr spent some dollars with the hotel staff to learn that her name was Carrie Lyle and that she was from L.A. The three men were from Milpitas, California, and they'd each given the same address on McCarthy Boulevard when they'd registered. Online, in the hotel's business center, he found that the Milpitas address was the headquarters of Null Space Integrated, a manufacturer of specialized graphics chips, and that the men were NSI's three most senior design engineers. Of Carrie Lyle he could find no trace at all.

A pro then, trolling for technical intel, or maybe for talent. It didn't surprise Carr, but the knowledge left him feeling somehow disappointed, as if such mundane loot wasn't deserving of her performance. Because it really was an exceptional performance—maybe the best he'd seen—subtle, unhurried, and finely calibrated to each member of her small audience. He saw it in her body language—the way she arranged herself at their sides—and he heard it in the snippets of conversation he'd managed to steal. She was tentative, almost shy, with the tall man; coltish, nearly awkward, with the bald one; and with the blond Buddhist she was ethereal and dreamy. Three women, beckoning.

It didn't seem much work for her to reconcile her various selves when she entertained the three men at once. It was a matter of small adjustments as far as Carr could tell from his corner of the patio—something in her laugh, her posture, the way she touched her hair. A matter of little intimacies bestowed like candies: a fingertip on the back of a hand, a tanned thigh pressed for a moment against a pale one, a tanned foot sliding on a pale ankle, a hand on a nervous hip. The skinny men were like cats under a full moon, and at his shaded table Carr himself felt a lunar itch and an urge to howl.

So, mystery solved. Carr sighed heavily at the squandering of talent and hoisted himself from his seat. He headed toward his room and wondered what he and Declan might not get up to with someone like her on their crew. They'd been talking about recruiting someone with that kind

of knack—a roper, a honeypot—but neither of them could come up with a likely prospect. Carr slid his key into his door and wondered if Carrie Lyle, or whatever the hell her real name was, might do. And then a gun was in his back and a hand was on his neck, pushing him inside.

The man didn't wait until the door had closed. "The fuck you want, motherfucker?" His voice was American and nervous.

Carr turned slowly and took a slow, deep breath. The man was maybe thirty, and wore jeans and a polo shirt. He had short, black hair and a narrow frame, and something about his tapered head, and the way it swayed on his neck, reminded Carr of an otter. The man was sweating and breathing hard, and a vein throbbed at his temple faster than Carr's pulse was racing.

"The fuck you want with her?" the otter said, and Carr sighed with relief that this was about Carrie Lyle and not some older piece of business. He studied the damp face. He didn't think he'd seen the otter around the hotel, but he knew he wasn't perfect when it came to those things.

"Want with who?"

"Don't screw with me, asshole. You're fucking bird-dogging her, and I want to know why."

The gun was a little S&W, and Carr didn't like the way it jumped around in the otter's hand. "You mean the redhead? Take a look at her, brother—what do you think I'm interested in?"

The otter almost spit. "Right—that's why you duke the desk guy a hundred bucks to see all those registration cards."

Carr nodded slowly. She'd set up trip wires. She'd had someone watching her back. Carr was impressed, even if her guard dog was a lightweight. She'd known someone was trailing her and still she hadn't broken stride. Carr took a half-step closer. The otter didn't notice. "I wondered what she saw in those geeks," he said. "A girl like that—I couldn't figure it. I still can't."

The otter swallowed hard. "Bullshit. What are you—NSI security? Something private?"

Carr took another step forward and put a quaver in his voice and a frightened look on his face. "Seriously, I'm not anybody," he said, and he raised his hands in the air. "I'm just here on vacation from—"

Carr jabbed his thumb into the otter's throat, then into his eye, and then he took the otter's gun. The man gagged and put his hands to his

face. Carr pushed him backward into a chair. He tried to get up and Carr pushed him down harder and flipped him over. The otter had a wallet in his hip pocket and Carr took it, and slapped the back of his head when he tried to resist.

According to his driver's license, his name was Kenneth Kern, from Van Nuys, California, and according to his business card, he was a partner and senior investigator with Victory Security Services, Inc. Carr tossed the wallet at Kern's feet.

"I don't work for NSI," Carr said. "And I could give a shit what you guys are up to. I just want five minutes of her time—a quick chat, and nothing else." He emptied the S&W while he spoke, and put the bullets in his pocket. Then he popped the cylinder out of the gun and tossed what was left into Kern's lap. He held up the cylinder. "She comes to see me, I'll give this back."

She showed up around midnight, wearing a gray linen shift and an expression of impatience and disdain. She looked years older than she had poolside, and even ignoring the little automatic in her hand, she was about as seductive as the taxman.

Valerie's voice was flat and without accent. "Your five minutes started fifteen seconds ago, so if you've got a pitch, make it now."

Carr handed her the S&W cylinder. "I promised your boss I'd give this back."

She snorted. "Kenny's barely the boss of his shoelaces," she said, and dropped the cylinder into her purse. She looked at her watch again.

Carr nodded and said his piece. Two days later, after she'd e-mailed the specs for NSI's next mobile phone chip to her client in Shanghai and shorted a thousand shares of NSI stock, Valerie arrived for lunch in Chamela. Her expression was wary when Carr greeted her at the door of his casita, and warmed only slightly when Declan offered her a drink.

His phone is jittering on the bedside table, and Valerie is shaking his arm. Carr wipes a hand across his face and gropes for the light. Seven people have his number: the three men he was at dinner with hours earlier; the woman he's in bed with now; Mr. Boyce, who rarely calls; Declan, who's dead; and Eleanor Calvin. The caller ID shows a 413 area code, and Carr calculates the time in Stockbridge—five twenty in the morning. He takes

the phone into the bathroom, turns on the light, and shuts the door on Valerie's curious gaze. He runs water in the sink, and when he speaks his voice is thick and distant.

"Mrs. Calvin, what's the matter?"

She's seventy, about the shape and size of a hockey stick, but despite the early hour her voice is blue jay bright. "It's not a good night for him, dear. He's been walking the floor for hours, and now he's calling for you."

"Calling me for what, Mrs. Calvin?"

"You know how hard he can be to follow. He's talking about your summer break, and a job—an internship, I think—at the State Department. I'm missing part of it, I'm sure, but I think he's angry because you're supposed to call someone about it, but you haven't."

The light in the bathroom is harsh and broken, the surfaces too shiny, and it all feels like sand in his eyes. In the mirror, his features are pale and smudged—a lost boy look, Valerie would say. Emphasis on the lost, Carr thinks, and for an instant Declan's voice flashes in his head: *Neither sober nor quite drunk enough.*

"That was a dozen years ago, Mrs. Calvin."

"It's not a good night for him."

"Would it help if I spoke to him?"

"It would help if you came for a visit."

"Soon, Mrs. Calvin. Did you tell him I'll be back there soon?"

"I did, dear, but honestly I'm not sure the ambassador knows who I am right now."

Carr lets out a long breath. "He wasn't an ambassador, Mrs. Calvin."

"Of course not, dear. Now wait just a minute and I'll get your father."

6

It is raining in the Berkshires, a warm patter from a low sky. The waxy leaves shudder, branches bow under the gray weight of water and humid air, and the odors of damp wood, moldering paper, and rodent piss rise from the clapboards and curling shingles of his father's house. Carr stands on the front porch and feels the old lassitude creep over him like a fog. It's been years since he's spent more than a night or two in the sagging Victorian pile, but its musty gravity is insistent.

The reek of long neglect and decay is the perfume of Carr's adolescence—of the year he spent here with his father and mother following their abrupt, chaotic decampment from Mexico City, and of the boarding school holidays he endured in the years after his mother's death. The creeping torpor—the feeling of lead in his bones, cotton wool in his skull, and breath coagulating in his lungs, of life coagulating around him, even as it surges ahead in the world beyond the slumping stone wall—is what has kept him away, except for days here and there, since the morning he left for college. Part of what has kept him away.

Eleanor Calvin is at his side, her wiry, freckled hand on his arm. She wears paddock boots, pressed jeans, and a rain slicker—a bright yellow flame against the overcast. Carr eyes the knee-high stacks of newspapers and magazines that run the length of the porch. Calvin follows his gaze.

"It's hard to keep up," she says. "He has so many subscriptions, they accumulate faster than I can get to recycling."

The piles of *The New York Times*, *The Wall Street Journal*, the *Financial Times*, *The Washington Post*, *Foreign Affairs*, and *Foreign Policy* are yellowed and dissolving. To Carr they look no different from the ones he saw the last time he was here.

"I told him he can get them all online," Carr says.

Eleanor Calvin nods sadly. "It's difficult for him sometimes, remembering the passwords. And then he gets angry."

"Nothing new there—angry is his usual state."

Calvin frowns and shakes her head. "It's because he's scared of what's happening to him." She pats Carr's arm. "It's what the doctor said, dear—there'll be good days and bad, and over time more of the bad ones. But today he's good, and you should enjoy it. I told the ambassador you were coming, and he's looking forward to it."

Carr sighs, but doesn't correct her.

Inside the light is gray, as it always is, regardless of weather, time of day, or season of the year. Arthur Carr is in the dining room, at the head of a long table that is layered in newspapers, folded laundry, and heaps of unopened mail. He looks up from his *FT,* blinks his gray eyes, and pushes half-glasses into a still dark hairline. His face is long, angular, and academic-looking, the skin of his cheeks pink from shaving, the fine nose veined from drink. It isn't Carr's nose, which is twice broken but otherwise unmarred, and the eyes are different too: Carr's are hazel, like his mother's, but still the resemblance is pronounced. Which always startles Carr and makes him uneasy.

"You're sunburned," Arthur Carr says. "How do you manage that from behind a desk? Or do they have you in the field now?" Still the Ivy League drawl, but higher-pitched now—an old man's voice.

Carr isn't sure which *they* his father means. He's left his employment status vague since being fired from Integral Risk, adopting Declan's usefully elastic *consultant* when pressed. It's been months since his father has pressed. "I had some vacation time," he answers.

"Well, don't waste it here," his father says. He points a long finger at the dining room window and the neon yellow form of Eleanor Calvin standing on the porch. "I told her not to bother you, but she gets so damned dramatic."

"It was no trouble—I'd planned to come next week. I just moved things up a little."

Arthur Carr turns back to his newspaper, rattling the page. "At any rate, you must be glad to get out of that sewer."

Carr has been vague about his living arrangements too. His father believes that he's still in Mexico City. "It's not so bad," Carr says.

His father snorts. "Long as you don't need to breathe the air, or drink the water, or drive ten blocks in under an hour. I don't know how you stand it."

"It's not so bad," Carr says again.

"*Not so bad?* You don't know what you're talking about. Twenty years down there, I could never stand it."

Noxious shitholes was the phrase his father favored, and he used it often—more often with a few drinks in him. Carr remembers him red and fuming, a glass in one hand, the other gesturing at a broad window, and the low, smudged skyline—of what city Carr can't recall—that lay beyond, hunched under a shelf of smog. He remembers his mother too: pale and still and quiet before his father's wave of complaint, always in a dress and heels, always with a cigarette. He doesn't remember the details of his father's rants, but the broad strokes were all the same: the wrong political connections, the wrong family ties, the wrong school ring; the inept boss, the paranoid boss, the vengeful boss; favors and grudges; being passed over, and passed over again. Thwarted. And so it went in Lima, São Paulo, Buenos Aires, Asunción, Quito, San Salvador, Managua, Ciudad Juárez, and Mexico City.

Carr remembers his father's rising voice, his mother's massive silence, and his own clenched dread. It was a swooping, taloned thing that seized his chest, seized his voice, and chased him through the houses that blended one into the next.

They were different, it seemed, only in their addresses. Always walled and gated, with leafy courtyards and burbling fountains, their rooms were cool and quiet, their furnishings heavy, dark, and carefully arranged—like store displays, and just as lifeless. Carr can still recall the sour odor of spilt wine that lurked in the sofa cushions, and the smell of singed fabric—the remnants of one of his parents' parties, or maybe of a prior resident's. Not their sofas, of course, and not really their houses: they were just the latest in a long line of temporary lodgers—in and out in two years, maybe three. The attendant cooks and gardeners and maids, always dark and wary, had greater claims on those places.

He made friends from time to time, other Foreign Service brats, and he remembers his quiet envy of the houses that they lived in. Not very different from his own in shape or size, they'd been transformed by an alchemy unknown to his family from anonymous showrooms into homes, with photos on the mantel, bicycles in the drive, and a carved pumpkin at Halloween. They made wherever he was living seem like a rented van.

Arthur Carr wasn't an ambassador; he wasn't even close. The highest he'd climbed in nineteen years was to the number three spot in the Economic Section of the embassy in Mexico City. That was his final posting, and he'd lasted barely ten months.

His father is up now, leaning at a sideboard that is littered with white plastic grocery bags. A flock of ghosts, Carr thinks, and they make a noise like dry leaves as his father brushes them aside to find a rocks glass. Carr checks his watch as his father pours an inch of scotch and swirls it around.

"You look like your mother when you look like that," Arthur Carr says.

"A little early, isn't it?"

"Is it?" his father asks, and lets his reading glasses fall to his nose. "And just what the hell do I have to wait for?"

The rain has lightened to a mist when Carr returns to the porch, and the air is warmer and more cloying. Eleanor Calvin is staring at the treetops and the leaden sky.

"There's a salad for lunch," she says. "There should be enough for both of you. And there's roast chicken for dinner, and some new potatoes."

"I booked a room at the Red Lion," Carr says. "I can eat there." Eleanor Calvin sighs, still looking up. She's waiting for something. "Do you need a lift home?" Carr asks.

She shakes her head. "It's just a mile, and hardly raining."

"It's no trouble, Mrs. Cal—"

"Do you remember my daughter, dear?"

Carr recalls a rangy blond girl, a few years younger than he. A rider, he remembers. "Annabeth, right? She went to law school down south."

"She's still there, in Atlanta. She had a baby six weeks ago, her second little girl."

Something frozen drops into Carr's gut. "Another granddaughter—I had no idea. Congratulations."

Eleanor Calvin takes a deep breath. She looks at Carr, who is looking at the floorboards. "She wants to go back to work, dear, and she needs help with the children. She's got plenty of room, and she's asked me to move in."

Carr is focused on his breathing, fighting the light-headed feeling. He flexes his fingers, which are suddenly cold. "I had no idea," he says again, softly. "Look, I know he's difficult. If it's the money, I could—"

Eleanor Calvin frowns. "It has nothing to do with money," she says sadly. "You've been more than generous, dear. And you know how fond I was of your mother. But Annabeth and her girls need me now, and truth be told these winters get longer every year."

Carr is still staring down, shaking his head slowly. "When?" he asks.

"Two or three months, I think. I've listed the house. I've got some cleaning up to do before they can start showing it, but I can go before it's sold."

"I need time."

"Of course you do, dear. It's a big change. It'll be a big adjustment for your father."

"That woman who filled in for you—the one who came when you went to Florida—could she come on full-time?"

A pained look crosses Eleanor Calvin's weathered face. "But, dear, I thought you understood—your father needs more than home care now. Atlanta aside, I don't know that I could do for him much longer. It's getting more . . . complicated."

"Complicated how?"

A blush spreads across her lined cheeks. "He's . . . he's starting to have bathroom problems, and last week the police picked him up at ten at night, a half mile down the road from here. He didn't have shoes on and his feet were bleeding. I wish I could do more, dear, but really the ambassador needs a different sort of care."

"He wasn't an ambassador," Carr says, but only to himself.

Eleanor Calvin gives him three months, and leaves Carr on the porch, figuring furiously. Some of his figuring is about timing: three months is bad. He has scheduled thirteen more weeks for the job, including a one-week contingency. Three months would fall at the endgame—the close of the

third act. It couldn't be worse, and he'll have to beg or bribe her for an extra two weeks.

But most of his figuring is about money. His father has next to none, and Carr has been paying for his care for several years: every month an envelope stuffed with used hundreds to Eleanor Calvin. The arrangement works well for both of them: a tax-free income for her, and the anonymity of cash for him. But cash won't fly with a nursing home. They will have forms to fill out, contracts to sign, and bank accounts, employment, and income to verify—and all in his actual name. Which is, of course, impossible.

And which assumes he can even find a place that will take his father. Eleanor Calvin had done research and pressed some papers on him—a list of websites with information on facilities for the elderly, and on Medicare, Medicaid, and Social Security, is folded in his pocket, along with a list of nursing homes in the Berkshires. He scanned them once, twice, but they turned to Greek.

Arthur Carr calls from the front hallway: he wants his lunch. Carr goes inside and finds Eleanor Calvin's salad, and watches his father eat it and drink more scotch. Clouds thicken in his head as he listens to his father's monologue, which skips like a stone from war to stock markets, to the decline of the West, to Eleanor Calvin's cooking, to her designs on the family silver.

Eleanor Calvin thought Carr should tell his father sooner rather than later about her move, but Carr has no stomach for the conversation. His father's talk grows angrier and more tangential with each refill, and as the day fades Carr wonders if his father will sleep soon, or if he should start drinking too. Instead he walks across the hall into the living room.

It's dimmer than the dining room, and more chaotic, with newspapers and magazines and precarious stacks of books on nearly every surface. There's an upright piano against one wall, a block of ebony and dust, and on top, in tarnished silver frames, lying facedown, are photographs. Carr stands them up.

They're desiccated and yellowed behind their smudged panes—ancient-looking, like bugs in a collection. His grandparents—his father's parents—starched, pale, and unsmiling beside a long, dark sedan. His father, young and smirking amid a group of distant cousins. They are gathered by a pine-edged lake, all in dark shorts and white shirts, like

campers or a Bible study group. His father again—older, taller, in cap and gown and an already bitter smile, the Battell Chapel and a bit of New Haven street behind him. And then, in the most tarnished frame, the photo he is looking for, of his mother, her black hair loose, her eyes shining, her white teeth and a curl of smoke visible between her parted lips.

He called the picture by different names as a child, because he didn't know where it was taken or what she was doing in it, and so he made up different stories about it. *En el jardín. En la fiesta. En el baile. In the garden,* because his mother stands before well-tended hedges, with a bed of blue flowers visible over her shoulder, and a vine with red blossoms winding up a trellis. *At the party*, because she wears pearls and a floral dress, and holds a champagne flute, and because she might be laughing. *At the dance,* because her hair is sweeping past her shoulder, her neck is long and curved like a dancer's, and she might be looking at someone—a partner—outside the frame. He still doesn't know which of those stories was the right one. Maybe all of them.

His father says something from the dining room, but Carr can't make out what. He waits for more, but nothing comes. After a while he sweeps a pile of magazines from the sofa and lies down.

The phone, burring in his pocket, wakes him from a clammy sleep. It's dark now and he turns on the porch light as he steps outside to answer. The air is like a cool cloth on his face. Mr. Boyce, who almost never calls, is calling.

"You're not in California," he says. His voice is heavy and smooth, an amber syrup. "You're supposed to be in California today, and you're supposed to be out here tomorrow."

"I'll be there. I'm flying out of Boston first thing."

"Is there a problem?"

"No. No problem."

7

Backlit on the fourteenth tee, Mr. Boyce is a slab of granite escaped from the quarry, or spare parts from Stonehenge. Carr walks up the cart path, and from fifty yards features emerge in the monolith: massive arms and shoulders, a corded neck, a shaved head, black and gleaming against the blue sky. *Rockefeller Center*, Carr thinks, *the statue of Atlas.* He thinks it every time he sees Boyce. Carr stops walking as Mr. Boyce sets up over the ball. The driver is like a blade of grass in his hands, and though Carr has seen him play many times before, he is always amazed that the heavily plated torso can coil and release with such ease. There is a slashing noise, a gunshot, and Mr. Boyce looks down the fairway and nods. Then he beckons to Carr.

This is the twenty-second time they have met, and their twenty-second meeting on a golf course, though never on the same course twice. Today they are in Wisconsin, just outside Madison, at a private club set beside a lake, amid hills drenched in green. As he was the first time Carr saw him, in Atlanta, under a punishing August sun, Mr. Boyce is wearing tailored black. And, as always, he is golfing alone, walking the course, and carrying his own bag.

Which isn't to say he is without retainers. There are two of them today, trailing behind in a golf cart: a large man in khakis and sunglasses, with short red hair, whose name Carr has never learned but who drives Mr.

Boyce's cars, and next to him Tina, who is slim and white-blond, whose oval face is as smooth and empty as a mannequin's, and who, Declan once told him, kills people for Mr. Boyce. Tina looks up from a glossy magazine through dark, rectangular glasses and smiles.

A frisson of tension ripples through Carr's gut as he walks down the fairway and cuts through the dull throbbing in his head. Ahead, Mr. Boyce seems too large for the landscape. It's an illusion, Carr knows, though not of the light off the lake, nor even of Boyce's considerable mass. Rather, it's the aura he casts—of power barely controlled, of destructive potential contained, but just for now.

"Like a chainsaw," Declan said that first time in Atlanta, "or a crate of blasting caps. You want to walk careful around him, young Carr. You want to keep a little distance."

The menace is palpable, but always implicit. In all their meetings, Mr. Boyce has never been other than exact, economical, and watchful. Still, he's the only man Carr knows of who made Declan nervous.

It was a long drive, three hundred yards at least, and the ball sits on the right side of the fairway, at the bend of a dogleg left, not far from the rough. The green is uphill, 150 yards away, and ringed by bunkers. Mr. Boyce walks slowly around his ball. In person his voice is even deeper— the rumbling of an earthquake.

"I expected you earlier," he says, "by the ninth hole."

"My flight was delayed."

Boyce nods. "Thunderstorms over New York, I know." The wind is gusting off the lake and Boyce studies the treetops and the distant flag. He scatters bits of grass from his fingertips and watches them fly.

"What do you think—blowing left to right, about twenty miles an hour, a little less on the green with that stand of trees. You make it a seven iron from here?"

"You know I don't play," Carr answers.

Mr. Boyce shakes his head. "Too bad. There's a lot you'd like about it. The precision, the planning—everything just so."

"Maybe in my retirement."

Boyce chuckles, which sounds like an air horn. "I admire your optimism." He pulls a seven iron from his bag and takes an easy practice swing. "Everything fine with your father?"

"Sure," Carr says quietly.

"Sure," Boyce repeats, and then all his attention is on the ball. Again there is the slash, the gunshot, an arc of cut grass in the air, and the ball bounces on the green—once, twice, now rolling toward the pin. Boyce turns back to Carr. "So tell me how you're spending my money."

And for the next two holes Carr does exactly that, pausing only for Boyce to strike the ball. On the seventeenth tee he finishes, and Boyce asks questions.

"Where are the stones now?"

"Here."

"On you?"

"They're in the trunk of your Benz, in the first-aid kit, underneath the cold packs."

A rueful smile crosses Mr. Boyce's face. "You broke into my car?"

"I'll need them in the Caymans. I need you to hold them for me till then."

"And what about the cash?"

"I'm using it for expenses."

"I want receipts," Boyce says.

"You'll get them."

Boyce looks down the fairway. It's a short par four, 330 yards, and he takes the driver from his bag. "You think three's enough to buy you in?" he asks.

"More would be better, but the right references and the right introduction should convince him there's a steady supply."

"And Bessemer is the guy to introduce you?"

"He's the best bet."

"You're sure of that?"

"Of course not. But he's known Prager for years, he's been referring clients to him, one way or another, for a while, and he's approachable. He's the best bet."

"It's your call," Boyce says, and tees up his ball at the tips. "And what about the woman—Chun?"

"Valerie has a good feeling about her."

"*Good feeling?* I like to base my investments on a little more than that."

"If we want to add six months to the timetable, then we can look elsewhere. If not, then Chun's our girl."

Boyce shakes his head. "Let's hope it's a *great* feeling," he says, and

another gunshot echoes across the lake. The ball hits the fringe and bounces onto the green. Boyce nods slowly as it rolls, then he turns to Carr and leans his hip against his driver, as if it were a cane.

"So Valerie's doing all right?" he asks.

"She's doing fine."

"And Mike and Bobby, and the kid?"

"Dennis. They're fine too."

"Must be an adjustment for them, not having Deke there. A different rhythm for them—a different style."

"This isn't the first time we've been around the block together."

"But you're not part of the crew anymore. You're the boss now. Management."

Carr pinches the bridge of his nose and looks at Mr. Boyce, whose eyes are like black stones. "It's all good."

Boyce taps the toe of his golf shoe with his driver. "Deke ran a tight ship—very firm, very hands-on. He wasn't worried about being liked—"

"He didn't have to worry—everybody liked him."

"Regardless, that wasn't his focus. His focus was on having his orders followed. He was a good soldier that way—a good platoon leader. It's not an easy job, and not everyone's built for it. Some people need to be liked; some people get lazy or stupid."

"Which one of those do you think is my problem?" Carr says.

The wind subsides for a moment, and the smells of grass and loam and trapped heat rise up, as if the ground has opened. Mr. Boyce straightens, and Carr takes a step back. "You'll know when I think you have a problem," he says, and Carr can feel the bass rumble in his chest. Boyce looks at him for a while, sighs, and drops his club into his golf bag.

"You have anything for me?" Carr asks.

Boyce points at Tina, who is already headed for the tee with something tucked under her arm. "She'll fix you up," Boyce says, and he turns toward the green.

Carr and Tina sit on a bench off the cart path, in the heavy shade of an oak. The air is cool here, and Tina's legs shine white in the shadows.

"The new stuff's at the last tab," she says, and she opens the latest British *Vogue* while Carr opens the latest edition of Curtis Prager's dossier.

Carr remembers the first time he read it, six months back, in a hotel bar in Panama City, and remembers Declan's whiskey-furred voice as he slid it across the table. *Last job of work we'll need to do, boyo. It's the feckin' sweepstakes.* The lined red face split in a grin. Carr has read and reread it countless times since then—all but memorized it—but still he looks at every page.

A picture comes first, Curtis Prager years ago, emerging from the back of a black car. He is lithe, tanned, and shiny, his features finely sculpted, his hair like blond lacquer on his neat head, his shoulders square. An Apollo of finance, Carr thinks—a gilded man for a gilded age. All that's missing is a laurel wreath.

After the photo are the puff pieces about him that appeared in financial trade rags in the United States and Europe with great regularity before the crash. In tone they run a narrow gamut from fawning to sycophantic, and they all tell the same tale: of the tow-headed prodigy, homeschooled in Cincinnati until age sixteen, then off to Princeton, Harvard B-school, and Wall Street after that. By age twenty-five, he was the youngest managing director in the history of Melton-Peck; by twenty-eight he was the head of all trading there; and by thirty he was out the door—off to seek his fortune as a hedge fund manager, with a very large fortune in bonus money already in hand, and a flock of investors following behind him, all eager to pay for the privilege of having the wunderkind manage their money. •

And so the birth of Tirol Capital, which from the first charged staggering fees, made a mania of secrecy, and cultivated an air of exclusivity to rival any Upper East Side co-op or private school. The formula worked well for Prager and, along with the outsize returns he reported year after year, helped make Tirol one of the fastest growing funds of the new century.

Besides the money, and the truckloads by which it arrived at Tirol's Greenwich, Connecticut, doorstep, the articles discuss Prager's many good works. There are lists of scholarship funds, endowed chairs, research laboratories, and hospital pavilions that bear his name, and pictures of Prager and the missus—tall, blond, disdainful—at an endless series of charity events. Black ties, white ties, polo shirts and sunglasses—the dress code varies, but never the smiles, which are tight and entitled. Smiles of any sort are in short supply in the next set of clippings—the ones from the trials.

There were two of them, the first just before the markets collapsed, the second just afterward, and despite the torch-and-pitchfork temper of those times, both ended in hung juries. The press attributed this to the complexity of the government's case against Prager—the difficulty of making money-laundering and conspiracy charges stick, the arcane financial instruments involved—though some in the U.S. Attorney's office grumbled darkly, and not for attribution, about jury tampering.

The feds were about to have a third go when their only witness, a former Tirol compliance officer named Munce, drove his Lexus off a dark road in Litchfield County, and through the frozen skin of the Housatonic River. His blood alcohol level was twice the legal limit, and there was ice on the roadway, but still the feds had both Munce and his car stripped down to their frames. The autopsies found nothing, though, and the most they could do to Prager were a dozen stiff fines for a dozen obscure record-keeping violations.

But the mere fact of his indictment, along with the implosion of the markets, had already dealt much worse punishment to Prager and his firm. Tirol was losing investors at a slow bleed before the first trial began, and like a broken hydrant afterward, and by the time the feds imposed their fines, the firm was down to a measly billion or so in assets under management, and a handful of clients in Florida, Latin America, and the Caribbean.

News coverage of Curtis Prager dropped off sharply four years back, after the fines—a mention in the *Greenwich Time* of the sale of his North Street estate, another in the *New York Post* of his divorce and exodus to the Cayman Islands. After which the press had bigger, more blatant frauds to cover, and the entries in the dossier switch from press clippings to what Carr recognized on first reading as intelligence reports.

"Where does Boyce get this stuff?" he'd asked Declan at the time.

Declan had shrugged and, typically, answered a different question. "He likes to keep an eye on the competition." Carr stopped asking about what other lines of business Mr. Boyce was in, though he's never stopped wondering.

About Curtis Prager's business, the reports leave little doubt. With a labored dispassion typical to the genre, and with no mention of sources or methods, they describe how Prager, having relocated to the Caymans, closed down what was left of Tirol Capital and established Isla Privada Holdings, a firm whose ostensible business is the acquisition, consolida-

tion, and management of small banks and trust companies in the United States, but whose actual purpose is to deliver financial services to organized criminals.

A comprehensive list of services too, according to the reports, especially for a relative newcomer to the field: bulk cash processing, foreign exchange, electronic funds transfer, access to a network of overseas correspondent banks, provision of fully documented shell corporations, asset management, even tax consultation—everything a crime syndicate might require to launder large sums of money, move them around the world, invest them, and bring them home clean.

The reports say that Prager is still building his business, and that his client base is still small—a Mexican drug cartel, a Colombian cocaine syndicate, a smuggling ring out of Panama, and a Salvadoran private army that expanded from death-squad work into regional arms supply. But he has grander things in mind, and his marketing efforts have recently spread beyond the Caribbean and Latin America to Central Europe and Asia. The list of Prager's clients stopped Carr in his tracks the first time he read it. He peered across the table through the smoke from Declan's Cohiba.

"We know some of these guys," Carr said. "We hit them twice, they're going to take it personally."

"It's not them we're hitting, boyo, it's their banker. Deposit insurance is his problem."

"You're thinking about a cash shipment?"

Declan shook his head. "Keep reading."

The lightbulb went on two paragraphs down, in the midst of a dry discussion of the common back office used by the banks that Isla Privada owns. The centralized processing system gives Curtis Prager ready access to all of the accounts in all of the banks in Isla Privada's portfolio, and—with the help of an obedient, well-paid, and meticulously incurious operations and accounting staff—makes it a simple matter to commingle licit and illicit cash and hide dubious funds transfers in a forest of legitimate ones.

Carr had looked up at Declan, who was grinning like a shot fox. "That back-office system of his is a fecking magic lamp," Declan said. "The great Prager rubs away, wishing for some clean money, it spews a bit of smoke, and *poof*—out pops a wire transfer! Any given time, he can move a hun-

dred million at least with that lamp, boyo. I say we do a bit of wishin' of our own."

"You say something?" Tina asks him. She's lifted her glasses off her nose, and her gray eyes are motionless. Carr shakes his head. "You sure you're okay?" she asks. "'Cause you look like a fucking ghost."

"I'm fine," Carr says. He flips past the profiles of Prager's staff—his security chief, his tame accountants and auditors—and leafs through the technical section. Floor plans of Isla Privada's offices on Grand Cayman and of Prager's beachfront compound, the makes and models of alarm systems, registry listings for Prager's sloop and his motor yacht, the tail number of his G650—Boyce's people are good at this sort of thing, and it goes on for pages.

Carr squints at a column of figures and rubs his head. He turns to the last tab and scans the latest updates.

There are pictures of a party by a long swimming pool, at night—men in linen trousers, women in gauzy shifts, waiters in starched jackets, and in the background a line of luminous surf. Carr recognizes it as Prager's Grand Cayman beachfront.

"These are from his party last week?" he asks. Tina doesn't look up from her magazine, but nods. "You bought yourself one of the caterer's people?"

"Rented," she says.

"Another fund-raiser?"

Tina nods again. "For a local grade school."

"Prager schedule the next one?"

"Just before Labor Day—right before he leaves on his prospecting trip."

"Still off to Europe?"

"And Asia now. Lot of money to be washed out there. He'll be gone about five weeks."

"So, Labor Day—that's about eleven weeks."

"Ten," Tina says, and turns another page of her magazine. Carr keeps studying the party photos.

"I don't see Eddie Silva here."

"Next picture," Tina says.

It's a photo of a fifty-something man, thick, with a salt-and-pepper buzz cut. It's a daytime shot, and he's coming out of a bar. His eyes are

smeared and his face is like pitted pavement. "He's off the wagon?" Carr asks.

Tina nods. "Again."

"That's what—the third time in five months?"

"That's what I make it."

"Hell of a thing for the head of security."

"Nice for you though."

There are more photos at the back of the folder, and the very last one stops Carr. It's another shot of Curtis Prager, and like the first picture in the file it shows Prager climbing from a car, though this car is a Bentley, and the street, sunny and white, isn't in New York, but in George Town, on Grand Cayman. Prager is wearing jeans and a guayabera. His hair is long, curling, bleached from the sun, and his mouth is open, as if he's about to speak.

Carr flips to the front of the file and then to the back again. There can't be five years between this photo and the first one, but in the interim Prager's face has aged fifteen years at least. His skin is hide brown, seamed, and pulled too tight over the fine bones. The cords of his neck are like rigging, and his eyes are adrift in a sea of lines and shadows. His mouth looks wider and hungrier—weathered, but avid too, Carr thinks. Prager's thrown off the collar and found himself some appetites to indulge— found that indulgence agrees with him. So, more a pirate than ever; more Bacchus than Apollo now. Carr shakes his head. They hated this kind of thinking at the Farm, and his trainers dinged him for it more times than he could remember. Projection, they called it. *Don't impose a narrative, for chrissakes—let them tell their own stories. An agent gets an idea there's something particular you want to hear, all he'll do is sing it to you. He'll have you chasing your tail right up your backside.* Still, he looked like a pirate.

Tina is holding a flash drive and looking at him. "File's on here," she says.

Carr closes the dossier and pockets the drive. "You have anything else for me?"

"Anything like . . . ?"

"It's been four months, for chrissakes."

"I told you, it's slow going. We don't have a lot of friends down there."

"So four months of digging and nothing to show?"

Tina closes her magazine and places it on her lap. "Not exactly nothing," she says.

Carr draws a hand down his face. He is awake now, fully, for the first time today. "Exactly *what*, then?"

"Not a hundred percent sure. A guy one of our few friends knows met another guy who pilots for a vineyard down there. He flies in and out of an airfield near Mendoza. His brother works part-time at the same field, doing maintenance on the prop planes. The rest of the time, the brother works at a private field northwest of town, a dirt strip on an *estancia*."

"Bertolli's place."

Tina nods. "Works there on Tuesdays and Fridays. And word is he told his big brother that one Friday morning, four months back, before he could even get his truck parked, the foreman waved him off. Told him *hasta la vista*—go home, no work today. No explanation besides there was a party going on at the ranch that night, which seemed weird to the mechanic because he knew that Bertolli was away in Europe for two weeks. But the foreman gave him a day's pay anyway, for doing nothing, so he didn't ask questions. He did notice something as he was driving out the gate that morning, though: a truckload of men driving in."

"What men?"

"He'd seen some of them around the ranch before, but they scared him and he always kept his distance. Bertolli's hard boys. The mechanic tells his brother they looked like they were there to work."

Carr stands slowly and puts a hand on the back of the bench. "Which Friday morning was this?"

"Four months back, the second Friday of the month. That makes it the morning of the twelfth."

After a while, Carr clears his throat. "That's the morning of the day before," he says.

"Mr. Boyce says not to read too much into it."

Carr looks down at Tina, and at his own face, black in her black lenses. "It doesn't take any reading," he says quietly. "They knew he was coming. They were waiting for him."

8

At 9:35 a.m. Howard Bessemer will leave his blue, Bermuda-style cottage, turn right on Monterey Road, turn right again on North Ocean Boulevard, and drive south, past the Palm Beach Country Club, to the Barton Golf and Racquet Club, there to meet Daniel Brunt for a ten o'clock court. He will play no more than two sets of tennis with Brunt, and afterward drink no more than two iced teas, and then he will shower, dress, get in his car, and drive across the Royal Park Bridge for lunch in West Palm Beach. This is Howard Bessemer's routine on Tuesdays and Thursdays, and this being 9:33 on a Tuesday, Carr knows that Bessemer will soon appear. Because if Carr, Latin Mike, Bobby, and Dennis have learned anything in the weeks they've been watching him, it is that Bessemer is a man of routines.

Tuesdays and Thursdays: tennis and lunch. Mondays and Wednesdays: golf and cocktails. Friday mornings: sailing. Friday afternoons: more cocktails. And Friday nights straight through Sunday afternoons: high-stakes poker, cocaine, and whores—two, sometimes three, at a clip—all in a basement below a Brazilian restaurant, not far from the medical center. They can set their watches by Bessemer, and they love him for it.

The garage door opens, and the blue BMW pulls out. Bessemer has the top down, and his thinning blond hair is a tattered pennant in the breeze. Right and right again, and Bobby waits another fifteen seconds

before he pulls the gray painter's van away from the curb. Carr calls Latin Mike.

"We're gone," he says into his cell.

"We're in," Mike replies, and in the side mirror Carr sees Bessemer's front door swing shut.

This stretch of Ocean Boulevard is flat and straight—a corridor of stucco walls, hedges, and gated drives, whose usual quiet is deepened by a sense of off-season abandonment. Traffic is sparse, and Carr can see Bessemer's BMW blocks ahead, shimmering in the heat. The Atlantic appears to their left in flashes, in the alleys between properties—white, heaving, covered in sunlight.

Bobby tugs his painter's cap lower. "Got another doughnut?" he asks. Carr hands him a powdered sugar, rolls down his window, and lets in the salt breeze and the smell of ripening seaweed.

Bessemer is nimble for a thickset man. He tosses his keys in a neat arc to a valet in a pink polo shirt, hitches his tennis bag on his shoulder, trots up the steps of the Barton, and disappears into its Spanish colonial facade. The valet slides into the BMW and wheels the car around the crushed shell drive. On another Tuesday he would head due west, fifty yards down a service road to the club's parking lot—but not today. Today, half of that lot is being resurfaced, and only the cars of Barton members are being parked in the other half. The cars of staff, and of guests like Howard Bessemer, go around the corner, to the unattended lot of an Episcopal church. Carr and Bobby are parked across the street when the BMW arrives.

The valet drops it into a slot next to a Porsche and sprints off toward the club. Carr takes a black box smaller than a deck of cards from the backpack at his feet.

"Two minutes," he says, but he doesn't take that long. When he returns he has another small box in his hand, like the first but caked in mud and dust.

"Korean crap," Bobby says, disgustedly. "Second one that's died on me this year. The fucking Kia of GPS trackers."

Bobby drives around another corner and down an alley. They park beside a dumpster and Carr takes a camera from the backpack. He sights through the viewfinder, and through a gap in the green court windscreen, and finds Bessemer and Brunt on their usual court. He has plenty of pic-

tures of Bessemer—the benign, round face, the watery, perpetually astonished blue eyes, the ingratiating smile—and of the tanned and simian Brunt, but just now Bessemer is talking to someone Carr hasn't seen before, a tall, knobby man, awkward and embarrassed-looking in tennis whites. Carr takes half a dozen photos and checks the results on the camera's little screen.

Bobby picks through the doughnut box. "Used to be, a guy like Howie did a little time, laid low awhile, then hooked up with a charity board," he says. "Raised money for cancer or something. Now he can't even get membership in a fucking tennis club—has to be like a permanent guest. Fraud and embezzlement—you'd think he was skinning live cats. I guess that fucking Madoff really queered it for guys like him."

Carr smiles and passes the camera to Bobby. "Do we know this guy?" he asks.

Bobby looks at the screen and speaks through a mouthful of Boston cream. "Howie had a lunch and a dinner with him last week. I call him Ichabod. Don't know his real name."

"Time to find out," Carr says.

Time, in fact, to pick Howard Bessemer's pockets and rifle through his sock drawer, down to the lint and the last stray pennies. The dossier from Boyce has given Carr and his crew a head start: the basics of Bessemer's story. The early chapters are straightforward enough: a young man of mediocre intellect and even less ambition—not to mention a DWI arrest on his eighteenth birthday—finds a spot at the university that generations of his family have attended, and where his grandfather has recently built a gymnasium. Not much new there.

The middle passages are similarly predictable: a degree after five and a half years, a record distinguished only by his term as social director of his fraternity and three more DWI arrests—though no convictions—and yet Howard still wangles a place in the training program at Melton-Peck, where his great-uncle was once a board member. A job as an account manager in the private bank follows, as does a marriage, a promotion or two, a co-op on the Upper East Side, a baby, and finally a rancorous, pricey divorce. Again, nothing novel, except that it is during this period that Bessemer met Curtis Prager. They overlapped at Melton-Peck by two years, and when Prager started up his first hedge fund, Bessemer referred clients to him—and eventually became one himself.

It's in the later chapters that things get more interesting, and that the Bessemer story plays out in the New York newspapers, and in the records of the U.S. District Court, Southern District of New York. It becomes the tale of an affable private banker who for years poached funds from the accounts of certain customers to bolster the investment returns of certain others. A banker who, when caught knee-deep in the cookie jar, sang long and loud to the feds about the inner workings of an elaborate tax evasion scheme that involved several of his well-heeled clients and a pair of Swiss bankers, and featured hundreds of large wire transfers that somehow managed not to appear on anybody's suspicious activity reports.

Cooperation and a guilty plea bought Bessemer a reduced sentence—eighteen months in Otisville—but he could've gotten off with even less. The feds had dangled another offer before him, just before his trip upstate: a suspended sentence in exchange for testimony against Curtis Prager and Tirol Capital. But Bessemer declined. Mr. Boyce's dossier dryly lists two possible reasons, neither of which involves Howard's unwavering loyalty.

One hypothesis is that, despite his friendship with Prager, Howard was never a Tirol insider, so he simply didn't know enough to be useful to the feds. Another—a favorite of the prosecutors, and encouraged by the conspiracy theories of the ex–Mrs. Bessemer and her frustrated lawyers—is that Howard knew plenty, but kept quiet because Prager had helped him hide assets during his divorce. Eighteen months of medium-security time, their reasoning went, was more appealing to Howard than writing off five million or so in hidden funds.

Bessemer did his time without incident, and when he was released, two years back, he settled himself in Palm Beach, in the Bermuda-style cottage he'd inherited from his grandmother, and with a modest income from a trust she'd left.

A good start, but not enough for Carr's purposes. Nor is his own research—not yet. Seventeen days of arm's-length observations have given Carr the routines—the tennis, the lunches, the poker, and the whores—and the comfort that Bessemer does almost nothing to safeguard his home or his person, but Carr needs more than that, and for more he needs to get close.

So Dennis and Latin Mike are even now in Bessemer's cottage, with an hour to work before the maid arrives for the weekly cleaning—time

enough to plant the microphones and cameras, tap the landline, skim the mail and the garbage, and for Dennis to work his dark magic on Bessemer's laptop: sniffers, keyloggers, screen scrapers—enough spyware to turn Bessemer's computer into a digital confessional every time he switches it on. Carr checks his watch. Time enough.

Bobby wipes his chin and opens the van door. "Give me the Nikon," he says, as he unzips his painter's coveralls. He brushes stray crumbs from the AT&T logo on the polo shirt he's wearing underneath, tosses the coveralls in back, and straps a phone man's tool rig around his waist. Carr hands him a palm-size camera from the backpack, and Bobby drops it in the pocket of his cargo shorts.

"The last jelly's mine," he says, and Carr watches him shamble down the alley to the Barton's small loading dock.

For the job of following Howard Bessemer around Palm Beach, Bobby is Carr's first choice. Valerie is distracting, and besides, she is otherwise occupied in Boca Raton, and Dennis is too jumpy. He sweats and fidgets whenever he has to playact, and his anxiety glows like neon. Latin Mike is poised and utterly capable but, with Carr at least, sour and taciturn. His shuttered face and silent disapproval wear on Carr and remind him of his father.

Bobby is easier to take, especially without Mike around. Without Mike to impress, he's more relaxed and accommodating—funnier, and less inclined to carp or balk. More likable. Carr knows that Bobby isn't as comfortable with him as he is with Latin Mike—Carr lacks Mike's working-class credentials—but one-on-one, Bobby gives him the benefit of the doubt. And, most important, Bobby likes to talk.

A steady stream of it has issued from him as he and Carr have tailed Bessemer—a miscellany of profanity-laced observations on Bessemer's choice of car and clothing, the latest heartbreak served up by Bobby's beloved, despised Mets, the crappy house he, Mike, and Dennis are staying in, the ass of any woman who crosses his line of sight, his Brooklyn boyhood, his truncated air force career—McGuire Air Force Base, Ramstein, Aviano, and back to McGuire for the court-martial—his shrew of an ex-wife. A grab bag, but short on the topic that interests Carr most— the topic that has circled his thoughts like a scavenging bird ever since his last conversation with Tina.

Carr tries to keep in mind his long-ago training, incomplete though it

was, on agents and their early cultivation. *Walk softly. Come at it obliquely. Keep your shopping list to yourself. Let them broach the topic first, but change the subject the first time they do. Change it the second time too.* But he was impatient at the Farm—one of his many failings—and he's been impatient in Palm Beach too, and in neither place did it help his cause. His instructors scowled and shook their heads, and so did Bobby.

Another truck, another alleyway, three days before.

"For fuck's sake," Bobby said, "you ask about this I don't know how many times. What else is there to say about it?"

Carr put on a pensive look. "I've got no one else to ask, Bobby. Valerie wasn't there, and Mike won't say shit about it."

"Well, you know it all already. Deke thought it was a layup, but it wasn't. Bales of cash sitting in a barn on Bertolli's ranch. No real security besides a little local talent, and the ranch being at the ass end of nowhere, and all we have to do is drive in, deal with the locals, load up, and drive away—straight through to Santiago. Deke had a flight lined up out of Los Cerillos. The driving-in part was fine; after that it was a shit storm."

"You had two trucks."

Bobby sighed. "Two vans—Fords—four-wheel drive conversions. Ray-Ray lined 'em up in B.A., and we drove 'em north. Me and Mike in one, Deke and Ray-Ray in the other. You know all this."

"Deke decided who rode where?"

"Deke decided everything. Ray-Ray was the best driver, then me—so he split us up."

"And he rode with Ray."

"He always got a kick out of the kid."

"Everybody did; he was a good kid. So you drove in the main gate?"

Bobby squinted at him. "You not listening the first ten times I told it? We came up a service road—three miles of washboard in the pitch-fucking-black—and clipped the chain on a cattle gate. It was another two miles from there to the airstrip and the barn."

"And then you hit trouble."

"Soon as we got out of the vans. They came around back of a tin hangar on the other side of the strip—four big four-by-fours—and fucking fast."

"You didn't get into the barn?"

"Didn't get closer than twenty meters. We got out of the vans and they lit us up like fucking Vegas."

"They seem like regular security, or something laid on especially for you guys?"

"The fuck should I know? All I know is they could shoot."

"Deke said there wouldn't be much opposition."

"That was the intel."

"Where'd he get it from?"

"Might as well been from a cereal box, for what it was worth. He'd been looking at Bertolli a long time, I know that, but he always played his sources close to the vest. He was big on that *need to know* crap."

"You guys put up a fight?"

"It was like pissing in the wind. We had MP9s; they had like a dozen guys with AKs. Mostly we ran like hell."

"But not in the same direction."

"It was Deke's call—split up and regroup in Mendoza. We had a fall-back off the Avenue Zapata, near the bus station. He and Ray-Ray went out the main gate, me and Mike went out the way we came."

"And only you and Mike made it."

"Only by the hairs on our asses, lemme tell you—those motherfuckers were serious. Two-plus hours hard running down Highway Forty, and those bastards were bouncing in my mirrors the whole time. We could barely put a mile between us and them. Half busted an axle, and my rear panels were like Swiss cheese. Wasn't till we got to town that I could shake 'em."

"Just the one truck after you guys, though—just one of those four-by-fours."

"One was enough."

"So the other three were on Deke and Ray-Ray?"

"The fuck should I know? All Deke said was that they were on his ass. He didn't say if that meant three trucks or one."

"He called just once?"

"And I could barely hear him then. The service isn't great out there."

"He didn't say that he wasn't going to Mendoza? That he was making for Santiago instead?"

"He said they were on his ass, and that was it. If he'd said anything about Santiago, or not showing up at the fallback, we wouldn't have spent two days waiting in that fucking hole, peeping through those moldy curtains, and jumping every time a toilet flushed."

"So no idea how Deke and Ray-Ray ended up westbound on Highway Seven?"

Bobby ran a thick hand down his face. "Come on, Carr—enough already with this."

"You were there, Bobby—you must have an idea."

"Like what—they were cut off, couldn't get back on Forty, took one of those horse trails to Seven, and got tagged in the mountains? You don't like that story, make up one of your own. You know as much as I do about what happened."

"You were there."

"And you weren't, and you don't know how to give it a rest. Look, everybody gets that you never liked the deal—you and Val both. Not enough planning, too rushed, whatever. You guys made it clear, and it turns out you were right. Nobody thinks it's your fault, Carr. Nobody holds it against you, except maybe you."

"I'm not holding anything. I just want to know why it went bad."

"There're a million reasons. Crappy planning, crappy intel, crappy roads, crappy luck—take your pick. Who knows why, and who the hell cares? Deke is gone, and so is Ray, and picking at the roadkill won't bring 'em back. You feel guilty, find yourself a priest. Talking to you about this is like talking to my Irish grandma, for chrissakes, or talking to a cop."

Carr had smiled at that. He hadn't been talking like a cop, but he'd been listening like one. That was the sixth time he'd gotten Bobby to tell the story, the third time since his talk with Tina, and every time Bobby had told it just the same way, down to the pitch-fucking-black, the bastards bouncing in his mirrors, the half-busted axle, and the moldy curtains. Always the same details—never more, never less, never different. Every time. The same.

Bobby comes up the alley, wiping the corner of his mouth, and Carr comes back.

Bobby unhitches his tool belt and tosses it into the van. "Ichabod's name is Willis Stearn," he says. "I got more pictures. I got a number and an address too. And I knocked over the kitchen for a tuna on white with the crusts cut off. Fucking master criminal, huh?"

Carr nods. "Nobody better, Bobby."

9

In the maze of machines and shining bodies, it is her shoulders that he finally recognizes. They're angular and broad for a woman, with well-defined deltoid muscles and a faded scar—a ragged-edged dime of unknown origin—over her left scapula. It appears and disappears beneath the edge of her sweat-darkened tank top as she works the fly machine. Carr forces himself not to stare, but to keep drifting around the perimeter of the vast gym.

It has taken him ten minutes of drifting to find Valerie, and no wonder. Her hair is shorter now, and expensively tinted—a champagne and honey cap with bangs swept to the side—and her skin is biscuit brown. But the hair and tan are just window dressing, sleight of hand. The real transformation runs deeper, and Carr is no closer to working out the trick now than he was in Costa Alegre.

So she is older today—thirty-five, maybe forty—and very fit. But also tired, though not from the exercise. It's a longer-term fatigue, a kind of erosion—the product of a beating tide of disappointment, wrong choices, bad luck. Its etchings appear at the corners of her mouth and around her eyes, in her dye job, and in the concentration she puts into her workout. They tell a story of assets carefully managed but dwindling nonetheless—an inexorable spending of the principal. Carr has stopped and is staring again, and now she knows he's here.

This is another bit of magic he can't work out—some radar she possesses. Her look is fleeting—less than that—the barest flick of her eyes on the way to glancing at the wall clock, but Carr reads the anger there. He drifts back to the lobby, out the doors, and across Mizner Park to his Saturn.

In twenty minutes Carr is at the Embassy Suites, in a pale blue room with a view of some dumpsters and of planes departing the Boca Raton airport. Forty minutes after that Valerie is at the door, in flats and a sleeveless orange dress. She smells of honeysuckle, and her hair is still damp from the shower. She walks past Carr and sits at the end of the bed.

"What the hell were you doing there?" she says. Her voice is tight with anger, and Carr hears something else in it—the hint of a twang, a whisper of Texas or Oklahoma.

"I told them I was interested in a membership," he says. "They let me walk around."

"I don't give a damn what you told them. What the hell were you doing? We were supposed to meet here. You want to fuck this up while we're still at the gate?"

"Was Amy at the club?"

"She had a yoga class this afternoon; she left half an hour before you showed up. But that's not the point. The point is I don't want you there. I don't want to be seen with anybody there. Jill's supposed to be on her own."

"You take the yoga class with Amy?"

Valerie's lips purse. "Monday. I join the class Monday."

"You talk to her yet?"

"In the locker room, to say hello," Valerie says, and slips off her flats. Her bare feet are tanned; her toenails, like her fingernails, are pale pink.

"She knows who you are?"

"She knows I'm Jill. She's heard me talk about being new in town."

"That's not much."

"It's enough for now. Get this for me," she says, rising and turning her back to Carr. He slides her zipper down.

"You have a better read on her?"

"I know she takes care of herself. Yoga, spinning, weights, laps in the pool—she's at the club every day. She spends money on her hair and nails, and serious money on her wardrobe. St. John, Carlisle, Akris—nice stuff.

Low-key, but classy. And that handbag of hers is no knockoff. Twenty grand, easy. She's a loner, though. Never says more than a word or two to the staff, or to another member. Never has guests."

"But she says hello to you."

Valerie nods, and lets her dress fall in an orange pool at her feet. She wears no bra, and her panties are sheer orange silk. "I'm sociable," she says.

She throws the spread off the bed and pulls down the blanket and top sheet. Carr leans against the desk. His heart is pounding and his words catch in his throat. "You see the video Dennis and Bobby shot of her house?" he asks. Valerie nods. "What did you think?"

"It's modern—lots of glass."

"I meant about the security."

"No surprise: she's president of a bank, and it's a pain in the ass. She's in a gated community, so there's the gatehouse, the authorized visitor lists, the prowl cars, and lots of rent-a-cops—who, by the way, are all strapped. Bobby said the house itself is wired pretty good too—not that it slowed him much.

"On top of that, there's the bank's security people. She's got a retired sheriff's deputy that drives her everywhere in that nice black Benz, and her office, her car, and her house all get swept weekly for electronics."

"On a set schedule?"

She shakes her head. "That'd make life too easy. And as far as her work laptop goes, Bobby says it rides to the office with her in the Benz and comes home the same way, and when she stops at the gym, it waits in the car with her driver."

Carr nods. "Dennis send you anything from her personal computer?"

"He spiked it, and he's supposed to send me her e-mail and her browser history. He confirmed it doesn't have the Isla Privada software on it, and none of the security hardware to access their network." Valerie sits cross-legged on the bed and pulls a pillow onto her lap. "You think I'm not doing my homework?"

"Maybe you saw something I didn't."

Valerie shakes her head. "It's what we thought: we want access to Isla Privada's network, we need their hardware; we want access to that—to Amy Chun's equipment, anyway—we need somebody who can hang out in her house. And that would be Jill."

Carr nods slowly and sits up on the desk. "How's your apartment working out?"

She shrugs. "Mid-nineties generic. Lot of corporate types in the building, on long-term business trips, plus some divorced dads with cars they can't afford. I can see a slice of the Intracoastal from the balcony. It's right for Jill."

"We could've met there."

Valerie narrows her eyes. "No we couldn't," she says, scowling. "I told you: Jill's on her own."

"Yeah, I got that. You color in any other parts of Jill's life?"

"I'm waiting for the take from Amy's computer," she says. Valerie looks Carr up and down. "You're perched on that desk like it's a lifeboat. We sinking or something?"

"I'm trying to figure out if you're going to keep snapping at my ass. I'm thinking maybe I can hide behind this thing."

Valerie is still for a beat, and then she sighs. "Yeah. Sorry. It takes me a while to let her go. I can't switch her off just like that." She snaps her fingers, like a branch breaking. "Jill's pretty much had it with men. She's a little angry."

"I get that."

Valerie sighs again, longer and more heavily. "Not me, though. I'm not angry." She pats the mattress beside her, and Carr crosses to the bed.

Afterward, covered in gooseflesh and the sour breath of the air conditioner, Valerie pulls him back from the edge of sleep. Her head is on his chest, and her fingers comb gently through his pubic hair. Her voice is husky.

"Let's play geography," she says.

Carr sighs. He can't remember who started it, or when they started playing, but it's become a fixture of the long stretches the crew spends together in cars, in vans, in darkened rooms—a way to relieve the monotony of sitting for hours with earpieces jammed in their heads, watching, listening, waiting. Dennis called it retirement geography, and it was simple to play: tell a story about what you're going to do once you've made your nut, and where you're going to do it—your dream of life afterward. Which, Carr thought, told you a lot about a person.

Bobby's ideal retirement changed venues now and then—shifting from Nassau, to Vegas, to Macao, to Monte Carlo, and back to Nassau again—but regardless of the particular locale, it was always the same: a high-roller suite at a high-end gambling resort.

"These new villas, they have private elevators right down to the casino floor, and private hostesses who spoon-feed you caviar and wipe your ass with silk. I'll make sure they all have pictures of my ex, with orders to shoot on sight." A simple man, Bobby, with a simple plan.

Latin Mike's vision of his golden years was also straightforward, if less gilded: he wanted off the grid. "A thousand acres in the high desert. I put up a wind turbine, solar cells, and a tall motherfucking fence. I have a few horses, maybe a goat, and nobody needs to send me a Christmas card."

Ray-Ray had a second career in mind—a ski school in British Columbia, with a bar attached. "I'll run the tourist babes up and down the mountain all day, and at night I'll ply their sore little bods with alcohol."

And Dennis dreamed of setting up a venture capital shop on Sand Hill Road and financing the next Google. Bobby always laughed at that. "You're a fucking pure breed, Denny; you're geek to the bone."

Carr didn't play the game, and neither did Valerie. He would simply shake his head when his turn came around; she chose deflection.

"I'm falling off the map, boys," she said, the last time Bobby tried to goad her into it. "Over the edge, like those ships when the world was flat."

Bobby laughed. "C'mon, Vee—that's not how you play."

"Fuck you—you think I want you guys showing up on my doorstep, looking to borrow money?"

Of all of them, Declan liked the game best, and he was best at it. It called to some Celtic storytelling gene in him, and he would spin elaborate yarns about his retirement by the sea. Over the years he'd had several shores in mind: Hoi An, in Vietnam, and Hua Hin, in Thailand, La Barra, in Uruguay, was a favorite for a long while. He would talk about them at length and in detail—the weather, the waters, the cuisines, and local real estate markets. Carr remembers him hunched over binoculars, waxing poetic about asado and fish empanadas, while the smell of his cigar filled the van.

"Yer young now, but you'll see, when yer all wizened bastards like me, you won't want to be working or whoring or—forgive me, Mike—roasting in the feckin' desert. You'll want a cottage by the sea, I'm telling

ya, and a boat, and maybe a garden with a fruit tree. And who knows, but maybe you'll want to do some breeding yerselves. Me, I'm hoping the local publican has a daughter of marrying age, or maybe the baker—a homely but grateful girl. That's the ticket, lads." The gravel whisper went on and on about the meals he'd cook, the wine he'd drink, the darts he'd play, and the dog he would buy.

Carr rubs his eyes and sits up in bed. "I thought you didn't like that game," he says.

"I didn't," Valerie says, "when it was just a game. Now it's less abstract. Come on—you show me yours . . ."

Carr shakes his head. "I have nothing to show. I haven't given much thought to afterward."

Valerie sighs and settles herself again, her cheek on his thigh. "Bobby said you were talking to him about Mendoza. Asking about what happened again."

"And?"

"And it worries him."

"Worries him how?"

"He thinks you're picking at something, and he doesn't know what. He's worried you're taking your eye off the ball."

"Screw him. He should keep his mind on his own goddamn job, and let me take care of mine."

"He says you feel guilty."

"Bobby's a psychiatrist now? That's a sure sign of the apocalypse."

"I don't like what happened down there either. It was a waste, and I was as broken up about it as anybody—but I don't feel guilty."

Carr shakes his head. "No offense, Vee, but I'm not sure you're the best yardstick."

Valerie sits up and pulls a sheet over her breasts. "If I wasn't such a cold-hearted bitch, I might take offense at that," she says with a bitter laugh. "Maybe I didn't know those guys as long as you, but I trusted them with my life more times than I can count. I trusted them to back me up, and they didn't disappoint. Not ever. Ray was like a kid brother, for chris-sakes, and Deke . . ."

She looks at the ceiling and breathes deeply—once, twice—to steady her voice. "We told Deke what we thought about that job—you and me both. We said everything there was to say about the planning, the intel,

the risks—everything and then some. Maybe you remember, he was pretty pissed at us when he left. I thought the two of you were going to come to blows. You tell me, what else were we supposed to do?"

Carr shrugs. "We should've been more convincing."

"Right—'cause Deke was always so open to suggestions."

"He listened to me."

"He listened when he felt like it, but he didn't listen then. And really, how many ways can you say *bad idea* and *stupid fucking plan*? I think we tried them all."

Carr runs a hand through his hair. "Maybe it wasn't just the plan that was bad. Maybe something else was going on."

Valerie sits up and looks at him. "What the *fuck* are you talking about?" Carr shrugs again, and Valerie's hand is on his biceps. "*Something else* like what?"

"I don't know. Bertolli might've gotten wind of something."

Valerie shakes her head. "Are you for real with this? What was Bertolli going to get wind of? The only guy as insane about operational security as you are was Declan. You really think he got sloppy with that?"

"Maybe somebody got sloppy for him."

"You're not serious with this paranoid shit, are you? You think Bobby or Mike dimed him out? Or maybe you think it was me?" She slides her palm up his arm, over his shoulder, to his neck. The smell of honeysuckle is strong. Her voice softens. "Guilt does that, you know—it makes you paranoid. You feel bad, you feel responsible, so you feel like there's a bill coming due. Then you're looking over your shoulder every other minute, waiting for it to arrive. Paranoid."

Carr rolls away from her, out of bed, and goes into the bathroom. He turns the water tap, drinks from a cupped hand, and looks in the mirror. The angular face, the cropped black hair, disheveled now, his mother's hazel eyes, smudged with fatigue, the wiry frame, the white sketch marks of scars here and there, are somehow unfamiliar to him—pieces he can't assemble into a working whole. He stands in the bathroom doorway. Valerie is sitting cross-legged, the sheet down around her waist.

"Our being down there wouldn't have changed anything," she says, "except maybe we'd be dead on the side of a road too. So we were someplace else—so what?"

"I know where we were," Carr says, his voice rising suddenly above the drone of the air conditioner. "I know what we were doing."

Valerie laughs, and there's a note of satisfaction in it—a long-held theory finally confirmed. Jill's twang reappears in her voice. "So you feel bad about that too—that we were in St. Barts, fucking, while it was going on. You sure you weren't raised Catholic, or maybe Jewish? 'Cause, baby boy, you got the guilt down cold."

"You and Bobby can talk it out in your next session. Compare notes."

"That might be deep water for Bobby," Valerie says, and throws off her sheet. She pushes past Carr into the bathroom and runs the shower.

Carr watches as she steps in—the muscles in her back, her brown ass, her skin flawless but for the ragged-edged dime on her scapula. "Why the hell are you talking to Bobby about this anyway?" he says.

Valerie works her fingers through her water-darkened hair. "I thought you wanted me to—that you wanted my help with these guys. To take their temperature—make sure their heads were on right. I thought we both wanted this job over and done with, and done right. Then, if you want, we can work out that guilt and whatever other little bugs are crawling around your head. We could have ourselves some fun afterward."

Valerie builds a creamy lather on her arms and breasts and belly. She beckons to Carr, and through the scrim of water and curling steam her smile is bright.

The sky above the hotel parking lot is gray, and it's heavy with car exhaust and the metal heat of the fading day. An erratic breeze sends a paper cup back and forth across a patch of cracked cement. Sitting in the Saturn, Carr is similarly restless. He doesn't know why he started talking to Valerie about what happened in Mendoza, or why he stopped. Maybe he was fishing for something—for her to tell him to forget his suspicions, call them paranoid shit, and remind him to keep his mind on the job. He thinks about the game she tried to play—retirement geography, and all those stories of *afterward*. He hears his own voice—*I haven't given much thought to afterward*—and wonders if maybe he should.

Certainly, *afterward* is easier for him to think about. Easier than thinking about how Bertolli's men came to be waiting for Deke in the dead of night. Or why Bobby always tells the story just the same way. Easier than dealing with Mike's snide comments and hostile silences. Or finding a useful handle on Howard Bessemer. Or thinking about Valerie and Amy Chun. Easier by far than thinking about his father, and the tar pit of

brochures, applications, and FAQ pages Carr has drowned in every night for nearly three weeks. Assisted living facilities, nursing homes, dementia units—the nomenclature sticks to his arms and legs, and fills his ears with static. Eleanor Calvin has left messages—six, eight, Carr has lost count—but he hasn't returned a one.

So *afterward*. The problem is, Carr doesn't know much about *afterward*—with Valerie, or with anyone else.

His relationships with women haven't lasted long—a few weeks, a month or two—no longer than the gaps between his jobs with Declan. But there was a sameness to them all, a sense of melancholy that suffused them from the start—the feel of a beach in midwinter.

The women themselves were not much alike, not at first glance anyway. Hannah was from Seattle, a filmmaker shooting a documentary on the Costa Rican rainforests and staying in the same hotel as Carr, in Puerto Viejo. Ann was from Zurich, a geologist with ABB, analyzing core samples taken off the Belize coast and drinking at night in a bar in San Pedro that Carr also favored. Brooke was a UNICEF pediatrician from Toronto, on vacation in Antigua between a stint in Haiti and a posting in Phnom Penh, and she and Carr dove the same reefs.

The list went on—different ages, different nationalities, different professions and appearances, but still, a sameness. They were all nominally married, but they were solitaries by nature—self-sufficient, emotionally reticent, even prickly. They were all obsessive about their jobs, and chronically exhausted by them. And they all possessed a certain brand of low-key intellectual charisma—a smart-girl glamour—that pulled at Carr like the moon pulled the seas.

The other thing they had in common, of course, was Carr himself. He understood something of his own appeal. Yes, he was attractive enough, enthusiastic and inventive enough, articulate and reasonably amusing when he had something to say, and smart enough to keep quiet otherwise. But his main draws, he knew, lay elsewhere. He was convenient. He was unburdened by backstory. And he was, without question, impermanent. It made him the perfect time-out from the rest of their lives—ephemeral, essentially anonymous, as disposable as the aliases they knew him by. And it left Carr entirely ignorant of *afterward*.

His thoughts find no forward traction with Valerie, and inevitably they slide back, to St. Barts. The vast, glassy plain of Flamands Bay, the

crescent of bone-white sand, the white umbrellas, like a line of portly nuns, and their rooms overlooking it all. Their rooms that they never left. All that time working together, and St. Barts was their first time. And there, amid the ravaged bedding and the ruins of room service trays, was the first time it occurred to Carr that perhaps things didn't have to be quite so temporary.

Then the calls came in. The first was at five a.m., local time. Bobby's voice was low and flat and affectless, difficult for Carr to understand. It wasn't until after he'd hung up that Carr realized Bobby was in shock. The next calls, hours later, were from Mike, and they were confused and angry and scared. By then Carr had packed his bag and arranged his transit to B.A.

The heat has put him nearly to sleep, but there's movement across the lot, a flash of orange and short blond hair, and Carr wakes himself. He sees Valerie get into her Audi and drive off. He counts off thirty seconds and starts up the Saturn.

She takes Military Trail south and Palmetto Park east, to a stretch of stores and low apartment buildings. Valerie's building is glass and concrete, and as generic as she described. She pulls into the residents' lot, and Carr parks across the street. He doesn't see her enter, but in a while he sees a row of lights in some third-floor windows, and a slender orange figure crossing a room. In another minute he sees Valerie on a balcony, a glass in her hand, her face turned east, looking perhaps at a slice of the Intracoastal.

It is full dark when she goes inside again and draws the curtains. Carr watches her blank windows for an hour afterward, and then gets on 95 and drives back to Palm Beach.

10

No palms on this street—barely any green at all besides a runty saw palmetto, and its fronds are mostly gray. Bobby was right about the house; it's crap: a low concrete bunker the color of dishwater, with barred windows, a tin-roofed carport, and a sagging school yard fence. In a neighborhood where chipped breeze block and auto parts on the lawn make up an architectural school, it's still the worst house on the street. But the locals don't worry much about how the hedge next door is clipped, or if they do, they know better than to say. Which makes the house crap but also ideal. A jet passes low, directly overhead. It casts a broad shadow and shakes Carr's stomach, and leaves behind the tang of spent kerosene.

Carr has been here only twice before, but still it's more than familiar to him, a cousin to every workhouse they've ever used, in more bleak neighborhoods, by more airports, harbors, and rail yards than he can count. He knocks twice and waits. His head aches, the midday glare makes his eyes water, and, though he had nothing stronger than soda water the night before, he feels hungover. The kerosene smell settles in his hair and clothing. He can feel it on his skin. Dennis opens the door.

The lights are on in the living room, and all the shades are drawn. There's music playing, propulsive Colombian hip-hop, but it's fighting a losing battle with the air conditioner rattling in the wall. The living room furniture—a spavined sofa, a lumpy recliner, some battered kitchen chairs, a side table pitted with burn marks—is pushed up against the

walls, and the center of the space is dominated by two long tables with plastic tops and folding legs. Bobby and Latin Mike sit at one, peering into the same laptop screen. Dennis folds himself at the other, behind an uneven berm of equipment—laptops, printers, routers, modems, a laminating machine, and a tangle of cabling. Like every other workhouse.

Carr winces at the music and the odor—of cigarettes and burned coffee—and locks the door behind him. He places the white paper bag he's carrying on Bobby's table and tears it open. The smells of tomato sauce and grease waft up to mix with the entrenched aromas.

"Two meatball and two sausage and pepper," Carr says.

"Just in time," Bobby says. "Denny was starting to look like a plate of wings to me." Bobby reaches across, takes two of the foil-wrapped torpedoes, and passes one to Dennis. Latin Mike sighs and takes a long pull on his cigarette.

Bobby tears the wrapping off his sandwich and takes a bite. He makes small grunts as he chews, and red sauce runs down his chin. Latin Mike shakes his head. "You never heard of a napkin?" He reaches across Carr for a sandwich and carefully peels the foil away.

Bobby looks at Carr. "You not eating?"

Mike laughs. "*Jefe* don't need to eat with us. He's got that nice café by his condo. All those white tables, and the waitresses in their aprons, right, *jefe*? Not a place for workingmen like us, Bobby."

Carr looks at Mike, who smiles and eats his sandwich. There's nothing in the grin beyond his usual bullshit—the theater of labor versus management that he's compelled to perform every time he has to report progress. He did it when Declan was alive, and Carr has learned to bear it.

Carr smiles. "Yeah, they wax your Bentley with every meal. How about telling me what's up with Bessemer."

Dennis giggles behind his monitors. Mike wipes his mouth and hands carefully. "Well, it looks like Howie's got himself a job since gettin' out. And he's been busy at it. Eight days take from the wires we planted, and we got what we need. Howie's making valuable contributions to his community."

Dennis giggles again. "Real valuable," he says.

"A public servant," Bobby adds, laughing.

Carr sighs, and the throbbing in his head is more insistent. "Dennis, you want to turn down the music? And how about we skip the banter?"

Dennis kills the hip-hop. Latin Mike smiles and turns his laptop

toward Carr. "Look for yourself. This is off one of the cameras we put in his house—the one behind his desk."

A window opens on the laptop and fills with a murky image: the back of a leather chair, the surface of a desk—scuffed wood, a blotter, a green shaded lamp, a computer keyboard and monitor. Beyond the desk, beside a darkened window, is a pair of green leather club chairs. Howard Bessemer is in one, and Daniel Brunt, his frequent tennis partner, is in the other. Their voices are muffled but entirely intelligible, and they both sound slightly drunk.

"*Is her name actually Natasha?*" Brunt says. "*They can't all be named that, can they? And is she even Russian, or is she from Latvia or one of those other places?*"

"*I have no clue where she's from, Danny. Really, I don't ask.*"

"*But you know she's eighteen, right?*"

"*I know what they tell me.*"

"*Because the last thing I need, Bess, is underage issues.*"

"*You don't need any issues, Danny. Nobody does.*"

Carr taps the mousepad and the video pauses. He looks at Mike, who is smiling. "Whores? They're talking about whores?"

"Russian whores, *jefe.*"

"Howie takes Brunt to his poker parties?"

"Not that we've seen," Bobby says around a mouthful of meatball.

"So . . . ?"

"Howie is a *player, jefe.* This little Pillsbury *pendejo* is a *pimp.*"

Dennis clears his throat. "I think he's more of a pander, technically, or a procurer. I mean, the girls don't work for him."

"Whatever," Latin Mike says. "The point is, he's lining 'em up for Brunt. And not just whores."

"And not just for Brunt," Bobby adds.

Carr looks at the image of Howard Bessemer, frozen on the laptop screen—the round, unlined face, the high forehead catching the dim light. Carr shakes his head. "What else besides whores?"

"Danny here likes his Vicodin," Bobby says.

Latin Mike turns the laptop around again, and works the keyboard. "We got the best stuff from the cameras in his house, and the mics in his car and his tennis bag," Mike says. "They all know better than to put this shit in e-mails. This one's from the car." He turns the laptop around again.

There's no picture, but a voice comes on. It's lazy, low, entitled. Carr doesn't recognize it.

"*. . . more of that stuff you got last week? That was very nice—very mellow.*"

Carr stops the playback. "This is who?"

"Nick Scoville," Dennis answers. "Howie sails with him. He's got a smack habit."

Bobby laughs. "And his golfing buddy Tandy—he likes coke with his whores. He likes really fat whores, by the way. The other golfer, Moyer, is into ice, and lots of it."

"Nice friends," Carr says, and hits PLAY again. Bessemer's voice comes on.

"*I'll talk to my guys and see what they can do.*"

"*See what they can do with price, Bess. I mean, it's pretty shit but it's not cheap.*"

Carr hits STOP. "Who are these *guys* he's talking about?"

Mike takes the laptop again and brings up a photo. He turns the screen back to Carr. "They're brothers," Mike says.

There are two men in the photo, both stocky and dark, one muscular, the other just fat. The muscular one wears a gray suit and a white shirt, open at the collar. The fat one wears jeans, a black T-shirt, a rumpled blue blazer, dark glasses, and a three-day beard. Carr recognizes the backdrop: the frosted glass front of the Brazilian restaurant beneath which Bessemer spends his weekends.

"Mister *GQ* is Misha Grigoriev," Bobby says. "The dough boy is his baby brother, Sasha. Russkies, in case you couldn't guess. Came over when they were teenagers, by way of Jersey. Now they're local bad boys, with a little bit of everything going on. They own the Brazilian place and two others like it in Jupiter and Vero Beach. They got a string of high-end call girls here in town, and a couple of small-time dope guys on staff. They got a gambling joint down in Boynton Beach. Like everybody else around here, they got a construction business to pump the money through, though these days I can't see how that flies so well."

Carr looks sharply from Bobby to Mike and back. "Where'd you get all that?"

Latin Mike scowls and mutters something in Spanish. Bobby puts up his hands. "Don't worry—we didn't leave tracks. I bought drinks for a

stumblebum vice cop who couldn't find his own dick to piss with, and doesn't know me from Adam. And Denny did some crazy shit with a fed computer."

"A DOJ server," Dennis says, and smiles sheepishly. "And I made it look like all the traffic went in and out of Moscow."

Carr nods and looks at the Grigorievs on the screen. "Are they connected?"

Bobby shakes his head. "According to the feds they're independents."

"And Bessemer works for them?"

"He's a middleman," Bobby says. "A freelancer. He's buying the dope from the Grigorievs' people, marking up the price, and selling to his buddies."

"He's fronting the money?" Carr asks, and Dennis nods. "For the whores too?"

Another nod. "Yeah—with a markup. He relays the where, when, and how many to the Grigorievs' man, and the whores show up."

"He making much money?"

Bobby shrugs. "His margins look pretty thin. The Russkies aren't giving him any breaks on price. Play the one with Sasha, Denny—from Howie's car."

Dennis fiddles at the keyboard until another voice comes on. This one is deep and impatient, with a trace of an accent.

"*You have a problem, you talk to Willy, not me, right?*"

"*But this stuff isn't for me, Sash—you know that. It's for my friends, and the price—*"

"*I don't know about any stuff, and I don't want to know, Howard. You don't talk to me about this crap, you understand? What Willy says is what goes, okay? He don't know who this is for, and he don't care, right? All he knows is you, and shit costs what he says it costs, and that's it, right? What you do after that is your thing.*"

Bobby hits STOP. "He's whining about the price of coke. They charge Howie one-ten a gram, which is full retail and then some for around here."

Carr draws a hand along his jaw. "This is a lot of risk he's taking," he says, "especially for a guy with a record. What the hell's he doing it for?"

Latin Mike blows out smoke in a disgusted blast. "*Cabrón*, who gives a shit why he's doing it? It's enough we know what he's doing. Like you said,

it's a big risk for a guy like him, and that makes it a good handle. A handle like this, we pick him up and carry him anywhere we want."

Another jet passes, shaking the glass in the windows. Carr rubs a palm over his chin. "It's not enough. We get only one shot at Bessemer, and we need to make it stick. We need to know all the strings there are to pull. I want to know why he's doing it. Is it just money? Is it something else?"

"*Hijo de puta!*" Mike flicks his cigarette across the room and jumps to his feet. There's a burst of red against the cinder block, and a smoldering ember on the carpet, and Mike's chair tips back. He points at Carr. "The *fuck* is up with you? This thing is lined up like dominoes. What's wrong with knocking it over?"

When he finally answers, Carr's voice is quiet. "I said we don't know enough yet."

"I tell you what's not enough," Mike says, and he cups a hand around his crotch.

Bobby has stopped chewing, and Dennis is frozen at his keyboard. The room is silent but for the chugging of the air conditioner and the receding rumble of a jet. Blood rushes in Carr's ears as he stands. "I don't recall you ever making quite that argument to Declan, Mike."

Mike smiles and steps forward. "That's 'cause Deke had a pair."

Carr nods. "And most of the time he managed not to confuse them with his brains."

Mike steps forward until his chest is nearly touching Carr's. He looks down at Carr and smiles wider. "That's right, *pendejo,* I'm just a dumbass chicano. What the fuck do I know? What kinda dumbass thing will I do next?"

Carr forces his breathing down—*inhale, exhale, not too fast.* He can smell the cigarettes on Mike, and the coffee, and the cologne. He studies Mike's throat—the pulse in his carotid artery, the soft spot below his Adam's apple—and tenses his fingers. He nearly jumps at Dennis's nervous cough.

"I . . . I know what Valerie would say if she were here." Dennis's voice is cracking. "Something like *put 'em back in your pants.* Don't you think, Bobby?"

Bobby's laugh is too loud. "Yeah, or maybe *sit the fuck down.* Right, Mike?"

Mike shrugs, but his gaze never leaves Carr. "She's not here now. And

what the fuck does she care how long this takes? She's not living in this shithole. She's like Carr—got herself a nice apartment with a view of the water and everything."

"But that's what she'd say, Mike, and she'd be right." Bobby tries to catch Carr's eye and fails. "She'd be right, Carr," Bobby says. "We got to keep our heads in the work."

"She's not here now," Carr says quietly.

Dennis stands, still holding his sub. "For chrissakes, I didn't sign up for this kind of thing," he says, and backs away until he hits the wall. When he does a large meatball is ejected from the end of his sandwich. It lands with a wet thud on the carpet between his feet. All three men turn to look first at Dennis, and then the meatball.

Bobby's voice is low and grave. "Look at that—you made the kid shit himself."

And then, suddenly, air returns to the room and the four men are laughing. Carr's shoulders relax, and Latin Mike rights his overturned chair. "You better clean that up, Denny," Mike says. "I don't want to be steppin' in it."

"I don't know," Dennis says, "I think it goes with the carpet."

The men laugh again, and Latin Mike lights a cigarette. Carr moves to the door and turns the lock.

"I don't want this to take longer than it has to," he says, "but we need to know more. Give it a week—if we don't turn up anything else, we'll go with what we've got."

Carr closes the door behind him and hears someone lock it. He walks down the cracked path, through the rusting gate, and it is only when he's around the corner that he takes a breath.

11

His apartment is in North Palm Beach, on Ocean Drive, and even the parking lot has a water view. Carr locks the Saturn and stops to watch the flashes of lightning on the horizon. The sky is purple, going to pitch-black at the eastern edge. It's the verge of something that might ripen to a hurricane, or amount to nothing more than rain. The forecast is muddled with conditionals—colliding zones of warm and cold seawater, churning air masses, equivocal fronts from Canada, butterfly wings over Africa— too many variables. Carr can empathize with the weathermen.

Too many variables. Why is Bessemer doing what he's doing? Will his Russian friends care when he gets burned? Why is Mike such an unremitting asshole, and how does he know about the view from Valerie's apartment? Carr pockets his keys and pushes through the briny air to the lobby.

Here he is Gregory Frye, investor in distressed real estate, down from Boston for an indefinite stay. The doorman greets him by name and makes a joke about the Red Sox, and Carr smiles and nods and gets on the elevator.

He leaves the lights off in the apartment, pulls six beers from the refrigerator, and settles on the sofa, before the tall windows. He opens a bottle and drinks half in one pull, and he's watching the distant lightning when his cell phone burrs. Eleanor Calvin's number appears on the dis-

play, and he tosses the phone to the other end of the sofa, where it glows like a ghost light in a theater.

"Shit." He sighs.

He's been trying, since he left Stockbridge, to dredge up some warmth for Arthur Carr—to find a happy memory of his father or, barring that, any memory that isn't tainted by anger, disapproval, or disappointment. Maybe he's been looking for that for most of his life. The best he's done lately is La Plata, southeast of Buenos Aires, out in the Río de la Plata.

They were sailing then, just the two of them, in an eighteen-footer his father had rented for the day. The wind was from the east, the estuary was brown and choppy, and the sun was waning but still bright. Carr was twelve.

He remembers his father in a faded blue polo shirt, shorts, and bare feet, his arms ropy and brown, and his face shaded by a long-billed cap. They'd been running through man overboard drills for most of the after-noon, steering figure eights again and again to rescue an orange life vest that his father kept flinging over the side.

"There goes Oscar," Arthur Carr would say, and toss the vest again.

His father did the spotting and fished out the vest when they came alongside; Carr was in the cockpit, one hand on the tiller, the other on the lines.

"Bring her around—*quickly* now—the man *is* drowning, after all. Now come to his windward side—*his* windward—that's good. Now ease up on the sheets. Let them luff, for chrissakes—you don't want to run by him!" Carr had gone through it too many times to count that afternoon.

For the last drill of the day, his father wanted Carr to do it all—spot, sail, and haul in the victim. "Pretend for a moment that you actually had a friend, and it was just the two of you out here. Now what would happen if your friend went in? What would you do—watch him drown? You can't just sit there and watch." And over the side the vest went once more.

"You're on your own now," Arthur Carr said.

Carr's heart was pounding, but he kept his head on a swivel, kept his eyes on the bobbing patch of orange, and kept them off his father, who crouched in the companionway and stared at him like a baleful bird. He guided the boat away from the vest and, when he had enough room, tacked smartly. He panicked for an instant as the bow swept around and he lost the vest in the loping brown swells, but he found it again, and lined

up on its windward side. He came in on a close reach, and let his sails luff. As the boat slowed, he scrambled under the boom. He kept low, gripped a stanchion with one hand, and ducked under the lifeline. He leaned out, but the vest was just beyond his straining fingers. Carr slid his hand up the stanchion to the lifeline and leaned out farther. And then a big swell hit.

There was a forward pitch, a sickening drop, scrabbling fingers, rushing, flooding cold, and a blow to the head that ran through Carr's whole body. There was bubbling and roaring, and no time to call out, and no breath to call with. The shadow of the boat rose above him and began to fall again, and then Arthur Carr had a fist through the front of his life vest—was dragging him up through the brown water, up into the air, and dropping him on the cockpit bench.

Carr coughed and sputtered, and his father wrapped a blanket around him and studied his face. He peered into one eye and then the other, and put alcohol and a bandage over the gash on his cheek, where he'd slammed into the hull. Then he took the tiller, turned the boat back toward the marina, and shook his head in disgust.

"Now you're both dead," his father said flatly, "you and your nonexistent friend."

That's the best he can do: an afternoon more than two decades back when his father hadn't actually flown into a rage, had instead been only casually cruel, but had cared enough to pluck him from the river. Though he wasn't sure about the caring part—saving him might simply have been easier than explaining his absence to Carr's mother.

Carr takes another pull on his beer and empties the bottle—his third somehow. Blue light is rippling through the sky, and a red light is blinking on his phone in the corner of his sofa. Mrs. Calvin has left another message. He opens a fourth beer, takes a long swallow, and hears his father's voice again: *You can't just sit there and watch.*

But watching is what he's best at—what he's always been best at, from when he was very small: the comings and goings of neighbors; the shopkeepers in their storefronts, sweeping, chatting with customers, hectoring clerks; the deliverymen; the embassy drivers; the maids and cooks and gardeners; and his parents most closely of all. His father didn't like it—it made him edgy, he said—but his mother didn't mind. In fact, she encouraged it, nurtured it, made a virtue of it, and a game.

He remembers sitting on her lap, in the tall windows of one of their houses, looking out on a tree-lined avenue. Was he even five years old? She would place a pale finger on the glass and point, and he would follow her gaze. Then she would put her hand over his eyes. *¿Qué ves, mijo? What do you see?*

And he would tell her. A man with a dog. A lady in a hat. A blue truck. A green taxi. A grandpa at a café table. He remembers the softness of her palm across his brow, the smell of her hand—gardenias and tobacco. *And what is the old man doing?* Reading a newspaper. Smoking. Drinking from a cup. *What kind of cup? What color hat? How large a dog?* They would go on and on, in English, in Spanish, as afternoon went down to dusk. He would lean against her, sleepy, her voice warm and husky in his ear. *¿Qué color es el coche, mijo? And how many men are in it?*

When his father returned from work—always furrowed and simmering, his tie askew—the game would stop, and it was as if his mother had left the room. As if she'd left the house altogether. She took him from her lap, and her arms were stiff and cool. Her hazel eyes were narrow. She spoke quietly, and only in English, and she said very little. Mostly she listened to Arthur Carr's litany of irritations and slights, nodding without ever conveying agreement.

Carr remembers his father's voice—droning at first, and growing louder as the cocktails took hold. He remembers his father's rumpled shirts, damp spots under the arms, and his father's broad, sloppy gestures. He remembers his mother's rigid shoulders, a vein thrumming in her neck, her stillness otherwise. He would try to catch her eye sometimes—offer up a grimace or a conspiratorial smirk—but it was as if he wasn't there. Or she wasn't. Other times, he would perch in the window and continue their game on his own, but inevitably his father grew irritated.

"It's like living with a goddamn cat," Arthur Carr would mutter, pulling him from the sill. "Nobody likes a cat."

More lightning, another beer, and Carr thinks about his father's anger and his mother's distance, and he remembers the maps.

His mother was a great one for them. Maps and guidebooks and histories and almanacs—but especially maps. When word of a new posting would come, despite Arthur Carr's grumblings—or perhaps because of them—she would smile, haul out the maps, and study them.

"Should we just stumble around like tourists?" she would say to Carr.

"Get lost on our way to buy ice cream? No—we must know something about this place. We can't have people think you are *un hombre inculto*."

Carr remembers her at the dining table, half-glasses balanced on her nose, a cigarette burning in an ashtray, a cord of smoke twisting to the ceiling. The books were open in an arc in front of her, and the maps were unfurled. Her hair was pulled back and tied with a black ribbon.

"Here's where we will live, *mijo*," she said, pointing with a sharp red pencil. "And here is Daddy's office, and the new school." She made neat red check marks as she spoke. "Here is the museum, and the *fútbol* stadium, and the port, right here, and three train stations, and the main post office. Here is the airport, and the television studio, and the radio station, and the power plant. And see—here is the park, *mijo*, and the carousel."

And he remembers wandering the cities with her, remembers the narrow streets and the squares—cobbled, noisy, sometimes with a fountain, a dark arcade, or a looming church. His mother would hold his hand through the crowds, and buy him a lemon ice, a slice of melon, or a skewer off the grill. Then she would find a bench or little table and smoke and watch the people while Carr ate. They would sit for what seemed like hours to Carr, but he didn't mind. She would run her fingers through his hair, and sometimes, after he'd eaten, he would lean against her and doze.

Often, he recalls, she would meet someone she knew. Or they would meet her. And why not: the whole world seemed to stroll through those squares. Carr recognized some of the men and women, from embassy parties he thought, but most of them were strangers to him. They spoke mainly in Spanish to his mother, though some spoke in English and some in Portuguese. They would stop long enough to say hello, to talk about the weather, to shake hands and offer a cigarette or a book of matches. They all stared at him.

He remembers the heat of the stones, the smells of rotting fruit and grilling meat, the cool damp of the arcades, the drone of many footsteps on the cobbles, the feel of her dress as he leaned against her. Gardenias and tobacco.

And then there is a voice behind him, and a cool hand on the back of his neck.

"I thought you'd know better than to sit with your back to the door."

12

He jumps, and his beer goes flying, and Tina smiles.

"At ease, soldier," she says.

It's the first time he's seen her away from a golf course, the first time he's seen her without Mr. Boyce, and the change in context is disorienting. For an instant Carr wonders if she's come to kill him, but decides probably not. If she had, he would probably be dead by now. Probably, too, she would've worn something else.

She's dressed in black shorts—very short—a black tank top, and black flip-flops. Her black sunglasses are pushed into her white-blond hair. Her arms and legs are ghostly, and her hands, long-fingered and elegant, are raised. Her gray eyes are steady.

"The door was locked," Carr says.

"Guy like you should get better locks," Tina says, lowering her hands. "Sorry for the surprise."

"You could've called first."

"Don't like phones," she says. "Besides, I like to keep in practice."

Carr wipes his hands on his pants. "It doesn't seem like you need much. And somehow I don't think that's the only reason you're here."

She smiles thinly. "Mr. Boyce didn't want to pull you away, but he does want to know how things are going."

"And he doesn't like the phone either?" Tina nods. "So you're here to check up?"

"More like checking in."

"I don't remember a lot of checking in with Declan."

She shrugs. "Does it need explaining?"

"I'm not Declan—I get it."

Tina sits on the sofa, slips off her shoes, and folds her legs beneath her. "No need to pout," she says. "So how about we open a couple more beers, and you tell me what's what, and I do the same?"

Carr looks at her more closely, and his disorientation becomes bewilderment. Tina out of school is less guarded—relaxed, almost funny. Her voice is soft and liquid—intimate in the confines of a room. And her pale, oval face, always smooth and empty at those golf course meetings, has an appealing touch of irony at the corners of her eyes and mouth.

"You want yours in a glass?" he asks. Tina shakes her head.

Tina's had three bottles by the time Carr's made his report, and Carr has had two more. His head is cottony, and Bessemer's work as a procurer, though no less mystifying to him, is more amusing as he tells it to Tina.

"Maybe it's not all that different from private banking," Carr says, smiling. "It's all about keeping the clients happy."

Tina shakes her head. "Guy's a few cards short of a deck, for sure. It's a big gamble just to pick up some extra income. Can't blame you for wanting to find out why."

Carr shrugs. "And what about you? Anything new with our pal Prager?"

"Not much. His security guy, Silva, has fallen off the wagon again."

"Christ," Carr says, drinking the last of his beer. "It's a wonder he has a liver left."

"I'm not sure he does. And this time he's fallen off the radar too. He was on a tear in Homestead last week and we lost him."

"Probably staggered into the Everglades."

"We'll let you know if he staggers out again," Tina says. "You need any help with Bessemer, or maybe with his Russian friends?"

"If I do, what's it going to cost me?"

Her smile is chilly. "The deal doesn't change: we front your expense money, and we get paid back—plus finance charges—off the top. Services rendered are at cost plus."

Carr counts off on his fingers. "Expenses, finance charges, cost plus, finder's fee, management fee. You guys are fucking crooks."

Tina laughs, and it's surprisingly girlish. "We don't do pro bono." She drains her beer bottle and thrusts the empty at Carr. "But you want to do for yourself, fund your own expenses, save a little money, it's okay with us."

A frown darkens Carr's face. "That didn't work out so well for Declan." He takes Tina's empties and his own to the kitchen, and returns with two fresh beers. Tina is standing at the window, watching the distant storm.

"Speaking of which," she says. Carr takes a deep breath, trying to chase the wool from his head. He stands next to Tina. Their reflections are like ghosts in the glass. "We had a talk with somebody down there," she continues. "Somebody who used to work for Bertolli."

"*Somebody* who?"

Tina shakes her head. "Somebody who worked security for him, up until a few months ago—security in Mendoza."

Carr leans forward. "Did he say anything about how they knew Deke was coming? Who they got the word from?"

"He didn't know anything about that. He was strictly an order taker; he didn't ask questions, didn't even think about having questions."

"So what use is he?"

"Everything we heard about that night—everything we heard from you—says that your guys got tagged almost as soon as they pulled up to that little airstrip."

"That's the way it was told to me, every time—that they'd barely gotten out of the vans."

"And they never got inside the barn? Never laid eyes on the cash?"

"That's the way I heard it. I assume that you've heard something different."

She nods again. "This guy says that your people didn't get hit coming out of the vans; they got hit coming out of the *barn*. He says when it was all over that night, Bertolli was short almost two million euro."

In the glass, Carr sees Tina watching him. "And this guy is who?"

"I told you, he worked security for Bertolli."

"So he's what—some brain-dead kid with a gun? And your friends down there just tripped over him? Or did he volunteer his services?"

"He's no genius, but he's no walk-in either. Our friends worked hard

to turn him up, and they spent some money too. He was hiding out in B.A. Seems he'd had a falling-out with his crew chief up in Mendoza. Something about the chief's sister."

"And your friends believed him?"

"I did too."

"You spoke to him?"

Tina nods. "Went down there last week."

A jagged white line lights the horizon, and the afterimage flares behind Carr's eyes. He takes a long pull on his beer. "Two million euro," he says. "Maybe it burned with Declan's van."

"I asked about that. This guy said Bertolli had them sifting through the wreckage, looking for some trace. They didn't find one."

"There wasn't much left of that van," Carr says.

"If you say so."

Carr turns to look at her. "What's that supposed to mean?"

Tina keeps her gaze on the horizon. "You're the one had eyes-on. You were at the salvage yard; you were at the morgue. I wasn't."

"Eyes-on," he mutters, and the traces of lightning vanish from beneath his lids, replaced by twisted metal, blistered paint, melted upholstery, charred, fire-stiffened limbs, blackened flesh, and naked, shattered bone. And the smell, even days after, even in the air-conditioned bays of the city morgue . . . It comes over him in a wave, and the beer in his gut threatens to erupt.

"You okay?" Tina asks.

"That van was like a fucking shell crater. I'm not surprised they didn't find anything. They blew the hell—"

"Yeah, that's another thing," Tina says, cutting him off. "According to this guy they didn't run Declan off the road. According to him, they were hauling ass on Highway Seven, but Declan got way out in front. They lost sight of his van for like twenty minutes. They were thinking about turning around when they saw a flash up ahead of them, and a column of smoke. The van was wrecked and burning on the roadside when they got there, but they didn't see it happen."

"I saw the bullet holes—in the rear bumper, in the side panels. As twisted up and black as everything was, you could still see those."

"He didn't say they weren't firing at it—in fact, he said they chewed its tail up pretty good—he just said they didn't force it off the road."

Carr shakes his head, steps away from the window. "Am I supposed to make something of that? He said they shot up the van. Maybe it blew a tire. Maybe the gas tank was leaking and there was a spark. So Bertolli's men weren't around to see it go up—so what?"

Tina perches on an arm of the sofa and draws a knee up under her chin. She examines her toenails, which are perfectly manicured and glazed white. When she looks back at Carr, her gray eyes are as steady as ever. Her voice is vaguely amused. "A girl can't win with you. You bitch when we don't turn up anything, and you bitch when we do. You make what you want out of it, I'm just telling you what I've found.

"We're looking at this only because you said you wouldn't go on with the Prager gig otherwise—and it's the only reason Boyce agreed to split the costs with you. You don't like how we're going about things, you don't want to hear what we learn—that's cool. He's got other ways to spend his money, and I've got other ways to spend my time."

Carr looks at her for a long minute, and then smiles. "And here we were getting along so well."

She shrugs. "Honeymoons never last."

Carr sits at the other end of the sofa and puts his beer on the floor. "Two million euro. If it didn't burn in the van, and Bertolli's boys didn't pocket it themselves—"

"I seriously doubt that. Bertolli's got them terrified."

"Then where did it go?"

"I figured you'd have a theory."

"Your guy didn't see anyone else out there? No cars, no trucks?"

"I asked a few different ways; he said no. But it's remote as hell up there, with lots of twists and turns, and fucking dark. Somebody running without lights . . . who knows?"

Carr reaches for his beer, and looks through the brown glass at the dregs that remain. "Two million euro—it's not pocket change."

"Nope," Tina says. "Maybe you want to ask your boys if they've seen it lying around."

Carr drains the bottle. The beer is warm and mostly froth, and he nearly gags getting it down. He shakes his head at Tina. "I don't want to," Carr says, "but I will."

13

Bobby calls in the morning, to say that Bessemer has broken his routine.

"He's playing tennis with Stearn today—just the two of them, no Brunt. And they're having lunch afterward. That's new and different for a Thursday."

Carr's head is like bad fruit, but he drags himself to a sitting position and tells Bobby he'll meet him in an hour. He raises the shades and squints into the milky sky. Then he stumbles to the shower, where the blast of water hurts, and then helps.

Carr finds street parking and meets Bobby in the alley behind the Barton Golf and Racquet Club. Bobby has traded the painter's van for a gray sedan. He has the AC on and the cold air is like a second shower. Bobby is drinking a blue slushie from a plastic cup the size of a sap bucket.

"Howie's jumpy today. He got that way when Brunt called, and told him it was just going to be Howie and Stearn on the tennis court. Got more that way when Stearn called to invite him for lunch after."

"Stearn makes him nervous?"

"Haven't seen them alone together much, but I think so. He lets him win at tennis. Double-faults if he's about to beat the guy."

"He does the same with Brunt, and he lets those other guys beat him at golf. That's Howie's thing. We know what Stearn does for a living?"

"Rich and retired, like most of Howie's friends. Denny tells me he was

over in London for twenty-plus years, with an American bank—a portfolio manager or something. Got fired in a merger, and came here after that. On a couple of boards around town—the hospital, the art museum. On the board of a prep school, up north."

"He married?"

"Wife spends the summer in Maine. Kids are grown."

"Nothing obvious that would make Howie nervous."

"Come on, the guy looks like some kind of zombie scarecrow. He makes me a little tense."

Stearn wins the second set when Bessemer double-faults, and the men sling their racquet bags and walk to the clubhouse. Bobby pulls the car around and they follow Bessemer's BMW as it follows Stearn's Mercedes from the Barton.

Lunch isn't far. They travel south from the Barton, then east, then south again, on South Ocean Boulevard. Carr and Bobby are a hundred yards back when the Mercedes and then the BMW pull through the black iron gates of Willis Stearn's estate. Driving past the entrance, Carr catches a glimpse of lawns like carpet and, in the distance, a mustard-colored villa. He swears softly.

"We've got a mic in Howie's racquet bag," Bobby says, as they round the corner, "but I'm betting he leaves it in the car."

"Which means we're deaf and blind."

The properties here are large, and private, and the security patrols are not lazy. The closest parking spot Bobby finds is nearly half a mile away, a dirt patch at a construction site. It's beyond the range of the mic in Bessemer's bag, and just at the limit of the one in his car, but in any event there's nothing to hear besides distant traffic and the occasional growl of thunder. Bobby switches off the engine.

"The GPS will tell us when he moves," Bobby says. He reaches for a laptop on the backseat and balances it on the console between them. Then he settles himself lower behind the wheel and runs his straw around the bottom of his empty cup.

Carr takes a deep breath. "Dennis come up with anything else on Bessemer's friends?"

"He's looking. Mike's on it too, or will be when he gets back from Boca."

Carr turns in his seat. "What the hell's he doing down there?"

"Val needed a replacement for one of the cameras she's gonna use in Chun's house. Mike brought it down."

"Why the hell didn't she call me?"

Bobby puts up a hand and arranges his meaty face into as close as it comes to a conciliatory look. "She calls me direct sometimes. She's done it before. It's not a problem."

"It's a problem for me, Bobby. I want to know who's doing what, and where. And if she called you, how come you didn't go down there?"

Bobby clears his throat and suppresses a smile. "'Cause I'm here with you, looking at Howie."

Carr sighs and peels his shirt from the upholstery. "Run the AC."

Bobby does, and the two of them sit without speaking, watching some stonemasons build a long wall. They are shaping and fitting the rocks, and their hammers sound like gunshots to Carr. The air conditioner dries the sweat on his skin but does nothing for the throbbing in his temples. Tina's words reverberate there: *Bertolli was short almost two million euro.* Two million euro—Declan thought there'd be more.

They were in Port of Spain, in the bar at the Hyatt Regency. Wind was shaking the windows, and the city lights were lost behind low clouds. The place was empty, and they were all a little drunk. Declan was like a red-faced witch over a cauldron.

"The bastard doesn't trust banks or bankers," he said. "Oh, he uses them—he's got to with the feckin' money he makes on all that crap he smuggles in—but he likes to keep some cash on hand. Nothing big, mind you, we're talking three to five mil in euros—he prefers them to dollars. Keeps enough around for incidentals and traveling funds, in case he has to move in a hurry, which he's done a few times—out of São Paulo, out of Ciudad del Este, out of Argentina and back again. He's quite the jackrab-bit, Señor Bertolli is.

"I had this job lined up years ago—had it all worked out—but the fat fuck skipped on me. Hightailed it out of Argentina when a new govern-ment came in, with his wife, mistresses, and various bastards in tow. Got away about a minute before the PFA knocked down his door. Took all his cash with him too. But that party's gone now, and so Bertolli and his money have come home."

Carr was slow on the uptake. He'd been working on the Prager job all day—peering at floor plans and wiring diagrams. His eyes were gritty and his head full of numbers, and he didn't get the point right away. Declan was annoyed.

"Wake up, Carr—it's the feckin' expenses. The up-front costs on the Prager job are running twice what we expected, and they'll run higher still. I don't know about you, but I don't want to be paying such a big chunk of my take in finance fees to the grand Mr. Boyce. It's usury what he's chargin'! This deal is lovely—a quick in and out, three bucks easy, and then we don't need his feckin' financing."

That was all he'd had to say to convince Mike and Bobby and Ray-Ray, who were already antsy from too much planning, and who were never happy paying anyone for anything. Some part of Carr had known right there that it was a losing battle, but still he spent the next week in increasingly heated, increasingly pointless argument with Declan. He and Valerie both—though that night, in the Hyatt bar, she'd just stared into her drink and said nothing at all.

Carr's head drops, and he realizes he's been dozing. Bobby is watching him. "Up late?" he asks.

Carr wipes his chin. "Anything from Bessemer?"

"His car hasn't moved, and there's nothing on the mic but seagulls."

Bobby has a cooler in the back, and Carr pulls a bottle of water from it. He takes a long pull and looks at Bobby. He doesn't want to ask about it— doesn't have the energy today—and besides, he knows what the answer will be. But still . . . *Bertolli was short almost two million euro.* He clears his throat.

"At Bertolli's place that night," Carr begins, and at the mention of the name Bobby's face colors with surprise and anger.

"You're *fucking* kidding me with this!" he says, and then the laptop pings twice, loudly.

Bobby sits up fast. "Bessemer's moving," he says, and he throws the car into gear and guns it through the dirt lot. There's a curtain of dust around them; the laptop slides from the console and Carr catches it mid-flight. Bobby pushes through the side streets and they hit South Ocean Boulevard in time to see Bessemer's convertible pull out of Stearn's place. His top is still down and his thin hair is flying as they pass him going north.

"Fast lunch," Bobby says, and he slides the car through an easy U-turn and into the northbound lane.

"I'm not surprised," Carr says. "Did you see Bessemer's face? He looked like he was about to throw up."

Two miles up South Ocean Boulevard they watch him do just that, in a garbage can by the side of the road.

14

"A lot of phone time for Howie tonight," Dennis says, "and he didn't sound good."

They're at the workhouse—Carr, Bobby, Dennis, and Latin Mike—and the pent-up heat of the day is suffocating. Mike is tilted back in a kitchen chair, clean-shaven, hair slick from a shower. The half-smile on his face sets Carr's teeth on edge.

"He called the Caymans a few times," Dennis continues, "his pal Prager's number, but he never got past the help. Then he called his pimp. Took him four tries to go through with it. First three times, he hung up before anyone answered."

"Prager didn't take his call?" Carr asks.

Dennis shrugs. "The secretary said he wasn't in, but she had to go away and check before she said it. The second time, she told him Prager would get back to him."

"Has he?"

"Not yet."

Mike grins nastily. "I thought Prager was his friend," he says. "That's not so friendly, *jefe*."

"And the pimp?" Carr asks. "What was going on with the three hang-ups?"

"He didn't want to pull the trigger," Bobby says.

Carr squints at him. "Pull the trigger on what?"

Dennis shakes his head. "He didn't say on the phone."

"Who's the pimp?" Carr asks.

"Calls himself Lamp. Works for the Russian brothers."

Mike dangles a cigarette from his lip, but doesn't light it. "Howie's gotten whores for his friends before. How come he's nervous now?"

Bobby shakes his head. "The guy is freaked about something. The way he blew his lunch this afternoon—I thought his socks were gonna come up."

Carr looks at Dennis. "You find out more about Bessemer's friends?"

Dennis taps at one of his keyboards. "Plenty," he says, "though I'm not sure it amounts to anything. Brunt and Moyer are retired money guys, like Stearn. Moyer was a bond trader; Brunt was an investment manager."

"They all work at the same place?"

"Different companies, different places. Stearn was in London, Moyer in New York, and Brunt was in Chicago."

"And the other two guys?"

"Tandy is also retired. He was a partner in a law firm up in New York. He got downsized a few years back—him and half the firm. As far as I can tell, Scoville has never worked. Lives in the guesthouse on his mother's property, a few miles down the road from Stearn. Besides sailing and heroin, lying around the pool seems to be the only job he's ever had."

"Married?"

"Not Scoville, but the rest of them are."

"Any of them have records?"

"Scoville took a couple of possession busts in New York, one with intent to sell. He got probation and rehab."

"Any of them friends with Bessemer before he came down here?"

"Not that I can tell."

"So Howie is what to them—the only guy they know who knows the rough trade?"

Mike lights his cigarette and chuckles derisively. "We trying to get inside their heads now too? Who gives a fuck?"

Carr ignores him. "And we think Howie's doing this . . . why?"

Bobby sighs. "Same reason people do most things," he says, "for the money." He looks at Dennis.

"The guy's chronically short," Dennis says. "The divorce cleaned him out pretty good. His house is paid for, but his grandmother's trust throws

off barely enough income to cover the taxes and his liquor bills, and she set it up so he can't get at the principal."

"My *abuela* was a bitch too," Mike mutters.

"I thought Prager was hiding money for him," Carr says. "What happened to that?"

Dennis shrugs. "It's not in any of the accounts I can see, though I can't see into Isla Privada."

Carr shakes his head. "When's Howie meeting the pimp?" he asks.

"Monday," Bobby says, "outside the Brazilian place. I'll be there."

Carr looks at Latin Mike. "We'll all be there."

"Sure, *jefe*," Mike says, smiling. "All of us."

The night is close and the airport throws sheets of flashing light against the low clouds. The smell of the jet fuel, of the house, of Mike's cigarettes, and of his own sweat are caught in Carr's clothing, and he walks the long way around the block to get to his car. He's halfway there when he hears footsteps behind him and whirls.

Latin Mike chuckles from behind the glowing end of a cigarette. "That's slow, man. I want to hurt you, you be all the way hurt by now."

He steps from the shadows and Carr takes a slow, deep breath to quiet his pulse. "You going out again?" Carr says.

"Just for some air. Not enough in that dump tonight. And you?"

"To bed. You want something?"

"Me? No, I got what I need—but you're still looking for something."

Carr sighs. "We've been over this. I want to know more before we go at Bessemer. I want to know why—"

A barking laugh, and Mike blows smoke into the blinking sky. "I'm not talking about Bessemer. Bobby says you're still asking him about Mendoza. Says you did it again today."

Carr takes another deep breath. "And?"

"And I want to know what that's about."

"It's *about* what it seems to be about: I want to know what happened, what went wrong. Bobby didn't tell you?"

"Bobby tells me everything, *jefe*. But why you keep asking him about this? You think he's gonna tell you something new? You think he doesn't get what you're doing when you ask the same questions over and over? That you're calling him a liar."

"I didn't know it was upsetting him so much."

"Sure you did. So why don't you cut it out? You still got questions about what happened down there, ask me."

"Why, are you going to tell me something new?"

Mike barks again. "I'm gonna tell you to fuck off."

"So nothing new."

Another laugh. "You want new, maybe you need to get different questions."

"Maybe I have one."

Mike smiles and rolls out a line of smoke rings that break on Carr's shoulder. "Give it a try, *cabrón*."

"Okay. Did you get into that barn before Bertolli's guys turned up?"

In the long silence that follows, a car passes, a jet passes, someone shouts from somewhere in Brazilian Portuguese. Mike flicks his cigarette into the street. He shakes his head and laughs to himself. "Deke was always so hot on you—always talked about how smart you were, how good at planning, how you saw angles other people didn't, how you thought big. It was like you were his kid or something.

"Me, I never got it—and I told him so. More smoke than fire, I said. Too much complication. Too much bullshit. After a while, he didn't want to hear it: told me to shut up or move on. I thought about that a long time, and decided to stay. I liked Deke; I was used to him, and I liked the paydays, so . . . I didn't change my mind about you, but I kept my mouth shut. But when the old bastard bought it, I tell you I was ready to book. I would have too if this gig had been any smaller, and if Bobby and Val hadn't asked me—shit, they *begged* me—to stick it out."

Carr kicks at a piece of broken pavement. It skips and skids and ends up in a storm drain. He laughs softly. "I don't hear anything new, Mike, and I don't hear an answer to my question."

Mike's fists clench and his arms swell. "Here's my answer, *pendejo*—if you're running this thing, then *run it*, and if you're not, then shove off. 'Cause this is the last *fucking* job I'm doing, and if it turns to shit, it's *you* I come looking for. No one else—just you. So get your mind off Mendoza and Declan and Bertolli's *fucking* barn, *cabrón*, and get it on Bessemer and Prager."

Mike turns and walks back into the dark, and Carr sees his lighter flare as he fires up another smoke. "Was that a *yes* or a *no* about the barn?" Carr calls, but Mike doesn't answer.

15

They lean together like schoolgirls, flushed and whispering as they stroll the pink arcades around Mizner Park. They're not quite holding hands, but it takes a second look to be certain. Valerie—Jill—is in a summer dress: spaghetti straps and long, tanned limbs. On her day off, Amy Chun, president of the Spanish River Bank and Trust Company, wears a tan wrap skirt, a white T-shirt short enough to expose a narrow band of mid-section, and low sandals. She's in her mid-forties, slender, shorter than Jill by two inches, and more darkly tanned. Her straight black hair is done in a loose braid, and her sunglasses are sleek and smoky.

They pause at the window of a jewelry store. Jill points, Amy takes off her glasses, nods, and they both laugh. Jill walks on and Amy watches her.

Carr's chest aches and he realizes he's been holding his breath. He sighs and runs down the car window. A damp breeze wanders in. Not even two weeks since Jill joined Amy Chun's yoga class, he thinks, and already she's set the hook deep.

Valerie's voice was tired and raspy on the phone the night before, and she was reluctant at first to talk about Chun—like a magician asked to explain her very best trick—but Carr had insisted.

"She's better than I'd hoped," Valerie said. "Basically, she's got no life. She goes from work to her workout to her house, and then it's more work, into the night."

"No friends or family?"

"I haven't seen any friends, and the only family she's got are her parents, in Vancouver. No, it's all work for Amy. But the little time she's not grinding away, she spends online—and not just shopping, either."

"What's she doing—looking at pornography?"

"A little, but that's not what I'm talking about. Amy is a stalker—a cyber-stalker, anyway. I went through the take from Dennis's spyware—her e-mail, her browser history—and it's plain as day. She's keeping tabs on someone named Janice Lessig."

"Who the hell is she?"

"She runs a little company out in the Bay Area—makes organic bread and shit like that. She lives in Berkeley, plays the cello in a couple of amateur groups, has two daughters, and a domestic partner named Elaine."

"I repeat—who the hell is she?"

"She and Amy went to B-school together, twenty years ago, and they were pretty tight. I think maybe she's Amy's *road not taken*."

"They were lovers?"

"I can't say for sure, but they wrote some articles for their B-school review together, and their last year there, they were its coeditors."

"That doesn't mean—"

"Dennis dug up a copy of the school's student directory for their last year. The two of them lived at the same address off-campus. The same apartment number."

"And you think Chun still has a thing for her?"

"She visits Lessig's Facebook page every night, and the Radclyffe Hall Bread Company's website too—the pages with Lessig's pictures on them. Ditto the websites of the Piedmont Amateur Strings and the Shattuck Quartet. And it's not like these pages change very much. She even cruises the website of the private school Lessig's kids go to. It's got a picture of Lessig on it, from when she came in for career day. On top of which, Amy Googles Lessig a couple of times a week. I don't know how else to read all that."

"Is Chun in touch with her?"

"Not that I can tell. No e-mail to or from Lessig—and Amy saves her e-mail since like the beginning of time. She never posts anything on Lessig's Facebook page. Dennis found her Christmas card list on the laptop, and Lessig wasn't on it."

"Okay, Chun is still carrying a torch for Lessig. What do you do with that?"

"Use it to fine-tune Jill. So now she has red highlights in her hair, and her clothes are a little more crunchy-granola. Now she cooks, and wants to start a catering business. And she sings, and someday she wants to have kids."

"You cook and sing?"

"I do a lot of things."

Sitting in his darkened living room, looking at a distant light on the black ocean, Carr had swallowed hard. "What about Jill's backstory?" he asked eventually.

"The same," Valerie said. "She's still been through the wringer; she's still looking to change her life."

Carr shifts in the front seat and watches them. Her walk is new, he thinks—a bit less assertive, a bit more coltish—and her accessories are different too: dangly earrings, a looped necklace of colored glass beads, a row of thin gold bracelets. And there are tattoos now: a complicated henna braid around her right biceps and a narrower one around her left ankle. Carr slouches lower as they pass.

There are other people in the park: other couples, off-season tourist families, people walking dogs, but it is Jill and Amy who draw the eye. It's more than beauty, Carr thinks. Something about their attraction to each other, the simmering anticipation, the wisps of steam before a full boil. It's in the air between them, like a magnetic field—invisible, but palpable nonetheless.

Carr hears faint, intermittent music—a bossa nova spilling from one of the stores when its automatic doors slide open. It's a familiar tune but the door slides shut before he can place it. He watches the women and struggles to recall the tune, and he's taken suddenly by an aching loneliness—like the last student left at school at the start of a long holiday. The door opens, closes, opens again. The music seeps out, and Carr has it: Jobim playing "Lamento," and he hears another version of that song.

An infinitely worse version, the one he remembers—the scraping of a quintet that didn't know half the notes, and didn't care much for the rest. They were playing in a beachfront bar, and he and Declan were there with several bottles between them. They were two days gone from Bogotá, and the crew was $5.7 million richer for it—the take from the first job that

Carr had planned end to end. Carr felt like he'd just graduated from something, and Declan—creased and unshaven—was beaming. The sky was six shades of violet and the first stars were lit, and all was right with the world.

Declan lifted a glass. "Brilliant, lad—feckin' brilliant. They never saw us—never even dreamed of us." He'd said it before, but Carr didn't mind the repetition. He lifted his glass in return.

Declan laughed. "Those spreadsheets at Langley didn't know what they had, did they? Couldn't recognize a natural right there in their midst."

Carr never liked this subject, and he shrugged and looked away. "A natural what?"

"A natural spy, lad—a fella bred for the secret life."

"They would've disagreed with you."

Declan shook his head disgustedly. "What the hell did they know? I've run across my share of company men, and they're about as subtle as a dog humpin' yer leg. They think it's all about sales, fer chrissakes—that if you can charm Granny into buying an estate car, you can nick war plans from the North Koreans. Was that it, lad—you weren't enough of a salesman for 'em?"

Carr shrugged again. "They don't explain much."

"They must've said something."

"They didn't think I had the temperament for it. They said I had a problem with authority."

Declan smiled broadly. "And who doesn't that's worth a goddamn?" he said, and raised his glass in a toast. "And that was all? That was enough to shitcan you?"

Carr took a long pull on his drink. "They didn't think I'd be good with agents."

Declan squinted—indignant on his behalf—and refilled his glass. "What the hell does that mean?"

"They didn't think I'd be good at running them. They thought I had a tendency to see what I wanted to see and hear what I wanted to hear, and that when time came to squeeze them hard, or burn them, I wouldn't have the stomach for it. *Overly invested* they called it."

"Sounds like feckin' psychobabble to me."

"They were big on that," Carr said.

"Well, fuck 'em, I say! Big outfits like that, they don't appreciate the solitary man. Don't understand him. A fellow like yerself makes 'em nervous. You don't fit their molds—so they don't know what moves you, what levers to pull."

Carr filled his own glass, and Declan's too. "But you've got that figured out, have you?"

Declan drank and nodded. "To lead men, you must know what they love."

Carr laughed. "And that would be what?"

"For you, solitary Carr, I'd say it's being a ghost. You love drifting through the drab workaday mess—all the tinkers and tailors and doctors and bankers; you love watching their monkeyshines without actually being a part of 'em. You're in it, but you're not—not really. You're like a feckin' specter."

Carr hid his surprise behind another drink, and slid the bottle to his side of the table. "Now who's into the fucking psychobabble? You're hammered."

"It doesn't mean I'm wrong. You love flying above it all, looking down like yer on an airplane, or yer floating over a reef, watching the wee fishes. That was the appeal of Integral Risk, wasn't it—your clients, their lives, the things they got up to—it was like an aquarium, and you on the other side of the glass."

Carr looked at him for a while and nodded slowly. "Tell me you don't like that aspect of it—being apart from things."

"How else could I recognize it in you? 'Course I like it—I'm a solitary too, at heart, so I know the appeal. You feel invulnerable, somehow— you've no connections, no dependents, no hostages to be taken. Nobody can lay a finger on you, 'cause yer just not there. It's better than bullet-proof. But some advice from an aged bastard: you want to watch you don't get overly fond of it. You step out of the flesh and blood world long enough, it's hard to step back in."

Carr held the bottle up, saw the moon turn amber in it. "That assumes you ever lived there in the first place."

Declan laughed. "Ah, Carr, save yer tragic tale for the ladies, and pass me that feckin' bottle."

Sweat rolls down Carr's ribs, and his head is bobbing in the heat. He shakes off sleep and memory, and gets out of his car. Jill and Amy are a

block and a half away now, and he follows them down the arcade. They're window-shopping—clothing, handbags, shoes, more jewelry—pointing, laughing. They pause outside a furniture store, and again at a real estate office.

Carr trails them to an outdoor café. They take a table near a tiled fountain and order iced teas. The air is thick and the palms and bougainvillea hang in limp surrender, but Jill and Amy don't seem to mind. Even in the shade, their arms and legs are shining. Jill reaches for the sugar, nearly tips her glass, just catches it, and laughs nervously. Carr shakes his head at the performance.

It's the seamlessness that impresses him most, the integration of elements small and large into her fabricated persona. The endearing clumsiness, the slightly funky clothing and accoutrements, the accent and the diction, the attitude, the wear and tear: all Jill, all of a piece. He wonders how she's done up her apartment, what's in the glove box of her car, and what's on her iPod. Not a false note, he's sure.

The heat is a weight on his shoulders, and he finds a bench beneath a palm. He thinks back to Costa Alegre, to Valerie's easy shifts between the three engineers. He recalls the other men and women he's watched her seduce over the years, and the characters she's inhabited to do it— doctors, lawyers, Indian chiefs . . . He watches her sip tea, and something about the dappled light on her legs reminds him of Port of Spain, the perpetual overcast of the two months they spent there, laying the groundwork for the Prager job.

Declan installed them in one of the new glass towers on the waterfront, in seven apartments—Declan, Bobby, Ray-Ray, Dennis, and Mike on the seventh floor, Valerie and Carr on the ninth. After which Declan, Bobby, Ray-Ray, Dennis, and Mike developed a sudden fondness for cricket, and decamped most afternoons to Queen's Park, leaving Carr and Valerie squinting into their laptops. *Fucking Cinderella* was Valerie's grumbled gloss on the circumstances.

At first they worked separately—digesting Boyce's dossiers, ferreting out additional information, collecting technical data—and met in the evenings to compare notes and drink beer. Later they worked in Valerie's apartment, assembling and disassembling the framework of a plan, again and again, until they had something that might float.

He stared out her living room window a lot, at the highway and the

rush of cars, at the shipping containers stacked along the wharves, like the ruins of an ancient city, at the ocean like beaten lead. A pearly light filled her place, along with a perfume—something with lime and orange blossom and vanilla.

Valerie went to buy lunch one afternoon, leaving him there alone. Carr walked through every room and thought about looking inside her medicine chest and her closets, but didn't. He stared for a long time at the pile of books by her bedside. They were paperbacks, slim volumes by Borges, Fante, Akhmatova, Didion. He leafed through them, and when he heard her key in the lock he piled the books up again. He was standing at the living room window when the door opened.

Was it then that things began to simmer, or had it started long before? Either way, she leaned in closer after that, touched him on the hand or the arm often, didn't look away. Her apartment felt smaller, and Carr felt a surge of anger and disappointment whenever the cricket fans returned.

The phone shudders in his pocket and it brings him back to his bench. He looks down the arcade and sees Amy Chun, alone at her table. He reaches for his phone, and Valerie is on the other end, whispering angrily.

"I don't know what you think you're doing here," she says, "but you've seen enough for one day. Now clear the fuck out before you queer my play."

16

Monday noon is too early for Lamp. He grimaces at the sky, adjusts his sunglasses on his peeling nose, and fiddles with the visor on his open-top Jeep. Then he hoists up his iced coffee and takes another needy pull. He does it all very slowly, as if he's half asleep, and the other half is in some pain.

Carr watches from a wine bar across the street and decides that Lamp looks like his job. Not the pimp job, but the other one, which, according to Dennis, is owner and manager of Lampanelli's Surf n' Sport, in Riviera Beach. He's fortyish and tall, with sandy hair, a tan, and a gut edging toward sloppy. He's wearing a pink T-shirt and khaki shorts, and has a tattoo of a parrot on his left calf and a look of annoyance on his unshaved face.

Lamp glances around the parking lot. The Grigoriev brothers' Brazilian restaurant is closed today, and the lot is empty but for his Jeep. He checks his watch. Carr hopes that Lamp finds some patience, or is tired enough to stay put for a while. Bobby and Latin Mike have called to tell him that Howard Bessemer is en route, but moving slowly due to traffic and what seems to be a lethal hangover.

"Looks like he's been living on bad fish and toilet water," Bobby said, laughing. "We're about half a block back of him, and twenty-five seems to be his top speed today."

"Hungover or reluctant?" Carr asked.

"Both," Bobby said.

Definitely reluctant, Carr thinks, and for several days now also reclusive. Bessemer didn't leave his house for his usual weekend poker and whore festival, or for anything else. Lunch and dinner were delivered three days running, along with parcels from the local liquor store. And televisions were on around the clock in the kitchen, the living room, and the bedroom, though Bessemer watched none of them, but wandered from room to room drinking gin and smoking joints. When he did pause, it was to collapse wherever he was standing, and to sleep for a few hours. Then up again and back to work. The only other breaks in the action—besides his occasional puking—were when Bessemer tried calling Prager. None of his attempts was successful.

The waitress brings Carr another soda water. He watches Lamp drain his iced coffee cup. On the street beyond the far side of the parking lot, Carr sees the van where he parked it, long before Lamp pulled in. Dennis is in back, with a couple of laptops and wireless broadband cards. He looks for Bobby and Mike, but doesn't really expect to spot them. They're good enough that he won't see them climb into the van. There's movement in the foreground and Bessemer's BMW rolls into the lot.

Despite the clear skies, Howie's got the top up, and from Carr's vantage he's no more than a ghost at the wheel. He leaves a parking space between his car and the Jeep and kills the engine. And then he sits. And sits. Unmoving, with his white hands on the wheel, as if at any moment he might drive off again. Lamp is as puzzled as Carr, and after a while he holds his wristwatch out toward Howie's car and taps the face with his finger. Howie gets the point.

He opens the door slowly and cringes like a vampire in the midday sun. Lamp looks Howie up and down and shakes his head. Howie leans against the Jeep and starts talking, and Carr curses another conversation he isn't going to hear.

Whatever Howie's saying, he's saying it fast, and Lamp holds up a hand and looks irritated. Howie pauses, rubs a hand over his face, and starts again, more slowly this time. Lamp listens and begins to shake his head, and the look of irritation is replaced by one of vague disgust. Carr's phone vibrates.

"Me and Mike are in the van," Bobby says. "You see this?"

"I see it," Carr answers, "but I have no idea what he's saying."

"Whatever it is, Lamp's not crazy for it. You'd figure a guy like him has heard it all before."

Lamp is still shaking his head, and Bessemer is still talking, leaning more heavily now against the Jeep. Finally Lamp holds up a hand and points at Howie's car. Howie begins to speak again, but Lamp points once more and pulls a cell phone from the pocket of his shorts. He waits until Howie is back in his car, and then he makes his call.

"Who do you think he's calling?" Bobby asks.

"Wish I knew," Carr says.

Lamp talks for a while, glancing now and then at Bessemer. Then he nods his head and punches off. He rubs a hand across the back of his neck, rolls his shoulders, and punches in another number.

This conversation is longer, and Lamp walks around while he has it. He circles his Jeep slowly, inspecting bumpers and kicking tires. Finally Lamp pockets his phone and walks over to Bessemer's car. He raps on the window and Bessemer runs it down. Lamp leans over, props his forearms on the sill, and starts talking.

"Put this on speaker," Carr says into his phone.

And Bobby does. Lamp's voice comes on, hollow, choppy, but the New Orleans accent clear.

"You on for Friday night," Lamp says, "but don't let's make this a regular thing. This kinda product's not for me—too many problems. Too much fucking risk. Your pal want something like this again, you gotta go elsewhere, you get me, bro?"

Howie nods.

"And the folks that bring her, you pay them up front—in cash—or she don't get out of the car."

Howie nods again.

"And best not to fuck with these folks, Howie, you know? Or even talk to them too much."

Lamp doesn't wait for another nod, but climbs into his Jeep and drives away. A cloud of dust hangs over the asphalt, and Bessemer rests his forehead on his steering wheel. He sits this way for five minutes, and then he too leaves.

17

Bobby and Mike follow Bessemer from the Brazilian restaurant, and when it's clear he's headed home, they call Carr, who drives with Dennis to the workhouse. They open one of Dennis's laptops and bring up the mics and cameras in Bessemer's cottage. They watch Bessemer fumble ice into a glass, hold a bottle above the tumbler, and pour for a long time. Then they watch him wander to his office and drop heavily into a chair.

They both start when Bessemer's landline rings. Howie doesn't move, but lets the machine answer. It's Willis Stearn, nervous but excited.

"Just calling to see if you'd worked things out—if we're on for Friday, and if she's . . . if everything is per our discussion. Call me back."

Howie mutters to himself after Stearn hangs up, and finally he speaks out loud. "*Fuck!*"

Then he hauls himself from his chair, digs in a desk drawer, and comes out with a cell phone. He finds a number in its memory, presses a key, and sets the phone on the desk. A woman answers, her voice thin through the phone speaker, and Bessemer asks for Curtis Prager. And gets him.

It is the first time Carr has heard Prager's voice, and it's deeper than he expects, and calmer. It's an oddly denatured voice too, lacking any regional accent or twang—an anchorman's voice, but without the practiced affability. His pleasantries are mechanical and distracted, lacking any actual warmth—a sociable shell over an icy core.

"What can I do you for, Bess? I understand you've been burning up the phone lines."

Bessemer hems and haws for a while, and Carr hears him swallow hard. Finally, he comes out with it. "It's my money, Curt—I need my money back."

There is a long pause from Prager. "Where are you calling from?" he asks.

"Don't worry, I follow the rules—I'm on a prepaid cell, just like you said. It's been a very long time, Curt—years, for chrissakes—and I really need my money."

Prager chuckles patronizingly. "I heard you the first time. We've talked about this before, Bess. Often. You know it's not a simple matter."

Bessemer's voice is nervous but determined. "I know you always make it sound complicated, but I'm still not clear why that should be."

Again, the chuckle. "We've been over it again and again."

"A simple wire transfer—I'm not sure why it's more involved than that."

Another sigh, longer, more impatient. "How many ways can I say it?" Prager asks. "Transferring the money is the easy part. Provenance is the problem."

"But that's . . . isn't that *my* problem?"

"The hell it is," Prager says brusquely. "Who do you think will be the second person the feds want to talk to, as soon as they've eaten you for lunch?"

"We could break it into several transfers, in smaller amounts. I know you know how to—"

Prager's voice turns colder. "That's called *structuring*, Bess, or maybe you've forgotten. And the feds are always thrilled to find it. It tells them they're on the right track. I know they'd especially love to see it in your bank account."

"They're not still watching me," Bessemer says, with more hope than conviction.

"Really? Is that what all *your* security people tell you? Because *my* security people tell me something different. They say that the feds are still fascinated by what flows through your accounts, and that Tracy and her fucking lawyers do their best to keep them interested."

Dennis looks at Carr, puzzled. Carr shakes his head. When Bessemer speaks again, his voice is a white flag. "I need money, Curt," he says softly.

"I know," Prager says. "And believe me, I'm working on getting it to you. In the meantime, if you need something to tide you over, I'm sure we can work it out. We can do what we've done before: package it as a consulting fee, for client referrals. As long as we give it documentation, and keep it to small amounts, it should be fine."

Prager's reassurances are met with silence. A skeptical silence, Carr thinks, and maybe Prager thinks so too, because his next words are lower and somehow more threatening. "What's the matter, Bess—after everything we've been through, you suddenly decide you don't trust me? All these years, and I still haven't proven I can keep my word?"

Bessemer coughs and sputters, but his declarations of trust come too late: Prager has already hung up.

"What was all that about the feds?" Dennis asks. "We're the only ones following Howie around. And who the hell is Tracy?"

"She's Bessemer's ex," Carr says. "I don't know what the rest of that shit was about." Carr is still rubbing his chin when Bessemer makes a second call—this one to Willis Stearn.

"Friday night, at nine," Howie says when Stearn picks up. His voice is clipped, almost angry.

"At your house?"

"That's what you asked for."

"And she's—"

"It's what you asked for, Willis."

"How old is—"

"For chrissakes, Willis, she's what you fucking ordered!"

Bessemer hangs up, and Dennis stares at Carr, his Adam's apple twitching. They watch on the laptop screen for a while, while Howie drinks in silence

"Tell Bobby and Mike to come back," Carr says finally. "He's not going anywhere."

Bobby and Mike bring a lot of beer with them. They all sit around the folding tables in the workhouse, in the glow of the laptop screens. An oily, late-day rain beats at the windows.

"How much gin you think Howie's gonna put away tonight?" Bobby asks between swallows of beer. "I bet he makes it through the bottle, but doesn't hold it down. How about it—anybody want to start a pool?"

Mike drags on a cigarette. "Howie's delivering the goods to Stearn on Friday," he says. "We get video of that, we can put whatever kind of leash we want on him. What do you say, *jefe*—we ready to roll on this?"

Dennis slams his bottle down and some beer sloshes out the top. His face is red, and his reedy voice is trembling. "Video? Are you saying we're just going to sit there and watch while this shit happens?"

They all look at him, surprised. In the time they've known him, they've never heard Dennis raise his voice beyond a goofy laugh. Latin Mike shakes his head, and Carr leans back in his chair.

Bobby looks into his beer. His voice is quiet. "C'mon, Denny—we've seen bad shit before. Most of what we do is watch scumbags, and if they're not doing boring shit, they're doing bad shit. We've seen people get knifed, get shot, get the crap kicked out of 'em. Get killed. We've done a little of that ourselves."

"This is different. Those people were scumbags too, and they were all adults. Bessemer is talking about a *kid* here."

Mike laughs bitterly. "Jesus," he says, and looks at Carr. "Why don't you talk to him? Tell him to grow up or something." Carr doesn't answer, and Mike shakes his head. He turns back to Dennis. "We don't even know for sure what Stearn ordered, bro."

"Bullshit," Dennis says. "You *know* this girl they're talking about is a kid. Why else would Howie's pimp be so nervous—not to mention Howie shitting his pants?"

"And what do you want to do about it—call the *policía*? Or maybe you're gonna ride to the rescue yourself—go snatch her from Bessemer's place and leave her on the church steps, wrapped in a blanket."

Dennis stares at nothing. "I . . . I don't know what to do about it," he says softly. "I just don't want to sit there watching—*recording*—while shit like that goes down."

Mike snorts. "You want somebody else to work the video, so you don't have to see?"

"That's not the point."

"You sure about that, junior? Maybe your conscience just needs a little wiggle room."

"Fuck you," Dennis says to Latin Mike, and then he turns to Carr. "If we're going to roll Howie up," he asks, "what are we waiting for? Let's do it now—tonight."

"Which does what, *cabrón*—besides save you from seeing something

you don't want to see? The kid they're pimping out would be in the same shit regardless, on top of which we give up some leverage on Bessemer."

Bobby runs a hand through his hair and sighs. "We're not cops, Denny."

Dennis pushes his chair back from the table. "I'm not saying we are. I'm just saying . . . Fuck—I don't know what I'm saying."

Mike blows a plume of smoke at the ceiling. "So what are we doing, *jefe*?"

Carr studies his beer, thinking about Prager, recalling the threat heavy in the anchorman voice. *What's the matter, Bess—after everything we've been through, you suddenly decide you don't trust me? All these years, and I still haven't proven I can keep my word?* It had left Bessemer scared, but scared of what?

"There's something we're still not seeing," Carr says softly.

"*Hijo de puta!*" Mike shouts. "What else is there to know? And why the *fuck* do we need to know it?"

Bobby puts a hand on Mike's shoulder, but Mike shakes it off. Bobby looks at Carr. "He has a point: we've got video and sound of the guy buying and selling drugs, arranging hookers for his buddies, and come Friday we'll have him in the middle of who knows what kind of sick shit. What else do we need?"

Carr shakes his head. His voice is low and raspy. "The feds offered to let him walk away from eighteen months in prison if he rolled on Prager, and Bessemer turned them down. Prager's got a grip on him, and I want to know what it is. We get only one shot with Bessemer, and I want to go in holding all the cards."

"I thought he kept his mouth shut because Prager helped him hide money from his wife," Bobby says. "What else—"

Mike cuts him off. "We got the fucking cards already. We got Bessemer with his dick hanging out, and this time he won't be looking at some bullshit Wall Street summer-camp jail. He'll be looking at real prison for the shit we've got on him. There's no way he has the balls for that."

"There's something we're not seeing," Carr says again.

"You're saying you want to wait?" Bobby asks.

He shakes his head slowly. "I'm saying between now and Friday, I want to know what's going on."

"And how the hell we gonna find out?" Mike asks, disgusted.

"That's not your problem," Carr says.

* * *

On his apartment's balcony, Carr switches to rum. He puts his bare feet on the railing and tilts back in his chair, and his thoughts skid like bad tires. He thinks about the rain and the heat, and sees Bessemer, slumped over the wheel of his BMW, and wonders again what hold Prager has on him. He sees a light on the water, bobbing and blinking in the dark, and he wonders who might be out there—so far out—on a night like this. He leans forward and squints, but loses sight of it.

The wind shifts, and the smells of wet earth and decaying vegetation come in. He thinks about his father's house, the gray light, his father's eyes, the list of nursing homes Eleanor Calvin has given him, and the messages from her that he's continued to ignore. The light reappears on the water and vanishes again when he tries to fix on it—like a dust mote, he thinks, almost imaginary.

The wind shifts again and a sweet smell—some night-blooming flower—washes across the balcony. He thinks about Valerie—Jill—and Amy Chun leaning close, and wonders how they're spending this rainy evening. He thinks about Tina, curled like a cat on his sofa, about Bobby and Mike, and Bertolli's missing money. He thinks about the wreckage of the van, and Ray-Ray and Declan, and the morgue smell that still rises sometimes from his clothes.

And he thinks again and again about Dennis—his red face, his reedy voice, his disgust. *Are you saying we're just going to sit there and watch while this shit happens?* It seems to Carr he's been doing that for a while now, one way or another. With Declan, and before that with Integral Risk.

It was raining in Mexico City, a halfhearted drizzle on a warm spring day, when Carlos Morilla summoned him to his office tower out in Santa Fe. He was chairman and CEO of Morilla Farmacias, and Integral Risk's largest client in Mexico. Carr was the account manager.

Morilla's face was dark and shuttered as he told Carr to have a seat. His voice was rumbling, and his English without accent. There was not the usual offer of coffee. Morilla slid a blue Integral Risk folder across the desk.

"You are telling me that my Patricia is homosexual?" he said. "My only daughter—a lesbian? This is your finding?"

Carr took a deep breath. "The report draws no conclusions, sir. You

requested that we observe Patricia and her friend for a period of time and document their activities. That's what we've done."

Morilla frowned. "Is there another conclusion one could reach?" Carr said nothing and Morilla's face had grown even darker. Morilla sighed. "She is very young, Patricia, and she has led a sheltered life. She is very impressionable—susceptible to the influence of . . . of the wrong sort of person. So there is something else I would like you to take care of."

Carr thought he'd never gotten proper credit for the patience he'd shown. He hadn't interrupted Morilla's commands, even when the executive's voice had shaken, his face had reddened in a way that reminded Carr of his father's, and he'd snapped his Montblanc pen in two. Carr remained quiet and composed throughout, and when Morilla was done, Carr had taken a deep breath and explained things slowly and carefully.

"Integral Risk is a corporate security firm, sir, and while we deeply value the business we have done together, this is simply not the sort of job we can undertake. It is neither in your best interests, nor in ours. I think, with time to reflect, you might also see that this is not the wisest course for your family."

It was this last suggestion—that someone else, the hired help no less, might know what was best for the Morilla family—that Carr realized too late he should have kept to himself. Morilla had colored deeply, but said nothing for a long time. Then he picked up the phone and called the general manager of Integral Risk Latin America—Carr's boss's boss.

Carr hadn't minded the weeklong enforced vacation. He went to the seashore. He swam every day, and read and drank at night. What he'd minded was learning, when he returned, that Luisa Rios, an art student at UNAM, had had her face slashed from her left earlobe to the corner of her mouth and her right arm broken in three places.

The wind rises, and the sounds of the rain and ocean and thrashing palms merge into a great wave, and Carr's chair is slipping out from under him, falling backward, and Carr with it. The jolt knocks the breath out of him, and his glass breaks on the balcony deck. He carries the pieces inside and dries his face. Then he picks up his cell phone.

"You up for a road trip?" he asks when Valerie answers.

18

The cheerleader figure is sloppy now, and the etched features are blurred. Her skin is lined and lax, like her paint-stained jeans, and her brown eyes are wary. The avid smile—so much on display in the wedding announcements Carr found online—is nowhere in sight, and her hair, lacquered chestnut in those photos, is curled by the ocean air, sweat-dampened, and streaked with gray. The cheerleader's older sister, Carr thinks: wiser certainly, but angrier too, with little left in the way of expectations. He is certain that more than just time has worked these changes on Tracy Holland—six years of marriage to Howard Bessemer doubtless played a part.

Holland lays her roller in the metal tray, and wipes her hands on her T-shirt. She sweeps hair off her forehead and gazes at Carr suspiciously.

"We rang the bell," he says, smiling. "But no one answered."

Holland frowns and looks at Valerie. "You're the one who called yesterday, about the film? Megan . . . ?" Her voice is scratchy.

Valerie walks through the French doors. She steps around the ladder and the paint cans and extends a hand. "Hecht, Megan Hecht. Looks like we caught you in the middle of something."

"A place this age, there's always something," Holland says.

Carr nods. The white shingle pile, all porches and dormers, must be 150 years old at least. It sprawls against a hillside, above a rocky stretch of

Maine coast and a choppy sea—Townsend Gut emptying into Boothbay Harbor.

Valerie pushes her plaid sleeves above her elbows and looks around the dining room. She smiles appreciatively at the meticulous paint job—dove gray with intricate eggshell trim. "This looks like a pretty big project."

"Scraping and sanding were the hard parts; this is just boring," Holland says. She looks at Carr. "Who is he?"

"Brian," Carr says, putting out a hand.

"Brian helps me with research," Valerie says, "and scouting locations."

"And getting coffee," Carr adds, but still there is no smile from Tracy Holland. She wipes a forearm across her brow, drinks from a sweating bottle of Sam Adams, and moves through the French doors to the porch. Carr and Valerie follow.

"A documentary about Wall Street wives," Holland says, doubtfully. "Not the most sympathetic subjects in the world, are they? Probably do better with a reality TV show—some crap about a bunch of women you love to hate. That's more like it."

"You may have a point," Valerie says. "But as I mentioned on the phone, our director thinks women like you have some interesting stories to tell. A perspective on the crash that we haven't seen before."

"*Women like me*," she says. "I'm not sure what that means." Holland leads them to a pair of wicker armchairs. She and Valerie sit, and Carr leans on the porch rail.

"Do you mind if we tape?" Carr asks, and reaches for the camera case slung over his shoulder.

Holland frowns. "Yes, I mind. I'm still not sure if I want to be involved in this."

"Sure," Valerie says soothingly. "Talking is great."

"But why talk to me? It's not like Howard and I were boldfaced names in New York. The most coverage he got was when he got arrested."

"The kind of storytelling we do—it's about taking the particular experiences of individuals and finding the broader themes. You and your husband led a certain kind of life in New York: his job, the Upper East Side co-op, private schools, charity boards. Now that's all over—the market, his career, that whole life. And you seem to be a kind of refugee. There are other Wall Street wives in that spot. More than a few."

Tracy Holland sips some beer and looks out at the water. She chuckles again, more bitterly this time. "By which you mean what—women who made deals with the devil, only to find the devil couldn't hold up his end?"

Valerie's smile turns confiding. "Is that what happened," she asks, "a breach of contract on Satan's part?"

Holland smiles back. "Isn't that how those deals always end?" she says. "But you should probably talk to those other wives. It was a long time ago, and I don't think I'm typical of anything."

"No?"

"I'm pretty sure none of my old friends do their own painting, diminished circumstances or not."

"You keep in touch with many of them?" Carr asks.

She squints at him, surprised he has spoken. "No."

"What about your ex-husband? Do you think he was—"

The squint turns into a scowl. "My lawyers deal with him. I don't."

"I was just going to ask if he was typical of men who worked on Wall Street then."

"You think there was only one type—a bunch of Gordon Gekko wannabes in suspenders and slick hair? Kind of outdated, isn't it?"

Carr makes a conciliatory nod. "I'm sure they're all unique, but maybe they had motivations in common."

"You mean greed."

"It's what makes the markets go, and what inflates bubbles—according to popular wisdom, anyway."

Holland takes an angry swig. "You seem to know it all. I don't see why you need me."

Valerie looks at Carr and coughs discreetly. "I'm sure we know hardly anything," she says, "but I'm hoping you can educate us. What made Howard tick? What led him to Wall Street?"

Holland holds the beer bottle against the side of her neck and sighs. "He wasn't typical. Not one of those people who always had their sights set on a Wall Street career. Basically, most of Howard's trust fund was gone by the time he left college. He needed to work, and he didn't think he could get a job anywhere else."

"It's not like bagging groceries at the supermarket," Valerie says. "There was a lot of competition for those jobs."

"There still is. But Howard didn't have to worry about that—he had family connections at Melton-Peck."

"So it was the only firm that would hire him?"

"So Howard thought. He also thought it was the only thing he was cut out for."

"Banking?"

"He said he wasn't enough of a quant to be a trader, and that he didn't have enough energy to be in sales. He said that catering to the whims of people richer than he was was the closest thing to planning parties for his fraternity, and that was all he was ever good at. Hence private banking."

Valerie nods slowly. "Sounds like he gave it a lot of thought."

Tracy Holland sighs again, more deeply this time. "Another way Howard wasn't typical. Wall Street people aren't much given to self-reflection, not the ones I knew anyway. Howard was different that way."

"Introspective?"

"Enough to know his own failings, though not enough to do anything about them. Does that make him better or worse than the guys who never give it a thought?"

"Doing something is always the hard part," Valerie says. "What were they—his failings?"

"Jesus—where to begin? Always taking the path of least resistance? No impulse control? Chronic self-pity? How about his sense of entitlement? Or his whining about the burdens of growing up with the appearance and expectations of wealth, but without the actual money to back them up?" She takes another sip of Sam Adams and sighs. "You don't have the time, and I don't have the energy."

"Doesn't sound particularly appealing," Valerie says. "Or easy to live with."

"He wasn't."

"So why did you?"

"I found Howard kind of cute, at first—like a blond, blue-eyed teddy bear. He was funny and self-deprecating—more the class cutup than the quarterback types I usually went with, and I liked that. He was sweet, and easy to be with, and if I'm being honest, there was the economic factor too. Fading trust fund or not, Howard seemed to be at the start of a good career when I met him. And where was I then—a pre-K teacher at a private school, and filling in part-time at Sotheby's. That's what a fine arts degree got me—that, and my house painting skills."

Valerie nods. "So cute and funny didn't do it in the long haul?"

"They never had a chance: the longer he worked at the bank—the more time he spent with those people—the more drinking and whining there was, and the less there was of cute and funny. And having a baby just made it worse. He was useless as a father—well-meaning, I guess, but useless." Holland pauses and laughs bitterly. "Of course, the gambling, the drugs, and the hookers didn't help much."

"Are you serious?" Valerie asks, and Tracy Holland nods.

"Who do you mean by *those people*?" Carr asks. "Who was he spending time with?"

Another frown from Holland. "His clients, his colleagues—all those people."

"Was Curtis Prager in that group?"

The frown deepens, and an icy silence settles on the porch. When Holland speaks again, her voice is tight and low. "I'm the wrong person to talk to about him. Maybe I'm the wrong person to talk to altogether."

The silence expands until Valerie clears her throat and points at Holland's beer bottle. "You have another of those around?"

Holland is surprised, but after a moment she stands. Valerie raises a hand. "Brian can get it, if you tell him where."

Holland pauses and nods uncertainly. "In the kitchen, in the fridge."

Carr takes his time, going back through the dining room and down a hall. The kitchen, when he finds it, is another work-in-progress: new cabinets and countertops, raw wallboard where tiles will go, the smells of sawdust and paint still strong in the air. The old refrigerator is forlorn in a slot that's sized for a larger model. There are layers of paper stuck to it with magnets, and Carr flicks through them. Bills from a dentist, an electrician, a plumber, an invoice from a fuel oil company. There's a calendar too, with drawings of lobster traps and fishing buoys on it, and a dense scrawl of appointments in red ink. Beneath all these there are photographs of a boy.

They are badly rippled by the salt air, but still his resemblance to Howard Bessemer is plain. The same blond hair, though considerably more of it, the same round face and benign, guileless smile. The photos cover a range of ages: at six or seven he is dressed as a colonial soldier, trick-or-treating with a tricorn hat and plastic musket; at eight he's at the helm of a sky-blue sunfish; and at nine and ten and eleven, he's playing soccer—blond hair flying amid clouds of dust and turf. His face is a mask

of concentration and resolve. And then a door slams, and there are knobby footsteps behind Carr, and the boy himself is there.

He's twelve now, small and solid and still a soccer player. His cleats and knees are muddy, and his jersey is stained with grass and sweat. His cheeks are red and his thick blond hair is matted. His head is canted as he stares at Carr, and his face and eyes are without expression.

The eyes are dark and wide-spaced, like his mother's, and Carr thinks the camera missed what's important in them: the wells of suspicion, the watchfulness, the deliberation, and the stillness—the sense that the boy is always preparing for the ground to shift beneath him, or to fall away altogether, always waiting for another shoe to drop.

Carr smiles. "You must be Simon," he says. "I'm Brian."

The boy nods slowly, weighing Carr's words and his own reply. "Where's my mom?" Simon Bessemer asks eventually.

"On the porch, with my boss. I'm supposed to bring beer. What position do you play?"

The boy pauses again, considering. "Defense."

"Fullback?"

"Defensive mid."

"You must be fast," Carr says. The boy nods, and Carr points at his soccer jersey. It's blue, with a broad gold band across the chest. "Boca Juniors?"

Simon Bessemer raises an eyebrow and nearly smiles. "The home jersey."

Carr nods. "I've been to some of their matches."

The near smile turns skeptical, and the boy looks suddenly like his mother. "In Argentina?" Carr nods again, but the disbelief doesn't fade. "I watch them on satellite," the boy says, "on the soccer channel. You're a friend of my mom?"

"We're doing research, my boss and I, for a documentary about Wall Street. About banking."

The boy's forehead clouds with questions, but he doesn't ask any. "My dad worked in banking," he says finally, "when we lived in New York."

Carr nods again. "You must've been pretty young then. You remember much about it?"

Simon Bessemer studies Carr for another moment and shakes his head. "I don't really know him," he says. "I haven't seen him in a while." And he turns and leaves the kitchen.

His footsteps recede down the hall and up a flight of stairs. Carr looks again at the pictures on the fridge. Something in the boy's eyes is familiar, though he cannot say what at first. Something about the watchfulness, and the suspicion. Something about the deliberation. Later, after he has delivered a beer to Valerie and brought another one for Tracy Holland and excused himself again, it comes to him. He is in a hallway powder room, sluicing water on his face, and he looks up, into the mirror, and there it is.

19

"Portland to JFK at eight," Carr says as he comes down the wharf. "Then we pick up a rental and drive to East Hampton."

Valerie grimaces. "Eight *a.m.*? Do we have to be such fucking early birds?"

Carr smiles at her. She takes his hand, and they walk farther out. "There's a worm waiting for us," he says. "At least, I hope there is."

Valerie nods. "Tracy was pretty clear about it," she says. "The date it went from merely intolerable with Bessemer to call-in-the-lawyers bad. She knew when it was, and where he'd been, and she knew that whatever he was doing, he'd been doing it with Prager. Of course, the fact that it was the weekend of their fifth anniversary, and Howard was supposed to have been at home with her, probably helped it stick in her mind.

"Before that weekend—according to her—he was just a middling-to-bad husband and dad, out drinking with clients too often, paying no attention to her or the kid when he was at home, whining all the time. After that weekend was when it went south in a big way: the gambling and drugs and whores—usually with Prager as his wingman. Or vice versa."

"Sounds like a worm to me," Carr says.

What's left of daylight is sputtering out in the low brick skyline of Portland. The sodium lights along the wharf cast an amber glow on Valerie's face. Her hand is warm in his. She leads Carr to the railing, and they look out at the swaying boats.

"She didn't like you," Valerie says after a while.

"Yeah, I got that."

"You shouldn't take it personally—she doesn't like men. She's permanently angry."

"I got that, too. Is it all thanks to Howard?"

"He just finished the job. Her dad started it, and there were others in between."

"You got all that from a beer?"

"It was six beers, each, and it helped that you made yourself scarce." Valerie unwinds her hand and slips it around his waist. "Besides," she says, "I'm a good listener. People open up to me."

"So I've seen."

"Most people, anyway." She looks at the harbor again and starts to whistle something Carr almost recognizes.

He is fairly certain she isn't drunk—he's seen her drink much more than the beers she had with Holland and the bottle of wine he and she shared in the hotel lounge, and with no discernible effect. No, this evening she's something different—something open and unguarded, and seemingly without calculation. A Valerie he hasn't seen before? A performance he hasn't seen, anyway. She leans against him at the rail, and her scent mixes with the smells of diesel and low tide.

"You like the water, don't you?" she asks. "Diving, sailing—all of that."

"I do."

"You grew up around it?"

"I learned to sail when I was a kid."

"Who from?"

"My father."

"You were close to him?"

Carr looks at the bobbing lights and the water, nearly black now. He shakes his head. "I liked it in spite of him."

"An asshole?"

"Like Tracy Holland—permanently pissed off."

"At you?"

"At life; at the world; at my mother. I was a convenient proxy."

The wind picks up, colder now, and Valerie shivers beside him. Carr takes off his blazer and hangs it around her shoulders. Valerie rubs her hand up and down his forearm. "Poor baby boy," she says, chuckling.

"Are you making light of my troubled childhood?"

"Did they smack you around? Or each other?"

"No."

"Then we have different definitions of *troubled*."

"You have that kind of trouble?"

She looks up. Her face is flushed from the wine, and Carr can feel the heat rising from her. "I was too cute to get mad at."

"Even then?"

She nods. "Still, it sucks having an asshole for a dad. Probably sucks worse for a guy. Role models, and all that."

"You're watching too much daytime television down in Boca."

Valerie wraps his jacket around her and laughs. "It explains so much, though—Deke's appeal to you, his big, bluff paternal thing, why you're still picking at what happened in Mendoza like it's a scab."

Carr steps back from the rail. "Definitely too much television."

"Oprah can't tell me shit, babe. You think I can do what I do without knowing what makes people tick? Now tell me Declan wasn't a father figure to you."

"I can't say I've given it much thought."

Valerie laughs. "Of course not."

Carr takes another step back, and puts his hands in the air. "Deke had big plans, he ran a good crew, and he was a good soldier—disciplined, focused, a good motivator. He kept his head in the game, and he made us all rich. That's what I know."

"You're remembering a different guy," she says. "Yes, he thought big, and he ran a good crew—but disciplined? Focused? C'mon, Carr—that's what he had you for. And half the time, he didn't want to listen. Deke liked any excuse to light it up, and you know it. He got bored too easy, and deep down he was a fucking cowboy. Toward the end, it wasn't even down that deep. Personally, I think it was some sort of midlife crisis."

"That's bullshit. Besides Mendoza—"

"I'm not just talking about Mendoza, and you know it. There was César, and before that the Russians in Nicaragua. Before that, there was—"

"That's enough, Vee," Carr says, and his voice is icy.

"Don't go all Eastwood on me now—we were almost having a conversation."

"You were doing the talking."

She smiles at him, and there's a little pity in it. "Okay," she says softly. "But you're remembering a different guy."

She takes his hand again and leads him down the wharf, past a yellow cigarette boat, a chrome-heavy sport fisher, and a big white catamaran. She's whistling again, softly, and Carr sighs.

"What about you?" he asks. "No lingering mommy and daddy issues?"

She laughs. "You don't know anybody more mentally healthy than me."

"Most of the people I know are borderline sociopaths. Your parents stay together?"

Her laugh is sharp, and it echoes like a shot on the water. "They were both military, so they knew how to fight. It was like a nonstop cage match."

"But you have no issues."

She shakes her head and slips her arm around him. "It doesn't always have to be like that, you know—like my parents, and yours. Like the battling Bessemers."

"I haven't seen many examples to the contrary."

Valerie moves in front of him, and slides her hands under his shirt. They're cold and smooth against his ribs, and a shudder runs through him. "Maybe that's what we'll do afterward," she whispers. "You and me. We'll conduct a little research to find some happy couples. We'll be like archaeologists."

"You think we'll have to dig them up?"

Valerie laughs, and her mouth is hungry on his. "Early morning tomorrow," she whispers. "We should call it a night."

20

Carr arrives at the workhouse at three p.m. on Friday. He has swum, showered, shaved, and dressed in a blazer, jeans, and dark glasses. No one inside the house looks as good.

Bobby is bristled and fragile, and he's working slowly though a liter of Coke and an egg sandwich. Latin Mike is also unshaven, vaguely jaundiced, and unconcerned with anything beyond the cup of coffee on the table before him, the cigarette burning in his ashtray, and the bottle of Advil in his hand. Dennis is green, shaking death. Carr lets the door slam behind him and smiles when they wince.

"I see you've been busy while I was away," he says loudly. Mike ignores him, and Bobby flips him the bird over his sandwich. Carr chuckles. "How's our man Bessemer doing?" he asks.

Dennis wipes sweat from his forehead. "Pickled. He was at the gin again last night, and didn't get up until noon. Hasn't been out of the house yet today. Stearn called him an hour ago, to check that his party was still on for tonight."

"And?"

"Howie told him nine o'clock."

"Has he spoken to Prager again?"

"He's tried twice—yesterday and the day before—and got nowhere."

Carr nods. "And Amy Chun? How's she coming along?"

Dennis taps on his keyboard. "Good. I pulled some stuff from her laptop—her personal one, not the Isla Privada equipment."

"And?"

Dennis manages a smile. "She's been e-mailing Val—Jill, I mean. She talks about how she misses her, how much she enjoys hanging out with her."

"Fuckin' Vee," Bobby says through a mouthful of egg.

"Chun's also been searching for anything and everything about Jill Creary on the Web," Dennis says.

"No more stalking Janice Lessig?"

"Not for a while now."

"What's she finding on Jill?"

"Everything we put out there, everything Val asked for. Footprints in New York and in Boston. Modeling, PR, cooking school."

"Chun does all the looking herself? No professional help?"

"All by herself," Dennis says, and scrolls through some e-mail. "Her last note to Jill, she talks about the two of them going on vacation together."

Carr shakes his head. "That's fast."

Mike rouses himself from his coffee to smile bitterly. "A real heart-breaker, that Vee."

Bobby laughs, takes a bite of his sandwich, and wipes his mouth with the back of his hand. He looks at Carr. "You gonna say how your trip went?"

"It went fine, Bobby."

"Fine as in you had a nice little vacation, or fine as in you found something out about Bessemer?"

Carr smiles, but says nothing.

"Asshole," Bobby says, and he takes a long swallow of Coke. "What time do we set up at Howie's tonight?"

Carr's smile widens. "I'm thinking six."

Latin Mike scowls. "Why the hell we need to get there so early? Stearn won't show till nine, and the pimp's people won't be any sooner."

"We don't need to wait for them," Carr says. "We don't need them."

Dennis looks up. "What?"

"We don't need them. We're set for tonight, without them."

Confusion and relief play across Dennis's pale face. "What about Stearn, and Lamp? They're expecting—"

"Howie will sort them out for us."

Latin Mike shakes his head. "Guess *jefe*'s trip worked out okay."

Bobby looks at Carr. "How do you want to work it tonight?"

"We give Bessemer no time to think," Carr says. "I want fear, confusion, and compliance."

Bobby nods, and burps loudly. "You sound just like my ex," he says.

21

Water gurgles in the shower drain as Howard Bessemer presses a towel to his face, and then he hears his front door open. He leaves damp footprints on the tiles as he steps cautiously out of his bedroom, and a puddle forms where he stands frozen and stares openmouthed at the men in his entrance foyer.

Carr hands the laptop to Latin Mike. "Set it up in the living room," he says, and Mike nods and walks off. Carr looks at Bessemer. "You want to get your pants on, Howie, or are you good like that?"

Bessemer wraps his towel more tightly about his waist. His mouth closes and opens again and a sound comes out, but it's not a word.

"Pants, Howie."

Bessemer squints, and takes a step backward. "Wha . . . What?"

Carr points to the bedroom. "Pants."

"Who . . . Who the hell are—"

"Get your fucking pants on, Howie," Carr says, smiling, and he unbuttons his blazer and lets Bessemer see the Glock in his belt. Bessemer backs slowly into the bedroom, and Carr counts to twenty. When he walks to the bedroom door, he finds Bessemer holding the telephone handset, staring at it.

"Just out of curiosity, Howie, if the phone was working, just who do you think you'd call?"

Bessemer drops the phone and stumbles on the edge of his towel. Carr waits in the doorway while Bessemer dresses in Madras shorts and a polo shirt that's too tight across the gut. Then he walks him into the living room.

It's a long, bright space, with Persian rugs on the floor, equestrian sketches on the walls, and teak and rattan furniture that is old but still solid. Latin Mike is standing at a black lacquer cabinet whose doors are open to reveal barware and bottles. He pours two fingers of Glenlivet into a tumbler and offers the bottle to Carr.

"Not just now," Carr says. "You have the disk?" Latin Mike produces a DVD case and scales it across the room. Carr plucks it from the air. "Collect his cell phones. They should be in the office." Mike downs the scotch and nods, and Carr carries the DVD to the laptop that is open on a low teak table by the sofa.

"Have a seat, Howie," Carr says.

Bessemer draws himself up and takes a deep breath. "Just who the *hell* are you, and what do you think you're doing in my house?" The teddy bear face is damp and pink, and the voice is shaky.

Carr puts a hand on Bessemer's shoulder, spreads his fingers across Bessemer's collarbone, and digs. Bessemer cries out and collapses to one knee. "What the fuck!" His face is red and there are tears in his eyes.

Carr yanks Bessemer to his feet again. "On the sofa, Howie. Shut up, and watch the movie."

Bessemer perches unsteadily on the edge of the sofa and Carr slips a disk into the laptop. It whirrs and hums and a video starts to play. And Howard Bessemer goes pale.

Carr stands silent for several minutes, watching the video and watching the teddy bear split at the seams. When he sees Bessemer's hands tremble and his chin quiver, Carr clears his throat. "Guess it's true what they say about the camera, Howie—it adds ten pounds, at least. But still, it's easy to tell it's you. Easy to identify your friends too: Brunt and Scoville, Tandy and Moyer, and if you wait just a minute you'll see Lamp and the Grigoriev brothers as well. See—you can even make out their license plates. And the audio is good quality—nice and clean—you all sound like yourselves."

Bessemer moans, and Carr puts a hand on his shoulder, gently this time. "This is just the highlight reel, Howie. We've got hours more of you

guys—phone conversations, payments being made, dope being delivered, girls . . . lots of stuff."

Bessemer waves his hands, as if he's shooing away gnats. His voice is a frightened whisper. "You . . . you're cops," he says.

"Oh no, Howie." Carr laughs. "We're much worse than that."

22

Carr is sitting in an armchair, drinking soda water from a highball glass and leafing through a month-old copy of *The New Yorker,* when the teddy bear groans and lifts his head from the waste can. Carr places his glass on an end table and watches as Bessemer's gumdrop eyes dart about the room—ceiling to floor, wall to wall, lingering over the laptop, and coming to rest finally on the highball glass on its coaster and the Glock beside it.

Carr smiles benevolently. "All done throwing up? You want some water now?"

Bessemer shakes his head and sits back on the sofa. He runs a hand through his thin hair and across his mouth. His eyes dart some more, and then light on a brass clock atop the liquor cabinet.

"Yes, it is getting late," Carr says. "Time to call Stearn, and Lamp. Tell each of them that the other one has canceled on you. Tell them that you don't know why, and that you'll have to get back to them to reschedule. Best to be brief and vague." Bessemer looks at him and squints, as if straining to remember something. "Are you sure you wouldn't like some water?" Carr asks again.

"Who *are* you?" he asks.

Carr shakes his head and calls out: "Can we get Howie a phone?" Latin Mike emerges from the kitchen with one of Bessemer's cell phones. He tosses it to Bessemer, who jumps as if it's a hand grenade. Mike laughs.

"Stearn," Carr says, "and then Lamp. Then we'll talk."

"Who . . . ?"

"Make the calls, Howie."

And Bessemer does. He's both brief and vague, and all the time he talks, he never takes his eyes off the gun on the end table. When he's done, he hands the phone back to Carr and lies back on the sofa. He closes his eyes, presses his fingers to them, and opens them again. He looks surprised to find Carr still there.

"I'll have that water now," he says.

Carr goes into the kitchen and brings out a glass, with ice. Bessemer sits up and drinks it all. "Who are you?" he asks Carr.

"Gregory Frye," Carr answers, and puts out his hand. Bessemer's grip is soft and damp. "And I'm not a cop."

"Then what the hell are you doing in my house, acting like it's your goddamn house? Who *are* you, and what the hell do you want from me?"

Carr chuckles and finishes his drink. "I'm the guy who doesn't care what you're doing with Willis Stearn or Daniel Brunt or Nick Scoville, or Tandy or Moyer, or Lamp, or the Grigoriev brothers." Carr points at Bessemer's glass. "Refill?"

Bessemer blanches, and Carr wonders if he's going to vomit again. But Bessemer rights himself, smooths his hair, and sits up straight. "I don't know what you're talking about."

Carr shakes his head. "Let's not do *that*, Howie."

Bessemer wipes his forehead. "I'm going to call the police."

Carr sighs and hands him the telephone. "Really, Howie, the dramatics are a big waste. You pretend, I threaten, and round and round we go. Why put yourself through it? You must be tired after the past few days. All that worrying. All that running around. It's a long way from the Upper East Side, isn't it? From Otisville too—though maybe not quite as long."

"I don't know what you're—"

"It's hard to argue with video, Howie."

Bessemer sits frozen with the phone in his hand. His polo shirt is mottled with sweat, and his face is a crumbling mask of fear and confusion. His eyes race around the room again and come to rest on his Persian rug. He doesn't resist when Carr takes the phone from him.

"What do you want?" Bessemer asks softly.

"I want to meet a friend of yours."

Bessemer squints again. "Who—Willis? Nicky? Danny Brunt?"

"None of those guys."

"Well, I don't have any other friends. Not anymore."

"You've got at least one, Howie—an old friend."

He shakes his head. "I don't know who—"

"Curtis Prager. I want you to introduce me to Curtis Prager."

Bessemer straightens his shoulders, and lines of defiance appear around his eyes. "Who is—"

Carr sighs. "You steered investors to him when he was starting Tirol Capital. You put your own money in. He helped you hide some of it when your wife was divorcing you."

"He didn't—"

"Your wife's lawyers thought he did, even if they couldn't prove it."

Bessemer's mouth stiffens. "I don't know him."

Carr shakes his head regretfully, and his voice falls to a whisper. "I'll put up with a certain amount of drama, Howie. I suppose it's unavoidable. But I won't tolerate lying. And especially not this kind of thing—it's insulting. You might as well call me an idiot. My clothes, my grammar, my reading this magazine and bringing you water, may have given you the wrong idea about me. You may think I'm very different from Lamp and the Grigorievs and the other trash you've been hanging with, but in the ways most relevant to your health, I promise you I'm not."

Bessemer's body softens and slumps. Carr claps him lightly on the shoulder and carries his highball glass to the kitchen. He returns with it refilled and Bessemer looks at him.

"What do you want with Curtis?" he says.

"To meet him. To do business."

"I'll give you his number. You can call his secretary and make an appointment."

Carr laughs. "I had a more personal intro in mind."

Bessemer drinks some water and spills more down his shirtfront. He wipes his mouth with his fingertips, gathers his breath, and sits up straighter. "Listen, Mr. Frye, you might've done me a favor tonight—keeping me from doing something I wasn't looking forward to—so I'll give you some valuable advice, for absolutely no charge: I don't know what business you think you want to do with Curtis Prager, but whatever it is, you don't want to do it. Whatever it is—and I'm not asking what—I

tell you, it won't work out. It won't end well, for you or anyone else involved. Anyone besides Curtis."

"And who knows better than you?"

Bessemer slumps again. "What's that mean?"

"It means your own business with Prager hasn't panned out so well. It means he has your money and doesn't want to give it back, so now you earn your gambling, coke, and hooker money by dealing dope to your friends and procuring prostitutes for them. And call me Greg, Howie."

Bessemer blanches and swallows hard, and Carr smiles to himself. "Who are you?" Bessemer whispers.

"Wrong question. You should be asking, *What's in it for me? What can Greg Frye do for me?*"

"And what would that be?"

"I can get you out from under, Howie—out of the low-margin fetching and carrying you do for your pals, out of your grandma's bungalow, out of scratching at the doors of clubs that won't have you for a member. I can get you out of this life altogether. I can get your money back—your money and then some."

Howard Bessemer stands and shakes his head. "I . . . I want no part of that."

"No part of what, Howie?"

"If you're thinking about . . . I don't know what you're thinking about—all I know is I want no part of it."

Carr sits back in his chair. He nods slowly and drums his fingers on the armrest. "Not surprising, I guess. You heard that offer before, or something like it, just before they put you on the bus for Otisville. *Talk to us about Curtis Prager and get out of jail free.* But you didn't bite then."

Bessemer's eyes are wide now, and he's pointing. "You *are* a cop!"

"I'm not, Howie, and don't yell."

"*Then who the fuck are you?*"

"Again, wrong question."

"No—I don't *care* what you can do! Whatever you're thinking, forget it. You can't—"

Carr holds up a hand, cuts Bessemer off, and lets quiet descend on the room. He takes a deep breath. Time to climb the ladder, he thinks, and his own heart begins to pound. "If you don't care what I can do *for* you," Carr says, "then worry about what I can do *to* you."

"I don't—"

Carr cuts Bessemer off again. He works a hard look onto his face and an angry edge into his voice. "I'm not just talking about video of you and those country club shitheads doing lines, Howie. Drugs and whores are not even frosting on this cake."

"What—"

"And I'm not one of your ex-wife's asshole lawyers, either. I'm not stupid enough to think you kept quiet just because Prager sheltered funds for you. And I certainly don't think it's because you're a stand-up guy."

"I don't know what you're talking about," Bessemer says, so softly Carr can barely make it out.

Carr stares at him. Time to step onto the platform. "I'm talking about the hold Curtis Prager has on you, Howard—the reason you kept your mouth shut and did your time, and the reason you're still taking his shit today. I'm saying that *I know*, Howard. I know, and I have no problem using it."

"Really, Mr. Frye—Greg—I don't know—"

Carr takes a deep breath. Time to dive. "Sarah Cotter," he says evenly. "Sarah Cotter."

In the silent seconds that follow, the dive becomes a spinning, sickening free fall. Puzzlement supplants fear on Bessemer's face, and Carr is suddenly sure that he's gotten it all wrong—that he and Valerie somehow read too much into what Tracy Holland said, heard what they'd wanted to hear, and connected dots in East Hampton that formed no hidden picture at all, but were nothing more than . . . dots. Bessemer squints at him, and Carr feels his temples pound and a line of sweat slide down his spine. His mind races through unlikely alternate plans—a desperate landscape of threats and blandishments—as the silence expands. And then Howard Bessemer sways before him, his knees buckle, and he sits abruptly on the sofa, as if his spine has turned to water.

Carr breathes a long sigh and lets his voice soften. "After all these years, it's still an open case, but I guess that's no surprise. A young woman like Sarah Cotter—just twenty-three—hit and run so early in the morning, and not a witness to be found. No forensic evidence either—no paint transfer or tire tracks, nothing. The police out there don't get too many cases like that."

Bessemer is staring now, at nothing in the room. He's paper-white,

and his hands are shaking. "You're a cop," he whispers, and to Carr it sounds like a plea. He sits on the sofa and puts a hand on Bessemer's shoulder.

"I'm really not," he says quietly.

Bessemer looks at him—disappointed, Carr thinks. "It was so early," Bessemer says after a long while. His voice is low and exhausted. "The middle of the night really—no light in the sky at all—and there was fog too, like goddamn soup. I still wonder what the hell she was doing out there in the dark. Who rides a bike in the dark like that?"

"She was training for a triathlon."

"I read that in the papers. But still—what the hell was she doing there?"

"That time of night, the fog—it must've been hard to see."

Bessemer squints at him and shakes his head. "That's what Curtis said, when I drove back to his place—*even sober, you'd never have seen her, Bess.* Then he woke up his security guy and told me he'd take care of everything. And fuck me if I didn't believe him."

Bessemer hangs his head, and a shudder runs through him. Carr claps him on the arm. "You can't change the past, Howie, but you don't have to be a prisoner of it."

Bessemer shrinks from his hand. "What bullshit," he says. "What total bullshit. What you really mean is that I can trade one jailer for another—Prager for you."

Carr sighs, crosses the room again, and picks up his gun. He blows a speck of something off the barrel and slips it into his belt. "You're looking at it the wrong way. I've put a carrot *and* a stick on the table: you help me out and you get your money back and get out of this life; you don't help, and . . . well, we both know how that goes. With Prager, you get only the stick—and you've been getting it for years. I figure you've got to be a little tired of it by now."

Bessemer makes a sound halfway between a groan and a bitter laugh and pushes his hands through his thin hair. "I need something more than water," he says, and points to the liquor cabinet. Carr nods. Bessemer walks unsteadily to it, and finds a bottle of Bombay Sapphire inside. He pours some into a glass, drinks half, and coughs. He shakes his head slowly.

"You're planning on . . . on stealing from him?" Bessemer struggles

with the word *stealing*, as if just speaking it is enough to bring down thunder. Carr looks at him and says nothing, and Bessemer takes that as an answer. "If I got involved in this—if I helped you—and Curtis found out, prison wouldn't be the problem, if you know what I mean. Curtis and the people who work for him—the people he knows—they're capable of—"

"I know who they are, Howie, and what they're capable of. You get your money back, you can afford to go somewhere else. To be somebody else."

"What—an alias? A new identity?"

"You're really happy with the old one?"

"But I . . . I wouldn't know how—"

"It's not hard, Howie. I can show you."

Bessemer drinks the rest of his gin and massages his temples with his thumbs. He rummages again in the liquor cabinet. He comes out with a mirror, a razor blade, a silver straw, and a small white envelope. He taps a pile of white powder onto the mirror and draws it into six thin lines. He bends over the mirror and four of the lines disappear. He looks up at Carr.

"First Curtis, then Misha and Sasha, then Stearn, and now you," Bessemer says, sniffling. "I don't know why this keeps happening. Sometimes I feel like I have a sign around my neck—*kick me*, or something."

"The Grigorievs are squeezing you?" Carr asks, and Bessemer nods. "Stearn too?" Another nod.

"The brokering that I do—with the drugs and the girls—Misha and Sasha got me into it. I ran up a big tab with them—bigger than my cash flow could handle—and they suggested a way I could pay it off. *Suggested* isn't quite the right word actually."

"Insisted?"

"That's closer. Anyway, that's how it got started, but this thing tonight, with Willis . . . I've never been involved in anything like that before. When I found out what he wanted, I tried to beg off. I told him I didn't have those kinds of contacts, but he wouldn't hear it. He said I was getting a reputation around town, and that I needed to be careful. He said things could get awkward for me if rumors got back to the police." Bessemer offers Carr the straw.

Carr smiles. "Not just now."

Bessemer snorts another line. "You see, I haven't been lucky recently.

So how do I know, if I get involved with this, it won't turn out the same? What assurance do I have?"

Carr nods and smiles sympathetically. "Other than my word as the guy holding the gun, you have none. But you also have no choice. Not to put too fine a point on it."

Bessemer looks at Carr and then looks down at the mirror atop the liquor cabinet, at the last line of cocaine, at his own reflection. He bends, snorts the final line, and wipes his nose with the back of his hand.

"Who are you supposed to be?" he asks, sniffling. "When I talk to Curtis, what am I supposed to say?"

"I'm a guy you met in Otisville, a good guy, someone who helped you when you were inside. Say that we've stayed in touch, and now I'm in the market for a banker. We'll do the details later."

"And when you meet with him, then what happens?"

"I do a little business with him."

"You know it won't be that simple, right? Curtis checks. He checks on everything, very carefully, and then he double-checks."

Carr nods and finishes his soda water. "Don't worry, Howie. I'm double-checkable."

23

"He sounds like a whiner, and more than a little screwy," Tina says to Carr, as the tide runs over their bare feet.

Carr looks at her over the top of his sunglasses. "He's both of those, and a lush to boot. And a cokehead."

"Well, I feel much better." Tina laughs. "And I can't wait to tell the boss. He'll love it that your whole plan hangs on a guy like this." They turn and walk north through the creaming surf. The hem of her gauzy black skirt and Carr's rolled cuffs are damp with foam.

"I can't say I'm thrilled myself," Carr says, "but it's not like there were a lot of options, or a lot of time."

Tina shrugs and watches the ocean, glassy and orange in the late daylight. "How's Bessemer adapting to his new circumstances?"

"He's self-medicating on gin and blow, but he's behaving. I've got a babysitter with him all the time, and I think he likes the company."

"When push comes to shove is he going to cooperate? Is he going to stick to the script with Prager? Will he be convincing?"

"He'll get there. Right now he's mostly scared."

"Of who?"

"Of Prager; of me."

"Who's got the edge?"

"We're holding the same threat over his head, but I'm the guy in his living room with a gun. Plus, I've got the carrots."

"And he believes in them?"

"He wants to, but he's not sure."

"So maybe he's not completely stupid," Tina says, tracking a gull as it swoops above some flotsam. "That was a nice piece of research up north, by the way, with the Cotter thing. A big roll of the dice, for sure, but it worked out. You could be a cop."

Carr shrugs. "Bessemer's ex was the key. She gave us the where and the when. That made it a whole lot easier to figure out the what—especially since it happened in the off-season. It was a big deal for the papers out there—the only real news they had to report at the time. And the place they found her—that stretch of road—it was one of the routes you'd take if you were driving from Prager's place to the highway."

"Still, a risky play," Tina says. "It hasn't occurred to Bessemer that Prager can't rat him out without implicating himself in the cover-up?"

"He said he tried that line of reasoning once, and never again. Prager told him he could get a dozen people to swear that it never happened— that Bessemer drove off in the middle of the night and didn't return, and that Prager wasn't even in East Hampton at the time."

Tina nods, still following the gull as if she's taking aim. They come to a hotel beach, and a hotel bar with shaded tables. Tina points. "I need to get out of the sun."

Carr orders an iced tea, Tina a lime soda. She takes a sip and shakes out her hair. It shimmers like white tinsel. "When are you going to have him make the call?" she asks.

"In a few days. I want him to settle down a while longer, and I want to go over the story with him some more."

"Dennis fix up your past?"

Carr nods. "Bumped some servers at Justice and the Bureau of Prisons. Frye did federal time for receiving stolen property. Overlapped eight months with Howie in Otisville. Before that, a money laundering beef, with charges eventually dropped. Nowadays, he's based in Boston. Has a nice little online business selling jeweler supplies to the trade."

"Too bad it's bullshit—I bet he could get me a deal on some earrings. How are things going in Boca?"

Carr takes a long swallow of iced tea and looks into his glass. "Val says it's going well."

"Love is in the air?"

"She's got Chun locked in. She'll be all but moved in there soon, and

then she can plant whatever we want, and clean it up again before the security sweeps."

"She was a big help with Bessemer's ex, I guess. A regular Watson to your Holmes."

Carr nods. Tina rests her heel on the edge of her seat. Her skirt falls away and her bare leg is like ivory. She brushes sand from her bare foot. "You don't like talking about her," she says.

Carr's voice is carefully neutral. "Are there questions I haven't answered? Something you want to know that I haven't told you?"

"You and she have a thing going, once upon a time? Or maybe going on now?"

Carr's face is taut. "Who's asking—Boyce or you?"

Tina lowers one foot, raises another, brushes away sand. A tiny smile flickers on her lips. "You're a big boy, and nobody's playing chaperone. It's just not typically the best management technique. *Don't shit where you eat*, et cetera. Fucks up unit cohesion. Doesn't help command judgment much either."

The sun has dropped behind the hotel tower and the sky is washed in violet. Carr drops some bills on the table. "Let's walk," he says.

Carr heads for the shoreline. The sand is cooler, and he turns north again, for a jetty a quarter mile away. Tina is silent at his side.

"How are things in the Prager compound?" Carr asks eventually.

"Same same," Tina says. "He's getting ready for his prospecting trip to Europe and Asia. Silva still hasn't surfaced from whatever glass he's climbed into."

"Good," Carr says. He stops and digs a flat stone the size of a silver dollar from the sand. He launches it in low, spinning flight over the smooth water, and it bounces and jinks more times than he can count before vanishing into a gray swell. "And down south?" he asks. "Are we making any progress there?"

"Maybe. Our guys were in Santiago, trying to locate the pilot Declan made his exit arrangements with. They went trolling at the bars near Los Cerrillos—the pilot bars—and got a hit. Found a charter operator named Guerrero. He's got a light jet, a Hawker, and he's apparently used to working for cash, and with no questions asked. You know the name?"

Carr shakes his head. "Is he the guy Declan hired?"

"He told my guys he took a deposit from someone that sounds a lot like Declan."

"Declan's plan was to go to São Paulo. From there, there were a lot of options to get back to Port of Spain. Where was this Guerrero supposed to go?"

"He wouldn't say. He wouldn't say anything else without money."

"Your guys didn't want to pay?"

"My guys check with me first. I told them I'd come down and see for myself. I'm flying out of Miami tomorrow."

Carr stops and looks at Tina. The tide rushes up over their ankles and he sees a shiver run through her. "This is a lot of personal attention," he says.

Tina takes off her sunglasses and nods. "You got me interested."

Carr's phone burrs as he opens the door to his apartment. He answers without looking and Eleanor Calvin's voice takes him by surprise. She is just as surprised by his.

"I didn't think I'd actually reach you," she says. "I've tried so many times."

"I've gotten your messages, Mrs. Calvin, but things have been crazy at work."

"I'm sure, dear."

"How's your move coming? Are you showing the house yet?"

"I've got an offer on it—two, actually. The real estate agent thinks there might even be a third one coming. They all want to close soon."

Carr stands in the darkened living room and takes a deep breath. "Oh," he says.

"Have you settled the arrangements for your father, dear?"

"I'm working on it, Mrs. Calvin."

"I know it's difficult for you, but there isn't much time."

Carr walks to the window and leans his head against the glass. "I'm aware, Mrs. Calvin."

"I know you are, dear, and I didn't call to talk about this. The ambassador is a little agitated this evening, and he wants to speak with you."

"Agitated about what, Mrs. Calvin? I really don't have—"

"I'm not sure what's upset him, but he's insistent. He's been . . . difficult all day, and I'm afraid he's been drinking."

Carr sighs. "Put him on," he says.

His father's voice is scratchy and attenuated across the ether, and he

sounds to Carr like an old recording of FDR. Nothing to fear but fear itself. He seems at first more angry than drunk.

"She lies to me, you know. Tells me she's done things when she hasn't. Tells me she hasn't done things when I know she has. And she takes things. That's why I can never find a goddamn thing in this house."

"Mrs. Calvin doesn't take things, and she doesn't lie. She's not your maid either."

"You're taking her side."

"There's no side to this."

"You're just like her, you know."

"Like Mrs. Calvin?"

"Don't be thick. You're just like her—always watching—like a goddamn cat. Quiet like a cat, and arrogant—no one can tell you anything, oh no. And stubborn—goddamn stubborn—just like her. Everything on your terms, and you won't let go until you're goddamn good and ready."

"I don't know what you're talking about, Dad," Carr says, and he sighs heavily. "What is it you're upset over?"

"I can't find it. I spent all day looking. Looked in her room, in your room, even got up in the goddamn attic, and I can't find it."

"Can't find what?"

"The *plata*. I can't find her *plata*."

Carr puts his hand out in the darkness and finds the back of a chair. It fails to anchor him in the present.

Plata. Carr gave it that name, the family story went, when he was three or so, and speaking his first words of Spanish. They were in Lima, and the *plata* was an S. T. Dupont cigarette lighter, a tiny, weighty slab of silver that the young Carr liked to play with. It was a gift to his mother from her sometimes tennis partner, the courtly, ever-smiling Sr. Farías—commemorating not only their success in the Club Regatas mixed doubles tournament, but also his appreciation of Andrea Carr's help in landing the Spanish journalist an interview with the new American ambassador.

Hector Farías turned up all over Latin America, bouncing from country to country at least as often as the Carrs. And whenever they found themselves living in the same cities, Farías and Andrea Carr resumed their tennis. Carr's recollections of him are mostly blurred and, he knows, mostly composites. Farías in tennis whites, drink in hand, his hair wavy

and damp, his teeth like white tiles. Farías at a consular reception, his shirt like a cloud, his shoes like glass, smoke curling from his smiling mouth. Farías on the living room sofa, straightening his tie, tugging at his cuffs, grinning at Carr, while his mother, cheeks burning, stepped quickly to the window and smoothed her skirts. Which living room was that?

His clearest memory of Farías, though, is from a photograph in a Buenos Aires newspaper. It was already three months old when he saw it on his father's desk, and they'd been in Stockbridge for almost that long, sorting through boxes others had packed for them so hurriedly in Mexico City. The unannounced visits from the dark-suited, block-shouldered men, their long discussions with his parents—together and separately—behind closed doors, the trips his parents made to Boston and Washington, had all grown less frequent. It was a good photo—not grainy at all—Farías with a trench coat over his broad shoulders, flanked by a pair of uniformed policemen, his hands thrust awkwardly before him, the handcuffs snug around his wrists. *Un Espía Cubano* was the caption.

"I can't find it," Arthur Carr says again.

"Why do you want it?" Carr asks.

"It's none of your goddamn business why I want it. Maybe I want to light a cigar. Maybe I want to burn down the house. Why the hell do you care? I just want it."

Carr drops into the chair and looks out at the empty night. He sighs again. "You're not going to find it."

"Because she took it. I told you, she takes things."

"Mrs. Calvin didn't take it."

"Then where the hell is it?"

"It's in the . . . It's with her—with Mom. You buried it with her, Dad."

24

"A full boat," Howard Bessemer says to Bobby. "Jacks over eights." He sweeps the chips from the center of the dining table into the large pile already in front of him. "It's just not your night."

It is nine a.m., and sunlight is streaming through the windows of Bessemer's dining room, reflecting from the white plaster walls, refracting through the crystal ashtray, the highball glasses, the bottle of gin on the table, and the curtain of smoke above.

He turns to Carr and smiles. "Top of the mornin', Gregory," he says. Bessemer is a dissipated teddy bear today, in seersucker pajama bottoms, a New York Athletic Club T-shirt, and a three-day beard that is a dirty-blond shadow on his pudgy cheeks. His blond hair is bent at odd angles, his gumdrop eyes are red and shiny, and so is the new cut at the corner of his mouth. He picks a joint from the ashtray, lights it, and takes a long hit. "Deal you in?" he asks.

"Not just now, Howie," Carr says, and he hands Bobby one of the grocery bags he's carrying. "Let's make coffee."

Bobby follows Carr to the kitchen and empties the bag onto the counter. Egg sandwiches, bagels, fruit salad in a plastic tub. There's a TV on the counter and Carr switches it on and turns up the volume. He tosses Bobby a pound of ground coffee. "Late night?" Carr asks, his voice low.

"Howie couldn't sleep. He wanted to play cards, so we played."

"You get high too?"

Bobby yawns and flips him the bird. "Yeah, baby, I'm trippin' on Coca-Cola and potato chips."

"You hit him?" Carr asks. Bobby spoons coffee into the machine. "Bobby?" Carr says again. Bobby fills the coffeemaker with water and presses the button. He looks at Carr but stays silent. "Bobby?"

"It was nothing. Mike was a little torqued up, and Howie was whining about something and Mike told him to shut up. Howie got mouthy and Mike got pissed."

"And hit him."

"Barely."

"For chrissakes, Bobby, we need him in one piece."

"Hey, I broke it up right away. And it's not like we're keeping the guy around long-term."

Carr frowns. "While we've got him, we need him happy."

"I'm down like two hundred bucks to the guy. That's not happy enough?"

Carr shakes his head. "What's got Mike twisted up?"

"Who the fuck knows?" Bobby says, unwrapping a sandwich. "It's gettin' so he's almost as moody a bastard as you."

Bessemer has finished his joint when Carr carries a sandwich and a cup of coffee into the dining room, and he's stacking his chips into neat columns before him.

"I make it two hundred fifteen dollars I've taken off him," he says.

"He's good for it. Sorry about the bruise."

Bessemer shrugs. "Your other friend is kind of an asshole, Greg. No fun to hang with at all."

"He'll take it easy as long as you do, Howie. Everybody's a little stir-crazy, and the sooner we move things along, the better."

"Amen to that," Bessemer says, and takes a slug of gin. Carr takes the glass from him and slides the sandwich and coffee in front of him.

"Let's do breakfast now, Howie. Then we'll do the story."

It takes Bessemer two sandwiches, three cups of coffee, and a long shower before he's ready, and then he and Carr settle in Bessemer's office. Sunlight seeps around the edges of the shades, but Carr leaves them drawn. He sits at the desk and turns on a brass lamp. Bessemer sprawls in a studded leather chair.

"Take it from the top, Howie," Carr says.

And Bessemer does. He's got the facts down cold: how he met Greg Frye in Otisville, where Frye was serving out the last months of a federal sentence for trafficking in stolen diamonds; how Frye had helped him learn the ropes there, and avoid the predations of the rougher trade; how they've kept in touch over the years; and how Frye has come down to Palm Beach in search of a banker, and—possibly—a business partner. And his delivery is solid: offhand, uncomplicated, adorned with enough detail to be convincing, but not enough to be dangerous. Bessemer is an apt pupil—at home with deception—but Carr knows that drills are one thing and live fire something else entirely.

Bessemer yawns and rubs his eyes. "I might crash right here, Greg," he says.

"Not yet," Carr says. "You think Prager's going to be interested?"

Bessemer smiles. "You're asking me now? I thought you knew it all."

There's a drinks tray on the credenza behind the desk, and Carr pours a gin and hands it to Bessemer. "You actually know the guy."

Bessemer sits up, and curiosity sparks in his bloodshot eyes. He sips at the gin. "Curt will be interested enough to talk. Why wouldn't he be? I've referred clients to Isla Privada before, and even if he doesn't take them on, he always talks. Talking's free, he says. Besides, he'll like the synergy."

"Meaning?"

"Meaning a client who can broaden his business model is better than a plain old client to him. Curt will like the idea of taking your money—assuming there's enough of it—but he'll like the diamonds even more. Someone who can take cash in exchange for diamonds, and who can do it in quantity—that's going to appeal to him. Diamonds are a lot easier to move than cash. And if you tell him you've got a network of people around the world who can do the transaction in reverse—take in diamonds and pay out cash—well, that's a new model." Bessemer takes another drink and smiles at Carr. "Assuming your story is solid."

"It is."

"Because if it isn't—if it's not granite—"

"It is, Howard."

"You're confident," Bessemer says, finishing his drink. "That's good."

"You should be confident too. You should be thinking about what you want to do afterward, when you get your money back."

Bessemer sighs and looks at his empty glass. "I have been thinking about it."

"And?"

Bessemer furrows his broad brow. "I don't know. I'm skittish about making plans. Seems whenever I do, things never work out. Sometimes I think the best way for me to make sure that I *don't* do something is for me to make a plan to do it."

Carr shakes his head. "Kind of self-defeating, isn't it?"

"Self-defeat's my best thing."

"Maybe this is an opportunity to turn over a new leaf."

"That kind of plan is always the most disappointing."

"Then start small."

Bessemer nods slowly. "I could get myself cleaned up—lose some weight, ease up on this." He holds up his glass. "Maybe try to get fit."

"All good ideas."

"Then maybe I could spend some time with my kid. He's twelve now, and I haven't seen him in . . . a long time."

"Baby steps, Howie. Baby steps."

Bessemer stretches out on the office sofa and dozes. He shifts around occasionally and murmurs words that Carr can't make out. Asleep he looks younger, Carr thinks, and much like his son. Carr empties ashtrays and fills the dishwasher and makes himself another cup of coffee. He looks out the window, at a jet crossing the sky, and thinks about Tina, flying down to Santiago, and Guerrero, who may have been Declan's pilot. He thinks about Declan, and his hastily sketched exit plan from Mendoza, and he remembers Valerie's words on the wharf in Portland.

You're remembering a different guy, she said, and Carr knows she's right. Sometimes it seems that he's remembering several different guys. It's like a hall of mirrors, and everywhere there's a version of Declan— short, tall, skinny, fat . . .

There's the grinning red pirate who recruited him in Mexico; the wise mentor who taught him the ropes; and the tough, charismatic soldier who executed plans with precision and economy, improvised like Coltrane whenever things went sideways, and always led from the front.

Then there's the melancholy, whiskey-voiced raconteur, sitting in a

darkened bar, spinning out tales of his days in the service—in Ireland, the Middle East, and at unnamed stops along the Silk Road—of the hell he raised with other crews, and the swag he hauled away. And there is the weary campaigner, aging, aching, and contemplating retirement with a mix of anticipation and dread. Those incarnations didn't turn up often, and when they did it was always just before a job, or just after one.

And then there's the Declan Valerie had in mind—the erratic, reckless Declan, the willful, capricious one. It's hard—impossible, really—for Carr to reconcile her version with those others, but he can't say he hasn't seen them before. He has, in bits and pieces, several times over the years. And especially toward the end.

He hears Valerie's voice again: *There was César, and before that the Russians.* They were the last jobs they worked, before Mendoza, and she was right about them—Declan hadn't been at his best.

César was a transporter, and he'd ship pretty much anything to any-place, according to Mr. Boyce and Tina. He'd started out, like so many in the region, with drug shipments, and found natural synergies in the movement of small arms and cash. Then, in the early years of the new century, he diversified into transporting heavier weapons, hijacked elec-tronics, pirated software and DVDs, and human traffic headed north. Despite his success, or perhaps because he kept so busy spending its fruits on hookers, Ferraris, and thoroughbred horses, César had, over the years, underinvested badly in his own security infrastructure.

"I've seen 7-Elevens with tighter perimeters," Tina had said.

The perimeter she was talking about was in Puerto Barrios, Guatemala, around a waterfront compound where César kept an office, some odds and ends of his shipments—a pallet or two of flat-screen TVs, a crate of RPGs—a climate-controlled garage for some of his Testarossas, and $6.8 million in shrink-wrapped packs of hundred-dollar bills. The money was in a cinder-block annex to the Ferrari garage, and it should've been a simple job—three sleepy guards, a fence to scale, a video feed to interrupt, an alarm system barely worth the name, and a safe room that wasn't. In and out, unseen and unheard, in seventeen minutes flat. It should've been simple, but it wasn't, because Declan developed some-thing of a mania for César.

Not that that was difficult to do. César was unlikable in the extreme—a thug, a beater of women and children, a liar, a casual killer, and an all-

around swine. Though he was, in truth, no worse than any of the other people they stole from, Declan had for some reason decided that he was.

"I think it's his girth, boys," he confessed over beer one night in a Puerto Barrios bar. "He's such a fat fuck, and he dresses like . . . What's he dress like, Bobby?"

"Like an L.A. pimp, Deke, circa 1977."

"Not even that well, lad. And he's an insult to those cars of his. I just don't know how he jams his guts behind the wheel." It was a running joke through all their planning, and then, on the night of the job, in an instant it wasn't.

Carr was on the fence, and Declan, Bobby, and Ray-Ray had the safe room. Carr watched through the nightscope as Bobby and Ray-Ray came out, bags over shoulders, and headed toward him.

"Where's Deke?" Carr said into his headset.

There was a pause, a whispered chuckle, and then Declan's raspy voice. "Leavin' a little something for that feckin' sack," he said, and Carr saw him in the doorway of the Ferrari garage—saw him pitch something in under-handed, and then come running.

"Might want to add some quick, lads," he said, and then the night lit up with an orange flash, a muffled blast, a symphony of breaking glass, and a shock wave that Carr felt even fifty yards away. He tore the nightscope from his head.

"What the fuck?" Bobby and Ray-Ray shouted, nearly in unison.

Declan was laughing when he reached them, and laughing later that night, when they passed a bottle around in the cabin of a sport fisher, halfway to Belize.

"He didn't deserve those cars, the fat shite. All I did was restore order to the universe. And what the fuck was he gonna do with that box of pineapples anyway? Nothing so productive, I'll guarantee you." He looked at Carr. "Why're you being a feckin' old woman about it, anyway? It's fire-works is all—nothing to fret over. It's like a tonic."

Bobby and Mike and Dennis and Ray-Ray had laughed with him; Carr and Valerie had not.

Nobody was laughing after Nicaragua, though. The Russians were called Dudek, and they were actually from Ukraine—two cousins who cashed out of the army and headed west when the Evil Empire dissolved. And weapons were their specialty. They bought them, sold them, shipped

them, serviced them, and trained clients in their use. And unlike César, they did not leave piles of money about in cinder-block sheds. They did, however, keep some petty cash on hand—$5.1 million, more or less—in a safe in the back office of Dudek Air Charter, not far from the Managua airport. The safe was a serious one, as was the security around it, which relied less on technology than it did on the presence of many guys with guns.

Carr hadn't liked the job at first, hadn't seen a way of doing it that didn't devolve into a full-on firefight, but Declan had pushed, and eventually he'd come up with a plan. It relied on distraction, misdirection, and some painfully tight timings, but if it played as written, it would get them in and out without a shot fired. Carr was pleased with it; Declan less so. It was late, and they were sitting in the shitty kitchen of a shitty house, in a city—Managua—full of shitty houses.

"The way in is okay, I guess, but the exit is too clever by half. We'll have the swag in hand, fer chrissakes, we don't need yer feckin' floor show. We just head for the door."

"And do what," Carr had said, "shoot your way out? Those aren't rent-a-cops at Dudek, those are mercs—mostly kid mercs. They're not big on judgment or hesitation or worries about mortality—theirs or anyone else's. You light it up with them, it's not a halfway thing."

"I know who they are, boyo, and the last thing I need is a lecture on firefights. Not from you. I'm saying yer plan is riskier than it has to be because yer shy when it comes to heavy lifting—you always have been. You're delicate, so to avoid the shootin' you have us wastin' time in that stairwell, while you sing and dance. Well, I say that's a higher risk. I'd rather do the shootin' than wait around fer someone to do it to me."

"I'm talking about a series of flash-bangs on the other side of the building, to draw them off. I'm talking about a wait of a minute, ninety seconds tops. We make some noise, and then you leave, and if you do meet people on the way out, you'll meet fewer of them."

"So you say. But what're you so worried about, boyo—you'll be on the outside, out of harm's way."

"There are risks we can minimize, and risks we can't. The exit plan falls in the first category. If I'm worried about anything, it's that you don't see that. I'm talking about a minute, Deke, a minute and a half tops."

"You shy because they're kids? Is that it?"

They went back and forth like that, until the sky grew pale and everyone but Latin Mike agreed with Carr, and Mike stayed silent. Finally—peevishly—Declan folded. And then, three nights later, as he and Bobby and Mike were on their way out of the Dudek Air Charter building, he changed his mind.

No one laughed after that. Not Bobby or Mike, who had taken a round through his right arm and who Carr had never seen so pale, and not Declan, who'd taken a round in his left thigh and killed three child soldiers along the way. The wound didn't seem to bother Declan much on the drive west, from Managua to the Pacific coast, nor did it stop Carr.

"We had a plan," Carr said.

Declan's smile was thin and cold. "You know what they say about those, boyo: they don't survive the first shot."

"We all agreed on it."

"And since when was this a feckin' democracy?"

Carr stared for a long while, and then shook his head. "What the fuck is the matter with you?" he whispered. Declan stopped smiling, but had no other answer.

It's nearly nightfall when Mike arrives, and there are clouds in the darkening sky, and approaching thunder. Mike has a six of Corona under one arm, and a bucket of fried chicken under the other.

"Howie's still sleeping," Carr says, as he passes Mike in the doorway. "Don't hit him again." Mike starts to say something, but Carr keeps walking.

·

Dennis is eating dinner when Carr arrives, a Cuban sandwich and a beer. He's bent over a laptop, wearing headphones, and he doesn't look up when Carr opens the door. Carr raps on the table, and Dennis starts and pulls the phones off.

"I'm looking at the latest from Chun's place—the wires Vee laid down."

Carr pulls a chair alongside Dennis's. "And?" he asks.

Dennis colors. "It's good," he says. "Actually, it's great."

The image is clear, despite the low light: Amy Chun in her home office. The tiny camera is planted in a bookshelf behind her desk, and the view is over and above her right shoulder. She's wearing a sleeveless white shirt,

and there's a mug of tea steaming in a corner of her desk, next to her cell phone. She is pushing aside the keyboard of her home computer and opening up the laptop she carries every day to and from her office suite at the Spanish River Bank and Trust Company.

"Laptop keyboard is nice and clear," Dennis says. "Vee did a good job with placement."

Chun takes a fingerprint scanner from the desk drawer and plugs it into the laptop. From her purse she takes something like a keychain fob, with a tiny LCD strip down the center—an automatic password generator. A log-on window opens on the laptop, and she types in a password, one part of it from memory, and the rest from the screen of the password generator. Another window comes up, and Chun presses her thumb onto the fingerprint scanner. The laptop screen flickers and then her cell phone chimes. Chun picks it up, listens, picks up the password generator again, and keys a code from its screen into her cell phone. The laptop screen flickers again and she's into the network shared by the Spanish River Bank and Trust, and the rest of the banks owned by Isla Privada.

Carr shakes his head. "We knew how all that worked, we could save ourselves a lot of trouble."

Dennis stiffens beside him. His tone is frosty. "It's a virtual private network with multifactor authorization, including an out-of-band security feature, and I know exactly *how* it all works. What I'm missing is the checksum for Chun's thumbprint, the algorithm her key fob is using to generate those one-time passwords, and the authentication chip inside her laptop. If I had all that, *and* Chun's private password, *and* a phone on the network's call-back list, then we wouldn't need Vee in there at all, and I could log on to the Isla Privada network whenever I wanted. Give me Curtis Prager's private password on top of that, and we could all go home right now. Now *that* would save us trouble."

Carr suppresses a laugh. "I stand corrected," he says quietly. "We got Chun's part, though, didn't we?"

"We got it," Dennis says. "We got her password and we got account numbers."

"Nice job," Carr says, and claps him on the shoulder. "What else is on the tape?"

"Vee comes on," Dennis says, blushing. He fast-forwards several minutes, and a shadow crosses Amy Chun's desk. A moment later, Valerie's—

Jill's—hip leans against Chun's arm. She's wearing a short white T-shirt and panties with lace trim, and she's carrying a rocks glass. Carr can't tell what's in it, but he can hear the ice. Jill rests her arm on Chun's back.

"I'll miss you," Jill says.

"It's just a day," Chun says, looking up at her. "New York and back. I'll be home before eleven."

"You'll call me?"

"Why don't you meet me here?" Chun says, and she slides her hand beneath Jill's shirt.

Jill inhales sharply and her hips shift. Her voice is choked. "Hurry and finish," she says, and she exits the frame to the tinkle of ice.

"Christ," Dennis whispers.

Carr lets out a deep breath. "Is that it?"

Dennis blushes again. "There's more . . . in the bedroom. The light is low, so the picture's not great, and the AC is blowing, so the sound is—"

"Play it."

Dennis clicks on another video file, and a dim, sepia-shadowed image appears: a heap of pillows, a tangle of dark blankets, two pale blurs on a paler, rectangular field. There is the faint shifting of sheets, the sound of someone drinking, someone sighing.

Amy Chun's voice is a tentative whisper. "Have you been . . . *out* for a long time?"

Valerie—Jill—laughs. Her voice is sleepy and soft. "I never thought about it that way; I never was really *in*. I've known how I felt since grade school, and I've never pretended anything different."

"Your parents?"

"They were too busy fighting with each other to pay much attention to me. I was in college before they noticed."

"They didn't care?"

"If they did, I didn't notice, and pretty soon I was out of there."

"My parents would notice," Amy Chun whispers, "even from Vancouver. And they would care. So would my board of directors."

"It's your life, Amy, not theirs. Your one-and-only life, and your happiness."

"Coming out is no guarantee of happiness."

"Nope—I know plenty of unhappy couples—of all persuasions. But *not* coming out—that *is* a guarantee."

Sheets rustle and someone exhales slowly. There's a sound of ice in a glass. "I'm happy now," Amy Chun says quietly. "Happier than I've been. Definitely happier than my parents are."

"They don't get along?"

"Never."

"It doesn't always have to be like that, you know—like my parents, and yours."

There's more shifting, and a giggle. "No?" Amy Chun asks.

"Maybe that's what we should do, you and me," she whispers. "Go away together and conduct a little research, to find some happy couples. We'll be like archaeologists."

There's more sighing and rustling, and the clip ends. Dennis lets out a long breath and pushes back from the table. "She is good," he says. "Sincere. Believable. Like scary good."

Carr looks at the image frozen on the screen—two women, bare, clinging to each other in the wreckage of the bed. He nods but doesn't speak.

25

All subtropical financial districts look alike, Carr thinks. The broad, divided boulevards; the lush foliage at street level; the towers soaring above; the German cars at curbside, each with tinted glass and a large, watchful driver; the overcaffeinated, expensively suited young men who stride along, mesmerized by their BlackBerrys and chattering maniacally into the ether; the young women—stylish, tanned, with impossible heels, impossible legs, impossible self-possession. It could be Avenida Paulista, Avenida Balboa, or a stretch of Reforma, but it's not. It's Brickell Avenue in Miami, and Carr is walking north, following Valerie.

· He's kept his distance all the way down 95, but now she's out of her car and he's out of his, and he needs to be careful. The lunchtime rush helps and hurts: Carr hides in the crowd, but so does Valerie, and he's nearly lost her twice since she gave her car to the valet at the Four Seasons and set out on foot. It's clear today, and cooler than it has been, but that just means it feels like ninety-something. Carr's shirt is stuck to his back, but Valerie, when he catches a glimpse, looks cool and crisp in a pale gray skirt and sleeveless white blouse. She crosses Brickell and heads west on Tenth Street.

Bessemer's call to Curtis Prager that morning was anticlimactic. Sitting in his dim office, Carr at his side, Bessemer had phoned Prager's private number, only to learn that Prager is away until tomorrow, and please try

again. And so an unexpected day off for Carr. He'd consigned Bessemer to Bobby's care, driven down to Boca Raton, and phoned Valerie from a spot fifty yards from her apartment building. Where she'd lied to him.

"I could drive down," he'd said, "and take a room. We could have lunch at the beach."

Valerie had yawned loudly. "That sounds nice, baby—really nice—but I've got to get some rest. I've been up late every night this week, and I'm supposed to meet Amy again tonight. I've got the drapes closed, and I'm going back to sleep."

Carr wasn't sure why he hadn't believed her, why he'd waited in his parked car after she'd hung up, why he'd followed her little Audi, half an hour later, when it pulled out of the building lot and made its way to 95. Maybe it was because her yawn had been too elaborate, or because he could see from his parking space that her drapes were wide open. Maybe it was the memory of her conversation with Amy Chun, the night before, and what she'd said to him back in Portland. *Maybe that's what we should do, you and me—go away together and conduct a little research, to find some happy couples. We'll be like archaeologists.*

She turns north again at First Avenue and passes beneath the elevated tracks of the light-rail. She crosses the street, to a compact shopping plaza in the shadow of the Metromover, and goes into a coffee bar. Carr keeps walking on Tenth Street, enters the plaza from Miami Avenue, and stands in the shade of a stunted, bushy palm tree. The coffee bar is busy, but through the wide front window Carr can see Valerie slipping through the crowd toward the back of the room. He edges closer and sees her settle on a bar stool at a narrow counter along the side wall, in front of a keyboard, a mouse, and a monitor.

Carr can't make out the screen from where he is, but Valerie reads for a while and then types. She's at the computer for about three minutes, and then she pushes away from the counter and leaves through the back door.

Carr jogs into the coffee bar, shouldering past customers and ignoring the angry looks. A twenty-something man in linen pants, a Daddy Yankee T-shirt, and lots of body ink has a hand on Valerie's bar-stool when Carr steps in front of him.

"Hey, I'm sitting here, man," he says, and he puts his coffee cup on the counter.

"You definitely are," Carr says softly, "in about thirty seconds." Carr finds the browser icon on the desktop and clicks on it.

"I'm sitting here *now*, man," the twenty-something says, "so get the hell out of my way."

"Yep, absolutely," Carr says, watching the browser open, "I'm out of here."

"You talk, but you don't move your ass." The twenty-something puts a hand on Carr's arm and pulls, and his face seizes up in a grimace. Carr has his hand around the man's wrist and fingers and has bent them back at impossible angles. The twenty-something's face is pale and his knees begin to buckle, and Carr eases up on the finger lock.

"Another second," Carr whispers, and he opens the browser history. The screen is empty and Carr stares at it a moment and says: "Fuck." Then he hits the back door at a run, leaving the twenty-something rubbing his wrist and gasping and the few patrons who've noticed anything shaking their heads.

She's a block and a half down First Avenue, walking in the shade of the Metromover tracks, and Carr is just in time to see her turn east on Eighth Street, back toward Brickell Avenue. He sprints to close the gap.

She walks briskly down Eighth Street and crosses Brickell as the light changes. Carr waits on the other side of the street and watches Valerie disappear into a tower of white stone and green glass.

When Carr steps into the building, Valerie is nowhere in sight, and security is already eyeing him. And why not—no one else in the lobby is as rumpled as he is, or as damp with sweat. He walks over to the building directory and scans the list of tenants. Software companies, law firms, management consultants, but more than anything else banks and brokerages. And, Carr notices, mostly foreign firms.

"Can I help you, sir?" the guard asks. He's big and uniformed, and so is his hovering partner.

"Think I got the wrong address," Carr says, and he exits into the midday heat.

There's a Starbucks next door to the building, and a wine bar on the opposite corner. Carr likes the sight lines from the wine bar better, though neither are perfect: there are too many ways out of the green tower. Still,

he takes a window seat and orders a bottle of soda water and a ham sandwich on a baguette.

The traffic churns past on Brickell while Carr eats and watches and wonders. What was Valerie doing in the coffee bar, where she had no time to drink coffee, but time enough to delete her browsing history? Surfing? Sending? And if sending, then sending to whom? And why do it there, when she has Internet access back in Boca Raton?

Privacy and anonymity are the obvious answers, and both worry Carr. He and his crew are the only people in a position to eavesdrop on Valerie's laptop. What might she be doing online that she'd want to hide from them? And who might she be doing it with?

After an hour, the lunch crowd has thinned on the street and in the wine bar, and the air-conditioning has dried him off, but Carr has seen no sign of Valerie. He worries that he's missed her in the wash of people, or that she's left another way, and he pays the check and steps outside. The humidity is like a wet hammer, and Carr is sweating before the light changes. There's a shaded plaza beside the green tower, with white pergolas, razor-straight rows of palm trees, tables with umbrellas, and a view through the lobby glass of the elevator banks. Carr heads for one of the tables, and when he stops in his tracks he's not sure at first what it is that's stopped him.

Something in the corner of his eye. Something he knows. Broad shoulders held just so, a thrusting gut, an aggressive, pumping gait—a familiar bulk. In the lobby, in the shuffling clutch of people at the elevator doors. When Carr picks him out, there's a rush of noise in his head—gears grinding on one another—and he's frozen, flat-footed, in the plaza. He might as well be waving a flag. It's sheer luck that Nando doesn't look over.

"What the fuck?" Carr says to no one, and he steps behind one of the manicured palms.

Nando crosses the lobby and pushes through the doors. He's wearing a tan suit and an open-collared French blue shirt, and he's carrying a tan briefcase. He's thicker and darker than when Carr last saw him, years ago in Costa Alegre, and more prosperous-looking than ever. He's on his cell as he crosses Brickell and heads south. He's still talking when he enters another office tower, this one clad in brushed metal and gray glass. He's alone in the elevator when the doors slide shut, and Carr watches the numbers climb to eight.

Security in the gray building is lazy, and no guards brace Carr as he

scans the lobby directory. The assortment of firms is only slightly differ-ent here—more lawyers, fewer consultants—but there are still plenty of foreign banks. The eighth floor, in fact, is nothing but banks.

Nando is inside for about an hour, after which Carr follows him down Brickell to another building—gold glass this time. Carr can't tell which floor he's headed to—there are too many people on the elevator with him—but there is no shortage of banks here either. Nando reappears fifty minutes later. Carr is buying gum at a lobby kiosk and readying himself for another walk in the heat when Nando turns not to the Brickell Avenue doors, but toward the back of the lobby and the enclosed passage that leads to the building's parking structure.

Carr comes down the passage in time to see Nando board an elevator. It stops on the third parking level and Carr jogs up the stairs. He comes out of the stairwell and hears footsteps echoing, a car door closing, and an engine turning over.

"Shit," he whispers, and he waits at the stairs as Nando drives by in a white rental.

Back on the sidewalk, Carr looks up and down Brickell Avenue, but sees no sign of Nando's car, or of Valerie. He walks up the street to the gray tower with the lax security. Around the corner he finds the tower's four-level parking structure and, on its lowest level, the loading dock. There's security there—two guys in rumpled uniform shirts and sneakers—but they seem only semiconscious. Carr checks the block and climbs a low wall into the parking structure. He bounces hard on the fenders of three parked cars—Lexus, BMW, Rover—and their lights flash and their horns blare. He steps behind a wide pillar, and when the security slackers wan-der over to investigate the alarms, Carr slips into the loading dock and into the service elevator and rides to eight.

Three banks—all foreign—have offices on the eighth floor, but only one has a reception desk. The blonde behind it looks barely out of middle school, and she has a fizzy voice and a manic smile.

"How can I help you today?" she says.

Carr puts on a beaten look. "I'm hoping you can help me out with my boss," he says. "He's was in here a while ago, and he thinks he left his BlackBerry. Now he is rip-roarin' pissed—like it's my fault he can't keep track of his stuff."

The girl nods in solidarity and sympathetic understanding of irra-tional bosses. "I haven't seen anything lying around."

"He was in about two hours ago. Black-haired guy, big, dark, in a tan suit and a blue shirt."

The blonde nods. "New accounts," she says, and she picks up the phone. "Britty, you find a BlackBerry over there? That new client, Mr. Reyes—he thinks he might've left his here." She listens and nods and smiles at Carr. "She's checking," she tells him. Then she listens again and frowns. "Thanks anyway, babe," she says into the phone, and she shakes her head.

He is barely aware of the walk back to the Four Seasons, and surprised to find himself there. More surprised to find that Valerie's car is still in the lot. He gets into his own car and finds a spot with a view of the hotel entrance and waits.

The afternoon rush washes about him, and so do the questions. Mr. Reyes? New accounts? What is Nando doing in Miami? And what the *fuck* is he doing with Valerie? The questions spin around like water in a drain, and there's orange in the sky when he realizes he hasn't been watching the hotel, or anyway that he hasn't been seeing it.

A dinner crowd is arriving, and the valets cast long shadows as they dart among the idling cars. Carr watches them run, and watches the pretty crowd disappear inside, through the revolving doors. And then he sees a couple step out. The woman is first, and Carr recognizes Valerie right away, though her blouse is untucked now, and her hair is damp, as if from a bath. It takes him a moment longer to recognize the man, who pauses in the doorway and then walks forward, slips a thick arm around Valerie's waist, and rests a large hand on her hip. Mike.

26

"You're not yourself this morning, Greg," Bessemer says to Carr. "Need some more coffee?" He reaches across the kitchen counter and fills his mug.

Latin Mike looks at Carr with no expression, and Carr looks back. "I'm going now," Mike says, and Carr nods.

Bessemer squints at him, curiosity plain on his round face. "Rough night?"

And it hasn't ended yet, Carr thinks. The rum brought him no sleep, and even now there's a blur around the borders of things, and a hollow echo to every sound. His thoughts want to wander, to drift sideways, to skid. They steer the wrong way and then hit the gas until the skid becomes a dizzying spin.

They left the hotel separately—Mike first, then Valerie. Carr followed Valerie back to Boca, back to her apartment, then out again to Amy Chun's place. After an hour of watching dark windows, he left her there. Then he drove back to North Palm Beach and started to pace. Sometime past midnight the drinking began.

Drinking, pacing, replaying how many moments, again and again, in his head. Poolside at Chamela. Her apartment in Port of Spain. More workhouses and hotel rooms than he could count. And more questions. When did his suspicions begin? What set them off? When did she meet

Nando, and how? Why, along with the sensation of having missed a stair, does he feel something equally jarring—something a lot like relief?

Round and round he went, unable or unwilling to get to the middle of it, to get a purchase on the central problem: the dimensions of her betrayal. What has she done? What is she in the midst of doing? Who is she doing it with? Who can he trust, and what the hell should he do?

Howard Bessemer is still holding the coffeepot, still squinting at him. "Are we going to make that call today, Greg?"

Carr looks at him but says nothing.

Drinking, pacing, staring at the ocean. *What the hell should he do?* His options are limited to exactly two: finish the Prager job, or cut and run—and the second choice is more or less a nonstarter. Mr. Boyce has fronted a lot of cash on this job, and if Carr decides to fold, he's going to want it back—and with a nice return. Yes, Boyce is currently holding the diamonds the crew picked up in Houston, and they'll go some way to paying off the debt, but Carr has no intention of being stuck with the balance. Neither does he want to spend the rest of his life looking over his shoulder, waiting for Tina to appear.

Sometime before dawn, he decided he couldn't stand his apartment any longer, and he walked across the road to the beach, leaving his shoes at the edge of the sand but bringing the rum. The sand was cold, and in the moonlight the breakers looked like white smoke rolling toward him.

He thought of Tina and looked over his shoulder and laughed out loud at the notion of telling Boyce what was going on. Or rather telling him that *something* was going on, but that Carr didn't know exactly what it was. Not much of a thought, really—not much of an option. At best, Boyce would pull the plug on the job himself, and still want his money back. More likely, he'd decide the whole shit storm was an unacceptable breach of operational security—a terminal breach. And there, over Carr's shoulder, would be Tina again.

Walking down the beach, he stepped on something slippery and colder than the sand. A jellyfish. He braced for the sting, but felt nothing and kept walking.

The bottom line is, he needs Prager's money, needs what it can buy. A few months back he'd calculated that he had enough put away to do what he wanted for as long as he wanted, but that calculation is out of date. His father's situation and Mrs. Calvin's impending departure have thrown his cash flow assumptions to the wind. He needs the money.

Bessemer clears his throat once . . . twice. "I'm thinking that maybe you're not into this today, Greg—that your mind is elsewhere. Greg?"

So, finish the job. Easy enough to say, but it begs the question of who he can trust while he's doing it. He's been asking himself that since Declan's death, or maybe even before, but now it's acquired a particular urgency.

Working the paranoid calculus—that's what his instructor at the Farm had called it, an atypically neat turn of phrase from an otherwise lumpish fellow. Tracing the lattice of connections, mapping the shifting landscape of who-owes-who and who-owns-who, of loyalty, grudge, and pressure. Who's in bed with whom? Who's working what angle? Who benefits? Nando and Valerie. Valerie and Mike. If Mike, then Bobby as well? They were both in Mendoza, after all. And what about Dennis?

The answer—the short answer—is to trust none of them, not for a second, not as far as he can throw them, not even half that far. But nothing is ever so straightforward. The practical truth is, if he's going to finish the Prager job, then he needs them—all of them. And they need him. They have to trust one another to carry out their assigned work—to watch one another's backs. Like birds of a feather and bugs in a rug, arms linked in a chorus of "Kumbaya." Thick as fucking thieves—right up until the moment they transfer the money out of Isla Privada's accounts. Then the question becomes how to survive their success.

Dawn found him standing frozen at the shoreline, surrounded—as if in a minefield—by acres of clumped seaweed and the glistening bodies of jellyfish. His ankles ached with cold, and his head was filled with shuffling images of burned and broken metal, Declan's skewed grin and blackened limbs, and Valerie in the dark. He could almost summon her smell and the feel of her skin, but the rising light and the ocean breeze swept his conjuring away. Surprise? Sadness? Anger? Relief? Like the seaweed, they're tangled too thoroughly for Carr to pick apart.

Bessemer is standing now, a look of alarm replacing the curiosity on his face. "Are we calling or not?"

Carr looks at him. "Pour me another cup of coffee," he says, "and get the telephone."

27

They're followed from the airport on Grand Cayman—two men in a muddy blue Nissan, as inconspicuous as it's possible for a single-car tail to be. Carr spots them as he turns the Toyota onto Dorcy Drive.

"They were at the rental counter," he says, "but that's not a rental car." Bessemer starts to turn in his seat, but Carr puts a hand on his arm. "Use the mirrors," he says. Bessemer does, and his brows crease in confusion.

"The driver was outside passport control," Carr says, "but he wasn't on our flight."

"You think they're following us?"

"I know they are. You ever see them before?"

"I don't think so," Bessemer says, and there's worry in his voice.

"This a usual thing for Prager?"

Bessemer shakes his head. "If it is, I never noticed."

They're quiet after that. Bessemer watches the Nissan in the rearview. Carr watches traffic and looks at the landscape of the northern edge of George Town, which is flat, cluttered, and homely under a pale sky. Carr lowers his window and the smell of ocean rushes in, mixed with odors of asphalt and exhaust and brackish salt marsh. He glances at Bessemer, who is still looking in the mirrors, and whose face has tightened with fear.

"Strip malls and SUVs," Carr says. "Just like Florida."

Bessemer nods stiffly. "The north side's nicer. This your first time

down here?" Carr smiles but doesn't answer, and Bessemer's eyes dart back to the mirror.

"They're just watching, Howie. They're not going to do anything."

Bessemer's nerves have been fraying since the call to Curtis Prager, which, when it finally happened three days before, had gone as well as Carr could've hoped. Bessemer had stayed on script and had managed to sound convincing about it. And, because Prager doesn't like phones, he hadn't had to talk for long. Bessemer told Prager that a good friend, Greg Frye, was in town, looking for a money manager. *And when I heard about the business opportunity Greg's got, I thought of you right away, Curt.*

Prager asked how good a friend this was and how Bessemer knew him. When Bessemer explained that he was an Otisville friend, Prager went silent for a long while—so long that Carr wondered if they'd been cut off. When Prager finally responded, he was brief.

"You know I'm always happy to meet prospective investors, Bess. So if you've got the time, you and your friend should come down here. We'll hit some balls, we'll put some lines in the water, and we'll see what bites."

Bessemer started fretting as soon as he hung up. "I thought all you wanted was an introduction, Greg. I think I've held up my part of the bargain."

"So far, so good," Carr said.

"You never talked about a trip."

"It's a short trip, Howie."

"But you never said—"

"Prager invited both of us down. It would be a little awkward if I showed up by myself."

Bessemer paced and worried his lower lip. "It'll be awkward for me if Curtis thinks I've lied to him. Awkward as in dead."

"Don't be dramatic."

"*Dramatic?* I'm not the one holding somebody hostage in his own house, or blackmailing him into being part of some kind of scam. I'm not the dramatic one."

Carr had almost smiled. "Don't be so negative, Howie. This doesn't have to be complicated: we go down there, we hang out, and then we're done. Stay focused on what you get out of this: your money, your life back, a fresh start."

"I don't know," Bessemer said, shaking his head and walking to his liquor cabinet.

"The upside, Howie—focus on the upside."

They're on Tibbetts Highway now, the Nissan still with them, a quarter-mile back. They come up a gentle rise and on his left, beyond the big hotels, Carr sees the beaches, the ocean, and the cruise ships at anchor, each one as graceless as a Soviet apartment block. Away to his right, North Sound is like a pale blue plate, and the feathered wake of a powerboat like a fracture line across it. Closer on the right is the broad dome of a landfill, with a thousand white gulls wheeling above. Carr glances at Bessemer, who is drumming his fingers on the armrest and still staring at the mirrors. Carr understands nerves—his own are like confetti.

He saw Valerie the day before he left Palm Beach. She drove up while Amy was at work, and he took a room at the Marriott. She said not a word about Miami or Nando or Mike, and Carr managed not to ask. Managed not to speak much at all that afternoon, unless spoken to—and there wasn't much of that at first. Later, when the sheets and pillows were on the floor and they were sideways on the bed, Valerie had questions of her own.

"They're set up down there?" she asked.

"Dennis went yesterday. Bobby and Mike go tonight."

"They must be happy to get out of that dump."

"They were getting stir-crazy. Forward motion calms everybody down."

"Everybody, including you?"

"I want to get it done as much as anyone."

"And afterward?" she asked softly, and slid a bare foot up his calf. "You ever been to New Zealand? It's really something down there—Middle Earth, just like in the movies. I know a place where we could have a cottage to ourselves, just us, a few thousand acres, and some sheep. Nothing to see out the windows but cliffs and sky and ocean. What do you say— you take care of the airfare, and I'll pick up the tab at the Wharekauhau?"

"New Zealand's a long way."

"You can afford it. And besides, isn't that what you want—something far away?"

He had no answer for that, so he nodded vaguely and went into the bathroom. When he came out, Valerie was standing by the balcony doors.

She'd opened the drapes to the width of her shoulders, and she wore nothing but the long bar of light that came through the glass. Carr stared at her for some time, looking for he didn't know what. A mark? A sign? Some sort of clue? But there was nothing except that body, slender, wanton, tinted pale saffron by the streetlight. She turned to look at him, and her face, half in shadow, was suddenly exhausted.

"We moved a lot when I was a kid," she said quietly. "Base to base— never anyplace longer than a year or two. My mother was useless around the house, but my father could do things, and he'd always try to fix up whatever crappy billet we'd been assigned. He'd paint, hang pictures, plant a window box, that kind of thing. But those places weren't ours, and all the petunias in the world couldn't change it—couldn't make us belong somewhere. I get the feeling you know what that's like."

"I know."

"I'll be glad when this is done. I'm tired of hotels and furnished apartments and putting on these lives like somebody else's clothes. I want someplace I can sit still. Someplace that's mine." The air conditioner came on and she shivered in the breeze. She wrapped her arms around herself. "I want my skin back."

Carr swallowed hard, and Valerie stepped away from the window and began to collect her scattered clothes. "Something's on your mind," she whispered.

Did they show, he wondered—the questions that still spun through his head? He shrugged. "Prager, Bessemer, a bunch of things."

"You need help," she said. "Let me help you."

The resort grounds are vast: a golf course, clubhouse and marina on the sound, and, across West Bay Road, a curving, coral-pink hotel complex on Seven Mile Beach. The Nissan doesn't follow when Carr turns through the main gates, but any relief he feels is short-lived. There are two more men in the lobby, watching them from behind day-old newspapers.

28

They're in a fourth-floor corner suite—two bedrooms separated by a living room, a kitchenette, a wet bar, a terrace, and glary views of pool and ocean. While Bessemer explores the bar, Carr carries his bag to a bedroom and drops it on a luggage rack. He steps into the bathroom and runs water in both sinks. Then he opens his cell and calls Bobby.

"Not bad here," Bobby says. "You can practically smell the offshore cash."

"It's very fragrant," Carr says. "You guys clean when you came in from the airport?"

"Sure. Clean last night, clean today. Why?"

"Two guys were with us on the drive here, and another pair picked us up in the lobby. I see one of them down by the pool. I don't know where his partner is."

"You think they're Prager's?"

"I hope like hell they are," Carr says. "We don't need new players at the table."

"His security guy was supposed to be a joke."

"Maybe he's on the wagon again."

"Fucking drunks," Bobby says, "you can never count on 'em. I got your stuff; you want me to bring it over?"

"And you can check out the babysitters while you're at it. Howie and I

will take a walk around the grounds, starting with the bar by the pool. We'll meet you back here. You need a key to the suite?"

Bobby laughs. "Now you're just being a prick," he says, and hangs up.

The Caiman Lounge is a broad expanse of terra-cotta tile, bleached wood, and sliding glass doors that let the bar merge with the patio around the pool. Carr and Bessemer pause at the entrance. Carr doesn't see Bobby—doesn't see anyone besides a few off-season honeymooners sitting close. He and Bessemer take a table near a large aquarium. Carr orders an iced tea, and Bessemer a gin and tonic. Bessemer is transfixed by a green and blue triggerfish swimming lazily behind the glass.

"Ridiculous fish," he says. "Goofy-looking. It reminds me of my ex-mother-in-law."

"Triggers are aggressive," Carr says. "They'll take a chunk out of you if you get between them and the next meal."

"Definitely my ex-mother-in-law."

Carr nods, and then he spots the lobby men. One takes a seat at the bar and orders something. The other walks in from the pool patio, sits at a table in back, and studies a menu. Bessemer is rambling on about his former in-laws, and Carr tunes out to regard the minders from the corners of his eyes.

Polo shirts, thick necks, bristly haircuts, heavy, confounded brows, and a general air of unfocused anger. Corporate security types, he thinks—ex–law enforcement, ex-military—the kind of foot soldiers he used to hire and fire at Integral Risk. The waitress delivers their drinks, and Bessemer interrupts his ramble to clink glasses. Carr sits for another ten minutes, not listening to Bessemer, not looking for Bobby, and then he gets up.

"Let's walk, Howie."

And so they do, for half an hour or so: around the pool, down to the beach, back to the lobby, in and out of the pricey shops, and through the barbered gardens. And the two minders stroll with them—never obviously, not to Bessemer at any rate, never too close, but never really out of sight. Carr leads them on a final turn around the marina, then back across West Bay Road and through the lobby again. He and Bessemer are alone on the elevator to the fourth floor. When they return to their suite, Bobby

is there, drinking beer. He's got the blinds drawn, and a Marlins game on the big plasma screen.

Bessemer is in the doorway, about to speak, when Carr raises a hand to stop him. Carr looks at Bobby and lifts an eyebrow.

Bobby holds up what looks like an old-fashioned beeper with a stubby antenna on top. "It's okay," he says. "I swept it. It's clean."

A tentative smile falls from Bessemer's face. "What's clean?"

"The room, Howie," Bobby says. "And a pretty nice room too. First-class all the way with Greg, huh?" Bessemer nods vaguely, still confused.

"What did you see?" Carr asks.

"Just the two buzz cuts. They looked like a couple of water buffaloes, waddling around after you."

"What are you talking about?" Bessemer asks. "Who's a water buffalo? Are we still being followed?"

"It's all good, Howie," Carr says, shaking his head. He sits in a chair across from Bobby and opens the brown plastic grocery bag that Bobby has left on the coffee table. Inside, wrapped in a hand towel, is a holstered Glock, and beneath that a small box, about the size of a deck of cards. Carr opens it and empties the contents into the palm of his hand: three black, one-gigabyte flash drives.

"Gave you two extra, for backup," Bobby says. "Prager plugs it in and we're good to go."

"He doesn't have to open a file or read the directory?"

"Nope. All he has to do is plug it in and the worm loads."

"You make it sound easy," Carr says.

Bobby shrugs. "You're the guy who's got to get him to do it."

Bessemer's eyes lurch from the gun to Carr. "Do what? Plug what in?" His voice is brittle and shaky.

"Not to worry, Howie," Carr says, and then he nods at Bobby. "I'm going out, but he'll keep you company while I'm gone."

"Gone where?"

"No place far," Carr says. "We'll call Prager when I get back." And then he goes into his bedroom, rummages in his bag for a bathing suit, and opens his phone.

Tina's hotel is down the beach from Carr's—practically next door, she said, but it turns out to be a mile-and-a-half swim. The water is warm and clear, but there's rough surf around the reefs, and a powerful undertow at

a break in a sand bar, and it takes Carr almost forty minutes to make the trip. He's breathing hard when he pulls off his fins and mask and walks out of the ocean. His shoulders and thighs are burning.

Tina is waiting for him in a white canvas beach cabana, the last tent in a curving white line. She's lying on a lounge chair, wearing a black two-piece swimsuit and big black sunglasses. Her skin is pale and petal smooth, and Carr can feel her eyes on him as he crosses the sand.

She hands him a heavy white towel. "I'm impressed," she says, "but wouldn't driving have been easier?"

"Sure," Carr says, drying his hair. "Except I didn't think you'd want me bringing my minders along."

Tina sits up and pulls her glasses off. Her eyes are narrow. "What are you talking about?" she says softly.

"Minders. Two of them—big biceps, high and tight hair, milling around the lobby. Not to be confused with the pair who tailed me from the airport."

"Where did you leave them?"

"On the hotel beach, trying to pick me out of a few dozen people snorkeling offshore."

"At some point they're going to realize you're not coming in."

Carr shrugs. "They can tell the lifeguard."

Tina looks into the middle distance. "No idea of who sent them?"

"They've got that corporate look, but otherwise no clue."

"Prager's?"

"That's the optimistic interpretation."

"It seems awfully diligent for Eddie Silva."

Carr nods. "Surprises were inevitable down here: security immediately around Prager is what I know least about."

"Bessemer was supposed to be your ticket around all that."

"And Silva was supposed to be a useless lush."

Tina makes a sour face and raps her sunglasses idly against her lounge chair. "So much for theories," she says. "What did you do with Bessemer?"

"Bobby's with him, at the hotel."

"He and Mike and the kid settled in?"

Carr nods. "In a place on the sound, with a yard and a dock and a straight shot to the airport. They like it better than West Palm."

Tina gives him a speculative look. "You want the stones?"

Carr sits. "That's why I'm here."

"And I thought it was just to see me," Tina says. There's a canvas beach bag at her side, and she reaches in and pulls out a large nylon shaving kit, blue with a zippered top. She tosses it to Carr, who catches it and opens the zip. The diamonds are in three plastic bags inside. Carr takes them out and weighs each one in his palm. "Everything here?"

"Except what I used for belt buckles and toe rings," Tina says.

Carr smiles and makes a show of weighing the bags again. "As long as you left me enough to get Prager's attention."

"From the minders, I'd say you already have it."

Carr puts the stones back in the zippered case. He looks at Tina and gets another questioning look in return. "You worried?" she asks. "About these guys following you around?"

His first impulse is to laugh, and he almost does. Not because he isn't worried about being followed—he is. Out from behind the listening end of a microphone, outside of anonymous cars and vans, Carr feels naked. The minders have simply added a spotlight and pointing finger. No, the almost laughter isn't because the buzz cuts don't scare him, it's because they're at the end of a long line. In the crowded landscape of Carr's fear, they are mere foothills beside Valerie, Mike, and Nando, beside his galloping suspicions about what really happened on that bleak highway to Santiago, beside his dark fantasies of what might happen here afterward, if his crew is successful in stealing Prager's money.

His second impulse—and it surprises him—is to tell her. The idea of giving voice to his fears, saying them aloud, confessing them to Tina, makes him dizzy for an instant. Words well up in his chest. They bubble and rush and nearly spring forth, and then he remembers who he's talking to. The half-smiling woman on the lounge chair vanishes, replaced by a slender figure—a riding crop in a black dress—standing in the deep shade at the edge of a golf course. So Carr swallows the words with his laughter and shrugs.

"I'm not crazy about working the front of the house," he says, "being the face Prager sees, the one he'll remember."

"First time for everything."

"First and last time for this."

"You never know—you might develop a taste for it."

"Not going to happen," Carr says, shaking his head. "Last time I saw

you, you were headed down to Santiago, to have a look at Guerrero. How did that go?"

Tina sighs. "I wish I could say it was a breakthrough, but it wasn't."

"Guerrero wasn't Declan's guy?"

"He was the guy all right, but that was it. He had nothing to tell us."

"Nothing at all?"

"Declan—or somebody very much like him—put down a cash deposit to fly that Saturday night. He paid cash, and booked for four passengers, plus baggage."

"Going where?"

"São Paulo."

"Declan."

"Sounds like. Unfortunately, that's all this Guerrero had to say. The date came and went, the guy didn't show and didn't call, and Guerrero happily kept the cash. End of story."

Carr's jaw clenches. "Which leaves us where?"

"No place great," Tina says. "It takes us back to our two original questions: Who gave Bertolli's men the heads-up, and what became of Bertolli's missing money?"

"How about Bertolli's former security guy down there—the one your people turned up?"

"How about him?"

"We could go back to him—push a little harder, or sweeten the pot—get him to do some digging into who warned Bertolli."

Tina is doubtful. "The guy was pretty scared . . ."

"So that's it then? I've spent my money on dead ends?"

"You want to keep spending, I'll keep my guys working—knocking on Bertolli's man again, trying to turn up another source, whatever. But if we're going to do that, then we've got to work it from the other end as well."

"Meaning what?"

"Who knew Declan's plans, and who was in a position to leak them? And who might've benefited from doing it? Those are the questions—and I think you know who you need to ask."

A gust of wind blows through the canvas walls of the cabana. Carr hunches like an old man and pulls the towel around his shoulders.

* * *

Tina buys him a T-shirt and flip-flops from her hotel's gift shop, along with a beach bag for his fins, mask, and diamonds, and she drives him back to his hotel. They say little in the car, and she drops him at the roadside just past the resort's flower-draped gate.

Bobby is watching television when Carr returns, a Dodgers game now. Bessemer is snoring in his room, diagonal across the bed, one arm flung out in a desperate reach for something. Carr closes the bedroom door.

"He went down about an hour ago," Bobby says. "The guy is not looking forward to seeing Prager."

Bobby is gone when Bessemer teeters into the living room, wiping crust from his eyes and spittle from his chin—a bedraggled teddy bear. He squints at the television, and then at the evening sky.

"Jesus," he says. "What time is it?"

"Time to make a phone call, Howie," Carr says.

Bessemer's hair is a weed patch, and he pushes clumsy fingers through it. "Call to who?"

"Come on, Howie, wake yourself up."

"You want to call Curt now?" he asks. His voice is a rusty hinge. "I don't think that's a good idea, Greg. Really, I'm not my best."

Carr shakes his head. "Room service will fix you. Coffee and a club sandwich."

Bessemer waves his hands and drops onto the sofa. "No, really, Greg, now isn't a good time. How about I give you Curt's number? Just say that I told you to call."

Carr goes to the bar and fills a glass with crushed ice and Coke. He places it on the coffee table in front of Bessemer, takes a seat next to him, and drapes an arm across Bessemer's hunched shoulders. Carr's voice is low and intimate, almost a whisper.

"And how about I put your face through those glass doors, Howie, and drop you four floors off the terrace? Because unless you pull yourself together and remember who you're talking to, that's exactly what I'm going to do. And I'll be long gone while they're still figuring out which pieces of you go where. So drink your soda and have a think, Howie, but don't take too long. I'll get the room service menu."

Carr gives Bessemer's shoulder a friendly squeeze as he finishes, and he sets a cell phone down next to the sweating glass.

29

Isla Privada Holdings is headquartered in a six-story slab of concrete and tinted glass that would be anonymous in an actual city, but that in George Town is a soaring office tower. It's off Elgin Avenue, not far from a police building that looks like it's made of orange sherbet. Carr parks next to a Land Rover with a large man leaning on the bumper. He's wearing a dark suit and fiddling uncomfortably with his shoulder holster, and he gives Carr a hard look as he and Bessemer pass, but Carr knows it's just for practice.

It's not yet noon, but the asphalt is already soft underfoot as they cross the parking lot. Bessemer is shaved and combed and barely bloodshot, but his steps are hesitant.

"We take it nice and easy, Howie," Carr says softly as they approach the glass doors. "And we keep things simple."

Carr has said it before—spent much of last night saying it. "You introduce me, and you let me talk. He asks about Otisville, you stammer, look embarrassed, and you let me talk. Just do what you said you always do when you arrange these get-togethers—make the introductions and fade into the woodwork."

"Why are we doing it at his office?" Bessemer asked a dozen times or more. "He always has me over to the house. I've never even been to the office before. Curtis hardly goes there himself." And a dozen times or

more Carr replied with comforting noises, none of which he himself quite believed.

There's a security desk in the lobby, and cameras, but nothing more heavy-handed in the procedures than a glance at their passports, consultation of the visitors list, and a call upstairs. Carr fights the impulse to turn away from the cameras. Someone at Isla Privada approves them, and they're pointed toward a small elevator for a slow ride to the fifth floor. Bessemer is shifting from one foot to the other.

"You have to pee, Howie?" Carr asks.

"Among other things."

A woman, fit, brisk, and fiftyish, meets them at the elevator. She wears tan trousers and a sleeveless white blouse, and has a thick blond ponytail that barely moves as she leads them down corridors, around corners, and through a maze of low cubicles.

Isla Privada's offices aren't empty, but they feel that way—like a Saturday morning, rather than almost noon on a Wednesday—and the decor is decidedly low-key. The furnishings are as muted and generic as the building itself—slate and putty and taupe. The office artwork is visual pabulum: placating and instantly forgotten, surplus from a shopping mall or an airport lounge. Even the ringtone of the telephone system is muffled to a low burr that sounds to Carr like an electronic snore. The air is cool and smells like a new car.

This is not the back office—the centralized operation that processes the transactions of all the bank and trust companies in Isla Privada's portfolio and that enables Curtis Prager to wash and move so much money so efficiently and inconspicuously. Those offices, Carr knows, are two miles away, in an even blander building, wrapped in much more serious security. But looking over the cubicles as he passes, Carr sees no clue of the business being done here. Insurance? Consulting? Selling time-shares? It could be anything.

The woman leads them to a glass-walled conference room. She stands by the door and ushers them in with a sweep of her muscular arm. There's an oval conference table in the center of the room, and beneath the shaded windows a low credenza with trays on top. Coffee service, ice bucket, glass tumblers, and small bottles of soda.

"Sorry for the wait, fellas," the woman says. "Please have a seat." Her voice is husky, aggressively upbeat, and has a trace of Texas in it. Her skin

is tanned and grainy. "We'll get started in just a minute, but in the meantime we have refreshments." She crosses the room and carries the trays from the credenza to the conference table. Bessemer reaches for a glass and a bottle of ginger ale.

"And for you Mr. Frye?" She spreads her hands toward the trays, like a trade-show model presenting a dishwasher. "Please, help yourself," she says, and leaves, closing the door behind her.

Bessemer fills a glass with ice and ginger ale and empties it in one long swallow. He picks up a cocktail napkin and wipes his mouth and his forehead. Then he goes to the window and raises the shades. Carr sees the low rooftops of George Town, bright under the hammering sun, and the busy blue harbor. Bessemer turns and begins to speak, and Carr shakes his head minutely.

"Lots of boats," Carr says.

Bessemer nods. "Curt must be running late," he says, and begins to pace.

Carr stares until he catches Bessemer's eye. "Another drink, Howie?" he asks, and slides a bottle of ginger ale across the table. Then he reaches for a glass of his own.

Twenty minutes later, Carr his finished two club sodas, and the hairs have risen on the back of his neck, though he doesn't know why. Bessemer is pacing again, but the little knot tightening in Carr's stomach isn't fallout from that. He swirls the ice in his glass and looks around the conference room, which has suddenly come to resemble a fishbowl.

"Does Prager usually keep you waiting long?" he asks.

Bessemer flinches, startled by Carr's voice. "He never keeps me waiting, and he never parks me in a conference room either. I feel like a salesman, for chrissakes."

"I know what you mean," Carr says, and he looks through the glass walls at the people in the their cubicles doing god knows what. "Have you caught a glimpse of him, walking around?"

"Walking around out there?" Bessemer says, flinching again. "No, I haven't seen anything." And the knot tightens more.

And then the blond woman is at the conference room door again, still smiling, though this time apologetically.

"Fellas, I feel *terrible* about this. I just now got off the phone with Curtis, and he's not going to be able to make it in today. He's on his way to the

airport—got a little emergency, and he's got to jump over to Nassau real quick. But he wants you to know he's *real* sorry for this, and he'd like to reschedule for Saturday—lunch at his place."

Carr looks at Bessemer, who is sputtering. "This is unbelievable," Bessemer says. "We came down to see Curt, not for a vacation. I'd have come in February if that's what I was after."

The blonde nods and her smile slides smoothly into a sympathetic frown. "And Curtis is *so* sorry. In fact, he'd like you to send over your hotel bill, so he can take care of it."

Bessemer begins to speak and Carr puts a hand on his arm. "That's all right," Carr says, smiling. "Things come up—I know how it is. And Saturday should be fine, don't you think, Howie? Give us time for some golf."

Bessemer looks at Carr and nods vaguely. "Golf, sure."

The blonde's smile returns. "Great—so I'll tell Curtis Saturday."

"Saturday," Bessemer says.

The blonde makes more noises of cheerful apology and leads them out of the conference room and through the office again. The knot in Carr's stomach moves into his chest. They pass the men's room, and Carr makes an abrupt right turn.

"I've got to make a pit stop," he says, leaning on the bathroom door. "I'll catch up at the elevators." Carr pushes through, and as he does he sees the blonde's face tighten with a look of annoyance.

The bathroom is small and gray and smells of disinfectant. Carr runs water on his hands and dries them and listens to the blonde's voice dwindle down the hallway. When it's gone he throws away his paper towel, steps into the corridor, and turns left. He walks down the hall, turns a corner, and stops when he sees the conference room, and the man at the conference table, who is sporting a crew cut, a polo shirt, and vinyl gloves, carefully placing Carr's drinking glass in a plastic evidence bag.

At the elevators, Bessemer is sweating, and the blonde is checking her watch. Carr smiles as he approaches. "Sorry to hold things up," he says, chuckling. "Too much club soda."

The blonde returns his smile and presses the elevator call button. "So we'll see you Saturday, Mr. Frye? Mr. Bessemer?"

Carr nods and puts out his hand. "You'll be there too, Ms. . . . ?"

"Oh, I'm sorry—I never did make a proper introduction to you fellas. I'm Kathy Rink."

"A pleasure," Carr says. "Are you Curtis's assistant?"

Kathy Rink smiles wider and laughs as she squeezes Carr's hand. "Oh, no, Mr. Frye, I'm his head of security."

30

"She's ex-DEA," Tina tells Carr, stirring the ice in her drink, but drinking nothing. "She left eighteen months back, after fifteen years there. Spent most of her time in the New Orleans district, in Shreveport and Baton Rouge, and her last three years down south, in Honduras. She came on about four weeks back, with a recommendation from one of Prager's clients. Word is she's still got plenty of friends in the agency."

"Shit," Carr says. His voice is low and cold.

They're alone on the terrace of a bar perched over a cove, at a table by the wooden railing. The tide is rolling in, slapping at the rocks below and casting up a briny mist. Carr has nothing in front of him but the strips of a shredded cocktail napkin that are being carried away, one by one, on the wind.

"That's all I've got so far," Tina says, "but I'm expecting another call."

"And is this call going to explain just what the *fuck* happened to your intel?"

"I don't like surprises any more than—"

"It's not your ass on the line."

Tina's face is without expression and as white and still as carved bone. Her eyes are invisible behind her dark glasses, and her voice is without affect. "You want me to say it's a fuckup? Fine—it's a fuckup. You feel better now?"

"No," Carr says. He presses his fingers to his temples. "If Rink's still got

federal wiring, then Greg Frye won't last. He's not built for that. He's good for a quick look-see—a criminal records check, or somebody trying to confirm that he and Bessemer were at Otisville together—but for somebody with fingerprints and access to AFIS . . ."

Tina nods. "She'll run right through Frye to you."

Carr looks down at the foam-covered rocks. "They took my prints when I applied, at every one of my interviews, on my first day at Langley, and a half dozen times afterward. Dennis is good, but he's not good enough to scrub all that away."

Tina leans back and chews on her straw. "Your minders still around?"

"We wouldn't be meeting here if they were. They were with us to Prager's office this morning, but not afterward, and they're not at the hotel."

"You left Bessemer there?" Carr nods. "How's he holding up?"

"He was nervous before we met Rink; he's bat-shit now. Bobby's probably scraping him off the ceiling, if he hasn't actually killed him yet."

"How's Bobby doing?"

"Pissed off, scared, ready to pack his bag."

And Bobby wasn't the only one. After parking Bessemer in the suite and phoning Tina, Carr had arranged a conference call with Valerie, Bobby, Mike, and Dennis. His story of what happened at Prager's office was met first with silence, and then angry, colliding voices. Bobby's was the loudest and most poetic.

"What the *fuck*? We pay Boyce for intel, and this is what we get—a steaming pile of dog shit? This is fucked, brother—up, down, and sideways—and I'm heading for the fucking airport."

Dennis had been slightly less noisy but no less upset, and Mike had done his yelling in Spanish. Only Valerie had been quiet, and Carr swore he could hear the gears turning in her head.

"Everybody else feel the same as Bobby?" Tina asks.

"What do you expect? The boss doesn't bring on a new security chief because he wants to keep things the same. So what we knew about Prager's personal security, and what we could infer because of Silva, is all subject to change now. The same with Isla Privada's network security, and even Amy Chun's protection—all out the window. And I didn't even tell them about the prints. Once they find out about that they won't even bother to pack."

"So don't tell them," Tina says. She looks out at the ocean, and Carr

watches the breaking waves in her black lenses. She tosses her straw into an ashtray. "Four weeks isn't a lot of time in a new job," she says. "It's barely enough to figure out what changes you want to make, much less to make them."

Carr squints at her. "You think Rink hasn't changed anything yet?"

"She hasn't even been there a month."

"That's a fucking big *maybe*—and let me point out that we saw some changes today."

"We'd have to take a second look at things, of course—verify that nothing important has—"

"And you think we'll get it right on the second look? Or maybe the third? Come on, Tina."

She takes off her sunglasses. Her gray eyes catch the light and glitter like broken glass. "So your bag's packed too, is that it? I just want to make sure I get it right for when Boyce asks me."

"I don't know that there are any other options here."

"Bags packed—yes or no, Carr? 'Cause if it's yes, I've got to get the accountants working on what you owe us. And by the way, I'm going to want those diamonds back, as a down payment."

"I'm not pulling out on a whim, Tina, or because I decided it was all just too much work. This is about the wheels falling off because of an intel fuckup. *Your* fuckup."

"No one's arguing that, and trust me there's a certain lazy bastard who has a date with the inside of an oil drum, but when Boyce asks me if I think this whole thing is irretrievably screwed, I'm going to tell him *no*."

Carr's laugh is bitter. "Everybody in the stands gets an opinion. They just shouldn't confuse watching with being on the field."

"Is that really how you want to approach this?" Tina says quietly. Her smile is thin and chilly and doesn't reach her eyes. After a moment Carr looks away.

There's a gull hanging in the breeze above the terrace, eyeing the paper scraps on the table and, Carr thinks, eyeing him. He waves a hand at it, but the bird is unimpressed. He looks back to Tina. "Even if Rink hasn't made many changes to Prager's security—and even if we could verify that—there's still the issue of my prints. A day or so from now, she's going to know I'm not Greg Frye. How do you make that go away?"

"*I* don't," Tina says, and then she picks up her phone and walks to the far corner of the terrace.

She's on for a long while, walking a tiny square while she talks. The wind carries her voice in pieces. Carr can't make out the words above the beating of the surf, but her tone is tense and urgent. Her face, when he can see it, is blank, and her shoulders are rigid. The longer she speaks, the tighter his chest becomes.

Tina closes her phone, leans against the terrace rail, and looks out at the waves. For a moment Carr thinks she might throw the phone into the sea, but she slips it into her pocket instead and walks back to the table.

"Boyce?" he asks. Tina nods. "And?"

"We have to wait and see."

31

From half a mile out, from beneath the canopy of an open fishing boat rocking gently on flat water, the Prager compound is impressive even to the naked eye. The sweep of sand is like a quarter-mile curve of new snow. The bordering palms are lush, lithe, and synchronized in the breeze. The stone stairs, terraces, and retaining walls are meticulous gray lines. The boathouse, at the end of a spidery pier, is a trim, white chapel. The three-hole golf course is like a velvet swag across the east end of the property, and the corner of a house, visible between palm trees at the west end, is like a slice of pink cake.

"Let me have the binoculars," Carr says, and Bobby passes them over. Carr adjusts the dial and details emerge in the bobbing frame. Shadowed foliage becomes careful landscaping, dense green with generous dollops of color—hibiscus, bougainvillea, ixora, and red ginger. A swimming pool casts a shimmering web on a striped awning. A gust of wind swirls tennis court clay into a thin red cloud that settles at the edge of a croquet lawn. The slice of cake turns out to be the corner of a guesthouse—a pink stucco confection with a satellite dish. Of the main house, only a section is visible—an acre or so of terra-cotta barrel tile, a length of colonnaded portico, and a line of French windows that catch light off the ocean.

"We got them curious," Bobby says. "On the beach, at the bottom of the stairs."

Carr scans the binoculars from west to east and sees them, two security grunts: crew cuts, polo shirts, dark glasses, and earpieces—first cousins to the minders at his hotel. "Didn't take long," he says. He drops his sunglasses back on his nose, pulls his ball cap down low, and hands the binoculars back to Bobby.

"I make it six minutes."

Carr nods. "Me too. Get a head count."

Bobby peers through the binoculars and Carr steps around the center console, keeping his back to the shore. He fiddles with the fishing rods and the lines that run off the stern.

"I got five," Bobby says. "The guys on the beach, one more by the guesthouse, and two at the pier, who look like they're coming to say hello."

Carr glances up and sees two men donning float vests and pulling at the lines of a red-hulled Zodiac moored near the boathouse. "Plus the two we saw on the gate," he says, reeling in the lines.

"And who knows how many inside," Bobby says. "That's seven-plus on a weekday afternoon, with nothing much happening. With a party going on, it could be twice that."

Carr stows the fishing rods and returns to the console. He flips a switch and the twin outboards start. There's a puff of pale exhaust at the stern, an upwelling of foam, and a throaty rumble that echoes across the inlet. He lifts the binoculars and sees thick faces turn, can feel their sharpened interest. The men are climbing into the Zodiac now, and Carr hears their outboard whine.

"I don't need any more," Bobby says. "How about you?"

"We've seen what we came to see," Carr says, and he pushes the throttle, turns the wheel, and carves a long white crescent in the ocean.

What they've seen is bad to worse, and it's been the same everywhere they've looked the past two days—since Carr agreed with Tina to make a hurried reconnaissance of Isla Privada's security arrangements. In George Town, at Isla Privada's back office, the new guards are practically tripping over the old ones. From Boca Raton, Valerie called to report that Amy Chun's lethargic driver is due to be replaced in the coming week by an armed one, and that her house will be swept even more frequently for unwelcome electronics. Curtis Prager's personal protection has gone from one paunchy ex-cop to three muscular crew cuts. And here at his

compound on Rum Point Drive, the household detail has grown from four to something north of seven. Only Dennis has yet to report in, on the all-important state of Isla Privada's network security. If that has changed, Carr told Tina, it's game over.

Carr has the boat planing now, and just coming even with the jagged peninsula that marks the western edge of Prager's property. He looks back along their wake. The protected inlet is dwindling behind them, and so is the red Zodiac, which has barely made it to the reef, two hundred meters from shore. Carr begins a wide curve around the rocks. He sees the Zodiac slow and then turn back. He looks ahead, and in the misty distance he can make out Rum Point.

Bobby calls to him over the engine and the rush of wind and water. "You want a beer?" Carr shakes his head. Bobby reaches into an ice chest beneath his seat and pulls out a bottle of the local brew. He takes a long swallow and sighs. "This stuff sucks."

"It's what they had at the store."

"No wonder," Bobby says, and takes another drink. "This Rink chick has been busy."

Carr nods. "Seems that way."

"She's got people nervous."

"I know, Bobby."

A third swallow and he pats his mouth with the back of his hand. "I fucking hate surprises."

It's pretty much all Bobby has said for two days—how much he hates surprises, how fucked up Boyce's intel was, and that they should be thinking about packing it in. And Carr has explained, over and over, that if they can't get a handle on what changes Rink has made, or if she's changed anything material to their plans, then they would indeed call it a day. The message has a half-life of about five minutes in Bobby's brain. Dennis is even more anxious but, mercifully, more inhibited about saying so, and Carr is glad he took Tina's advice and made no mention of Rink taking his fingerprints.

As wearing as Bobby's and Dennis's worry is, Valerie's and Latin Mike's seeming lack of nerves is somehow even more so. After his initial outburst, Mike has uttered no other word of complaint or concern, but simply set about reconnoitering—an uncharacteristically cooperative soldier. Valerie has yet to say anything.

They are approaching Rum Point, and there are other fishing boats ahead, pushing north out of the sound, and swimmers closer to the beach. Carr eases up on the throttle and turns the wheel a couple of points northwest.

Bobby pulls off his T-shirt, wipes his brow with it, and leans back in his seat. His body is thick and white, a fish from a different sea. "Could be twice the security when he has a party, could be three times—we really don't know," he says. "We're just guessing at what Rink might've changed. We don't know shit."

Carr sighs. "There was a lot we didn't know when Silva was in charge."

"We knew he was a lazy drunk, and that was . . ." Bobby puts up his hands, searching for a word.

"Comforting?"

"There you go," Bobby says, raising his beer bottle. "We're just feeling around in the dark now, and I like it better with the lights on."

"Like I said, Bobby—if she's changed anything important to our plans, then we don't go. If all she's done is add muscle—"

"You sound like Mike now."

"Yeah? I haven't heard Mike say much lately."

"Well he's saying the same shit as you—how it's all manageable, how we should keep on keepin' on. Personally, I think his perspective's fucked."

"Which means that mine is too?"

Bobby shrugs. "You can't like a job so much you lose sight of the basics. You can't get locked in. You gotta be willing to cut your losses if it's the smart thing."

"And you think I'm not willing?"

"Hey—I want to finish this as much as anybody. I got the same time in—the same sunk costs. But there'll be other jobs."

"Not too many others this size, Bobby."

"See what I mean—locked in," Bobby says. "That's the kind of attitude that gets you killed, brother." He drains the rest of the beer, pulls a fresh one from the locker, and holds the bottle against the side of his face. He closes his eyes.

Carr swings the boat farther north. They pass day-sailers and catamarans coming out of the sound, and divers massed along the reefs of Stingray City. When the sea around them is empty of other boats, Carr cuts the engines and lets them drift.

Bobby sits up and looks around. "What—we fishing for real?"

Carr shakes his head. "You know, I had a talk like this with Declan, just before the Mendoza job—"

"Oh for chrissakes!"

"About getting hung up on a job, and losing sight of the fundamentals."

"Motherfuckin' Carr—"

"You think that kind of attitude got him killed, Bobby, or was it something more specific?"

"I thought for sure we were done with this crap."

"We're done when I say so, and I'm not there yet. But here's where I am, Bobby: I'm down to the short strokes on the last job I ever want to work; I've had a nasty surprise with bad intel; and whenever I've asked a question in the last four months about what happened in Argentina I get answers that are at least fifty percent bullshit. So I'm nervous. And I don't want to be nervous anymore. I'm fucking tired of it. I'm tired of wondering who's got my back and who's going to stick something in it. If I'm going to finish this job, I need to know what's what, Bobby, and you're going to tell me."

Bobby shakes his head slowly. "Mike said—"

"Mike isn't here, Bobby. You're going to tell me."

Bobby chuckles and opens his beer. He takes a long swallow. Then he looks over his shoulder at the empty ocean. "Or what—you're gonna make me swim back?"

"We're pretty far out, so let's not have it come to that."

Another drink. "What the fuck do you want me to say, Carr?"

"I want to know what happened that night."

"Jesus, I've told you—"

"Talk to me about the barn. Talk to me about the money in the barn."

Bobby looks up. He shakes his head and laughs softly. "Mike thought you knew. In fact, the fucking guy thought I told you."

Carr sighs and looks at the sketchy clouds. He nods and smiles minutely. "Well, now he's right."

"Aw fuck!" Bobby barks. He pushes his sunglasses into his hair. His eyes are bleary and buried deep in a nest of lines and folds. "You fucking prick. That was bullshit, Carr—total fucking bullshit. What are you, practicing to be a cop?"

"Yeah, really sorry, Bobby. I feel just awful about betraying your trust. Now talk about the barn."

"Fuck you."

"So you're going to try the swimming?"

"Fuck you," Bobby says again, but there's less to it now. He lets his sunglasses fall to his nose, and he takes a deep breath. "Everything I told you about our run up to Bertolli's place, and everything I said about our running out again—all that was true. The only bullshit part was about the barn. They didn't hit us before we went in; they hit us after—after we came out."

"Who's *we*, Bobby? Who went in?"

"All four of us—me, Mike, Ray-Ray, and Deke. It was pitch-fucking-black, like I said, and cold—cold enough to see your breath if it wasn't so dark. We came up real quiet—coasting in at the end. There was a chain on the sliding door, and we clipped it. Then we popped the door lock and went inside.

"The goddamn place reeked of dirt and horse shit—it came out like a big cloud—but there were no horses. No, it was just like Deke said it would be—a long row of empty stalls, and one at the end that was outfitted as a strong room. Steel wall panels, a big reinforced door, this giant fucking lock that was about as useful as skates on a pig, and some really stupid wiring. We snipped the wires, jacked the door frame right off the wall, and opened her up like that." And Bobby snaps his fingers.

Carr starts at the sound, and it breaks a spell he didn't realize Bobby had woven. The darkness, the oiled weight of weapons and tools, the rich, humid scent of earth and horses, the metal tang of adrenaline on the tongue—Carr could taste it and smell it and feel it all. He could practically see Declan, hulking but somehow graceful as he moved through the shadows. Bobby is watching him, looking worried.

Carr tugs at the bill of his cap. "And inside?"

Bobby drags a hand across the back of his neck. He's staring at his feet, at the beer bottle, empty now, at anyplace but Carr. "Inside was money—bricks of euros, banded and shrink-wrapped, very neat. It was like Deke said, just not quite as much of it."

"How much?"

"We took out about two."

"Two million?"

"About. In two duffels. Ray-Ray had one, Mike took the other."

Carr nods slowly. "Split evenly—a million in each?"

"Pretty much."

"And then what?"

"And then we came out to the vans, and it was like I told you—they came around that hangar and lit us up."

"As you came out of the barn?"

"As we were getting back in the vans."

"And Mike still had the duffel?"

"He had one; Ray-Ray had the other."

Carr nods again and watches a cruise ship churn across the horizon to the north. "Then what happened?"

"Then it was lights, camera, action: yelling, shooting, hauling ass out of there—exactly like I said."

"Except you left out the part about hauling ass with a bag full of money."

"Yeah, well, the driving was the same, and so was the shooting."

"And the safe house, and the call from Declan—were those the same too?"

Bobby blots his face with his balled-up T-shirt and looks at Carr. "I swear to Christ, that was straight up—all of it."

"But you and Mike decided not to mention the money. Why?"

"It was Mike's idea," Bobby says, slouching in his seat. "After Mendoza, we didn't know what the fuck was going on—if the Prager job was still on, who was gonna run things, hell, we didn't know if there was gonna be anything to run. And Mike said it was us who almost got our asses shot off—not you or Val or Dennis. We'd earned the money, and why the hell should we pay into the kitty for a job that might not happen."

"Except, as it turns out, the job is happening—and it's been happening for a while now. But I guess you two never revisited your original reasoning."

Bobby sits up and sticks out his chin. "It was us—"

"Who almost got your asses shot off—I heard you the first time. So, you lied about the money. Anything else you want to clear up?"

"Fuck you. Nothing else."

"No? You didn't kill Declan then? You didn't sell him to Bertolli?"

Bobby's face and fists clench tight. "You keep talking like that, ocean or no, you're gonna catch a beating."

Carr shakes his head. "So what was the take?" he asks.

"I told you—we got about half."

Carr pulls off his sunglasses. "Don't give me this *about* crap, Bobby. How much exactly?"

Bobby reaches into the ice chest and pulls out a fistful of crushed ice. He sits down and runs it over his neck and shoulders. "One point two even."

"And what happened to it?"

"In a bank—banks—finally, and what a pain in the ass that turned out to be. That much cash—it's a fucking albatross. Took forever to get it moved, converted to dollars, give it an acceptable past, and get it deposited. I see why we pay Boyce to handle all that crap. Mike needed help to get it done."

Carr is standing now, out from under the canopy. "Help from who, Bobby?"

Bobby smiles and reaches into the ice chest for another beer. He pulls the cap off and takes a long drink. "That's a funny story," Bobby says. "Nando fixed it for us—set us up with a couple of friendly bankers in Miami. Remember Nando? It was a real blast from the past when Mike told me he was in touch. He knows all about this shit now. Guess he's come up in the world."

32

The dream leaves him sweating and breathless, grasping for the story line even as it fades in the predawn light. Something with his father. Something with his mother. The courtyard in Caracas, the bedrooms in Mexico City. The beds empty. A booming, piratical laugh. Carr wakes holding nothing more than sheets.

He runs water on his face and walks into the living room. The walls are bathed in shifting blues and yellows from the television, playing silently to Latin Mike, who is stretched out on the sofa. A shopping channel from the States—makeup and jewelry that is not quite gold.

"You buying, Mike?" Carr says quietly.

Mike yawns widely. "Maybe the eyeliner."

Carr nods at Bessemer's bedroom. "Howie sleep tight?" he asks.

"Went in there with a bottle about midnight," Mike says. "Hasn't come out since."

Carr opens the bedroom door and looks inside. Bessemer is a snoring mound in a landslide of pillows and blankets. A bottle of Bombay Sapphire lays on its side, on the end table. Carr closes the door. "The guy puts it away," he says.

"More every day," Mike says, and he stretches and scratches and wanders to the terrace doors. He looks out at the glowing pool and the gray ocean. "You want to watch that. He's got to be upright for Prager."

"He will be." Carr walks to the bar and fishes in the little refrigerator for a Coke. "You're good to stay the morning?"

Mike nods. "You think Dennis got anywhere last night?"

"We'll find out."

A new salesman appears on the screen, with a pitch about a moisturizer.

Mike points and laughs. "Should buy some of this shit for Bobby. Guy looked like Larry the Lobster when you brought him back."

Carr nods. "I told him to use sunscreen."

Which is a lie. Carr had watched as Bobby drank beer and grew ever more pink, but he had said nothing about getting burned. What he had done was make Bobby repeat his story several times more, and answer questions about Nando and Valerie.

About Nando, Bobby had said little, besides that Mike had kept in touch with him over the years, and that the fee Nando had charged for helping them launder money "wasn't robbery." About Valerie he'd said less.

"She's never asked about the money, and I've never told her. If she knows something, she heard it from Mike."

"Mike tell her a lot of secrets?" Carr had asked, and he'd gripped the canopy rail tight enough that his fingers ached.

"Fuck should I know?" Bobby had said, but he'd looked away.

A silence followed, during which Bobby drank another beer and Carr replayed his afternoon in Miami against the new backdrop Bobby had painted. It was Bobby who'd broken the silence, with a decorous belch and an observation.

"Mike won't put that money in the pot."

"I'll save him the trouble—I'll just deduct it from his cut. From yours too."

"He won't like it."

"And how about you, Bobby?"

Bobby had shrugged. "I'm not crazy about it, but I wasn't crazy about the sneaking around, either. I figure if we're gonna do this job, then let's get it done. I want this fucker over with. But that's me—Mike's another story."

"I'm not going to lose a lot of sleep over it."

"So, am I supposed to tell him about this, or what?"

"Do what you want, Bobby."

It doesn't seem to Carr that Bobby has yet told Latin Mike anything, though with Mike it wouldn't necessarily be obvious. Maybe Bobby has been too busy tending his sunburn.

Bessemer is still asleep when Carr leaves the suite, and Mike is still on the sofa. Carr is careful on his way through the lobby, and watchful, but there is no reappearance of Kathy Rink's men. The sky is painted pearl gray as he crosses the visitors' parking lot, and already the day's heat is building beneath it. There's a rumble of thunder off to the east as he climbs into Mike's SUV and drives away.

The workhouse is at the end of a quiet lane, on a canal that feeds into North Sound. It's a stucco box in faded blue, with a tiled roof and plaster embellishments around the windows. From the street, Carr can see into the sandy backyard. There's a metal dock there and the fishing boat is tied up alongside it. Dennis opens the door. A week on Grand Cayman and he's paler and thinner than ever—a red-eyed, unshaved reed. He puts a finger to his lips.

"Bobby's still crashed," he says softly. Carr follows him in.

The main room is white and raftered, and the big front window has a view of unkempt hedges, milky sky, and planes angling toward the airport. The furnishings are a hodgepodge of hotel castoffs: fraying slipper chairs, sagging leather and chrome armchairs, water-stained end tables, and the ashtrays of a dozen defunct lounges. Dennis has three laptops open side by side on a chipped glass dining table, behind a stack of high-speed modems, coils of cable, and a platoon of empty soda cans.

"You want coffee?" he asks Carr. Carr nods and Dennis disappears into the kitchen, reappearing with a steaming mug.

Carr takes a drink. It's bad. "When's the last time you slept?" he asks.

Dennis's smile is skewed and slightly goofy. "A while ago."

"Hope you were doing more than just surfing porn sites."

A blush spreads up Dennis's neck. "Not just porn."

Carr puts his coffee aside. "So what's new in the virtual world of Isla Privada Holdings?"

"That's a nontrivial question," Dennis says, rubbing his chin and taking a seat before one of the laptops. Carr girds himself: Dennis gets

pedantic when he's tired, and he's tired now. "Security on their VPN wasn't totally stupid to begin with. I mean, aside from the happy gap we want to exploit, the multifactor authorization is pretty cute. And the rest of the stuff—it may be textbook, predictable, maybe even lazy, but it's not *totally* stupid. It's good enough, for instance, that if you look at it too hard—look *actively*, I mean, poke around too much—they're going to know you're there. And they're going to poke back." He looks up at Carr, his eyes shadowed but earnest. "We don't want that."

"We don't," Carr affirms.

Dennis opens four packs of sugar over his coffee mug, stirs with a pencil, sips at it, and smiles. "So, a nontrivial question—how do you look inside the box without taking the lid off? Not so easy, unless . . ." Dennis taps a forefinger lightly on his temple.

"Unless you're you—I get it. So what's changed?"

Dennis drinks more coffee. His fingers beat a droning drumroll on the tabletop. "A few things. They've upgraded their routers; they've implemented better filtering on inbound and outbound packets; and they're scanning their servers better. Still textbook, but at least a more recent edition. In fact, if I was going to mount a denial-of-service attack on them, I might actually have to spend more than ten minutes planning it."

"I didn't think we cared about that stuff."

"We don't."

Carr counts to ten and struggles to keep the impatience out of his voice. "What's changed that we care about, Dennis?"

"For the moment, nothing—at least from what I see. The network access protocols and authorization layers are the same. The out-of-band component, to the user's cell phone, is still in place. Last night, I walked through video of Chun as she was logging in yesterday, and I synchronized it with the sniffer logs. Everything looks the same."

"And our gap?"

"From what I see, it's still there. Once you pass through the authorization layers—the password generator, the thumbprint scan, the call back to the cell phone with a second password—and you get onto the network, access to Isla Privada's processing system is by password alone. And there's still no cross-check between the network access and processing system. So if I've got Curtis Prager's processing system password, then that system thinks I'm Curtis Prager, and it lets me do everything

Curtis Prager can do, even if I've gotten onto their network using Amy Chun's ID."

Carr sighs. Something loosens in his chest, but it tightens again when he looks at Dennis. "There are a lot of qualifiers in what you said, Dennis—'for the moment,' and 'from what I see.' They're not particularly reassuring."

Dennis's fingers drum faster on the table. "They shouldn't be. I can't see too far into their network without hitting trip wires, but I've seen enough to know that their environment is changing. They haven't fixed the hole that we want to climb through yet, but I'd say it's just a matter of time."

Carr sighs again, but there's no relief in it. "How much time?"

Dennis shrugs. "Ask Kathy Rink."

Tina's hotel room overlooks a garden, with lavish beds of jacaranda, frangipani, and hibiscus massed around a weathered stone fountain. The garden is empty and the flowers are limp and restless in the humid breeze. Carr turns from the window.

"You should be smiling," Tina says from the sofa. "It's all good."

"You call it good; I call it fucked up, though maybe not completely fucked up. *Maybe* not. There's a difference."

"Semantics."

"Call it that when it's *your* ass hanging out."

Tina chuckles and unfolds herself from the sofa. She wears a simple gray skirt and a short black T-shirt, and her white-blond hair is pulled into a short ponytail. She pads barefoot across the room to refill a glass of ice water from a pitcher.

"Come on, Carr—the system stuff hasn't changed, security's tighter but still manageable, and your prints came back to Kathy Rink with Greg Frye's record attached—and only his record: that's good news." Carr looks at her and raises an eyebrow. "What?" Tina says.

"I'm just wondering how you managed it—the fingerprints, I mean."

"*I* didn't."

"Boyce, then."

"I don't ask, and he doesn't tell." She smiles at Carr but he doesn't return it.

"This is more than just ordering off-menu—more than calling in a

favor here and there. This is pulling some serious weight, and I have a hard time believing you don't know shit about it."

Tina returns to the sofa, folds her white legs beneath her, and smooths her skirt. "I know about gift horses, and where not to look."

"I'm serious, Tina."

"So am I. I'm not talking about this anymore, and if you've got half a brain you won't either." Her eyes are flat and icy and unwavering, and finally Carr turns back to the view of the garden. "How's Bessemer holding up?" Tina asks.

"He's pickling himself in gin."

"He going to keep his shit together for Prager?"

"Mike was worried about the same thing. He will."

"And Mike, and the rest of your crew—how're they doing?"

Carr takes a deep breath and turns around. Tina's eyes have lost some of their chill, and that makes it easier. "I found out what happened to Bertolli's money," he says, and he tells her about Bobby's confession, and about the afternoon he spent in Miami, walking up and down Brickell Avenue. Tina is perfectly still; her face is without expression while Carr speaks and in the squirming silence that follows. Finally, she clasps her white hands together and puts them in her lap. Her voice is soft.

"Well, they're busy beavers, aren't they? Maybe you're not giving them enough to do. Too much time on their hands."

"I'm sure that was the issue."

Tina frowns. "There's plenty here for me to be pissed at—like the fact that I'm only just now hearing about this—but I'm doing my best to rise above it, and so should you." Carr nods and Tina continues. "Assuming Bobby's not full of shit, this explains where some of the money went—though not all of it."

"Bobby said Declan had the rest. If he did, then it went up with his van."

"Maybe. You buy that Bobby and Mike had only half the cash?"

"Why lie about that? He's no more of a shithead for walking off with the whole take than he is for walking off with half of it."

"Maybe," she says again. "And what about tipping off Bertolli? You don't think those two had anything to do with that?"

"I think Bobby was telling the truth about that."

"And you've proven to be such a good judge."

Carr bites back his first response and rubs his chin. "They sell Declan

to Bertolli, they sell themselves in the bargain. They were all getting shot at together."

"If you buy Bobby's version of events."

"What about your witness—Bertolli's runaway gunman—did he have orders to shoot at only two out of four guys?"

Tina shakes her head. "Maybe Bobby and Mike were willing to roll the dice—warn Bertolli and take a chance that in the ensuing shit storm Declan would get iced and they could split with the cash."

"That's a hell of a chance, Tina. Takes large brass balls to make that bet, or a tiny little brain."

Tina shrugs skeptically. "Mike and Bobby don't fit that profile? Well, you'd know better than I.

"But what about Fernando—what the fuck is he doing with these guys? Last I heard he was slapping up condos in Cabo or something. Guess the real estate market's driven him back to a life of crime." She shakes her head. "And Valerie in on it too—who'd have guessed she couldn't be trusted?" Tina looks at Carr and smiles thinly.

"I don't know what she's in on, or since when."

"Ask her—I'm sure she'll give you a straight answer."

Carr looks at the garden again. The wind has picked up and the flowers are shaking their heads at the darkening sky. "You don't think she would?"

Tina's laugh is like a blade. "It's what you think that matters. Do you trust her—do you trust any of them—to do their jobs? This late in the game, that's what it comes down to: honor among thieves."

"Fuck trust—I'll have their money. They need me if they want to get paid."

"Now *that's* a working relationship," Tina says, nodding. She shifts on the sofa, stretching out her legs. "And speaking of which—what about our little project down south?"

"What about it?"

"The unanswered questions—who tipped Bertolli, and what happened to the rest of the cash—you want to spend more money on them? Should I keep asking around?"

There's a rumble of thunder outside, and fat drops of rain against the glass. The garden is dark, the flower beds a uniform gray.

"Keep asking," Carr says.

* * *

The wind is gone and the rain falls straight and heavy; the short sprint from parking lot to lobby leaves Carr soaked. He shivers as he steps into the elevator and presses the fourth-floor button. He's alone in the car and the door is nearly shut when a hand slides in and bumps it open again. And then Valerie is there, wet from the rain. She presses the button for three, waits for the door to close, and presses her mouth against his.

33

Howard Bessemer is a vision in seersucker: clear-eyed, pink-cheeked, hair slicked and shining—an altogether healthier vision than his recent diet should allow. He sits erect and alert in the passenger seat, scanning the approaching coast, the whitecaps, the immaculate sky, as Carr bears left off Frank Sound Road onto North Side Road. Bessemer's window is down and his face is turned into the salt breeze, and he reminds Carr of a dog out for a ride.

"Day like today, you see why people move here," Carr says.

Bessemer smiles. "Wait till you see Curt's place. It's not quite San Simeon, but it's a hell of a spread."

Carr nods. "Prager live there all by himself?"

"Him and the staff. Every now and then he sets up a girl in the guesthouse."

"Girl as in girlfriend?"

"As in hooker," Bessemer says, smirking. Carr lifts an eyebrow. "Always pricey, though. Very high-class."

"No doubt," Carr says.

They ride on in silence, Bessemer watching the sea, and Carr, despite their destination and the mounting tension, failing to keep his mind from the night before. Lack of sleep casts a dreamlike scrim over his memories of the evening—burnishing the images and shuffling their order.

Even from across the room, Valerie's voice was close in his ear. "You want this job done, and so do I. I did what I had to do."

Her hands were cold under his shirt. Her hair was wet and smelled like lilac and an airplane cabin.

"All I know about what happened down there is what Bobby and Mike told us. The first Mike said anything to me about euros was the day before we went to Miami."

Her mouth tasted of airline wine, and it seemed to be everywhere at once.

"Bobby and Mike talked about Nando sometimes, and so did Deke, but I never met him until that day in Miami."

Her dress was wet, and it peeled away like a shedding skin. She left it in a pile beside the minibar.

"Amy's gone for two days, up in New York. I'm booked on the first flight back to Boca tomorrow morning."

Her legs were smooth and slick, and the hollows of her neck were full of rain.

"Mike was going to pull out of the job if I didn't help him wash his money—and he was going to take Bobby with him."

Her room was on the third floor, overlooking treetops and a loading dock. She kept the lights off and opened the drapes.

"Bobby told Mike that you knew, and Mike told me, and then I got on a plane down here. I didn't want to talk to you about this on the phone."

Her lips were searing.

"The e-mail from that coffee bar? That was to Nando. He said no cell phones—messaging only. He was superparanoid."

In the dim light, her skin was like matte gold.

"That afternoon, with Mike, that was the only time. You want this job done, and so do I. I do what I have to, and I'm not going to apologize for it."

The rain grew heavier, and it made a tearing sound as it fell through the leaves.

"Have you thought any more about afterward—where you want to go, what you want to do? 'Cause if you haven't, I've got ideas."

North Sound Road becomes Rum Point Drive, and Bessemer clears his throat. "We're coming to it," he says, and a surge of adrenaline drags Carr from his reverie.

Prager's property announces itself to their right, with a wrought-iron fence and high, dense shrubs that obscure the ocean view. A while longer and they reach the gate.

It's tall and steel and topped with cameras, and adjoined by a green pastel bungalow. There are two men inside and Carr recognizes one of them from the airport tail. The man comes out wearing a trained smile and a Glock on his hip. He's carrying an iPad and Carr sees two pictures on the screen: his own and Bessemer's. The guard glances at the photos and at them and rests a hand on the car roof.

"Mr. Frye, Mr. Bessemer, welcome. Mr. Prager will meet you at the main house. Just stay on this drive—you can't miss it." As he speaks, the gate opens and he steps aside and waves them in.

The drive is crushed shell and it's bordered by close-cut lawns and ironwood trees sculpted by the constant winds. It curves gently west and rises up a hillside that he knows, from the broader topography, must be man-made. Another curve and they're at the top, where the drive empties into a wide circle of pavers, set in a herringbone pattern. There's a fountain in the center, marble, pale pink, like the inside of a baby's ear. A marble fish stands on its tail within, and the braid of water falling from its mouth makes a prosperous sound. Across the circle is the house.

Its architectural pedigree is indeterminate—an uneasy hybrid of Italianate, Spanish Colonial, and Georgian—with *big* the only unifying principle. Beneath the tiled roof, its stone walls are yellow—goldenrod in the main parts, going to a butter color for the arched colonnades and the ornament work around the windows and doors. There is a portico in front, and two glossy black doors. They stand open, and Curtis Prager is in the threshold, in sandals, linen trousers, and a pale pink polo shirt. Kathy Rink is at his side, in a green golf skirt and with a smile fastened on her face.

Carr glances at Bessemer, who is smiling oddly and humming softly, tunelessly. Carr wonders if he's taken something. "Shit," Carr whispers, but when he pulls up to the portico, Bessemer sharpens.

Bessemer is out of the Toyota before Carr has switched off the engine, a big smile and a big hand extended. There's a clumsy hug and biceps squeezing, and then Prager holds Bessemer at arm's length. He's taller than Carr expected, with more ropy muscle on him. He seems to dwarf Bessemer.

"Jesus, Bess, you look like shit. What the hell have you been doing to yourself?"

Bessemer grins and ducks his head almost shyly. "Just the usual misdemeanors. But what about you—you keep a special portrait in the attic, or something? Drinking pints of virgin's blood? You look twenty years younger."

"*Virgin's blood.*" Prager laughs. "That's the pot calling the kettle. I just do a day's work once in a while, and then I get on a tennis court or in a boat. Get some oxygen in my blood, instead of pure ethanol."

Prager claps Bessemer on the shoulder once more, and Bessemer ducks his head again, and it occurs to Carr that he's witnessing a sort of theater: an imitation of camaraderie, an acting out of Bessemer's subordination. He's not sure who the intended audience is. Maybe himself. Maybe they do it for each other.

There's a final lockjaw laugh, and Prager turns to Carr. His eyes, in his lined, brown face, are the color of sleet. His hand is cool and wiry. "And you must be Mr. Frye—at long last. Sorry for the scheduling screwup, but this week has been one fire drill after the other."

"There are worse places to kill time," Carr says. "And call me Greg."

Prager nods. "I'm Curt. Now, I hope you'll bear with me a bit longer, Greg, before we sit down." He looks at Kathy Rink, who looks inside the house and beckons.

Two men appear, both stocky with crew cuts, one holding something that looks like an old-fashioned walkie-talkie. He smiles politely and approaches Bessemer, while his partner waits, eight feet off.

"Mr. Bessemer, if you could spread your feet apart and hold your arms straight out from your sides, I'll sweep you down real quick. Mr. Frye, you'll be next."

There are platters of shrimp, crab legs, and scallops on crushed ice, a tureen of ceviche, bowls of gazpacho, frosted pitchers of iced tea, and plates of sliced fruit, all on a linen-covered table, under a wide awning. Beyond the awning, there are trees with songbirds in them, and a hillside descending in terraces to the beach and the swaying sea.

"Kathy insists on a frisk," Prager says, smiling across the table at Carr and Bessemer. "Personally, I think she likes it."

Rink smiles just as brightly. "It's what you pay me for, Curt, and I'm sure Mr. Frye—Greg—understands."

Carr nods and raises a glass of iced tea. "I'm all for hobbies."

Howard Bessemer squeezes a lemon wedge over his plate. "That other fellow you had—what was his name—he never saw the need to have me felt up."

Carr watches over his glass as Rink seeks out Prager's eye, and Prager nods to her minutely. "See what you were missing?" Prager says, and he dips a shrimp in red sauce and eats it.

"When it comes to security, Howie, it's smart to change things up now and then," Carr says. "Otherwise your boys get stale." He looks out at the ocean, the sand, two patrolling guards; then he looks at Prager. "Your private island?"

Prager smiles. "Not an island, but private."

"It's nice, but don't you miss home?" he asks Prager. "The States, I mean."

Prager eats another shrimp. "This is home to me. It's the only place I miss."

"But there's no issue with you going back stateside?"

"I go back when I need to," Prager says. "And what about you, Greg? And you are Greg today, right—not Glenn Freed, or Gary Frain, or Craig Farley? Is Boston still your base, Greg, or are you resettling in Palm Beach?"

Carr knows he's supposed to be impressed that Prager knows Greg Frye's aliases, and intimidated, and he lets his face tighten. "I do business in a lot of places. People come to me if they need to, and they don't seem to care much where I am or what I call myself, as long as I meet my obligations. Palm Beach is okay, though. The real estate market's still plenty soft."

Kathy Rink pats her mouth with a linen napkin. "That what you're doin' there, Greg, bottom-feeding?"

"That's real estate, right? Making money off somebody else's stupidity. Or their shit luck."

"Too true," Prager says approvingly. "But property's just a sideline for you, isn't it? I mean, you didn't come to talk to me about mortgage financing?"

"I need a banker. And maybe it's possible a banker could need me."

Prager's smile is indulgent. "They always need customers, otherwise they'd have no business. But strictly speaking, I'm not a banker, Greg—I

run a holding company. And I don't have customers, per se, I have investors—typically, quite large ones. That said, Isla Privada does own several financial institutions in Florida. If you need an account set up, I'm sure we can help you out."

Carr spears a fat scallop on his fork. He dips it in a dill sauce and pops it whole into his mouth. "I really like your paranoia, Curt," he says, chuckling. "But it's a fucking conversation killer. Would it help if she pats me down some more? Maybe a cavity search?"

Kathy Rink's laugh is throaty and loud. "Can it wait till after lunch?"

Carr winks at her and looks at Prager. "I think you have some idea what I do, and what I'm looking for. I came here to do business, not to hang out by the pool or tiptoe around."

Prager shrugs. "As I told Bess, I'm happy to listen. But doing business is something different, Greg. The truth is, I don't know you from Adam."

"Howie's not a good reference?"

"You're here only because of his introduction. But with all due respect to Bess—and he knows I love him—an introduction is not quite the same as a reference. Bess doesn't actually do business with you, whatever that business is—he can't vouch for you that way. So you don't come with the same kind of pedigree most of my new clients come with."

"The fingerprints didn't tell you enough?"

Prager glances at Rink. "They tell names and dates and places, Greg," Rink says. "Which could add up to somebody interesting, or could be somebody who's a little vulnerable."

"Vulnerable to what?" Carr asks.

"To being squeezed."

"Squeezed? By who?"

Rink chuckles. "It's a long fucking list of acronyms. We'll run out of daylight before I get through 'em all."

Carr smiles and works some incredulity into his voice. "You think I'm a cop?"

Prager smiles back. "I don't know enough about you to think anything at all, Greg. That's why, for now, it's better that I just sit and listen. If what you have to say is interesting, I may decide to spend the time and money to find out more about you—pretty much all there is to know. If not, we will have had a pleasant lunch and we'll say good-bye."

Howard Bessemer partly stifles a belch. He looks at Carr and shrugs. "I think that's your cue, Greg."

34

They leave Bessemer with the remains of lunch, and they walk as Carr talks—he and Prager in the lead, Kathy Rink trailing. It's a slow saunter around the grounds, and they stop occasionally to admire the horticulture or the view, but throughout, Prager and Rink maintain a careful silence. No questions, no comments, not even a sigh. Carr has waited a long time to make this pitch, and he knows Frye's business as well as Frye himself might, if he weren't fictional.

"It's a simple operation: I'm basically a middleman, a wholesaler. I buy stones in quantity—sometimes large quantities, sometimes smaller lots—and I resell them to other middlemen, or to retailers. The nature of my suppliers is such that I pay significantly discounted prices, so I can offer merchandise to my buyers at a price point way below other wholesalers, and still maintain a very fat margin. As you'd expect, it's a cash business, end to end: my suppliers want only cash, and I take only cash from my buyers.

"I started out regional—the Boston area, and New England—but, my trip to Otisville aside, I'm good at what I do and I've been successful. I can handle quantity in a hurry in either direction—buying or selling—and I can ship it, so now I've got suppliers and buyers all over the United States and abroad. Like I said before, they come to me, and I can do business anywhere. I keep my overheads low, in part by contracting whatever services I need—security, transpo, storage, whatever—so, no employees. I

spend a few months here, a few months there, but I'm based pretty much nowhere, and that's how I like it.

"I figure my banking needs are nothing new to you. I've got cash to move, and to put on deposit somewhere—with somebody who's not going to file a whole lot of paper. I want to invest what I deposit—build a diversified portfolio, nothing too aggressive, but with some international exposure. China definitely, maybe India—we can talk about it. And I need someone who can help me repatriate my assets—give them a boring history, something I can pay taxes on, though not too much. But something that'll stand up to an audit. And of course I want access—cash on demand, wherever I happen to be, in the States or abroad.

"In terms of quantity, I've got ten bucks I'd want to place up front, and I'd be looking to place maybe two bucks a month afterward. Maybe more sometimes."

Carr pauses as they approach Prager's pink guesthouse, waiting for some reaction but getting none. The guesthouse has a wall of French windows on the ocean side that open on to a patio. There are two tables there, with umbrellas and chairs, and Prager sits in one and watches the surf unfurl. Rink sits next to him and looks at Carr, who continues.

"What's different about my setup—where maybe there's an opportunity to work with somebody like you—are my buyers overseas. I have a lot of them—in Europe, Latin America, Asia, all over—a whole network of gray market independents. And all they do, all day long, is buy and sell stones—for local currency, for euros, for dollars, for pretty much whatever you want. Cash goes out, diamonds come in; cash comes in, diamonds go out—all day long, and no questions asked. And they all know how to ship."

Carr pauses again, waiting for a response. And he gets one, after a fashion: Prager looks at him for a long while and raises an eyebrow before he stands and strolls away. Carr follows, and Kathy Rink follows him. They pass a greenhouse and a low cinder-block building painted the same pink as the guesthouse. It's the size of a two-car garage, and it has a tin roof and roll-down metal door. The door is open, and two young black men are inside, talking, laughing, and doing something with the gardening equipment ranged around the walls. They fall silent as Prager passes. The path curves toward the beach again, and when they hit the sand, Carr continues.

"Stones are a lot easier to move than bulk cash," Carr continues, "and

a whole lot harder to trace. They're easier to store and secure, and easy to convert to cash when you need to—especially with a network like mine at your disposal. How much simpler does your operation become if you don't have to worry about moving cash—if you can move diamonds instead? Or better yet—if somebody is moving the diamonds for you? How much does that improve your margins? And how much more can you charge your clients for access to this kind of network?"

Carr finishes as they climb the stairs that lead from the beach to a vast blue swimming pool. They cross flagstones, headed toward more glass doors. Carr sees Bessemer, still at the table under the awning. Bessemer raises a hand in salute, and Carr waves back and looks for cameras, remembering where they're mounted, figuring the blind spots. The three remain silent as they go into the house, down a paneled hallway, past what looks like a wine cellar, and up a flight of stairs.

At the top of the stairs, past a study, a game room, a music room, through an atrium, and down another paneled corridor, is Prager's office. It's white and glass, minimally furnished in an aggressively modern style—a monk's cell with Barcelona chairs, a pair of Rothkos on the wall, and a view of palm trees and a Caribbean garden. Prager takes a seat behind a brushed aluminum desk that looks like a knife blade and that is bare but for a laptop, a large, wafer-thin monitor, and a phone. Rink takes one of the guest chairs. Carr takes the other and tries not to look at the laptop or at the thumbprint scanner plugged into it. Prager clasps his hands behind his head, leans back in his chair, and sighs.

"You're a guy off the street, Greg. Yes, you know Bess, and you have a little story to tell, but basically you're a guy off the street." Prager says it quietly, with a faint smile that is almost regretful. Carr says nothing.

"You could be a big deal, or a big waste of time," Kathy Rink says. "Or you could be something worse than a waste of time. How're we supposed to know?"

Carr shakes his head. "I'm confused. Are you saying no, or that you want to know more?"

It's Rink who answers. "Maybe he's saying you haven't sold him yet."

Carr shrugs and looks at Prager. "I'm not a salesman. It seems to me you're either interested or you're not."

"I don't know if I'm interested," Prager says. "I don't know if you're anything besides talk."

Carr lets a silence descend, and then he nods his head. "How about I get something from the car?"

Prager nods to Kathy Rink, who picks up a phone. In a moment a crew cut appears. "Take Mr. Frye to his car, and then bring him back," Rink says. "Anything he brings with him gets scanned."

The crew cut leads Carr out. When they return, Carr is carrying a slim metal attaché case.

"You checked it?" Rink asks, and the crew cut nods and leaves. Carr places the case on the desk and turns it so that the latches face Prager.

"I take it I'm supposed to open this," Prager says, and Carr nods. Kathy Rink comes around the desk to stand beside her boss. Prager looks at her and she lifts the lid.

Prager is silent for a moment, and then smiles thinly. "Very dramatic, Greg. They for real?"

"You expect me to say they're not? But I'm going to leave them with you, so you can check them out yourself."

"How much is here?"

"In carats or in dollars?"

"Dollars."

"Loose like that—three bucks, plus or minus. A lot more when you turn them into earrings and bracelets. But I figure you'll check that too."

"This a big lot for you?"

"Nope."

Prager leans back and sighs again. "So you're a guy off the street with a story and props—albeit, expensive props."

"Which makes me more worried, not less," Rink says. "Not many folks can afford this kind of window dressing. Assuming they're even for real."

Carr reaches across the desk and closes the attaché case. "I guess this is where I say thanks for lunch."

Prager puts a hand on the lid. "If you were in my shoes, would you do it differently?"

"It would depend on how much I wanted your business," Carr says.

"The dollar amounts you're talking about are rounding error," Prager says, shaking his head. "Not even that."

"Then I guess it would depend on how interested I was in access to this network—what kind of problems it could solve for me, what kind of new revenue streams it could bring."

"And if you were interested?"

"I'd ask you to open your kimono—at least a little."

Kathy Rink clears her throat and frowns. Prager ignores her and nods slowly. "And if I ask?"

Carr rubs his chin and looks at Prager. "Open the briefcase. Look in the lid pocket."

Prager lifts the lid and lowers it again. He holds a black flash drive between thumb and forefinger. "What's this supposed to be?"

"My kimono," Carr says.

35

Carr walks into the suite, and Latin Mike and Bobby look at him like children at a Christmas tree. Bobby's face is red and peeling. "Did he take it?"

Carr closes the door behind Bessemer and nods. "He took everything. When I left, the jump drive was sitting on his desk, right next to his computer."

Latin Mike sighs. Bobby smiles and puts out a fist. Mike taps it lightly. "So now we wait," Bobby says.

"We'll know as soon as it's plugged into anything with an Internet connection," Carr says.

"When what gets plugged in?" Bessemer asks from behind the bar.

"Gotta be the next day or two," Mike says, ignoring him. "He's got that party next weekend, and afterward he's on his road trip."

"Prager invited us to the party," Carr says. "I want to be far away by then."

"What's supposed to get plugged in?" Bessemer asks again.

"I gave Prager some information on a jump drive—information about my business, and some of my colleagues abroad. It should give him a better idea of what I've got to offer." Which only seems to make Bessemer more nervous. Bobby and Mike exchange looks, and Carr smiles thinly.

"Why don't you sit in the sun a while, Howie," he says. Bessemer shrugs and carries his gin and tonic to the terrace.

Bobby shakes his head. "Seriously—how long will that shit hold up?"

"Not long," Carr says. "The names are real, and they're really diamond dealers, all over the world, all active in the gray market. But only one of them—a guy in Singapore—knows the name Greg Frye, and that's because he's been paid to know it. I told Prager that the Singapore guy's the only one with approval to talk about my business. I told him if he likes what he hears, I'll okay the others to talk too."

"And this Singapore guy—what's he gonna say?"

"Something plausible. Given what Boyce is charging us, it better be. With a little luck, though, Howie will have done his thing and we'll be gone before it's an issue."

Latin Mike looks out at Bessemer, and then looks at Carr. "How did he do today?"

"He was fine," Carr says. "Kept it together, didn't speak unless he was spoken to, focused mainly on the food."

"And you think he'll keep on keepin' on?"

Carr nods. "He has only one more thing to do, once Dennis tells us the drive's been plugged in."

"So I guess it doesn't matter that he's asking a lot of questions," Mike says, nodding. "'Cause pretty soon it won't matter how much he knows."

"He's my problem, and I'll take care of him."

"He's everybody's problem if you don't, *jefe*."

"I said I'd take care of him."

Mike looks at him, and doesn't look away when Bobby clears his throat. Bobby puts a hand on Mike's shoulder. "Once that thing's plugged in, we zip up and get out, *amigo,* so we better start packing."

Bobby and Mike depart, and Carr collapses into an armchair. The two of them seemed to take up more than their usual share of space and oxygen, and Carr is relieved to be alone. His breath leaves him in a long sigh, and the tensions of the day—Prager's relentless skepticism, Rink's barely veiled hostility, the constant fear of a wrong word from Bessemer, the constant feel of cameras on him, like a finger tapping incessantly on his skull, and all the pumping adrenaline—hit at once. His shoulders cramp, his legs tighten, and the sweat that stayed away, even through the day's heat, rises suddenly through his shirt. A bitter taste washes through his mouth. His stomach twists, and for an instant he feels his lunch coming up. And then his cell burrs.

"You're answering the phone," Tina says. "That's a good sign."

"I've got all my fingers and toes too, at least so far."

"Prager was interested?"

"We'll see just how much."

"No word from Dennis yet?"

"Not yet."

"What's taking so long?"

"Prager's a busy guy. I assume he's got some other things to do before he gets around to researching me."

"You'll call when you hear?"

"I'll call."

To stay in the chair is to sleep, Carr knows, so he hoists himself up and goes to the bar. He fills a glass with crushed ice, club soda, and limes, and looks at Bessemer on the terrace. He's numb in a lounge chair, his head to one side, a leg dangling—a puppet without strings. His round face is empty, and Carr thinks again of Bessemer's son, Simon—his watchful eyes, his suspicion. Bessemer's glass is balanced precariously on his belly, in the grip of limp fingers. Carr opens the terrace door and retrieves it. Bessemer mutters something he can't make out.

Carr showers and changes his clothes, and when he steps into the living room again, he finds the daylight fading and Bessemer sprawled on the sofa. His shoes are off, and his shirt is untucked, but he's out just as cold. Carr shakes his head and picks up the room service menu.

He's just about made his choices when his phone rings again. Carr crosses the room at a run.

"You don't call?" Valerie says. "I've got to depend on Mike to let me know? What's the matter, you tired of me?"

He sighs. "I figured you'd call me."

"I guess you figured right. It went well?"

"So far so good, but he hasn't done anything with the drive yet, and that's what matters. Chun is back from New York?"

"Yeah, and she has no trips planned for a couple of weeks."

"And her security?"

"Nothing new since last time," Valerie says. "You going to let me know when you hear something, or am I going to have to keep chasing you?"

"I'll let you know."

There's a long pause, filled by the soft hiss of the ether, and then Valerie sighs. "It's just around the corner now. You come to any decisions about what you're going to do with yourself afterward?"

"I'll let you know."

Carr looks at Bessemer and can't imagine him going anyplace, and decides against room service. He has a light dinner in one of the hotel restaurants, and afterward he kicks off his shoes and rolls his pant legs and walks along the shore. The beach is empty but for a few couples, strolling arm in arm, and Carr gives them a wide berth. The sea breeze has turned cold, but a tropical lassitude still trails him across the sand.

Too long on the roller coaster, Declan called it. "Yer jacked up so long, you get used to it—used to the fright and paranoia, and then you get stupid. You know you're supposed to stay scared, to stay alert, but you can't seem to care enough to make it happen. Too tired and bored to save yer own goddamn life. And it always comes at the worst feckin' time—right at the end, when you need to be on top of the game."

Right at the end—it's where Carr is at last: Dennis says the word, Howie makes his call, and then it's Valerie's turn, a matter of little more than typing. And then . . . what? A flight north, to watch his father disintegrate? A flight south, to watch Tina's men sift ashes? A flight into the sunset with Valerie? One too many options to settle by the toss of a coin, and Carr wonders if it really matters which he picks. *Too tired and bored to save yer own goddamn life.* Too tired, certainly. He thinks about Bessemer, in a heap on the sofa, and of Latin Mike's admonition: *He's everybody's problem if you don't . . .* His throat tightens and a clammy sweat breaks out across his forehead.

The incoming tide is lapping around his ankles when his phone goes off, and he answers without looking at the number.

"Dennis?"

"Who's Dennis?" Arthur Carr asks, and Carr can tell right away that his father's been drinking.

"Someone I work with. Is everything okay?"

"I'll call some other time, if you're working."

"It's fine. Are you all right?"

"All right?" Arthur Carr snorts. "You know she's leaving, don't you?"

"Who's leaving?"

"Eleanor Calvin—who else would I be talking about?"

"She told you she was moving away?"

"The question is, Why didn't you tell me? She said you've known for weeks. Is this privileged information? Maybe you think I'm a security risk."

"I didn't want to say anything until I'd made new arrangements."

"*New arrangements*—what the hell do I need *those* for? I didn't like the old arrangements you made, and now that she's walking out, I don't need any goddamn new ones. The hell with that disloyal bitch."

"Is she there?"

"What if she is?"

"Put her on the phone."

His father's laugh is jagged. "Well, she's not here. She walked out on me. Said I could fix my own dinner if I didn't like her cooking, and that if I was going to curse—"

"What did you say to her?"

"I had no idea her sensibilities were so—"

"What did you say?"

"Nothing much, and I can't imagine she hasn't heard the word *whore* before."

"For chrissakes!" Carr says, and he realizes he's shouting, and that the few people on the beach are staring.

Arthur Carr laughs again. "In fact, I'm sure she's heard worse."

Carr sighs and walks toward the jetty that marks the edge of the hotel property. "You can't talk to her that way, Dad," Carr says softly. "You can't expect her to put up with it."

"Do you have any idea what *I've* put up with?"

"You can't talk to people that way."

"*People?* She's not people—she's my goddamn wife, and I'll talk to her any goddamn way I please."

The breath catches in Carr's throat, and there's a rushing noise in his ears. When he speaks, his voice is soft and even. "We're talking about Mrs. Calvin, Dad."

There's angry silence on the other end, and then an embarrassed cough. "What the hell are you saying? I know who we're talking about."

A wave catches Carr as he reaches the jetty, lifting him and banging his knees on a rock. The sound of surf against stone drowns out the sound of his father's hasty good-bye.

"Fuck," Carr says aloud.

When his phone rings again, he thinks it's his father calling back, but it's not.

"Jesus, Dennis, I've heard from everybody *but* you today," Carr says, leaning against a rock. "Please give me some good news."

"I would if I could."

"The fucking thing's still not plugged in?"

When he answers, Dennis's voice is thin and tired. "I got the message ten minutes ago. It's plugged in all right, just not into Prager's computer."

36

Bobby has exhausted his many variations on *fuck this*. He hunches forward on the sofa in the sunny front room of the workhouse and runs his hands though his hair. When he looks up at Carr, he looks as though he's come through a hurricane.

"It's the worst fucking Plan B I've ever heard," Bobby says.

"No argument," Carr says. "It sucks. So give me an alternative." He looks at Latin Mike, who stares longingly at a jet dwindling in the sky.

"It's for shit," Mike says, "but I got nothing better."

"You can get the hardware?" Carr asks Bobby.

"That's not the problem. I've got the boat; a couple of WaveRunners won't be an issue. The problem is all the fucking variables."

"And the putty?"

Bobby shakes his head. "I know where I can get it, the det cord too—equipment's not the problem. The problem is too many variables—too many places where the fucking wheels can fall off."

"Let me worry about those."

"That's not a lot of comfort," Bobby says. "No offense."

"Then give me an alternative," Carr repeats.

Bobby shakes his head and puts his hands through his hair again. Carr looks at Dennis, who is thinner than ever—a ghost-eyed wheat stalk. "And you're sure it'll load, even if the screen's locked?"

"Screen locked, power-saving mode, waiting for a password, whatever—I'm working down below the operating system. If the computer's switched on, it'll load. Fifteen seconds, max. The LED will blink green."

"What if the computer's not switched on?"

"Then switch it on—it'll load. It'll just take a little longer—a minute, maybe."

Latin Mike gives up on the airplane, lights a cigarette, and blows smoke at the ceiling. "What about Bessemer—can he handle it?"

"It's a party—mostly he has to handle eating and drinking. He's good at that."

"He'll have to say his piece to Prager in person. You think he can do it?"

Carr nods. "A case of nerves will make him more plausible."

"Long as he doesn't crap his pants, *jefe*."

Carr stands and stretches. He hasn't slept and his eyes feel like an ashtray. "I'll let you guys start putting it together."

Still bent forward, Bobby laughs bitterly. "You don't know what they're going to do with a party going on. How do you know they won't call the locals? I don't want to find myself playing hide and seek with a coast guard cutter."

"Rink won't do that," Carr says. "She's still new. She wants to prove herself."

"You don't know," Bobby says, shaking his head. "You don't know shit."

Carr shrugs and walks to the door. "No argument there, Bobby."

There's a tin-roofed shack, painted bright blue, on the side of the road to the airport, where the fat counterman serves fresh fish-and-chips and cold beer, and where Carr meets Tina. It is well past lunchtime, and they're the only ones sitting at the open-air counter. Carr drinks an iced tea and eats fries from Tina's plate, which is otherwise untouched.

Tina watches heat rise from the asphalt. Her voice is low and tight. "Isn't that your job, to plan for these things?" she says. "To have a fallback when shit goes wrong?"

Carr laughs. "I did plan for it. Of course, my plan assumed that Eddie

Silva was still running security, and I didn't find out he wasn't until I was standing in Prager's offices. Remind me again who's responsible for that triumph of intel."

"Fuck you," Tina says, without much conviction. "You think this will fly?"

Carr shrugs. "The bigger question is whether Greg Frye will last until the party."

"It's not much longer."

"Yeah, but Dennis tells me Rink's been busy. She's poring over what was on the flash drive, Googling like mad."

"Doing it herself?"

"Apparently."

"I'll call Singapore—make sure our guy remembers his lines."

Carr nods. "If he does, and if Rink stays focused on the info on the flash drive, Frye might last. If she starts digging deeper into his criminal record—trying to talk to arresting officers or prosecutors—we're hosed."

Tina's jaw clenches. "Just a few days more," she says, and she jabs her fish with a fork.

Carr has a laptop open and aerial photos of Prager's property spread out on the coffee table. He's looking at a floor plan of Prager's house when Howard Bessemer walks in. Bessemer is fresh from the hotel spa, wrapped in spa terry cloth, shod in spa slippers, and admiring his new spa manicure. He stops when he sees Carr and stares at the coffee table.

"That doesn't look like packing, Greg," Bessemer says.

"Don't worry, Howie, we're going home—right after the party."

Bessemer's spa glow vanishes, replaced by a nervous pallor. "You said we were leaving before then."

"Change of plans."

Bessemer looks down at his terry-cloth slippers, and then at the tabletop again. "That can't be good."

"It'll be fine, Howie," Carr says, and he returns to his work.

"What do we—"

"It'll be fine," Carr says again. "Just think about what you're going to do afterward. It'll be fine." Bessemer looks at him skeptically and Carr ignores him until he goes away.

Thick as Thieves

Carr isn't lying to Bessemer. An uncharacteristic calm settled over him the night before, as Dennis delivered the news, and it hasn't abandoned him yet. The adrenaline started pumping as he began laying flesh on his skeletal fallback plan, and it's built with every detail he's added, but it hasn't jangled him. In fact, there's something oddly comforting about it.

He studies the photos and drawings, memorizing points of entry and egress, camera fields and blind spots, alternate routes and dead ends, and it reminds him of his training days at the Farm. His heart rate is up, his fingers are drumming on the table, and there's a hum in his gut that he recognizes as eagerness. Carr can almost hear the rough brogue and smiles to himself. *Roller coasters*—after all this time, here, on his last job, he's finally developed a taste for them. Declan would be proud.

The call comes in the empty night, when it seems even the ocean is still. The voice on the other end is held together with tissue paper and trembling breath, and Carr almost doesn't recognize it as Eleanor Calvin's. When he does, he's certain she's calling to report a death, but he's wrong.

"He is . . . I don't know . . . I can't find him anywhere. I came over this afternoon and . . . the ambassador was gone."

37

Carr ignores the phone twitching in his pocket for the third time in ten minutes, for the hundredth time since dawn, and focuses on the Stock-bridge cop shifting nervously on the porch steps. He's young and earnest, and every time he speaks his Adam's apple jumps behind the collar of his uniform shirt. He reminds Carr of Dennis.

"There's nothing new since the Lenox PD called this morning, to say they found his Volvo in the town lot. They haven't found anyone who saw the ambassador park it yet."

Carr bites back the reflexive correction and nods. "My mother is buried in Lenox. He may—"

"Mrs. Calvin told us. Lenox has a man doing drive-bys in case he shows up there, but they haven't seen him yet."

"Did they check the local inns?"

"Lenox checked the inns in town, the Staties checked the motels along Route Seven. Nobody's seen him."

"How about the car? Did it look like he'd slept in it? Did it look broken into?"

"Broken into?"

Carr sighs. "Is it possible it was stolen from someplace else and dumped in Lenox?"

The cop reddens. "I . . . Lenox didn't say anything special about it, but I can ask them."

"I'll ask myself, when I go up there. What about the temperature last night?"

"The temperature?"

"How cold did it get up there?"

The cop squints, and then it dawns on him. "No, no—he would've been okay. It was in the low sixties last night."

Carr nods. "You'll tell the Lenox PD I'm coming up?"

"Sure, Mr. Carr," he says. "Did you have any luck finding his cell phone, sir? Because if it's turned on—"

"It was in his sock drawer. The battery is dead."

The cop's Adam's apple leaps, and he shakes his head regretfully. "We'll be in touch then," he says, and he walks down the path to his cruiser.

Carr rubs his palms over his face, which feels thick and numb. His eyes are sticky and he smells like airports and rental cars.

Eleanor Calvin is inside, red-eyed, sniffling, smaller. "Tim Binney," she says. "He's a nice boy. I just wish he had more to tell us."

"Uh-huh," Carr says. Even with the shades up and all the windows open, the house is gloomy, and it reeks of food and heat and mildew. Carr swallows hard, tries not to breathe too deeply or to look too closely at anything.

He fishes his phone from his pocket and scans through a long list of missed calls. Mike, Bobby, Bobby, Mike, Valerie, Valerie, Valerie. He turns the ringer on, and as soon as he does the phone burrs. Valerie again. He turns the ringer off.

"Your phone is always ringing."

"Work," Carr says. He looks up at Eleanor Calvin. She's crying again. "Mrs. Calvin, it's not your fault."

"Yes, it is. I knew he was upset. I knew he was confused. I just never thought he would . . . I lost patience with him."

"He has that effect on people."

She shakes her head. "No. I was stupid. He was upset and confused and frustrated, and I shouldn't have argued with him. I didn't know that Volvo still ran. I didn't think he had the key."

"I took it away last year, but he must've had a spare. He was upset even before he found out that you were moving?"

She nods. "He's been agitated for weeks, on and off."

"About anything in particular?"

"He's been talking about your mother."

"Why?"

An embarrassed look crosses her face, and she looks away from Carr. "Her birthday is coming up, dear—next Tuesday. She's always on his mind, this time of year."

"What does he say?"

Eleanor Calvin's cheeks redden. "He curses sometimes, the way he cursed at me—but I don't think he means anything by it. Other times, I can tell he misses her. Just a few days ago he was talking about . . . I don't know, I suppose it might've been a vacation the three of you took. And there was something about a fairy tale—King Midas, I think, and a maze. Honestly, I couldn't follow most of it. Does it mean anything to you?"

Carr looks at her and shakes his head.

The Lenox Police Department is headquartered in a reassuring brick building with columns and dressed stone trim that dominates the south end of Main Street. But when Carr steps through the heavy doors, into the heat and glare of the afternoon, he is not reassured. The Lenox force is no larger than its Stockbridge counterpart, and its strengths run similarly to directing traffic and protecting weekend homes. Manpower is stretched thin in this high season of outdoor concerts, dance recitals, and outlet shopping, and though the stocky, gray sergeant promised they were doing all they could, Carr knows it's not much.

There's a bench outside headquarters, in the shade of a wide oak and with a view of cars streaming toward a concert at Tanglewood. Carr takes a seat and sighs. His bones are leaden.

The sergeant had led him out back, to where the Volvo had been towed, and let him look over the car. There wasn't much to see. The doors had been unlocked when the Lenox cops found it, but there were no signs of a break-in. It was as mud-spattered and pollen-caked as it had been when Carr had seen it last, decomposing in his father's driveway. Inside, it was bare and sour. No motel keys or gas receipts or maps with circled destinations. The sergeant had told him his patrols would keep an eye on the lot where the Volvo had been found, in the event Arthur Carr returned for it. Carr had nodded and thanked him.

What had he expected them to do about a man who'd simply gotten in

his car and driven away? Did he think they would organize a posse? Call out the bloodhounds? Dredge the Stockbridge Bowl? And really, what had he expected to accomplish up here himself? What the hell was he doing?

Latin Mike had asked a similar question, in a call Carr had made the mistake of answering in the Miami airport, while he waited for a flight to Boston. "Forty-eight hours to game time, and you *fucking* disappear on us? The fuck's the matter with you, *cabrón*? This job's not hard enough as is—you got to walk off in the middle of the night?"

"I told Bobby that I'd be back in time."

"I don't give a shit what you told him—I want to hear it for myself, *pendejo*. I want to hear about this *personal business*—or maybe you just lost whatever balls you pretended to have."

"I'll be back before the party, Mike."

"That's all you got to say? I got money sunk in this thing, asshole—I got *plans*—and if you fuck them up—"

Carr had hung up then, and had answered only one call since, from Valerie. He was about to board the Boston flight, and her voice was soft and worried. He could barely make it out over the announcements.

"Bobby said you had an emergency. Are you okay, baby? Can I do anything?"

"Just keep people calm," Carr had said. "I'll be back soon." If Valerie had said anything in reply, he hadn't heard, and he couldn't bring himself to talk anymore. Bobby, undaunted, had turned to texting. His last message summed it up nicely: "4 q s hole."

A bus rolls by, leaving behind a cloud of diesel and an impression of wrinkled faces and wispy white hair at the windows. Carr hoists himself from the bench, rubs his eyes, and drives to his mother's grave.

The cemetery is two miles outside of town, off a pitted road and behind a leaning wrought-iron fence. There's a chapel by the gate, with black shutters, peeling white clapboards, and a steeple with no bell. Carr doesn't come here often, and when he does, his heart pounds. It's pounding now, as he follows the path that climbs the hillside, and his face is warm, though not from exertion.

Her grave is near the top, by a stand of maples and a white stone bench, and with a view of distant woods and a nameless blue pond. It is

not a family plot—no relatives lie to rest nearby—it is simply a place his mother picked out when she learned that she was dying. He wasn't sure what about the site appealed to her. Maybe it was the pond, or maybe it was the company of strangers.

Her stone is granite—Dark Barre, from Vermont, Carr recalls from a corner of his exhausted brain. The chiseled inscription is simple: *Andrea de Soto Carr*. No dates; no epitaph; no embellishments of any kind. Carr rests a hand on the curved top. He doesn't fight the hammering in his chest or the burning in his eyes, doesn't resist the vertigo. It's a much diluted version of the feeling he'd had, at age fourteen, when his father told him she was gone. The rushing in his ears, the ground opening beneath him, the free fall, the sense that there was no bottom. There's something consoling in the memory of that initial terror. He'd survived it once; he could do it again.

The time between her diagnosis and her death was short—a matter of months—and Carr spent it sleepwalking. His vision, it seemed, worked only on things very close—his hands, his feet, a book—or very far away, but not in the middle distances, no place other people might occupy. Other people were an abstraction—like shadow puppets. Most of what they said seemed irrelevant or garbled, and he himself said very little in response.

What he remembers best of his mother from that time are her hands, white and narrow, strong until the end. She took up knitting again, something she said she'd done when she was younger. He remembers the white hands working, the skeins of dark wool, the click of the needles, the pieces she made that were neither scarves nor hats, but simply long, dark panels. He remembers too the streaks of gray that appeared, overnight, in her jet-black hair, and how her collarbones became so pronounced—the bones of a ship, laid bare by a storm. *Denial* was not a word he knew in this context, but later someone explained.

He can't look for too long at the stone, and so he focuses on the flowers placed beneath it—a wilting bouquet of gladiolas in yellow, pink, and white. Her favorite flowers, in her favorite colors—the same as the bunch he's holding now. He guesses that the older ones have been here for a day.

38

It's the white stone bench that does it. He sits on it, in the shade, for some time, looking at the flowers on her grave—the ones he brought and the ones his father left there. He runs his hand over the smooth stone, lets the coolness seep into his fingers. He studies the veins and seams—like threads—in the marble. He remembers her knitting, the coiled wool. He lets his eyes close and listens to the patrolling bees. He lets Eleanor Calvin's voice echo. Something about a vacation, about a fairy tale—King Midas and a maze. And then his eyes are open again, and he's up from the bench, trotting down the hill toward his rental car.

There are still lawn tickets available for the Boston Symphony Orchestra concert, and Carr buys one, but declines a program. The music will not start for hours, but the manicured lawns of Tanglewood are already busy with concertgoers spreading blankets on the grass, laying out picnics, pursuing their wandering toddlers. Carr sticks to the gravel paths and makes his way south and west, toward the formal gardens. It's been nearly thirty years since he was last here, but somehow he remembers the way.

The gardens are bordered by boxwood hedges, as high and thick and dark as they are in Carr's memory: looming green walls; gnarled, intricate roots; and, cut at intervals in the hedge, portals so narrow that even children must stoop to pass. Carr turns sideways and ducks low, but branches catch at his shirt.

It is quiet on the other side of the hedge, and the air is still. The box-

woods are shorter inside the garden, but high enough that the aisles between them seem narrow and clutching. Certainly Carr remembers them that way, remembers running headlong down those corridors in the fading light, remembers the thrill and fear, the sensation of walls closing in, the blind curves, sharp turns, dead ends. Remembers it as a maze—a labyrinth, his father called it.

Mrs. Calvin heard it wrong: not *Midas*, but *Minos*—King Minos, of Crete. Not a fairy tale, but a myth. He remembers his father's voice, chasing behind him, calling, in a bad imitation of Boris Karloff: "Beware the labyrinth. Beware the Minotaur." Carr was six. His father had been thinking about leaving the Foreign Service and was interviewing with the Economics Departments of several colleges in New England. They'd made a family trip of it. He'd never seen his parents so relaxed before, or ever again.

He's moving at a run when he comes to the white marble bench. It's at the far side of the garden, where two boxwood lanes empty into a clearing. It's broad and smooth, with a high curved back and a worn inscription, and it's cracked and stained by weather and much use. His father sits at one end, one leg crossed over the other, arms folded in his lap. He's studying the lawn, and he's so still and pale he might be made of marble himself.

Arthur Carr looks at his son without surprise, and with a faint, wry smile. "Minotaur chasing you again?"

"What the hell do you think you're doing?" Carr says, catching his breath. "Where the hell have you been?"

His father scratches his head and narrows his gray eyes. "Have you eaten lunch? I could use a sandwich."

At the diner, his father orders a roast beef on rye. He tries to order a scotch with it, and has some trouble with the waitress's explanation that beer is the best she can do. In the end he has a Heineken. Carr orders tuna fish, and goes outside to make phone calls.

He watches his father through the window while he talks to the local police and to Mrs. Calvin, and makes arrangements for the Volvo to be towed to a garage. Carr glances at his missed calls list, and sees more messages from Valerie and Mike, and one—an hour earlier—from Tina. He goes back inside.

Arthur Carr's reading glasses are perched on the end of his nose, and

he's scanning the ads and the children's games printed on the paper place mat. "Calling the office?" he asks, as his son slides into the booth. "I expect you'll be getting back soon."

"It wasn't work. It was about you."

"Not a particularly compelling subject," his father says, chuckling. "Who's interested in that?"

"Mrs. Calvin, for one. She was worried sick."

"Damned dramatic. Doesn't she have anything better to do? Shouldn't she be packing?"

"For chrissakes, you can't just take off like that."

"Nonsense—people do it all the time. They're here, and then—poof—they're gone, just like that." There's a connect-the-dots picture on the place mat, and his father moves his finger from number to number. "Christ, some people can vanish while they're standing right in front of you. They're in the very same room, but it's like they're not there at all. She had that trick down cold."

"Mrs. Calvin?"

His father looks up and scowls. "Don't be thick—you know who I'm talking about. You're just like her, for chrissakes—playing dumb when you want to, but taking it all in. She was a hell of a poker player, you know."

"I didn't know that."

His father squints at him behind his glasses. "So, maybe not taking it *all* in," he says, and a sly smile—as at a private joke—crosses his face. "It's her birthday coming up. Did you remember?"

"On Tuesday."

"It was always hard to shop for her. Who knew what she wanted? Nothing I had to offer." The smirk again, angrier this time. "For example, I never knew her taste in cigarette lighters. And I was never much of a tennis player, either. Always hated doubles."

Carr takes a deep breath. His father mentions Hector Farias only rarely, and when he does the reference is always oblique. And always he baits his son to respond—to ask about his mother and Farias, to offer some comment—but Carr never does. He's relieved when the waitress brings their food.

Arthur Carr is hungry, and in short order half his sandwich is gone, and so is half his beer. He pats his mouth with a napkin and sighs. "Her cooking isn't so remarkable," he says. "I'll take a few meals here every week and be just fine, and the hell with her."

"Don't start again," Carr says. "She won't be around for much longer, but for the time being, you've got to make this work. You've got to be civil, at least."

"Silence is the best I can manage," Arthur Carr says, and drains his beer. He turns his attention to the connect-the-dots picture again.

Carr shakes his head. "She does a lot for you."

His father looks up. His eyes are unfocused and confused for a moment, and then they sharpen. He crumples the place mat into a small white ball. "What exactly did she do for me, besides end my career and turn me into a cuckold and a laughingstock? Am I supposed to be grateful for that?"

Carr's jaw tightens. "I was talking about Mrs. Calvin," he says softly.

"I told you not to do that—pretend to be stupid. You know damn well who I'm talking about."

Carr looks around the diner. It's nearly empty, and he takes a deep, unsteady breath. His voice is a raspy whisper. "You want to have a conversation about her? Fine—let's have at it. You want to know what she did for you? For one thing, she put up with your crap for all those years. She put up with your absences and your anger and moving house every other year, and she still managed not to kill you. I'd say that was a fair amount. So she had a lapse in judgment—can you really blame her? She tried to find some happiness, and didn't think it through. She's not the first one."

Arthur Carr lifts his half-glasses off and pinches his nose between his thumb and forefinger. "*Some happiness*—is that what you tell yourself? Is that what you really believe?" His words are slow and his voice is quiet, and his expression is like a flickering candle, shifting from surprise to triumph to regret. "All that watching, and you never saw anything."

"I saw you red in the face, and heard the endless griping about your career—as if your failings were somehow her fault. You and your goddamn career."

"My career . . . Jesus." His father shakes his head. "You *are* an idiot."

"So much for conversation," Carr says, and he picks up his tuna sandwich.

"All that watching . . . ," Arthur Carr says, and he lowers his voice. "Don't you understand? If it wasn't for *my* career, she wouldn't have had one."

"Had one what? What are you talking about?"

"I'm talking about her career."

"Her career? She didn't have a career—she never even had a job."

Arthur Carr's laugh is bitter. "She *always* had a job," he says. "My job enabled her job, for chrissakes. It was her *cover*. *I* was her cover. *You* were her cover. *Her cover*—do you understand it now?"

There's a rushing in Carr's ears, a step he missed. "What? What are you talking about?"

"You insist on being dense. She was Agency, your mother—in the Directorate of Operations. You understand what I'm saying?"

There's vertigo, a feeling of the ground opening beneath him, and it's hard to get the breath out of his lungs. His fingers are splayed on the table. "What the hell . . . ? What are you saying?"

His father looks suddenly tired. His voice is a dry whisper. "Your mother was with the Agency, for chrissakes. She was a CIA officer."

Carr doesn't remember getting the check, or paying it, or leaving the diner, but somehow they're in the parking lot and he's grabbing his father's arm. It's thin and light—a bird's bone. Carr hears his own voice, but it's far away and attenuated—a radio in a distant room. "I don't know who you think you're talking about, but it's not . . . You're confused, Dad—you're seriously confused."

Carr stares into his father's face, into those gray eyes, but try as he might, he can't find confusion there—can't find anything but exhaustion and regret. He tells himself his father can't keep a thought straight any longer—can't find the thread, much less hold on to it. He doesn't know the difference between Mrs. Calvin and his own wife half the time. He tells himself these things, but his voice is tinny and remote and in his heart he knows it's full of shit.

A woman's voice cuts across it all. "There a problem, mister? You need a hand?" It's the waitress, calling from the diner door. She's holding a telephone, scowling at Carr, and staring at his hand on his father's arm.

Arthur Carr waves with his other hand and smiles. "We're fine, thanks. My son's just driving me home."

On the way, Carr's head is wrapped in cotton wool, and he can't tear it loose. He pulls over just before Lee, when he realizes he's not seeing the road. His father is unsurprised, and looks out the window at a crow picking at a flattened squirrel. The light is lengthening, tinted at the edges with orange, and a hum of insects rises from the woods. Carr draws a deep breath and his father turns toward him.

"Hector Farias," Carr says softly.

His father nods. "He was one of her sources, one of the agents she ran. He was her prize."

"She . . . she knew he was Cuban intelligence?"

"Of course—that's what made him so valuable. He was one of their senior guys; he was connected everywhere in the region. He was a star, and she had turned him and was playing him back to Havana. In theory, at least."

"And in reality?"

"He was playing her."

"The whole time?"

"The whole time."

"It was years that she knew him . . . all those places we lived. She never suspected?"

Arthur Carr sighs and turns to the window again. The crow draws a strand of gut from the dusty carcass. His beak is glossy, and so black it's nearly blue. It's an eternity before Arthur Carr speaks, and when he does, his voice is like dry leaves. "That's what the record says."

Carr turns in his seat. "What does that mean?"

Carr's father runs a forefinger down his long nose, to his mouth, and to his chin, which has begun to quiver. "She wasn't stupid. Your mother had her flaws, but that wasn't one of them."

The rushing grows louder in Carr's ears. "You're saying she *knew* she was being played? The whole time?"

"She sussed it out early on."

"She *knew*? She told you that?"

Arthur Carr studies the crow, hopping around the squirrel. After a while, he nods.

Carr can't seem to fill his lungs, and he throws open the door of the rental car and stumbles out into the road. The driver of a passing truck leans on his horn and yells, and leaves a cloud of dust in his wake. The crow flies off. Carr walks slowly to the edge of the woods, and slowly back, the whole way watching the ground. When he returns, his father has the passenger door open and is sideways in his seat.

Carr looks at him. "She *knew*, but she let it happen—she participated in it. She . . . she was a traitor." The word sounds strange in his ears—something foreign or archaic.

Arthur Carr makes a tiny, rueful smile. "Well, yes," he says.

"Why?"

"Why do you think?" his father says. "She loved that son of a bitch, and she thought that he loved her. Who knows, maybe he did."

Carr gazes at the treetops, the orange clouds, the coming twilight. "But that's not in the record, you said. That's not the official story."

"No."

"Why not? Why didn't the Agency come after her? Why didn't they prosecute? Put her in jail? Jesus Christ—why did they ever let *me* in the door?"

"The counterespionage people wanted to come after her. They were embarrassed and angry, and they wanted a full investigation and some-one they could burn at the stake."

"What stopped them?"

Arthur Carr stretches his legs in front of him. He massages his right knee. "I did," he says softly. "I vouched for her. I pulled what strings I had left at State. Finally I threatened to go public if they didn't let her be. It wound up costing me every chit I'd ever collected over twenty-plus years, and my pension too, but eventually they decided to call it incompetence rather than treason. So that's how the record reads." He flexes his knee and looks up at his son. "The only thing the Agency hates worse than being embarrassed by the opposition is being embarrassed by them in public. You'd think they'd be used to it by now."

Carr watches him rub his bony thighs and flex his aching fingers. He looks thin and brittle—like a leaf the wind might carry off. Another truck passes, another dust cloud settles. The crow returns and curses at them.

It is six a.m., and Carr is in Terminal A at Logan, waiting for his Miami flight, still waiting for the spinning to stop. He's at the gate, watching but not following the highlights of a baseball game on the wall-mounted TV, when someone steps into his view. She's wearing a black dress and dark glasses, and her bare arms are paper white. Her lips barely move when she speaks, and her voice is flat.

"He wants to talk to you," Tina says. "He wants to know if there's some reason you don't answer your phone." She takes off her glasses and makes a tiny flick of her eyes. Carr looks over her shoulder, down the long row of gates. Even at a distance, Mr. Boyce looms like a cliff.

39

They've gone over it once. They've gone over it twice. Now, as darkness settles on the workhouse and wind sweeps through the palms in the front yard and bumps the boats against the metal dock out back, they go over it a sixth time. Carr makes Bobby walk it through: the sequence, the timing, the signals, the routes in and out, the alternate routes, the rendezvous, the alternate rendezvous, and the contingency plans—meager though they are.

"And the minimum window is?" Carr asks when Bobby pauses.

"Five minutes. Five fucking minutes. How many times do I have to repeat it?"

"No less than five between the opening and the finale. Longer if you've got a receptive audience, but no less than five."

Latin Mike snorts from the sofa. "You don't know how many guys they're gonna have in the house, for chrissakes. You don't know if this is gonna distract them."

Carr answers without looking at him. "Loud noises get attention." Mike snorts again, and Carr ignores him. He turns to Dennis. "What's the weather forecast?" he asks.

Dennis is pale and skittish behind his laptop. He glances at the screen. "Mostly sunny and breezy tomorrow, with heavy surf from the storm. Weather service says it should hold off until after ten tomorrow night, and even then we should only get the edge of it."

"They downgraded it?" Carr asks.

Dennis nods. "Tropical storm Cara now."

"Is it gonna fuck things up at the airport?" Bobby asks.

"We get out before ten we should be okay," Dennis says.

"So let's get out before ten," Mike says, lighting a cigarette.

"That's the plan," Carr says. Mike snorts again. Carr looks at Bobby. "The surf's going to be rough. You okay with that?"

"We're good."

"Good," Carr says. "Let's go over it again."

It's eleven when they stop. Dennis buries his head in a computer. Mike grabs a whiskey bottle, plugs a cigarette into his mouth, and goes outside.

Bobby stretches and yawns. "Howie still sober?" he asks Carr.

"He was when I left him this afternoon. You were good with him."

Bobby shrugs. "Babysitting gave me something to do. He was jumpy without you."

Carr rubs his grit-filled eyes. "Nice to feel wanted."

Bobby looks at him, laughs ruefully, and shakes his head. "Fuckin' Carr," he mutters.

Mike is sitting on the front steps, drinking from the bottle, blowing smoke, looking at the sky. Carr walks around him.

"Guess you've given up tryin' to be like Deke," Mike says. "No pregame party tonight, right? So I got to make my own."

"Make it a small one. It's an early day tomorrow."

"I'll try to fit you in—unless something else comes up. Maybe I got to get my teeth cleaned or something."

"Give it a rest, Mike. I was gone for, what, a few hours?"

"It was more than a day."

"And now I'm back, so spare me."

Mike is fast—up and at Carr almost before the whiskey bottle hits the dirt. One hand goes to Carr's neck, his thumb in the hollow of Carr's throat. The other hand holds a knife. "If I didn't need you whole, *pendejo*, you wouldn't be," he says. "*¿Está claro?*"

"Very clear," Carr says quietly. "You feel better now that you got that off your chest?"

Bobby calls from the steps. "It's nice you boys are so glad to see each other."

"Piss off, *cabrón*," Mike says, but there's not much to it. He doesn't resist when Bobby hooks his arm and hauls him away.

"You know the world is fucked when I'm the voice of reason," Bobby says, turning Mike toward the house, "but maybe we should all just keep our minds on the job and save the rest of the bullshit for later."

It was, Carr thinks, driving back to his hotel, the same advice Mr. Boyce had given him in Boston.

Tina had stayed at the gate while Carr followed Boyce into the first-class lounge. It was empty, the attendants conveniently on a break. Carr was too tired to speculate on the coincidence. Even off the golf course Boyce was dressed in black, and he seemed much larger.

"Family," Boyce said, as he settled into an armchair. "What are you going to do with them?" Carr had no answer, and Mr. Boyce shook his head. "But that's no excuse. Pros don't make excuses. You have problems, I have problems—everyone has problems. But so what? You do your job, and *then* you deal with your problems. Get it the other way around, and you're no good to anyone. You want to look after your father, you'll keep your goddamn head in the game."

Boyce's words and rumbling voice had filled the room, and Carr had nodded in the right places. He kept nodding later, back at the gate, where Tina had reported in a low voice that Kathy Rink had called her man in Singapore.

"She was on the line for nearly an hour, listening to him talk about Greg Frye. Our guy thinks she went away satisfied."

Carr nodded. Tina had looked at him and hadn't liked what she'd seen. Before she left, she'd gripped him hard by the arm. "You better get a coffee or a searchlight or something, and get your head out of whatever fog bank it's in. You go sleepwalking into Prager's place, you won't walk out again."

Even now he can feel her fingers on his wrist.

Carr pulls through the gates of his hotel, and into a parking space. He shuts off the engine and sits in the dark and silence.

You want to look after your father? Look after him—it turned out he didn't even know him, didn't know either of them, and never had. *All that watching and you never saw anything.* What was it he had seen for all those years? What he'd wanted to see? What he'd needed to see?

Carr had driven back to Stockbridge on autopilot, and Arthur Carr had dozed the whole way. Carr helped him up the porch steps; he weighed

no more than a handful of straw. His father stretched his legs on the sofa as soon as they got inside and closed his eyes, and Carr had walked around the room. Though maybe *walked* wasn't quite right. *Wandered* might be closer; *staggered* closer still.

The vertigo that had come on in the diner, along with the news about his mother, was back again, and as he moved about the living room he had to reach for things—a doorknob, a windowsill, the dusty furniture—to keep from falling or floating away. Eventually he fetched up beside the piano.

The photographs were still there, in their tarnished frames, and Carr stared at them while his head swam and his father snored gently. His father at the lake; his father in cap and gown; his mother in a garden, or at a party, or at a dance. He'd spent his life looking at these pictures, and now it was as if he'd never seen them before. The people behind the dirty glass were strangers to him, and what he thought he'd known about them was less than smoke.

Carr switched on a lamp and gazed at the photo of his father at the lake, and suddenly the small, pale face seemed to wear not a smirk, but a shy grin. And in the commencement picture, Arthur Carr's smile didn't look bitter—it looked nervous, but excited and even hopeful. Carr shook his head and picked up the photo of his mother.

The dark hair, blurred by movement, the luminous skin, the graceful neck and white teeth, the finger of smoke between lips that were just beginning to smile, or to speak to someone out of frame—he knew the pieces, but he couldn't make them whole. Carr closed his eyes and tried in vain to retrieve another image of her, to hear the sound of her voice again, and the words she'd whispered as they peered from the windows, to feel her hand around his again. He breathed in deeply, straining to catch a trace of gardenias and tobacco, but found only the musty smells of his father's house and of the humid night. An ache burrowed deep in his chest—deeper than bone—a wound where something had been excised badly, and with a dull blade. It was like losing her again. It was worse. His throat closed up and his eyes burned.

He looked up to see his father, watching him from the sofa.

"What are you doing?" Arthur Carr asked.

"Looking at pictures," Carr whispered.

"What pictures?" Carr held up the photo in its frame. His father squinted at it. "I didn't know that was up there."

Carr rubbed his eyes. "Where's it from?"

His father shrugged. "That picture? Someone's wedding, I think. I don't remember whose. It was before you were born."

Carr cleared his throat. "You saved her. You said that you saved her from . . . from a full-blown investigation."

"That's what I said."

"But you didn't say why—why you did it. After everything she did—all those years—why did you protect her?"

Arthur Carr shook his head. "Why did I . . . She was my *wife*, for chrissakes—your *mother*. What was I supposed to do? I wasn't going to let them . . ." He shook his head some more, and then he sighed and closed his eyes. "I told you—don't be thick."

Sitting in the hotel parking lot, Carr reaches for his wallet. The photographs are inside, creased and antique-looking alongside Gregory Frye's fabricated identifications. His father by the lake and at commencement, his mother at some forgotten wedding. They are part of a narrative—the story of his parents, his father the embittered bully, his mother the brave, long-suffering victim—that is undone now: unraveled and debunked, like Santa or the Tooth Fairy, but even more ridiculous. Carr lays the pictures on the dashboard, smooths them out, and looks at them for a while. Then he folds them up again and tucks them away with the rest of his false papers.

40

Despite the sun and the honeyed breeze, Carr's fingers are cold and white. His elbows are stiff and his legs heavy, and when he moves them they feel clumsy. His chest is too small for his lungs, and too brittle for his hammering heart. It's fear, he knows, and adrenaline. He takes a slow breath in and lets it slowly out again, then shifts the champagne flute to his other hand. He flexes his fingers until the blood comes back, and he watches Curtis Prager grab a waiter by the arm.

Prager points at the carpaccio on the silver platter. "That's wagyu beef," Prager tells a banker from Panama City, "and what those bastards in Miami charge for it makes me think we're in the wrong business. Clearly, the real margins are in cows." The Panama City banker laughs as if it's funny, and so does everyone else within earshot, and Prager moves on through his guests. Carr hangs back, pretends to sip his champagne, and looks at the crowd.

It's an off-season party—not as large, Carr knows, as some of Isla Privada's charity events, but still a good-size turnout of local dignitaries, favor-seekers, would-be business associates, and other sycophants. It's a handsome crowd too, expensively dressed in regatta casual: the men in variations of Prager's outfit—white ducks, linen blazer, and deck shoes— the women in gossamer, bare arms, and sandals with intricate straps. Like birds, Carr thinks, all plumage and bright chirping. All appetite too. They

flock around the white-jacketed waiters as they emerge from the caterer's base camp in the guesthouse, swooping on trays of sushi, sashimi, oysters, and high-margin carpaccio.

Except for its lawns and patios and first-floor bathrooms, the main house isn't open to unescorted guests, so the crowd has flowed mostly to the beach. Carr is at the east end of the beach, near the boathouse pier, leaning against the red Zodiac that has been pulled up on the sand. He watches as his host makes his way slowly, convivially, westward. Handshake, peck, nod, chuckle. Shoulder squeeze, smile, nod, move on. There's a quartet set up on the guesthouse patio. They're laboring over a samba, and it seems to Carr that Prager has matched his movements to their rhythms. Peck, nod, chuckle.

Kathy Rink prowls in Prager's wake, like a pilot fish in an orange muumuu. Her eyes scan restlessly over guests and staff, her head pivots left and right, and her cell phone is constantly at her ear. Carr can understand Kathy Rink's nerves: this is the first of Prager's periodic soirees to take place on her watch. She wants it to be a smooth afternoon, as seamless and unblemished as the breezy blue sky. Carr allows himself a tiny smile and hopes it will be the worst day of her life.

He takes another pretend sip and scans the crowd for Howard Bessemer. He spots him at a bar set up in the shade of a palm. His jacket is hung over his arm, and he's laughing at something a heavyset redhead has said. Given the sweating and fretting of the morning, Carr thinks he looks improbably relaxed.

"I don't feel like going to a party," Bessemer had whined from beneath his blankets. "I feel clammy. I think I'm coming down with something."

"That's a hangover, Howie," Carr called to him. "Have some coffee, and it'll go away."

"I don't see why I have to go anyway. What do you expect me to do there?"

"I expect you to eat and drink, and when I tell you, to ask Prager to do that favor."

"But I don't feel—"

"You do it, Howie, and we're headed home tonight."

Bessemer leans against the bar and laughs some more. Carr shakes his head and checks his watch. He checks the empty ocean north, and the jagged peninsula to the west. He can't see them, but he knows Bobby and

Mike are out there now, beyond the rocks. They'll call when they're ready, and then they'll wait for his say-so. He checks his watch again. Time to lift the latch.

Champagne flute in hand, Carr crosses the beach and climbs one of the stone stairways. He cuts across the croquet lawn toward a fieldstone patio and the main house. His heart pounds harder as he walks, and his legs are reluctant. He passes two women headed for the beach. They smile at him and giggle as they teeter by. The taller one reminds him of Valerie, though she's not as arresting, and for a moment he wonders where Valerie is and what she's doing and if he'll see her tonight. He touches his ear, but there's no earpiece there, no whispering voice, no breath that he can almost feel. Then his mind comes back as he approaches a pair of glass doors. Laughter, music, the chatter of the crowd, all fade behind him. He takes a deep breath and doesn't look at the camera mounted above. He pulls at a handle and hears Declan's brogue in his head. *Nothin' like a house in the dark, lad.* Nothing like one in broad daylight, either, and filled with security guards.

The hall is quiet and the air-conditioning sends a shiver down Carr's arms. His footsteps echo on the polished stone floor. He has spent hours squinting at the floor plans of this house, and on them he's found three places he might enter when the time comes. Today, after walking the grounds, counting and recounting the guards, watching the flow of guests and staff, and visiting several bathrooms, he has narrowed his list to one.

Down the hall, on the right, is a powder room. It's small and windowless, and Carr has already been there once today. Just past the powder room, around a corner to the left, is a stairwell, with stairs climbing up. Past the stairs, across the hall, and three paces down is Carr's way in.

It's a rectangle labeled LAUNDRY-2 on the floor plans, but it's not the room's function that interests Carr, it's the small window set in its wall. It's in a casement-style frame, and because of its size and ground-floor location, and the dense hibiscus growing just outside, it has no view to speak of. What it does have, by Carr's careful calculation, is a position outside the view of any of Prager's security cameras.

As on Carr's prior visit, one of Rink's security crew cuts appears at the end of the corridor, to make sure he doesn't wander too far afield. Carr raises his champagne glass.

"Toilet?" he asks the guard.

"Of course, sir," the guard says. "Right here." He points toward the powder room. Carr steps in and locks the door. He lifts the toilet lid and pours his champagne down in a thin, noisy stream. Then he sets his glass on the edge of the sink and starts unrolling toilet paper.

"A little help," Carr calls, as he steps out of the bathroom.

The security guard comes down the stairs and around the corner, and almost slips on water that's begun to flow across the powder room's threshold. "Oh Christ," the guard says.

Carr smiles sheepishly. "I think it's clogged," and he points his glass at the toilet and the water and bits of toilet paper flowing from the top of the bowl.

"You think?" the guard says impatiently, a look of disgust on his face.

"I tried jiggling it," Carr says, and raises his hands helplessly. He looks down at the spreading water and moves out of the way, careful to keep his shoes dry. The guard steps gingerly into the bathroom, and Carr backs away.

The guard shakes his head. "Christ," he mutters.

When the guard emerges from the powder room, his knuckles are skinned from wrestling with the jammed water valve under the toilet tank, and his trouser knees are soaked. The hallway is empty, and the patio door is just swinging shut.

Outside, crossing the lawn, Carr feels the sun's warmth for what seems the first time. He takes a deep breath and at last there seems to be some oxygen in it. The music returns, coming to him on the warm, gusting breeze. His shirt, he realizes, is stuck to his back. He's suddenly thirsty, and he heads for the bar set up at the edge of a terrace looking over the beach. He orders an ice water and checks his watch and his phone vibrates.

"We're all right," Bobby says. His words are indistinct against the background noise of water and wind. "We're getting bounced around in the chop pretty good, but we're ready to rock. And you?"

"So far, so good. It should be soon."

"Soon would be aces."

Carr pockets his phone and looks out at the ocean. The sea is boiling around the reefs offshore, and platoons of whitecaps stagger drunkenly this way and that across the bay, to fling themselves on the sand. To the east, the sky is painted with a milky wash. Carr shakes his head and wonders how long the weather will hold.

He walks along the terrace and scans the beach, looking for Prager and Rink. He spots Prager, surrounded by a knot of petitioners and making his way east from the guesthouse. He doesn't see Kathy Rink immediately, but knows she can't be far behind. Suddenly, Howard Bessemer is at his elbow.

"Are we almost done?" Bessemer asks. He's pink from heat and from drink, and there are damp circles under the arms of his blue button-down shirt. His blazer hangs over his shoulder like a drowned thing.

"Soon, Howie."

"We're going to get some of that storm, you know. Sometime tonight they said on television, maybe sooner."

Carr nods and looks again for Kathy Rink. "Thanks for the update. You should head back to the beach and get something to eat. And switch to soda water."

Bessemer grimaces, unfastens another button on his shirt, and wanders off.

Carr picks out Prager again—smiling, nodding, drink in hand—walking up a shaded path. He sees no sign of Rink and checks his watch once more. It would be better, he thinks, if they were down by the water, but the thrashing surf and the sky and the tightening in his stomach tell him there's no point in waiting. He pulls out his phone.

"I'm headed in," he tells Bobby. "Put three minutes on the clock and go."

"Three it is," Bobby says over the wind. "Clock is running."

Carr finishes his ice water, places his glass on the bar as he passes, and heads back toward the main house. He rounds a corner and there's an orange blur to his right. Kathy Rink drops a thick, manicured hand on his arm.

She squints up at Carr. "Been lookin' for you, Frye. What the hell have you been up to?"

Carr looks at her, at the security man at her side, and at Curtis Prager, approaching from the beach. Carr smiles and shrugs. "Enjoying the view, enjoying the hospitality, and wondering if that's all I'm here for, or if somebody wants to do business."

Rink's squint turns into a scowl. "Jury's still out when it comes to business, but we want to talk more. And now's the time."

"Great," Carr says, smiling. The knot in his stomach tightens, and there's a ticking sound in his head.

41

Curtis Prager grips Carr's arm and steers him back toward the terrace bar. Rink and her security man fall in behind them. Prager's face is flushed and shining and fixed in a wide smile. Rink's scowl deepens.

Prager sweeps his arm in the direction of the beach. "Not bad, eh? Raising how much today, Kathy?"

"About two hundred thousand," Rink says.

"For who?" Prager says.

"Hospital," Rink answers. "Kids' wing."

"Kids' wing." Prager chuckles. "I'm a hero. *They* ought to pay *me* to grip and grin with this crowd for so long. Be a relief to get on the plane tomorrow."

Carr nods appreciatively. Prager leans on the bar and orders a ginger ale from the barman, who pours it into a tall glass and disappears at some unseen signal from Rink.

"Kathy spoke to your man in Singapore," Prager says.

Carr smiles and manages not to look at his watch. "How'd it go?"

"It went fine," Rink says. "He says you're tough, and reliable, and discreet, and smart, and that you generally walk on water. Which I'm guessing doesn't surprise you. It would've been pretty stupid to point us at someone who wasn't gonna say good things."

Carr shrugs. "So besides learning I'm not stupid, it was a waste?"

Rink starts to speak, but Prager shakes his head. "Not a complete waste," he says, "but we don't know this guy. We don't know any of the names you've given us so far. The bottom line is, Greg, we need to talk to someone we know. Someone we know, who also knows you. You understand—we need a reference."

Carr hears an engine drone, and for a moment he thinks it's Bobby and Mike, but it's too fast and too far off—an airplane. Carr nods. "I get what you're saying—I just don't know what to do about it. I don't know about you, but most of the people I deal with don't want their names traded back and forth."

"So maybe there's nothing else to talk about," Rink says, and she drums her fingers impatiently on the bar. Carr appreciates the sentiment.

Prager shakes his head. "Or maybe Greg can think about some of the people he buys stones from. Maybe we can talk to some of them."

Carr nods, as if he's actually considering it, as if he's thinking of anything besides getting to the house. And then he hears another engine drone.

It's two engines, this time—close, throaty, rough running, like dirt bikes—coming from the water. His three minutes are up. Prager glances toward the beach and knits his brows.

Carr clears his throat. "I'll think on it," he says, nodding, and the engine sounds grow louder. And now the ambient chatter of the beach crowd changes. A collective chuckle rises, and then a gasp.

Prager shakes his head and peers down at his bay, and his party guests, gathered on the sand. Carr leans left and catches a glimpse of two WaveRunners chasing each other through the whitecaps, rooster tails flying, engines stuttering and echoing across the bay. Bobby is on the red one, Mike the gray. Both of them wear flowered trunks, muscle tees, and aviators. They weave in close to shore—fifty yards or less—and Carr can hear their whooping and hollering and see the bottle of beer that Bobby is waving around. It's a nice touch, but Prager doesn't appreciate it.

He turns to Rink, and his face has darkened. "What's going on, Kathy? Who are those assholes in my backyard?"

Rink is blushing, and already on the move. She waves to the security man at her side, pointing him to the shore, and she puts her cell phone to her ear, but it's all too slow for Prager, who strides angrily toward a stair-

way that leads to the beach. Kathy Rink hurries behind, saying something into her phone. All Carr catches is "boat in the water," and then she's gone. He checks his watch and heads toward the main house.

He tells himself not to run, but it's hard to listen. On his way across the lawn, he sees a pair of security guys who have no such inhibitions: they're in full sprint toward the beach, with their radios squawking. Carr sees the fieldstone patio ahead, and before he comes within range of the camera, he veers right.

He is quick across the patch of lawn at the corner of the house, and quick into the stretch of heavy plantings. He keeps low as he moves between the greenery and the house, and stifles a yell when two red birds dart screaming from the bushes. He fights to keep his breathing under control, and when he reaches the dense hibiscus and kneels by the window whose latch he has broken from inside, he has to struggle to hear the buzzing of the WaveRunners over his own gasps. But there they are, along with exclamations from the crowd. Carr looks at his watch and figures that Mike and Bobby have begun their game of chicken.

Carr peers into the laundry room, takes a last look around the grounds, and sees no one. He dries his hands on his sleeves, works his fingers around the frame, and swings the window open. He checks the flash drives in his pocket again and climbs quietly in.

Carr closes the window and stands between the washing machine and the utility sink, listening. He hears the cycling of the air conditioner, the gurgle of water in pipes, the pounding of his heart, and nothing else. He looks at his watch again. Bobby and Mike have promised him a minimum of five minutes, of which two are gone. He crosses the room, drops to the floor, and looks through the gap beneath the door. There's no one in the hall, and he stands and opens the door a crack. A blade of air slips in, and cools his face. Behind it come voices.

They drift down the stairwell—men speaking and, through a screen of radio static, the voice of Kathy Rink. Carr can't make out her words, but her anger is unmistakable. The men find it funny.

One voice is Southern and deep: "Pine and Colley don't get that fucking Zodiac going, the old broad's gonna swim out there herself—turn those drunks into chum."

The other has a Midwestern twang: "Sounds like she's gonna make chum out of Pine and Colley. For chrissakes, how hard is it to flip a fuckin'

starter switch?" Carr smiles to himself. They can flip all they want, he thinks, it won't do much good with the battery unhooked.

The laughing voices recede, and Carr opens the door wider. He touches the flash drive in his pocket again, like a charm, takes a deep breath, and climbs the stairs.

He is in a wide, windowed hall with white paneled walls and a view onto a courtyard garden. Too much glass—not a place to pause. To the left is the game room, and Carr can see green felt—the corner of a pool table. To the right is the music room, and the gleaming lid of a grand piano. Carr goes right, the floor plans unfurling in his head—music room, hallway, office. His ears are straining; the muscles in his legs are quivering.

The music room is an exercise in monochrome—black piano, white rugs, black leather chairs, white leather sofas—but still too much glass for Carr's comfort. His footsteps are silent on the rugs, and he crosses quickly to the opposite door. And freezes.

A maid comes from behind the curving staircase, and it is only the basket she carries, and its high pile of linens, that saves Carr. He drops beside a white leather settee, crams his heart back into his chest, and listens as she climbs the stairs. Sweat runs down his face and along his ribs, and when he stands again it's like lifting a boulder. Somehow he manages to place one foot before the other.

He cuts across a sunny atrium and makes it to the final hallway. He pauses, listens, and hears voices in the library. It's at the end of this same hall, across from Prager's office. Which means it's on the ocean side of the house, and has an ocean view. The voices are low, and Carr is trying to decide whether they belong to the security staff when a radio squawks and answers the question.

Carr checks his watch: his five minutes are gone—he's in overtime now. So, wait or go? The radio chatter cuts in again—an angry, urgent blast: something's happening on the water. Something worth watching, Carr hopes. And then, behind him, there are footsteps approaching. So much for waiting.

Six paces down the hall. Six paces through quicksand. Through wet cement. Six paces without air or sound, and with his vision a narrow tunnel, the office door at the distant end. And then he's in. He doesn't bother to check if anyone else is there, but no one is. His shuddering sigh is

almost sexual, and for an instant he's giddy and light-headed. The windows are big and bright and full of palm trees and sky. The Rothkos rise above him like twin suns. He's transfixed by them, and imagines lifting them from the wall, prying them from their frames, rolling the canvases. He takes a deep breath, laughs, and shakes his head.

Carr reaches into his pocket for the flash drive and steps to the aluminum desk and stops. He stares at the desk, and at the flash drive in his palm. He squints and his eyes run over the desk, from end to end. He walks around it, and looks beneath it. He looks around the starkly furnished room for a drawer to search, or a cabinet, but there are none. He returns to the desk, thinking he must somehow have missed it. His gaze returns to the nearly bare surface. *Phone, monitor, cable.*

"Fuck," Carr whispers.

Prager's laptop is not there.

"Fuck," he says again. Only the voices in the library keep him from shouting it.

He puts the flash drive in his pocket and rubs a hand across the back of his neck. Where would Prager take the thing? Not to the Isla Privada offices—he doesn't go there. So where else? He probably takes it on trips. Trips like the one he's making tomorrow, to Asia, by way of Europe. Leaving tomorrow, so packing today. So he's packed the laptop and left it . . . where? Where's his fucking luggage?

Two places jump off the floor plan: a cloakroom, just off the main entry hall, and Prager's bedroom. Going to the cloakroom means crossing the entire main floor of the house; going to the bedroom—the master suite—means going upstairs. So, the bedroom first.

Carr doesn't remember the trip down the hall and back across the atrium to the curving staircase, but somehow he's climbing the stairs. There are footsteps below, and voices, and radio chatter. Carr hurries to the top.

Upstairs, the polished stone floors and raised white paneling give way to glossy wood and silk wallpaper. Carr passes a line of bedrooms, each one done in a different ocean color: sea foam, turquoise, aquamarine, and each with an ocean view. The maid is in the last one, a silhouette on a balcony, watching the action on the bay. Carr doesn't realize she's there until he's already passed.

"Shit," he says to himself.

The master is at the end of the hall, behind a pair of teak doors with gleaming brass hardware. The doors aren't locked, and the mechanism is almost silent. Chest heaving, Carr closes them behind him.

He's in a sitting room, with a fireplace, a big ocean view, and none of the austere minimalism of Prager's office. The sofa and chairs are fat and silk-covered, in blue and gray stripes, the rugs are Persian, the low tables are teak, and the pictures on the wall are tinted engravings of sailing ships. Outside, through glass doors and beneath a green awning, there is a large balcony that wraps around all three of the suite's exposures. And in the corner, near the fireplace, there is luggage: two large leather suitcases and a leather duffel, open and half-packed on folding stands. Pressed shirts, balled socks, but no laptop.

"Shit," Carr whispers. He looks at his watch. Nearly nine minutes since the show began. He walks into the bedroom.

It's like the sitting room, but with a king-size bed instead of a sofa and chairs, and a small teak desk near another set of balcony doors. Carr sighs deeply and smiles. Like the sitting room, only infinitely better: Prager's laptop is open on the desk.

He nearly laughs aloud when he touches the space bar and the screen lights with a message asking for a password. He pulls out the flash drive, feels for a USB port, and plugs it in. And then Carr hears the almost silent mechanism of the teak doors, and his heart lodges in his throat.

He drops low, peers into the sitting room, and sees a door swing open and the maid walk in. She's dark and serious-looking behind the basket of folded laundry. She crosses to Prager's bags, picks through the basket, and places a stack of underwear on a table beside the luggage.

Carr looks behind him, at the open doors of Prager's walk-in closet. He looks at the flash drive. Fifteen seconds to load, Dennis said, and the LED would blink. How long has it been in? Did the light blink? *Fuck!* The maid stacks undershirts on the table and lifts the basket, and in two quiet steps Carr is in Prager's bathroom.

It's like an old-fashioned bank—chrome and marble from floor to ceiling—and Carr stands behind the door, trying not to breathe. He watches through the crack as the maid stows clothing and glances out the window at the bay. She glances out often, as if something new is happening, and now she goes to the balcony doors. When she opens them, Carr can hear the buzzing of the WaveRunners along with a new sound—the angry sputter of an outboard. The Zodiac is running.

The maid stands in the open doorway, watching, shaking her head, and from down the hall Carr hears a voice.

"Yo, Sylvie!" a man calls.

"In here," the maid answers.

"Shit," Carr says to himself. He looks around the bathroom. It's huge, with a soaking tub, a steam shower, double sinks, and views of the garden. And straight back, its own pair of glass doors to the other side of the wraparound balcony. He looks through the crack again, and sees two crew cuts headed down the hall. One waits at the doorway to the master suite, the other—the one whose khakis have damp knees—comes in smiling.

"You watching the circus out there, girl?" he says. "My boss'll have a stroke if we don't chase those boys away." He steps onto the balcony and runs his hand over her back.

She giggles and knocks his hand away. "And so will my boss, she finds you up here wasting my time." The crew cut laughs and slides his hand lower, but Carr is watching his partner, who still stands in the doorway.

The maid giggles again and points at the water. "Your boss got her wish. They've run away behind the rocks. Show's over, I guess—no more circus."

Carr's whole body tenses and the crew cut on the balcony says something, but his words are lost in the flash and the *whump* and the rattling of windows. Carr feels the shock wave in his chest, and the maid is screaming now, and both crew cuts are on the balcony yelling *what the fuck,* and Carr steps into the bedroom. He stays low and pockets the flash drive, and then he's back in the bathroom, through the glass doors, onto the balcony, and over the rail.

42

Offshore explosions have a muting effect on parties, and Prager's party is not immune. The jetty screens his guests from seeing the blast itself, but they hear it and feel it and see the smoke. There are cries of surprise, then silence, then a milling confusion. And then the rush to be as uninvolved as possible.

Amid the hunt for valet tickets and the hasty good-byes, no one notices Carr's sweat-soaked shirt, or the scratches on his face and hands from the pindo palm that broke his fall. No one notices him listening intently to a voice on his cell phone. No one notices his smile as he puts the phone away.

Carr glides weightless through the crowd, with Dennis's words still echoing: *It's loaded, boss, nice and clean.* He touches the flash drive in his pocket, and tells himself to slow down, to focus. Now it's Declan's voice he hears: *Don't fall in love with yer own genius, lad—there's no greater arse than the one gets shot while he's staring in the mirror. Yer not home till yer home, and maybe not even then.* Carr runs a hand down his face and wipes the grin off.

He finds Howard Bessemer by the guesthouse, holding a glass and staring at the jetty. He's pale and sweating and shaking his head. "Now's the time, Howie," Carr says.

Bessemer swallows hard. "Jesus Christ," he whispers. "Did you see

what happened? Did you hear that noise? Did you see who it was on those things?"

"I know, Howie, everything's fine. It's time now—just like we went over. And then we go home."

Carr has worried this part to death. Would Howie balk? Would he freeze up? Would he fold altogether? For an instant, Bessemer tilts sideways, threatens to buckle, but the prospect of *home* has a bracing effect on him. He steadies himself on Carr's shoulder, nods curtly, and reaches into his glass for a chip of ice.

"Where is he?" he says, chewing.

Prager is outside the main house, smoldering. He's accepting quick, embarrassed farewells—one after the other—from his guests, and Kathy Rink is standing several paces off. She is paler even than Bessemer, and maybe more jumpy. Her shoes and the hem of her floral dress are wet, as if she's been in the water. When she speaks it's to bark at her men. When Prager speaks, she twitches.

Bessemer hangs back while Carr says his good-bye. Prager's eyes catch for an instant on a scratch on Carr's face, but he's got other things on his mind. They shake hands quickly.

"The police are on their way," Prager tells him, irritation swelling in his voice. "So you'll want to be on yours. Unfortunate we didn't get to talk more, but as you can see," his eyes flick to Kathy Rink and then to the cloudy sky, "this day has gone to hell." Carr nods. "Give her your number," Prager says. "We'll arrange a secure call while I'm on the road, and after you've had a chance to think some more." Carr nods again and moves off. When the line of departing guests ebbs, Bessemer steps up.

His shirt is dotted with sweat, his jacket is a limp balloon, and his tie has surrendered. He pushes a hand through his thin hair and puts it on Prager's arm. His head bends close. Carr can't hear what he says, though he and Bessemer have been over it enough that Carr knows it by heart. But he has no trouble hearing Prager's reply.

Prager shakes Bessemer's hand off, and his face is an aggravated red. "For chrissakes, Bess—this can't wait until business hours? What the hell do you think I am, a fucking teller?"

Rink, the guards, the parking attendants, and the few guests who remain turn their heads. Prager doesn't seem to care, and neither does Bessemer. He's a determined petitioner, and his hand goes to Prager's

shoulder. This time Carr catches some fragments of his speech—*serious guy* and *wants it yesterday* and *not kidding*.

Prager shakes his head, but his expression slowly cools from anger to a resigned acceptance of what seems to be his fate today. "All right, already," Carr hears him say wearily.

When he gets into the passenger seat, Bessemer's hands are shaking. Carr looks at him, and Bessemer answers before the question is asked. "He said he'd do it soon. He said he'd call when it was done."

Carr pats his knee and drives through the gate.

They rendezvous off Rum Point Drive, beside a snack shack damaged by some long-ago storm and never repaired. The parking lot is weedy and cracked. The nearby cove is empty but for the open fishing boat, rocking at anchor. Bobby and Latin Mike stand on the narrow, shingle beach. They're in blue shorts, polo shirts, and ball caps, watching the clouds and drinking beer.

Bobby turns when the car pulls in. "Man of the hour," he says, smiling. He lifts his beer bottle in a toast. "From the motherfucking jaws of defeat."

Mike smiles too. His teeth are very white. "You like the show, *jefe*? You like the time we gave you?"

Carr sheds his jacket and shoes and socks. Something loosens in his shoulders. "I liked it fine, Mike," he says, smiling back. "You guys were fucking amazing." He's surprised by how much he means it.

"And Howie?" Bobby asks. "How'd he do?"

Bessemer laughs nervously. "I was fucking amazing too."

"Fuckin' a," Bobby says, and there's laughter all around. Bobby passes out more beers and they toast. Mike takes a long pull and wipes his mouth. "What's *soon* to Prager?"

Carr shrugs. "Howie told him it had to be today, and he's flying to London tomorrow morning, so . . ."

"Phone charged up, Howie?" Bobby asks.

"A hundred percent," Bessemer says, and Bobby nods approvingly.

They watch a boat go by, east to west, a mile or so out. Carr can see flags, many antennae, and a big radar array. He turns to Bobby. "The WaveRunners?" he asks.

"Wiped clean, in pieces, on the bottom," Bobby says.

Carr nods, and the boat passes from view. He takes a long swallow and exhales and all the air seems to leave him. He can already feel the beer. He

closes his eyes and listens to the wind in the ironwood trees, the waves against the shingle, and Bobby, Mike, and Bessemer laughing at something. The water washes over his feet, and he's not sure if he can move again.

Carr stands this way for he doesn't know how long, and when Bessemer asks for another beer, he opens his eyes. Bobby hands the beer over and Bessemer's phone rings.

Bessemer freezes, and Carr takes the bottle from his hand. "You should see who that is," he says quietly.

Bessemer reaches into his pocket. He stares into the phone's display. "It's him."

Bobby shakes his head. "Soon was soon," he says.

Carr nods. "Nice and easy now, Howie."

Bessemer swallows hard and thumbs a button. "'Lo, Curt," he says. His voice is brittle and high. Head bowed, he listens intently. Carr sees his fingers whiten around the phone. Finally, Bessemer nods. "I can't thank you enough, Curt—you're a lifesaver. Have a great trip, and I'll call when—"

Bessemer takes the phone from his ear and looks at it. "The bastard hung up on me."

"Fuck that," Mike says. "Did he do it?"

Bessemer nods. "Thirty-seven thousand transferred from Isla Privada to my Palm Beach bank."

Bobby and Mike exchange high fives just as Carr's phone burrs. He steps away and answers. Dennis's voice is a shaking whisper. "We got it," he says. "Prager's password. We got all the parts now."

"Nice work," Carr says quietly. "You finish cleaning up; those two will be back to give you a hand." He closes the phone and turns around. Bobby, Mike, and Bessemer stare at him—eager and frightened. Carr nods and smiles.

They don't sigh in unison, but there is something in their collective silence that feels that way—relief, release, deflation. They look at one another and smile and shake their heads in disbelief. And then they are in motion. Mike wades out to the boat. Bessemer heads back to the Toyota, and Carr takes Bobby's elbow.

"Nice and clean at the house, Bobby, and nice and easy at the airport."

Bobby laughs. "I know—we're not done yet."

"Almost, but not quite. So let's not—"

Bobby laughs harder. "I know, for chrissakes—*yer not home till yer home.*"

Carr smiles at him. "So let's get there in one piece."

Mike starts the engine and calls to Bobby. "Come on, *cabrón*, this weather's not holding, and I want to make the earlier flight."

Bobby looks at Carr, and behind him, at Bessemer. "What about your housekeeping?"

Carr's stomach knots and a prickle of sweat breaks on his forehead. "It's covered, Bobby."

"We could take care of it here and now."

"I said it's covered."

Bobby shrugs. Mike brings the boat in close, and Bobby climbs in, and they roar off toward Rum Point. Carr stares at the clouds stacking in the east.

Bessemer is behind the wheel on the way back to the hotel, driving carefully, and Carr is in the passenger seat making calls. His first one is to Tina.

The tension is plain in her voice, and so is the relief when Carr tells her. "Christ," she says chuckling, "you couldn't have called sooner?"

"I waited until I knew for sure."

"The way you were at Logan, I figured hearing from you today was at best a sixty-forty thing."

"Happy I could disappoint you."

"Your guys are buttoning up?"

"And flying out, assuming this storm doesn't shut things down."

"They should be okay."

"Watching the Weather Channel, are you?"

"What else am I supposed to do while I'm waiting for you to call?"

Tina asks about flight times and arrivals and when he expects to be in Boca, at Amy Chun's place. Carr answers, but his mind is already on his next call.

Valerie's voice is a taut whisper. "You fucking asshole. You know how long you left me hanging? What the fuck happened?"

"It's done."

There's silence on the other end, and then a long breath. "Don't bull-shit me."

"I'm not. We've got it."

Another silence, longer this time. "So that's it then," she says finally.

Carr glances at Bessemer, whose gaze is fixed on the roadway. "Almost. I'll call you when I get in. How are things there?"

"I'm at her place now. She should be home in a couple of hours."

"We'll see you there tomorrow."

"And then what?"

"What do you mean? And then we're done."

"I'm talking about afterward. You made any decisions about that? 'Cause I know where I'm going; I just want to know if I'm going there alone."

"I haven't had much time to think about it lately."

"How much time does it take? You either want to or you don't."

Carr glances at Bessemer again. "Can we talk about this later?"

"Not too much later—Amy will be back. Or were you asking for more time than that?" Carr is still searching for an answer when Valerie hangs up.

Bessemer packs quickly, humming to himself while he does it. Afterward, he goes behind the bar and mixes a gin and tonic. "For the road, Greg?" Carr shakes his head, and Bessemer raises his glass to the room. "I'll miss the old place," he says. "Such fond memories."

Carr smiles and shakes his head. "Best to have none at all of these past few weeks, Howie. Best to get on with whatever it is you're going to do."

Bessemer looks at him for a long moment, and then he finishes his drink. "Do I have time for a shower before we leave?" Carr nods and Bessemer disappears into his bedroom.

Carr reaches into a duffel and pulls out the Glock. He drops the clip out, checks the load, and works the slide. Then he snaps the clip back in. He can hear the shower running in Bessemer's bathroom, and Bessemer singing badly. He thinks about Bobby and Mike—*He's everybody's problem if you don't*—and he thinks about Bessemer's son—*I don't really know him*—and he slides the clip out again.

"Fuck it," he says aloud. He opens the balcony door, drops the clip into a stand of dense foliage below, and feels as if a piano has been lifted from his chest.

Carr looks up at the shrouded sky. He thinks about flight delays, and the connections from Miami to Palm Beach. He thinks about his mother and father, and the house in Stockbridge, and about Valerie. He goes inside and picks up his phone.

He tries her three times but gets no answer, and wonders if Amy Chun has come home already, or if Valerie is simply ignoring him.

Bessemer emerges with wet hair and fresh clothes. He drinks a final gin and tonic and watches with amusement as Carr wipes down the rooms. Top to bottom, back to front. Carr makes Bessemer close the door. On their way to the elevator, Carr wipes off the empty Glock and drops it behind the ice machine.

They pause beneath the portico when they come out of the lobby. Rain is falling, in fat, erratic drops, but the sky promises more. It's dark now, and the trees are swaying. The lights in the parking lot are on and shaking on their poles. Bessemer curses softly, and they trot across the asphalt.

Their car is at the far end of the lot, in a space beside a light pole. As they approach, Carr notices that it's the only light not lit. There's a sedan parked in the next space that wasn't there before. It's dark—black or blue—and it's familiar to Carr, though he's not sure from where. A few steps closer and he sees that it's a Nissan, and Carr stops in his tracks. Bessemer jogs ahead and Carr calls out, and there are footsteps behind him.

Carr drops his bag and whirls, and headlights come on, and catch him full in the face. A hand clamps on his wrist and tries to fold it into a come-along hold. Carr pivots and throws his elbow up and something crunches. A voice yells *motherfucker* and the hand falls away, and Carr pivots again, out of the light, as another voice yells *stand clear*. Carr hears a pop, feels a sting on his back, hears a hissing sound. And then the sky lights up, and so do his arms, and legs, and skin, and bones. And then it all goes dark.

43

There's blood in his mouth when he comes to. He tries to feel it with his hand, but can't because of the restraints. They're the stiff plastic kind, and they're tight behind his back. And then there's the matter of the hood. Someone yanks it away and Carr is blinking into a hard white glare.

There are shapes behind the lights—charcoal figures pacing, pointing—and when the rush subsides in Carr's ears, he can make out voices. Men's voices, and a woman's.

"What's your name?" Kathy Rink says. "We know it isn't Greg Frye."

"I don't give a shit about his name," Prager says. "I want my fucking money back."

Carr's having trouble with the words—their meanings don't keep up with the sounds. And he hasn't taken any money—not yet. He tries to look at his watch, but again the restraints stop him. He hasn't taken any money. The air is damp and smells of newly turned earth.

There's a noise to Carr's right, something between a groan and a sob. He turns and sees the hood torn from Bessemer. His head lolls to one side. His face is white and wet with tears, and there's a triangle of blood spreading from his nose down across his mouth and chin.

"And you, you fat lying fuck!" Prager shouts. "I trusted you."

There are shuffling feet and urgent whispers behind the lights, and Carr tries to look around. He sees a concrete floor beneath him, and open

space above. To his left, half in shadow, there is a workbench covered with empty terra-cotta flowerpots, coils of garden hose, and sacks of potting soil. To his right, in a sodden heap in the corner, he sees what's left of his and Bessemer's luggage. Everywhere there is the clatter of rain on a tin roof. Bessemer groans again.

"Not me," he mutters.

"Anything broken, Howie?" Carr says softly.

Prager steps from behind the wall of light. He's in shirtsleeves, and his hair is wet and wiry. Cords pop in his neck, and veins pulse. Carr is fascinated by them. Prager grabs him by the collar, and Carr can smell his sweat and his fear. "What the fuck did you say? Come on, say it again."

"Curt, please," Kathy Rink says sharply. "Let me do my job." She emerges from the glare and puts a hand on Prager's arm.

He flicks her away like a bug. "I keep waiting for you to start," he says disgustedly. "Find my money. Find out what the hell he did to my system."

Carr blinks his eyes, trying to clear them. Maybe it's the lingering effects of the Taser, or his collision with the pavement afterward, but his mind is split into several pieces. One piece is trying to establish a basic fact set, and to make it sit still. Someone has hit Isla Privada, ahead of schedule. Prager has found out about the theft. Prager has found out about him. Prager is going to kill him.

Another piece is a storm of questions. How did Prager find out? Was there a camera he hadn't seen, a switch he'd tripped? Was he spotted in the house? He doesn't think so, but anything's possible. The biggest question—who has stolen Prager's money—Carr scarcely needs to ask, even in his fractured state. It's someone in his crew. Maybe everyone in his crew.

Yet another part of him tries to figure the timing. How many hours passed between Dennis reporting that his spyware had scooped up Prager's passwords, and Carr being tasered in the hotel lot? Enough time, certainly, for Dennis to call Valerie. Enough time for Valerie to sit down behind Amy Chun's desk. Enough time to do any number of things, if the people doing them had discipline and a plan. Carr tries to look at his watch again and strains against his plastic cuffs.

The last scrap of his mind is the busiest—a panting, scrambling thing, searching every inch of this arena of light, probing the shadows at its boundaries, looking for a way out. Flowerpots, garden hoses, potting soil,

an upside-down wheelbarrow, what might be a spade, what might be a rake, a garden tractor that is missing a wheel—he's struggling to turn any of it into a key. Kathy Rink isn't letting him think.

She's sitting on a stool now, her face close to Carr's. "I said, 'What do I call you?' " Her skin is grainy, and there are deep lines around her mouth. Her breath smells of old coffee.

"My name's Greg Frye, but call me what you want."

"But that's not your name, is it?" Carr tries a smile, but the cut in his mouth hurts. "Though your diamonds are for real, and your prints came back as Greg Frye, which—I gotta admit—gives me a scare. You some flavor of cop, Greg?"

Carr shakes his head. "You seem to have your mind made up about things."

"Your prints come back as Greg Frye, and there's a file for Greg Frye with the Bureau of Prisons, but after that . . ." Rink shrugs. "How'd you manage that?"

"If you think I'm a cop, shouldn't you be a little more careful with the merchandise?"

Rink holds his Greg Frye passport up. "Not so much, Greg. You and Bessemer checked out of your hotel, and the last anyone heard you were headed for the airport. I want to, I can have a couple of guys with your names on a plane to the ass end of nowhere, just as soon as the airport opens up again. Your handler'll think you two ran off together.

"Now, how 'bout you tell me where your buddies are—the ones who put on the little show this afternoon?"

Carr smiles again. "It seems like something's happened here, and you think I'm involved."

"*Something's happened here?*" Prager calls from the shadows. "My whole system is locked up. I might as well be fucking *blind.*" Kathy Rink looks sharply at him, and then turns back to Carr.

"I know a lot of people," Carr continues. "Let me make some calls. Maybe between the two of us we can figure out what's going on."

Kathy Rink produces Carr's cell phone from somewhere. "Who do you want to call, Greg? Give me your password, and I'll ring 'em up for you. And speaking of phone calls—who do you think would call Curt, out of the blue, with a heads-up about wire transfers? What reason would they have, and why would they throw your name around?"

"There are people up in Boston who don't like me much."

"They're not alone," Rink says, smiling, and she pats the side of his face.

There's a noise behind Rink—a metallic complaint, like a rusty garage door—and the sound of rain grows louder and a breeze blows in. There's movement beyond the lights, and a man steps into the arena. It's one of Rink's crew cuts, carrying several rolls of duct tape. His nose is packed and bandaged, and there's dried blood on his polo shirt. He glares at Carr through blackened eyes.

There are two other men with him, and they don't have crew cuts. One is a suntanned fireplug, with a peroxide ponytail, a camo wife-beater, and tattoos from his collarbones to wrists. He's got towels over his shoulder and a slant bench under his arm, and he smiles at Rink with crooked teeth. His colleague is small and slim and shaved egg-bald. His skin is the color of oatmeal, and he's wearing dark glasses and pressed fatigues. He's got a plastic water jug in each hand—the five-gallon kind that go on water coolers—and he sets them down in front of Carr.

"I tol' him we didn't need so much," the fireplug says to Rink. His accent is deeply Southern. "When does it take even a gallon? But he don't listen."

"I like to be prepared," the egg says. His voice is soft, his accent from nowhere.

Kathy Rink tosses Carr's phone and passport into the corner, onto the remains of his luggage. "We won't waste a lot of time going round with threats, or any of that *we can do this hard or we can do this easy* crap, okay? We both know you're not gonna say shit unless you have to—and even if you did, I wouldn't believe it. Besides, after what you did to me today, there's no way I'm gonna miss this opportunity."

The fireplug laughs and puts the slant bench down. He kneels and begins to adjust the angle. Howard Bessemer moans. "Jesus Christ," he says, his voice a choked whisper. "This wasn't me. None of this was me."

Rink turns to him and frowns. "My problem with you, Howie, is I'm not sure what you're good for. I mean, I don't need to put you on the board here—I could just smack you in the head and you'll tell me whatever it is you think I want to hear. So what exactly do I need you for?"

Bessemer cranes his neck, trying to see beyond the glare. "Curt! Come on, Curt!"

And then the lights go out.

Prager's is the first voice Carr hears. "Son of a bitch!" he shouts. "Son of a *fucking* bitch!"

"Flashlights!" Kathy Rink calls. "Somebody get some lights here."

There's scraping, stumbling, cursing, and then two thin, shaky beams cut the black. A pool of light spreads at Kathy Rink's feet, and another at Prager's, and then there are radio voices in the air. Someone calls from the darkness: "Power's out at the main house too." To which Prager responds: "You're *fucking* kidding me."

Two more flashlight beams emerge from the dark. Two crew cuts, wet with rain, emerge behind them. "It's a blackout, sir," one reports. "The whole north end of the island's dark."

Prager's voice quivers with anger. "Which is why I have emergency generators and two big tanks of diesel. So where the hell are my lights?"

"They're trying, sir. There's a problem—with a fuel line, they think. They're working on it, but it's slow going in the dark." Prager curses fluently, and Carr stifles a laugh.

There's throat clearing, and then the fireplug's voice. "This isn't the kind of thing you want to do by flashlight, Kath. I'm up for it if you are, but truth is, we might drown the fucker without meaning it."

Rink curses under her breath. "How long till we get the lights back?" she yells.

There's whispering and radio static, and then an answer. "An hour, maybe two."

"Fuck!" Prager shouts in the dark.

For a moment there is just the rain, hammering at the roof, sweeping through the foliage, and then Rink speaks. "I'm thinking we should take a break, Curt—wait till we have light to work by." There's no response from the darkness, and she tries again. "Curt?"

There's an embarrassed cough, and one of the crew cuts answers nervously. "He left, ma'am. I think he went up to the house."

"Shit," Rink whispers, and then, in a louder voice: "Let's button it up for an hour, boys." She points at two of her crew cuts. "Colley, Marco— you two are outside." And she looks at the fireplug. "C'mon, Vic, I'll buy you and Amory a beer."

The fireplug nods, and the egg smooths his fatigue pants. "I want Pepsi," he says.

44

There are footsteps, and the beams of light tremble and diminish, and the garage door scrapes down. The sound of rain is muted, the breeze vanishes, and the darkness is complete.

Bessemer sobs. "Is this part of it? Leaving us in the dark."

"It's a blackout, and let's hope it lasts."

"I don't even know where we are."

"There's a shed next to the greenhouse, with garden equipment in it. I'm pretty sure this is it."

Bessemer sobs again. "What the hell did you get me into?"

"Now's not the time, Howie. Now we get the hell out of Dodge. Can you walk?"

"Walk? I don't know if I can stand. My face hurts like a son of a bitch; I think they broke my nose. Besides, where am I supposed to walk?"

"I'm leaving, and you'd better come along."

"Are you kidding? I'm not going anywhere—you think I want to get in deeper?"

"It doesn't get deeper than this," Carr says, and he stands and shuffles slowly forward, navigating from memory. Around the slant bench, the water jugs, the light stands, toward the tractor. His shin smacks into something smooth and metal.

"What are you doing?" Bessemer says.

Carr turns around and stretches his arms back. "I hope I'm turning on a light," he says. He runs nearly numb fingers across a landscape of plastic textures—pebbled, cross-hatched, tacky, and smooth—until he finds the ridges of the tractor's little steering wheel. Then he reaches down and scrabbles over knobs and switches until he touches a key. Carr turns it, and the tractor's headlights come on—sickly beams that barely cross the room. To Carr, they are flares in a mineshaft.

Bessemer's voice is a frightened hiss. "They'll see!"

"The only windows are in back, Howie—those narrow slits near the ceiling. No one will see."

Carr follows the light to a workbench on the wall. He peers at the tabletop, then turns around and strains his arms back until his fingers catch the garden shears. "Stand up," he tells Bessemer.

"Why?"

"Because that way there's less chance I'll slash your wrists."

"What?"

"And for chrissakes stand still."

It takes two tries, back-to-back with the shears, and though Carr doesn't slash Bessemer's wrists, he does slice through his trousers and a chunk of his belt.

"Now cut mine," Carr says.

Bessemer cuts the plastic in one clean pass, and Carr massages his wrists and cold hands. "Now what?" Bessemer says.

"Now sit down again, and put your hands behind your back." Carr carries his own chair to the back of the room and places it beneath one of the narrow windows. He goes to the workbench, retrieves a pry bar from a hook on the wall, and stands on his chair.

"What are you doing?" Bessemer says. "We can't get out that way."

"No?"

"Maybe you can fit through, but I can't. Are you going to leave me here?"

Carr reaches up and slips the pry bar between the cinder-block wall and the window's aluminum frame. He grunts with effort and then there's a sound of rending metal and breaking glass, and he looks down at Bessemer. "Better sound the alarm, Howie."

And Bessemer does. Loudly. Loud enough to be heard over the lashing rain.

The metal door rolls up and two flashlight beams catch Bessemer in mid-yell. "The *bastard*, the *son of a bitch*—he left me here. That fucking prick went out the window and left me here!"

The lights dart and circle and find Carr's chair, and the broken glass and mangled window frame on the floor. Rain is blowing through the rectangular gap.

"Shit," the taller crew cut says. He draws his Glock and crosses to the window. His partner draws his gun too, but stays in the doorway, and Carr takes him first—the pry bar to the crotch, to the kidney, to the back of the head. There's an explosive bellow and the taller crew cut turns, is frozen for an instant, and brings his gun up.

And Carr is on him at a run. He clamps both hands on the Glock, forces it down, and drives his shoulder into the crew cut's chest. The crew cut goes back against the wall and the gun goes off and Carr snaps his head down hard on the bridge of the crew cut's nose. There's a crack and the crew cut's grip loosens. Carr tears the Glock free as the crew cut hits him with the flashlight. It catches him on the shoulder and bounces hard against his ear, and Carr hammers the crew cut again and again on the side of his head until he goes over.

Carr is breathing hard as he strips the guards of flashlights, guns, radios, cash. He goes to the corner and runs a light over their wrecked bags. He picks through the pile and retrieves their wallets and passports.

Bessemer is still sitting, gripping the seat of his chair. "Jesus Christ," he whispers. "Are . . . are they dead?"

Carr rubs the side of his head and stands in the open doorway. "Not yet," he says, "though Rink might change that. We better get a move on; someone probably heard that shot."

Outside they are drenched in an instant, and their flashlight beams are swallowed whole.

"Christ!" Bessemer says, struggling to keep up. "Is this even a path?"

"It'll take us to the boathouse," Carr says, "assuming we can stay on it."

"What do we do there?"

"Get in a boat."

"In this? Are you crazy?"

"I don't like it, but I don't like cutting across the property either, much less making it over the fence. I don't know how many men Rink has here, but it won't be long before they're all out looking for us. They're not going to look for us out there."

The wind gusts and twists, shoving them sideways, shoving them forward, shoving them back. Palm fronds snap past them and sand scours their faces. The ocean is a flailing, howling thing, much too close in the dark.

"The money," Bessemer shouts, though he is right at Carr's back. "I thought nothing was going to happen until we were in Florida."

"That's what I thought too," Carr says, and he pulls his mind away from a thousand questions about who did what, and when they did it, and where they are right now. There's a squawk on the radio, and Carr stops and holds it to his ear.

"Dammit," he says. "Someone's calling the guys at the toolshed."

"What do we do?"

"Go faster."

But they're not fast enough. They're not halfway to the boathouse when a ribbon of light appears behind them. "They've got power in the guesthouse," Carr says, and he looks up through the whipping trees. "And in the main house too."

"And there," Bessemer says, pointing. There are lights at the boathouse, and more lights moving down the path.

Carr looks back. "They're coming from the greenhouse too," he says. He grabs Bessemer's collar and hauls him off the path, through bushes and branches, onto wet sand. The surf is white and frenzied before them, streaming across the beach and past the line of palm trees. The bay is boiling ink.

Carr drops the guns and radio to the sand. "Take off your shoes," he shouts.

Somehow Bessemer's face finds new terror. "What?"

"You a strong swimmer?"

"*What?*"

"It's a simple choice: stay here and die, or take our chances out there."

"There is no chance out there."

"We'll head west, around the jetty. There should be some protection in the bay, but we need to stay clear of the rocks."

"We . . . we could hide."

"They're going to search every inch of this property until they find us, Howie, and when they do, they're going to torture us and kill us. So now's the time."

Carr wades in and the cold is like a fist clenched around his lungs. He

loses his breath and nearly loses his footing, and in two steps he's up to his neck. "Now, Howie."

Bessemer looks around wildly and sees lights approaching. His chest heaves as he kicks off his shoes, and he's fighting for breath when he calls to Carr. "Wait up!"

45

Carr is badly wrong about the bay: there is no protection—not from wind or wave or hungry currents, or from the constellation of debris that swirls and collides just below the angry surface. The lights from shore dim with the first swell, and disappear altogether with the second, and suddenly he's fifty meters out. Or is it a hundred and fifty?

The sea heaves in every direction, and the wind makes shrapnel of the whitecaps. Carr's feet tangle in what feels like plastic netting, and something hard—a fence post swept from somewhere—glances off his thigh and leaves his leg numb and useless. A sheet of drywall—peeling, dissolving—shatters across his back. There's a roll of carpet, a shipping pallet, chicken wire, and a drowned chicken. It's like swimming through a landfill, or in Dorothy's twister, though actual swimming is all but impossible. Carr flails and twists and tumbles, coughing, spitting, wrestling for breath, and the only thing louder than the wind and rushing sea is his hammering heart.

Bessemer vanishes immediately, carried off without a cry, and Carr doesn't see him for what seems a choking eternity—until he spots a white arm rushing past, struggling vainly against the riptide that he himself has just escaped. Carr sees him spin away—the white arm, the benign, round face, the sad, thin hair like sea grass—and then he calls Bessemer's name, fills his lungs, and kicks out after him.

The rip takes hold of Carr again—shoving, pulling, twisting him around—and he loses Bessemer behind a wall of water. He manages a sloppy breaststroke, but can't keep the ocean out of his mouth. He calls out, but the wind tears the words from his throat. He sees a shape that may be an arm, or a leg, or a tumbling body, and he lunges forward, through a breaking wave.

His fingers hook on something and he takes hold of an ankle. Bessemer is floating facedown. He finds his belt and flips him over. Carr slides an arm under Bessemer's arm and across his chest, and Bessemer's head rolls back against Carr's shoulder. Even in the dark, through the spray, Carr can see the ashen face, the blood flowing down his cheek, and the deep, depressed gash at Bessemer's left temple. He puts his ear to Bessemer's mouth and hears faint, uneven breathing.

"Howard," he yells, again and again over the wind, and Bessemer mutters weakly. The rip is pulling them out and under, and pulling Bessemer from him. Carr strikes out perpendicular to the current—to what he thinks is the east.

The current is twisting them, and he fights to keep Bessemer's face out of the water. His legs and shoulders are cramping, and his fingers, wound in Bessemer's shirt, are numb. He closes his eyes and concentrates on his breathing, on coordinating it with his kicks and his sculling arm, on ignoring the lead in his thighs and the weight clutched against his chest. And finally he finds it—the metronome he's been straining to hear, the rhythmic four count that silences the wind and the flailing sea: his heart, his lungs, in, out.

Carr loses himself in the cadence and loses track of time, and then, suddenly, the outbound surge is gone. They're free of the rip. Carr keeps kicking and realizes that another current, a lateral one, is pulling them slowly eastward. He lets it carry them, lifting his head to look for lights or land or anything at all, but he sees only darkness. They're well out of the bay now, he's sure—well beyond the reefs—and the waves are larger here and even more chaotic. One lifts them up high, and for an instant Carr sees a light, or thinks he does, and then another wave breaks across them, nearly tearing Bessemer from his grasp. Carr catches his arm, pulls him close again, and gets a better grip across his chest, and it is only then he realizes that Howard Bessemer has died.

46

From this height there's no trace of the storm—just pale sky, turquoise sea, and the edge of Cuba—brown and green and wrinkled as a fallen leaf. No trace, but he can still feel it moving in his arms and legs, and in his gut: a surge, a lift, a queasy drop. He can still hear the roar. Or is that the jet's engines? Carr signals the flight attendant and asks for another coffee and a blanket. Half a day since he came out of the water, and still he can't get warm.

He doesn't know how long he was in. Hours, certainly. Long enough for the lateral current to carry him miles to the east. Too long for him to hang on to Howard Bessemer's drowned and battered body. A wave finally tore it from his grasp, and some time afterward—he didn't know how long—Carr's foot found a sandbar, and eventually the shore.

It was a spur of rock off Old Robin Road, and there was a house under construction nearby, and a trailer to shelter in, once Carr had kicked in the door. He collapsed on a sofa, slept, and dreamed of nothing. In the drizzly morning, he'd hitched a ride with some housepainters to George Town.

A barefoot man in damp, salt-stained clothes hadn't raised as many eyebrows as Carr had expected. Maybe the locals wrote it off to the exigencies of the storm, or the eccentricities of tourists. Maybe it was Carr's still-wet cash that preempted their questions. In any event, it got him a

ride to the strip mall, where he bought clothes and a toothbrush and a prepaid cell in a discount store. He washed up and changed in the store's bathroom, then sat on a curb and made phone calls.

The first one was to his father, and the relief he felt when he heard Arthur Carr's voice—*Why the devil are you calling? You never call*—took him by surprise. The next ones were to Valerie, and Bobby, and Dennis, and Mike, and Tina, and they all went unanswered.

Two tries, three tries, and then he'd taken a taxi to a cruise ship pier. He'd invested in sunglasses and a ball cap there, with a smiling pirate turtle stitched above the bill, and joined a large group of tourists riding a shuttle bus to the airport. He'd spotted two of Rink's men in the terminal, but he stayed with the crowd and kept his ball cap low, and he didn't think they'd seen him. At the gate he'd made more phone calls, but with no more success.

The operational puzzles—clothing, transpo, evasion—had kept Carr's mind focused, anchored to the present and to the next step. When they were solved, and his pace slowed, other questions had crowded in. Questions about timing, about passwords, about access to Amy Chun's laptop. About where the fuck the money was. Carr had no answers to them, but he didn't mind that they filled his head. They gave him something to do and left no room for his anger, or for the images that seemed to rise up whenever he closed his eyes—of Howard Bessemer, white and drowned and dropping through black water.

Carr wakes with a start, and for an instant Bessemer's soft round face floats before him. He squeezes his eyes shut and opens them again and looks out the window. In the distance he sees the towers of Miami.

It's blue dusk when he arrives in Boca Raton. The rendezvous is on a quiet street of breeze-block homes in earshot of 95, and just two exits from the airport. Like every other house in the neighborhood, it's a neat, one-story rectangle, with a shallow pitched roof, a carport, and a brown lawn. It's painted some pastel shade, maybe pink, maybe yellow, though in this light everything is gray to Carr. He drives past the house and turns the corner three blocks down.

The whole ride up from Miami, he's thought more about the timing—how tight it was, how rapid the sequence of events. Dennis gets Prager's

password. Prager's money is stolen. Prager gets a call, telling him he's been robbed by Greg Frye. Prager grabs them from the hotel lot. All in the space of not quite three hours. By then, Dennis, Bobby, and Mike would've been in the air, en route to Miami—according to the plan, at least. But no one seemed to care much about the plan these days—not about Carr's plan, anyway.

He's thought about Dennis too. Young Dennis, skinny Dennis, pimply Dennis, tentative Dennis, genius Dennis. It's hard for Carr to believe that he's involved, but impossible to figure a way that he's not. Dennis and Valerie both. Dennis had Prager's password, Valerie had access to Amy Chun's hardware. They couldn't do it on their own, but they could do it together, and Valerie could be very persuasive.

He drives past the house a second time. The carport is empty; the shades are drawn; no lights—the house has a buttoned-up look. The streets are quiet. Few cars and no pedestrians. He turns the corner, parks two blocks down, and sits behind the wheel for forty-five minutes, until night has finished falling.

There's a tension in his stomach as he walks down the empty sidewalk, and it winds tighter as he vaults the alley fence into the darkest corner of the house's backyard. No lights back here either, and no open windows. Buttoned up. He's soft and quiet moving up on it, but that's more habit than anything else. He has the feeling he could launch fireworks and no one would care. The house has that look.

He stands against the back wall, by the screen door, and listens. A chorus of night bugs, a television playing in Spanish, half a block down, and the ceaseless whisper of 95. Nothing from inside. He takes out his cell and punches Dennis's number once more and holds the phone away from his ear. He rests his head against the door, and hears—very faintly—a ringing from inside.

"Fuck," he says aloud, and he cuts off the call and punches Bobby's number. Again, faintly, a ringing inside. "Fuck," he says again. He snaps on plastic gloves, takes a flashlight and a screwdriver from his pocket, and wishes he had something more substantial.

He slides the screwdriver into the frame and the back door opens with a whisper, and the smell hits him right away. It's one that's familiar, but still, his stomach nearly empties. He rubs his eyes and pulls his shirt up to his nose and steps inside.

It's a small house, and the smell has filled it to bursting, and so have the heat and the flies. It takes no searching to find them: they're in the living room, Bobby sideways on the sofa, Dennis genuflecting by a card table. Carr can't tell how long they've been dead.

He stands over Bobby's body and runs the flashlight up and down. There's a beer bottle on the cushion next to him, and the remains of a cigarette that scorched his pants and the flesh underneath. The flies buzz and hover and Carr shoos them away from Bobby's head. He can see the entry wounds then—one to the back of the neck, one to the back of the head. He can't tell if there are powder burns.

Dennis also has two wounds, also to the head and neck. His laptops are missing, but his clothes are there, still packed in a duffel, as are Bobby's. Mike's are not. Carr stands stock-still as a van drives slowly past, and then he leaves. He waits until he's in the alley, two blocks away, before he throws up.

47

There's only one place left for Carr to go, but it isn't late enough yet, and he needs a shower. He takes a room at a Fairfield Inn near the airport and stands under the spray for a long time. He uses all the little bars of soap and all of the shampoo, but still it's not enough. Wrapped in a towel, lying on the bed, he tries to work the puzzles—the efficient double taps in both bodies, the lack of struggle, the missing laptops, no Mike—but nothing will sit still. He sees Dennis, dumped like lost luggage beside the table. He sees Bobby's wry, irritated, tired face. *Fuckin' Carr*, he hears him say. He can hear the flies and feel them lighting on his hair and arms.

Amy Chun's gated community has decent security, but the golf course abutting it does not. The cart path that runs along the sixth fairway is bordered on one side by palms and lush plantings, and on the other side by an eight-foot wrought-iron fence. Amy Chun's house lies just beyond, across an empty street. Crouched on the golf course side, Carr watches. Just past midnight, just after the security cruiser makes its half-hourly run, he climbs over.

The house is modern and glass, all planes and angles, and the landscaping is all about privacy—tall bamboo, fanning palmettos, and long ornamental grasses. Path lights pick out a white gravel walk that disappears into the foliage.

All the windows that Carr can see are dark. He crosses the street quickly, finds heavy shadows, and waits. Nothing moves, nothing but bugs make a sound. Carr is quiet approaching the front door. It is massive and metal clad, and there's a discreet sign nearby, warning of alarms and armed response. Carr would be more concerned if he couldn't see the control pad through the door sidelight, and the status indicator glowing green, for disarmed.

He follows a path around the back to a long deck. It looks out on a man-made pond and a garden of rocks and combed gravel. In the dark it looks to Carr like the surface of the moon. Glass doors run the length of the deck, but the glass is dark, and Carr can see nothing inside. He takes out his phone and tries Valerie's number, and then Mike's. He gets no answer, and hears nothing from inside. He's not sure if he's relieved. Then he punches Amy Chun's number.

The phone is loud through the glass. It rings five times, and then the voice mail kicks in. Amy Chun's voice is crisp and businesslike, and her message is brief. Carr closes his phone and pulls on his plastic gloves. He turns on the flashlight, takes out the screwdriver, and takes a deep breath.

Amy Chun's air-conditioning is efficient, but the cool temperature doesn't mask the odor. It hits Carr harder this time, and he has to hold the door frame until his head stops spinning. He turns on the flashlight, shrouds the beam with his hand, and follows the smell.

Through the living room, down a short hall, to a frosted-glass door, half-opened and marred by a jagged crack. Amy Chun's office. Despite the overturned chairs, the crooked pictures on the wall, and the books and papers on the floor, Carr recognizes it from Dennis's spycam video. The desk is askew, but Chun's Isla Privada laptop is there, along with the other hardware—the password generator, the fingerprint scanner, and Chun's cell phone. And there is blood too.

It's on the edge of the desk, and the arms of the chair, but most of it is on the floor, in the corner, around Amy Chun's body. Her back is against the wall, and one bare leg is bent beneath her. The other is straight out in front. Her arms are at her sides, and her hands lie palms up on the floor—a supplicant's hands, Carr thinks. Her head hangs down, and her long black hair hides her torso. Carr is grateful he can't see her face.

The smell is stronger here, and Carr's head is spinning again. He can't look away from her hands, her pleading fingers, and he feels

embarrassed—as if he's come upon her in the midst of something deeply private. The flashlight seems a terrible invasion, and Carr turns it off, but even in the dark he can see her hands.

He remembers her walking with Valerie beneath the arcade, their heads bent close, their fingers brushing. He remembers the bar in Houston, the green paper lanterns hanging, the smell of beer and cigarettes, Bobby and Dennis watching Valerie. He sees Howard Bessemer's pale hands, and his pale, round face drifting away. And suddenly, desperately, he needs air. Carr turns and the beam hits him full in the face.

It's a hard blue light, and he can't see who is behind it, but the glint of the chromed gun barrel is unmistakable, and so is the bass rumble of the voice. Like thunder, but not at all distant.

"Where are you rushing to?" Mr. Boyce says. "And where the fuck is my money?"

48

Inhale, exhale, not too fast, Carr tells himself, and he shifts carefully in the long grass.

November is early summer down here, but to Carr the predawn sky looks like winter, and the ocean—dead calm—looks frozen. The beach below is like a field of ice, and the sun—still a waxy splinter on the horizon—looks coated with frost. Carr knows the forecast calls for another warm day, but there's nothing warm about the ground he's lying on, and nothing soft about the grass. It feels like winter ground to him.

Carr moves the binoculars slowly along the coastline, but there is little to see. Some fishing boats to the north; to the south something larger, and farther out at sea. A tanker maybe, or a cargo ship. The beach is empty but for a stray dog worrying a carcass—a gull's perhaps—a quarter mile away. He can hear a jet far off, but can't see the lights. The only other noise is the wind. Of the ten armed men ranged along the hilltop with him, he sees and hears nothing. Even the man beside him is practically invisible, which is a considerable achievement given his size.

"Watch the flare off the lenses," Mr. Boyce whispers. Carr nods and scans the binoculars down, to the house at the bottom of the hill, at the edge of the sand.

It's a modest house by local standards, a cottage really, without the cantilevered decks, sweeping windows, or vast infinity pools common to

its newer neighbors. But still, a nice house. Thick, whitewashed walls, red tile roof, fences and patios of rough local stone, a vegetable garden in back. Carr studied the site survey at the records hall, in town, and knows it sits on nearly a dozen acres—from beachfront to the top of this hill. Nice, and not cheap.

A yellow light appears in a window—a kitchen window, Carr knows. Boyce sees it too. "He a morning person?" Boyce asks.

"I don't know what he is," Carr says.

Nearly three months of tracking him—tracking both of them—following money and rumors and bodies across half the world, and Carr still doesn't know. He knows they were damn smart, though—that he knows without a doubt. The web of wire transfers that emanated from the initial one—the one that relieved Curtis Prager of one hundred million dollars—was intricate and broad, similar in concept to what Carr had planned, but more complicated.

Prager's money was quickly split into fifty separate transfers of two million each, and sent to fifty different banks around the world, into accounts owned by fifty shell corporations. Within hours of the theft, while Prager was still struggling to get Isla Privada's systems working again and to notify his correspondent banks that something was amiss, those accounts had themselves been emptied by still other transfers. The layering and structuring of electronic payments continued for days, until the money came to temporary rest in banks in Luxembourg and Switzerland, in accounts owned by yet another set of shell companies.

Then came the cash withdrawals. There were nearly forty of those, over the course of five days, in Zurich, Basel, and Luxembourg—in amounts ranging from one million to three million euro. They made for heavy briefcases, but nothing a healthy courier couldn't handle. Once in cash, the money became nearly impossible to trace. Carr suspects it didn't travel far—to banks down the street from the banks it came out of, most likely, and into another set of accounts.

It was elaborate, and it must've taken at least a year, and a fair amount of money, just to set up the shell companies and open the bank accounts. A lot of planning, and more discipline than Carr would've expected from him, but maybe that was her influence. There's motion on the beach, and Carr shifts the binoculars. The dog is in the water now, snapping at sea foam, his jaws closing on nothing. Carr knows how he feels.

Three months of staring at account numbers, wire transfer logs, bank statements, flight manifests, and security camera footage have left him feeling alternately like an accountant and a cop, and both of them empty-handed. But dead ends, bleary eyes, overcaffeination, and exhaustion notwithstanding, he hasn't minded the work, or even Boyce's microscopic scrutiny of him while he does it. In fact, he's welcomed it—welcomed anything that occupied his brain, and left room for nothing else. Not for thoughts of how blind he was, how foolish, or how wrong. Not for guilt or hungry rage.

Mostly, the job has fit that bill, but even amid the columns of numbers, the megabytes of data, and the stacks of paper, there's been downtime. The flights are the worst, and commercial or private makes no difference. Something about the long sleepless stretches, or the darkened cabins, or the dead, cold air, or the unceasing grind of the engines, or maybe all of those things together—something summons them. Memories of Bobby and Dennis in the workhouse, in Boca—the flies and the smell—of Ray-Ray in the morgue, in Mendoza, his blackened bones and clawing fingers; of Howard Bessemer, white and bloated and spinning through the waves; of Amy Chun's hands—

"Kitchen window," Mr. Boyce whispers.

Carr shifts his binoculars and sees a silhouette moving in the yellow square. "Can you tell who?" he asks.

"No," Boyce says. He touches the mic on his neck and whispers something. They watch in silence, and after a while the shadow disappears from the window. After another while, Boyce sighs and lowers his binoculars.

"You called your father last night?" he asks Carr.

"You know I did."

Boyce nods imperceptibly. "How is he doing?"

"He's okay. I'm sure you know that too."

"I don't eavesdrop."

"Your distinctions are too subtle for me."

Boyce smiles. "How's he getting along with Margie?"

"As well as he does with anyone. Which is not well."

"She was an army nurse for twenty years—I think she can handle it. Margie can stay on with him, you know. She likes it up there."

Carr shakes his head. "After this, I go back. That was the deal—that, and the money. Nothing's changed."

"I just want you to know you have options."

Carr points down the hill. A door has opened near the kitchen window, and a rectangle of yellow light falls on the patio stones. A shadow—the elongated shape of a man—fills the rectangle. The shadow is still, and Carr finds that he's holding his breath. The door closes again and Carr sighs.

Boyce chuckles softly. "He's like a dog, sniffing the air. His hackles are up, but he doesn't know why."

Carr looks at his watch and looks at the sky. Three months, and the end is a hillside away. He feels his heart rate rise, and a tightness spread through his shoulders and down his arms. "He'll know soon enough."

Boyce turns to look at him. "You're sure about going in alone?"

"I'm sure. You'll be cleaning up with sponges otherwise."

"And you don't want to bring anything?"

"The wire is enough," Carr says. "There'll be more than enough guns in there." Three months.

Mr. Boyce reads his thoughts. "It's been a long time," he says in a quiet rumble. "A long time chasing. A lot of time to think. To brood. I know a little something about disloyalty, but now's not the moment to get impatient or sloppy or . . . emotional."

Carr's laugh is quiet and rueful. "I thought I was just tired."

"You are. Anger is tiring."

Carr rubs a hand across the stubble on his jaw. "The light's coming up," he says.

Boyce checks his watch and whispers something into his mic. He waits for an answer, and then looks at Carr. "It's time then."

Inhale, exhale, not too fast.

49

Carr is quiet down the hillside and across the patio, but when he opens the door he knows he hasn't been quiet enough.

Declan is looking up from a newspaper spread on a long table. He's holding a pair of reading glasses in one big hand, and a Taurus nine-millimeter casually—almost carelessly—in the other. Neither one of them moves or speaks, and blood rushes madly in Carr's ears.

Then Declan smiles. It's huge and crooked, and it engages every crag and freckle on his ruddy face. His eyes gleam, and Carr would swear the light gets brighter. "You got grass stains on your knees, lad, and you look like pickled death. You better have yourself a coffee." The brogue is stronger than ever.

Carr nods slowly. "Coffee would be good."

"I just put the pot on. There's breakfast too, if you like. Fry up some eggs?"

"Just coffee, I think."

"Coffee then," Declan says. He slips the gun into the waistband of his pajamas and pads barefoot across the tile floor. He takes two mugs from a cabinet. "And would you close the door, lad—unless your friends are comin' too."

Carr shuts the door. "Not yet."

Declan smiles. "Not yet," he repeats.

"You lost some weight," Carr says. "And I like the beard—even with all

the gray. You look good." Actually, he looks older to Carr—leathery, smaller, and somehow desiccated, like an old boot.

"Death agrees with me."

Carr smiles. "You don't seem too surprised."

"Had a feeling the past few days. Not even a feeling—more like an itch I couldn't reach, or a yen for something, but I didn't know what. So, not entirely surprised."

"Surprised it's me?"

Declan shakes his head. "When I heard you'd gotten yourself away from Prager, I figured if it was anyone, there was a better than even chance it'd be you." He points a thumb across the open living room, at what Carr knows is a bedroom door. "I told her that. And I told her yesterday that something was up. But she wasn't havin' any. She said I was paranoid—*an old woman* was how she put it. She can be . . . unkind."

Carr nods. "Yes, so I've seen."

The coffee is ready, and Declan pours it out and carries the mugs to the table. He fetches a can of condensed milk from the pantry, shakes it, and punches the top with a can opener. "I remember you like this stuff," he says. Carr pours some milk in, stirs, and takes a sip. Declan smiles. "I can see you're feeling more spry already."

Carr nods, but actually he's more exhausted than ever. He studies Declan across the table and tries to find some other feelings. Rage? Hatred? Disgust? He's harbored them all over the long months— nurtured them, savored them sometimes—but now they've abandoned him. He tries to conjure them up, recalling images of Bobby and Dennis, of Howard Bessemer's white face and Amy Chun's pleading hands— images that he's run from for three months—but it's like turning out empty pockets. There's nothing there.

Or almost nothing. He looks at Declan's shoulders, slumped in striped pajamas, his gray-streaked beard and graying hair, the little gold hoop— that's new too, and even more ridiculous than the beard—his reading glasses and bloodshot eyes, and finds a speck of something. A grain of . . . pity? It confuses Carr, and he's relieved to have questions to fall back on.

"So, how was it supposed to work?" he asks.

Declan drinks some coffee and smiles ruefully. "Not to put too fine a point on it, lad, but you weren't supposed to walk away from Prager's."

"It was hardly a walk."

"I can only imagine. But if you'd stayed put, it would've looked like

your crew had fucked you, and then fucked one another: three down and the other two in the wind, and no one to say different. Boyce could beat the bushes for them as long as he wanted, but in the end who would he find?"

"And of course no one would be out looking for you."

Declan smiles. "Death benefits."

"Which, I gather, was the point of the theatrics in Mendoza."

"I needed room to move, yes, and also some extra operating capital. Setting up that pipeline wasn't cheap."

"It was goddamn expensive for Ray-Ray."

Declan's face darkens for a moment. "Don't think I was happy about it—I wasn't. I'd planned for him to drive with Bobby and Mike on the way out, but things were a little crazy."

"No crazier than you wanted, though. I mean, it was you who gave Bertolli and his men the heads-up about the raid, right?"

Again the smile. "They were more eager than I expected."

"They didn't shoot you off that road, though. That was you again, right?" Declan nods modestly. "And you had a ride waiting out of there?"

"A four-by-four. I drove off-road after that, back to Mendoza, and it was hell on my kidneys."

"And the body alongside Ray-Ray's?"

"The fellow that brought me my four-by-four."

Carr shakes his head. "What did you do in Mendoza?"

"I laid up for a couple of weeks, then made my way to Mexico. Short hops, nice and easy."

"Home free, while we were weeping at your grave."

"From what I heard, you two weren't doing much weeping—you and Val."

Carr's throat tightens. "You didn't worry we'd scrap the job?"

Declan laughs. "Walk away from that payday? I knew you a lot better than that." He points his thumb at the bedroom door again. "She was worried about it, though—worried about you running things, frankly—but I told her you were the man for the job. Told her to help you out too—lend a sympathetic ear, and so forth."

"Thanks for the vote of confidence," Carr says softly. He drinks some coffee and struggles to get it down. "Bobby and Mike didn't share your faith. They didn't like my management style. Half the time they were

ready to walk. So was I, for that matter. The rest of the time I was thinking that they'd sold you to Bertolli. That's why I made a deal with Boyce—told him I'd stay on only if he'd look into what happened down there. But I guess you know all about that."

"I was touched when I heard, lad—really."

"But not worried."

Another rueful smile. "Well, no—there was never much chance you'd find anything I didn't want found. And you know my thoughts about idle hands—I figured the more you had on your mind, the less opportunity there was of you getting into anything too troublesome. Bobby and Mike and their money-laundering shenanigans were a surprise, it's true—those feckin' pirates—but it helped to keep you busy.

"And in the end, you pulled it off! It was a knotty piece of work, with all sorts of unexpected shite falling on your head, but you made it happen. A true classic!"

Carr shakes his head. "Then I went and fucked things up by not letting Prager kill me."

"You left us scrambling, yes, but I was still a dead man, and we had faith in the pipeline we'd laid down, and that we'd left no trail to this little hidey-hole. And so I must ask you, lad—what brought you to our doorstep? It wasn't following the cash, was it?"

"No, you covered those tracks too well. We did find Mike's body, out in the 'Glades, and we found that guy you dropped in Lake Worth—the Russian kid. He was what—your computer guy?"

"He was no Dennis, but he was good enough to steal Prager's password off the server Dennis's spyware sent it to. Of course, we did tell him where to look, didn't we? But he was good enough to bring Prager's systems down for close to a week. That was a help—a nice head start."

"We found one of your couriers too, in a landfill outside Frankfurt."

Declan snorts. "And he deserved every screaming second of it, the suited prick—running off with my luggage like that. I'd kill the bastard again if I could."

Carr nods. "I'm sure. Anyway, he's about as far as we followed the cash."

"Then how did you manage it?"

"It was the real estate."

"What—this place?"

"You used to talk about this neck of the woods, once upon a time, when you played retirement geography—you and Bobby and Mike and Dennis and Ray-Ray. You used to talk about Punta and José Ignacio and La Paloma—this whole stretch of coast. How wide the beaches were, the blond sand, the fishing. And then, about two years back, you stopped talking about it. You just dropped it—never mentioned it again. You talked about plenty of other places afterward—in Vietnam, in Thailand—but not here."

"Fuck me. I didn't think anyone was paying attention."

"I was. It was your favorite place, and then it wasn't. Was that when it started, the planning for all this—two years ago?"

"Who keeps track?" Declan says, smiling. "A pretty slim reed, though, wasn't it—some game we used to play?"

Carr nods. "It was grasping at straws, for sure—but what else was there to do? The money trail was cold. So I looked for purchases of private homes—beachfront property only—made by foreign individuals or companies where payment was in cash. Anytime in the past two years. Anywhere from Punta, north to Costa Azul. It was a shot in the dark, but this stretch of coastline isn't all that long. Hell, the whole country isn't that big. Turned out there weren't so many purchases to sort through. And, of course, Boyce has the resources."

Declan's face darkens and he shakes his head. "Doesn't he though, lad—a whole feckin' empire at his feet. And have you finally sussed out who it is you're working for?"

"It didn't take much figuring. All that access, all that data, the intel reports . . ."

"Your old dad will be pleased to know you're serving your country again."

"I'm a consultant," Carr says, frowning. "A subcontractor."

Declan's laugh is bitter. "That's what you tell yerself. That's how it starts. The bastard doesn't want Prager's money, you know—he never did. He wants Prager himself—his very own bent banker as a pet, and all that intel on Prager's clients, current and future. He was going to squeeze Prager—threaten to rat to his clients that a hundred million of their money had walked out the door—if Prager didn't roll over."

Carr nods. "Which is what he did. Boyce squeezed, and Prager rolled over."

"So things worked out fer him after all—that's grand."

"Don't kid yourself—Boyce is out of pocket one hundred million plus some hefty expenses. He wants his money back. And I want mine."

Declan's laugh is full of irony. "Ah, young Carr, is that what all this is about to you—nothing more than money?"

Carr pushes his mug across the table. His face is hot. "I could ask you the same. Was this just about money to you? Was it worth the fucking body count?"

"Don't moralize, lad. I'm a thief—same as them. Same as you."

"I didn't slaughter the men I worked with."

Declan stands quickly and runs a hand through his hair. "You think that's what I set out to do?"

"I think you have an amazing ability to rationalize just about anything. That firefight at Bertolli's place, being out there in the dark, blasting away, making it up as you go—I think you love shit like that. It's right up your alley. I think the only thing you love more than money and yourself is risk—and fuck the collateral damage. If there are bodies in the street, it's their own damn fault for getting in the way."

"They knew the downside of this work, same as you. They knew what could happen."

"Bessemer didn't know it. Amy Chun didn't know it."

"Bessemer was never going to make it, and Chun was questionable."

Carr's jaw aches from clenching. "And what about our own guys? Did they know that their biggest risk was the man they were working for? For chrissakes, they trusted you!"

"Trust? You naive ass—you think they wouldn't have sold you out? You thought they'd ratted me to Bertolli. You thought they were going to do the same to you—and they might've, lad, given half a chance. Look what they did in Mendoza: ran off when the shooting started—with a chunk of my money, mind—and then lied to you about it. They're professional liars! You're telling me you trust men like that?"

Carr shakes his head in disbelief. "You don't seriously believe that, do you?"

"You should thank me for opening your eyes. They were thieves and killers, not my feckin' kids. You were on borrowed time with them, same as me—only I had borrowed more."

"So that makes it okay, then? We were going to fuck you eventually, unless you fucked us first?"

Declan waves a hand, as if he's shooing a fly. "This is a young man's

game, and I was too long at it. It was just a matter of time, and that bastard Boyce wasn't going to let me retire. He won't let you go either, you'll see."

Carr pushes away from the table and looks out the window. Light is swelling in the sky now, and the ocean is yellow and scored with whitecaps. He looks at Declan—a grizzled old man in rumpled pajamas, with a gun in his hand. He reaches once more for those feelings, but it's just empty pockets.

"I can't even follow your bullshit anymore, Deke. It's too convoluted, or I'm too tired. It's all just noise."

Declan squints at him and at the Taurus, and slides the gun onto the table. His smile is thin and tired. "Maybe the simple answer's the best, then. Maybe I did it for her."

Carr laughs coldly. "You did it for *love*?"

"You sound shocked."

"I expect cynicism from you, not delusion."

Declan's smile is tired. "Not a believer, lad?"

"In a love that has you killing your own? I don't call that love."

"You think it's all paper hearts and stolen kisses? You're not *that* young, Carr. You've read a book or two."

Carr sighs. "I hope she's worth it."

Declan laughs bitterly. "Too soon to tell, lad," he whispers.

Then the bedroom door opens, and Tina walks through. She's wearing fatigue pants, a black T-shirt, a black plastic holster under her left arm, and another on her right hip. Her platinum hair—longer now—is tied in a tight braid. She slams a clip into a Glock as she crosses the living room, and slides the gun into her shoulder holster.

She shakes her head in disgust. "If I have to listen to much more of this, I won't wait for Boyce to shoot me. I'll do it myself."

50

There is heat in Carr's face again, and a rushing sound in his ears, and the feelings that eluded him with Declan come surging back now. He looks at the Taurus on the table, and has to make a fist to stop himself from reaching for it.

"Long time, Tina," he says.

She purses her lips. "Not long enough, if you know what I mean," she says, and looks at Declan. "You pat him down?"

"Jaysus, girl, he's not come here to throw down. If that's what he wanted, he'd have done it already."

"That's your view. Pat him down."

Declan rolls his eyes and puts up his hands in mock despair. "Indulge her, lad," he says. Carr stares at Tina for a moment, and then he stands and puts his palms on the table and spreads his legs. Declan is quick and thorough, and there's only the slightest hesitation when his fingers find the mic taped between Carr's shoulders. He smiles at Carr and looks at Tina. "Like a baby," he says.

Tina goes to the kitchen window and looks up the hill. Then she turns to Carr. "Great. Now if you two are through catching up, we can—"

"Not quite through," Carr says softly.

"What, more questions? Let me guess—Valerie?"

"I want to know what happened to her."

Declan coughs nervously. "Come on, lad, you—"

Tina cuts him off. "He knows what happened to her. He knows."

Carr nods slowly, as his chest tightens. "It was at Chun's place?"

"She never saw it coming, if that makes you feel better. And it was clean. And fast."

The floor is shifting beneath him and Tina's voice is faint. Carr sits down again, carefully. Declan is staring at the floor, and Tina is back at the window. "I shouldn't have let Chun see it happen, though," she continues. "That was a mistake. The woman went fucking ape-shit—put up a hell of a fight."

"Where?" Carr says. His voice is small and choked. "Where is she?"

"Valerie? Burial at sea, due east of the Boca Beach Club, four miles out or so. I don't know the GPS coordinates or anything."

The room seems to darken, and Carr's knees shake. "Christ," he whispers, and he closes his eyes and there is Valerie in Napa, the candlelight on her arms and neck, her hair coming loose from its braid, her smile. And there she is in Portland, the dying orange light on her face, her hands cold under his shirt. *Maybe that's what we'll do afterward, you and me. We'll conduct a little research to find some happy couples. We'll be like archaeologists.* And there is her amber voice, close in his ear, intimate. *Afterward.* And there is the weight of her, above him, the heat of her body washing over him. Carr's chest aches, and his bones are lead.

"Regret's a bitch," Tina says from somewhere far off. "You spent all that time wondering about her, but she wasn't lying to you. You ask me, I think she liked you. She put up with your whining, which was more than I—"

"Stop talking," Carr says. He is surprised to find himself on his feet, his chair overturned. He wants the Taurus, but Declan has a hand over it and is shaking his head.

Tina looks at Carr. "At last, something we agree on: enough fucking talk. How many men out there?"

"Too many," Carr says.

"I count seven," Tina says. "Am I right?"

Declan chuckles. "You planning on a war, love?"

"I'm not planning to go anyplace with Boyce."

"Darlin', I think they've got us fair and square."

Tina crosses her white arms on her chest. "The hell they do. We've got Carr. If they want him back in one piece, they'll let us walk."

Carr's laugh is jagged and loud. "You think anyone on earth cares if I'm in one piece?"

"You better hope Boyce does," Tina says. "Otherwise this is going to be a mess, and you'll be the first stain." And she slips the Glock from her shoulder holster and points it at Carr.

Declan laughs. "We have a better negotiating position than that, girl. Boyce wants his money, for chrissakes, and recovery's easier with us than without. In fact, it's impossible without us."

Tina's mouth puckers in disgust. "You think I'm going to deal away my money?"

"It's not just *your* money."

"Whatever."

Declan smiles and walks around the table. He puts a hand on Tina's shoulder. "I like to mix it up as much as the next fellow, but it's nice when there's at least the ghost of a chance. You know Boyce as well as I do, love. He leaves no daylight."

Tina shakes off his hand. "You *are* a fucking old woman. After all that work, the time we put in, all the goddamn bridges we burned—you're ready to deal it away? Well, I'm not." She turns the Glock on Carr again. "How many men out there?"

"I forget."

Declan's smile is unwavering. "Who says we have to deal it all away? That's what negotiation is about. I'm sure Boyce will agree, recovering some money is better than recovering none at all." He puts his hand out again.

She steps back and keeps her gun on Carr. There are pink spots on her cheeks, the first time Carr has ever seen color there. His mouth is dry and he looks again for the Taurus, but he can't see it on the table.

Tina shakes her head at Declan. "You're mister diplomat now? Sure, Boyce might negotiate—and then he'll hose us once he has the cash. And then where will we be? I'm getting tired of asking, Carr—how many fucking men?"

"Two. Four. A hundred. Go out and count them yourself."

Declan drapes a big arm on her shoulder. "We'll still be alive, love. Even a shit deal is better than dead."

Tina ducks from beneath his arm and draws the second Glock from her hip. "The hell it is. If you think I'm—"

Declan hits her with the Taurus on the side of the head, and Tina

crumples to the floor. He kicks her guns away, kneels beside her, and checks her breathing and her pulse. Then he slides all three guns across the tiles to Carr. "Better than dead," he says, and he picks Tina up and carries her to the sofa.

Boyce and five of his men are on the patio when Carr opens the door. The men go inside. Carr hands Boyce the guns. "You hear it?" Carr asks.

"I heard. I'm sorry about Valerie."

"So am I," Carr says, swallowing hard. "It wasn't a surprise, but . . ."

"Knowing it is different."

Carr leans heavily against a whitewashed wall, dizzy for a moment in the morning air. "You'll deal with the money?"

Boyce nods. "Why don't you sit down?"

Carr waves him off. "I'm fine."

Boyce looks at him for a moment and then puts out a massive hand. They shake and Boyce goes inside, and Carr walks through a gate in the stone fence and down to the beach.

He keeps walking until the sand is firm beneath his feet, and then he stops and watches the ocean, and the waves unfurling. The stray he'd seen at dawn is back, rolling and splashing in a tidal pool. His coat is heavy with water, glistening like a seal's, and he's holding a piece of driftwood in his mouth. A boy comes down the beach now, with a leash and a yellow tennis ball. The boy whistles; the dog attends. Not a stray then. Carr looks north and sees a lighthouse in the distance. He thinks about walking there, but finds that he's kneeling in the sand and that he cannot move.

Epilogue

It is February, and Stockbridge lies under a blanket of new snow. The storm that spread it moved on before dawn, and the morning sky is blue and painfully bright. Carr wears sunglasses to shovel and salt the drive, the front steps, and the stone walk out to the mended gate, and he keeps them on while he drinks a cup of coffee on the porch and watches a town plow throw pillars of snow into the air. When his coffee is gone, he stacks bales of newspaper into his pickup—yet another load for the recycling center. The bed is nearly full when a black Mercedes pulls into the drive. Carr pushes his sunglasses into his hair and takes off his gloves.

A liveried driver walks carefully around the car and opens the rear door. Mr. Boyce emerges, too large to have ever fit inside. He squints in the glare, turns up the collar of his black overcoat, and smiles.

"I thought I might be too early," Boyce says. His deep voice is somehow muffled in the snow.

"I'm up with the chickens," Carr says. "But I wasn't expecting visitors."

"I thought I'd tell you in person that the money's finally settled."

"About time."

"Declan doesn't make anything easy."

Carr nods and crosses his arms on his chest. "Tell me the final numbers."

"After expenses, et cetera, the recovery netted seventy-eight five, of

which a third stays with me, and two-thirds—that's fifty-two million and change—goes to you. Per your instructions, ten of that goes to Bessemer's kid—"

"Simon."

"To Simon Bessemer, of Boothbay Harbor, Maine; another five to Maureen Shepherd, of Eugene, Oregon—Dennis's mother; and five more to Elaine Geller, of Bethpage, Long Island—Bobby's sister."

"What about Mike?"

"There might be an aunt in San Diego. We're still looking."

"And Valerie?"

Boyce shakes his head. "Daniel Finch and Dawn Schaffer—the mother went back to her maiden name—both deceased, no siblings."

Carr lets out a breath that hangs in the air like a ghost. "Finch," he says quietly, "that was her name? Valerie Finch?"

"*Anne* Finch," Boyce says. "That was her real name. Anne Elizabeth Finch."

Carr swallows hard and stares for a while at a snow-covered fir. "Her parents . . . do you know where they're buried?"

"In Texas, at a place near Austin."

"Both of them, in the same place?"

"Same place. Why?"

"I want to get something—a stone or something—near her parents. Could you—"

Boyce nods. "What do you want on it?"

"Just her name," Carr says.

The plow passes again, going in the other direction, and the chains sound to Carr like sleigh bells. He and Boyce watch as it recedes down the road, and then Boyce takes an envelope from his coat.

"It's a statement," he says. "It lays out the recovery, the expenses, the split—everything."

"What about the tax situation?"

"That too. You're square there—with the feds and the Commonwealth of Massachusetts—all documented and paid up, as far as they're concerned."

"Thanks," Carr says, and tucks the envelope in his back pocket. "And thanks for the courier service."

"I figured I'd see for myself how you're doing."

Carr shrugs. "I'm still racking up the frequent-flyer miles at the dump and the recycling center, and they throw rose petals at my feet at the hardware store."

"How's your dad?"

"Some days he reads to me from the *FT,* other days I read to him, and then there are the days he craps his pants. It's up and down, but the general trend is down. He's dying."

Boyce nods gravely. "And the help situation?"

"A new one started Monday. She's a few years out of nursing school, worked in a dementia unit, over in Springfield. Nice kid, very eager. I figure she'll last two weeks."

"Say the word, and I'll have Margie back tomorrow. She did fine with him before, and it would give you a break for a while. A little time to do something else."

"Something else?"

"I've always got something else that needs doing."

"I have my hands full here," Carr says.

"Any thoughts about what you might do . . . afterward?"

Carr tenses at the word. "Not a one."

"A man's got to do something."

"Maybe not. I've got a lot of money now."

"I don't see you as the idle type."

"I just need some practice."

Boyce smiles and shakes his head. "You sure about Margie—about taking a break? This sort of thing . . . it can be long, and none of it is easy."

Carr shrugs again. "He's my father."

Mr. Boyce nods and grips Carr's hand. He walks to his car, and the driver comes around to get the door. Boyce pauses and turns back to Carr. "You never ask about them—about Declan and Tina. Not once."

"There's nothing I want to know," Carr says, and Mr. Boyce folds himself into his Mercedes and is driven away.

Carr brings his coffee mug inside. The front hall is warm and smells of soap and floor wax and fresh paint, and the living room smells of apple wood from the fire he built the night before. He raises the shades and white winter light pours in and pools on every polished surface—the floorboards, the andirons, the silver bowl on the mantel, the silver frames atop the gleaming black piano.

Thick as Thieves

The frames are empty still—the photographs of Carr's parents lost in Prager's toolshed, or in the storm, or maybe to the sea—and the glass panes are like black windows. Arthur Carr has assured him that there are other photos of them—*just as damned blurry*—in a box somewhere in the attic, but Carr has yet to look. It's freezing up there now, and there are dozens of boxes to search, and Carr knows that in these matters his father is not reliable.

Carr straightens the frames on the piano, carries his coffee mug to the kitchen, and raises every window shade along the way.

A NOTE ON THE TYPE

This book was set in Minion, a typeface produced by the Adobe Corporation specifically for the Macintosh personal computer, and released in 1990. Designed by Robert Slimbach, Minion combines the classic characteristics of old style faces with the full complement of weights required for modern typesetting.

Composed by North Market Street Graphics,
Lancaster, Pennsylvania
Printed and bound by Berryville Graphics,
Berryville, Virginia
Designed by Virginia Tan

THE
VALIANT KNIGHTS
OF DAGUERRE

I HAD SEEN *them depart on their great mission, those valiant knights of Daguerre, Amfortas–Stieglitz, suffering from acute pictorialitis; Gurnemanz–Keiley, his faithful friend and adviser; Titurel–Steichen, whose pictures were not quite immaculate enough to prove him the best photographer in the world; and young Parsifal–Coburn, who but recently started from Ipswich in quest of the Grail—I had seen them depart, fully armed with kodaks and cameras, on their perilous journey over the Allegheny Mountains to open the Secession Shrine at Pittsburgh, leaving me behind with deep yearnings in my heart. Imagine my ecstatic joy when I received a telegram which read as follows: "The Shrine will be opened tomorrow. Take the next train and join us. Money enclosed. We can not do without you. We need somebody to write us up." So I sharpened my pencil, took my dress-suit out of pawn, packed both into my suit-case which had led a dream-like existence in the garret, as my traveling of late consisted largely of "L" trips in the rush hours, seized it with a grim grip, bade farewell to my wife and offspring, and set forth on my nocturnal pilgrimage.*

SADAKICHI HARTMANN, 1902

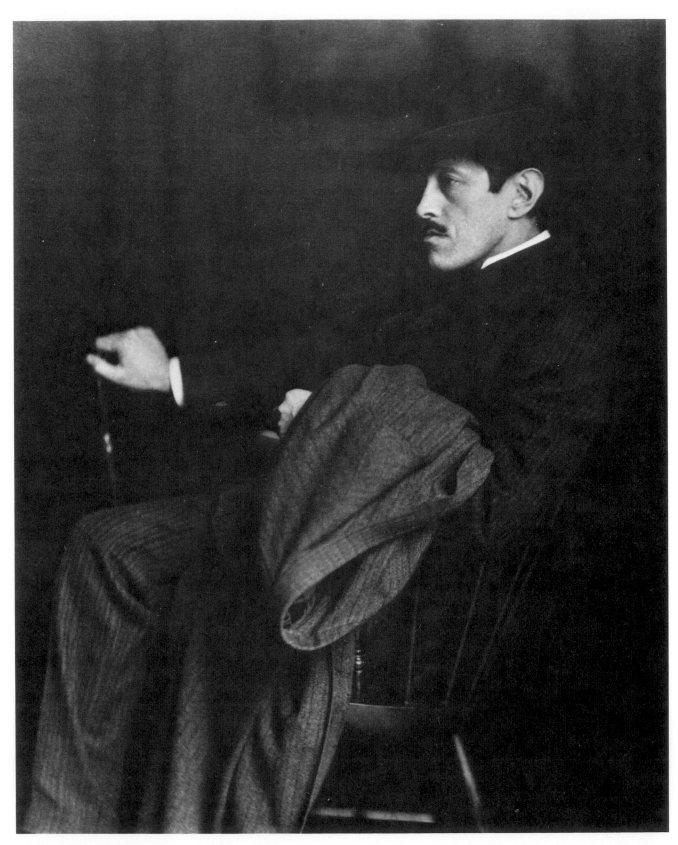

J. C. Strauss: Sadakichi Hartmann, 1911. whl-ucr.

THE VALIANT KNIGHTS OF DAGUERRE

Selected Critical Essays on Photography
and Profiles of Photographic Pioneers

BY SADAKICHI HARTMANN

EDITED BY HARRY W. LAWTON AND GEORGE KNOX
with the collaboration of Wistaria Hartmann Linton

FOREWORD BY THOMAS F. BARROW
BIBLIOGRAPHY COMPILED BY MICHAEL ELDERMAN

UNIVERSITY OF CALIFORNIA PRESS   Berkeley · Los Angeles · London

University of California Press
Berkeley and Los Angeles, California

University of California Press, Ltd.
London, England

ISBN 0-520-03356-6
Library of Congress Catalog Card Number: 76-47987
Printed in the United States of America

1   2   3   4   5   6   7   8   9

CONTENTS

Selected Critical Essays on Photography

Profiles of Photographic Pioneers

FOREWORD

$\mathcal{J}$HE FORTY–SIX essays in this volume by Sadakichi Hartmann, originally published between 1898 and 1913, are filled with prescient observations on photography by one of its most important critics to date. I am certain they will stimulate further research into Sadakichi Hartmann's almost forgotten contribution to photography's critical literature. Such further investigations will be greatly abetted by the comprehensive Sadakichi Hartmann archive at the University of California, Riverside, which is part of the recently acquired Wistaria Hartmann Linton Collection. The essays presented here are an accurate sample of what the archive contains in depth: the writings of a critic of the visual arts that have, many years after their origin, significantly more than a clinical, archaeological interest. Hartmann is an excellent example of an author who can be read with great pleasure while he is informing us about art, the process of making art, and the act of assuming a critical position.[1]

During the last seventy years of photographic history, it has been a continuing question whether the critic is a necessity or a pernicious luxury. It may be hoped that the pieces that appear here will indicate the necessity of critical work like Hartmann's. When any art form is in its youth, an individual who can establish benchmarks for the judgment of quality is invaluable. Hartmann did this and did it well in large part because he *knew* art; not merely the relatively narrow area encompassed by photography (which, with a conviction shared by few of his contemporaries, he truly believed to be an art), but much broader areas that included printmaking, painting, and sculpture. And while one is always aware of his enormous respect for American art, he consistently paid homage to European and Oriental accomplishments. This broad understanding and catholic sensibility were reflected in his 1903 article "On Pictorial and Illustrative Qualities"[2] in which, after an intelligent discourse on the somewhat cloudy boundary between painting and illustration (with reference to Callot, Corot, Alma-Tadema and Gérôme, among others), Hartmann turns the entire discussion specifically to printmaking and photography, stating:

> Illustration and the various black and white processes . . . can express *everything* that happens in actuality or in imaginary worlds with impunity; they have, in regard to choice of subjects, no limitations, although etching, lithographs, etc., that treat an exceptional pictorial moment with painter-like concentration, like Whistler in his etching of a young girl, will always evoke the remark: "What a pity to waste such a motive on a monochrome process." Photography has, as we all know, its mechanical limitations, but aside of these it enjoys the same liberties as the other graphic arts, with the difference perhaps—as it lacks manual spontaneity in its manipulation—that painter-like effects are even more desirable than purely illustrative ones.

Throughout his writing career, Hartmann acknowledged and explored the very real relationship between photography and printmaking in an informed manner with numerous references to specifics in the history of art. Given the unevenness of photographic criticism at the turn of the century (with the significant exceptions, in addition to Hartmann, of Roland Rood and Charles Caffin), Hartmann's comparative analyses alone would have been important; but he also displayed a special understanding of the unique possibilities inherent in the photographic medium and the divisive problems it would create for the artist. In an 1898 article, Hartmann outlined many of the dichotomies that separate amateur and what he called "artistic photography."

> Since amateur photographers are as plentiful as bicyclists, the more astonishing it seems to me that those men who really produce something artistic can be counted on the fingers of one hand.[3]

In fact, the entire article might serve as a palimpsest for the illumination of the recent attempts to establish the amateur's snapshot as photography's taproot. Strangely, as is the case with many of Hartmann's writings of importance, this article has not been widely read and seems virtually unknown even among photo–historians. In the same article, questions of major aesthetic import are posed, for example "Why does a man photograph?", and answers are given that are still germane to all creative endeavors. Hartmann often seems to have possessed an almost intuitive comprehension of the photographic medium, as in the following observation: "In higher stages photography can reflect all the subtleties of a man's mind; but then it is no longer a pastime, but the strenuous study of a lifetime."[4]

Another way of appraising Hartmann's unique critical quality might be through his idea that "The essential point is that the photograph should be seen *as a photograph* and not be judged by the formalist rules of the other arts."[5] And yet somehow it was precisely those formalist rules that gave him the concepts and vocabulary with which to discuss the images of a process that continues to confound critics.

There are no quick or easy answers as to why Hartmann understood so much so early. There can be no question that his ideas would be as valuable today as at the turn of the century, but he was fortunate in the time that he wrote. He did not suffer from the restraints of any "New Criticism." It was possible and necessary for him to know an artist personally and enter into his life and his working habits. This appears to have been an enormous asset in his creation of the amalgams that inform us so clearly today. Hartmann's intimate manner of working was not without its weaknesses.[6] But when his writings are viewed in anything approaching their totality, they maintain an extraordinarily strong sense of lasting quality in art. This sense was greatly supplemented by the enthusiasm with which Hartmann availed himself of the constantly expanding cultural resources that existed in New York City.[7] His friendship with men of brilliance equal to his own, James G. Huneker for one, also assisted his evolution as a critic. All of the preceding and many, many more aspects of Hartmann's remarkable life (see Editors' Introduction) add to the substantial prophecy of his work. In a more romantic vein, perhaps his German extraction helped make the entire body of his writing, in Goethe's words, "fragments of a great confession."

THOMAS F. BARROW
UNIVERSITY OF NEW MEXICO
ALBUQUERQUE, NEW MEXICO

ACKNOWLEDGMENTS

$\mathcal{T}$HE EDITING AND compiling of *The Valiant Knights of Daguerre* was made possible by the knowledge and assistance of a multitude of people and institutions.

Many of the photographs reproduced here have been made from original negatives or by copying images in the collections of the International Museum of Photography at George Eastman House, Rochester, New York; the Art Museum of the University of New Mexico; the photo library department of the Museum of the City of New York; the department of photography, Museum of Modern Art, New York City; the photography, prints, and photographic division, Library of Congress, Washington, D.C; the Smithsonian Institution, Washington, D.C., and the Wistaria Hartmann Linton Collection, special collections, Library of the University of California, Riverside. These photographs are indicated, respectively, by the letters IMP-GEH, UNM, MCNY, MOMA, LC, SI, and WHL-UCR. We gratefully acknowledge the assistance of these institutions in making this book possible and for giving us permission to reproduce photographs. Unfortunately, the editors were unable to locate the negatives or original images of some of the photographers represented in this volume—if such works still exist. It was therefore necessary to copy these photographs as faithfully

as possible from the reproductions in the original magazine articles. In some instances, we could not secure a satisfactory copy of a photograph from the magazine. Occasionally also, a Hartmann article was published without accompanying illustrations, even though he might refer to specific examples of the photographer's work by title. In the latter two cases, museums were rarely able to find the photographs we desired. We found it necessary to accept substitutes from museum collections or copy other examples of a photographer's work from magazines of his period. This may prove disappointing to a reader intrigued by Hartmann's description of Breese and Eickemeyer's portrait of Yvette Guilbert, "Le Désir," for example, but hopefully some of these missing prints will eventually be discovered now that attention is focused upon them. For assisting us with copying, we wish to express our thanks for the very generous help provided by Herbert Quick, senior photographer, and Thomas Neff, photographer, of the photographic service, University of California, Riverside. They did the best job possible, working with magazines that were frequently brittle with age and stained by users.

The editors also wish to acknowledge the conscientious assistance and major contributions made to research on Sadakichi Hartmann by Michael Elderman, formerly a graduate student in the English department, University of California, Riverside, and Brent Sweeney, also a former graduate student in English at the same institution. Mr. Elderman began our bibliographic file on Hartmann while in graduate school, and has continued to maintain it since that time. He is primarily responsible for the thoroughness of the bibliography of Hartmann's photographic writings which appears in this volume. Mr. Sweeney served as a diligent research assistant, ably assisting in the preparation of the notes and an index.

We particularly want to acknowledge our great indebtedness to the photo-historians, who were as liberal with their encouragement as their knowledge: Beaumont Newhall, visiting professor of art, University of New Mexico, Albuquerque; Thomas F. Barrow, associate professor of art, University of New Mexico; Peter Bunnell, McAlpin Professor of History of Photography and Modern Art and director of The Art Museum, Princeton University; John Szarkowski, director of the department of photography, Museum of Modern Art, New York City; Jerald C. Maddox, curator for photography, prints, and photographs, Library of Congress, Washington, D.C.; Van Deren Coke, director of The Art Museum, University of New Mexico; and Joe Deal, assistant professor of art, University of California, Riverside, who while visiting the International Museum of Photography at George Eastman House, Rochester, New York, made many of the photographic selections for this volume. We are also deeply grateful for the assistance of Roger P. Hull, associate professor of art, Willamette University, Salem, Oregon, who has carried out pioneer research on Hartmann's role in photography and in the politics of the Photo-Secession.

In addition, we wish specifically to express our appreciation to Miss Georgia O'Keeffe for permission to use material from the Stieglitz Archive at Yale University and to the late Donald C. Gallup, curator of the Yale Collection of American literature, who rendered invaluable assistance in making material from the archive available. We are also most grateful to those persons who undertook special missions in behalf of this volume or rendered helpful suggestions, editorial advice, or other assistance: Richard Morris of Mountain View, California; James L. Enyeart, executive director of Friends of Photography, Carmel, California; Christine Hawrylak, photographic print service, International Museum of Photography at George Eastman House; Marshall Van Deusen, professor of English, University of California, Riverside; Jon Bosak, photographer and editor, Riverside, California; William Purcell, photographer, Riverside, California; Thomas Pelzel, associate professor of art history, University of California, Riverside; Richard G. Carrott, associate professor of art history, University of California, Riverside; Eugene Ostroff, supervisor and curator of graphic arts and photography, The Smithsonian Institution, Washington, D.C.; Dorothy Norman, New York City; Edward R. Beardsley, associate professor of art, University of California, Riverside; Roberta De Goler, photographic print service, International Museum of Photography at George Eastman House; Keith Macfarlane, associate professor of French, University of California, Riverside; Sarah Greenough, graduate student in art history, University of New Mexico; Vicki Hearne, Wallace Stegner Fellow in Poetry, Stanford University; Gerald Ackerman, associate professor of art history, Pomona College, Claremont, California; Clifford R. Wurfel, associate librarian, University of California, Riverside; Charles Gregory Robbins, library assistant in special collections, University of California, Riverside; Richard L. Tooke, supervisor of rights and reproductions, Museum of Modern Art; Susan Bokanovich, editor of *Mosaic,* University of California, Riverside, who has assisted in cataloging the Wistaria Hartmann Linton Collection; and our wives, Mrs. Elizabeth Knox; and Mrs. Georgeann Lawton. Various librarians and libraries which cooperated in the search for Hartmann materials are acknowledged in the bibliography. Mrs. Clara

Dean, Mrs. Margaret Good, and Jo Ann Bickel assisted us with typing and manuscript preparation. We are also most deeply grateful to Wendy Cunkle Calmenson, who served as production editor and designer on this book and made many excellent suggestions.

Finally, we wish to acknowledge the dedicated efforts of Hartmann's daughter, Mrs. Wistaria Hartmann Linton, who has closely worked with the editors both on this book and on earlier and ongoing research on her father. Her friendship has meant as much as her collaboration.

FOR BEAUMONT NEWHALL

who first charted the territory

and left for the rest of us the discovery of new trails

EDITORS' INTRODUCTION

You have never had much literary discrimination, but you must have instinctively felt I was the right man of the period.

—SADAKICHI HARTMANN TO ALFRED STIEGLITZ
LETTER OF MARCH 9, 1923

HE WAS ADMIRED; he was feared; he was detested. Among the pioneers of photographic criticism in America none exerted such direct personal influence on so many photographers as did Sadakichi Hartmann (1867–1944), the Japanese-German writer and critic. He began his career as a photographic critic by allying himself with Alfred Stieglitz and the cause of artistic photography, but he soon expanded his focus to include all aspects of the medium—artistic, professional, and amateur. Whereas Stieglitz's milieu was New York and the international scene of art photography, Hartmann's encompassed the backwater towns of America—where the ordinary photographer struggled to perfect his craft in the darkroom along the railroad track. A stimulus to talent at every level of photography, Hartmann also served as ambassador for Stieglitz in bringing the photographic revolution to the provinces.

From 1898 until shortly after World War I, Hartmann rampaged uncompromisingly through the photographic world, saying whatever he believed needed to be said, discovering and championing unknown photographers, sparking endless controversies, and serving as an unconventional speaker and outspoken judge at innumerable conventions and exhibitions. Under his own name and the *nom de plume* of Sidney Allan, he published two books and hundreds of essays on all phases of the medium in photographic journals throughout the country, at a time when the Kodak was a new craze and such magazines flourished in almost every large city. Photo-historian Thomas F. Barrow, associate professor of art, University of New Mexico, recently called Hartmann "the last really prolific, sensible, constructive critic" of photography.[1]

Quixotically Bohemian and whimsically cynical, Hartmann was a raffish orphan of the American *fin-de-siècle*. To John Ward Stimson, founder of the New York School of Artist-Artisans, he was "full of force, fire, and fearlessness."[2] Critic Benjamin De Casseres characterized him as "a man who belonged in Cellini's gang or with the rowdy geniuses of the Mermaid Tavern."[3] Usually he affected an aristocratic studiousness in photographic circles— as contrasted to the gypsy-like spontaneity of the Hartmann who frequented the *avant-garde* ateliers of Greenwich Village, where he reigned as self-proclaimed King of Bohemia. Yet his sense of the absurd and his loathing of sham and genteel convention were such that in moments of capriciousness or inebriation Hartmann might turn the most proper gathering into a Marx Brothers' comedy.[4]

Since Hartmann's forthright opinions on all matters concerning art sometimes made enemies, he was not an ideal companion for those intimate luncheons Stieglitz held for many of his colleagues at Holland House in the Prince George Hotel.

Hartmann resented the fact that Alfred Stieglitz recognized this and often maneuvered to keep him in the background, away from the pleasant social occasions of the Photo-Secessionists. Nonetheless, Stieglitz was one of the few who understood how Hartmann's diverse talents might be best employed, who commanded his full respect if not his full allegiance, and who had the patience to work with the unruly critic for more than a decade, despite several serious breaches in their relationship.

Because of a series of annual lecture tours across country, initiated in 1905 and extending intermittently until his death, Hartmann became better known to the rank and file of photographers outside New York than such outstanding critics as Charles H. Caffin and Roland Rood. He amassed followers in city after city, photographers who eagerly read and discussed his essays and awaited each lecture circuit to show him their latest work. Because Hartmann's sensibilities were wounded easily over trifles—often imagined slights—and he could be abrasively difficult over payment for his work, some photographic magazine editors published him reluctantly, only to satisfy the demand of their readers, men and women who relished being visited in their small-town studios by the cosmopolitan Sidney Allan.

At exhibitions Hartmann was a formidably aggressive judge, striding from picture to picture, denouncing slipshod workmanship with Whistlerian sarcasm that delighted or horrified gallerygoers, praising prints that met his exacting standards, and always tempering even his caustic outbursts with common sense advice. In 1906, a reporter from the *Des Moines Register and Leader* spent a morning trailing Hartmann about as he judged entries at the Iowa State Photographic Convention. To the reporter, Hartmann with his shock of long black hair and flowing cape, followed anxiously by photographers, was a "unique figure." "The photographers worship the ground over which Allan walks," he wrote. "He is harsh and brutal at times in his criticism, but he hits the nail on the head every time."[5]

Hartmann's influential role in the American art and photographic movement that began in the 1890s has generally been ignored or only partly comprehended by modern art historians. He is usually accorded a measure of praise which assumes that his reputation rested on several popular books on art: *Shakespeare in Art* (Boston: L. C. Page & Co., 1901); *A History of American Art* (Boston: L. C. Page & Co., 1902); *Japanese Art* (Boston: L. C. Page & Co., 1903); and *The Whistler Book* (Boston: L. C. Page & Co., 1910). All of these works, except possibly the last, were written hastily against contractual deadlines. The first and third of these works were written in less than a month with little research and a heavy reliance by Hartmann on his almost photographic memory. All were churned out in periods of desperate poverty to stave off creditors. *A History of American Art* has been recognized as a pioneering effort and once was a standard textbook. Despite incisive evaluations of many artists, however, much of the *History* is uneven, partly as a result of the cut-and-paste methods Hartmann employed in assembling the book from his earlier critical articles and reviews in magazines. Of these four volumes, the work on Whistler is the most durable and literate, exploring the affinities between different arts and using its subject as a base from which to examine the sources of artistic inspiration. Hartmann also wrote two instructive manuals for photographers: *Composition in Portraiture* (New York: Edward L. Wilson, 1909); and *Landscape and Figure Composition* (New York: Baker Taylor Company, 1910).

Hartmann's most impressive writing on the visual arts, however, lies buried in the art journals, photographic magazines, and newspapers of the 1890s and early twentieth century. Jerome Mellquist was the first art historian to assert that Hartmann had been a pathfinder, noting that among the "scouts and raiders" engaged in a continuous battle to crush prejudice against a native art "none had been more effective than Sadakichi Hartmann."[6] In his *The Emergence of an American Art*, Mellquist provided some sense of the kaleidoscopic range of Hartmann's interests:

> Sometimes he merely darted forward on a swift foray, naming Pictorial Photography as a possible source of stimulation to interior decoration. Again he nimbly sketched Steichen's studio, or memorialized a suicide sculptor, John Donoghue. Still later he cast a strange fragrance as he wept over the death of Whistler in *White Chrysanthemums*. But the main charges of this restless intelligence were elsewhere. As early as 1903, in an essay entitled *The Value of the Apparently Meaningless and Inaccurate*, he unforgettably identified the magazine [*Camera Work*] with an objection to the merely accurate in art. For, said he, "the love of exactitude is the lowest form of pictorial gratification." Thus he had already forecast the fighting lines of a decade later.[7]

More recently, Barbara Rose presented excerpts from two Hartmann essays in her *Readings in American Art Since 1900*, observing that Hartmann and Caffin were "two of the earliest apologists for modernism in America."[8] Hartmann first entered the arena for modernism with articles on new European painters in *The Boston Evening Transcript* in the mid-1880s. He was probably the first American critic to speak of Gauguin, mentioning him in an 1894 essay on French painters.[9] During the early 1890s, he was already corresponding with, or visiting the studios of, members of the future Ash Can School who would launch their revolt in painting in 1908 at the Macbeth Gallery. By the middle of the 1890s, Hartmann was reviewing the works of Robert Henri, Arthur B. Davies, Maurice Prendergast, George Luks, and many other young painters who were scarcely known to the American art world until the Armory Show of 1913.

Art critics usually become more conservative and entrenched as they grow older, but Hartmann's critical arteries failed to harden until the late 1930s.[10] When his contemporary, James Gibbons Huneker, once an apostle of insurgency, charged that the "Younger American Painters" show held at the Photo-Secession Gallery in 1910 was a "revolution that doesn't revolve," it was Hartmann who prophesied that the war cry of the future would be color and "palettes will pour forth a stream so rich and many colored that the death of the art of painting alone could dam it."[11] When almost every American critic joined the onslaught against Max Weber's first comprehensive exhibit in 1911, Hartmann rallied to the painter's defense, perceiving that Weber's work was not so mystifying and that he "merely dissects the human form into geometrical ratios and color patterns and apparently proceeds like a primitive bent upon conquering his own knowledge of visual appearances."[12]

But however sensitive to newer currents, Hartmann was not hypnotized by schools. Impressionism, symbolism, realism, cubism, vorticism, expressionism—all passed Hartmann's scrutiny at various periods, and all he evaluated in terms of the excellence of individual practitioners. For what was any movement really? "As is always the case when painting undergoes a change and is entering upon a new phase of development," he explained, "a score of men, perhaps entirely unconscious of each other's efforts, are bent upon solving the same problem, to unravel the intricacies of a subtler and more convincing method of representation and to find the safest and surest medium to convey this new view of life."[13]

Although Hartmann's ambitions were primarily literary—he was the author of numerous dramas, short stories, poems, and one novel—he earned his livelihood for more than three decades primarily as an art and photographic critic. His critical output was prodigious, but none of Hartmann's most significant essays on either art or photography were collected in book form during his lifetime. His work appeared wherever he could find a market—from the literate monthlies such as *Harper's* and *Forum* to the obscure quarterlies and promotional house organs of commercial firms. Since much of his criticism was written on demand, often tailored to a length predetermined by editors, the quality of his production is highly erratic. While Hartmann distinguished between his better essays—such as those which appeared in *Camera Work*—and his blatant hackwork, he was at heart didactic, forever at the mercy of sudden insights which he could not resist affixing like jewels to otherwise jejune material. For this reason even many of his lesser essays on photography contain illuminating ideas.

As a reviewer Hartmann's frequently sarcastic or ironical approach—as when he said he had "seen few men represent Nothing as interestingly" as the pictorialist Joseph T. Keiley—often precipitated feuds with artists and photographers.[14] Still, he had many partisans among them who believed that they profited from even his most acerbic stances. The painter William M. Chase considered Hartmann's art criticism always interesting, and in the domain of composition thought his views were "the sanest and most practical ones I have ever read on the subject."[15] Another painter, E. E. Simmons, once said: "Hartmann may be capricious and malicious, and rather careless at times, but he is, after all, the only critic we have who knows a good picture when he sees it and who is not afraid of expressing his opinion."[16] The critic Roland Rood, in an article he later repudiated, ranked Hartmann as one of the three important factors in the pictorial movement, stating that when Hartmann "lent his pen to the photographic movement he helped it as no other man could."[17] Rood rather extravagantly eulogized Hartmann's achievements in photographic criticism as follows:

. . . He was the first art critic who realized the possibility of photography being developed into a fine art. His were the first pictorial criticisms in the photographic world. It was Hartmann who first conceived the idea of writing about a photographer as an individuality. What Hamerton did for etchers, Hartmann did for photographers. His first series of [sic] Stieglitz, Käsebier, White, Eickemeyer, Keiley, Day, and Eugene (which latter one Hartmann discovered)[18] gave a new note to the art world, and was imitated in England by Bernard Shaw. If it had not been for Hartmann, many of these and others, too, would never

have been heard of, most of them would have been forgotten. He came between these artists and the art loving public, he explained to the public, he gave them courage. Hartmann fought their battles when all other critics passed by, or at best scoffed.[19]

Much of this goes too far and is not really accurate, but then Rood was apparently captivated at the time by the charismatic Sadakichi, who appears, in turn, to have been promoting the younger critic as a protégé.[20] Arguments as to whether there was a place for photography among the fine arts went back almost a half century in Europe, and continental resistance towards its aesthetic merit was fast fading before the turn of the century. In America, J. Wells Champney, Thomas Harrison Cummings, Darius Cobb, and William M. Murray—to name only a few—preceded Hartmann in discussing the aesthetic issue. Other critics also had written articles on photographers in a personal vein, including Ralph Adams Cram, Osborne I. Yellott, and Cummings. Although photographers may have embraced Hartmann as an art critic joining their ranks, he was not a member of the critical establishment of the American art world represented by such academy-sanctioned spokesmen as Kenyon Cox and the arch-conservative Royal Cortissoz. Indeed, from the standpoint of the art academy, his credentials were the shaky ones of the itinerant art scribbler.

Yet in some respects, Rood's evaluation mirrors truth. Hartmann, by exploring the aesthetic problem of photography more doggedly and on a more cerebral level than most of his predecessors, helped give photography a public exposure previously lacking in America. He took the controversy out of the realm of self-defensive quibbling among photographers in their own journals, forcing even painters to think about it, and confronted the American art world with the task of rendering a verdict. In the same way, although he never neglected the technical aspects of the medium in his interviews, Hartmann's essays on individual photographers lifted such sketches above darkroom shoptalk, captured something of the individual personality of each photographer, and dignified the solitary worker as artist and craftsman.

When Hartmann briefly turned upon Stieglitz in 1904, assailing him as the dictator of American photography, he wrote one of his blistering attacks under the pen name of "Caliban." The pseudonym was well-considered. Stieglitz, on the island of Manhattan, fighting against the isolation of the American artist, was indeed a Prospero with a magician's touch. Inevitably Hartmann's immense ego chafed under the feeling that he had become the creature of this man he envied and toward whom he nourished an unfamiliar awe. Like Shakespeare's Caliban, he believed that his master relegated him to the background, assigned him menial tasks, "whiles you do keep from me/The rest o' the island." Stieglitz undoubtedly knew or suspected the identity of the hidden sniper—Hartmann's rhetoric was inimitable—yet he was magnanimous when Sadakichi sought to resume their relationship.

As the prophet of an American art (and we will not concern ourselves in this introduction with his role as a photographer), Stieglitz's genius lay in being an emblem of courage for other artists and photographers, inspiring them by his example to keener efforts, bringing their works and those of foreign artists to attention at his '291' gallery, and serving as a translator between the arts. Although he wrote frequently about photography, Stieglitz disliked making value judgments on the work of colleagues. In Hartmann he found a spirited gadfly with the necessary sting, unlike such genteel critics as J. Wells Champney, whose reviews in *Camera Notes* were exercises in amiability and who could not bear to judge exhibitions for fear he might hurt someone's feelings.[21] As one commentator observed: "Stieglitz was in need of a man who could write up his disciples and at the same time criticize them in a manner which he, in the position of their patriarch, could not very well do himself. Hartmann performed this task with great verve."[22]

When Stieglitz resigned from *Camera Notes* and in 1902 launched the most remarkable publication

in the history of American art, *Camera Work*, he gave Hartmann a chance to broaden his range of expression. It was then that Hartmann discovered his most authentic voice. His gift was the seeing of aesthetic possibilities where none had been seen before, for analyzing subterranean influences and inter-connections between the arts, and for portraying the lonely fight of individual artists for recognition in a manner with which all artists could identify. Although Shaw, Maeterlinck, Galsworthy, Gertrude Stein, and other illustrious literary names appeared in *Camera Work*, Hartmann, Caffin, Keiley, and De Casseres were the mainstays among contributors during the magazine's fourteen-year span.

Every great magazine has a unique tone, shaped first by the vision of its editor, next communicated to his editorial and art staff, and finally realized best through the few contributors who can perceive and rise to the magazine's aspirations. *Camera Work* was a mixture of photographic and artistic reproductions and literary materials brought together through Stieglitz's exacting craftsmanship into a luxurious marriage of typographic art. Next to Hartmann the most frequent contributors in the magazine's first two pioneering years were Caffin, proofreader Dallett Fuguet, and columnist J. B. Kerfoot. During this formative period Fuguet was the most prolific of the latter three men with twelve pieces, chiefly short verse; Kerfoot indulged in light humor and satire; and Caffin concentrated mostly on distinguished appreciations of work by members of the Photo-Secession. In the first two years alone, however, Hartmann provided twenty contributions, two or more each issue. In these pieces, Sadakichi raged across the arts, kindling sparks and signaling to future contributors that here was an independent journal which did not follow beaten paths. In large measure it was Hartmann—the magazine's most prolific writer throughout its existence—who reconnoitered far afield from purely photographic contributions to give intellectual substance and variety to Stieglitz's most imperishable achievement.

II.

The photographer B. J. Falk once inscribed a portrait he made of Sadakichi Hartmann with the phrase "To a Beloved Vagabond."[23] Hartmann's tumultuous career can best be described as that of a vagabond among arts and letters, following wherever his myriad interests led him. In his last years, broken in health and drinking heavily, Hartmann often found temporary refuge when he was down-and-out with Los Angeles artist Peter Krasnow and his wife, Rose. Edward Weston lived just down the street from the Krasnows. Weston hadn't seen Hartmann for many years when he encountered him one summer evening in 1928 at the artist's home. Weston was shocked to discover a "sad old ruin . . . paying for a dissipated, malicious life."[24] According to Krasnow, Weston had never liked Hartmann and usually avoided visiting when Sadakichi was present.[25] One night soon afterward, Weston arrived late at a party at the Krasnows and found Hartmann dancing for the guests:

> I had never seen Sadakichi dance, though from time to time I had heard enthusiastic comments.
>
> I add my eulogies. He is a much finer dancer than a writer. His gestures and facial expressions were superb. He knows the dance. No woman dancer could have approached his feelings and understanding. Again the male in art transcends the female—and in a field almost monopolized by females.[26]

Hartmann was then in his sixties. More than forty years had passed since Sadakichi had studied dance in Paris—according to him, under Grille d'Egout. Many who saw Sadakichi's improvisations insist he was one of the great interpretive dancers of all time. The incident recounted by Weston illustrates the peculiar virtuosity of Hartmann, who not only wrote about most of the arts, including an early essay on modern dance,[27] but also attempted to master each art to better understand it.

The multiple facets of Sadakichi were such that he is difficult to approach outside the scope of biography. At the age of twenty-three, he wrote with mock seriousness: "Until now my life has been a romance; it promises to become a spectacular play, in which I shall play alternately the hero, the lover, and the clown, and in the last act I'll die a penitent death."[28] Except for the last act, he played out his script with Rabelaisian gusto. A grab-bag of human extremes, he was both idealistic and cynical, arrogant and obsequious, ruthless and gentle, parsimonious and improvident, deceitful and honest—a man who acted many roles. One of these roles was Sidney Allan—his alter ego as photographic critic—and it is to that role we will primarily confine this introduction.

Carl Sadakichi Hartmann was born in 1867 on the island of Desima in Nagasaki Harbor, then a European trading colony, foreigners still being barred access to the Japanese mainland. His father was a German merchant, Carl Hermann Oskar Hartmann, and his mother, Osada, was Japanese, probably of the servant class. After her sudden death in 1868, the father shipped Sadakichi and an elder brother, Taru, back to Germany, where they were raised by their grandmother in the household of a wealthy, retired Hamburg uncle, Ernst Hartmann.

The uncle was a connoisseur and patron of the arts. His house had an excellent statuary collection; many original paintings hung on the walls, including a fragment of a Veronese; and one bedroom was embellished with large photographs of Venetian scenes.[29] As a child Sadakichi spent many hours leafing through dozens of illustrated books on art from his uncle's library. When his brother and other neighborhood boys played cricket, Sadakichi preferred walking a mile or two to the library or art museum. He was fascinated by the stereopticon shows presented at the Theater Marieux, and he acquired his own magic lantern and gave shows for the household. The uncle expected the boy to be able to discuss both art and the theater with discernment. Years later Sadakichi dedicated his *A History of American Art* (1902) to Ernst Hartmann "whom I have to thank for my first appreciation of art."

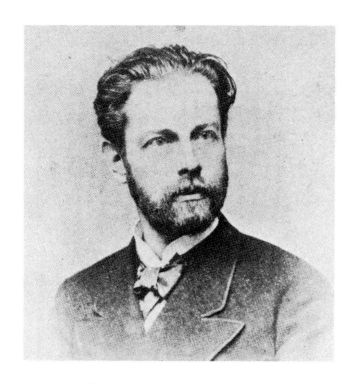

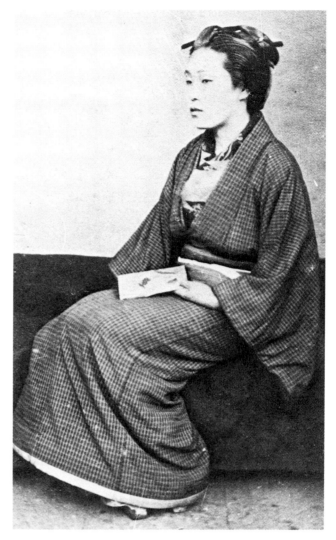

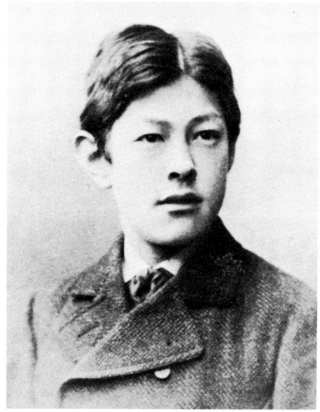

Above. Osada Hartmann, 1867, WHL-UCR.

Top left. Oskar Hartmann, n.d. WHL-UCR.

Left. Sadakichi Hartmann at the age of thirteen, 1880. WHL-UCR.

When Sadakichi's father returned from overseas and married a widow with two daughters, he placed the boy in a naval academy at Kiel. Sadakichi rebelled, ran away from the academy, and defied his father's attempt to send him back. Infuriated, the elder Hartmann shipped Sadakichi off to Philadelphia in 1882 to live with an aunt and uncle who had immigrated there. Soon after arriving in America, the teen-aged boy drifted away from his relatives to live on his own. In 1883 he worked for a short period for the lithographic firm of Wells & Hope, copying designs on stone; then as a stippler for another lithographic house; and finally as a negative retoucher for a Philadelphia photographer.

For a while, before he decided he lacked sufficient talent, Sadakichi entertained the hope of becoming an artist. At fifteen he took an evening drawing course at Spring Garden Institute, getting up early each morning in his cold garret to practice drawing before going to work. Sometimes he visited the landscape painter Carl Weber to seek advice on his sketches. In an effort to train his memory to be more rigorous, he spent his spare time in Philadelphia bookshops, where under the wary eyes of booksellers he would manage to browse through a hundred or so photographic reproductions of world art by the Soule Photographic Co. before being asked to leave. In this fashion he eventually managed to study most of the firm's fifteen thousand reproductions. He recalled that "even forty years later I was never at a loss to refer to pictures in this or that gallery which it had not been my privilege to enter."[30]

Meanwhile, prompted by an acquaintanceship with Walt Whitman, whom he occasionally visited at the poet's Camden cottage, Hartmann was also embarking on a literary and journalistic career.[31] He began selling free-lance articles—mostly on art, literature, and the theater—to newspapers in Boston, Philadelphia, and New York. Between 1885 and 1893 he made four trips to Europe, where he studied the theater and visited major art galleries in London, Copenhagen, Antwerp, Paris, Munich, and Berlin. He was still unsure how he would utilize the self-taught education he was acquiring, nor did he foresee "that for more than a quarter of a century I would be busy as a writer on art."[32] Instead, he viewed himself as something of an esthetic sybarite:

> . . . I wanted to see more and still more and remember what pleased me. The right way to go about it at the start. To fill up holes in the ground for a good foundation in art knowledge, to establish a high level of information advantageous for immediacy of judgement and vision.[33]

In 1892 Hartmann became staff writer for *The Weekly Review* in Boston. The earliest known article on photography which can be attributed to Hartmann is a brief item in the March 11, 1893 issue of that magazine. Since technological innovation interested Hartmann throughout his life, it is difficult to know whether a fascination with invention or a developing interest in photography motivated his report that William Kurtz, the New York photographer, has "lately done some photographic color painting that, when more perfected, threatens to oust Prang and lithography altogether."[34] The article is confined, however, only to a description of Kurtz' process of printing three negatives, each reproducing a still-life object to one of the primary colors.

When Hartmann in 1893 launched his own art and literary magazine in Boston, *The Art Critic*, he traveled up and down New England with a prospectus, taking advance orders from 388 subscribers. The magazine, one of the first *avant-garde* publications in America, with a heavy emphasis on the French Symbolist movement, lasted only four issues. Although it contained many articles on American and European art, photography is not discussed. Among the subscribers, however, were the pioneer theatrical photographer Napoleon Sarony and J. Wells Champney, both a painter and photographer.[35] During that same year Hartmann published his first play, *Christ*, which contained scenes in which the young Jesus was subjected to

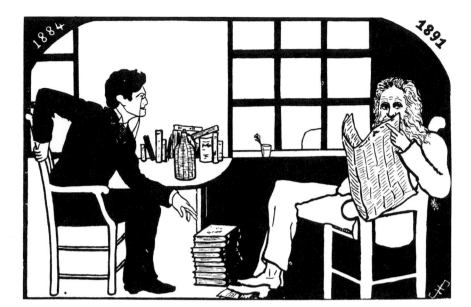

Caricature by Sadakichi Hartmann
of himself and Walt Whitman, 1895.

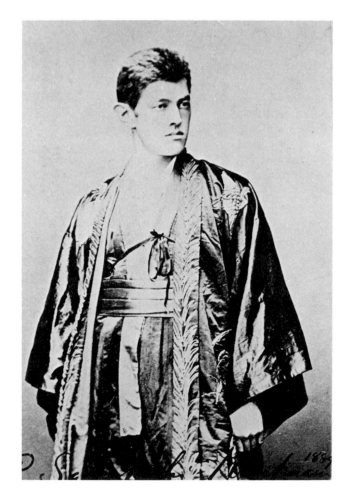

Sadakichi Hartmann as lecturer in Japanese kimona,
Boston, 1889.

sexual temptations by the harlot Queen Zenobia.[36] Although the play was fiercely moral in tone, it kicked up a stir in Boston and Hartmann was jailed on obscenity charges. The cost of attorney's fees and a $100 fine forced Hartmann to suspend his magazine.

After the failure of *The Art Critic*, Hartmann moved to New York, where for the next decade he was associated with the staffs of several magazines and wrote free-lance articles for many more. In 1896, he served as art critic for Richard Hovey's unique publication, *The Daily Tatler*, the only daily literary magazine ever published in this country. The magazine lasted thirteen days before the staff collapsed in exhaustion, agreeing it was an unfeasible venture.[37] Hartmann was probably the author of an unsigned editorial in one of the issues on the death of Napoleon Sarony, which noted "he took pride in his photography, and justly felt that he had raised it to the dignity of an art."[38]

Concerning his earliest involvement in photography, Hartmann himself wrote as follows:

There was a time, idyllic and serene, in my life when I was ignorant of the existence of such a thing as artistic photography, when I was only acquainted with the mechanical industry of the professional photographer, dignified by the name of portrait. Alas, those days are far remote now. One day I happened to meet Mr. William Murray, at that time one of the pillars of the Society of Amateur Photographers, who presented me with the admission card for some photographic exhibition. I went, and from that day on I have wielded my pen also as a critic of photography as well as of art.[39]

Assuming Hartmann's memory was accurate, his interest in photography probably began shortly before the consolidation of New York's two photographic clubs, the Society of Amateur Photographers and the New York Camera Club, which merged on May 7, 1896 to form the Camera Club of New York.[40] Much of Hartmann's critical writings during the 1890s was for the New York newspapers, where many of his *feuilletons* were printed without by-lines or under pseudonyms. If he was reviewing photographic exhibitions prior to the merger of the two clubs, these articles have yet to be found.

Hartmann's earliest known critical article on photography was published in German in the *New Yorker Staats-Zeitung* of January 30, 1898 under the title "Art Photography and its Relationship to Painting."[41] In the article Hartmann introduced the work of Alfred Stieglitz to America's German-speaking population. The essay revealed more than a superficial knowledge of the medium and its history, and thus suggests there may have been earlier articles. Noting that most artists considered the camera to be separated from the genius of the artist by a gaping abyss, Hartmann asserted that "one can with complete justification defend its artistic worth."[42]

The article was written soon after Hartmann's first encounter with Alfred Stieglitz at the old quarters of the New York Camera Club on Thirty-Eighth Street. Stieglitz had already taken over the

stodgy *Journal of the Camera Club*, and his first issue of the new magazine *Camera Notes*, appearing only a few months earlier in July, 1897, had astounded the photographic world with its quality. Letters of congratulation poured in on Stieglitz. A. Horsley Hinton, editor of England's *The Amateur Photographer*, wrote Stieglitz to say: "Strange we cannot do this sort of thing in England."[43] Even Alfred Dreyfus sent a tribute from Devil's Island: "*Camera Notes* is my only comfort in captivity."[44]

Opposite page top. Cover of *Camera Notes*, Vol. 1, No. 1, 1897.

Opposite page bottom. Frank Eugene: Alfred Stieglitz.

Below. Gertrude Käsebier: Alfred Stieglitz.

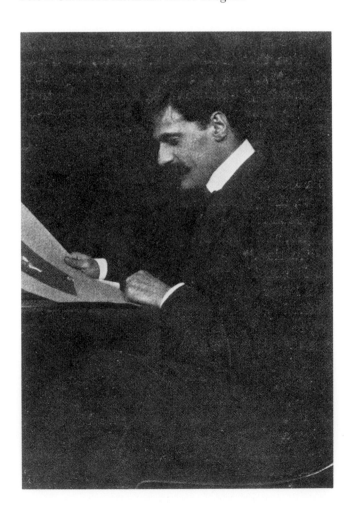

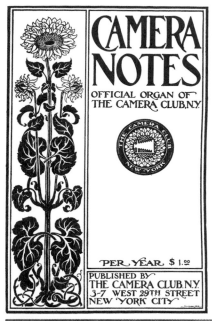

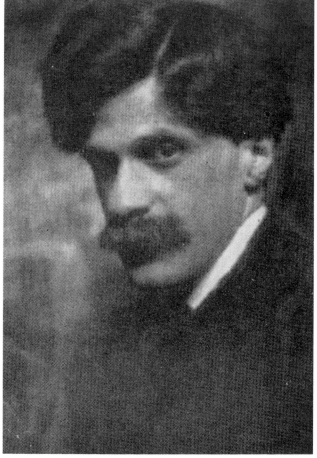

From the moment Sadakichi entered the offices of the Camera Club, where he immediately ran into his old friend William Murray, he sensed an air of vitality and seriousness. He was also impishly amused at the awe in which Stieglitz was held. None of the club members were willing to be interviewed. To every question Hartmann asked, they responded: "Wait till Mr. Stieglitz comes."[45] It reminded Sadakichi of his last visit to Paris in 1892, when mixing with the Symbolist crowd he often heard them speak of a school of poetry known as "Les Poètes Français," only to find on gaining access to this circle that it consisted of one poet, Charles Morice.

> When Mr. Stieglitz appeared on the scene, I was agreeably surprised. I had before me a man of the world of wide culture, very modest withal, but of rare diplomacy, an enthusiast to such a degree that even his voice changes its keynote as soon as he begins to talk of photography. I am not given much to eulogies of one man, but I am a hero worshipper in the truest sense. Any man who asserts himself in a certain vocation of life has my fullest admiration. There may be hundreds of amateur photographers in New York who do their very best to advance the art of Daguerre, but it would be absolutely foolish to deny that artistic photography in America would not have reached its present standard of perfection without Mr. Stieglitz.[46]

Hartmann's meeting with Stieglitz was propitious both for photography and for his own critical career. At the age of thirty, Hartmann was already embittered, haunted by a nagging sense of failure. Although he had been writing on aesthetic problems for more than a decade, the large circulation magazines had for the most part ignored his work and his criticism was scattered in a multitude of *avant-garde* and ephemeral little magazines. As Gorham Munson has pointed out, the major quarterlies of the 1890s were dominated by a clique of preacher-professors who consigned all that was original and vital in criticism to the cloudy limbo of fly-by-night magazines. Concerning Hartmann and two other forgotten critics of the period, Walter Blackburne Harte and Michael Monahan, Munson asserted: "These men should have been the powers in criticism of their day, but the times were against them. There were no giant critics to whom they might have allied themselves in a profitable warfare, nor was there any access to an adequate circulation for their thoughts."[47]

Through Stieglitz and the photographic magazines, Hartmann discovered a partisan readership and an outlet for his most seminal ideas on the arts. For more than two decades he threw most of his energy into writing articles for the photographic press. If national fame had eluded him, his alter ego Sidney Allan was at least a celebrity in the photographic world. Not only did the photographic journals provide Hartmann with a steady if slender livelihood, but his contact with their readership and active involvement in the affairs of photographers provided an audience that Sadakichi desperately needed.

Probably at their first meeting Stieglitz realized that here was a colleague who had thought deeply about the problems confronting American art, and who had a gift for analyzing its deepest dilemmas—as when Hartmann wrote of Puritanism as a force gone bad in America, "its tentacles, octopus-like, having entangled our very customs and manners."[48] Art historian Roger P. Hull has pointed out that of all Steiglitz's associates, the "one most similar to him in intellect, imaginativeness, temperament, and ambition undoubtedly was Hartmann."[49] Both men were of German ancestry, aristocratically Teutonic at times, yet committed to the democratic ideals of the new world; both shared a common sense of European cultural traditions and an awareness of the struggle that lay ahead before American art could aspire to parity with that of the Continent; both saw their role as championing and encouraging native artists in a materialistic environment that stifled the well-springs of creativity. Even Hartmann's outrageous Bohemianism probably appealed to a similar side of Stieglitz's nature. He was reasonably tolerant of many of Hartmann's foibles which alienated other members of the Stieglitz circle, seeming to understand that Hart-

mann saw himself as a latter-day François Villon, who might lift your purse even as he composed a sonnet in your honor.

Indeed, Stieglitz's letters often reveal a certain amusement at Hartmann's audacity and ingenuousness as a rip-off artist. Sadakichi had an endless series of tricks for upping rates on his articles retroactively or demanding payment for essays that mysteriously never reached their editorial destination. He wasn't above selling the same article more than once. (In fact, Stieglitz caught him selling an essay, "White Chrysanthemums," to Elbert Hubbard after it had already appeared in *Camera Work*.)[50] Sometimes Sadakichi sent a flood of telegrams to editors and friends announcing he was stranded in some remote city, unable to pay his hotel bill, a prisoner of management. This stratagem occasionally brought him enough money from concerned acquaintances—including those wise to his ways—for a month or more of high living. Increasingly, as Hartmann grew older, he considered patronage his due, and in his last sick years hundreds of patrons, including Ezra Pound and George Santayana, regularly sent him small contributions.

It may be said in Sadakichi's defense that editors were impressed by his professionalism. He was never at a loss for subject matter, he composed articles rapidly, he usually met deadlines, and he often helped an editor by turning out an article on the spot to fill a hole in the magazine's next issue. He was, as he often said, a "bread and butter critic," that is, a professional as distinguished from the many sporadic contributors to the photographic press. Although he tried desperately to support two families and twelve children (five by Elizabeth Blanche Walsh and seven by Lillian Bonham,) he frequently suffered from severe asthmatic attacks which incapacitated him for months. Thus there were many periods when he actually lived in dire poverty. Stieglitz never permitted himself to be conned by Hartmann, but he usually came through with help when he believed Hartmann's distress to

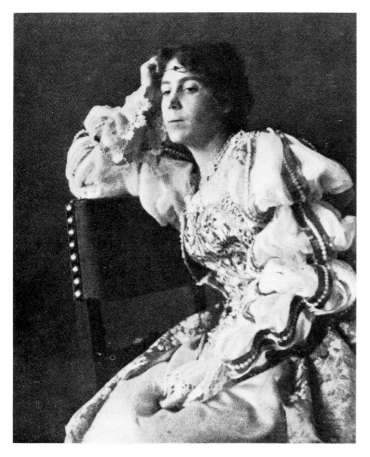

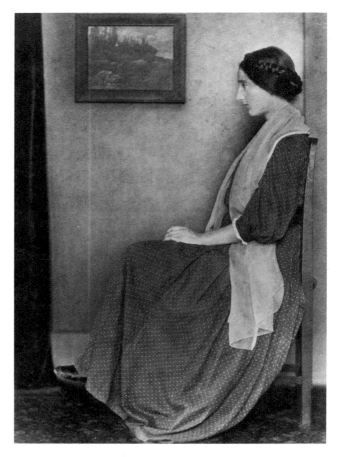

F. HOLLAND DAY: Portrait of Mrs. H., 1899. (Sadakichi Hartmann's first wife, Elizabeth Blanche Walsh).

CHARLES L. PECK: Portrait of Lillian Bonham, 1915. (Hartmann's second wife). Collection of Marigold Linton.

be genuine. Even so—as Stieglitz appeared well aware—his associate was incapable of being anyone other than the irrepressible Sadakichi, continually shattering his carefully manufactured image of the more serious and responsible Sidney Allan.

Although the extent to which Stieglitz concerned himself with the literary content of his magazines has been challenged,[51] the lengthy correspondence between Stieglitz and Hartmann fails to substantiate the view that Stieglitz left editorial policy in the hands of associate editors and was primarily interested in pictorial content. While he gave Hartmann considerable latitude in choice of subject matter, Stieglitz could not be maneuvered by Sadakichi into accepting essays on subjects that

did not appeal to him. His letters indicate that his was the firm hand in charting the course of both magazines:

> What's that about my giving you an order to write on the New Color Theory, as brought out by color photography, upsetting Goethe's, Newton's, and Chevreuil's theories; or a real critical review of Kandinsky's book? You amuse me. Why should I be interested in anything as serious as that. You do talk like a hayseed.[52]

Hartmann's first major essay on photography and the first of his long series of interviews with photographers, "An Art Critic's Estimate of Alfred Stieglitz," appeared in *The Photographic Times* in June, 1898. Probably Hartmann had already been tapped at this time as a contributor to *Camera*

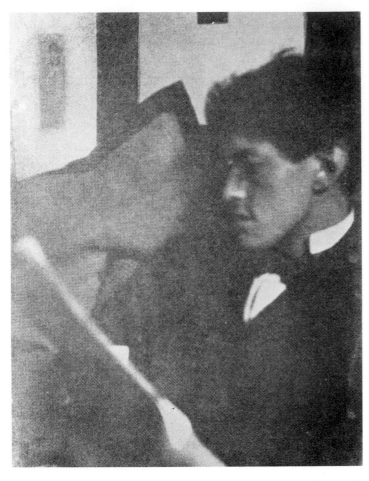

TOM HARRIS: Portrait of Sadakichi Hartmann, 1898. The earliest photograph taken of Hartmann by an artistic photographer.

Notes and Stieglitz preferred to see this eulogy to his own work appear in another magazine. *The Photographic Times* then launched a series of Hartmann portraits of individual photographers—Gertrude Käsebier, Frank Eugene, F. Holland Day, Rudolf Eickemeyer, Jr., among others—which ran for several years, only to be resumed later in other photographic journals. In this first article of the series on Stieglitz, one finds Hartmann setting forth a concept in some ways like Cartier-Bresson's *decisive moment.* That which separates Stieglitz's work from that of most artistic photographers, observes Hartmann, is his ability to select the right moment for his picture, to wait days or even years for it, and it is in the sureness of this instinct that "the photographer can show genius."[53]

In October, 1898 Stieglitz published Hartmann's first contribution to *Camera Notes,* "A Few Reflections on Amateur and Artistic Photography." In that same month Stieglitz called upon Hartmann to cover a photographic exhibition at the National Academy of Design. It was an indifferent show, marked by amateurishness and second-rate submissions—despite some excellent entries by F. Holland Day, Elias Goldensky, and Stieglitz—and it drew forth a devastating critique from Hartmann. The photographs, he noted, made an "adequate backdrop to the asters, grapes, and pumpkins" in the hall. He was particularly impressed by the framing:

> . . . It was a revelation to me. I have never seen an exhibition of photographs so excellently framed as this one. Why the composition of many of these frames and colored mats revealed more temperament, more pictorial quality, and more inventive handling of pure tone and color than many exhibitions of pictures which fate has had in store for me.[54]

Today such trenchant cuteness may appear excessive, but Stieglitz recognized that this was exactly what was demanded at the time, if photographers were to be aroused to strive for higher standards of aesthetic excellence. Only Stieglitz's associate editor Joseph T. Keiley could occasionally match Hartmann's bite, and the two men enlivened

Camera Notes by taking pot shots at each other. When Hartmann blasted the fuzzy tonality of an impressionistic print by Keiley as "pioneer work that opens up untrodden realms to general traffic,"[55] Keiley praised the misty quality in a print by Day, suggesting that it really ought to appeal to his friend Hartmann, who sought just such effects in his own pastel work.[56] Years later, after Keiley's death in 1914, Hartmann paid homage to him in a letter to Stieglitz:

> And so Keiley has fallen by the wayside, for what is life but a foolish endless pilgrimage! Brave, narrow minded soul that he was, so impossible from the Bohemian point of view and yet so subtle, pure, and appreciative. I wish there were more like him.[57]

As with all the arts he wrote about, Hartmann also sought assiduously to learn the rudiments of photography so that he might better understand its technical requirements. So far as is known he never exhibited any of his work, although one of his short stories, "The Broken Plates," suggests that for a while he nourished an intense ambition to master the art.[58] Although he lacked the requisite talent or drive to become a front-rank photographer himself, Hartmann—as he liked to recall—was the subject of more portraits by notable photographers than any literary figure of his period—a favorite model of hundreds of photographers from Tom Harris in 1898 to Cliff Wesselmann in the 1940s.[59] The unrivaled Steichen portrait delineated a stolid, Teutonic Hartmann, almost a grim academic. J. C. Strauss captured a Mauve Decade dandy, poised with a cane on a six-foot pedestal, proudly surveying the world. Käsebier realized a brooding luminous face, almost on the verge of sainthood. Eickemeyer's rugged, assertive-looking Hartmann in a great coat might well have been a longshoreman. The mobility of Hartmann's features lent themselves to almost any treatment until, as he said, "I was not sure any longer about my looks."[60]

Hartmann wrote under many pseudonyms, including Chrysanthemum, Hogarth, Juvenal, Caliban, and A. Chameleon; but his best known was

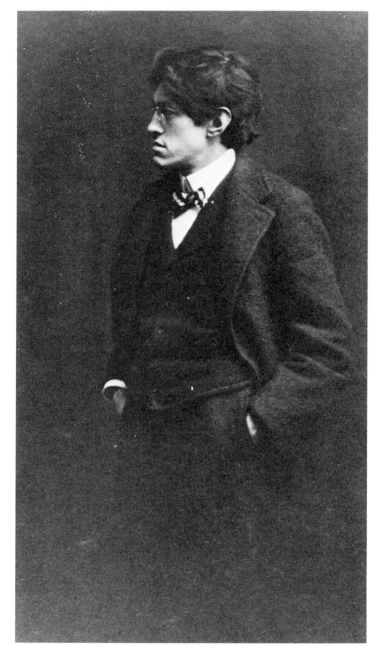

ZAIDA BEN-YÚSUF: Sidney Allan, 1898.

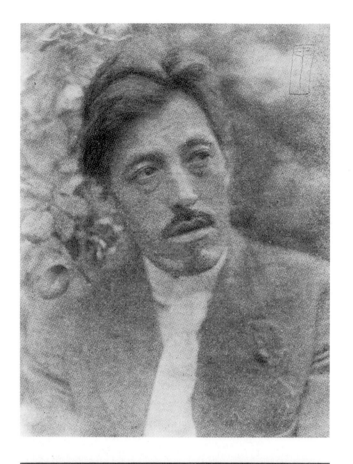

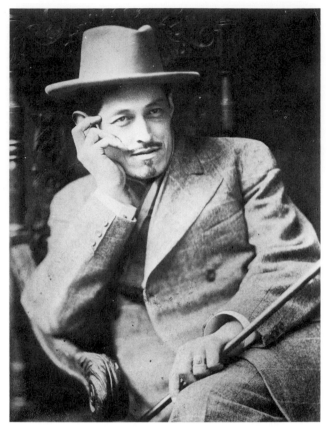

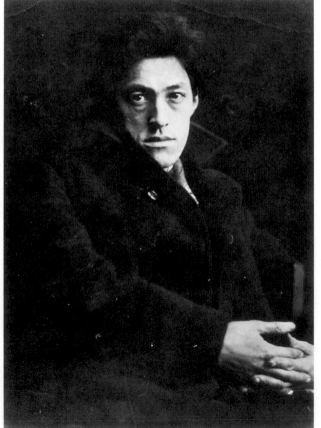

Above. B. J. Falk: Sadakichi Hartmann, 1907. whl-ucr.

Top left. Bessie Buehrmann: Sadakichi Hartmann, 1908. whl-ucr.

Left. Rudolf Eickemeyer, Jr.: Sadakichi Hartmann. whl-ucr.

Opposite page. Gertrude Käsebier: Sadakichi Hartmann, 1910. Collection of Peter C. Bunnell.

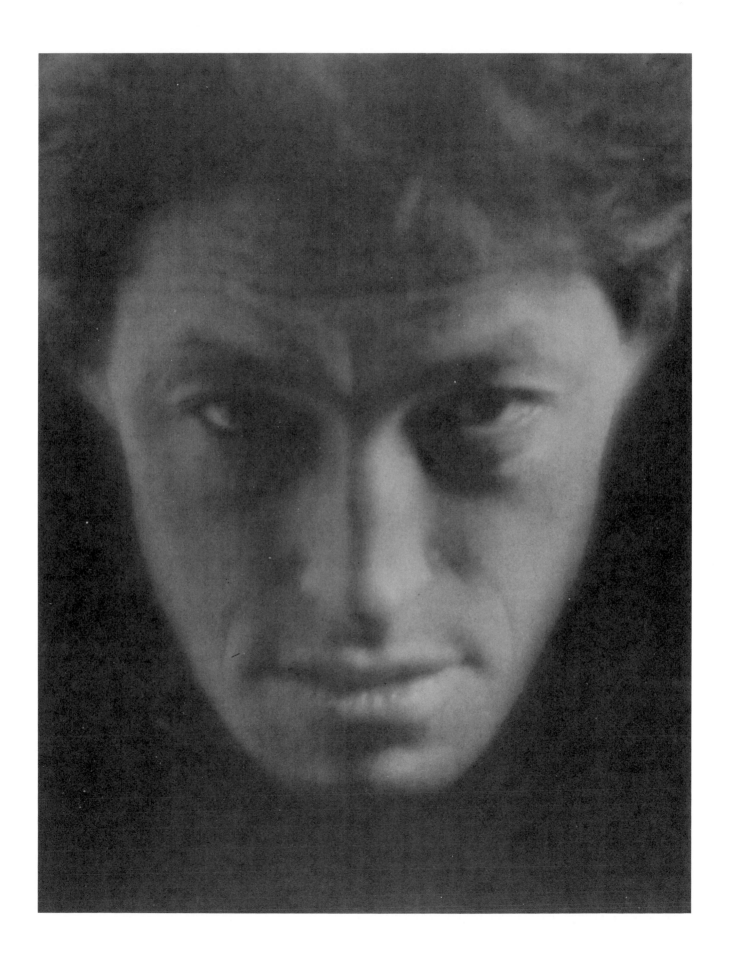

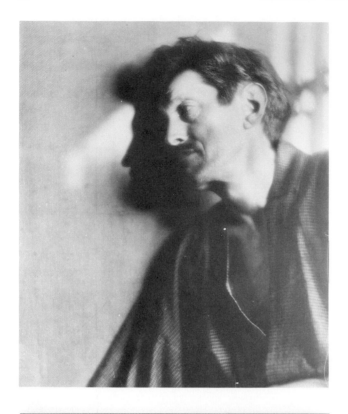

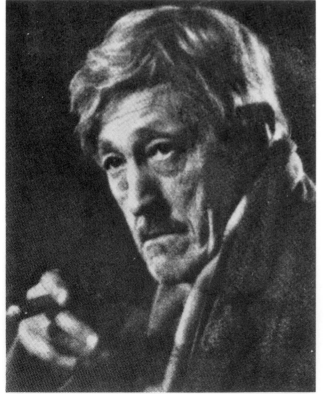

Sidney Allan, used only in his photographic writings. In a letter to Stieglitz in 1899, Hartmann expressed concern that two numbers of *Camera Notes* in succession were filled with his material.[61] Probably Hartmann's use of the pseudonym Sidney Allan was occasioned by Stieglitz and other photographic editors, who frequently used several of his essays in a magazine issue. He soon began employing the pseudonym as a lecturer also, and many newspaper reporters over the years interviewed him under that *nom de plume*, unaware he was Sadakichi Hartmann. As Sidney Allan he delivered his most applauded and reprinted lecture, "A Plea for Good Taste and Common Sense," the keynote address before the Twenty-Fifth Annual Convention of the Photographers' Association of America in August, 1905.[62]

In 1899, seeking a wider audience for the work of Camera Club members, Stieglitz launched a series of public one-man shows of the works of John E. Dumont, Charles I. Berg, Virginia Prall, Gertrude Käsebier, Rudolf Eickemeyer, Jr., F. Holland Day, Joseph Keiley and others. Hartmann's incisive reviews of many of these shows were ruthless, but tempered always by his effort to examine each work in the light of the artist's intention. In his reviews and portraits of individual photographers, his approach was impressionistic—an attempt to recreate the work in the minds of his readers through literary devices. Although he wrote numerous semi-technical and instructional essays, since such essays were popular with photographers, he was inclined to question their value. He believed that didacticism was permissible only in the highest order of criticism and photography was too young an art to command such a critic. What then was the primary task of the photographic critic? His answer was as

Top. EDWARD WESTON: Sadakichi Hartmann, n.d. WHL-UCR.

Left. J. E. MOCK: Sadakichi Hartmann, 1930.

follows: "The question is simply whether the artist has something to express and expresses it well, and it is the critic's business to tell his own impression frankly, without personal subterfuge, to his readers."[63]

Between 1898 and the turn of the century, the brilliant proselytizing for American photography of *Camera Notes*, the success of two international photographic exhibitions at the Philadelphia Salons of 1898 and 1899 (sponsored by the Pennsylvania Academy of Fine Arts), and the excellence of American entries at shows in Munich, Glasgow, and at the prestigious London Photographic Salon of 1898 focused attention both in the United States and abroad on the development of a distinctive American school of pictorial photography. The new school of photography hunted down fresh subject matter instead of time-worn clichés, favored bold highlights and dark shadows, experimented relentlessly with new techniques, and sought to formulate distinctive principles for photography apart from the other visual arts.

Amid a swirl of controversy generated by one of Sadakichi Hartmann's essays, F. Holland Day completed the "invasion" of the Continent in 1900.[64] Early that year Day began putting together a show of his own work and that of other American photographers—Zaida Ben-Yúsuf, Edward Steichen, Yarnall Abbott, Frank Eugene, Joseph Keiley, and others—which he offered to the forthcoming London Photographic Salon. Stieglitz, having reservations about the adequacy of the selections, hung back from supporting the show. The exclusive Linked Ring society, which Stieglitz had joined in 1895, rejected the exhibition for the salon. Day succeeded, however, in obtaining the sponsorship of the Royal Photographic Society and the show opened at Russell Square in October of 1900.

Hartmann's criticism had attracted attention in England as early as 1898, when the conservative *British Journal of Photography* reprinted one of his essays.[65] The journal now swung into a demolishing attack on Day's exhibition, republishing Hartmann's portrait of Day from *The Photographic*

Times, which depicted some of the photographer's eccentricities, including his fondness for smoking water pipes and wearing Oriental costumes.[66] From the British point of view, it all smacked of humbug and "the aesthetic craze of 20 years ago." Hartmann had referred to a Day portrait as "plastic psychological synthesis" of the person represented. When the exhibition opened, the British magazine ridiculed it as "Plastic Psychological Synthesis at Russell Square."[67] It rapped Hartmann for "oleaginous admiration" of the new school of American photography, dubbing him "appreciator-in-chief" of the "Cult of the Spoilt Print." The exhibit, argued the journal, upset "all the old-fashioned ideals of the English photographer" and had no redeeming qualities.

> . . . The wordy Hartmann deludes his neurotic dupes that these faked camera images are plastic psychological syntheses, and the authors of the things, at any rate, appear to believe him. . . . The little coterie which calls itself the new school of American photography is so wrapped up with a sense of its own importance that it has clean forgotten such men as Dudley Hoyt, Pirie MacDonald, Strauss, Falk, Bremer, and scores of other masters of American photographic portraiture. . . . But new or old, representative or the reverse, and with all its cleverness, its excellence, and its failures, the Russell-square show will not in the least advance the revealed ambition of Mr. Day and his two or three friends or get photography ranked as an art.[68]

As arguments over the show simmered through the next six numbers of the journal, Day's exhibition steadily attracted crowds and won converts. Frederick H. Evans urged an objective appraisal, free from the "feeble extravagances" of Hartmann's essay, although he later added that Sadakichi had said some "true and critical things" about Day's work.[69] If anything, the controversy generated by the "Plastic Psychological Synthesis" label helped draw attention to the show. The British press was generally enthusiastic, the exhibition moved on to a warm reception in Paris, and the American photographic breakthrough on the Continent had been achieved.

In 1902 Stieglitz resigned as editor of *Camera Notes*. For some time dissatisfaction had been building up in the New York Camera Club between two factions: those who viewed the journal as a house organ for the club and its interests, and resented or disagreed with the emphasis on aesthetics; and those who supported Stieglitz's battle for recognition of pictorial photography as a fine art. On February 17, 1902 Stieglitz and his supporters organized the "Photo-Secession," which was formally introduced to the public through an exhibition at the National Arts Club. The parting of Stieglitz from *Camera Notes* was managed amicably between both sides, and Hartmann later summarized the issues involved:

> Photo-Secession! The outsider is generally startled at the name; he does not know the exact meaning of the word nor in what way it is applied to this class of energetic and enthusiastic workers. People wonder what the Secessionists really want, and yet their aim is such a simple one. They want to be artistic, that is all. They want to see their work classed as an art; but this is only a secondary consideration, as recognition can not be forced; it must come by itself. Their first and last aim is to do artistic work.
>
> Why, then, all this mockery, noise, and opposition? Because it is a fight, after all. It is a fight of modern ideas against tradition, or more modestly expressed, a fight for a new technique. I am convinced that the better class of photographers also want to be artistic, not quite as much as the Secessionists, but to their best understanding. The whole trouble is that the two parties can't agree on the mediums of expression. It is a fight about conception, theory, and temperament. And the Secessionists, even if they accomplish nothing but the improvement of the average standard of photographic work, will remain victors, because they are more sincere and are willing to sacrifice everything to reach their end.[70]

Opposition to the new photography was not simply from the professionals, established in their commercial studios and worried that new ideas might overturn the skills they had spent a lifetime acquiring. Any popular conception that painters and sculptors in America were interested in the advance of photography was shown to be misguided by Hartmann in an article, "A Photographic Enquête," in one of the last issues of *Camera Notes*.[71] Taking along a portfolio of prints (contain-

ing the work of Steichen, Stieglitz, Day, Käsebier, Eugene, and others), he bearded the artists and sculptors in their studios. D. C. French, the sculptor, was one of the few who was in sympathy with the movement, but even he, turning over the prints in the portfolio, said: "No wonder that these men do such good work. I understand they are nearly all men of leisure, who photograph for a pastime." Most of the other artists interviewed—William M. Chase, Frederick S. Church, Childe Hassam, George de Forest Brush, D. W. Tryon, and Thomas W. Dewing—either argued hotly that photography was not an art or attributed every artistic effect to the mechanism of the camera or an accident. If the tide had turned in Europe, it was clear that the fight for pictorial photography was far from won in America.

When Stieglitz launched publication of his independent journal, *Camera Work*, in January, 1903, Hartmann was asked in advance to write for the magazine and he was listed as a supporter in an editorial in the first issue.[72] Hartmann was most active as a contributor during the magazine's first two years, when he also served as an ardent publicist of the Photo-Secession by writing articles on the movement for other magazines. Intermittently, his relationship became cool with Stieglitz and he ceased writing for the journal. When Stieglitz began to heavily feature other visual arts in 1910, however, Hartmann demonstrated renewed enthusiasm with eighteen contributions over a two-year span. Despite some lulls as a contributor, Hartmann was the magazine's most prolific writer, and forty-two essays and poems, both signed and unsigned, can be attributed to him.[73] Roger Hull, summing up Hartmann's accomplishments for *Camera Work*, was particularly struck by his prescience:[74]

> Hartmann's contribution to the intellectual tone of *Camera Work* was substantial. His proclamation of 1903 that "accuracy is the bane of art,"[75] in conflict with the entrenched realism of the American school, forecast the revelations of the European entries in the Armory Show of

1913 and anticipated a style of painting (emphasizing the beauty of the brushstroke, however random, and other apparently accidental effects) which emerged fully in this country only in the 1950s with Abstract Expressionism. On Cubism, Hartmann alone among critics understood and intelligently discussed the movement's analytical orientation, its geometric underpinnings, and its relationship to primitive art.[76] He wrote the only discussion in *Camera-Work* of the motion picture, predicting films with color and sound and the use of motion pictures as a "home amusement" and as "home portraiture."[77] He alone dealt with the aesthetic possibilities of the skeletal frame then beginning to supersede the bearing wall construction of New York's tall buildings and urged readers to study the alley-side of skyscrapers for the unadorned aesthetic of the future.[78] With Louis Sullivan, he was prophetic of the distilled style of Mies van der Rohe and, in the visual arts, Mondrian.

In the first two years of *Camera Work*, the Photo-Secession made up of forty-seven members from many different areas, consolidated its position under Stieglitz's leadership as the stronghold of the pictorial movement in America. It developed rigorous rules concerning exhibitions and permitted only the finest photographs of its members to be shown. Hartmann appeared to be at the center of things, covering many activities of the Photo-Secession, including the important show held at the Carnegie Institute in Pittsburgh in February, 1904, which he praised as in advance of all its predecessors and hailed as eclipsing the Chicago and Philadelphia Salons of 1898–1901.[79] He attended monthly dinners of the Photo-Secession and at the February, 1904 banquet at Mouquin's restaurant delivered a much-applauded satirical sketch. In the medieval role of "Klingsor the Magician," scribe of the movement, he dubbed the Pittsburgh show the "Secession Shrine" and described the quest of the "valiant knights of Daguerre" in pursuit of the Grail.[80]

In the midst of the ascendancy of the Photo-Secession, Hartmann seems to have been playing an underhanded game, however, which went beyond any obligation of an objective critic to keep himself informed on everything going on in the photo-

graphic world. At this late date it is difficult to evaluate how deeply Hartmann was involved in the intrigues of rival photographic groups that were preparing to challenge the Photo-Secession, to what extent he instigated their efforts, and whether his motives were solely revengeful. He had always been his own man and Stieglitz respected Sadakichi's independence and his impartiality in giving credit wherever it was due. In the case of the American Photographic Salon of 1904, however, Hartmann's role was clearly not that of an observer and must have entailed duplicity in his dealings with the Secessionists.

Stieglitz had been planning to organize a governing body for all of the national pictorial groups, which would include the Photo-Secession and encompass ties with The Linked Ring in England. He also envisioned a large international exhibition of pictorial photography to be held in New York in 1905. None of this came about. Instead, a rival group of pictorialists—the Salon Club of America, which had been quietly organized in December, 1903, led by Curtis Bell, a professional photographer only recently arrived in New York—stole a march on the Photo-Secession and announced plans for the first "American Photographic Salon" in New York to be held in December, 1904. The photographic press was filled with the attacks of Bell and his supporters on Stieglitz, whom they charged with trying to dictate the future of pictorial photography. Hartmann's stance was to appear neutral and aloof:

> It nevertheless sounds like an open revolt. And there may be opposition! A duel between Messrs Alfred Stieglitz and Curtis Bell would prove indeed a great attraction. There are none upon whose swordsmanship I trust more surely upon than that of these two gentlemen. It will stir up the stagnant waters of pictorial photography—they surely need it—and make us all more happy at the end.[81]

Hartmann was not a disinterested observer, however. Sometime in 1904 he had begun to detect what he believed to be a waning enthusiasm for his company on the part of Stieglitz. This he

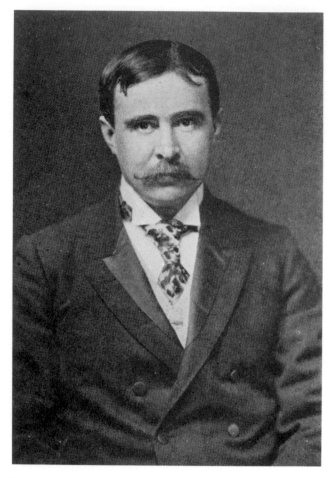

J. C. Strauss: Portrait of Curtis Bell,
Chairman of the Salon Club.

partly attributed to the return of Steichen from
Europe and his increasingly active role in the
Photo-Secession. Steichen, he was convinced, had
never liked him. In addition, Hartmann appears to
have been jealous of Roland Rood, the young critic
who was capturing more and more of Stieglitz's
attention, and who he believed was aspiring to the
press-agentry of the Secession.

All of Sadakichi's resentment poured out in a
letter he wrote to Stieglitz on September 2, 1904,
announcing that he had "wheeled over to the other
side."[82] No one, he insisted, had ever treated a loyal
worker "so shabbily" and he had "simply got tired
of your dictatorship." He was furious that Stieglitz
had invited him to a luncheon and then shown a

preference for the company of Steichen and Rood.
He was angry that he had not been invited to a
banquet honoring A. Horsley Hinton and that
invitations had suddenly ceased to the monthly
Photo-Secession dinners, which he charged was the
result of objections raised against him by Steichen
and Käsebier. Finally, he had asked for a $1
advance on an article and Stieglitz had humiliated
him by "shouting all over the place that you were
not my banker in the presence of Keiley and several
other gentlemen." He ended this diatribe on a
gracious note: "As far as your own work is concerned nevertheless always sincerely yours . . ."
He was now openly committed to Curtis Bell and
the Salon Club crowd. Caliban had found new
lords and would help them seize the island from
Prospero.

The charges of indifference on the part of
Stieglitz are difficult to substantiate. In the first
place, Hartmann was at the time being given more
space in *Camera Work* than any other contributor.
Secondly, Stieglitz's responsibilities had grown,
and he may not have been able to spend much time
assuaging his Bohemian colleague's easily ruffled
sensibilities. Furthermore, since Stieglitz was also a
master of preventing friction between co-workers,
he probably deemed it necessary to keep Hartmann
and some of his associates at bay.

On the other hand, Stieglitz may have become
perceptibly cooler to Hartmann in 1904 as a result
of the critic's own activities. Hartmann's was not
the straightforward position of undeviating loyalty
which he professed in his September letter. For
some time he had been involved in the counter-
attack that was building against the Photo-Secession.
In June of the same year, Hartmann had drafted and
personally signed the letters which the Salon Club
sent to German and Austrian exhibitors inviting
them to participate in the American Photographic
Salon.[83]

That rumors of Hartmann's association with
Curtis Bell and the Salon Club had reached Stieg-
litz is indicated by an undated letter from Keiley to
Stieglitz in which he reported that the "Hartmann-

Bell-Rood situation is most interesting" and that Rood had become pitted against Hartmann and Bell.[84] More damaging, however, is the fact that Hartmann was the author of several attacks against the Photo-Secession, written under the pseudonyms of Caliban and Juvenal, which began appearing in various photography magazines that fall and winter. One of these essays, "Little Tin Gods on Wheels," appeared in the September issue of *The Photo-Beacon*, which means Hartmann had written and submitted it prior to notifying Stieglitz that he was joining the other camp.[85] An eloquent piece of satirical invective, it charged the Secessionists with being a small clique who excluded the work of all who were "not *tony* enough to be expounded in the pages of the gray magazine . . ."

The first American Photographic Salon was held in December, and most of the critics found the exhibition of mediocre quality. Although the Secession had refused to have anything to do with the Salon, Stieglitz showed his impartiality with a diligent and fair review in *Camera Work*.[86] For a while, the Salon Club was dominant in photographic affairs in New York, but gradually it fell apart. One outgrowth of the feud, however, was that Steichen persuaded Stieglitz that the Photo-Secession needed its own gallery for exhibitions. As a result, two rooms adjoining Steichen's studio at 291 Fifth Avenue were leased, and on November 24, 1905 a new era in American art and photography was inaugurated with the opening of the "Little Galleries of the Photo-Secession." Through exhibitions of the most advanced art of the period, the "291" galleries, as they were known, were to effect a revolution in American art attitudes.

Meanwhile, Hartmann concentrated on writing for other photographic journals and assisted Charles Caffin with art reviews for the "Studio Talk" column in *International Studio*. He was in widespread demand as a lecturer on art and photography, and in 1905 began his first of a series of annual lecture tours. In that year alone, he spoke before the Ohio-Michigan Photographers' Convention, the Photographic Association of Wisconsin, the Photographers' Association of Pennsylvania, Maryland, and the District of Columbia, and at the annual convention of the Photographers' Association of America.[87] Through such lecture tours, he gradually became familiar with all of the major studios and haunts of photographers in America. In St. Louis he spent many convivial evenings with J. C. Strauss and his gang of Bohemian friends in the "Growlery" underneath the photographer's studio. He hung out at the Saturday night assemblages of photographers in the Cafe Thorndike in Boston, listening to the Armenian John Garo argue pictorial problems with Morris Burke Parkinson and Henry Havelock Pierce until the night turned grey. In San Francisco, he was accustomed to staying with Francis Bruguière, always eager to hear about Stieglitz.[88] As a speaker before camera clubs and conventions, he occasionally discussed art photography, but in general his topics were practical ones relating to the day-to-day problems of professional photographers. In 1912 he became the first critic ever engaged by the Photographers' Association of America to be available to members for three days at their annual convention for private criticism.[89]

Three years elapsed before Hartmann in his own words "swallowed my pride" and wrote to Stieglitz, begging him to forget what had happened. He did not apologize—he could not—but in a letter written on August 22, 1908, which he urged Stieglitz to destroy, he spoke of financial hardship and pleaded with Stieglitz to "lend a helping hand for old time's sake."[90] Stieglitz was generous, the breach was healed, and once more Hartmann embarked on a productive period of writing for *Camera Work*. Possibly his relationship with Stieglitz was reestablished on a sounder footing, since Hartmann was now aware he would never be a dominant force in the Photo-Secession inner circle. He could even joke with Stieglitz about it:

The people that still object to my presence should be poisoned. What a chance you miss. Your Holland luncheons could so easily gain genuine and lasting fame by being a little more like the banquets of Heliogabalus or a Borgia.[91]

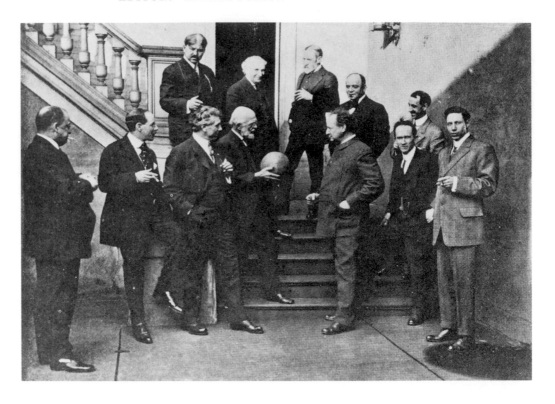

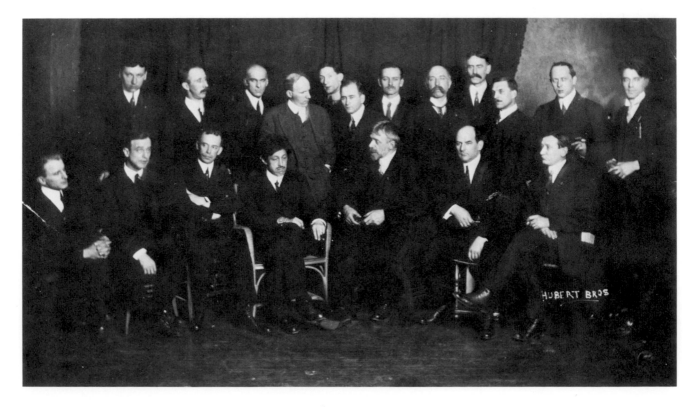

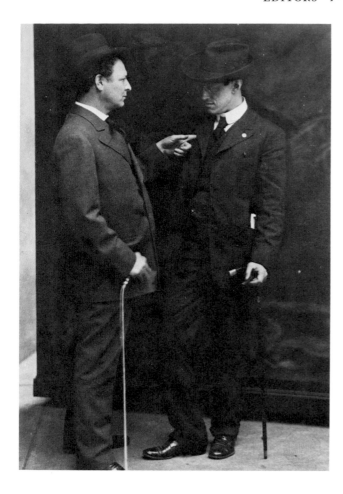

Above. J. C. STRAUSS: Strauss and Hartmann, 1905. (Note bulb release being held by Strauss). WHL-UCR.

Opposite page top. J. C. STRAUSS: In the Court, Strauss Studio. Upper row, reading from left to right: Henry Havelock Pierce, Boston; Lewis Godlove, St. Louis; William Crooke, Edinburgh; Judge M. N. Sale, St. Louis; Fred J. Feldman, El Paso; Lower row, reading from left to right: Frank A. Rinehart, Omaha; H. Walter Barnett, London; Frank Scott Clark, Detroit; A. J. Fox, St. Louis; E. E. Doty, Battle Creek; E. Swarzwald, Berlin.

Opposite page bottom. HUBERT STUDIO: Hartmann surrounded by members of Buffalo Section No. 6 of the Professional Photographers' Society of New York, after giving a lecture at the studio of Hubert Brothers on West Ferry Street, Buffalo.

Hartmann's last essays in *Camera Work* appeared in 1912, one of which was his prophetic pioneer article, "The Esthetic Significance of the Motion Picture." Although he continued submitting manuscripts, none of them proved quite suitable to Stieglitz; perhaps because Hartmann, having moved in 1911 to East Aurora, New York, was no longer in regular contact with Stieglitz and the direction of his thinking. Yet the two men kept in touch, possibly because Stieglitz felt that Hartmann as much as anyone continued to understand his aims. In December, 1911 he wrote to Hartmann:

> . . . Since you left a year ago I have undoubtedly had the most remarkable year in my career. Beginning with the Albright Art Gallery show it has been one crescendo culminating with a most remarkable three weeks spent in Paris. There I have had long most interesting sessions with or at Picasso, Matisse, Rodin, Gordon Craig, Vollard, Bernheim's, Pellerin's; finally winding it up with two days at the Louvre which in reality I saw for the first time. Then too I saw the various Salons beginning with the old one, then the Champs de Mars and the Salon des Independents, finally the Salon d'Automne. All this I did in the company of De Zayas or Steichen or both. De Zayas has developed remarkably and is a big fellow. Steichen too is growing fast. What a pity you couldn't have been with us . . .[92]

There were years of triumph for Stieglitz, followed by years of discouragement. At times Stieglitz wearied of the effort. Subscriptions to *Camera Work* dwindled. Photographers became increasingly indifferent to the emphasis given to modern art and literary experimentation in the magazine. The goal of making a nation receptive to modern art often seemed as far away as ever. This Hartmann could respond to with sympathetic encouragement, as in a letter of October, 1912:

> . . . The largest part of your work is done. And it has done its work. It has been beautiful, unselfish, and it will remain so to all who appreciate beauty. A year more or less will not add considerably to its merits. And yet—there is the trouble—art hungry men like you must always do something. Well, there are other ways. I know that you will never give up the fight . . .[93]

After 1912 Hartmann published few essays of a

serious critical nature on either photography or art. Although he remained astonishingly productive until 1919, his photographic writing was mostly journalistic—popular articles appealing to the professional or amateur, tips on how to arrange bridal dresses, advice on photographing domestic pets or guiding a sitter toward a natural expression, and series articles in which he analyzed the "good points" of prints submitted by photographers. To a whole new generation of photographers, Hartmann became better known for his expertise as a teacher than for his earlier role in championing the pictorial movement. Eventually it all bored him. He stopped writing for the photographic journals.

In 1923 Hartmann moved to southern California, where he cultivated the Hollywood motion-picture crowd. Between 1925 and 1931 he was Hollywood correspondent for an English theatrical magazine, *The Curtain*, reviewing films and describing Holly-

wood mores. He wrote the first motion picture script of *Don Quixote*, but was unable to find a producer. Douglas Fairbanks, fascinated by Hartmann's face, cast him in the brief role of the Court Magician in *The Thief of Bagdad* (1923). Although Sadakichi's acting was much acclaimed, his irresponsibility and unstable health during the filming of Fairbanks' classic made directors reluctant to take a chance on him for other roles.[94] His drinking became excessive, and he continued to act out a Bohemian charade that had now become *passé*. To many who met him in that period he appeared to be a grotesque caricature of the artist *manqué*—a fierce old man who told unbelievable stories of hobnobbing with Walt Whitman and bumming around Paris with Verlaine—in short, a charlatan.

In his last years he found refuge in a one-room shack which he built on the Morongo Indian Reservation, near Banning, California, adjoining

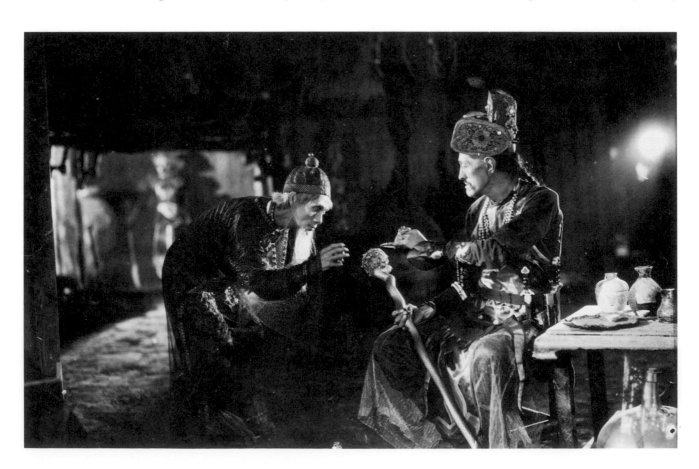

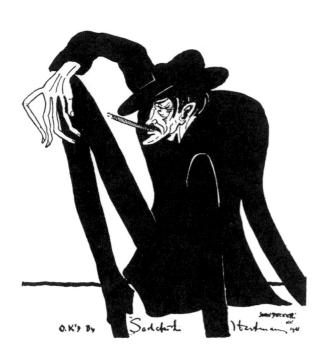

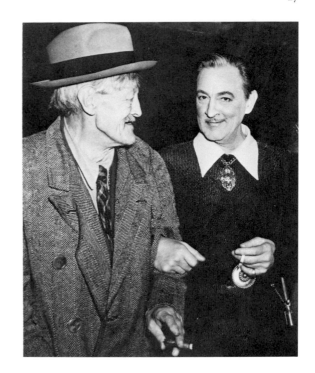

Above. JOHN DECKER: Sketch of
Sadakichi Hartmann. WHL-UCR.

Top right. Hartmann with John
Barrymore in Hollywood.

Right. "Opus to Sadakichi," by
American cubist BEN BERLIN, 1934.
Given by Berlin to Phillips Gallery,
1939. WHL-UCR.

Opposite page. Hartmann as Court
Magician in *The Thief of Bagdad*, 1923.

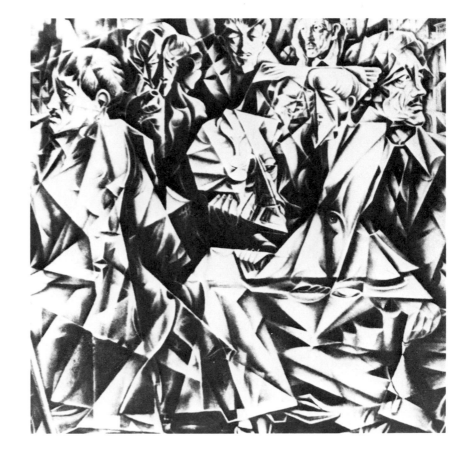

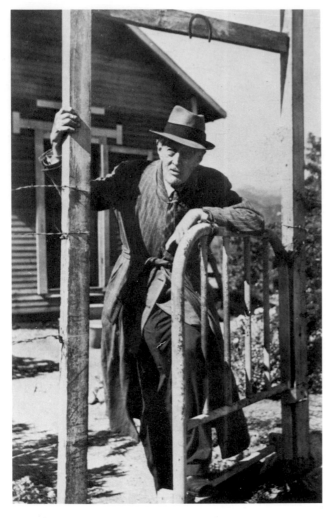

WISTARIA HARTMANN LINTON: Hartmann outside his Catclaw Siding shack on Morongo Indian Reservation, 1943.

the home of his daughter, Wistaria Hartmann Linton, who was married to a Cahuilla Indian cattle rancher. From the reservation he made frequent sorties to Hollywood, where he had become a drinking companion of the John Barrymore crowd, a group that met often in the studio of artist John Decker on Bundy Drive. Amid these cronies, brushing aside the skeptical quips of W. C. Fields, he displayed his mordant wit and cynical humor.

Occasionally, there was a letter from Stieglitz who, with some of his greatest photographic achievements still lying ahead, felt that his own career was also fading, yet, as he said, "Always fighting for photography—the same old fight."[95] Then, in one of his last letters, dated November 22, 1930, Stieglitz described the finality with which he relinquished the past.

> . . . A year ago in Lake George I burnt up negatives, prints, over 1000 copies of *Camera Work*, including a complete set—nearly a library of books—just to get rid of things. It was a great sight watching all these things disappear into the starlit night. I'm still in the ring—ever the damned Fool but alive.[96]

Hartmann, who had burned many bridges, as Roger Hull noted, could savor such a dramatic gesture.[97] "So you have turned into an Omar burning things . . . ," he responded. "Are you now tired of living among corpses? You and I are at least alive—and what did old Lake George think of that particular bonfire!"[98]

III.

Sadakichi Hartmann made his way across the continent by bus in November, 1944 to the home of a daughter, Atma Dorothea Gilliland, in St. Petersburg, Florida. He was seventy-seven years old and in a race against time—determined to gather material he had left with his daughter so he could complete a long-abandoned biography.[99] He died suddenly a few hours after arriving in St. Petersburg.

Behind him in a battered old trunk in his shack on the Morongo Indian Reservation, Hartmann left a portion of the manuscript for this book—several critical essays on photography and a series of semi-biographical profiles of individual photographers clipped from *Wilson's Photographic Magazine*, page-numbered in his own hand in the order he wanted them to appear. The essential plan of Hartmann's projected book was clear. When Hartmann put this manuscript together we don't know, but the dates of some of the essays suggest it was probably toward the end of his career as a photographic critic and maybe later than 1915. None of his early essays on photography were included (perhaps he had lost them in his wanderings), and there was little sense of historical continuity in the selection of critical essays. The manuscript suffered from an over-emphasis on the work of members of the Salon Club and inclusion of profiles of purely commercial photographers whose work has left little impress on the history of photography.

As editors we have not followed Hartmann's original outline, nor do we believe that he would have done so if he had had access to all of his writings on photography. The forty-six essays presented in this volume—many of which were in the Hartmann manuscript—were chosen only after we had reviewed all of Hartmann's available essays on photography. We began research for this book under the illusion that it would be a simple anthology to bring together, not knowing that Hartmann's boast of having written enough on

photography to "wallpaper a palace" would be confirmed by bibliographic research.[100] Wistaria Hartmann Linton's faith in her father's statement—and her childhood memories of his productivity—impelled us to expand the search beyond the boundaries of the photographic press and thus make many discoveries that would have otherwise been overlooked.

The first section of this book consists of nineteen critical essays on photography, followed by a second section containing twenty-seven portraits of individual photographers. Both sections present the essays in chronological order by year of publication. This arrangement was chosen to provide the reader with a sense of the historial progression of artistic photography between 1898 and 1915, an awareness of the conflicts that developed between rival groups such as the Photo-Secession and the Salon Club, and some idea of the evolution of Hartmann's own ideas on photography. Although Hartmann wrote on all aspects of photography, we have confined our selections mostly to essays dealing with artistic photography. While a few important commercial photographers who made contributions to artistic photography are included in the second section, the focus of the volume is on the work of the members of the Photo-Secession and other pictorialist photographers.

A few selections may appear curious to our readers, who will wonder why some essays of indifferent quality are presented at the expense of more impressive or influential pieces such as "A Few Reflections on Amateur and Artistic Photography" (1898) or "A Plea for Good Taste and Common Sense" (1905).[101] The latter two essays, significant as they were in their time, however, contain much that would be redundant in terms of other selections. Sometimes we chose an essay of lesser quality because it added to the historical continuity—such as the essay on the Salon Club—or contained data that has been generally neglected by photo-historians. One of our aims was to stimulate inquiry into areas that have been bypassed by photographic scholars. The Salon Club, for example, dominated artistic photography in America for several years before fading into obscurity, yet there has been little effort by archivists to secure examples of the photographic work of its members for museum collections.

In focusing only on photography, we were forced to exclude many of Hartmann's very finest essays—essays that are far more polished than most of his photographic writings. Hartmann gave more attention to literary style in his art essays than in his photographic writings, a notable example being his essay on Manet, "The Fight for Recognition."[102] Many of his best art essays—as noted earlier—appeared in *Camera Work* and other photographic publications, where they were read with equal interest by artists and photographers. His much-cited essay "The Flat-Iron Building—An Esthetical Dissertation" (1903),[103] for example, while concerned with American architecture, undoubtedly had an impact on photography. Such essays deserve an eventual volume of their own. So far we have developed only a rudimentary bibliography of Hartmann's essays on art, which may finally turn out to be more extensive than his photographic writings. The few art essays presented in this volume—such as the review of Marsden Hartley's paintings—were chosen because they also contain reflections on photography.

The second section of the book will prove of particular interest to photographers as well as students of photo-history. These essays provide an outstanding historical record of what it meant to be a photographer in those formative years between the turn of the century and World War I, when the language of the medium was continually being enlarged through the exploration of the camera's aesthetic possibilities and limitations. Some of the photographers depicted here, such as Zaida Ben-Yúsuf, one of the first women to become notable in American photography, have been almost forgotten. Edward S. Curtis, profiled in a brief essay, has emerged as the great photographer of the American

Indian, while the more realistic Frederick Monsen, who did not idealize his subject matter, is unknown today. A number of photographers, such as Rudolf Eickemeyer, Jr. and Elias Goldensky, have only recently been rescued from obscurity after many years of undeserved neglect.

Art criticism to Hartmann was "nothing but a peculiar mania for searching in every expression of art, and life as well, for its most individual, perhaps innermost, essence."[104] Since he believed art was largely a matter of individual temperament, Hartmann was fascinated by those qualities which differentiated the genius or talented man and woman from the multitude. In 1898, he set out to capture everyone he considered of importance in photography—to produce in a series of portraits a documentary record that would "reflect the character" of his subjects. Eventually, such a project proved impossible; there were too many converts every year to the ranks of artistic photography. Yet despite some notable omissions, such as Helmar Lerski and Edward Weston, whose works he reviewed but whom he never got around to depicting in character sketches, Hartmann was astonishingly successful. In some cases he provides almost the only knowledge we have of the personality, aspirations, and working habits of a particular craftsman.

In all, Hartmann wrote approximately fifty-five sketches of photographers, which were published between 1898 and 1916 in *Wilson's*, *The Photographic Times*, *Photo-Era*, *Camera Notes*, *Camera Work*, *The Camera*, and the *Photographic Journal of America*. The problem of selection posed many difficulties. In a number of instances, Hartmann wrote several sketches on a single photographer, each of which had merits. As a skillfully sustained mood piece, for example, an appreciation of John H. Garo, which Hartmann published in 1914, is far superior in literary style to the 1906 essay chosen for this volume.[105] Nevertheless, the former essay tells us less about Garo's background, his attitude toward his craft, and his working methods than the article selected for inclusion. Because this volume is intended primarily for photographers and students of photographic history, rather than readers of literature, the decision was made to select those essays richest in factual information.

Minor editing changes have been made in preparing the book for publication. Occasional typographical errors or misspellings in the original articles have been corrected. As an emigrant to America, Hartmann in his early years often had trouble with syntax. His photographic essays—often written rapidly—show less concern with syntax than his art essays. We have therefore sometimes taken the liberty of modifying infelicities in the service of readability: the misuse of prepositions, the entanglement of punctuation where confusing, and an occasional change in the paragraph structure for purposes of clarity. Notes have been provided to clarify statements understandable to contemporary readers which might puzzle readers of today. Photographers and artists mentioned by Hartmann—and occasionally celebrities of his time—are identified in the notes, except when they are as well-known as Leonardo da Vinci or Michelangelo. If we have bent slightly in the direction of over-identification, it is because we recognize that books on photography have a lay readership to which we also feel responsible. Where only a last name is given in fleeting references to personalities of the period and the context

is reasonably clear, we have omitted any note, permitting an entry in the index to serve for clarification. Photographers who are the subject of an essay in the book are not identified by notes when they are referred to in other essays.

Although over a half-century has passed since he wrote on photography, Sadakichi Hartmann's concerns in the essays that follow remain contemporary. The problems that absorbed him have obsessed photographic critics throughout the twentieth century.[106] He is, as others have observed, sometimes spiteful, occasionally careless of facts, gratuitously erudite, given to a chameleon-like style that ranges from slang to the academically *caduc*,[107] and often contradictory (usually as a corrective to photographic fads and with a gleam of self-mockery). Henry Holmes Smith has deplored the "lack of workable terms" with which to describe real differences between photographs, but the critical models he suggests for the future can all be found in Hartmann's earliest writings on photography.[108] Sadakichi's continuing relevance may, as art historian Peter Plagens pointed out, lie in the fact that among the trio of the finest art critics of his age—the others were James Gibbons Huneker and Benjamin De Casseres—Hartmann is not only the most compelling and tragic figure, but the only one who approached criticism with the vision of the artist.[109]

HARRY W. LAWTON
GEORGE KNOX
UNIVERSITY OF CALIFORNIA, RIVERSIDE

SELECTED CRITICAL ESSAYS ON PHOTOGRAPHY

1

Portrait Painting and Portrait Photography

"*I* WOULD CONSIDER it a great honor if you would allow me to paint your portrait," I overheard a painter say to Prince Peter Kropotkin during his recent stay in New York.[1] Kropotkin replied laughingly, "You will have to excuse me. First, it is very tiresome for the sitter; and second, one never gets a likeness. I have seen four or five portraits of Gladstone by eminent English artists. None looked like him. Artists have too much individuality. One cannot be a portrait painter and an artist at the same time."

This curious answer, valuable, as it came from a man—scientist, explorer, enthusiast, and egotistic altruist—interested in the expression of every human endeavor, but with a preference for those conditions that concern the welfare of the masses, and therefore looking at everything from an utilitarian point of view, contains more truth than one is at first willing to credit to it. It suggests many of those contradictions inherent in portraiture that have never been satisfactorily explained. In this article I shall endeavor to state the intricacies of the problem rather than to solve it.

Lessing,[2] who, with scientific accuracy in his *Laocoön* and *Hamburgische Dramaturgie*, laid down fundamental laws for modern art which will resist the tide of many a century to come, did not grant portraiture a very high rank in the art of painting, because portraiture, although allowing ideality of expression, must be dominated by the necessity of producing a likeness, and thus it can only represent the ideal of a human being, not the ideal of humanity at large.

Neither the Greek nor the Japanese—the two styles in which Western artists like best to mask their incompetence to create a new style of their own—cultivated portraiture in the sense we do.

The aim of portrait painting is to produce a likeness—a likeness that reveals in one attitude as much of the sitter's individuality as is possible in a flat surface view. Beauty of outline, correctness of drawing, harmony of coloring, truth of tonal values, division of space, the individuality of brush work, contrast of light and shade, virility of touch, variety of texture, all become secondary attributes, because first of all the sitter will demand a likeness, and ought to have one for the time and money he spends.

But that this is rarely the case, everyone knows who has ever sat for a portrait painter; consequently, I have come to consider it as a somewhat crippled branch of art, which cannot be brought into perfect harmony with the demands made on it by the public, on whom it is after all dependent. Portraiture as it is practised to-day is, when at its very best, nothing but an aesthetic enjoyment for the few who like to see a personality delineated as another personality sees it, and which enjoyment increases the oftener it is repeated. Who would not, out of sheer vanity, like to have himself painted by

Whistler, Sargent, Bonnat,[3] Boldini,[4] Lenbach,[5] Watts, etc.?

It seems a portrait becomes a work of art only when sitter as well as artist have a strong and decided individuality. If these conditions do not exist, the portrait invariably becomes a conventional interpretation.

To produce a likeness of an ordinary vapid being is impossible without ignoring the laws of art in some way or other, and, sad to state, a portrait that is a work of art is rarely a perfect likeness.

The cinque cento masters nearly all made a habit of portrait painting, but at that time portraiture was not exercised on its present democratic plan, when everybody who has a smattering taste for art and can afford it has himself painted. Portraiture restricted itself (largely by the conditions of the time) to men and women of prominence, of character or rare beauty, and such types as the artist himself thought worthy of delineation. For this reason nearly all Dutch and Italian portraits of the Renaissance show good workmanship. How far they are correct as likenesses is, however, beyond our capacity of judgment. I believe people were formerly more easily satisfied. Photography had not yet taught them how their faces looked on a flat surface, as it has to our generation. The demand for a likeness has thereby become much stronger and more difficult to satisfy than ever. The sitter himself, the members of his family, his friends and acquaintances, all have formed their opinions about his looks, and the portrait painter must possess the gift to discover and perpetuate those characteristic traits which appeal to the sitter's inner circle of friends.

Portrait painting, like modern art in general, is divided into three distinct phases. I can best explain them by mentioning three men who wield the brush to that purpose: Bonnat, Boldini, and Sargent.

Of all the Frenchmen, Bonnat was always the most congenial to me. He is a fighter for truth. His portraits are always brutally correct; they are like confessions involuntarily made by his sitters. His art

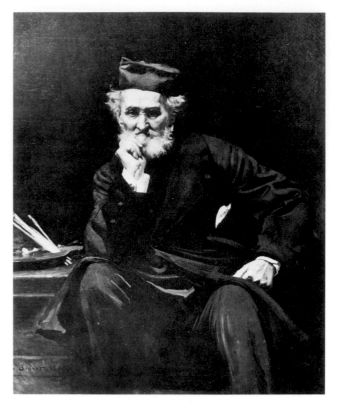

LEÓN BONNAT: Portrait of León Cogniet. Photo N. D. Roger-Viollet.

never lies; it is cold but sincere, and sometimes has a touch of grandeur. To represent man as he is, entirely, so to speak, dug out with the very roots of his existence, with all that blackish soil from which his personality has sprung up—for that Bonnat has striven in restless work and passionate ardor all his lifetime. With him painting approached science. He wanted to grasp the whole truth, theoretically apprehend it, and convince the world by painting the results of his investigations. Imagination had but little room in his art.

Eccentric Boldini is, at times, not less faithful to Nature, but in another direction. He paints the desires, theories, and dreams of a decaying civilization, the thirst for pleasure, the pessimism of a period of dissolution. His flowing lines, his grotesque poses, his instinct for the brilliant, capricious, sensuous charm of life are unexcelled. He

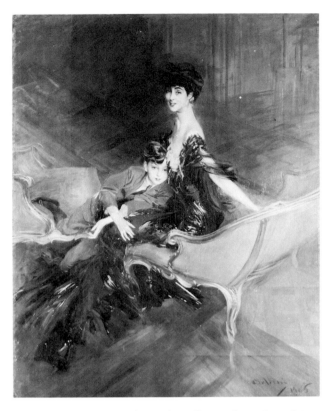

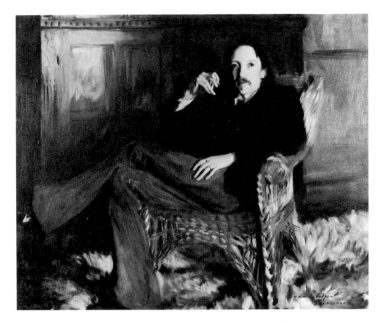

John Singer Sargent: Robert Louis Stevenson. Taft Museum.

Giovanni Boldini: Duchess of Marlborough, and Lord Ivor Spencer-Churchill. The Metropolitan Museum of Art, Gift of Consuelo Vanderbilt Balsan, 1946.

can, however, only paint highly seasoned personalities, like Whistler, the Count Montesquieu de Fezensac, and capricious *mondaines*. Just as Raffaelli,[6] the painter of proletarian socialism, can only depict tramps, indulging in his portraits even in the idiosyncracy of making men like Zola and Huysmans look like emaciated loafers on the verge of anarchism.

Paul Bourget once said, taking up the cudgel for the Psychological School of Literature, which began with Stendhal: *"La vie qui dépasse l'imagination en rutalités la dépasse aussi en délicatesses."* Boldini also believes in this. Like Henry Gervex,[7] Blanche,[8] Jan van Beers,[9] he symbolizes only in a superior, more clearly defined manner, our modern intellectual life, in which we find treasured up the whole wealth of the past, what millenniums have created. And despite our soaring ambition to create

something new, we know no better than to waste our time by playing and flirting with the stored up treasure of dead ages, and exclaiming in hours of despondency: "Oh, could we but forget all we have learnt, be naive again like children, open to all new impressions, without everlastingly thinking of what has happened before us!" It is the disease of the century, and Boldini is one of the artists who endeavors to represent it.

The third phase is represented by John S. Sargent, expressed in the resistless desire to attain a perfect technique that has taken possession of all studios. We all know his breadth of method, his ostentatious brushwork, his dashing schemes of color, his masterly handling of accessories, tapestry, silk hangings, etc. His ambition is to permeate every stroke of his brush with color and virility, independent of an idea, a work of art in itself. Every picture was merely a step forward in attaining this ideal. Sargent is a fanatic of technique, who sacrifices even facial characteristics to suit his own taste. He does not care a jot about the sitter's individuality if it does not harmonize with the decorative fancies of his marvelous execution. Whoever wants a sober, characteristic portrait should surely not go to Mr. Sargent.

The man who combines the characteristic faculties of these three men is James McNeill Whistler, in my opinion with Chavannes,[10] Manet,[11] and Monet[12] the greatest artist of this century. He combines the fanaticism of a perfect technique, the search for truth, and the refinement to create new sensations. Boldini also is curious to analyze what the French call *La Modernité,* which in one word expresses our breathless, nervous modern life with all its intricate desires; but he merely courts it, Whistler masters it. His art revels in the realms of imagination unknown to Bonnat's realism, and Sargent's pyrotechnical displays of technique look crude and barbarous in comparison to Whistler's unobtrusive, unerring brushwork, which masters all the optical illusions of this world with wizard-like dexterity. Are you acquainted with his Paganini? That is not the Paganini of ordinary life, nor is it the one we know from the concert hall. The artist has attempted to give us the whole atmosphere that surrounds an artistic genius. And how has he accomplished such a task? By a male figure in an ordinary dress suit with shimmering shirt front, the outlines of which are lost in a space of vibrant emptiness.

In his masterpiece at the Luxembourg Whistler does not merely represent his old mother. He endowed this old woman, sitting pensively in a gray interior, with one of the noblest and mightiest emotions the human soul is capable of—the reverence and calm we feel in the presence of our own aging mother. And with this large and mighty feeling, in which all discords of mannerisms are dissolved, and by the tonic values of two ordinary dull colors, he succeeded in writing an epic of

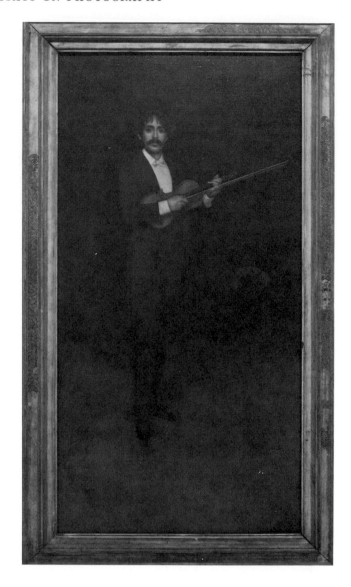

Above. JAMES McNEILL WHISTLER: Arrangement in Black: Pablo de Sarasate. Museum of Art, Carnegie Institute. Pittsburgh.

Opposite page top. CLAUDE MONET: Springtime. Walters Art Gallery.

Opposite page bottom right. PIERRE PUVIS DE CHAVANNES: The Toilette. (c) Arch. Phot. Paris/S.P.A.D.E.M.

Opposite page bottom left. EDOUARD MANET: The Balcony. (c) Arch. Phot. Paris/S.P.A.D.E.M.

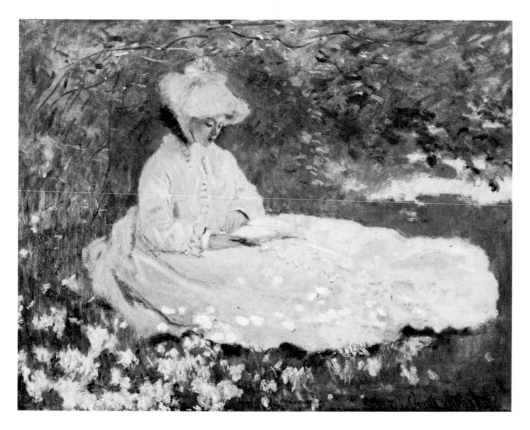

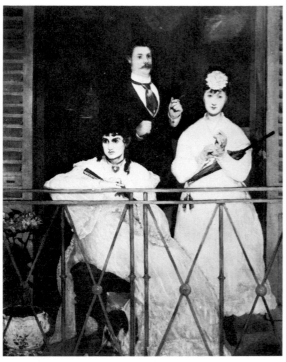

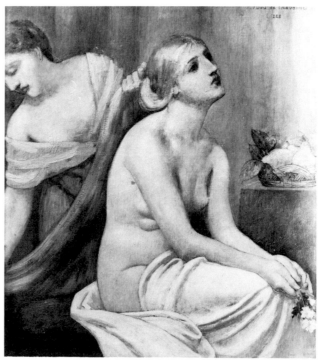

superb breadth and beauty, a symbol of the mother of all ages and all lands, slowly aging as she sits pensively amidst the monotonous colors of modern life. Nothing simpler and more dignified has been created in modern art.

Two other interesting phases of portraiture are expressed by George Frederick Watts[13] and Franz von Lenbach. Since Leonardo da Vinci nobody has expressed the soul life of a human being in a face as well as Watts. It shines from the eyes with an intensity that is appalling. Watts seems to concentrate all his feeling upon them. Take his Burne-Jones. Does not everything that is valuable in that man seem to radiate from the eyes and exist in their direct and searching glance? Color is not his strength. As delightful as his deep greens and browns and dull golds sometimes are, so unpleasant at times is his flesh painting. Even his vigorous drawing is secondary to his breadth of conception,

which neglects all outside characteristics in order to reveal the inner life. All his portraits—I may mention his Sir Panizzi, Stuart Mill, Dr. Martineau, Spottiswoode, Lord Shaftsbury—suggest the grandeur of mental labor, the peculiar noble traits of their specific characters, be they men of action or study, scientists, political economists or philanthropists. In this lies the intrinsic value of Watts' art, and also its limitation. He is the painter of the human soul.

The keynote of Lenbach's portraits is intellectuality. He is an exceedingly faithful reproducer of facial characteristics, but unsatisfied with merely copying them, he invariably makes his lines, so to say, a commentary on the sitter's personality; they are his means of telling what he thinks about them. Every turn and bend of his lines bristles with thought; that is his claim to originality. And with these lines—the other qualities of his technique are

G. F. WATTS: Burne-Jones.

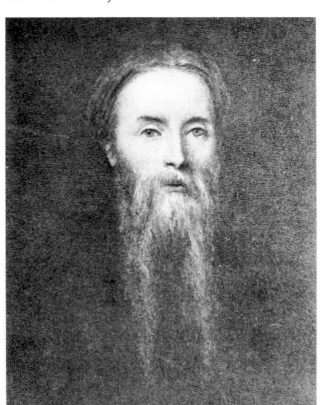

FRANZ VON LENBACH: Portrait of Bismarck. Städtische Galerie im Lenbachhaus, München.

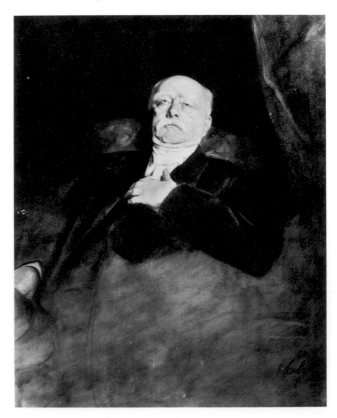

rather too dependent on the old masters—he endeavors to write history, and as he has created for himself the opportunities to paint more representative men than any other portraitist living, he has succeeded to some extent; the more so as he, realizing that it is well nigh impossible to do justice to and exhaust individualities like Bismarck, the Pope, or Duse[14] in one picture, has made various commentaries on each person. His portraits of Bismarck will become trustworthy documents, because he has painted the statesman so often that future generations will be able to deduct from them a reliable composite likeness.

On this occasion I also want to mention two of our American painters, who even among such illustrious company fairly hold their own. It afforded me a special pleasure to note that the two best portraits at the last portrait show—one of those peculiar institutions where only personages of the

F. P. VINTON: Wendell Phillips, 1881.

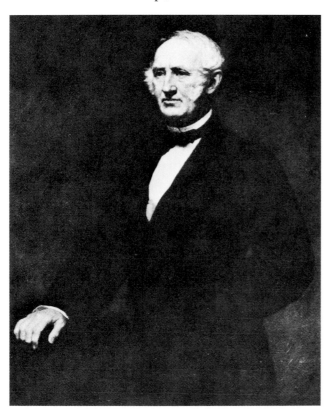

most exclusive circles are hung on the line—were painted by two Americans, F. P. Vinton[15] and Thomas W. Dewing.[16] Vinton is our American Bonnat; his vigor and power of characterization of men are marvelous, while Dewing is to me, with Stevens,[17] the most remarkable depictor of ladies of the elegant thinking world. He is the interpreter of aristocratic womanhood. A painter cannot describe the melodramatic situations of a woman's life in colors; his brush can only dwell upon her sensuous, flirtatious charms, and the atmosphere and the environment in which she lives. This Dewing has accomplished. His best pictures have something so curious and delicate about them as almost to suggest the vague dreams and aspirations of womanhood. With what sentiment can that man imbue the texture of a simple gown! And what chaste voluptuousness can he suggest in some lady's languid face or furtive movement of her hands or neck!

My particular favorite among modern portrait painters—although he is little known in the vocation—is Bastien-LePage.[18] Of all the great naturalists who have enriched painting since Courbet and Manet seized the pallette, Bastien-LePage was the greatest, because his naturalism disdained all pose, always possessed simplicity and dignity, and still was something beyond mere faithfulness to nature, for which we usually seek in vain among the ardent followers of this creed. Also Manet and Courbet[19] loved truth, but not so much for truth's sake as to affront conventionality and the old methods. Bastien-LePage was a naturalist, neither by intention nor theory, and least of all for effect, but because he had to be one; with him it was unconscious intuition, the natural way of expressing himself.

I have seen four of his portraits—his Albert Wolff, André Theuriet, Prince of Wales, and Sarah Bernhardt. His remarkable—one might almost say clairvoyant—power of characterization, which saw the most minute details, as well as his superior traits, made him change his entire method of brushwork with each sitter. In the first portrait his style is coquettish, capricious, brilliant, and intellectual, like that of the famous Parisian art critic; in

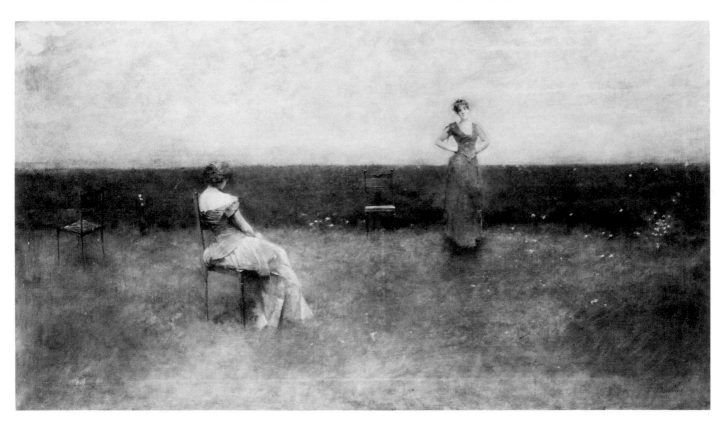

THOMAS WILMER DEWING: The Recitation. The Detroit Institute of Arts, Purchase, The Picture Fund.

the second reticent in gesture and of bourgeois dignity; in the third, loud, lavish, aristocratic, and ceremonious, and at last grotesque, nervous, electric-like genius. Bastien-LePage's Sarah Bernhardt is one of the few portraits which are likenesses and works of art at the same time. Observe the purity of the profile, the elegance of the nervous hands, the originality of the attitude, the virility of the line of the back! And the variety of texture! Dress, face, hair, background, statuette, each treated differently. And in regard to conception, is it not Sarah Bernhardt as we imagine her in her private life— bizarre, exotic, enigmatic, the supreme of artifice? Looking at this picture, we might come to the conclusion that there was, after all, a possibility for a harmonious union of art and portraiture.

Yet we cannot overlook the fact that even Bastien-LePage and all the other artists mentioned, Whistler included, find it impossible to adapt themselves to more than half a dozen types congenial to them, or to men and women of striking individuality. They all have produced numerous clever pieces of painting, and often masterpieces, but only on the rarest occasions, however, a likeness, and then generally of a personality of whom the public has always formed an ideal conception.

There is a great danger for portrait painters in being too individual. Boldini shows this most clearly. In short, nothing is rarer than a portrait painter who has the power simply to repeat nature and thereby produce a work of art. I only know of one who could take any ordinary human being—the first best one he meets—and, simply by studying the color and modeling, accomplish an interesting and artistic likeness. That is Anders Zorn.[20] He simply paints what he sees. He desires to reproduce nature as far as it is possible.

M. Chartran[21] remarked to me one day: "I have

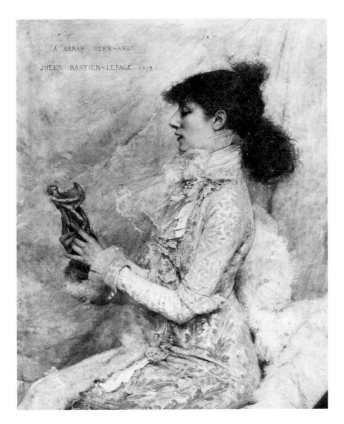

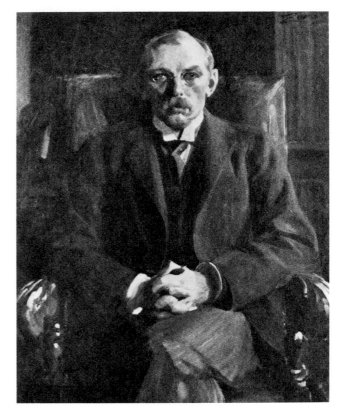

JULES BASTIEN-LEPAGE: Sarah Bernhardt. (c) Arch. Phot. Paris/S.P.A.D.E.M.

ANDERS LEONHARD ZORN: Bank Director, Marcus Wallenberg.

no patience with artists who say that 'such and such persons have no interest for me, I can't paint them,' for in every person burns a flame that appears now and then at the surface." Chartran thought that a portraitist should not have too much individuality in his technique, but that he should be a man of individuality enough to find something of interest in every person. Now, as much as I despise Chartran, and as little as he can claim his "say" for himself—his portraits are like poems dedicated to the sitters; there is nothing genuine in them, yet one accepts them smilingly because they flatter one's vanity—he was perfectly correct in his statement (which proves that a bad artist can be a wise critic at times). There is undoubtedly something of interest in the physiognomy as well as pathognomy of everyone, of my grocer or coalman, for instance, however insignificant and faint it may be, which at times flares up and can be reflected on the canvas.

Well, Anders Zorn can do that, but he fails when he attempts to paint a striking personality; then he gets nothing but virility and color and a general outside resemblance, nothing of the inner man. There lies the rub. It is his individuality to comprehend the appearances of ordinary life.

To have the power to comprehend all types of humanity, to grow enthusiastic enough about them, and to paint them faithfully, subordinating one's flights of fancy to the necessity of the moment, would take a man of Whitman-like love for humanity. If such a man would appear, he would undoubtedly be a stronger individuality than all these others. And individuality makes an artist, as I have shown above, unfit for getting a likeness. And that art without individuality is no longer art is equally clear.

Yes, Kropotkin made an approximately true statement when he said: "A man cannot be a portrait painter and an artist at the same time."

The aim of portrait photography is also likeness, and the camera is capable of producing it. True enough, not one lens is like the other, and each camera has therefore a certain individuality of its own, but in certain things it is always correct; for instance, a man with a Cyrano de Bergerac nose will never be represented by any lens as having a Roman or Grecian nose, as at times happens in portrait painting.

The reports of the cameras in producing a portrait might differ, for instance, in the facial expression. But as it is impossible to take the same subject with several cameras at the same time and from the same point, and as the subject and the light are continually changing, one cannot know precisely how much is the work of the camera and how much that of its manipulator.

And the majority of us are such bad observers of facial expression. Not only the Chinese all look alike to us; no, we do not even remember the lines and plastic peculiarities in the faces of the members of our own family. How little one man knows another was shown by the remark of Mr. Keiley,[22] who so gracefully crossed swords with me in *Camera Notes*, Vol. II, No. 3, in which he was pleased to call me "a man who never laughs." Now I believe there are few men who laugh and smile more than I do, for I do it all the time, on all occasions. It is a racial trait, as Lafcadio Hearn[23] has so deftly explained, that unconsciously plays its part in my facial expression. The reason why I looked so glum in Mr. Keiley's presence was his own peculiar sanctimonious appearance, which dampened within me all feelings of joy in so forcible a manner that I did not even dare to smile. And such gentlemen want to photograph each other and produce likenesses! No—a careful, intelligent system of posing, lighting, and retouching is not sufficient.

A portrait photographer should be even a better character reader than a portrait painter. He should put into practice the theories of physiognomists like della Parta or Lavater, Piderit, Claus Harms, or Shyler,[24] as he is continually confronted by people he has never seen before. He cannot get acquainted with them like a painter, who commands numerous sittings; he has to rely on his general judgment.

There is no art which affords less opportunity to execute expression than photography. Everything is concentrated in a few seconds, when after perhaps an hour's seeking, waiting, and hesitation, the photographer sees the realization of his inward vision, and in that moment he has one advantage over most arts—his medium is swift enough to record his momentary inspiration. Right at the start I must confess that I have never met such spontaneity of judgment in a man, who was a competent character reader, artist, and photographer in one person.

At present the art of portrait photography can be divided into three distinct classes, the amateur, the professional, and the artistic photographers.

About the first class, consisting of all those hundreds of thousands who press the button or hide themselves under the focusing cloth for their own amusement, I have nothing to say. The second class, made up of those who are willing to photograph us for money, from 25 cents upwards, figure very prominently in the thoroughfares of our metropolitan life. But they have, excepting two or three, nothing whatever to do with art. They merely reproduce our face and figure in the most inane aspects, and retouch the plate until all resemblance is lost. Hollinger,[25] with his delicate modeling of half tones in light tinted grays, is one noteworthy exception.

The third class is the one which interests me. They endeavor to make photography an independent art, a new black and white process to represent the pictorial elements of life. There is much agitation among them. There are clubs and leagues and societies of artistic photography, and lectures and debates on the subject. There are dozens of

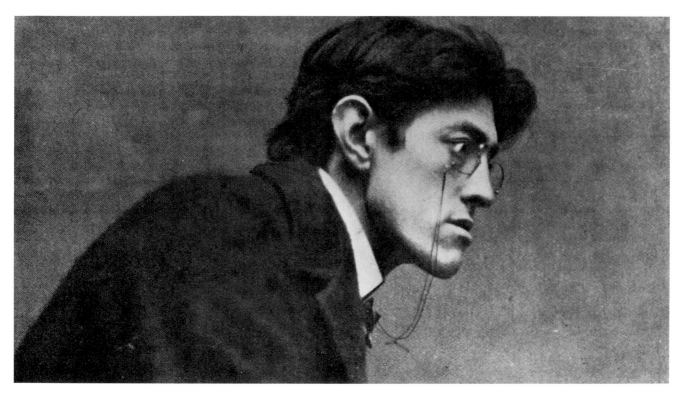

Zaida Ben-Yúsuf: Sadakichi Hartmann, 1899.

magazines exploiting artistic photography, and exhibitions galore. An artistic photograph is, nevertheless, the rarest thing under the sun.

The majority of these ladies and gentlemen represent objects indiscriminately, or take bad painters as models for their compositions, and the results, of course, are dire. Others imitate, by all sorts of trickery, black and white processes, and the pictorial side of painting in general, and produce something which in my opinion is illegitimate.

There are a number of artistic photographers in town, who devote themselves to portraiture, and make you look like a Holbein or a Dürer drawing, like an etching, like a reproduction of a painting, or like a Japanese ghost, all wrapped up in mist. I had the pleasure of being photographed by one of these ladies—Emmeline Rives,[26] Anthony Hope,[27] and Rosenthal[28] were posing for her in the same week, so I was in good company—and the result was a

print that she pronounced one of the best she ever made. True enough it was an excellent likeness, but the position of the head, bending forward, was so peculiar that nine out of ten of my acquaintances asked me if I had lately become a bicycle fiend, for the picture looked very much as if it had been taken by a snapshot when I was scorching away from some picture exhibition which had done its best to make me melancholy. Now this lady is one of the best artistic photographers we have, and my portrait is one of her best efforts. That, it seems to me, does not speak very well for artistic photography.

I also do not like their peculiar attitude. Instead of simply managing their business like ordinary professionals they avoid advertising, and act as if money is of no consequence to them, and yet contradict themselves by charging twenty-five dollars per dozen. They bother celebrities to come to their studio, as they would be ever so proud to focus the author of such and such a book and give them, after long waiting, two or three prints as a reward. These photographs are shown to the other customers, and, of course, if this great man had himself photographed by so and so, why should not the humble Mrs. X have herself depicted by the same photographer for twenty-five dollars?

Equally absurd it seems to me is that a limited number of prints of a photograph should make it more valuable. The producing of prints from a plate is an exceedingly delicate art, but after all, a mechanical process. One can make several hundred just as well as one (perhaps not all up to one's standard, but they can be made), and it would therefore fall into the vocation of photography to exercise its influence in an unlimited instead of a limited edition. A good photograph does not get less valuable because a hundred other copies of it are scattered throughout the world. With a painting or even a general drawing it is quite different; that can't be repeated, just as little as a photographer can pose a sitter twice in exactly the same way. But after the plate has once been made, the rest should be an ordinary printing process. That the plates have not yet reached the state of perfection to accomplish this may be an excuse for the present mania of retouching. I have a great weakness for artistic photography, but I must confess that I do not like its present ways of asserting itself, although I give due admiration to works of such portrait photographers as F. H. Day, Mrs. Gertrude Käsebier, J. T. Keiley, and Frank Eugene.

F. H. Day, apparently a man of wide aesthetic culture and of genuine, highly-developed, artistic insight, has the peculiar gift to render everything decorative. Sensitive to a high degree (I fear even oversensitive), he can only satisfy his individual code of beauty by arranging and rearranging his subject with all sorts of accessories and light effects, which show an extensive knowledge of classic, as well as contemporary, art. There is no photographer who can pose the human body better than he, who can make a piece of drapery fall more poetically, or arrange flowers in a man or woman's hair

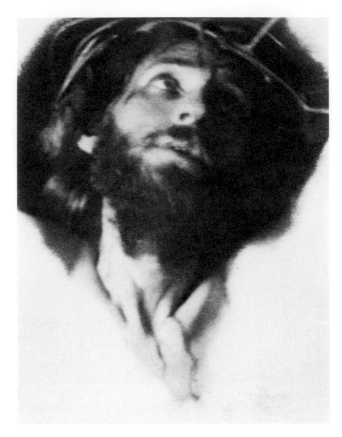

F. Holland Day: The Seven Last Words, I: "Father, Forgive Them, They Know Not What They Do," 1898. LC.

more artistically. He would have made (seriously speaking) an excellent manager of the supers of a dramatic company like the Saxon-Meininger.[29] Even Irving[30] could learn something from him. There are passages in his portraits which are exquisite, but all his representations lack simplicity and naturalness. He has set himself to get painter's results, and that is from my view-point not legitimate. He has pushed lyricism in portraiture as far as it can be without deteriorating into a mannerism; even his backgrounds speak a language of their own, vibrant with rhythm and melody; they are aglow in the darkest vistas. Day is indisputably the most ambitious and most accomplished of our American portrait photographers.

Lately he has managed to astonish the photographic world by making a series of photographic

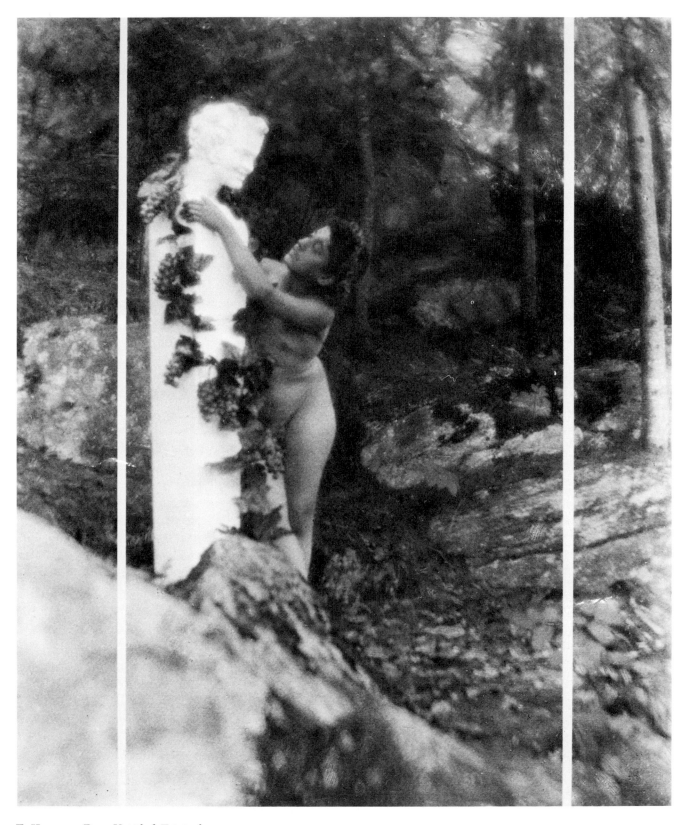

F. HOLLAND DAY: Untitled Triptych. LC.

representations of the Crucifixion, of scenes at the Sepulchre, and the dies of Christ's head. In depicting this extremely difficult subject he has followed, as far as conception goes, absolutely conventional lines; I mean he has not interpreted Christ in a new manner, as, for instance, Uhde[31] and Edelfelt[32] have done. For such an innovation he had probably neither the inclination or the nerve. His is, nevertheless, an innovation in the photographic field worthy of unlimited praise. Anything to deliver us from the stagnancy of commonplace, stereotyped productions! And Day took a step, however short and faltering, toward Parnassian heights. Pictorial representation of a classic subject on classic lines has spoken its first word in artistic photography, and no one knows where it may lead to.

Mrs. Gertrude Käsebier brought her art to a degree of interpretive perfection which it never before attained. She *imitates* (Day does not imitate but adapts) the old masters with a rare accuracy. Her management of tonal values is at times superb; she also understands the division of space and the massing of light and shade. But she is absolutely dependent on accessories. Without a slouch hat, or a big all-hiding mantle, a peculiar cut and patterned gown, a shawl or a piece of drapery, she is unable to make a satisfactory likeness. She utterly fails to master the modern garb; only in rare cases, as for instance her "Twachtman," or the "Girl with the Violin," she succeeds, and solely because the sitters have themselves individuality enough. It is, comparatively, an easy task to get a good portrait of a personality, as the camera is sure to produce some of the individuality without the aid of the photographer. People will say that merely her "Mother and Child" pictures are free from these mannerisms, yet they have many fine qualities; but I, for my part, associate maternal joy rather with an outburst of gay sunlight than the stifling artificial atmosphere in which Mrs. Käsebier places them. Her skillful schemes of light and shade lack luminosity. Besides the subject in itself contains so much poetical charm, it suggests poetry even without the help of the artist.

Such people as Mrs. Käsebier depicts are very scarce on our streets, and whenever they appear they do it to the great sorrow of the rest of humanity. Why should a respectable citizen be transformed into an eyesore? But Mr. Day, as well as Mrs. Käsebier, pre-eminently wish it so, as they are eminently fit to represent that class of human beings who wear slouchy drapery instead of tailor-made costumes, and carry sunflowers, holy Grail cups or urns, filled—I presume, with the ashes of deep thoughts—in their hands. People do not seem to comprehend that it may suit an idol-woman like Sarah Bernhardt to be represented with a statuette in her hand (besides she is a sculptress herself), but that it would be absurd to represent an ordinary society girl (third generation of a parvenu who married a washerwoman) in the same way. It merely shows the incompetence of the photographer to tell character.

I do not believe in Maeterlinckism, I mean by that a combination of all that is suggestive and modernizable in the old arts—as one can trace, for instance, in Maeterlinck the influence of Greek simplicity, Chaucer's fancies, Japanese laws of repetition, of Shakespeare, Virgil, etc.—our modern life is beautiful enough, and our modern garb in no way less picturesque or less absurd (just as you like) than that of Holbein's or Velasquez's time, and yet these men succeeded in rendering it artistically without taking refuge in Assyrian and Egyptian fashions.

There is no sap of life in such art. It is still-born. The seeking of inspiration in the old masters without utilizing it in an original manner constitutes no creation. The intentional fabrication of a photograph to look like a Holbein drawing has nothing in common with the nobler aspirations of our age, and it is an insult to the colossal genius of that man who rooted in his time and mastered it.

Leave the work of those great men undisturbed, except in hours devoted to a silent admiration! They have contributed their share to the history of art, and if you could only produce the epigrammatic suggestion of an original idea, such as they have created, you would deserve and gain your little niche in the Pantheon of fame!

Frank Eugene is a painter of remarkable versatility, who has taken recently to portrait photography, and not for a moment does he deny his original profession. He strives for the same picturesque muddiness in his plates as in his painting. He relies largely on his instinct. Mr. Day and Mrs. Käsebier use a good deal of premeditation to arrange their subjects. Mr. Eugene knows at one glance what he can do with a sitter. He fakes up an artistic background out of gobelins, faded foliage, flowers, etc., throws some drapery over the lap or shoulder, lets somebody hold a mirror to throw a reflection on the face, and takes the picture. All the others *think* to accomplish their results; he *feels*. Look, for instance, at his portrait of the Misses H. I have never seen anything so nonchalantly artistic in

photography before. The accessories are marvelously interesting without hurting the importance of the figures. Not a master in the exercise of his new profession, he makes many technical mistakes, but he understands how to cover them up. He scribbles and scrawls and scratches on his plates in a manner to which Mrs. Käsebier's "stopping out" processes, sprays, washes and baths are mere child's play. These corrections are not legitimate, but they are always right where he puts them, right for him and in the right place. He is a virtuoso in blurred effects, and understands values like few; his faces and shirt fronts have never the same values. He is little known to the photographic world at present, but I predict that his planned exhibition at the Camera Club next fall will be a revelation to many. He is, to my knowledge, the first American painter who has become a portrait photographer.

GERTRUDE KÄSEBIER: Mother Nursing Child. IMP-GEH.

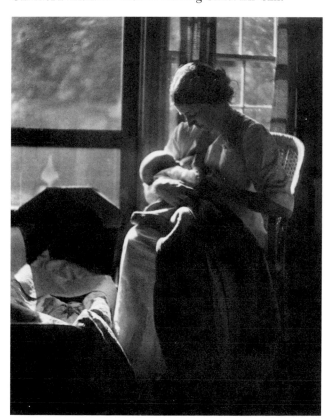

FRANK EUGENE: Hortensia, 1900. The Metropolitan Museum of Art, The Alfred Stieglitz Collection, 1933.

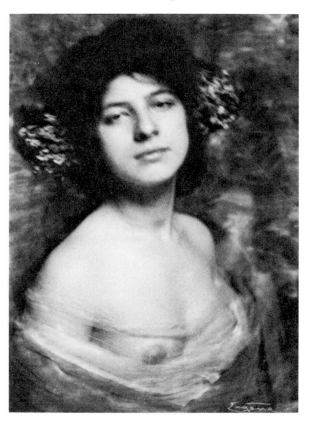

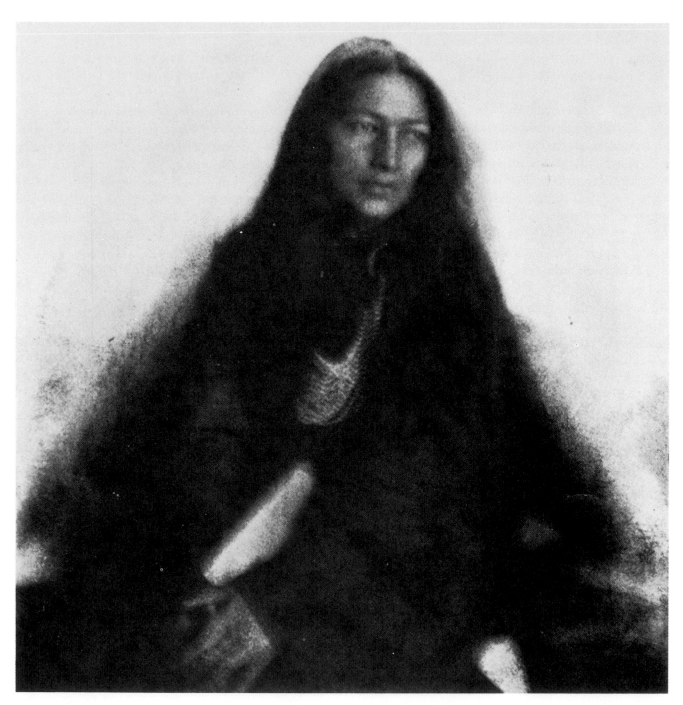

JOSEPH T. KEILEY: Study of an Indian Girl, 1899. IMP-GEH.

J. T. Keiley represents the Japanese phase in photography, which, for certain reasons, is very sympathetic to me. The "crazier" other people think them, the better I like them. It only shows that other people understand heartily little of the spirit of Japanese art, which the majority professes to admire so much. His blurred effects, his losing detail here and discarding it entirely there, and yet suggesting it frequently by an entirely empty place—you see a line and yet it is not there—are truly Japanese. The values of a beautiful head of hair are interesting enough, without the profile, neck, and shoulders, particularly if they are so delicately and poetically treated as Mr. Keiley at times succeeds in doing. If I were a Herrick I would write a villanelle to his "Japanese Coiffure." Yet these fragmentary outbursts of his muse can hardly be called portraits; they are studies (he wisely calls them so), and even if they should reproduce a complete face and neck, and not merely the vision of a shoulder, the broken silhouette of a seven-eights view, or the fragile values of the sternoclido mastoid music, they will play frolic with the face of the vicarious sitter, who may be delighted, nevertheless, to know how he looks when conventionalized by Japanese codes of line, space, and tonal values.

The four artists (artist is the right expression for them; they are too much artists and not enough photographers—Mrs. Käsebier's ingenious signature alone shows that) have one grievous fault in common, they all overstep the limitations of photography. We may pardon a Wagner for ignoring the fundamental laws of music, but not a Mlle. Chaminade.[33] All four experiment. They are modifiers of the half truth the camera is capable of telling, for retouching is nothing but an artful destruction of the light and modeling done so graciously by Dame Nature herself—a covering up of technical mistakes, and the suppression, modification, accentuation, etc., of uncongruous details, until the picture looks no longer like a photograph, but is an hermaphroditic expression of one of the graphic arts. A plate on which retouching is necessary is not a perfect plate, that is all I have to say about it.

These photographers I am going to mention now, I believe they are all—perhaps not as fanatically as myself—adherents of photography "pure and simple." They disdain the assistance of retouching, by which Demachy[34] in Paris, and Einbeck[35] in Hamburg have attained some of their most marvelous results. They realize that artistic photography to become powerful and self-subsistent must rely upon its own resources, and not ornament itself with foreign plumes, in order to resemble an etching, a poster, a charcoal or a wash drawing, or a Käsebier reproduction of an old master.

Miss Zaida Ben-Yúsuf, G. Cox,[36] R. Eickemeyer, Jr., and I believe also C. H. White, work in that direction. They are less burdened with aesthetic lore, and for that reason better adapted to photography. They want likenesses, and that alone can make portrait photography great.

Of C. H. White I have seen only one print, his "Mrs. H," which alone ranks him among the best portrait photographers. A modern girl in a summer dress, conventional even to the crease in front, that is all. The figure is as well posed as a Sargent. The tonal quality is admirable in its delicacy and clearness. The only faults I have to find are that the parasol is not rendered as interestingly as it could be, and that the picture on the wall would have improved the portrait if it had been a landscape or Japanese print instead of a head.

Miss Ben-Yúsuf, of all the photographers I know, relies most on her camera. She is wise enough not to retouch. She is a fairly good character reader, and understands posing. She composes her pictures with the simplest means, without applying any special artistic arrangement; good taste and common sense seem to her sufficient. Her simplicity of purpose, the absence of affectation and of the display of great stores of knowledge is refreshing. She pursues her art on the right lines. It is only to be deplored that her work at present is so frightfully uneven. Many

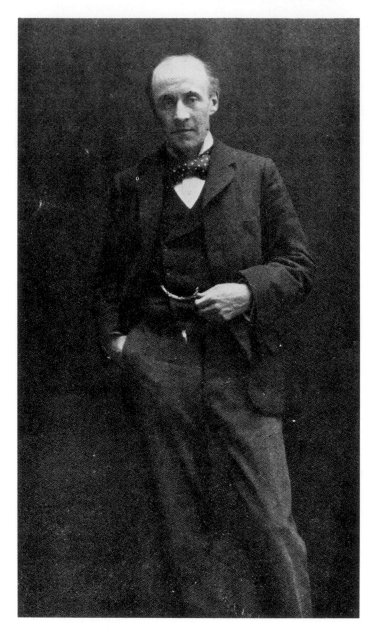

ZAIDA BEN-YÚSUF: Anthony Hope.

of her portraits are as bad as those of a Bowery photographer, while others, for instance her Anthony Hope (standing), is one of the most masterly plates in existence. The initial portrait of this article is a fair likeness; she got the swing of my body, although she knew me scarcely an hour then. The arm akimbo and the background on the left, however, are uninteresting.

Cox has taken several remarkable portrait heads, among which the head of Whitman belongs to the best. There we have a strong, straightforward handling, that knows what it is about; no wayward caprice—a simple, decided, and genuine method. One can speak neither of elegant taste, nor individuality of characterization but the unity, simplicity, and breadth of his execution is beyond praise. It is Whitman unmistakably for all those who have known the "good gray poet" when he was in the "sands of seventies," by far more enjoyable than Alexander's[37] portrait in the Metropolitan.

Breese[38] and Eickemeyer have produced one plate that deserves unstinted recognition—the portrait of Yvette Guilbert[39] called "Le Désir," which shows that they only meant it to be a study. Although this picture contains enough of a certain phase of Yvette Guilbert's art, a certain wanton forgetfulness characteristic of this "Lady of Vain Virtue" (as Rossetti might call her), it is not, and could not be, a portrait. We Americans have never known the real Yvette Guilbert—the "female faun"—and all on account of her wearing a wig here, while in Paris she appeared with her own carrot-red hair. In New York she was a naughty pre-Raphaelite maiden, while at the "Concert Parisien" she represented Ugliness singing the misery and frivolity of modern society. Nor was I aware that lilies of the valley expressed desire; lilacs would have been more appropriate. Or did the Carbon Studio[40] wish to convey that nervous Yvette Guilbert fell into a trance by inhaling the pure innocent odor of the lilies of the valley—a combination of refinement and naiveté, as we see in Chavannes' mural decorations? I hardly think so.

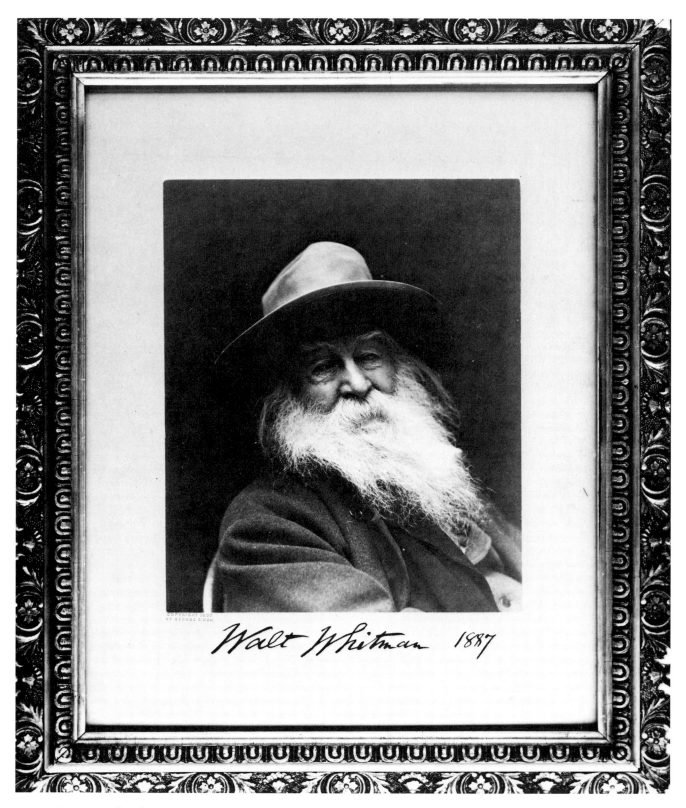

George C. Cox: Walt Whitman, 1887. LC.

Much more to the point, though less curious, are Eickemeyer's study of a ranchman and the portrait of his father. That is portrait photography. There is no transfiguring, magnifying, and generalizing of reality. Exactitude is in no way violated. And they are not accidents. Eickemeyer is only too scientific; he may be naive in the symbolism of flowers, but not in his technical methods. Read his "How a Picture Was Made," and you will know what hard and severe training he has gone through, and what strenuous study he has made. He also is on the right track, although a little more temperament would not harm him.

About Alfred Stieglitz as a portrait photographer I am not equally certain. We all know that a student of photography could not have (in references to technical usages) a better master than he. He is a fanatic of simplicity, but has done too few portraits, and these not individual enough to make an estimate. In his "Mr. R"—exact and cold like science, which may be a merit as it happens to represent a professor—he has succeeded very admirably indeed. The monotonous line of the left arm and the veins of his right hand, however, disturb my enjoyment. At all events it is a valuable object lesson, and as such worth hanging up where students congregate.

Letting all these artists pass in review once more in my mind's eyes, it seems to me that after all the genius of the painter, comparatively speaking, is more successful in getting an artistic likeness than the mechanism of photography. This is largely due to the fact that, with a very few exceptions, only mediocre talents have been drawn to the rubber bulb and focusing cloth. Artistic temperaments have avoided photography in fear of its restrictions, and so it has come to pass that until now the word genius could never yet be applied to any craftsman in this special branch of artistic photography.

The range of the technical expression of photography, in comparison with painting, is indeed very limited. First of all it lacks color. It controls line only as far as it is produced by broad opposite lights and shade (of which Mr. White's print is such an elegant example); it is impossible to accentuate any special part, as, for instance, Bastien-LePage has done in the back of Sarah Bernhardt. One cannot produce a clear, unhesitating line full of life from beginning to end. Also in representing texture, photography is handicapped. Of course the camera reproduces only too faithfully certain unimportant details, but the surface is always the same, unless where you retouch it so cleverly that it will suggest variety. It commands, however, tonality, but that other arts also convey equally well, and if photography is ever expected to assert itself as one of the independent—probably for a long time to come—minor arts, it has to develop that quality which no other medium has in common with it. The beauty of blurred lines, produced by the action of light, for photography does not draw lines but rather suggests them by painting values, may be compared in importance to the linear expression of etching or wood engraving,* and the massing of black (viz., Goya) and the moss-like gradations of gray (viz., Whistler) in lithography. These arts, although allowing big scope to creative power, are exposed to a certain restriction in regard to subjects. This is not the case with photography, as it has the power to express *movement,* for instance the spontaneity of facial expression, which no other art can do in the same degree and with the same ease.

What artistic photography needs is an expert photographer, who is at the same time a physiognomist and a man of taste, and great enough to subordinate himself to his machine; only a man thus adequately endowed could show us a new phase in portraiture, with which even the eye and hand of the painter would find it difficult to compete.

However, only when color photography has been

---

*Also pen and ink, and the various processes of engraving have given expression, but etching and wood engraving are capable of expressing tonality at the same time. Copper and steel engraving do this only to a limited degree, and besides lack the freedom of expression, which restricts them largely to reproductive purposes.

made possible, and kinetoscope photography in the hand of artists has developed to that extent that full justice can be done to the spontaneity of *actual* movement—to the continuous, almost undiscernible changes in a human face, the delicate nuances in the evolution of a smile, or any other human sentiment, passion, or common every-day expression of routine life—will artistic portrait photography fulfill its highest vocation. For would we not prefer a fragment of our children's life represented in actual movement, just as if they were alive, to any representation of one stereotyped position by a painter, no matter how skillful? A child looking roguishly at us, quickly changing its facial expression into a smile, would mean infinitely more (and it could be equally artistic) than if a Sargent would place the same child like a big doll under a still bigger vase in a hall vibrant with emptiness (viz., Sargent's "Hall of the Four Children"). And a characteristic gesture, a pensive attitude, or furtive movement of one's wife, as expressed by the kinetoscope of the future, would be much more valuable than the rare aesthetic pleasure of letting Watts wrap her up in a pre-Raphaelite soul-mist, or Lenbach draw her picture in lines worthy of a Herodotus, or Boldini make her look like a languid bachantee of modern joy.

But artistic kinetoscope photography in color is so far off! We have to deal with the present, have to make the best of the existing conditions, and form from them, if we possess the power and are unselfish enough, those foundations on which the photography of the future will construct itself.

—1899

2

A Plea for the Picturesqueness of New York

$\mathcal{A}$T EVERY EXHIBITION I am astonished at the limited range of subjects which the artistic photographers attempt to portray. One invariably finds numerous portraits and studies of heads or draped figures, a number of landscapes, interiors, and out-of-door- snap-shots, and a few—very few—serious compositions, mostly genre subjects, which can claim a general pictorial quality. This paucity of ideas is really embarrassing to the lover of art, who is interested in the sights and scenes of our own times.

Occasionally an artist seems to have resolved to be new and a few brilliant efforts are made, but, considering all, little has been done by the average amateur to exchange cheap portraiture and studio orientality and mediaevalism for a style more true to his existing surroundings. The passions of life and the passions of art are not the same to them.

They seem unaware that the best art is that which is most clearly the outcome of the time of its production, and the art signifying most in respect to the characteristics of its age is that which ultimately becomes classic. To give to art the complexion of our time, boldly to express the actual, is the thing infinitely desirable. What artistic photography needs most is a Steinlen,[1] who has succeeded in expressing in his weekly illustrations for the *Gil Blas* supplement[2]—as valuable as any Japanese wood cuts—the heat, the hurry, the vexations, the lurid excitements and frivolous graces, the tragedies and comedies of Parisian life, and in a more perfect manner than Zola[3] has in his long-drawn series of novels.

All these years our artistic photographers—and painters and sculptors as well—with a few exceptions have been mumbling old formulas, and have apparently combined in a gigantic trust of imitation. The dignified vigor of the old masters, the restless desires of modern art, the incomparable suggestiveness of the Japanese, have all been mortgaged. No past effort has escaped their versatility for reproducing. Everything seems to have struck their fancy, even that which is only questionably good.

I know that a large majority will object to my arguments: those who do not feel that there is an imposing grandeur in the Brooklyn Bridge; who do not acknowledge the beauty of the large sweeping curves in the new Speedway, which would set a Munich Secessionist[4] wild; who do not feel the poetry of our waterfronts, the semi-opaque water reflecting the gray sky, the confusion of square-rigged vessels with their rusty sides and the sun-burnt faces peering from the deck; and who would laugh outright if anyone would dare to suggest that Paddy's market on Ninth Avenue or the Bowery could be reduced to decorative purposes.

Such men claim that there is nothing pictorial

and picturesque in New York and our modern life, and continue their homage to imitation. The truth is that they lack the inspiration of the true artist, which wants to create and not merely to revive or adapt. They are satisfied with an incongruous mixture of what they know and see with what they have learned in school and what comes to them easily, no matter whether at second or at third hand; it saves them experiments and shields them from failures. They work as do the journalists, who write of things they know nothing about, and whose superficial knowledge is concealed by the rapid succession of publications. But for that reason their work can also be likened to the wake of a ship—it foams a little to be seen no more.

To open new realms to art takes a good share of courage and patience. It always takes moral courage to do what the rest of the profession does not; that of course the man possesses who starts out to conquer the beauties of New York. It takes actual physical courage to go out into the crowd with your camera, and to be stared and laughed at on the most inopportune occasions. But that even Mr. J. G. Brown[5] braved; why not you? It takes also a marvelous amount of patience to stand for hours at the same spot, perhaps in very bad weather—in rain, snow, or even in a thunder-storm—until at last one sees before him what he considers essential for a picture; or persistently to return at every opportunity to a subject—perhaps to something that may recur only once in a year, as the "May Festival" in Central Park—until he has at last mastered it. And even after one has succeeded, there is no harvest of praise to reap, for all those who are in quest of beauty will experience that the very people who said there could be no beauty there will later on point out that it undoubtedly was there long before it was discovered.

But what does it matter? The true artist works for himself, and does not care a rap for the opinion of others, as long as he knows—if that should be his aim—that his work has been infused with the spirit of to-day, with something unmistakably the out-come of the present. I would like to make his acquaintance; I might feel inclined to become his Ruskin.

I am well aware that much is lacking here which makes European cities so interesting and inspiring to the sightseer and artist. No monuments of past glory, no cathedral spires of Gothic grandeur, no historic edifices, scarcely even masterpieces of modern architecture lift their imposing structures in our almost alarmingly democratic land. Despite this, I stick to my assertion, and believe that I can prove its truth. For years I have made it my business to find all the various picturesque effects New York is capable of—effects which the eye has not yet got used to, nor discovered and applied in painting and literature, but which nevertheless exist.

Have you ever watched a dawn on the platform of an elevated railroad station, when the first rays of the rising sun lay glittering on the rails? This Vance Thompson[6] compared to the waterways of Venice in pictorial effect. The morning mist, in strange shapes and forms, played in the distance where the lines of the houses on both sides of the street finally united.

Have you ever dined in one of the roof-garden restaurants and watched twilight descending on that sea of roofs, and seen light after light flame out, until all the distant windows began to glimmer like sparks, and the whole city seemed to be strewn with stars? If you have not, you are not yet acquainted with New York.

Then take Madison Square. Place yourself at one of its corners on a rainy night and you will see a picture of peculiar fascination: Dark silhouettes of buildings and trees, surrounded by numerous light reflections, are mirrored in the wet pavement as in a sheet of water. But also in daytime it is highly attractive. The paths are crowded with romping children, and their gay-colored garments make a charming contrast to the lawn and the foliage of the trees, to which the Diana's tower and the rows of houses with windows glittering in the sun form a suitable background.

The Boulevard has many interesting parts. The rows of trees in the middle, the light brick fronts of the new apartment houses, and the many vehicles and bicyclists on a Sunday afternoon offer ample opportunity for snap-shots.

Comparing New York with other cities, it can boast of a decided strain of gayety and vitality in its architecture. The clear atmosphere has encouraged bright colors which, when subdued by the mist that hovers at times over all large cities, afford delightful harmonies that can be suggested even by the photographer's black and white process.

Almost any wide street with an elevated station is interesting at those times when the populace goes to or returns from work. The nearer day approaches these hours, the more crowded are the sidewalks. Thousands and thousands climb up or down the stairs, reflecting in their varied appearance all the classes of society, all the different professions, the lights and shadows of a large city, and the joys and sorrows of its inhabitants.

In Central Park we meet with scenes of rare elegance and dignity. Many a tourist will find himself transported to the palace gardens of the old world, as his eyes gaze on these quiet lakes peopled with swans and on the edifices shimmering in the

Joseph Byron: Cornelius Vanderbilt House, Fifth Avenue and 58th Street. The Bryon Collection, mcny.

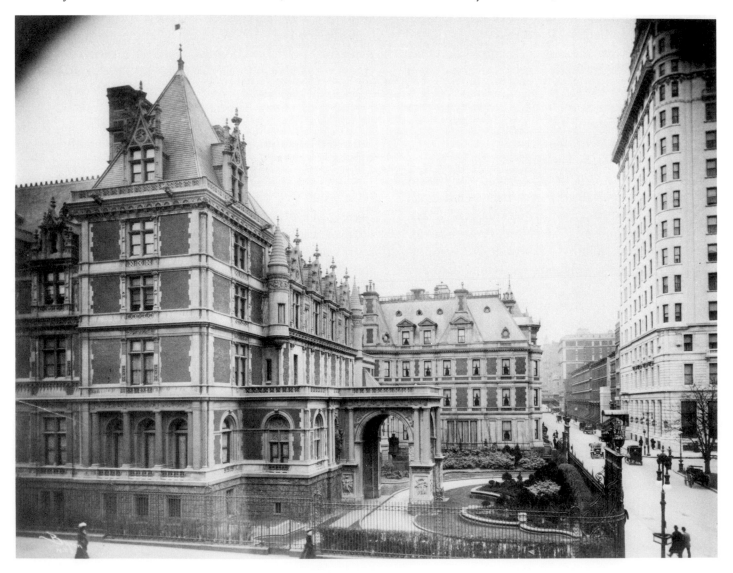

sun and rising from the autumnal foliage into the sky.

A peculiar sight can be enjoyed standing on a starlit night at the block house near the northwest entrance of the Park. One sees in the distance the illumined windows of the West Side and the Elevated, which rises at the double curve at One Hundred and Tenth Street to dizzy heights, and whose construction is hardly visible in the dimness of night. A train passes by, like a fantastic fire-worm from some giant fairyland, crawling in mid-air. The little locomotive emits a cloud of smoke, and suddenly the commonplace and yet so mystic scene changes into a tumult of color, red and saffron, changing every moment into an unsteady gray and blue. This should be painted, but as our New York artists prefer to paint Paris and Munich reminiscences, the camera can at least suggest it.

A picture genuinely American in spirit is afforded by Riverside Park. Old towering trees stretch their branches towards the Hudson. Almost touching their trunks the trains on the railroad rush by. On the water, heavily loaded canal boats pass on slowly, and now and then a white river steamboat glides by majestically, while the clouds change the chiaroscuro effects at every gust of wind.

JOSEPH BYRON: Skating in Central Park, 1894. The Byron Collection, MCNY.

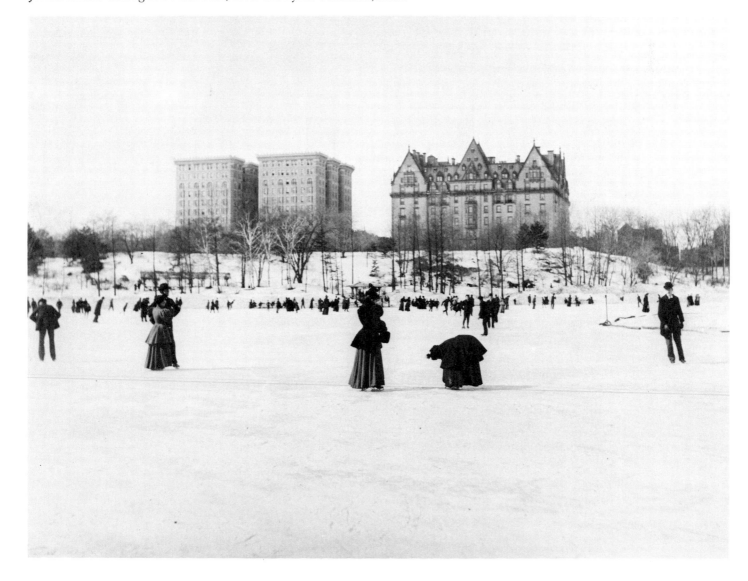

Another picture of surprising beauty reveals itself when you approach New York by the Jersey City ferry. The gigantic parellelograms of office buildings and skyscrapers soar into the clear atmosphere like the towers, turrets, and battlements of some ancient fortress, a modern Cathay, for whose favor all nations contend.

The traffic in the North and East rivers and the harbor offers abundant material; only think of the graceful four-masted East Indiamen that anchor in the bay, laden with spices which recall even in these northern climes quaint Oriental legends, of indolent life under tropical suns. I am also very fond of the vista of the harbor from Battery Park, particularly at dawn. How strange this scene looks in the cold morning mist. There is no difference and no perspective; the outlines of Jersey City and Brooklyn fade ghost-like in the mist; soft shimmering sails, dark shadows, and long pennants of smoke interrupt the gray harmony, and are in their uncertain contours not unlike the fantastic birds which enliven at times the background of Japanese flower designs.

Whoever is fond of panoramic views should place himself at the Highbridge Reservoir and look northwards. At sunset this scene—the wide Harlem River sluggishly flowing through a valley over which two aqueducts span their numerous arches—reminds one involuntarily of a landscape by Claude Lorrain.[7]

For the lovers of proletarian socialism—who like Dudley Hardy[8] and Gaston Latouche,[9] and would like to depict the hunger and the filth of the slums, the unfathomable and inexhaustible misery, which hides itself in every metropolitan city—subjects are not lacking in New York. Only it is more difficult to find them than in European cities.

Rafaelli,[10] the French painter, once asked me to show him the poorest quarters. I took him through Stanton, Cherry, Baxter, and Essex Streets. I could not satisfy him. But when he saw a row of dilapidated red brick houses with black fire-escapes covered all over with bedding, clothes lines, and all

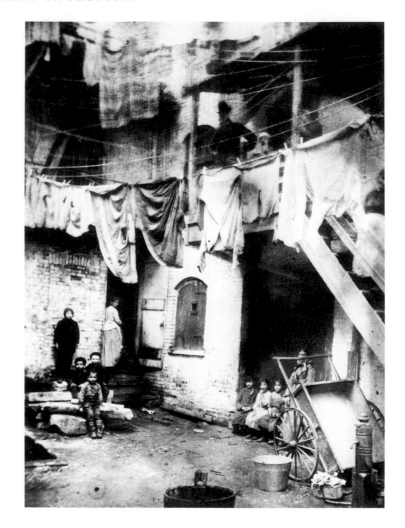

Above. JACOB RIIS: Baxter Street Court. The Jacob A. Riis Collection, MCNY.

Opposite page. JACOB RIIS: Five Cents a Spot, 1889. The Jacob A. Riis Collection, MCNY.

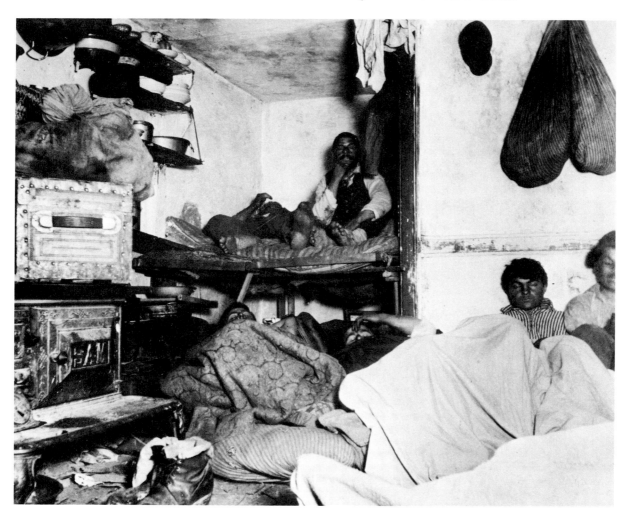

sorts of truck, he exclaimed: *"C'est fort curieux!"* and like a ferret ran from one side to the other to take a number of snap-shots.

True enough we have not such scenes of extreme poverty as Rafaelli found in the outskirts of Paris, at least not so open; but one only needs to leave the big thoroughfares and go to the downtown back alleys, to Jewtown, to the village (East Twenty-ninth Street), or Frog Hollow, to prove sufficiently that many a portfolio could be filled with pictures of our slums, which would teach us better than any book "how the other half lives."

From there you should go to the Potter's Field, on Hart's Island, that ragged little island where the nameless dead are buried in long trenches, each of which is marked by a stone to record that one hundred and fifty paupers lie below. And out beyond the sandy shore gleam the shimmering waters of the Sound.

But you can find mortuary themes in New York, without boarding at 6 A. M., the Fidelity, that sad little charity steamer which plies between the Morgue and Hart's Island. There lies in the very heart of the city, in the midst of a block bounded by Second Avenue, the Bowery, Second Street, and Third Street, a little neglected graveyard, as romantic as anything of that nature I have ever seen. The gravestones are sadly dilapidated, and almost

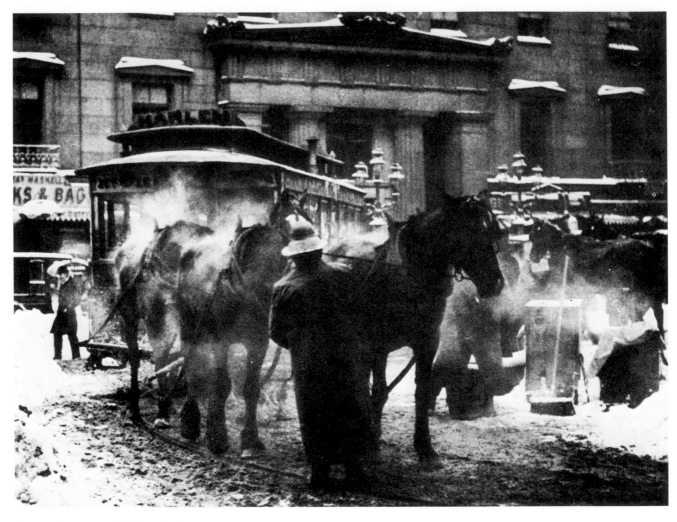

ALFRED STIEGLITZ: The Terminal. IMP-GEH.

disappear in the wild flowers that sprout in great abundance from the untrimmed grass and weeds. Clotheslines cross this desolate spot everywhere, and on week days long rows of linen flap gayly in the breeze. More than half a century has passed over these graves and left plain traces of the flight of the years. A Hamlet-like mood takes me at the sight. There the two gravediggers might dig up Yorick's skull and prepare the grave for the fair Ophelia.

Vereschagin[11] was particularly interested in our telegraph poles, now largely a thing of the past, and the net of wires that is spread all over the city.

Wherever some large building is being constructed, the photographer should appear. It would be so easy to procure an interesting picture, and yet I have never had the pleasure to see a good picture of an excavation or an iron skeleton framework. I think there is something wonderful in iron architecture, which as if guided by magic, weaves its networks with scientific precision over the rivers or straight into the air. They create, by the very absence of unnecessary ornamentation, new laws of beauty, which have not yet been determined and are perhaps not even realized by the originators. I am weary of the everlasting complaint that we have

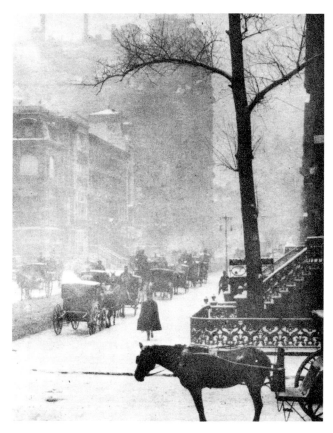

ALFRED STIEGLITZ: The Street. IMP-GEH.

no modern style of architecture. It would indeed be strange if an age as fertile as ours had produced nothing new in that art which has always, more than others, reflected the aspirations and accomplishments of mankind at certain epochs of history. The iron architecture is our style.

I still could add hundreds and hundreds of suggestions for pictures, but I fear I would tire my readers, I will therefore only mention a few haphazard. There is the Fulton fish market, a wonderful mixture of hustling human life and the slimy products of Neptune's realm, at its best on a morning during Lent; then the Gansevoort market on Saturday mornings or evenings; the remnants of Shantytown; the leisure piers; the open-air gymnasiums at Stryker's Lane and the foot of Hester Street; the starting of a tally-ho coach from the Waldorf-Astoria on its gay drive to Westchester; the canal-boat colony at Coenties Slip; the huge storage houses of Gowanus Bay. Another kind of subjects now comes to mind—the children of the tenement districts returning from school; or the organ-grinder, and little girls showing off their terpsichorean skill on the sidewalk to an admiring crowd.

But really what would be the use of specifying any further? Any person with his eyes open, and with sympathy for the time, place, and conditions in which he lives, has only to take a walk or to board a trolley, to find a picture worthy of depiction almost in every block he goes.

I am perfectly aware that only a few of my readers endorse my assertions and see something in my ardent plea. In thirty years, however, nobody will believe that I once fought for it, for then the beauty of New York will have been explored by thousands.

But who will be the first to venture on these untrodden fields and teach New Yorkers to love their own city as I have learned to love it, and to be proud of its beauties as the Parisians are of their city? He will have to be a great poet and of course an expert photographer.

May he soon appear!

—1900

3

On Plagiarism and Imitation

"To be free is not to be independent of any form,
it is to be master of many forms."

—SIDNEY LANIER

I HAVE ALWAYS endorsed Heine's defense of plagiarism, that it is permissible to steal entire columns and porticoes from a temple, providing the new edifice one erects with their aid is great enough to warrant such violent proceedings. The history of art has proven this somewhat surprising statement to be true.

What is the *Marguerite Gauthier* of Dumas but a modernized version of L'Abbé Prévost's *Manon Lescaut?* Did not Balzac in his *Père Goriot,* Turgéniev in his *King Lear of the Steppes,* and Zola in *La Terre,* make use of the same tragic theme as Shakespeare in *King Lear?* Is the story of the three rings in Lessing's *Nathan der Weise* not taken from Boccaccio's *Decameron,* which has served more writers with plots than any other book in the world's literature? And did Boccaccio himself not gather this collection of a hundred stories from every available source, often merely embellishing an old legend with the concise beauty of his style? Has it not been proven that Milton copied a large part of his *Paradise Lost* from the Dutch poet van den Vondel?[1] And did not Shakespeare take whole passages from Plutarch, simply changing them into blank verse and inserting them, for instance, in his *Antony and Cleopatra?*

To transform history into art is surely not a sin. In all those cases mentioned, the artist has freely borrowed material from predecessors, but has at the same time understood how to imbue it with his own individuality and to lend it new vitality through the vibrations of his own soul.

That is re-creation, which is almost as admissible as originality, if the latter is possible, and not, as in most cases, merely a new combination of the work of previous generations. For no artist is so self-sufficient that he will shape his course unaffected by, and apart from, what has been done before. It is impossible to wipe one's mind entirely clear of what one has seen and read and heard in intercourse with other beings. Every work of art must necessarily bear influences of previous accomplishments.

We are heirs of the ages, but the heritage bequeathed to us should merely be the basic soil for future growth, and reveal itself unconsciously. Otherwise it becomes mere copyism, a danger into which many a young artist, through an absorption of all that is best in the past and present, has fallen. It should widen, not narrow, our sympathies. Symonds[2] has well phrased it when he said, we modern men are in the need "of self-tillage, the ploughing and harrowing of self by use of what the ages have transmitted to us from the work of gifted minds."

It is logical for a young American comedy writer to imitate the so-called "paper chase" invented by Sardou,[3] in which the losing of an object is used to

64

tangle up all the characters, and thereby produce most unexpected and funny situations. But it is also offensive to our code of ethics if he slavishly reconstructs each situation with slight changes in the characters, perhaps merely Americanizing them, and yet gives out the result as his original work. Burglaries of this kind are committed often, and furnish ghastly examples of intellectual impotence and degeneracy.

But if a man remodels an original after a classic pattern, he may be accused of copyism, which however, is no serious reproach. To copy intelligently shows good taste and does not absolutely bar inspiration, invention, and creative power.

If Mrs. Käsebier would only study the play of light and shade in the old masters to give a deeper artistic value to her photographs, I would heartily endorse her methods. But when she attempts an exact reproduction of a Holbein drawing, I consider it the most futile kind of art plagiarism. The same objection holds good if Mr. Eugene puts a man in mediaeval armor and lets him pose like one of the famous Innsbruck figures. What is the use of it? Every intelligent art lover would pronounce it at once an imitation and would surely rather possess an ordinary photograph of the original than a sort of reconstruction at second-hand.

Still more deplorable is the fact that so many photographers rely entirely on what they have seen of paintings and illustrations for the composition and arrangement of their subjects. They take a fancy to a picture, pose a model in the same or a similar way, photograph it, and think they have accomplished something wonderful. Of course the photographer has to go somewhere for inspiration, and nothing is more natural than his turning to pictorial art in search of ideas. But what satisfaction can there be in repeating in a new medium what has been done so much better in another?

The commercial spirit prevalent in all matters seems to have set aside almost all scruples about plagiarism and imitation. A well-known sculptor told me one day. "The easiest way to make a good monument is to copy one of the masterpieces of European sculpture, only to make it a little better." That is an absurdity, for a man who will descend to copying of that sort belongs to that class of thinkers whose thought crystallizes into what is known as art.

Allow me to cite a few of the many cases of appropriation, or art plagiarism, that have come to my notice.

In art circles, for instance, it is generally known that the figures of a certain artist's stained glass windows can easily be found in illustrated books on medieval art, yet nobody accuses him of stealing, for the color of his windows is so wondrously beautiful that we forget all criticism. A pity only that he did not do it more cleverly, for the stealing of ideas that is not found out is not stealing to the idea of the world, but merely a matter that the artist has to fight out with his own conscience.

Yet there are cruder forms. If you are acquainted with Boldini's[4] work you probably remember the portrait of a *mondaine,* who is seated in a nervous, almost grotesque attitude on the edge of a lounge. Now, I saw at one of the Philadelphia Academy exhibitions a picture by an American painter, given out as an original work, which represented the identical figure in the identical attitude, only the color scheme was changed. That was outright theft and should be legally punishable.

A similar case I witnessed in a New York studio, when I saw a picture by a well-known English painter reproduced in every detail, only in a smaller size. The artist had the audacity to ask me if I did not consider the composition original. I was dumbfounded and thought I might, after all, be mistaken. But no, there was the whole scene that I knew so well, as its simple composition had made a decided impression upon me.

In my wanderings through the studios I had opportunity to witness many queer proceedings, and I found the sculptors as guilty as the painters and illustrators. I pride myself on my knowledge of contemporary art, and the ability to trace adapta-

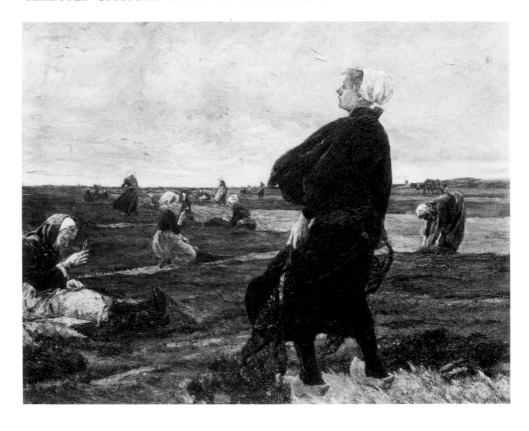

Max Liebermann:
Net Mender.
Hamburger
Kunsthalle,
Germany.

tions and *adeptations* back to their original source, but from time to time I have come across cases of undeniable plagiarism which even puzzled me. Years ago I saw the painting of a female nude by a Frenchman, his name has escaped my memory, which immediately attracted my attention by the dignified and graceful recumbent pose. The same pose I saw later on, depicted by Clifford Grayson[5] and by another American painter. Still greater was my astonishment when I saw a clay model by Sir Frederic Leighton,[6] entitled "Iphigenia," of the very same subject. And to show that it has entered every branch of art, I may add that I recently saw it again in a photograph after the nude by Frank Eugene. Will anybody kindly tell me which of these gentlemen has the most claim to originating the pose? Is it mere coincidence, or did they all appropriate the Frenchman's idea? Or did they perhaps all use the same model, whose form was seen to the best advantage in this position, or is the pose itself so beautiful and natural that one after the other discovered it?

Another incident I experienced with Mr. Blashfield's[7] "Angel With the Fiery Sword," one of his most forceful pictures. Looking over a French illustrated magazine, I discovered an initial letter, the design of which contained the same figure which I had admired so much in the painting. Now did Mr. Blashfield elaborate the designer's idea, or did the designer copy Mr. Blashfield's figure? In the first case it would be justified adaptation, in the second, rank stealing. In this case it would be difficult to make an accusation of borrowing, and it is a sad fact that very often accusations are made when there is no cause or evidence whatever.

Artistic photography offers such a case. Mr. Stieglitz exhibited his well-known "Net Mender" in Germany and was at once accused by several critics that he would never have thought of treating the subject if Liebermann[8] had not painted it. Now

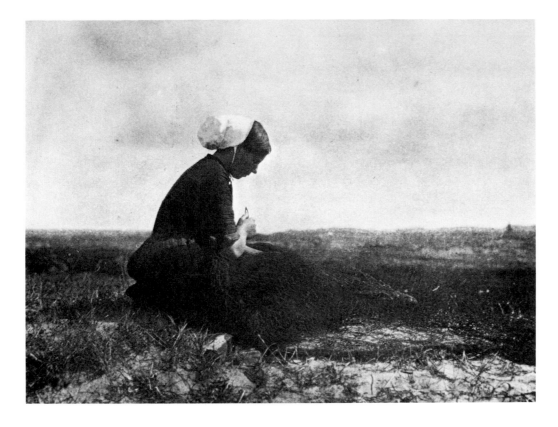

ALFRED STIEGLITZ:
The Net Mender,
1894. IMP-GEH.

Mr. Stieglitz states that although he is acquainted with Liebermann's work, he has never seen a painting resembling his "Net Mender" and that Liebermann's representation of Dutch fishing folk had never entered his mind. The critics consider it a foregone conclusion that if one of the two derived anything from the other it must necessarily have been the photographer. The general public is not yet sufficiently acquainted with artistic photography to know that it can rival other arts in originality and beauty. Much less do the artists realize this fact. They would unscrupulously make use of any photograph suitable to their line of work, and not for a moment consider it stealing, as to them photography is merely a helpmate, without any claim to artistic merit.

The similarity in this case is merely a matter of coincidence. Each in his respective medium has worked conscientiously to gain a certain effect, and both have accomplished it. But even if one of them were obliged for the idea to the other, it would be of no consequence. Both productions are works of art of a high type, and any indebtedness in this case would be owing to the creation of one masterpiece by the suggestion of another. And of that every artist is guilty.

Heine is right, borrow as much as you like. But be certain that you master the accumulations and accreted experiences of others to such an extent that they have become your own, only that you can rear on the understructure of precedent accomplishments still higher and more imposing monuments of beauty.

—1900

4

Random Thoughts on Criticism

*"The good critic is he who narrates the adventures
of a soul among masterpieces."*

—ANATOLE FRANCE

*T*HE POOR PHOTOGRAPHERS! They no longer work in sylvan quietude. Also their efforts are now exposed to the utterances of harsh criticism, in the same way that sensational books, music-hall artists, and prize fights are.

I do not know whether the photographic profession considers this an advantage or a disadvantage. I believe they are, in this respect, very much like the painters; they like to be talked about, but they do not like adverse criticism.

They fail to see that we live in an age of advertisement and that no matter whether a notice is *pro* or *con,* it is of value. Of course the artistic photographer does not desire the adulation of the mob, he is mostly an amateur, and not dependent on his art for a livelihood. But he would like to establish his name, to become well known to the profession and the art-loving public. And for that the press, unfortunately, is indispensable. Good work alone is not sufficient. If a man is but little known to a community like ours, he is apt to be entirely forgotten; as it is, he has to make his reputation over again every five years. Naturally, if a man stands so high above common mortals that art is all to him, and that he entertains an utter and honest indifference to the public, he may also shrug his shoulders at criticism. I am certain that such a man would be amused by intelligent blackguarding. But too high an opinion of oneself bars every improvement.

The art critic is the agreeable means of intermediation and conciliation between the artists and the public. And the best criticism is, after all, nothing but an individual, carefully considered estimate of a man of taste, and, in rare cases when it is at its best, the concentrated opinion of a certain part of the public. Professional men should appreciate the difficult position of the art critic in a country which is as stagnant, commonplace, and businesslike in art matters as America is in this year of grace 1899. And in Europe conditions are not much better. There the production of paintings has reached such alarming conditions that Emile Bergerat,[1] the "Caliban" of the *Figaro,*[2] exclaimed in despair, "I return from the Salon and am dumbfounded; painting is no longer an art—it is a vice." It is well nigh impossible for a critic to sift the hundred thousands of prints which artistic photography produces and do justice to others and to himself. For is it not the critic's duty to enter an artist's individuality, to discover his intentions—intentions of which the artist himself is perhaps unconscious—so as to judge how far he has realized them, and then to determine what place he occupies in contemporary art?

The trouble with photographic criticism at present is that it is maudlin and insignificant, without the slightest pretense to any educational or inspirational power.

The so-called criticisms that appear now and

then in the professional magazines are written either by photographers who have a special view to defend; or worse, by amateurs who consider photography, as well as the writing of the article, merely a pastime, or by clerks of wholesale houses of photographic material. That such concoctions are not worth serious thought is quite natural. They are merely ordinary writers, without any knowledge or discrimination about art, who indulge either in cheap praise or unjustified fault-finding. Some merely enumerate and write biographical notes, while others fill pages without venturing a single straight-forward opinion. Apollo be merciful to them!

The only branch in which something has been accomplished is in general technical criticism. I, however, know of no work on photography which would compare in clearness of purpose and expression with Philip Gilbert Hamerton's[3] etchers' handbook. But an account of processes can hardly be termed criticism, and criticism of individual methods becomes too easily didactic to be of much use. We all like to know how a man does a thing, but it is futile to advise him how to do it. The critic is not necessarily a pedagogue, although the majority of them possess that philanthropic disposition. When they visit a photographic exhibition they equip themselves with a big bag of regulations, and woe to the poor photographer who dares to violate one of these. They pursue with indefatigable advice, pity, and hostility all who are obstinate and endeavor to search for truth in roads different from those they consider right.

There is, in reality, only one kind of criticism which is just to all, and the man who practices it must be willing and able to understand and absorb the artist's idea and judge his work from the artist's point of view. No matter whether a photographer depicts New York models as Weeping Magdalenes, or himself as Christ, scientific foreground studies or Fifth Avenues in Winter, Japanese ghosts or morose Old Masters; no matter how he exposes, retouches, and paints; whether it is over or under exposure, whether he dodges or applies chemical baths,

etches on the plate or lets it take care of itself; whether he prints light or dark, on platinum or on aristo—all that is but little consequence. The question is simply whether the artist has something to express and expresses it well, and it is the critic's business to tell his own impression frankly, without personal subterfuge, to his readers.

Only in the highest order of criticism is didacticism permissible—that is, in the laying down of universal rules for one or another art, as Lessing[4] has done for painting, sculpture, and the drama, and Boileau[5] for poetry. These critics do not bother with individuals and specimens of work unless they serve the purpose of proving one of their theories. Ruskin, who endeavored to establish rules for a certain school of painting, the Pre-Raphaelites, unnecessarily limited his field of labor, so that his theories now seem partial and already, in most cases, hopelessly out of date. They will be forgotten unless his style saves them.

Photography is still too young an art to command such a critic. The time has not yet arrived to write a history of artistic photography à la Taine.[6] The material would not warrant it. The majority of photographers do not consider their profession an art. Even a Demachy[7] and Stieglitz feel very sceptical about it. What, then, can be expected of the critic!

Looking over the list of the prominent art critics of to-day, I could not mention a single one who has occupied himself seriously with artistic photography, except in now and then launching an anathema against the mechanism of photography, which is received with great satisfaction in artistic circles, for the painters and illustrators, who do not disdain to use photography as a help, are very reluctant to give it a place amongst the fine arts.

And, sad to state, the general mass of production is quite unworthy of the critic's attention. The majority of amateurs seem to imagine that composition and chiaroscuro of a degree of badness which nobody would tolerate in a painting somehow becomes allowable in photography; that because no clearly-defined laws exist for the art of Daguerre, a photographer is at liberty to set at defiance all the known laws of nature and art; that the mere pressing of the rubber bulb implies in itself a cleverness, elevating the practitioner above the common canons of criticism.

There are a few able artistic photographers, a very few, however, and, of the quantities of prints which are turned out every year, nine out of ten are not only valueless, but a nuisance, doing much harm by propagating and confirming those false conceptions of the art which are still generally prevalent.

Here is, indeed, room for criticism, but hardly for that which demands printer's ink and paper. Verbal criticism, such as is practiced at private lantern slide exhibitions in the clubs, is by far preferable. There is no use analyzing nonentities for the public. The critic can only give his attention to exhibitions of the work of men that command universal atten-tion. Even then his scope will be very limited.

No, indeed, the critic of artistic photography has no easy task. Very few of the exhibitors have a striking individuality, which would be as easy to handle as that of some European celebrity in the world of art. The critic of artistic photography has to dispense with brilliancy of style and striking metaphor. Instead, he has lovingly to pick out those more modest qualities deserving praise, to strengthen feeble knees and encourage the flicker-ing blaze, and at the same time continually to contend against prevalent prejudices.

However, one satisfaction is undoubtedly con-tained in it; that of having been a pathfinder and roadbuilder when the victory at last is won. And I can only state, for my part, that it would be one of the greatest satisfactions of my life to see artistic photography occupy its proper place in the world of art.

—1900

5

On Composition

A FRIEND OF Jean Léon Gérôme[1] came one day to the painter's studio, when he was busy with the composition of a new picture. One sketch after another appeared upon the canvas, only to be rubbed out again. In the afternoon the friend happened to call again, and seeing that the painter was still occupied in the same fashion as several hours before, exclaimed: "Still laboring at your composition?" "Oui, il n'y a que ça," answered Gérôme—"Yes, there is nothing else but that."—not meaning that the composition is the only quality of importance in painting, but very likely holding the opinion that it is the most valuable of technical accomplishments, as it determines the character of the entire work.

To Gérôme it has meant even more. It has saved his work from the clutches of absolute mediocrity. He is one of the men of whom the young art students say: "Pshaw, Gérôme, he is so old-fogyish; but he knows something about composition."

He is one of the few painters to whom composition is still a science, not merely a decorative scheme of handling a certain space in a way that does not offend the eye. Study his sketches, "Conspiracy" and the "Death of Marshal Ney," how, by continual alterations, he gradually improved the pictures, and you begin to understand why the constructive element played such an important part in the creations of the old masters.

It will only be necessary to mention some really genuine work of art, like Leonardo da Vinci's "Last Supper," Raphael's "Sistine Madonna" or Titian's "Entombment of Christ," to prove how sound principles of composition transfused and enabled all their mode of expression. The whole success or failure of their work, the sentiment, the character, the triumph of the soul over matter, hinged on composition in those times.

How marvelously do all the lines in da Vinci's picture converge to the central figure of Christ—he made the laws of perspective the laws of composition. Raphael composed in an entirely different manner—he applied the typical geometrical forms of nature with preference—the triangle, the circle, and the ellipse—giving them full sway to reign in supreme beauty and significance over the creations of his brain. Titian proved that an accurate juxtaposition of colors and the relations of their tones can be just as valuable for the making of a perfect picture as perspective and geometry. Michelangelo regarded architecture and the plastic element of sculpture as the foundations of great paintings, and Rembrandt believed that the massing of light and shade was sufficient to produce a masterpiece.

Each of these men excelled in his style of composition, which had become a part of their individuality; and one was as good as the other.

The situation has somewhat changed in modern

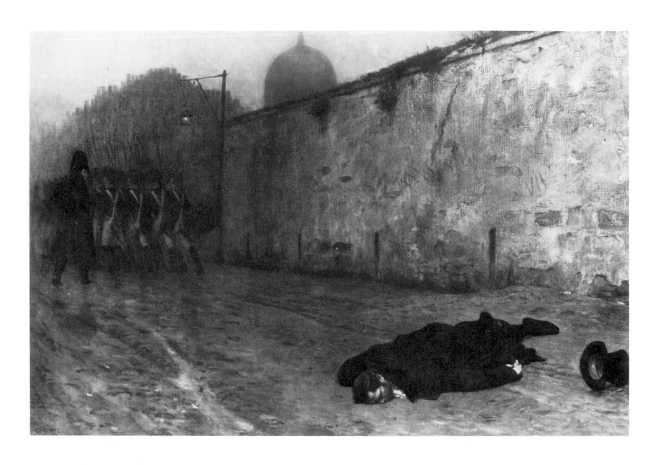

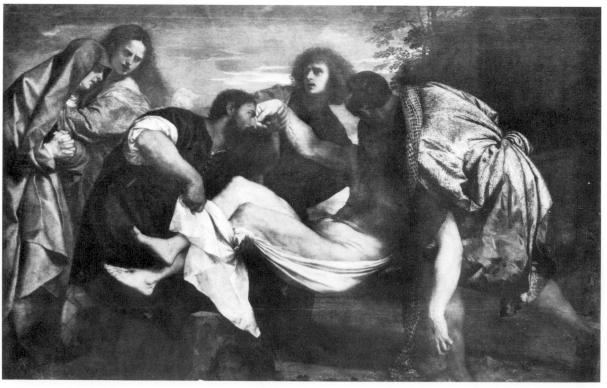

times. Composition is no longer considered absolutely essential. It is even disregarded by the realists and impressionists, or at least subordinated to other qualities. They want to represent life as it is, and claim that nature cannot be improved upon. A faithful reproduction of what they see before them is all they desire. They claim they work on broader principles than hitherto, principles derived from the habits of the eye to note transient effect—largely produced by instantaneous photography of movement, and to compare the values of color-patches with each other and to arrange them in a harmonious ensemble. They even assert that composition is no necessity; that there are no iron cast laws to go by, and that the true artist works out his salvation unconsciously.

I beg to differ on that point.

True enough, composition cannot be narrowed down to a few laws, which assure success to everyone who slavishly follows them. There are no definite laws for the composition of a portrait, a landscape, or an historical picture. But it has taken men like Chavannes and Whistler to prove that the decorative treatment of comparative values, or a solemn, low-toned key of color are as effective as the elaborate technical resources of the old masters. These men are geniuses who have beaten their own track through the labyrinthine thickets of modern art. Yet I doubt very much if they are not just as dependent on certain principles of composition as their predecessors, the only difference being that they proceed in a less scientific manner, and work more unconsciously—not because they know less, but, on the contrary, more. They have seen everything that art has ever produced, and their knowledge of composition really embraces the entire history of art: ancient, mediaeval, and modern, Oriental as well as Occidental.

Opposite page top. JEAN LÉON GÉRÔME: Death of Marshall Ney. By permission of the City of Sheffield.

Opposite page bottom. TITIAN: Entombment of Christ. (c) Arch. Phot. Paris/S.P.A.D.E.M.

Every great artist makes his own laws of composition by studying the methods of his predecessors, and by giving infinite time and trouble to the elaboration of their ideas on the subjects. The mastery of composition is the final result of patient study of everything that is available in life and art.

And who can deny that the elements of Japanese art, the parallelism, the continual repetition with slight variation, the wayward caprice of losing detail here and scorning it there, the rhythm of line and the harmony of space proportion have influenced modern western art to such an extent that nearly every artistic production of the last thirty years shows a trace of one or another of its peculiarities. We believe that by adopting Japanese methods of composition we have discarded science and become more intuitive. But it is an illusion. Nobody who has studied the rigid canons of Japanese art will make such an assertion, for he will have found out that the fundamental process of so-called space-art and the putting together of lines and masses is as scientific as the theories of Leonardo da Vinci and the Renaissance, and the academic rule of French artists.

As for the photographers, I do not believe that even the best have ever bothered themselves much about composition. Of course, they cannot do without it. But they have never taken it half seriously enough. They have simply imitated the painters in a more or less careless fashion.

It will be interesting to see how far they have succeeded.

There are four styles of composition in vogue at present: line composition, light and shade composition, space composition, and tone composition.

Eickemeyer is principally a story-teller of the old school, and his composition is largely a deduction of the methods of genre painters; he is at times very good in detail, but lacks fundamental principles. His pictures very seldom show concentration. Stieglitz excels in space composition (*viz.*, "Fifth Avenue," "Scurrying Home," or "A Decorative Study"). Also Day, in his "Miss Devens," for instance, and Käsebier, in several of her portraits,

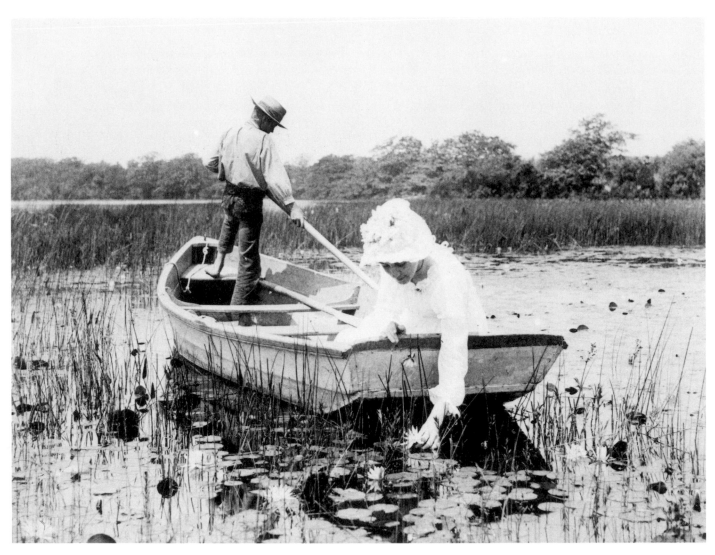

RUDOLF EICKEMEYER, JR.: The Lily-Gatherer, 1892. SI.

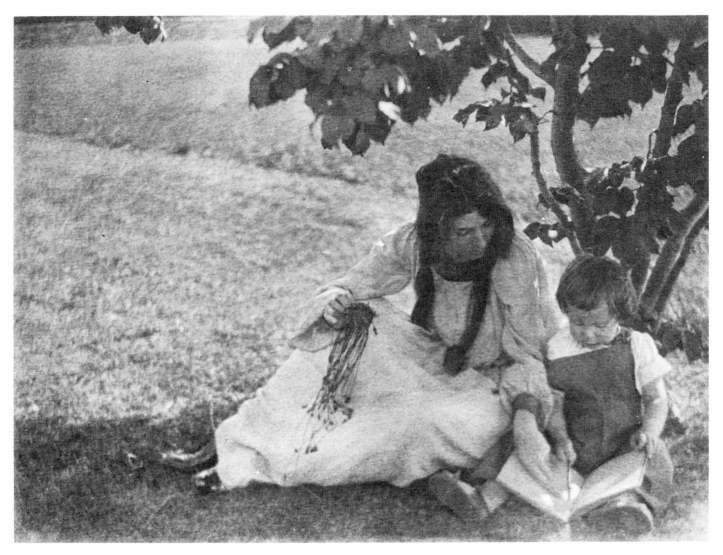

GERTRUDE KÄSEBIER: Mother and Child. IMP-GEH.

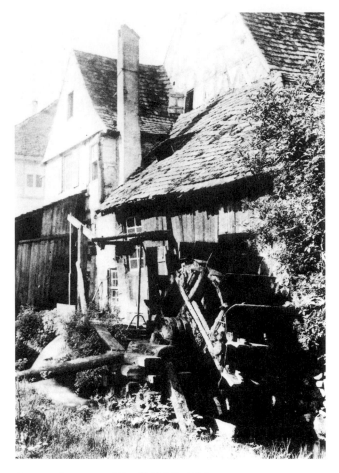

ALFRED STIEGLITZ: The Old Mill, 1894. UNM.

show how cleverly space can be broken up into parts of various shapes.

Light and shade composition (in the sense of Mauve[2] or Corot[3]) is rarely accomplished in photography. The distinction between light and shade in photography always lacks vigor and, what is more, proportional value. The first shortcoming is a mechanical one, the second due to the ignorance of the art. Stieglitz's "Old Mill" is a fair specimen of light and shadow composition (although from the point of subject, a sentimental platitude). A better one, because more rhythmic in its massing, is Käsebier's "Mother and Child." Line composition is still rarer. The only photograph I know that can claim this quality is Stieglitz's "Decorative Study." White at times makes weak attempts at it. So do

others, but in most cases it is largely due to the model when they succeed in suggesting it, as in Eugene's "Miss Lillian." Keiley[4] is the only exception; he was wise enough to study A. W. Dow's[5] book on composition, and whenever he fails he at least knows why.

In tone composition our artistic photographers celebrate their greatest triumphs. Day, Käsebier, Keiley, and White are all ardent competitors for the harmony of tonal effects. I give the palm to Day and White; Day's tonal nuances in his portraits of Ethel Reed,[6] Mrs. Potter,[7] and some of his foreign types are so subtle and fugitive that any painter could be proud of them. I believe even Whistler would appreciate some of his prints in that respect. White's tonal schemes are managed with such delicacy of sentiment that they lend a peculiar poetic charm to all his work.

There is really not much else to say about composition in artistic photography—that is, of what is actually done. Volumes could be written about what should be done, but I doubt if it would do much good. As I have said before, every artist of any independence of thought must make his own laws of composition. The photographer must go outside his profession and enter the province of the painter. The wielders of the brush must be his teachers.

The great painters, in the course of their practice, have authorized a sort of conventional language of composition, which every photographer ought to know, and apply whenever he possibly can. You are astonished that I, who otherwise always clamor for individuality, give such advice. You argue that your originality would be sacrificed by the use of such conventionalism. Pardon me; do not. Authors of books use combinations of words which have been in use for centuries, and yet display their originality, when they have any. Do they not enhance the beauty of their style by such knowledge?

It is the same way with composition. It has certain qualities which are understood by all who have studied art. And it is wiser to express one's

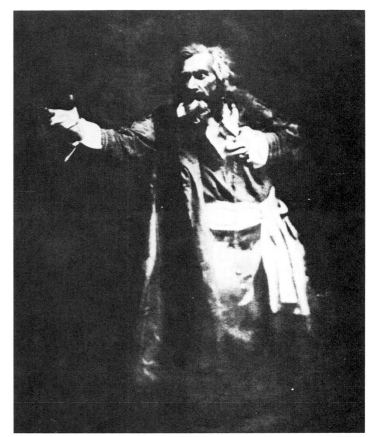

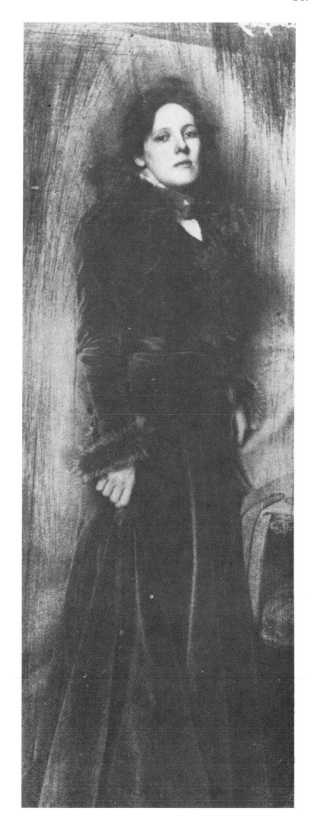

Above. JOSEPH T. KEILEY: Shylock, 1901. IMP-GEH.

Left. FRANK EUGENE: Miss Lillian.

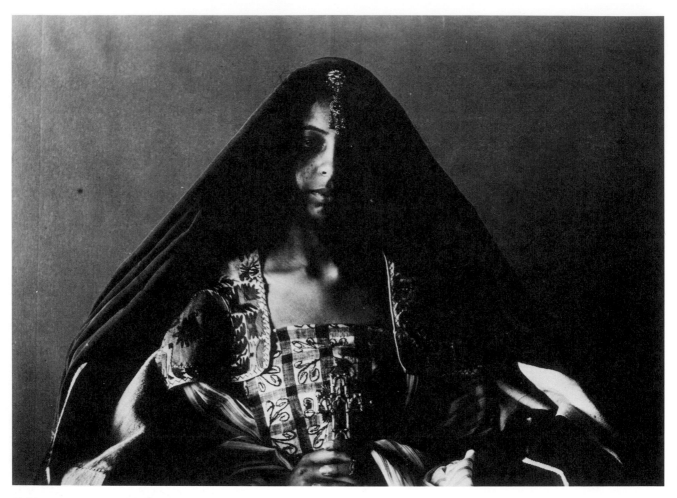

F. Holland Day: Study of Drapery. lc.

own ideas, with such modifications as may be necessary, in this language, than to make the vain attempt to form a new one, or to talk incoherently.

If you are still young and do not aspire as yet to be ranked among the artistic photographers, amuse yourself for a while in trying different methods. Should you ever feel a decided preference for one or the other, have faith in your preference, for it is suggested by your own mental constitution, and practice your selected method till you succeed in it.

Les photographistes arrives must work out their own salvation, for they won't listen any more to well-meaning advice; they know it all, or at least the largest part of it.

—1901

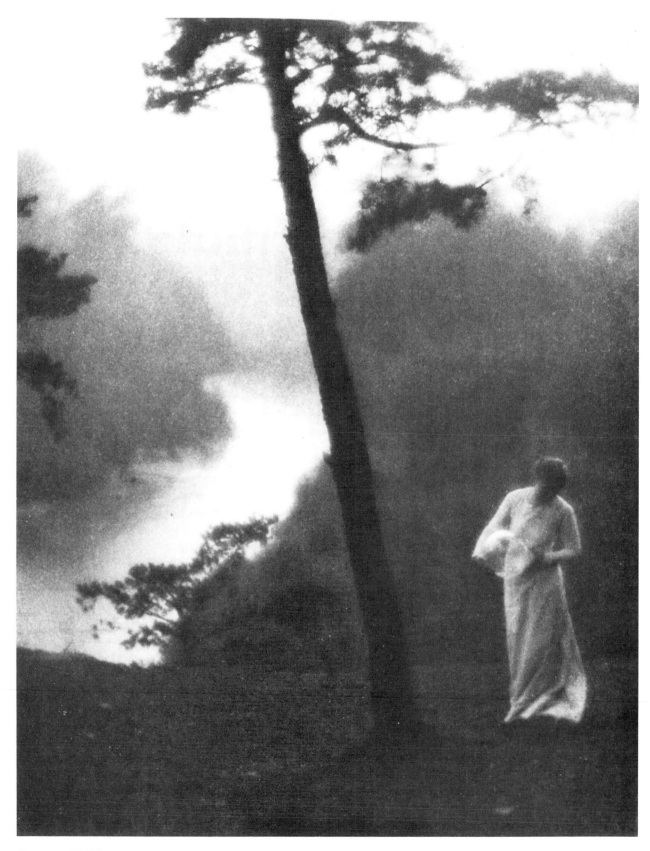

CLARENCE H. WHITE: Morning. IMP-GEH.

6

On Genre

GENRE SUBJECTS have always enjoyed more popularity with the general public than any other branch of the art of painting. The wielders of the brush however have always looked upon story telling in painting as something unworthy of the highest ideals of their profession. By this they do not altogether mean that minute study of details and exact presentation of facts make their productions conspicuously uninteresting as works of art, but rather that they lack those qualities which are associated with the most advanced phases of modern art.

This hatred for genre subjects has always seemed a rather futile agitation to me. Nobody with any pretense to taste will deny that those painters who devote the utmost care to the most insignificant objects (and who are still considered by the large majority the pillars of art, because their shortsightedness is relative to the ordinary seeing capacity of the crowd), are artistically inferior to those who master touch and technique, the problems of tone and color, and the decorative side of painting.

But how about the little Dutch Masters, who were genre painters in the strictest sense of the word, and who nevertheless understood to invest the true likeness of their subjects with a charm and fascination far beyond ordinary graphic powers and force of draftsmanship? And cannot also the paint-

ings of a Fortuny[1] and Knaus,[2] for instance, be defended on the same grounds?

You may say that such men are exceptions, that the harmonious concentration of vision, peculiar to them, lifts them above minor talents—painters like Defregger,[3] Vauthier,[4] and Mosler,[5] whose pictures are like pages torn from a popular novel. But if there are exceptions, the fault can hardly lie in the choice of subjects, and the question whether a genre painter paints artistically or not is reduced to a large extent to personal opinion.

Let us investigate this matter a little more closely. First of all, it will be necessary to ascertain of what material a genre picture is constituted, an extremely difficult problem, as it is well nigh impossible to draw the boundary lines with indisputable precision. The standards which guide the painters in their judgment have assumed no definite shape, they are mostly a matter of personal feeling and the traditional "ism" of some special school, and consequently not to be relied upon. Moreover they are full of paradoxes.

Take for instance a painter like Defregger. No matter how this painter might treat a group of peasants, we would classify his picture at once as *genre*. On the other hand if we are confronted with a peasant by the hand of Isräels[6] or Liebermann[7] we would hesitate and prefer to call their produc-

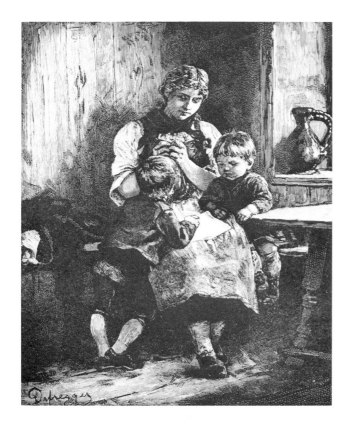

Left. FRANZ VON DEFREGGER: Sister and Brothers.

Below. MAX LIEBERMANN: Workers in the Beet Fields, 1876. Niedersächsisches Landesmuseum Hannover.

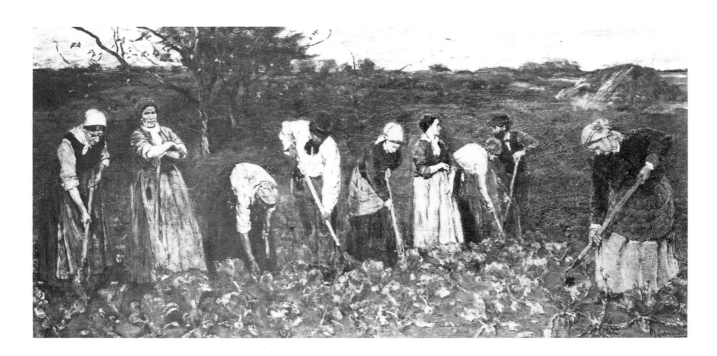

tion "a study." And yet there is in both the same careful study, the same striving to get at the secrets of certain types of humanity, the same desire to record completely and definitely their special traits.

The whole difference seems to lie in the conception, for it cannot be denied that both pictures tell a story. The one is told à la Dickens in a popular way, the other in the style of a writer of the modern realistic school, which may be some day just as popular as the other one.

But the problem is still more difficult. For how shall we classify a single finished figure of Meissonier[8] or Zamaçois![9] We might be inclined to call it a study, as long as the figure is merely placed against a background without any special occupation, while we would designate it as genre as soon as the figure is represented as playing chess, looking at a

piece of statuary, etc., or in other words approaching the anecdotal style of painting. On the other hand who would deny that the women of Stevens,[10] who are generally depicted in interiors and employed in one or another phase of domestic or social life, do not show the same subtle refinement and psychological insight as the ladies of Aman-Jean or Dewing, who sit in attitudes of pensive grace against backgrounds that are nothing else but color arrangements?

True enough, but Stevens is an exception, he is a psychologist and a colorist of the first order, somebody will argue. He is infatuated with anything feminine which suggests to him harmonies of tone, in which the richer color chords shine like the faint lustre of ancient gems in a twilight atmosphere.

If this argument holds good, then the subject is not the point at all, but the treatment alone.

THOMAS WILMER DEWING: In the Garden. Hartmann states in his unpublished autobiography that the painting represents three views of a woman he identified only as "Ruth," whom he met in Boston in 1888 and courted until his excessive ardor cooled her interest in him.

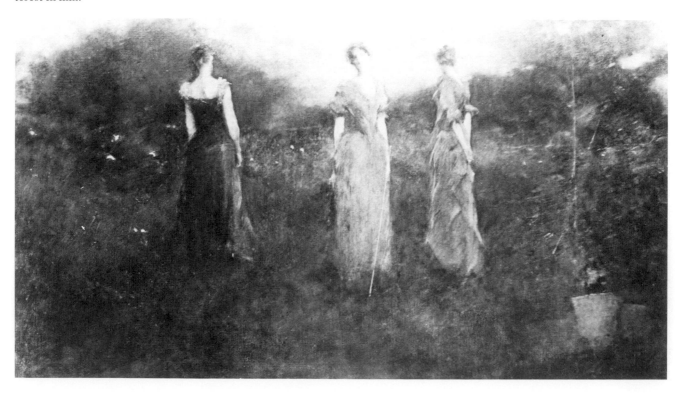

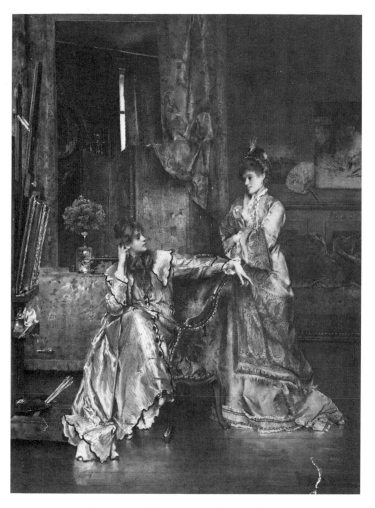

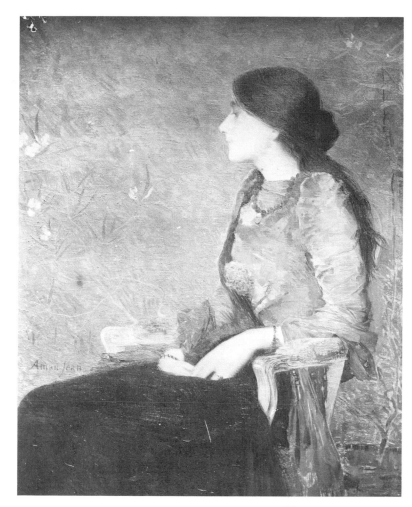

ALFRED STEVENS: The Visit. Sterling and Francine Clark Art Institute. Williamstown, Mass.

EDMOND AMAN-JEAN: Study. Photo N. D. Roger-Viollett.

Although story telling is, in my opinion, rather unaesthetic in the pictorial representation of human figures, as long as these are seen separately and individually and not *en masse*, as by the impressionist painter, I see no reason why genre subjects should be tabooed altogether, as it depends entirely on the way they are treated. In ideas Fortuny has hardly more to tell than Gérôme[11] for instance, but how differently he tells it! To him life is a masquerade, ebullient and capricious, where every detail glitters like a piece of jewel-clustered brocade. All that should be avoided in pedantic realism, which busies itself with every little thread stealing out of a buttonhole, and which can see only things detached in detail and not as a harmonious whole.

In artistic photography the situation is a similar one, the same fight is on and almost the same arguments could be used in regard to the works of Dumont,[12] Eickemeyer, Stirling,[13] White, Käsebier, and Steichen. However there is one difference. A painting, no matter how trivial or prosaic its subject may be, can still charm by technical qualities, in which certain characteristics of the artist may be reflected, while a photographic genre picture à la Defregger or Vauthier, no matter how cleverly composed is always hopelessly inartistic. It depends too largely on the models and their ability to pose, and to remain natural looking while a long studio exposure is taking place. It is almost a physical impossibility.

Eickemeyer's "The Dance" was a most ambitious attempt to overcome these difficulties; he had the proper models and studio outfits on hand, he thought out the composition night and day, altered it frequently, made study after study until he finally succeeded in getting a faultless picture from the photographic point of view. Artistically it is of no more interest than a reproduction of a painting by Diehlman.[14] The same might be said of White's "Ring Toss." The means of modification do not seem to be sufficient to generalize the facts which the camera tells with such unrelenting bluntness. The more artistic a photographer is, the more he will see in an object what he looks for, but the camera will never fail to remind him that there are forms in nature which the mind at the time did not perceive. A study of these two prints will give a fair estimate of the limitations of the photographer's craft. Elaborate genre scenes in which several figures are introduced are practically impossible, and to strain after effects like these means to invite failure and to join hands with mediocrity. One and two figure subjects lend themselves more easily to photographic treatment as Dumont and White have successfully proven, but their efforts are hardly more than finger posts in the right direction. They lack virility and *esprit,* and excite as pictures hardly more than a passing interest.

Steichen and Eugene are as far as I know the only ones who might possibly succeed in discovering and expressing in photographic genre some of that "painter" element which we admire in the works of Liebermann or Isräels. For those who are not initiated into the painter's technique it very much resembles the pursuit of the impossible, an occupation which they should leave to people of less discretion than they are supposed to possess.

—1902

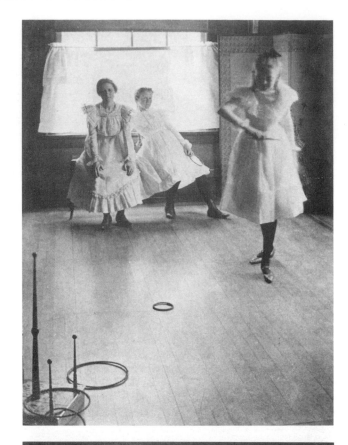

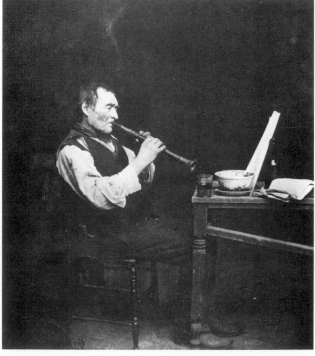

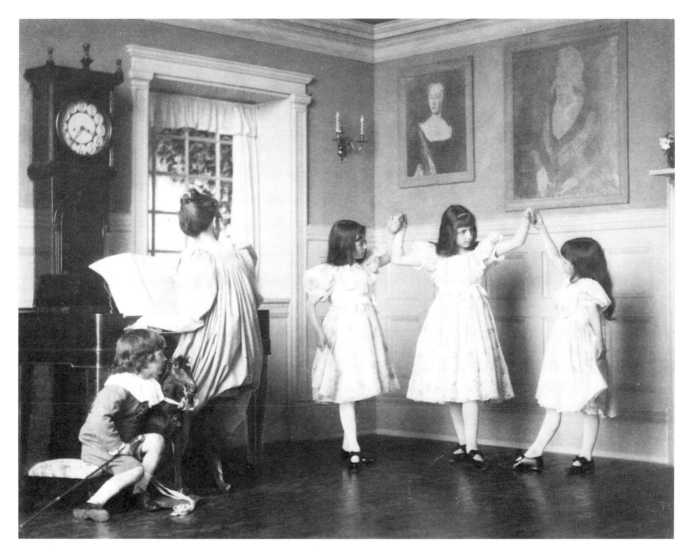

Above. RUDOLF EICKEMEYER, JR.: Dancing Lesson. SI.

Opposite page top. CLARENCE H. WHITE: Ring Toss. IMP-GEH.

Opposite page bottom. JOHN E. DUMONT: Clarinet Player. IMP-GEH.

7

A Photographic Enquête

Ever since i became interested in artistic photography—which is now more than six or seven years ago—I have been curious to gather the opinions of artists on the aims and methods of the new graphic art, and often during studio visits broached the subject instead of other current topics. I found the large majority rather ignorant of the subject, as they are to this day. They knew very little of what had been accomplished in recent years, and only in rare cases knew anything about individual workers—Mrs. Käsebier, on account of her showcase on Fifth Avenue, being perhaps the best known.

To most of them—the illustrative in particular—it still seems impossible to disassociate photography from the prevailing ideas, that it can claim nothing—interesting as it may be from many points of view—but the virtues of a mechanical industry. They are apt to attribute every artistic effect to the mechanism of the camera and to accident, and entirely to overlook those points which in fairness should be allowed to be due to personal influence of the worker and the direct control of a tool which otherwise would take a different direction. The opinion of such men, indoctrinated with the fixed idea that nothing higher, nothing better is capable of being done by the photographer, can be of but little value to the profession and will not be

mentioned on this occasion, although I have fought them in many a bitter battle.

The sole object of this photographic *enquête*—as I may call it—is to state the opinions of such artists as are capable of receiving an innovation without prejudice, or who at least feel that the recent efforts of artistic photography involve a claim which is honestly put forward, and deserve at least an honest and impartial examination.

The selection was difficult. Artists are, as a rule, not very good talkers. What can one do for instance with a man who has nothing but ejaculations, like "This is a bird," or "That's a peach," for words of approval! And those who express their opinions more fluently are often mediocrities, and therefore hardly desirable for quotation.

My choice has fallen on those of our leading sculptors and painters who had something individual to say, even if they treated the subject of photography with the amused condescension of men whose conception of art seems outraged by "so much resemblance and yet so great a difference."

I generally jotted down our conversations a few hours after they had taken place, and can therefore in most cases vouch for the correct wording (with the exception of course of awkward or unquotable mannerisms of speech). I also must mention that I often found it necessary to show them my portfolio of prints (containing the work of Ben-Yúsuf, Käsebier, Stieglitz, Eickemeyer, Day, White, Eugene, Steichen, and others) in order to get them interested and to put them in the mood to talk on the subject.

Fragments of the various conversations with commentary notes follow at random:

D. C. French,[1] the sculptor, is one of the few who is in absolute sympathy with the movement. His appreciation of artistic photography is long standing and he seems to realize the excellence of some of the work accomplished. Several prints decorate the walls of his studio, and I remember him saying years ago, when my knowledge was still rather limited, "that photography of this kind should be cultivated, for it was undoubtedly of great assistance in promoting the study of nature and in fostering a sound artistic taste."

Recently he rather amused me by saying, while turning over the prints of my portfolio: "No wonder that these men do such good work. I understand they are nearly all men of leisure, who photograph for a pastime. They have no cares, and have to make no effort to *please*. They do not seem to care a rap for the opinions of the public. That is delightful! And as for the mechanism of photography, of which people talk so much, I don't think it can be compared with that of sculpture. Think of the casting and recasting, the construction of skeleton forms and of iron pipes, etc., and all the dirt connected with it. There is mechanism enough for you. The photographers surely get their effects much more easily."

G. G. Barnard,[2] the talented disciple of Rodin, an idealist of the first water, who always clamors for high art in his conversations, was rather evasive at the start in expressing an opinion.

"I have not given more than a passing attention to the graphic arts." But when I pressed him he ejaculated, with a faint smile on his lips, "What does it all amount to! It must be awful for you to write about such things. Yes, there may be certain beauties of tone, now and then a pleasing picture; but what of that! *Cela n'en vout pas la peine.* Have they made any pictures of lasting value? What does not remain in one's memory and insist on being permanent is not worth remembering. They imitate and do not get beyond the elementary considerations of type, composition and detail. I really do not see any chance to do great work in that line. You say they are honest and sincere in their efforts. These are merits that I appreciate. Perhaps a sculptor could after all learn something from them."

"Yes, to be sure, they do clever work," remarked W. M. Chase[3] to me in his studio at Boussod Valadon, the walls of which are lined with stacks of pictures of which comparatively few are his own, and which make it look as if the great technician was as much an art dealer as a painter. "Look at these photographs by an amateur, a Miss F_____, are they not wonderful? This one looks just like a Velasquez. They are full of suggestion."

"But this technique is abominable," I interjected, "The young lady knows nothing about developing nor printing."

"That may be, but they are artistic nevertheless, and without any pretense of being called works of art. Photography of that sort is a great help to a painter. You probably are aware that Lenbach never painted a portrait without the help of photography."

"But do you not think that a photograph itself can be a work of art?"

"Oh! awfully clever work is done, no doubt; but I would make this discrimination; I would call them artistic and not works of art. And I for my part prefer unpretentious amateur work. Take for instance the case of the young lady. She enjoys making her photographs and her family and her friends enjoy them; it improves the taste all around, and even an artist can look at them with benefit.

Photographers in my opinion should rest content with being amateurs, and they have a pretty wide field before them without extending the sphere of their activities."

"I want to have your opinion on artistic photography," I said to F. S. Church,[4] the painter of the "Surf Phantom," the last time I called upon him. Laughingly he rejoined, "I know nothing of the subject, I know only the more I study painting the more ignorant I feel. But so much I can say in favor of photography that whenever I open a magazine I like those pictures best which are photographs. That is, as long as they reproduce actualities; for instance, scenes of the Boer war. No illustration can touch them. Every photograph means something, tells you something, instructs you; the illustrator merely gives you some imaginative fancy, which in such cases, where you want to know the truth, is absolutely valueless."

"But that is merely the lowest form of art, similar to reporting. What do you think of the chances of the camera for imaginative work?"

"I think the process too mechanical for a successful realization of the picturesque fancies of an artist. This would take away the power of the artist to give shape to his own convictions and to present them in persuasive guise, and would make the efforts of the artist photographer ineffectual. To expose his imaginings to the uncertainties of a mechanical process would be to destroy their credibility, to make them affectations."

"You mean you could not photograph a picture like your 'Surf Phantom.'"

"Nor a picture like Ryder's[5] 'Flying Dutchman.' You may depend on that."

"Of course they can only do certain things. But you can't deny that the works of a White or a Käsebier show a decided imaginative strain?"

"I won't deny that, they have talent. But it also takes talent to be a good shoemaker—which is perhaps more satisfactory, as he can realize what he wants to do. The photographer can't, and the more artistic talent he has, the less he can realize. The subjects which the camera can master are mightily limited, I fear."

Childe Hassam,[6] the impressionist and street painter *par excellence,* took great pleasure in looking over my collection.

"It is astonishing what they do. But at the same time I can't comprehend why they strive so much for high finish. Photography surely could produce impressionistic scenes more easily than they can be rendered in other mediums. The camera is so inaccurate in its work. Think only of the chances of accidents, often marvelously artistic. I do not say this because I am an impressionist myself, but because the camera has the advantage, that its reproduction of instantaneousness—there is a work like that, isn't there—is mechanical."

George de Forest Brush[7] I met one day when he was just leaving the house with his two eldest children to take them to the circus.

"What have you there?" he asked, pointing to my portfolio. I handed it to him, he looked it over hastily on the stoop, then handing it back to me we walked down the street together, and he said:

"These are queer times. Perhaps we shall have to accept new ideals of beauty. Maybe the East River bridges will be aesthetically attractive to the man of the coming generation as the Parthenon appeared all-sufficient to our forefathers, and that the convention of monochrome will be deemed more satisfying than painting."

"Yes, it is a risky thing to speculate on a contemporary's chance of future fame," I remarked.

"To-day is essentially a time when mean things are done so finely that future ages may refer to it as a period when the minor arts attracted the genius and energy diverted, by modesty or timidity, from heroic enterprises. So as we collect Whistler's lithographs, and pay thousands for a piece of porcelain or some other article, it may be other ages will pass by our pictures and poems with a smile of contempt, and collect artistic photographs such as these with keen interest. And nature, who is herself perfect in trifles as in entities, is not wholly wronged thereby. But there is my car; we will talk another time more about it, I hope."

With D. W. Tryon[8] I had several conversations on the subject. These are some of the things he said:

"Eugene knows how to get color, but he absolutely lacks repose. Some of his portraits are more interesting than any I have seen in the recent painters' exhibitions, but that doesn't say much, as most of these are so ridiculously bad."

Then referring to Day's, White's, and Käsebier's work: "I don't see why they reproduce such unsympathetic types. There is no spirituality and but little intelligence in them. It is a real conspiracy of ugliness. I also do not like their modes of modification. Photography surely aims at something else than draftsmanship and all which that word implies. And yet I do not fancy the ordinary photograph either. Do you remember Leighton's tree studies? In them no detail was stinted, nothing skimped, from the stem to the uttermost leaf; every part in succession records equal interest, and yet the whole is not devoid of a large quality which brings it together in a harmonious whole, so that it is as much the study of a tree as the study of each separate item composing one. Photography can't do that.

"Every good artist fully appreciates the value of different mediums. The photographer has one decided advantage, he gets at the very start so much what we artists can only gain by strenuous work. But that is perhaps also his greatest drawback. He can only retouch what he has on hand. He cannot gradually grow into the subject, and imbue it with a strong personal note. He has no equivalent for the individual touch of the artist, to make the arm, the wrist, the finger-tips do what the eyes see and the soul dictates from minute to minute, from day to day until the ideal is realized. The artist is, above all else, very human; herein lies his great charm. The photographer can never be in such perfect sympathy with his subject as the artist.

"I always considered it possible that some day the dislike of color may grow so strong—from a too subtle perception of it—that artists, despairing of ever putting down the light and vibration of natural color, will prefer to leave it to the imagination of students of their work. A new graphic art would be necessary for that, but I do not think that photography could ever take that place. Photographs seen in masses, even the very best, are awfully fatiguing, for they all lack subtlety, they never *vibrate*."

With Thomas W. Dewing, who as a painter of women has no rival, unless it be the famous delineator of feminine charms, Alfred Stevens—I had one of the hottest arguments.

"Do not these points demonstrate that beauty of form, color, design, and draftsmanship, exquisite balance of line arrangement, and consummate skill of handling, are all possible in a photograph?" I argued, trying to be as enthusiastic as possible.

"What you have shown me to-day is more promising than anything I have seen before. But, hang it, it is the model that does everything in photography. It is surely clever arrangement; that is all it amounts to. If you have a model that knows how to move, you can make a good picture—there you are!"

"But do not you also need a special type of model for your pictures?" I queried, throwing a side glance at his model, one of those long-necked ethereal looking girls of thirty, which he never grows tired of painting.

"Naturally, but the photographer cannot get away from his model; he will always get something which will resemble the model, a *banale* inaccurate likeness, so to speak, while I merely use one as a suggestion. No, I don't admire pictures that simply look like something because the photographer happens to know a good looking model. The true artist gets his effects he does not know how."

"But if a man like Whistler would take to photography?" I asked.

"He might do something; but it is absurd. A man like Whistler would never have the patience to photograph. And if he had bothered with photography, when he was a young man, he would never have become a Whistler afterwards. The practice of photography would induce a man to shirk certain duties, as to make life studies, etc. But a Whistler would have done something original and not imitated paintings, the old masters. Don't they know better? It is a dangerous play that has wasted the time of painters for about two centuries."

"But you like some of these pictures, you said so yourself a few minutes ago."

"Yes, they show taste, they are clever—they are better than the pictures of many artists—but they are just like reproductions on the surface, dead! You know yourself that they do not suggest any emotions or recall any memories of past experiences, of love, poetic thoughts, etc. They have nothing new to say, so they look at a landscape or pose a beautiful model and think they have done something wonderful."

"They at least help to improve public taste," I argued.

"Nonsense! Hang the educational value business altogether," exclaimed Mr. Dewing, impatiently. "We've heard enough of that kind of rot lately to last us for the rest of our natural lives. What is the value of art, anyhow? Nothing but the pleasure of making it. If it gives them pleasure to make such stuff, well and good."

"Then what do you think a photographer should photograph?"

"Real life. All that the painter cannot do or only with great difficulty. Likenesses not only of faces, but of the actual forms. Movement, character, energy, all that which the realistic painters depict, subjects which really have no longer any place in painting. They could render the prosaic phases in a more artistic manner. The ordinary illustrations raised to a higher standard, that is what their aim should be, and it is a very high one. They could make it a true art, which everybody had to admire, and which would in no way interfere with imaginative art, which is the domain of poetry and painting."

—1902

8

The Influence of Artistic Photography on Interior Decoration

THE ELABORATE way in which the artistic photographers mount and frame their prints has attracted attention everywhere and called forth critical comment, favorable as well as the reverse, from various quarters. Nobody can deny that they go about it in a conscientious, almost scientific manner, and that they usually display a good deal of taste; but the general opinion seems to be that they attach too much importance to a detail which, although capable of enhancing a picture to a remarkable degree, can do but little toward improving its quality. The artistic photographers differ on this point. They argue that a picture is only finished when it is properly trimmed, mounted, and framed, and that the whole effect of print, mounts or mat, signature, and frame, should be an artistic one, and the picture be judged accordingly.

This is a decided innovation. In painting, frames only serve as "boundary lines" for a pictorial presentation, similar to those to which we are subjected in looking at a fragment of life out of an ordinary window.

The frame clearly defines the painter's pictorial vision, and concentrates the interest upon his canvas, even to such an extent that all other environments are forgotten. At least, such was the original idea. But it seems that we have grown oversensitive in this respect; we would also like to see the frame harmonize with the tonal values of

the picture it encloses. But up to date, very little has been done in this direction. The official exhibitions still insist on the usual monotony of gold frames, and the painters seem to have neither any particular inclination nor the opportunity to create frames of lovely forms and well-balanced repeating patterns of their own. The frame-makers and art-dealers are masters of the situation, and their interests are strictly commercial ones.

"Attractive enough at first sight; hopelessly inartistic on further inspection," is the verdict which one has to give of the average frame of to-day. Tryon,[1] Dewing,[2] and Horatio Walker[3] are the only painters I know who seriously oppose the mechanically manufactured picture-frames. They have their frames specially designed for each picture—Stanford White[4] being the designer of quite a number of them. Their frames are wide and flat without corners and centerpieces; the repeating pattern is generally a simple, classic ornament, with a tendency toward vertical lines. The coloring is gold, but tinted and glazed by the painter himself until it corresponds with the color keynote of the special picture the frame was designed for. This method will undoubtedly find favor with many of the younger men, but a radical change can not take place until the despotic "framing" rules of exhibitions have been abolished.

The artistic photographers, on the other hand, had no rules to adhere to. All they wanted were artistic accessories for their prints. They could allow their imagination full sway. They obeyed every impulse and whim, and indulged in any scheme as long as it was practical and specially adapted to the print for which it was planned. Every frame was made to order; they ransacked the frame-maker's workshops for new ideas and revolutionized the whole trade. The result was much that was bizarre and overfastidious (some photographers apparently mistook their packing paper mounts for sample-books of paper warehouses), but also a fair average of sterling quality was produced. The mounting and framing of the leading artistic photographers of America was simple, tasteful, and to the point; they go far ahead in this respect of all other black-and-white artists, and can proudly claim that they are the best mounters and frame-makers of the world.

Their style is largely built up on Japanese principles. The Japanese never use solid elevated "boundary lines" to isolate their pictures, but on the contrary try to make the picture merely a note of superior interest in perfect harmony with the rest of the kakemono,[5] which again is in perfect harmony with the wall on which it is placed. The Japanese artist simply uses strips of beautifully patterned cloth to set off the picture, and endeavors to accentuate its lines and color-notes by the mounting and the momentary environments, which is easy enough, as the mounting is generally so artistically done that it fits in anywhere. (I refer, of course, only to Japanese homes.) Pictures in Japan are merely regarded as bits of interior decoration. The Japanese art-patron does not understand our way of hanging pictures in inadequate surroundings; he does not disregard the technical merits of a picture (which is to us always the most important point); on the contrary, he is very sensitive to them, but he always subordinates them to his inherent ideas of harmony. He would never hang a picture if it did not harmonize with the color of his screens, the form of his lacquer cabinet, etc.

The artistic photographers try to be like the Japanese in this respect. They endeavor to make their prints bits of interior decoration. A Käsebier print, a dark silhouette on green wall-paper in a greenish frame, or a Steichen print mounted in cool browns and grays, cannot be hung on any ordinary wall. They are too individual; the rest of the average room would jar with their subtle color-notes. They need special wall-paper and special furniture to reveal their true significance.

That is where the esthetic value of the photographic print comes in. It will exercise a most palpable influence on the interior decoration of the future. People will learn to see that a room need not be overcrowded like a museum in order to make an artistic impression, that the true elegance lies in simplicity, and that a wall fitted out in green and gray burlap, with a few etchings or photographs, after Botticelli or other old masters, in dark frames is as beautiful and more dignified than yards of imitation gobelins or repoussé leather tapestry hung from ceiling to floor with paintings in heavy golden frames.

We have outgrown the bourgeois beauty of Rogers[6] statuettes, and are tired of seeing Romney[7] backgrounds in our portraits and photographs. The elaborate patterns of Morris[8] have given way to wall-paper of one uniform color, and modern furniture is slowly freeing itself from the influence of former historic periods and trying to construct a style of its own, based on lines which nature dictates. Whistler and Alexander have preached the very same lesson in the backgrounds of their portraits. Everywhere in their pictures we encounter the thin black line of the oblong frame which plays such an important part in the interior decoration of to-day, and which invariably conveys a delightful division of space.

The artistic photographer has elaborated on the black frame and white mat. He has created in his frame innumerable harmonies of color, form, and material, and if there shall ever be a demand for them, and if they shall ever serve as suggestions for interior decoration, we shall surely be able to steer clear of monotony; for I must confess that if the majority of rooms were furnished in the Whistler fashion (as suggested in "His Mother" and "Carlyle"), it would be as unbearable as the present museum style.

Also, the advanced professional photographers, slowly falling in with the steps of the artistic photographers, help the cause. The former way of mounting photographs on stiff board, which could only be put in albums or bric-á-brac frames on mantelpieces, etc., had no artistic pretense about it whatever. Their present way, mounting the print on large gray sheets of paper with rough edges and overlapping covers is really nothing but an invitation to buy a frame for the print and hang it on the wall. The professional print has acquired a pictorial significance.

But it is, after all, an open question whether these efforts will be crowned with success. We are too much interested in the utilitarian equipments of our homes ever to give, as the Japanese do, first consideration to harmony. And harmony, perfect harmony, is necessary to adapt their style of interior decoration successfully, the elaborate details of which in turn are lost in the background, which is impossible with our present system of house-building. As long as door-jambs and window-sills and mantelpieces are manufactured wholesale, and as long as our rooms are infested with stereotype chandeliers, registers, etc., a burlap-wall, with a few "Secession" prints will not save us. And to go to the extreme, as some esthetes are apt to do—and they have to go to extremes from our view-point— will always be regarded as an eccentric, visionary accomplishment.

I personally have never been sensitive to my surroundings; I like a general harmony of effect, but would tire of any room that carried out a distinct line- or color-scheme, and I would find it rather ridiculous to build a special sanctuary for a Whistler etching, a Dewing silver print, or a Steichen print. In Japan, furniture is scant and the interiors of the houses generally kept in a neutral tint, to which the details lend the color-notes. If our interiors were as simple and artistic as the Japanese ones, we should have a good basis to work on. As it is, the photographic prints are finger-posts in the right direction. Whether we can pursue the indicated path to the very end is a question which the future has to decide.

—1903

9

Repetition With Slight Variation

THE QUESTION, "What is the leading characteristic of Japanese painting?" has often been put to me, and I have invariably answered, "Repetition with slight variation."

Of course, there are other qualities to consider, as the peculiar color-distribution, the calligraphic dexterity of brush-work, the willful neglect or exaggeration of detail, the grotesque division of space, and the economic manipulation of backgrounds which apparently look empty and yet enhance the pictorial aspect of the picture to a rare degree. But more important than any of these peculiarities of composition seems to me to be their laws of repetition with slight variation, because a composition of that order possesses the two principal elements of pictorial art: It is decorative and yet true to life. Its object is not to execute a perfect imitation of reality (only bad works of art do that) or a poetic resemblance of life (as our best painters produce), but merely a commentary on some pictorial vision which sets the mind to think and dream.

If the Japanese artist wants to depict a flight of cranes, he draws half a dozen or more which at the first glance look alike, but which on closer scrutiny are each endowed with an individuality of their own. He foregoes perspective and all other expedients; he simply represents them in clear outlines in a diagonal line or sweeping curve on an empty background, and relies for his effect upon the repetition of forms. A Western artist would have

expanded this at least into a picture with a landscape or cloud effect as background; to the Japanese artist, working in the narrow bounds prescribed by custom and taste, any such attempt would appear futile; he knows that such an event can not be expressed more forcibly than by simply depicting the objects with only a slight variation in their representation.

The first form introduces us to the subject, its appearance, and action; the second accentuates the same impression and heightens the feeling of reality by the slight variation in the appearance and action; and every following form resembling, at the first glance, a silhouette is simply a commentary upon the preceding one; and all together represent, so to say, a multiplication of the original idea.

And in the same manner as they respect lines and masses, they vary color-schemes, which often resemble each other, but are nevertheless endlessly varied in shade and line. The French illustrators and the German designers of the "Secessionist" School[1] have *adopted* this method with considerable success. The painters, however, have been rather reluctant about following their example. They probably realize that their plastic style of painting would not harmonize with the idea of repetition, which is strictly decorative and specially adapted to flat-surface work.

I know of only two men who have successfully adapted this law in their composition and created something like a new style. They are Puvis de Chavannes,[2] and D. W. Tryon,[3] the American landscape-painter. Both, however, were wise enough to avoid repetition in a diagonal direction or in a curve arrangement. Chavannes, in his mural painting, is very fond of the parallelism of vertical lines. Not only the trees, but also his human figures are constructed in that fashion. His aim is to express dignity and repose, and nothing can accomplish it better than an architectonic arrangement of vertical lines, as, for instance, in his "L'Hiver."

Chavannes composes at *largo* while Tryon is satisfied with *adagios* and *andantes*. The latter was addicted for years to the parallelism of horizontal lines. Undoubtedly he went a step in the right direction, as the principal line-idea in all natural scenery is necessarily horizontal, and a painted landscape, where this parallelism is accentuated and elaborately worked out (balanced by vertical-line work and oval shapes), will convey the idea of vastness and level expansion more readily than those in whose composition a horizontal monotony of lines has been neglected.

In artistic photography I have not yet encountered any attempt at repetition with slight variation, and I would advise no one to take it up without devoting some profound study to it, and even then I believe it should only be utilized when life or nature spontaneously suggests it. I do not believe that it can be forced into photography without looking forced; but that the photographers have to decide for themselves. Whoever wants to make a study of it must learn to appreciate its various ways of application, and thereby get down to the very essence of its esthetic value, will find ample opportunity, not only in painting, but also in the other arts.

In musical composition it is very frequent. The

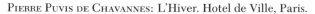

PIERRE PUVIS DE CHAVANNES: L'Hiver. Hotel de Ville, Paris.

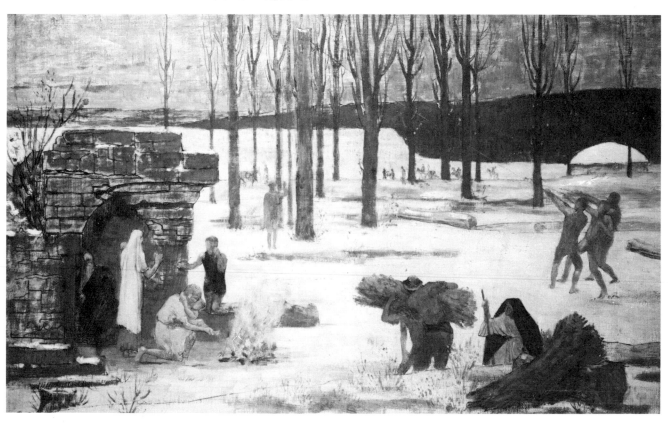

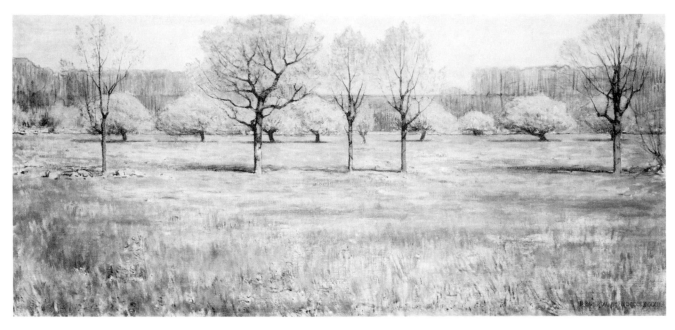

DWIGHT WILLIAMS TRYON: Untitled. Freer Gallery of Art.

pieces which treat variations of one theme are innumerable. In Western literature we find it in the refrains of ballads, in Poe's poems, and the work of the French symbolists, and above all else in the writings of Maurice Maeterlinck,[4] this quaint combination of Greek, medieval, and Japanese art reminiscences. In architecture it has always been one of the leading elements, only with the difference that in Western architecture everything has to be subservient to symmetry, while the Eastern world also recognizes (at least in the ornaments) the right of unsymmetrical composition. In the Gothic style one can study the parallelism of diagonal line, and in the Baroque and Rococo the repetition of curves. In dancing, the arrangement of a ballet, nearly everything depends on repetition; many figures are nothing but repetition *without* variation. The performers themselves substitute the lack of too frequent changes in movement and action.

Even the variety stage affords at times good opportunities for study. I realized it when I saw the Barrison Sisters.[5] They were an object lesson that should have interested any student of art. There were five pretty, gay ladies of fascinating leanness

and awkwardness *a la* Chavannes, who could neither dance nor sing, but who, simply having been drilled by a manager to expound in coquettish movements and attitudes a French-Japanese code of frivolity, unconsciously expressed the Japanese law of repetition with slight variation. But no other American critic at the time dwelt upon their esthetic values, and I may, after all, have been mistaken in my judgment.

Nature and every-day life, of course, are in this instance past-masters. One only has to keep one's eyes open to discover the raw material which the artist utilizes.

But there is still another side to the question—at least from the Eastern point of view. Not only the composition of Japanese artists is guided by the law of repetition, but also their inventive power. As inexhaustible as it seems, one will find that they have always treated a certain line of subjects. For instance, they have painted a crow sitting on a snow-covered fir-branch with the full moon behind a thousand times; but every painter who has handled the subject has tried to lend it a new individuality. Only the subject remains the same;

treatment and conception are invariably charged with the personality of the artist.

We Occidentals do not seem to be capable of this; our aim is above all else to be original; like Richard III, we roam through the fields of art and say: "An original idea! An original idea! My life for an original idea!" forgetting that originality does not consist of something that has never been done before, but rather in new ways of expression. And nothing tends more to the very opposite of the conventional and commonplace than to find a new variation of an old subject. Thousands of mother-and-child pictures have been painted by the old masters, but artists like de Forest Brush,[6] Abbot Thayer,[7] Tompkins,[8] and Mary Cassatt[9] have understood how to lend the time-worn subject a new note of interest.

The craze for originality is really the curse of our art, as it leads nearly always to conventionalism and mannerism. The artistic accomplishments of the Japanese are due largely to the fact of their never-tiring study of variation. They have realized that a beautiful idea always remains a beautiful idea, and that it takes as much creative power to lend a new charm to an old theme as to produce and execute an apparently new one, which, after all, may prove an old one.

—1903

10

The Photo-Secession Exhibition at the Carnegie Art Galleries, Pittsburgh, Pa.

WHEN TWO YEARS ago (it is hard to believe that it is only two years) a few artistic photographers founded the Secession, the outsiders—largely the profession, a few artists, and that small part of the public interested in photographic matters—smiled rather incredulously at the attempt and wisely shook their heads and offered all sorts of cheap advice. Love's labor lost, they thought; that might do for painters, etchers, wood-engravers, but for photographers—ridiculous!

But the Secessionists were not to be discouraged; they listened to no advice; they had convictions and persevered. Then came their first exhibition at the National Arts Club, at New York, which taught such a practical lesson to many a publisher, painter, and art-student. "It has met with success simply because of its novelty," the wiseacres remarked, "but wait awhile! It is just like a new play, everybody wants to see it merely to talk about it, then the interest will cease."

What have all these now to say after the triumph of the Secession ideas at the Corcoran Art Gallery in Washington and at the Carnegie Art Galleries in Pittsburgh?[1] Will they still be able to find excuses, or will they suddenly, as is usually the case in such matters, come over to the enemy's camp, proudly asseverating that they have fully believed, from the very start, in the principles of this movement.

Fortunately the Secessionists care little for pop-ular approval, insisting upon works, not faith, and believing that their share having been done in producing the work, the public must now do the rest. A few friends, and these of understanding mind, a few true appreciators, this is all they expect and all they desire.

The Photo-Secession Exhibition at Pittsburgh is indisputably the most important and complete pictorial photographic exhibition ever held in this country. I must confess to no special fondness for the ordinary run of photographic exhibitions, but the Pittsburgh show is so far superior to anything of its kind I have ever seen before, that I consider it a privilege to have viewed it and to have found real pleasure in my task of studying it. With exception of the background, which was red in color and dilapidated in appearance—a state of affairs over which the Secession had, unfortunately, no control—the arrangement, the lighting of the galleries, which concentrated the light upon the pictures and left all else in semi-darkness, was particularly effective and seemed incapable of improvement. The hanging, at best a thankless task, was done with untiring energy and exquisite taste by Mr. Joseph T. Keiley. The exhibit is exceedingly well grouped; the framing of the pictures up to the usual high standard; and the catalogues arranged by Stieglitz himself, especially the illustrated edition de luxe with cover-design by Steichen, which contained seven gravures, may all be regarded as models of good taste.

Thanks to those who selected the collection, fully two-thirds of the exhibit of three hundred frames is of a superior kind, masterpieces, of course, being as scarce here as everywhere.

Nearly all of the pictures contained some artistic note that lifted them above the commonplace. The exhibition was national in its character, fifty-four photographers being represented. Only Day, Lee,[2] Maurer,[3] and Genthe, for some reason or another, could or would not participate. The large bulk of the exhibit was by the members of the Secession.

Photo-Secession! The outsider is generally startled at the name; he does not know the exact meaning of the word nor in what way it is applied to this class of energetic and enthusiastic workers. People wonder what the Secessionists really want, and yet their aim is such a simple one. They want to be artistic, that is all. They want to see their work classed as an art; but this is only a secondary consideration, as recognition can not be forced; it must come by itself. Their first and last aim is to do artistic work.

Why, then, all this mockery, noise, and opposition? Because it is a fight, after all. It is a fight of modern ideas against tradition, or, more modestly expressed, a fight for a new technique. I am convinced that the better class of photographers also want to be artistic, not quite as much as the Secessionists, but to their best understanding. The whole trouble is that the two parties can't agree on the mediums of expression. It is a fight about conception, theory, and temperament. And the Secessionists, even if they accomplish nothing but the improvement of the average standard of photographic work, will remain victors, because they are more sincere and are willing to sacrifice everything to reach their end.

It sometimes seems to me as if this fight were not at all about esthetics, as the Secessionists seem willing to accept almost anything, so long as it contains a spark of artistic merit. They object only

to such commercial work as is produced for no other purpose than to suit a sitter or a publisher. They wish to be independent artists and not time-pleasing speculators. That was really the cause of their revolt. And the Secession was created for no other purpose than to foster and cultivate this genuine art feeling, which must be found at the root of every work of art.

The best which the exhibition had to offer, and so far as my personal feelings are concerned the best which the Secession has produced, are the prints of Steichen. None can deny his power. He stands in a class by himself. That which he shows us is not always photography, but it invariably belongs to the domain of art. He sacrifices everything to painter-like qualities and conception as well as treatment, and with astonishing precision he realizes the ideas which he wishes to convey. Like a

EDWARD STEICHEN: In Memoriam, 1904. MOMA.

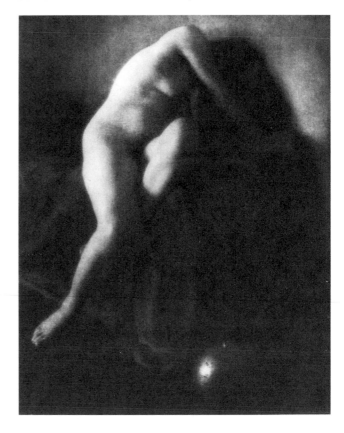

highwayman he lies in wait for beauty, seizes her, and drags her away as she passes. He steps straight into her path and, like an *Espada* whose reputation would be lost had he to make a second thrust, he settles the whole question with one clever stroke. To him life is a sojourn in darkness, illuminated by innumerable streaks of lightning. These he tries to grasp. Every object he endeavors to imbue with beauty, and even the simplest, a vessel or a branch of flowers, sets him to dreaming about some big artistic problem, and he at once makes the effort to transform it into a pictorial revelation.

Just his very opposite is Joseph T. Keiley. He, too, sees the beauty of detail, but finds it so beautiful in itself that he forgets all artistic possibilities. He lingers over details so long and lovingly and discovers such a wealth of beauty in them that he grows confused. When he photographs a beautiful

woman, he hesitates to show her in the full bloom of her youth, but tries to subdue her charms. And as beauty must be wooed in a more ardent fashion, she often evades so cold a lover; but when he succeeds in holding her she reveals herself in one of the most tender moods. His work conveys an effect like the ringing of an old church-bell. A deep, mysterious sound in the bass and above it a very light ethereal one, so fugitive that it seems to vanish at every moment. His "Spring," Corot-like and evanescent like spring itself, plainly sounds these two notes and is one of the gems of the exhibition.

Stieglitz, as usual, holds his own. His older work seems just as strong and interesting as it did years ago, and nearly every picture he adds comes near to being a masterpiece. In his "Hand of Man" he shows that he is still the same accomplished artist as in "The Net-Mender," "Watching for the Return,"

JOSEPH T. KEILEY: Spring. IMP-GEH.

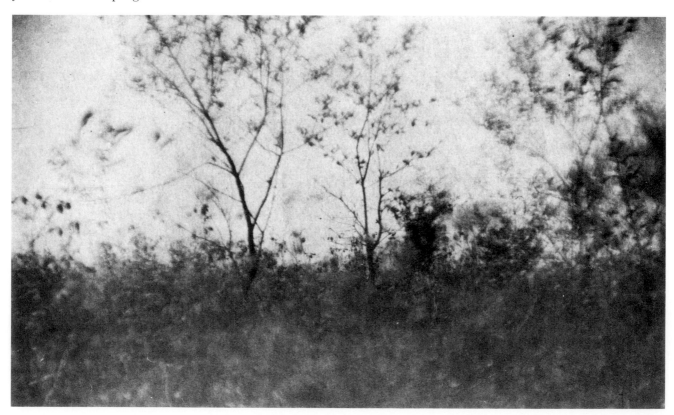

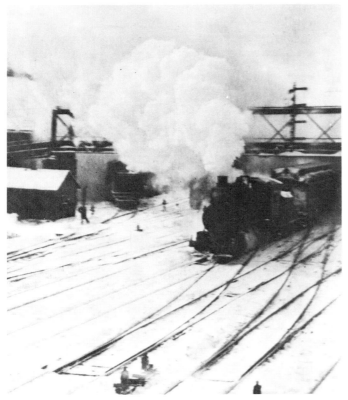

Left. ALFRED STIEGLITZ: Untitled (Variant of "The Hand of Man"), 1910. Collection of Eleanor and Van Deren Coke.

Below. ALFRED STIEGLITZ: The Hand of Man, Long Island City, New York, 1902. IMP-GEH.

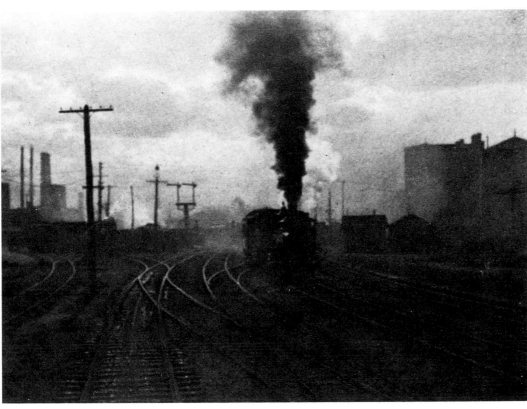

and "Winter on Fifth Avenue." In it he betrays a decided step in advance, as he has undertaken to imbue it with a feeling of mystery which his earlier pictures have lacked. We all know how indefatigably he has worked for the Secession, and I know no better word of praise than to apply to him what I have said about St. Gaudens[4] and American sculpture: "It owes the best, if not everything, to him; without him American artistic photography would be a myth."

A very welcome newcomer is Alvin Langdon Coburn. During the last two years he has made wonderful strides. The first exhibition of his pictures that I ever saw rather bored me, though his personality interested me, reminding me of the French symbolist poet Emmanuel Signoret[5] (whom he strongly resembles in appearance), who said of himself at the age of twenty: "I am young; I am a poet, for youth is poetry." But now matters have changed. He is on the way toward becoming a full-fledged personality. He has begun to see objects, insignificant in themselves, in a big way. His "Ipswich Bridge" is one of the strongest pictures in the exhibition. He displays a decided feeling for the decorative arrangement of masses, and his composition, strongly influenced by the Japanese, via Dow,[6] is at times exceedingly clever, as shown in "The Dragon."

Clarence H. White, a sincere, straightforward talent of rare refinement and never-tiring student in quest of beauty, has convinced me more than ever that his is a rather limited field, but that he stands absolutely unique as a photographic illustrator. His illustrations for *Eben Holden*[7] and "Beneath the Wrinkle"[8] will not be easily surpassed, the only man at times approaching him in the power of characterization being Edmund Stirling.[9]

A note, not exactly new, but nevertheless praiseworthy was struck by W. F. James.[10] He is the pictorial reporter *par excellence*. He displays a fine conception of atmosphere and of moving crowds, and his "Christmas Shopping" appeals to me even more than Stieglitz's well-known "Wet Day on the Boulevard."

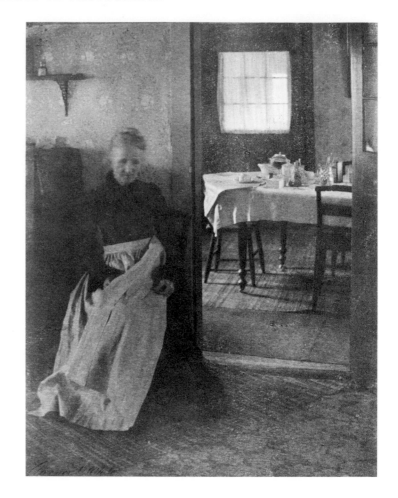

Above. CLARENCE H. WHITE: Illustration for "Eben Holden." IMP-GEH.

Opposite page. ALVIN LANGDON COBURN: The Bridge, Ipswich. IMP-GEH.

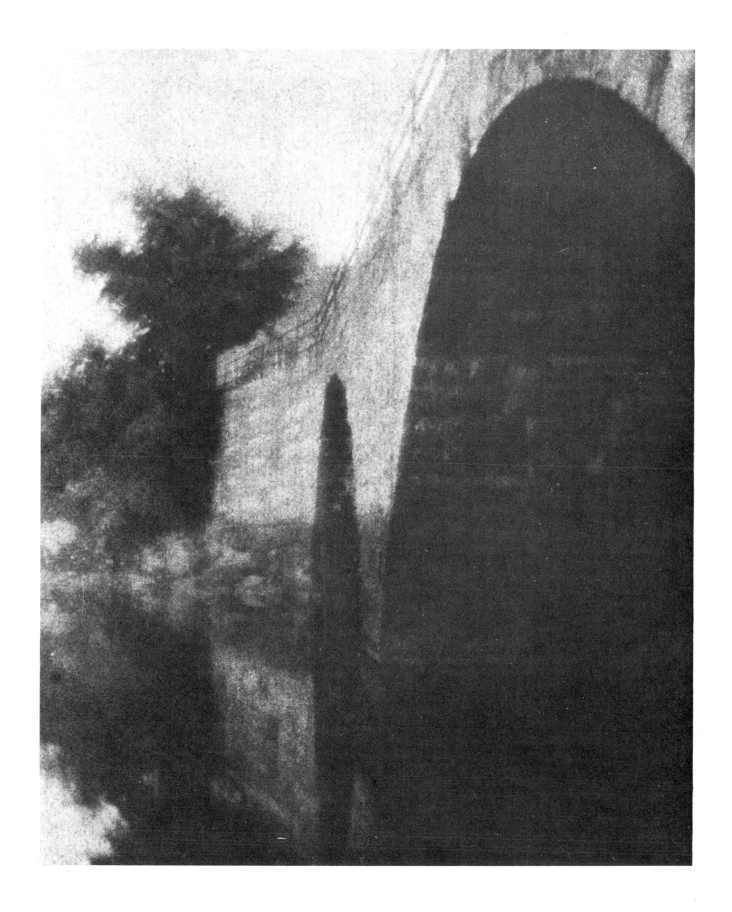

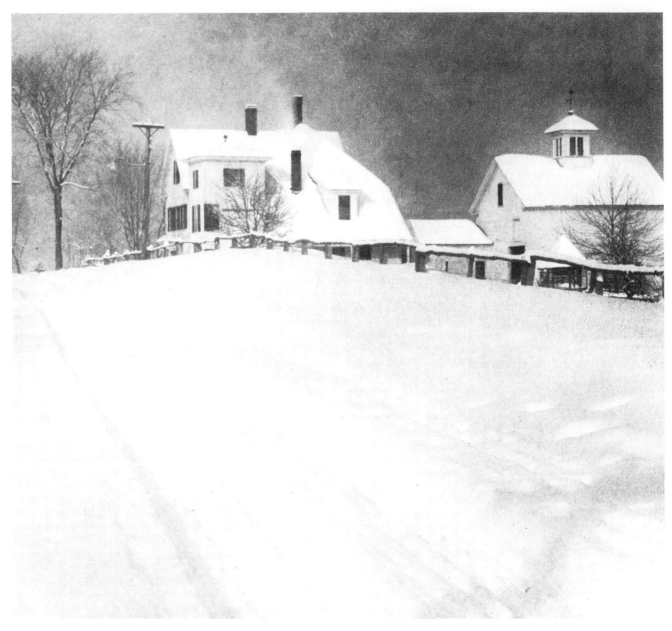

W. B. Post: Winter Weather. IMP-GEH.

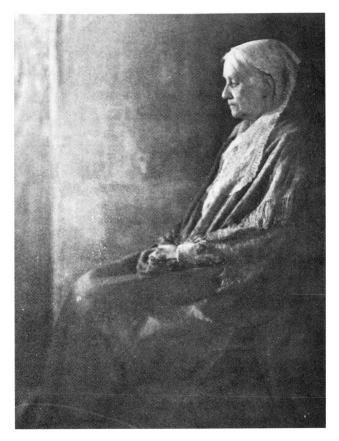

ELIZABETH FLINT WADE and ROSE CLARK: Madame G.

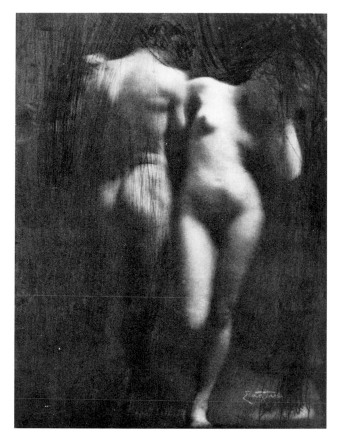

FRANK EUGENE: Adam and Eve. IMP-GEH.

A very satisfactory group of pictures is furnished by J. G. Bullock,[11] W. B. Post,[12] whose winter landscapes are perhaps a little too white and barren, and Rose Clark,[13] whose portraits, though not great, possess a refinement and vague pictorial old-masterlike charm that is exquisite.

Eugene has nothing new to show. Strange that a man with so much talent, with such an overabundance of talent—in his application of painter-like qualities he is second only to Steichen—should at times do such slovenly work. And yet one is forced to admire him, and his "Adam and Eve," in spite of its shortcomings, is one of the few great pictures artistic photography has produced. His art is like a flower which, though its leaves are withered and crumpled, still retains its perfume.

Mary Devens,[14] judged by her pictures in this exhibition, impresses me as being the strongest woman photographer we have just at present. Gertrude Käsebier's newer work does not appeal to me in the same way as her older, and is lacking in spontaneity and virility. Pictures like "The Manger" and "Blessed Art Thou Among Women" hold their own as of old in the best of company. Yarnall Abbott[15] and Rudolf Eickemeyer are rather inadequately represented. By having failed to show their most representative work they have missed a rare opportunity—or is it possible that the very high standard of this exhibition has made their work look less important?

But it is not my intention to criticize all the exhibits in detail—though I should still like to mention Dyer's[16] "Nude" and "Dinah Morris," Willard's[17] "Oenone" and "The Veil," and Herbert

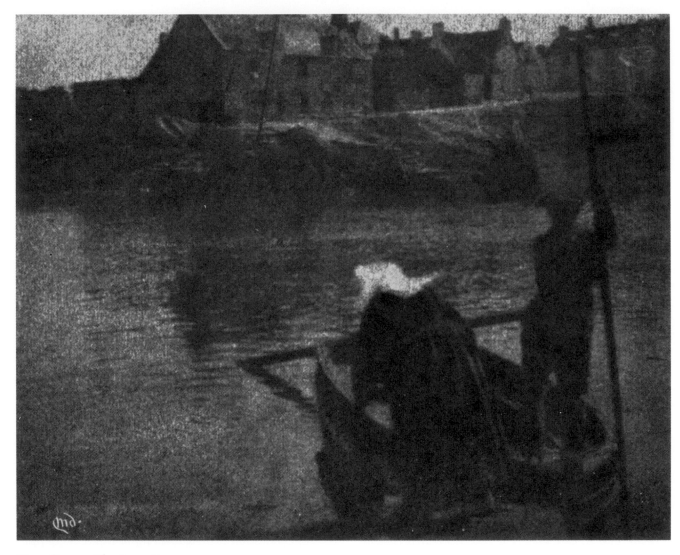

MARY DEVENS: The Ferry, Concarneau. IMP-GEH.

G. French[18] who, all by himself, holds up the banner of artistic photography in the large city of Cincinnati—I merely wish to prove that there are quite a number of photographic workers who have succeeded in making camera-work "a distinctive medium of individual expression." The best proof of this assertion is that nearly all the prominent Secessionists have imitators galore. There were decided indications of this in the exhibition. There are two ways of looking at it. One might say, here we have the proof that true reformatory work is never in vain, that genuine invention always produces an effect. But do these imitators really follow in the footsteps of their masters? Do they not merely strive for the form and not for the idea as revealed in Secessionist work? Do they not merely imitate certain lines and certain peculiar effects because others have applied and successfully applied them? And therein lies, to my way of thinking, the great danger of the Photo-Secession movement. Mannerism means the decline of all art. To substitute one mannerism for another surely is not their

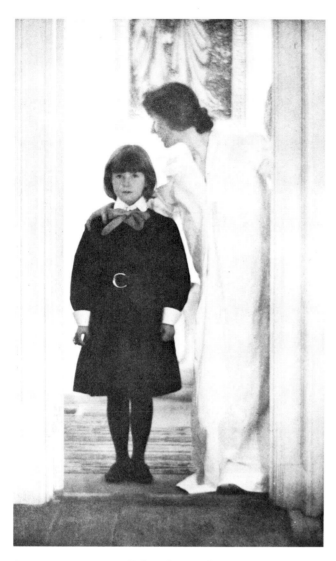

GERTRUDE KÄSEBIER: "Blessed Art Thou Among Women."
IMP-GEH.

aim. As soon as beauty is imitated or produced at second hand it ceases to be beautiful, and is at best but pretty, clever, or effective. There is no sincerity in it. It has deteriorated into mere play. It produces its effect not by its own merit but by reminiscences. To copy Hollinger or Histed[19] can surely not lead to the beautiful, no more than you can achieve beauty though you imitate Steichen, Eugene, or White.

In its future exhibitions, the Photo-Secession must guard against routine, imitation, and mannerism. Is this a complaint or a piece of advice? Neither. Complaint were unjust, and advice is not needed. The older Secessionists have long ago realized what I have just said. They can not hinder the influence of their individuality, though at the same time they know that the real fight has only just begun—a fight in their own ranks between the true and the false Secession.

With every human being a new world is born which did not exist before he saw it, which will never exist again when death closes his eyes. To represent the world, which is nothing but life as seen by the individual, is the aim of the artist. They are the story-tellers of some foreign land which they alone have seen and which they alone can depict for the benefit of others. To listen to the inner voice, to be true to themselves, to obey nobody, that is their law; and only those who in this fashion work out their own individuality, their own innermost convictions which they share with no one else; those who work it out in a convincing manner, without looking out to please or to succeed; they alone are true Secessionists. And if they produce others of the same caliber, pitilessly ignoring and casting aside all who adhere to time-serving aims, then the Photo-Secession will be the beginning of a great movement that will have a permanent value in the annals of American Art.

—1904

11

A Plea for Straight Photography

THE EXHIBITION of the Photo-Secession, which opened on Saturday, February 6, at the Art Galleries of the Carnegie Institute, Pittsburgh, Pa., affords a most unique opportunity of comparing the styles and methods of applying photography to artistic ends. It consists of about three hundred prints, contributed by fifty-four exhibitors.

The average merit of this collection is distinctly in advance of all its predecessors. It has eclipsed the Chicago and Philadelphia Salons of 1898–1901, the exhibition at the National Arts Club, New York, in 1902, and the recent Photo-Secession show at the Corcoran Art Gallery, Washington, not only in number but also in excellence of workmanship, and may be safely described as the most interesting and most representative exhibition of pictorial photography which has ever been held. The jury consisted of Messrs. Alfred Stieglitz, Joseph T. Keiley, and Edouard J. Steichen, who also supervised the hanging.

As was to be expected of an exhibition selected and arranged by three pictorial extremists, who lay more stress on "individual expression" than on any other quality, the majority of pictures showed a certain sameness in quality and idea, as well as in the character of the mounting and framing. And yet, at least three-fourths of the exhibits gave evidence of personal artistic intention, and clearly and unmistakably reflected the taste, the preferences, and the imagination of the individual maker.

It is only a general tendency towards the mysterious and bizarre which these workers have in common; they like to suppress all outlines and details and lose them in delicate shadows, so that their meaning and intention become hard to discover. They not only make use of every appliance and process known to the photographer's art, but without the slightest hesitation—as Steichen in his "Moonrise" and "The Portrait of a Young Man," and Frank Eugene in his "Song of the Lily"—overstep all legitimate boundaries and deliberately mix up photography with the technical devices of painting and the graphic arts. Both men are guilty of having painted, more than once, entire backgrounds into their pictures. Steichen's highlights are nearly all put in artificially, and Eugene invariably daubs paint and etches on his negatives to realize artistic shadows.

There is hardly an exhibitor, Photo-Secessionist or not, who does not practice the trickeries of elimination, generalization, accentuation, or augmentation; and many of them, who have not the faintest idea of drawing or painting, do it in a very awkward and amateurish way. But the striving after picture-like qualities and effects is the order of the day, and throughout the pictures hung—al-

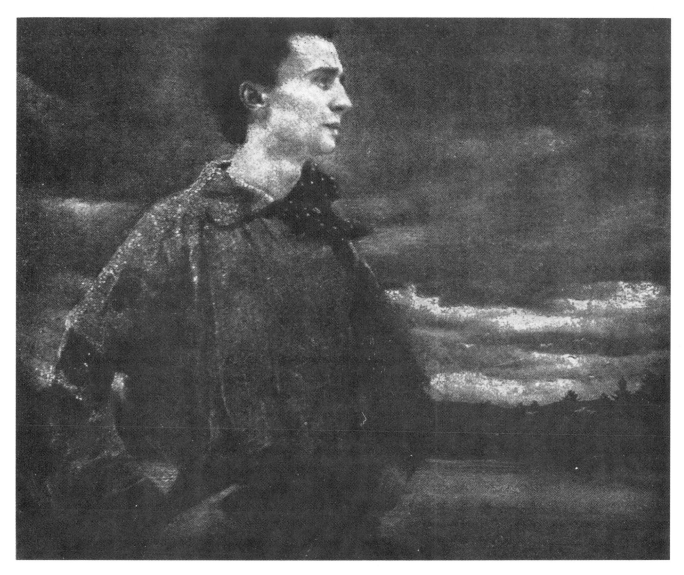

EDWARD STEICHEN: Portrait of a Young Man. IMP-GEH.

though practically nothing wantonly eccentric or repellant in its artificiality had been admitted—there was hardly one which was not influenced by the prevailing clamor for high art. Even in their titles they try to carry out this idea. Why, for instance, did Yarnall Abbott[1] call his nude with a background of trees (almost commonplace in treatment) "Waldweben"? What has a meaningless pictorial fragment to do with Wagner's realistic tone-picture? Are such proceedings not slightly misleading and somewhat pretentious?

And yet nobody can deny that their work, as a whole, is the outcome of intelligent and consistent effort. Grace and subtlety and a fair share of imagination it possesses without doubt, and its exponents put so much enthusiasm into their work that its very earnestness compels respect, even if it does not always command admiration. But the question (or rather the problem) is whether such pictorial work still belongs to the domain of photography. Are those people not doing injustice to a beautiful method of graphic expression, and at

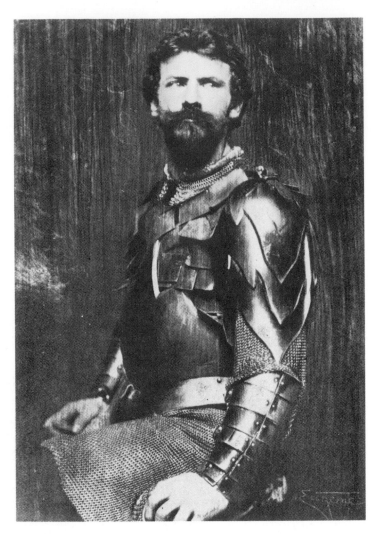

FRANK EUGENE: Man in Armor.

times debasing the powers which sixty years of photographic research and progress have established?

This is very difficult to answer. It depends entirely on circumstances and on the spirit in which one approaches such a picture. Should I, for instance, visit a rich man's art gallery and somewhere on the walls run across Steichen's "Lenbach" in which a number of lines have been etched, several high lights accentuated and half tones painted in by brush, or "A Charcoal Effect" by Mary Devens,[2] it would probably affect me with a special and unique expression of pleasure; I would care little and very likely not even notice whether it were a monotype, a charcoal drawing, an etching, or a photographic print. But when I go into an exhibition of photographs and encounter the very same prints, the situation is changed. I at once ask myself: What sort of photography is it? How is it made? Why does this part look like a hand painted monotype, and that one like an etching or a charcoal drawing? Is it still photography, or is it merely an imitation of something else? And if it is the latter, what is its aesthetic value?

Surely every medium of artistic expression has its limitations. We expect an etching to look like an etching, and a lithograph to look like a lithograph, why then should not a photographic print look like a photographic print? Etching, true enough, is capable of imitating other arts, and a clever etcher might produce an etching which is like an engraving, and another which is like a mezzotint, and a third which is almost like a black and white wash drawing. But if we saw nothing else but the imitations—and we rarely see them and never by master etchers like Jacque,[3] Appian,[4] Veyrassat,[5] Meryon,[6] and Whistler—we might be inclined to say, "Well, this is really very wonderful, but now suppose the etcher would imitate an etching!" As the etching needle is the great expressional instrument for sketchy line work, so legitimate photographic methods are the great expressional instrument for a straightforward depiction of the pictorial beauties of life and nature, and to abandon its superiorities in order to aim at the technical qualities of other arts is unwise, because the loss is surely greater than the gain.

By "a straightforward depiction of the pictorial beauties of life and nature," I mean work like Stieglitz's "Scurrying Homewards," "Winter on Fifth Avenue," "The Net Mender," etc., or his recent "The Hand of Man." "They also have been manipulated," the Photo-Secessionists will argue. Yes, I know he has eliminated several logs of wood that were lying near the sidewalk when he took the snapshot of his "Winter on Fifth Avenue," took out a rope that disturbed the foreground in his "Scurrying Homewards," lightened the sky in "The Net Mender," and darkened the rails in "The Hand of Man." Why not? Surely that is permissible, as it is really nothing but the old-fashioned retouching. If "dodging" is wrong, then also Eickemeyer, and nearly all pictorial photographers, have to be condemned. But if you allow elimination, why do you object to accentuation, do not all retouchers accentuate their highlights? Sure enough, but only where it is indicated on the negative and not willfully, wherever it happens to look well. The whole pictorial effect of a photographic print should be gained by photographic technique, pure and simple, and not merely a part of it. It is surely not legitimate to let the camera do the most difficult part, for instance the reproduction of a figure, and then after embellishing it with a few brush strokes or engraved lines (a comparatively easy task for a man used to painting) claim that it is all done by photography. Surely a figure can be placed and surrounded so artistically—just as nature at times composes itself so beautifully—that the result would be a picture which would even satisfy a secession jury, and necessitate no faking devices.

The strictly straight prints of these pictorial extremists—like the "Theobald Chartran" and "Solitude" of Steichen, the "Portrait of Miss Jones"

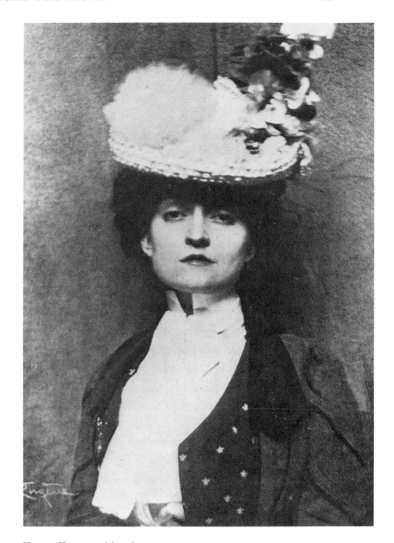

FRANK EUGENE: Miss Jones.

of Eugene—prove it. They are just as beautiful as their other work; why then make all in the same manner? It would be more difficult. But these men are all in other respects so painstaking and conscientious; why not also in their attitude towards photography itself, whose interests they wish to further. I fear they will never "compel the recognition of pictorial photography, not as a handmaiden of art, but as a distinctive medium of individual expression" so long as they borrow as freely from other arts as they do at present. Photography must be absolutely independent and rely on its own strength in order to acquire that high position which the Secessionists claim for her.

But all preaching is in vain, and judging from the present condition of things, it will take years before this latest phase of pictorial photography will be replaced by a more normal one, as it will render necessary a total readjustment of the ideas as to what art photography really is.

It may be interesting to investigate how this change in photographic taste evolved. At the start it was merely the outcome of a revolt from the conventional photographic rendering of sharp detail and harsh contrasts. This was refreshing, as the old-fashioned work had but little claim to beauty and none whatever to art. Stieglitz, Eickemeyer, Dumont,[7] at that time did some remarkable work. Then some new technical methods were introduced which completely revolutionized photographic work. The first was the gum process[8] introduced by Demachy[9] and carried to its utmost possible limit by Steichen, the second was the glycerine process, as practised by Keiley, and the third the manipulation of the plate, the so-called process of photo-etching invented by Eugene.

It is difficult to state which of the three processes has done the most mischief. In the meanwhile Alfred Stieglitz, who has become the champion of artistic photography in America, continually clamored for more "individual expression." And as "individual expression" in straight photography is extremely difficult to attain, the artistic photogra-

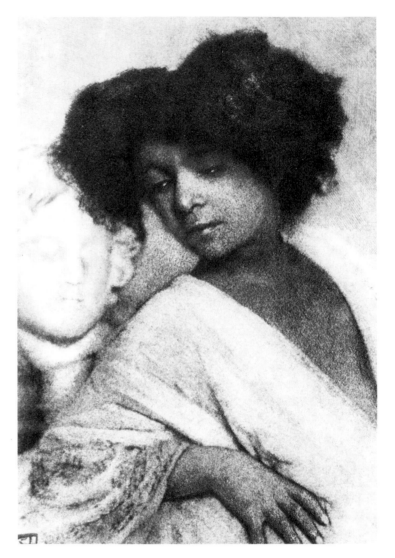

Robert Demachy: Contrasts. imp-geh.

pher began to imitate the artist. "Individual expression" became synonymous with "painter-like expression," and as the three processes mentioned facilitated their efforts in that direction, they were adopted by all the camera workers of the new movement. Alfred Stieglitz suddenly saw himself surrounded by a lot of men and women who professed to be artists in their life as well as in their work. The final results were a foundation of the Photo-Secession society in 1902, and the exhibition at the Carnegie Institute, Pittsburgh.

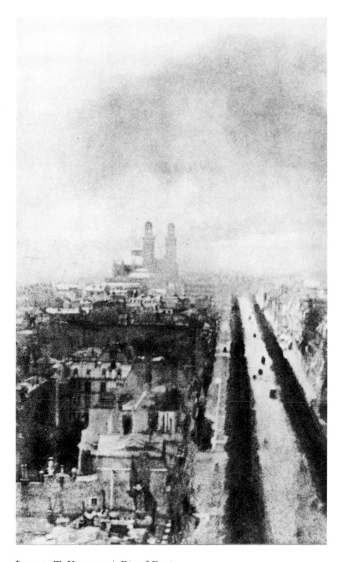

JOSEPH T. KEILEY: A Bit of Paris. IMP-GEH.

In the various groups exhibited one could clearly trace the evolution of the movement. It began with Eickemeyer; then followed in rapid succession Gertrude Käsebier (an expert in dodging processes), F. Holland Day, Clarence H. White, Eugene, Keiley, and finally Steichen and Alvin Langdon Coburn. Although Stieglitz reflects all the different phases, strange to say he remained a straight photographer in all his work.

All the other photographers could not resist the temptation of trying themselves in gum and gly-cerine or applying the Eugene-Steichen method of augmentation. It became the fashion to blur objects, and the so-called "cult of the spoilt print" set in. The results were often far from being satisfactory, largely because the majority of the workers could boast of no art training, and had no skill in the handling of brush and etching tools. The fun that was everywhere poked at the "fuzzy print" was not quite unjustified.

Of course no critic has the right to be absolutely positive that the work which he fancies is absolutely the only work that is in the right vein, and that everything else is only working and studying in order to make him laugh and have fun. He must be able to think independently of any tradition, of any set idea of what is right and wrong, and be ready to try and understand what the photographic workers have to say.

The glycerine development, especially when employed with mercury, is full of possibilities. It has qualities entirely its own and need not borrow by imitation, but why need it be invariably utilized for fuzzy effects. Why do they obstinately insist on carrying mediums farther than they go?

Yet I cannot deny that I have also seen very beautiful, convincing as well as self-explanatory specimens in this line of work. The Pittsburgh Exhibition was in many respects a revelation to me, and I would be the last to discredit the merits of enthusiastic workers as John G. Bullock,[10] Rose Clark,[11] Mary Devens, Wm. B. Dyer,[12] Herbert S. French,[13] Mary M. Russel,[14] Eva Watson Schütze,[15] Edmund Stirling,[16] S. L. Willard,[17] etc. But I claim and am absolutely convinced that still greater triumphs can be achieved in straight photography, and that they have been achieved by these workers whenever they applied the simple methods of straight or almost straight photography. It hurts me to see gifted persons like Gertrude Käsebier and Coburn, for instance, waste their talents on methods that have no justification to exist, and that have—mark my word—no permanent value and no future. The more so as they all can work straight, and are at their best when they work straight.

"And what do I call straight photography," they may ask, "Can you define it?" Well, that's easy enough. Rely on your camera, on your eye, on your good taste and your knowledge of composition, consider every fluctuation of color, light, and shade, study lines and values and space division, patiently wait until the scene or object of your pictured vision reveals itself in its supremest moment of beauty. In short, compose the picture which you intend to take so well that the negative will be absolutely perfect and in need of no or but slight manipulation. I do not object to retouching, dodging, or accentuation, as long as they do not interfere with the natural qualities of photographic technique. Brush marks and lines, on the other hand, are not natural to photography, and I object and always will object to the use of the brush, to finger daubs, to scrawling, scratching, and scribbling on the plate, and to the gum and glycerine process, if they are used for nothing else but producing blurred effects.

Do not mistake my words. I do not want the photographic worker to cling to prescribed methods and academic standards. I do not want him to be less artistic than he is to-day, on the contrary I want him to be *more artistic*, but only in legitimate ways.

The present movement has done an infinite amount of good, as it has awakened an interest in the artistic possibilities of photography, and proven beyond doubt that it is capable of distinct individual expression. But that it cannot continue in the present way, even Mr. Stieglitz realizes. The total suppression of almost every quality which we customarily associate with photography must cease. The photographer is not justified, as Mr. Steichen claims, in the striving to obtain results of the painter, the etcher, and the lithographer. And I am convinced a reaction will set in which will refuse all (at the very best only feeble) imitations of the material technique employed by any of these arts.

To me the Photo-Secession movement is merely the extreme swing of the pendulum which is necessary ere a reaction in photographic work will bring it back to a normal, but at the same time much higher, artistic plane than it has ever occupied before.

I myself have been concerned with this movement from the very start; I have stood by it through thick and thin because I realized that my ideal of straight photography could only be reached by making concessions and by roundabout ways. But now as the time for a reaction has come, I sincerely hope that my words will have so much weight with some of the workers that they will read this plea for straight photography and give it serious consideration; for it is my innermost conviction that there must come a change if we do not want to sacrifice all we have gained. I want pictorial photography to be recognized as a fine art. It is an ideal that I cherish as much as any of them, and I have fought for it for years, but I am equally convinced that it can only be accomplished by straight photography.

—1904

12

The Broken Plates (A Short Story)

THERE WAS A time when I also hoped to become one of the leading artistic photographers.[1] But the quest for fame or recognition of any sort is futile. Its realization depends on so many minor circumstances utterly beyond human control. At least it has been so with me.

My father was a painter of some reputation; from him I have inherited my artistic instincts, a keen sense of appreciation. But being by nature a dreamer—the foretaste of the future always robs the dish before me of its savour—I had neither the patience nor the perseverence to undergo a severe training of hand and eye. I drifted into photography largely in the hope that its mechanism might supply what I had failed to acquire. I soon learnt that I was seriously mistaken; the action of mechanism and accident which plays such a capricious part in photography had, however, a strange fascination for me. The contention of the artist that nothing artistic could be produced by the camera filled me with indignation, and I courageously set to work. Years of voluntary toil followed; I was determined to conquer. Yet the world, which looked so beautiful in my waking dreams, seemed dull and cold on paper. The spontaneity of my pictorial vision was invariably lost in the translation. Only once I came very near to my ideal. But the failure, due to an ungovernable accident, shattered all my hopes of ever realizing it.

The story I have to tell is without plot and exciting incidents; as simple as the most common every-day occurrence of which men hardly take any notice. And yet to me it seems more important than any story ever written.

It was somewhere on the coast of Maine. The name of the place is as of little consequence as the name of my heroine. We had summered in the same hotel, at the outskirts of some quaint old fishing village. The other guests—a rather dull, puritanical set, who had no idea how life should be enjoyed—had but little in common with our inclinations; we gladly dispensed with their company and tried to enjoy each other's. Our favorite excursion was, of course, to the dunes. We both felt the same desire to wander off; to venture out in the heat of the sun; to scour the beach and surrounding country. We passed our time in discussing art and literature and the morals of modern society. She continually poked fun at my ambition of becoming an "artistic" photographer. I was used to that, and did not mind her. I knew that my chance would come some day, and I was determined that my fair *moqueuse* should be instrumental in my final success. We had grown quite fond of each other. I was enamored with her passionate frankness and keen intelligence. Even the notes of discord in our characters—like all young people who walk the path of love, we quarreled and excited each other unnecessarily at the slightest occasion—made her only the more precious to me. She pleased me in her rebellion when she held her ground against me.

On that day, when my simple story was enacted, she wore a white serge coat and skirt, with a biscuit-colored shirt-waist, and a ribbon of the same shade around her sailor-hat. She sat watching me, busy with my stupid old machine, the endearing term which she was pleased to bestow upon my camera, her feet drawn up and her hands clasped below her knees. It was a beautiful October afternoon. The sun had warmed the old rocks, and the wide horizon stretched out under a dazzling sky. The sedges were swaying their slim, green bodies with the melody and the wind, and the ocean rippled and whispered to the pebbles on the shore. Conversation had been at a standstill. Presently I began:

"This day seems to me like a realization of my dream. I, after all, did well to stay true to it. It has blossomed through the years into a plant of wondrous growth, filling all my life with fragrance. And now the hour has come when the harvest can be gleaned."

"You are incorrigible. You possess the fatal quality of seeing objects in a halo of entrancement to a remarkable degree."

"But don't you see how perfect the conditions are for producing a masterpiece such as has never been made before? Look how clear and still the water lies against the shore; only by the brighter tint of the covered pebbles can the margin of the sea be told. It is like a land of legend, and you are like the fairy-queen which animates the scene."

"Are you quite mad to-day?" she asked, gazing at the topaz hills beyond the bay. The stain of duller red upon her cheek should have betrayed to me some quickening of her thoughts, but I was so engrossed in the lines and values of the scene that I merely saw her as a passing shimmer, a flash of whiteness in my composition.

"Oh, I am merely intoxicated with the beauty of this day," I replied, making a sweeping gesture with my arm. "Life has at last brought me what I

thought. I am, after all, no knight of the futile quest, as you have called me. This time I'll grip the dream before it flies away."

"Well, let us see if your dream will come true," and she rose, with a weary smile on her lips, and looked toward the sea.

"Remain in that position!" I enthusiastically cried. I saw her at that moment as if a curtain had been suddenly torn aside which had hidden her beauty. With her long, tapering limbs, her strong, slender body clearly outlined against the sky, her skirts fluttering in the wind, she seemed to me like an embodiment of youth and buoyant life.

That was the dream which I had guarded in the sanctuary of my heart. All my life I had hungered for such a vision of fresh, blooming, fragrant youth. And the calm October day, the translucent sky, and the deep blue sea formed a harmonious background to her beauty. I worked with feverish haste. I do not know if merely for minutes or for hours. I had lost the sense of time. I changed my position at every moment to scan some new pictorial wonder. And, although she was the center of all my enthusiasm, I seemed to have forgotten her actual presence. She appeared to me like the cloud-maiden of some fairy-tale, gliding before the wind in gowns of snowy whiteness, with tags of golden sunlight. And yet I had noticed at intervals that she was watching me with an interest that gradually became annoyed.

"There, it is done!" I cried. "I have accomplished it."

"You act as if you had never taken any pictures before."

"I haven't either—not like these," I cried. "They will be astonished. They don't think me capable of it. But it is done." And I wanted to catch her in my arms and press a kiss of gratitude on her lips; but she evaded my grasp.

"Are you not glad that I succeeded?"

"Yes, of course; but I am no judge of such matters." Her words had a peculiar, grievous sound, but I was still too happy to catch its full significance.

"Oh, you are!" I exclaimed. "But is it not wonderful that there is a whole world around us to look at for years and years? And yet we are never aware of it, we never see it till some happy moment suddenly reveals it to us. And I owe it all to you!"

"By ignoring me," she said, reproachfully.

I acted as if I had not heard her words. It was merely one of her moods. She would get over it. I packed my things and we started homeward. A chill wind blew across the dunes. The sun was rapidly sinking into the darkened sea. The whole scene, so joyous a moment before, seemed discolored and hopelessly monotonous. The magic had passed. Would she come to my help, I wondered, with a laugh or light word, or would disenchantment set in and furnish the aftermath for my triumphant hour? She remained silent and her glance looked away past me across the bay.

Traveling becomes difficult when every step onward is a slip down hill. We picked our way carelessly and silently side by side to the beach. On an intervening ledge her balance wavered, and I stretched forth both my arms to support her. In doing so the case with the plates, which I had carelessly slung over my shoulder, slipped and fell and struck the ground with a dull thud. I stood aghast. They had struck a rock. I jumped down. No lover of jewels, in fear of robbers, has ever opened his caskets with more feverish haste than I my case, filled with the treasured plates. They were all broken, smashed to fragments.

My dream was over. I could have sat down at the very spot, buried my face in my hands and wept. I looked at her. There was a strange glimmer in her eyes; it passed away as quickly as it came, but it seemed to me as if it had been the vague expression of malicious joy over the accident.

"Oh, I am so sorry!" her lips murmured.

"Are you, really?" I asked scornfully. "You have no idea what this loss means to me. You do not understand."

I looked inquiringly at her darkened features. A word with some touch of tenderness might at last have saved our love from the wreckage of my art. But she chose not to say it. Perhaps it was her diffidence which decided, perhaps her pride. She merely answered, "I dare say." Then, drawing herself together, she added in a hard voice, "Will you escort me, or have I to go home alone?"

What more is there to tell? Her indifference at that disastrous moment had deeply offended me and gradually killed all my affection for her. Also her feelings toward me had changed. The art, in which I was destined never to accomplish anything of lasting value had formed an insurmountable barrier between us.

I still belong to the little class of faithful workers, and occasionally turn out a clever bit. I still live in the kingdom of dreams, but am convinced more than ever that nothing will bring them to fulfillment. You may ask why I lack the courage to try again. Oh, I have tried again, but it is all in vain. The conditions will never be as perfect again as on that day. True, I may find another woman who will seem to me as beautiful as she did in that hour, and, if I am patient enough, also another October day may assist me with all its radiant, Indian summer charms, but can I conjure up the same emotions that inspired me? You may argue that I am too exacting, that the harmony of that scene was half imaginary, a vision softened by the ecstasies of love. I doubt it. I believe that in that hour the corresponding notes of our two natures were sounded to their very depth, and struck a full harmonious accord, and that her beauty was as much influenced by my presence as my inspiration was by her. But even if your argument were true, I could not rouse sufficient courage to live life over again. And that is final for me.

My fame was buried with the broken plates. And if you would realize, as I have done, how many vague hopes are shattered by just such uncontrollable accidents and influences, how many demonstrations of genius are buried before they have seen the light of day, you would agree with me that the quest for fame is the most futile of all futile quests.

—1904

13

The Salon Club and the First American Photographic Salon at New York

ABOUT TWO YEARS ago two solitary pictorial workers in the middle West—the one Louis Fleckenstein,[1] of Faribault, Minn., and the other Carl Rau, of La Crosse, Wis.—discussed the advisability of forming some kind of organization which would encourage the younger generation of pictorialists. Everywhere new talents were cropping up, but finding it somehow difficult to assert themselves and to gain the recognition they considered due to their efforts, they felt rather discouraged and disillusioned.

The two camera artists mentioned above realized the situation, and after carefully amassing the opinions of pictorialists throughout the country (west of the Mississippi River), came to the conclusion that it was time to make a move of some sort to bring the younger generation of pictorialists to the front. The result was the Salon Club of America, which was quietly organized in December, 1903, by eleven pictorialists whose work had successfully passed the Salon juries of recent exhibitions at Philadelphia and Chicago—namely, Mrs. Jeanne E. Bennett,[2] Louis Fleckenstein, Walter Zimmerman of Philadelphia, Curtis Bell,[3] Carl Rau, W. G. Corthell of Wollaston, Mass., J. W. Schuler of Akron, Ohio, Ralph E. Berger of Reading, Pa., J. H. Field of Berlin, Wis., the Parrish sisters of St. Louis, and Herbert A. Hess of Crawfordsville, Ind. Since then Carl Bjornerantz, Nellie Coutant, Zaida Ben-

Yúsuf, Adolph Petzold[4] and Henry Hall, and (just as we are going to press) the two Washingtonians, C. H. Claudy and C. E. Fairman, have joined the ranks of this enthusiastic little guild of camera workers.

The trend of their work can perhaps be best judged from their monthly portfolio. This portfolio idea is a very good one, as it keeps the various members, residing all over the country, in continual touch with each other. It is carried out in this fashion. Each member prepares several mounted prints monthly and writes a brief description of them for insertion in a monthly portfolio, which is forwarded by the Director with a list of members, according to the most convenient route for making the circuit quickly. Each member receiving the portfolio writes a criticism for mutual advantage and instruction on the blank accompanying each print, and forwards it to the next member.

I had the opportunity to see one of these portfolios at Miss Ben-Yúsuf's studio.

The work is very promising. It is not yet exactly what the French call *arrivé*. The majority of the Salon Club members is still experimenting and searching for a manner of expression in which the characteristic qualities of photography may be most perfectly exhibited—and, I hope, its limitations most loyally respected. Nearly all seem to be possessed by a clear idea of the things they want to say. Many of their prints show strong and individual

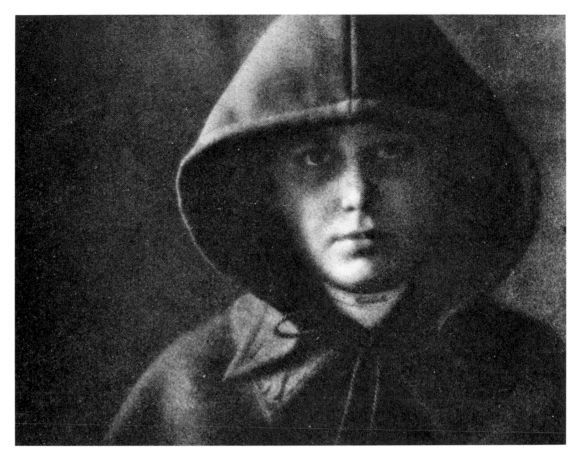

JEANNE E. BENNETT: La Fille au Capuchon, 1904.

workmanship, while others still lack that technical finish which we have become accustomed to in photographic prints. Their range of subjects is a very wide one, and they are particularly strong in landscape work.

The four most accomplished members of the Salon Club are Jeanne E. Bennett, Walter Zimmerman, Curtis Bell, and Adolph Petzold.

Like most of the Salon Club workers Jeanne E. Bennett is a newcomer. Her special realm is Brittany, and she apparently never tires of depicting little hooded girls at the ferry, fetching water at the brook, roaming through the fields, or busy with some domestic occupation in old-fashioned interiors. Her work is at times wonderfully vital, and always subtle and delicate. Each of her pictures has a meaning, and is handled with beautiful skill and rare artistic feeling.

In seriousness of work Walter Zimmerman can not easily be surpassed. He has rarely been seen in print, but his work is easily remembered, since all that he does shows the thoughtfulness of the artist whose work represents the pictorial as well as the photographic quality. He has contributed but little to current exhibitions, but whatever he has shown publicly is powerful, studied and noteworthy. His "Church Interior, Brittany" is an admirable piece of work, in which difficulties that would stagger even the most accomplished of pictorialists have been successfully subdued and mastered.

Curtis Bell is a very versatile talent. He is equally efficient in popular genre like his "Ravvy and Caddy," in children portraits—his "As Big as Mamma" is one of the best I have ever seen—and in landscapes, in which he effects a simple, quiet style. Pictures like his "Coming Storm" and "A Boyhood

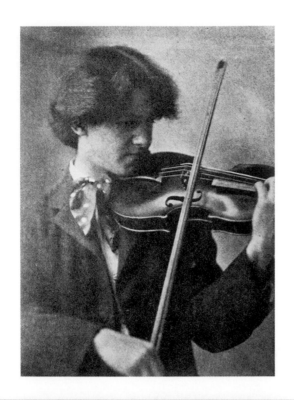
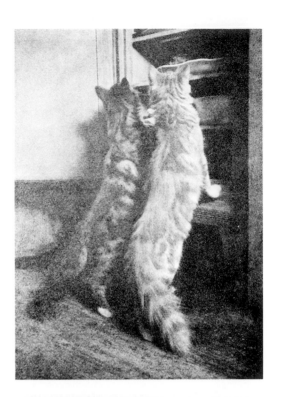
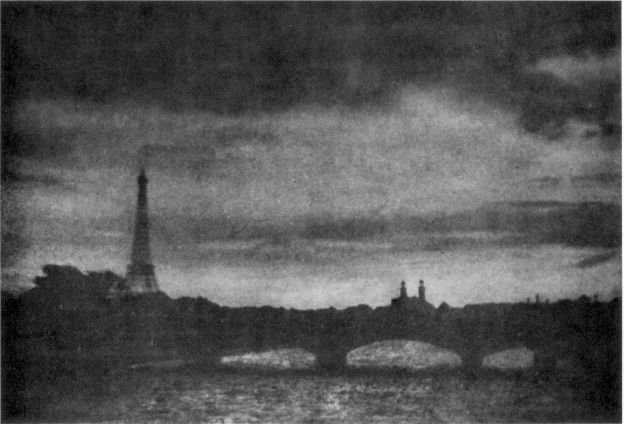

Memory" (the picture of an old country fence) hold their own in the best of company. His "Boat House" shows what can be done with material essentially modern and supposedly unpicturesque.

Among our American landscape photographers Curtis Bell, Adolph Petzold, and J. H. Field occupy a unique position.[5] They do not believe that it is the duty of a landscapist to see everything according to decorative formulae. They have the faculty of disengaging the practical significance of the commonplace object and fact. Curtis Bell sees everything in a minute pictorial way, as some American landscape painters interpret nature. Petzold's early work was also careful and elaborate, but he has gradually made his way to far greater simplicity and far greater power. The massiveness of his "Winter Twilight" is characteristic of his most

individual mood of working. J. H. Field is less direct and bold; his strength is nervous, delicate, and refined. He sees nature with the eyes of a lyrical poet.

The products of the two founders of this organization are of a very original sort, Louis Fleckenstein is as versatile as Curtis Bell, his popular genre pictures are rather weak and commonplace, but his landscapes and interpretations of children are

Opposite page top left. WALTER ZIMMERMAN: Adagio Sostenuto.

Opposite page top right. CURTIS BELL: Ravvy and Caddy.

Opposite page bottom. WALTER ZIMMERMAN: Pont Neuf, Evening.

Below. ADOLPH PETZOLD: The Butterfly.

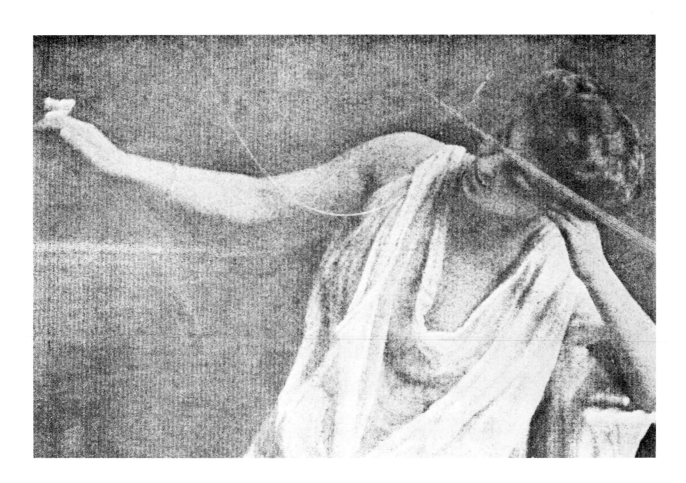

worthy of all attention. His capricious, piquant, and virile imagination, as displayed in his "Song and Danseuse" and "The Pastoral," is unique in our photographic art. Who would ever think of depicting a little girl in a chaste attitude with the frivolity of a Boldini.[6] It may be a trifle morbid, but what of that, as it is at least original and of excellent workmanship. Make any kind of picture you like my dear pictorialists, so long as they be beautiful pictures.

Carl Rau has an individuality in a field of work which is little cultivated. He tries his talents in symbolistic genre. His themes are very ambitious—in his "Mill" his art even assumes epic propor-

tion—but his technical or rather his pictorial skill does not always prove sufficient to carry out the idea. In his "At St. Mary's" he wished to convey "not so much a picture of a Catholic form of worship, but rather a symbol of peace, of rest, away from the busy world." A praise-worthy task, but does the picture really give us the impression of peace? I fear not—but I may say so much that whatever Rau puts in his work, it still remains interesting. His studies of old men's heads, on the other hand, leave me rather indifferent.

The Parrish sisters of St. Louis are newcomers in the literal sense of the word. They are, I have heard, hardly more than two years at it. Their work still

J. H. FIELD: May Morning.

J. H. FIELD: The Alley.

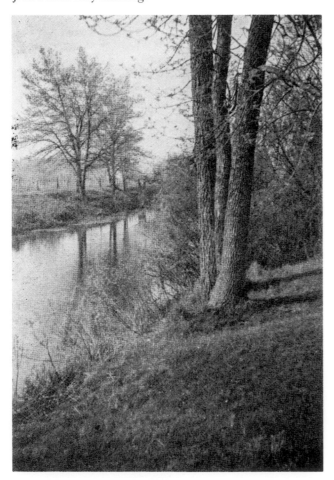

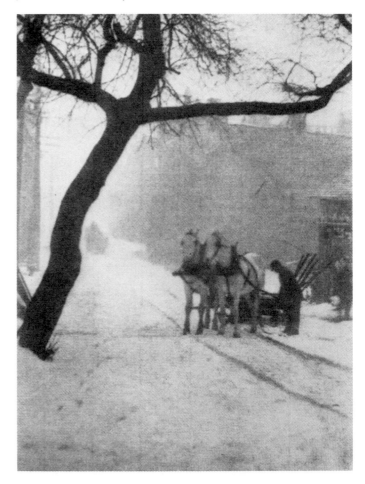

bears the earmarks of dilletantism. Their "Sleepy Girl," however, shows decided talent. One might say of it—for it is pleasant at times to drive a tandem of three adjectives—that it is brilliant, ambitious, eloquent, and melodramatic. The Parrish sisters are no doubt young ladies *plein d'avenir*. I expect a great deal of them. But at present were it not that they were young, their prints would not interest one very much. I should have glanced them over in the mood of Heine's hero who cried thrice "Tirily" and having tirilied, spun around on his heel and went his way. The day will come however, when I will have to pay full homage to their impeccable mastery of art.

The works of Nellie Coutant—the "little wooden shoe" pictorialist—of Zaida Ben-Yúsuf, whom I have always considered our leading portraitist on semi-artistic lines—and of Herbert Arthur Hess, our American "von Gloeden"[7] are too well known to be specially discussed. Also Carl Bjorncrantz, an excellent young worker; Ralph E. Berger, particularly fond of flat tone interpretations; J. W. Schuler, a clever landscape worker; Geo. Donehower, C. H. Claudy, and C. E. Fairman have done and do interesting things, but whom the lack of space at this occasion must deprive of further comment.

Two pictorialists, however, who can not be omitted from the briefest sketch are Henry Hall

LOUIS FLECKENSTEIN: A Pastorale.

W. and G. PARRISH: The Haunted Room.

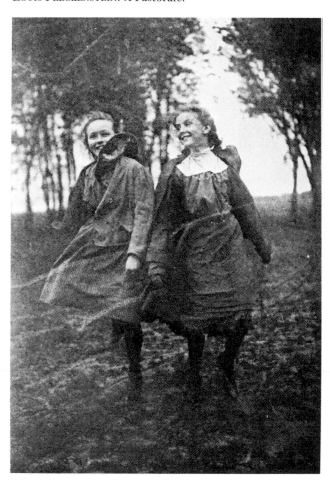

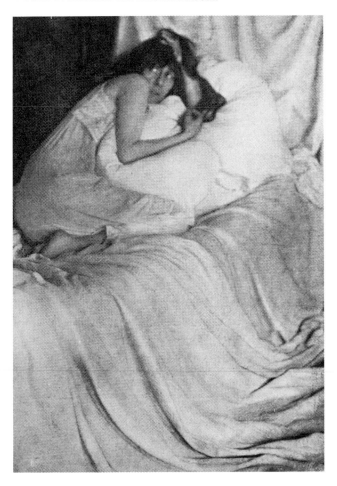

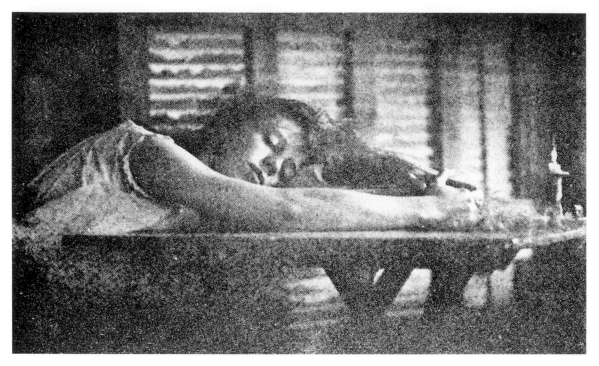

W. and G. Parrish: Sleeping Girl.

and W. G. Corthell. Hall seems to have made a specialty of child life. He represents really a marvelous amount of individuality in each of his little men and women. His "Rough and Ready" is a masterpiece. My friends Albert L. Groll,[8] the landscape painter, and Roland Rood, a critic of many moods and modes of thought, both agreed that "it was the best in the whole bunch." Corthell undertakes to lend to each of his prints an air of refinement, which alone lifts his work far above the mediocrity of these scores of busy little pictorialists who tinker values and solder tonalities and thereby consider themselves great artists.

Well, in December we will find out what stuff they are really made of, for then the Salon Club workers will make their debut before a New York audience at the First American Photographic Salon. This exhibition will be a memorable one in many respects. Let us glance over the prospectus to learn more about it.

In it we read that the management of the First American Salon at New York City cordially invites the cooperation of all artistic photographers in America and throughout the world, that it is the First Photographic Salon to be given in the Metropolis and the first of national scope under the control of a committee from all sections of the United States, that consequently an exhibition of the highest order is expected. There will be no favors to any and no discrimination against any. All work, whether from the famous or the comparatively unknown artist, will be exhibited equally, and the jury will not know the names of contributors until after the selection has been made.

No one "school" or "fad" will command precedence. The standard of judging will be the artistic quality of each print submitted.

On the page of "Conditions" we are furthermore instructed that the jury is composed of artists, who have been requested to act as judges of the artistic character of the work to be submitted (a list of excellent names is furnished. I know them all

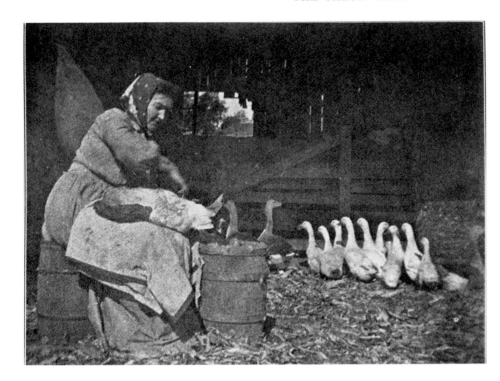

Right. NELLIE COUTANT:
The Goose Picker.

Below. J. W. SCHULER:
The Bridge.

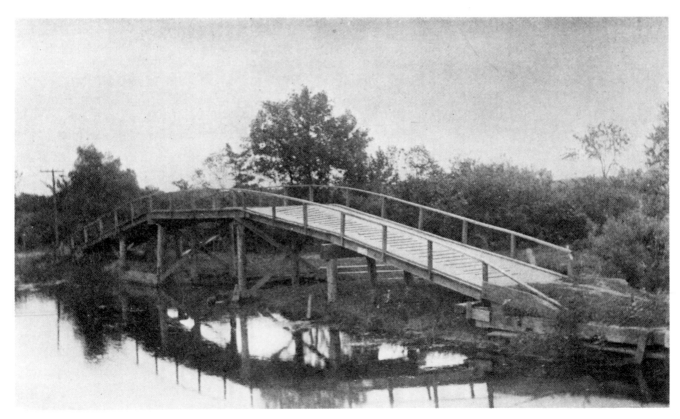

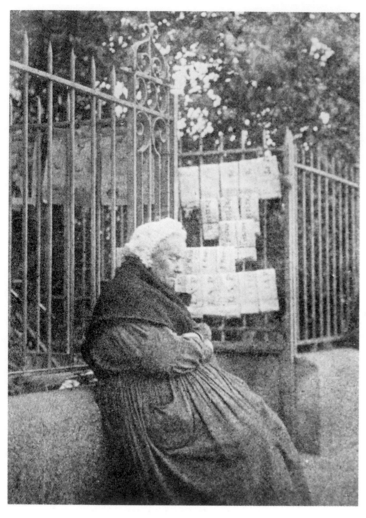

WENDELL G. CORTHELL: The Noon-Day Nap.

personally and by reputation, but how many of them will actually serve?); that "only those photographs which give distinct evidence of artistic feeling in subject and execution will be accepted"; and that "all amateur and professional photographers throughout the world are requested to forward work of the character described"; and that "there will be no invited work, and all prints forwarded will be examined by the jury."

I may add that the same exhibit will, later on, be shown at the Chicago Art Institute, the Corcoran Art Gallery, Washington, and the Boston Museum of Fine Arts.

All this sounds like open revolt! But far from being lawless, it is merely the expression of new laws. For each generation there is a different standard. Old forms and old perfections wither. Out of the old symbols the color fades day by day, and it is the younger generation's business to create new ones.

It nevertheless sounds like an open revolt. And there may be an opposition! A duel between Messrs Alfred Stieglitz and Curtis Bell would prove indeed a great attraction. There are none upon whose swordsmanship I trust more surely than that of these two gentlemen. It will stir up the stagnant waters of pictorial photography—they surely need it—and make us all more happy at the end.

—1904

14

Recent Conquests in Night Photography

THE NIGHT SCENE has given a new note to pictorial representation. It is a comparatively new achievement. Of course, we are all acquainted with the Nativities of the Old Masters, but they were ideal representations and had little in common with the nocturnal life of that period. The Dutch painters were the first realists. Van der Neer[1] is celebrated as a painter of conflagrations through the gloom of night, and oftener still of moonlight spreading itself in reddish-brown harmonies over lonely dunes. And Schalcken[2] who painted Dutch tradespeople selling their ware, illumined by candle light, was one of the first to reveal to us the charms of artificial light.

Night gained a deeper pictorial significance only with Whistler's nocturnes, and the various delineations of street scene painters. Most of us who dwell in the larger cities must have been struck some time or other with the charm which certain places display after daylight has taken its departure and artificial lighting reigns supreme, also the curious effects one sees on a wet night when the pavements endeavor to reflect to the best of their ability the lights which illuminate them.

New York is at all times picturesque, but never is it more so than when the daylight has faded and the street lamps are lit. Then it becomes another city entirely. Out of the darkness, like some magical effulgence, merges a dazzling shower of light, a myriad of beaming sparks. Buildings and objects that were of no pictorial consequence in the daylight may assume quite the first place in our favor, and ugly things, not to be dodged anyhow by day, most kindly retire out of sight, or else are turned into things of beauty. Of course, sometimes the opposite state of things prevails, and a subject picked out in the day as being particularly attractive may in the evening show all sorts of awkward lines, etc., the existence of which was quite unsuspected before.

Everywhere loom large bulky forms shrouded in mystery, suggestive, conducive to poetical imagining. Emerging from the gloom are weird shapes like outstretched limbs against a confused glare of light, and beyond an impenetrable depth of shadows. Optical sensations, discordant effects which we are not accustomed to in art, but which succeed in stirring the very depth of our nature.

This branch of photography until quite recently seems to have somewhat been neglected. I mean nocturnal photographs, depicting streets and other public places at night and which convey to the mind a true impression of night as we see it under its various conditions, and not to the daylight pictures "faked" to represent nocturnal impressions.

The "moonlight effects" which appeal so strongly to some amateurs, are in most instances merely sunlight exposures, taken facing the sun generally while its direct light is cut off by a cloud.

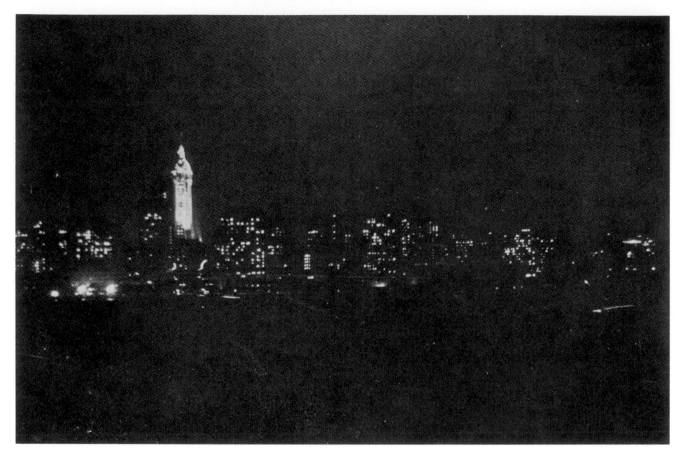

WILLIAM VAN DER WEYDE: The Plaza, New York.

They are grossly under-exposed in order to get most of the landscape and not a little of the sky itself, mere blackness, and the result, as is well known, is labelled "moonlight." It is obviously hopeless to include the moon herself in night pictures, for the longest exposure possible by which one may attain an unblurred image of the earth's satellite is several seconds, and this of course, is all too short for the registration of a strictly moving object.

Probably the reason for this neglect is that many considered it a hopeless, if not an impossible task, whilst others who have taken this work in hand have been deterred by fear of the consequences arising from standing about in the cold or wet or from perilous ascents to inaccessible places to gain a favorable viewpoint.

It offers nevertheless a good scope to those anxious for pastures new and sufficiently generous to consider the waste of innumerable plates as a stimulation to the trade. First and foremost a good stock of patience and perseverance is necessary. The exposures are apt to be so unreasonably long that they would tire out the pluckiest enthusiast.

Alfred Stieglitz, one of the pioneers of night photography in this country, achieved his results ten years ago only by exposures of half an hour or more, even when assisted by the reflection of snow on the ground. With the continual improvement of plates, lenses, and shutters, the material has become more and more flexible, and exposures of a few seconds have become possible.

The representation of life, traffic, moving fig-

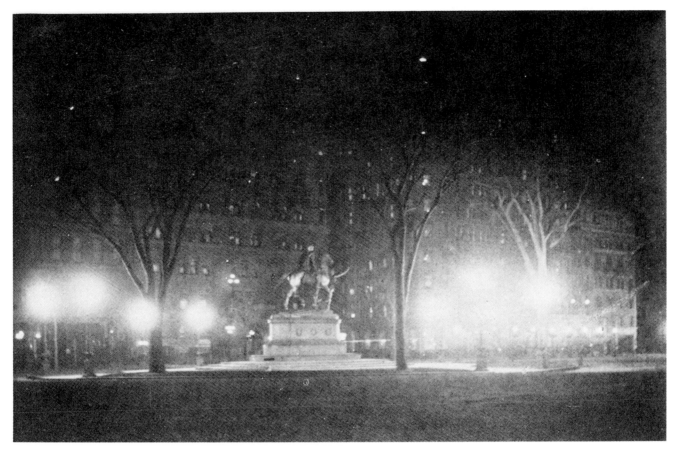

William Van der Weyde: The Singer Building.

ures, however, on account of the long exposure required, is rarely attempted. This is a shortcoming but a mere temporary one, as we seem to be within measurable distance of the time when the rendering of these subjects will be possible.

There are certainly some parts of our city that look satisfactory when portrayed without figures; but Broadway, for example, without vehicles or people, would—well, it would not be Broadway. For years the fine effects of the electric light and the moving traffic in this particular thoroughfare and the adjoining streets have fascinated every visitor and no doubt many photographers have had a great longing to photograph it, but always felt that a sufficiently long exposure to record the effect of the light on the buildings would result in a mere blur

for the traffic, and a short enough exposure to suit the traffic would give nothing worth having on the plate.

But there exists an endless variety of scenes in every large town that will yield the desired novelty of sensation. Every night as the darkness comes on and all the electric lights and places of amusement are lighted, a new world of solemnity, beauty, and mystery lies before our gaze, and every record looks to us at present like a new conquest.

Different subjects will require different treatment, and that is a matter which to a great extent will be left to the judgment of the operator. Some subjects will look good on moonlight nights, but one can safely say that snow or wet on the ground will no doubt be a great improvement in either case,

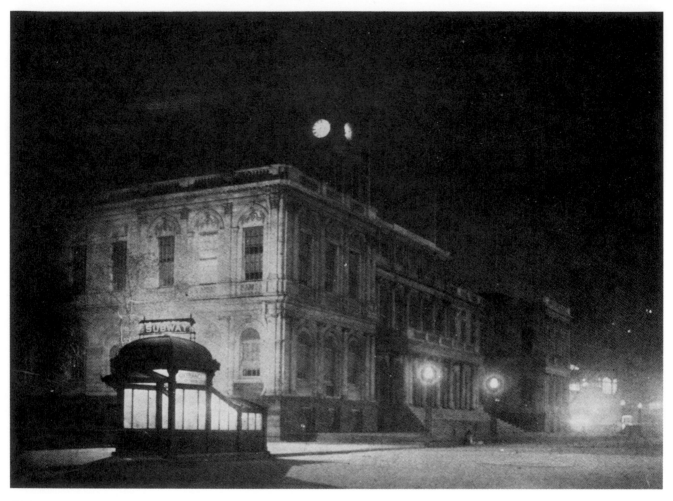

WILLIAM VAN DER WEYDE: The New York City Hall at Midnight.

and it is in this direction that formerly the most pleasing results were obtained.

But lately a new style of night photography has made its appearance. It deals almost exclusively with the bewildering confusion of light as seen from high viewpoints. Railway terminals, city squares, bridge scenes, torch light processions. illuminations, all sorts of artificial lights, vast vistas of lit-up skyscrapers, have become the topics of the hour, pictures that are perhaps less pictorial than a deserted street or a church in moonlight, but which are more realistically true of the restless flimmer and flare, the blaze and radiance of nocturnal life.

They are not mellow harmonies, these night pictures. The greatest extremes meet. Blinding light and absolute darkness. Vague darks here and there accentuated by vivid spots, flickering sheen, and unsteady scintillations, It is an expressive drama of conflicts. The lighted objects issue painfully out of shadow, they surprise us with their vehemence of lustre, and the eye is startled from them to noticing gradations of obscurity in the universal duskiness that surrounds them. We have to discipline our eyes for these surprising contrasts.

Along this line W. M. Van der Weyde[3] has made some notable achievements. He probably has taken more night pictures than anybody else. They look what they are. In fact, the striking realistic result is one of the most astonishing things about the pictures. Not only are they night pictures but they look like night pictures. The shadows are a dense black it is true, but the blackness is not more than is required from truthful rendering. The rendering of the actual light is remarkable, the haze around the lights being no more than can be seen by the eye.

It is only fair to add that the results are in no way faked; here and there an obtrusive light may have been toned down, but substantially they are straightforward photographs, and as such may fairly be regarded as amongst the most remarkable that have been published.

The reader may wish to know the *modus operandi* and apparatus necessary for the accomplishment of such facts, and no doubt will be astonished to hear that the photographer uses an ordinary simple hand camera that will brave the elements, an ordinary lens and sensitive plates.

Most night photographers use rapid isochromatic plates and are particularly careful to have them well backed. They wish to avoid the effects of reversal and undue halation. They still adhere to the old theory that all lights should be outside the field of the camera.

To include the source of illumination, gaslight surfaces, and particularly electric lights may at first appear an insurmountable difficulty, but it will be found that practically it is *nil*, as halations, and light seen in drizzling rain or spreading mist, really add to the pictorial effect. Ordinary rapid plates are more apt to produce a true realistic impression of the "ghostly joyousness of night" than isochromatic ones.

Those who are enamored with the artificial light of the night want it as it is, with all its breaks, supernatural radiance, hectic glow and gleam amidst opaque recesses and intensest darks.

A new era for after-dark workers in town has set in, and many bits of genuine and effective realism, and unknown harmonies of light and shade will be brought to light, which would have been scouted altogether not so very many years ago.

The life of large cities has found a new mode of expression that can reflect its energies and activities, its impulses and diversities, its light and beauty in virile and individual emotions. Herein consists the latest picturesque attainment; and it is one of the mediums through which the language of illustration nowadays can most powerfully address the modern mind.

—1909

15

On the Possibility of New Laws of Composition

THE WEALTH OF reproductive processes has enlarged our visual appreciation of form and general aspect of things to a marvelous degree. Photography, no doubt, has furnished the strongest impetus. It is the most rapid interpreter known to pictorial expression, and has given the person of undeveloped mind, of little skill and few ideas, an opportunity to become a picture maker. The results of photography permeate all intellectual phases of our life. Through the illustrations of newspapers, books, magazines, business circulars, advertisements, objects that previous to Daguerre's invention were not represented pictorially have become common property.

Former ages offered no opportunities to the common people to acquire this facility of discerning accurate representations of life on a flat surface in black and white. The draftsmen and stone cutters of primitive times, realizing that their delineation was a simple form of picture writing, had no thought of any more forceful delineation than that which sufficed people to clearly understand the meaning of figures and symbols. They had no conception of what modern artists call "effect," the pictorial study of appearances, which even the most ordinary newspaper illustration can claim. On one hand we see figures in pure accurate outlines, facts of easily legible forms; on the other hand delineations on the round, with the application of life and shade, perspective, environment, which demand a more delicate knowledge of appearances.

Photographic illustration has become a new kind of writing, and it would be strange if this evolution in our sight perception had not been accompanied by some changes in composition. Composition, tersely expressed, is the complete unity of parts. If we wish to emphasize any one part of the representation it cannot be done without subordinating the other elements. Only in this way will we succeed in concentrating the attention upon the principal figure without any embarrassment to the rest. The more pronounced our intention is in conveying a certain idea, the more careful must we be in balancing the other parts. This general principle will be true for all time. The symmetrical art of the Occident based on geometrical forms, and the unsymmetrical arrangement of Oriental art based in rhythm, are guided by the same idea.

A new spirit of composition, however, may arise in periods of increased esthetic activity. The relation between artists and the world at large is reciprocal. New laws cannot be elaborated by the mere will of a single individual. The composition of the Old Masters, used for centuries, has passed through its first decadence and by constant application has degraded into conventionalism. It grew more and more stereotyped, until impressionist composition—which explores obscure corners of modern life, which delights in strangeness of observation and novel view points (strongly influenced by Japanese art and snapshot photography)—gave it a new stimulant.

In photography, pictorial expression has become infinitely vast and varied, popular, vulgar, common and yet unforeseen; it is crowded with lawlessness, imperfection and failure, but at the same time offers a singular richness in startling individual observation and sentiments of many kinds. In ordinary record-photography, the difficulty of summarizing expression confronts us. The painter composes by an effort of imagination. The photographer interprets by spontaneity of judgment. He practices *composition by the eye.* And this very lack of facility of changing and augmenting the original composition drives the photographer into experiments.

Referring to the average kind of photographic delineation, we perceive how composition may exist without certain elements which are usually associated with it. A haphazard snapshot at a stretch of woodland, without any attention to harmony, can only accidentally result in a good composition. The main thoroughfare of a large city at night, near the amusement center, with its bewildering illumination of electrical signs, must produce something to which the accepted laws of composition can be applied only with difficulty. Scenes of traffic, or crowds in a street, in a public building, or on the seashore, dock and canal, bridge and tunnel, steam engine and trolley, will throw up new problems. At present the amateur has reached merely the primitive stage.

The most ignorant person will attempt a view or a portrait group out-of-doors. Even children will strive for accidental results. The amateur has not yet acquired calligraphic expression. Like the sign painter who takes care to see that his lettering is sufficiently plain to be understood at one glance, the amateur only cares to make statements of fact. As we examine amateur photographs as they are sent in to the editorial offices of photographic magazines, we now and then will experience a novel impression. We do not remember of ever having seen it done just that way, and yet the objects are well represented and the general effect is a pleasing one. I have seen trees taken in moonlight that were absolutely without composition and yet not entirely devoid of some crude kind of pictorialism. It was produced by the light effect. Such a picture cannot be simply put aside by the remark that we hear so frequently, "That is a bad composition." It may be poor art but it is physically interesting.

Climatic and sociological conditions and the normal appreciation of the appearance of contemporary life will lead the camera workers unconsciously to the most advantageous and characteristic way of seeing things. The innovations which will become traditional will be transmitted again and again, until some pictorialist will become the means of imposing the authority of the most practical manner upon his successors. In this way all night photographers, good or bad, will help to discover and invent a scheme or method that will be suitable for the subject and consequently become universally applicable. And so it will be with every branch of pictorialism, may it be in the domain of foreground study, of moonlight photography, of animal or flower delineation, of portraiture, figure arrangement, or the nude.

The most important factors in these discoveries will be those qualities that are most characteristic of photography as a medium of expression. The facility of producing detail and the differentiation of textures, the depth and solid appearance of dark planes, the ease with which forms can be lost in shadows, the production of lines solely by tonal gradations, and the beautiful suggestion of shimmering light—all these qualities must be accepted as the fundamental elements of any new development. Photographic representation, no doubt, will become addicted more and more to space composition, to the balancing of different tonal planes and the reciprocal relation of spaces. This may be an advantage from the point of physical optics. Beauty is chiefly concerned with the muscular sweep of the eye in cognizing adjacent points. It is generally conceded that the impression is more gratifying if these points are limited to a few. Every spot requires a readjustment of the visual organs, as we can only observe a very small space at a time. Too many spots, as may occur in modern compositions, no doubt will prove wearisome and fatiguing; but if the spotting is skillfully handled, it after all will represent the fundamental principle of esthetic perception, and the sense of sight will adjust itself gradually to the necessity of rapid changes.

Also the relationship of lines, so confused and intricate in scenes like a railroad station or a machine shop, factory, derrick or skeleton structure of a building, will need special consideration. The variety and the irregularity of such lines, in which the straight and angular line will predominate, may be compared to the unresolved discords, unrelated harmonies, little wriggling runs, and all the external characteristics of the modern French composers. Debussy mastered these apparently incongruous elements sufficiently well to construct novel combinations of sound that, after all, are pleasing to the ear.

If new laws are really to be discovered, an acquaintance with the various styles is prejudicial rather than advantageous, since the necessary impartiality of ideas is almost impossible, inasmuch as the influence of study and the knowledge of preexistent methods must inevitably, although perhaps undesignedly, influence new creations and ideas. All natural objects have some sort of *purpose*. And the photographer should strive primarily for the expression of the *purpose*. Each object (like the free verse of Whitman) should make its own composition. Its forms and structures, lines and planes should determine its position in the particular space allotted to the picture. More than ever must the artist be gifted with a happy appreciation of beautiful proportions, which often are sufficient to bestow a noble expression on a pictorial representation.

Much will depend on the amateur who by sheer necessity will work unconsciously in the right direction. His knowledge will increase and his ambitions soar higher. And as he grows in esthetic perception it will react upon the artist and urge him to attain a new and more varied, subtle and modern (though not necessarily more perfect) state of development.

—1910

16

Unphotographic Paint: The Texture of Impressionism

$\mathcal{A}$T THE BEGINNING of May a small collection of paintings by Marsden Hartley[1] of Maine found shelter at the hospitable Little Gallery of the Secessionists.[2] They were examples of an extreme and up-to-date impressionism. They represented winter scenes agitated by snow and wind, "proud music of the storm"; wood interiors, strange entanglements of tree-trunks; and mountain slopes covered with autumn woods with some island-dotted river winding along their base.

The depth and distance across the valley to the mountain, the plastic modeling and faithful detail, the hardiness and vigor of representation showed knowledge of form and sincerity of sentiment. It was the color scheme, however, that startled the beholder. It produced a strictly physical sensation. It irritated the retina and exhausted it. After leaving the gallery, Fifth Avenue looked more grey than usual. A melancholy vocation for such a robust phase of art!

Hartley's technique is interesting, though not necessarily original. It is a version of the famous Segantini[3] "stitch," of using colors pure and laying them side by side upon the canvas in long flecks that look like stitches of embroidery. I overheard some artist remark: "Lots of young painters in Germany paint in this crazy fashion." This may be true. Hundreds of painters all over the world are busy experimenting to expand and improve the original

impressionist technique, and there is no reason why somebody else should not lay on the paint in a similar way to Marsden Hartley. As long as the latter applies his colors in a temperamental, self-taught manner, he is above the reproach of imitation. I for my part believe that he has invented his method for himself, up there in Maine amidst the scenery of his fancy, and that only gradually has he learnt to reproduce nature in her most intense and luminous coloring.

Yet neither his courage nor the sincerity necessary to accomplish such a task, nor any understanding and mastery that he may possess, put my mind in an analytical mood and induced me to write this article, but rather the peculiarity and freshness of his viewpoint. Why do people paint this way! This simple question asserted itself again and again and called for an explanation. Why do painters more and more renounce the conventional ways of handling colors? Is it solely for the one supreme purpose of getting the effect of vibrating color, of light in motion!

It is an acknowledged fact that impressionism has heightened the key of tone throughout the studios of the world. It has given us an intenser and more varied study of illumination, a higher pitch of light. One thing is certain, the dramatic element has vanished. It no longer knows the mysterious harmonies of a Leonardo or the soft sparkling

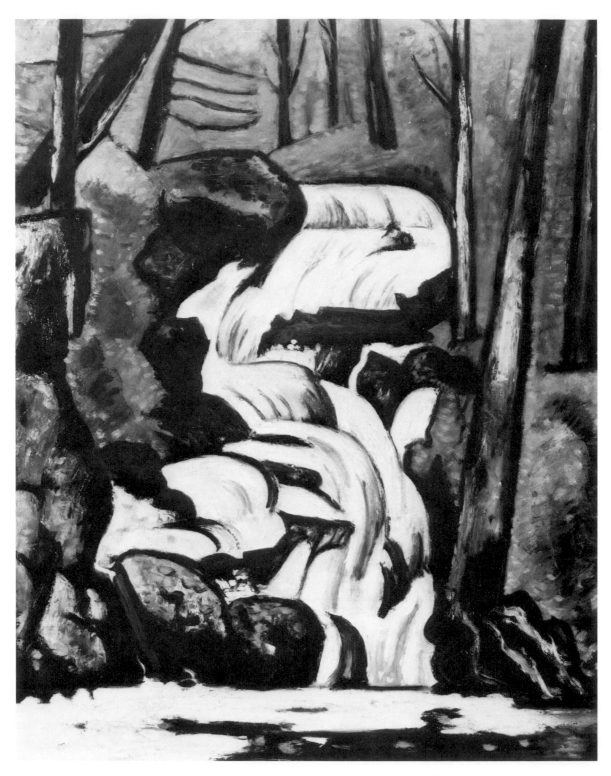

MARSDEN HARTLEY: Smelt Brook Falls, 1937. The St. Louis Art Museum. Purchase Eliza McMillan Fund.

shimmer of a Rembrandt. Light has lost its gleam and glitter as if vibrant with gold dust. The glamor of romance has faded out of it. In its stead we have the poetry of lighting that the days and hours bring to a single scene, as Monet has so loyally demonstrated in his series of haystacks, poplar trees, and the Rouen Cathedral. Whether these high-pitched light and color notations are a fair equivalent for the sudden spiritual light bursts that quiver through the gloom of medieval art, future art historians will decide.

The modern painter, treating different pictorial motives than his predecessor, felt the need of a new technique. The impressionist prefers to suggest form rather than to actually draw it, he desires to envelop figures and objects in space and atmosphere. A blurred definition ensues, in which the minutiae and subtleties of line are often lost. To accomplish this aim he invented a looser and more broken touch that neglects drawing (unless the painter possesses the sense of plasticity to a marked degree) and the old standards of composition.

But why this revolution of *facture*, this strange technique of squeezing on color thick, giving the canvas a tapestry or mosaic effect. Is it solely for the purpose of letting the eye look at the picture from a distance, to mix and melt the colors together on the canvas, and thereby give an effect of more air, more light, and truth? Were these effects not possible with a smoother surface and more uniform continuity of texture!

The paintings of Franz Hals and Goya, the foremost representatives of *bravura* brushwork, look smooth in comparison with an impressionist canvas. Monet's large flowing touches recall Velasquez. Even Monet's earlier work in small broken touches was still related to the cross hatching of pastel and stippling of water-colors of Watteau and his followers. Only gradually the painters began to lay the paint on thicker and thicker until the texture had an actual structural tendency, as in many of Segantini's works. Also Rembrandt at times encrusted his canvas a quarter of an inch

thick with color to imitate jewelry and strongly illuminated objects. Among modern painters, Monticelli[4] and Ryder use a rough dough-like impasto, and Mancini[5] while painting his shadows very thinly, models the lighted form with paint like a sculptor. With these painters it is merely a vehicle of momentary inspiration. They do not proceed scientifically. With the impressionist the regulated patch or stroke of plastic color, laid one beside the other, has become a professional mechanism, just as the smooth brushmarks must have been to a Guido Reni[6] or Andrea del Sarto.[7]

I believe that the artists individually have very little to do with the new development. It is nothing but a natural consequence of the modern tendency of art. And even as great an artist as Segantini deceives himself when he makes the statement that "this secret of technique, nowadays an approved fact, has been perceived by painters of all times and all countries (the first of whom was Beato Angelico)[8] and that it came to him through his loving and earnest study of Nature, and as something personal and individual."

Modern art prefers to be realistic. And in this ardor to express the fleetingness of things just as the eye sees them, artists have turned scientists (or at least try to see objects in a more scientific way), and for this purpose selected and developed a more *realistic* technique. The Old Masters tried to create an illusion, to reproduce the actual roundness of things and the esthetic possibilities of the three dimensions, and did not wish to interfere with the produced impression by any violence of texture. The main object of the impressionist, on the other hand, is to create an impression by suggestion and he asks assistance from the very medium he employs. The plastic aspect of color, no matter whether executed in the commas of Monet, the dots of Pissaro,[9] the irregular patches of Sisley,[10] the cross hatching of Degas or the stitches of Segantini, have to help physically to construct the image in the eye.

The result was a curious one. The canvases began

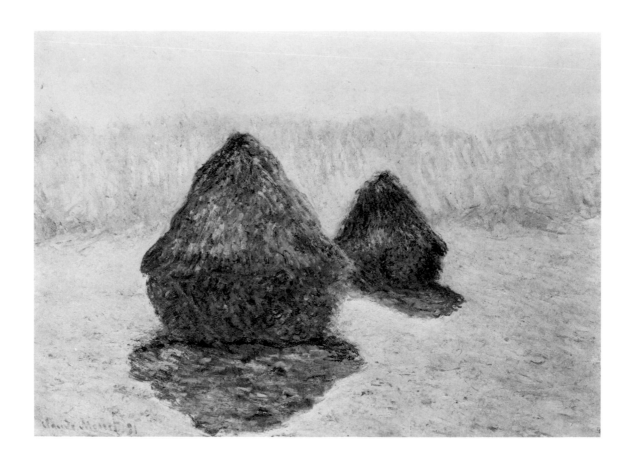

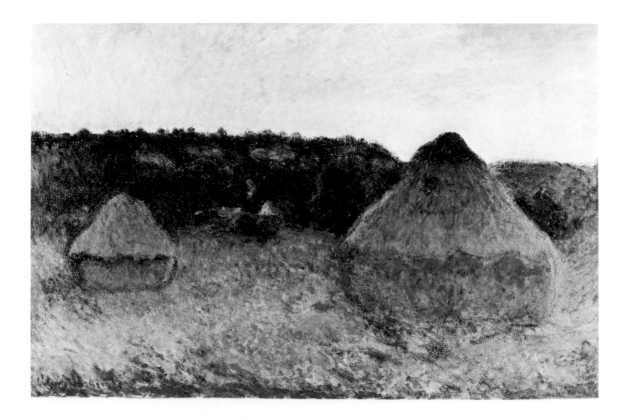

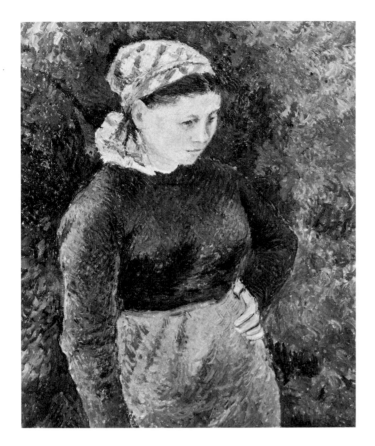

Opposite page top. CLAUDE MONET: Haystacks in Snow, 1891. The Metropolitan Museum of Art, Bequest of Mrs. H. O. Havemeyer, 1929. The N. O. Havemeyer Collection.

Opposite page bottom. CLAUDE MONET: Two Haystacks, 1891. Courtesy of The Art Institute of Chicago.

Left. CAMILLE PISSARO: Peasant Woman, 1863. Chester Dale Collection. National Gallery of Art, Washington, D.C.

Below. ALFRED SISLEY: The Banks of the Oise, 1878. Chester Dale Collection. National Gallery of Art, Washington, D.C.

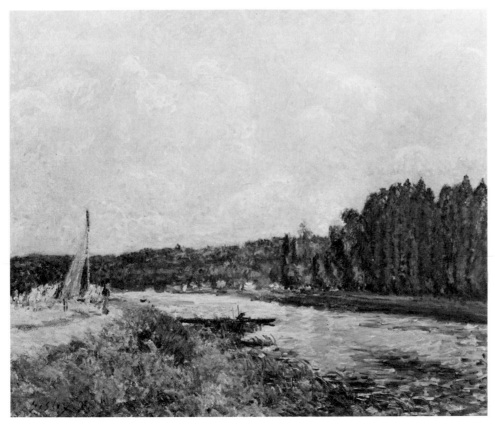

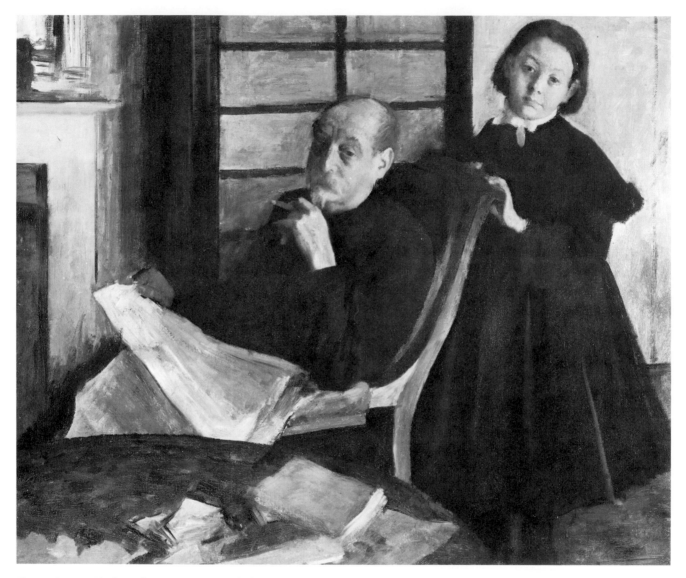

EDGAR DEGAS: Uncle and Niece. Courtesy of The Art Institute of Chicago.

to resemble wool, pottery, mineral surfaces, and oriental carpets; and through this very peculiarity of texture combined with color themes, they acquired a decorative tendency that was not anticipated by its originators. And this transformation of a realistically conceived technique into one of idealizing quality was largely due, as I hope to prove, to the choice of subjects.

The impressionist painters adhere to a style of composition that is strictly photographic. It apparently ignores all previous laws. They depict life in scraps and fragments, as it appears haphazard in the finder or on the ground glass of the camera (viz Renoir's "On the Terrace"). The mechanism of the camera is essentially the one medium which renders every interpretation impressionistic, and every photographic exposure, whether sharp or blurred, really represents an impressionist composition. The

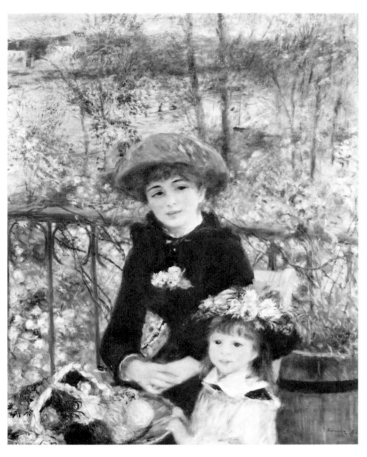

Pierre Auguste Renoir: On the Terrace. Courtesy of The Art Institute of Chicago.

lens of the camera taught the painter the importance of a single object in space, to realize that all subjects can not be seen with equal clearness, and that it is necessary to concentrate the point of interest according to the visual abilities of the eye.

It is a curious fact that all compositions of the Old Masters were out of focus. True enough they swept minor light and color notations into larger ones, but there seldom was any definite indication in their work whether an object was in the foreground or middle distance. Their way of seeing things no doubt was a voluntary one—they had a different idea of pictorial interpretation. In their pictures, as in nature, we continually allow our attention to flit from one point to the other in the endeavor to grasp the whole, and the result is a series of minor impressions, which unconsciously influence the final and total impression we receive from a picture.

The artist of the new school endeavors to reproduce any impression he has received, unchanged. He wants the impression to explain itself, and wants to see it on the canvas as he has seen and felt it, hoping that his interpretation may call forth similar esthetic pleasures in others as the original impression made on him. And it was largely the broadcast appearance of photographic images that taught him to see nature in a new light, as the human eye sees it in ordinary practice. At the same time the increasing popularity of these images emphasized in them the smoothness of texture which we were accustomed to for ages, and which is so peculiar to the photographic print that even artistic hand manipulation can not entirely overcome it.

Delacroix was the first to recognize in photography a serious competitor. And thus the young men of his period began to fight the imaginary danger; they experimented and within a score of years succeeded in developing a structural technique that guaranteed a vivacity and intensity of aspect. By this argument I do not mean to convey that photography was the sole cause of this technical innovation. Japanese art, color lithography, and scientific researches into the principles of color interaction all played important parts in it. But the influence of photography on painting is undeniable, and no doubt proved a most vigorous and beneficial stimulant in that direction.

In the meanwhile photography, in order to assert its esthetic possibilities, strenuously strove to become "pictorial"; this endeavor produced in recent years the singular coincidence that while men of the lens busied themselves with endowing their new and most pliable medium with the beauties of former art expressions, those of the brush were seeking but for the accuracy of the camera plus a technique that was novel and—unphotographic.

—1909

17

The Daguerreotype

A DAGUERREOTYPE:—There it lies in its case among old papers, letters and curios. A frail encasement of wood covered with black embossed paper. We cannot resist the temptation to open and glance at it. The clasp is loose: the old case almost falls apart. A weird tapestry-effect on the inside of the lid greets our eye, and opposite it is a gray blurred image set in a gilded frame with an oval or circular opening.

What a strange effect, this silvery glimmer and mirror-like sheen! Held towards the light, all substance seems to vanish from the picture: the highlights grow darker than the shadows, and the image of some gentleman in a stock or some lady in bonnet and puffed sleeves appears like a ghostlike vision. Yet as soon as it is moved away from the light and contemplated from a certain angle, the image reappears, the mere shadow of a countenance comes to life again.

What is there so attractive about it? Even if we find it hanging among Stuarts[1] and Sullys,[2] on the wall of some old-fashioned mansion, we are sure to stop for a moment in vague and wistful thought. Is it naught but the mystery of age that attaches itself to relics of the past—the haunting smiles of persons whose originals have lain in their tombs for generations, dreamfaces that call up love-led days? They look old, these daguerreotypes, as belonging to a far-remote period that has become estranged from us. But are they really so old as all that? People "in

the sands of seventy" may still own some of these images that represent them as they looked in their infancy. Octogenarians may remember the incident even, when they sat for them in a room admitting blue light through colored window-panes. Blue light, long exposures of five to twenty minutes, and the shifting silvery flare of the image—those are the unmistakable characteristics of the genuine daguerreotype, its signs of authenticity. Whenever younger persons tell you that once upon a time they were daguerreotyped, do not trust them implicitly: they are probably misinformed.

The reign of the daguerreotype was an exceedingly short one. The time following its invention was an active one in photography. One new process supplemented the other. There was the ambrotype which supplemented glass-plates for metal-plates, and the ferrotype which made it possible to make a picture on paper. Besides there were any amount of other "types," as the colotype, cyanotype, chrysotype, amphitype, chromotype, fluorotype, and behind all these loomed the wet-collodion process which was in practical working-order as early as 1851 and came into general use all over the world in the fifties. It was probably one of these more commercial processes that the younger set refer to, and in many instances they may have been merely "tintyped"—tintype being the colloquial name for a ferrotype—an amusement which, in our own recollection, played quite an important part at summer-resorts, cheap amusement-places, and county fairs.

The daguerreotype was in vogue, or perhaps better expressed, in general use for practical portrait-purposes, only in the forties and fifties. It never became really popular.[3] By the time the process had gained recognition, it was already discarded for quicker, easier, and cheaper methods. It was too expensive, painstaking and scientific a manipulation for the workman; and to sit quietly for five or seven minutes, even on the brightest day, was surely no inducement to public favor after the charm of novelty had once worn off.

This is the reason why daguerreotypes are becoming more and more of a rarity. These shining sorceries, on which light plays as on moonstone or mother-of-pearl, are attracting the attention of collectors and will steadily increase in value. A daguerreotype by John W. Draper,[4] the first Amer-

ican who made a portrait by this method, may bring exceptional prices at future auction sales. Professor Draper's subject was his sister Catherine,[5] who, with her face thickly powdered, patiently sat in the sunshine for half an hour, the time that her brother considered necessary for the exposure. The Smithsonian Institute in recent years has paid special attention to this branch of photography, and a younger generation, desirous to keep home- and family-memories alive, has become quite eager to have old daguerreotypes enlarged and reproduced. Quite a trade has sprung up in consequence. A genuine daguerreotype is surely as choice and precious an heirloom as any other, and the desire to duplicate these images is one of the few opportunities to display a feeling of reverence and ancestral pride.

In the early forties photography was still hailed "as one of the most surprising discoveries," and the

MAKER UNKNOWN. Daguerreotype made in 1849 at Harford, New York of Elizabeth Snyder, age eighteen, sister-in-law of Robert Bruce Pierce. Collection of Pamela Stern.

ABRAHAM BOGARDUS: Portrait made in 1848 in New York City of Robert Bruce Pierce, age seventeen. Collection of Harry W. Lawton.

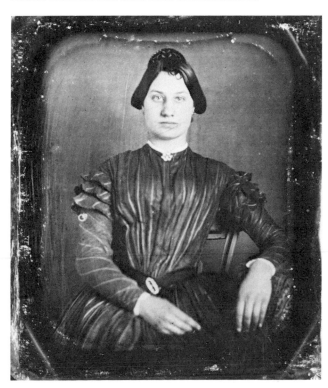

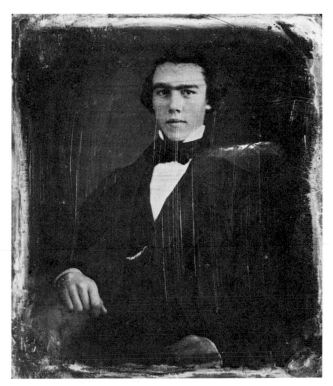

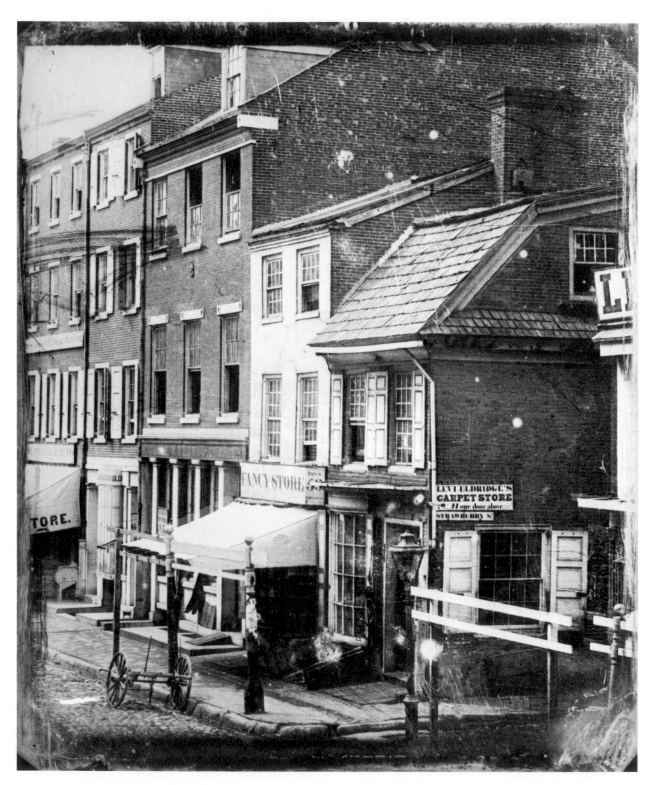

Maker Unknown: Chestnut Street, Philadelphia, 1844. imp-geh.

inventor L. J. M. Daguerre,[6] a scene-painter by profession but of little renown, who had frequently met the wolf of need at his doors, succeeded in selling the secret of his process to the French government. "For the glory of endowing the world of science with a new mechanical pictorialism," he received a pension of 6,000 francs for life, and the son of his former partner Niépce[7] one of 4,000. This may seem a small compensation now, but at that time few "prophets and visionaries" realized what this new pictorialism would eventually mean to the world; thus Daguerre and Niépce must be classed among the lucky inventors, in as far as Fortune rarely smiles more generously upon this precarious and most disappointing of intellectual occupations.

The scientific world had hoped for such a discovery, but had given up all expectation of the hope being realized. Ever since the Middle Ages, men had bartered peace and quiet in pursuit of the ideal of a sun-drawn picture. Not until the beginning of the eighteenth century did the dream take any definite shape. About this time a humble lithographer with the high-sounding name of Joseph Nicéphore Niépce used in his business for the reproduction of drawings a transferring-process which contained some of the vital elements of photography. Daguerre and Niépce met and entered into a partnership. They were looking for a convenience of reproduction merely, and they agreed to pursue their investigations and experiments in common and share the profits, whatever they might prove to be. No particular progress had been made when Niépce died in 1833, and Daguerre, with the grit that struggles to survive, continued to experiment along his own lines, finally achieving success in 1838. With the proud arrogance of the French bourgeois he announced publicly the full details of his invention before the Academy of Sciences on August 19, 1839.

It aroused interest everywhere. It shook the art-world with its fresh romance. Delacroix, the great French painter, exclaimed, "From this day, painting is dead!" However, he continued to paint.

Others took a deep interest in these sun-kissed products and, by the time the inventor had made known the process whereby his beautiful pictures were reproduced, in various countries men of scientific bent had taken up the idea. A New Yorker by the name of Wolcott,[8] an instrument-maker by trade and a philosopher in leisure hours, took out the first patent for a camera for portraiture. The products of these years were still in the experimental stage; but it did not take many months before some "men of science" were taking likenesses for money.

Readers who have retained a slight chemical knowledge from their college days may be interested in a short explanation of the actual process. They were not really positives but reversed images, negatives of exceeding thinness, almost transparent, "backed" by the mirror-like surface of the silver, very much like an ordinary kodak film that is held against a dark object and in that way brings out the picture. Daguerre used a polished plate of silvered-copper on which a very thin film of silver iodide was allowed to form, by exposing the shiny surface to the vapor of iodine. This coated plate was then exposed in a camera and developed by the action of metallic mercury vapor. Fixing was accomplished in a solution of common salt.

The chemicals were cheap enough, but the substance they had to work upon was sufficiently expensive to frighten away the most enthusiastic amateurs. To buy a dozen plates at that time amounted almost to the same as to invest in a dozen solid-silver cigarette cases to-day, and each of these expensive plates would yield only one picture. The newness of the manipulation, no doubt, also caused many disasters of over-exposure and under-exposure, and, frequently, no exposure at all. So if one desired to take to this new pastime in a whole-souled fashion, one had to be either a mine-owner, or some sort of Cassio who could follow Iago's advice. Nevertheless it made its way, and the semblance of all the celebrities of that period, such as John Jacob Astor, the elder Booth, Jenny Lind,

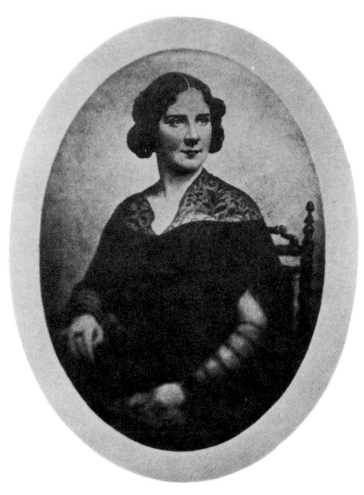

JENNY LIND (copied by Mary Carnell).

Charles Summer, Andrew Jackson, Webster; distinguished visitors like Kossuth, Dickens, and the Prince of Wales; and our early authors, Irving, Cooper, N. P. Willis, Halleck, Bryant, and Poe, have been preserved to us in daguerreotypes.

In order to take pleasure in these portraits of sixty and seventy years ago, it does not seem to be necessary to have known the persons whom they represent. To us their value consists in their faithful portrayal of fashions, environment, and personalities of another age, and, at the same time, by their finish, they reveal the character, the conscientiousness, and reach of that age. "People are inclined to smile because we praise the daguerreotypes of our grandfathers," said a prominent photographer recently, "but I want to say that the photograph of the present day is no improvement on it for artistic delicacy and subtlety of likeness." It is doubtful whether photographic portraiture of to-day will reflect our time in the same satisfactory manner. Its interests are, perhaps, too diversified, also, in most cases, too imitative of painting. Skill of execution is admired more than loyal interpretation.

The daguerreotype portraits show that their maker gave considerable thought to outward appearance and fashion. Portraiture was to them largely a matter of some person of means wishing to test this new style of image-making, who, naturally, desired a smart likeness of himself in colored vest, stock, flapping frockcoat and, if possible, a beaver on his head. Or it meant her ladyship in patterned gown, with bonnet and ribbons, short waist and puffed sleeves. Both of them had clean faces, new clothes and engaging smiles. Everybody had an air of tailoring and good breeding, as though born to a polite and comfortable life. The poses were the simplest imaginable, generally full-face views, as if they were looking at themselves in a mirror. There were no arrangements, no creeds of tone or pictorialism. They were too busy with the mechanical side of the sitting to delineate people at their best or what they, or their patrons, thought best. The papier-mâché furniture and other gallery-horrors, with the exception of the venerable headrest, had not yet been thrust upon an indulgent public.

The result was simplicity mingled with a certain primitive awkwardness. There is, however, in these pictures a fundamental quality which will never pass out of fashion, but will be appreciated always by those who love artistic things. For although these portraits show the originals dressed in a way that strikes us as absurd, or though the setting of the figures—to say nothing of the attitudes and expressions—often seem to us ridiculous, they are nevertheless the work of men of enthusiasm and taste. We feel that they embody, in many instances, the vision of an artist's eye, and that in their faces there is a vitality which none but keen observers of human nature could have rendered. The names of these early photographers will remain unknown. Their signatures were not recorded. They apparently could not persuade themselves that it was worth any man's while to sign his name to what seemed to be then little more than a scientific pastime.

How truthful they are to nature is difficult to say. No retouching was possible, and facial blemishes could be modified only by a touch of color on the cheeks. This was really in their favor. During the long suspense while the face passed into the solarized condition, the modeling was lost to a certain extent and the fleshtints were deadened, but these very deficiencies produce a delightful breadth of representation, as we have since learned to admire in the paintings of Manet and Whistler. And yet, at the same time, the detail of texture as, for instance, the sheen of a satin waistcoat, is copied with surprising beauty. They were composites of facial expression that were more trustworthy than those of the following period; for when more rapid exposure came into practice, the expression became more instantaneous, more restless, the shadows deepened and became opaque.

The daguerreotype will always be loved for its suavity of expression, its tempered technique, and its convincing grace. Truth of substance was wed-

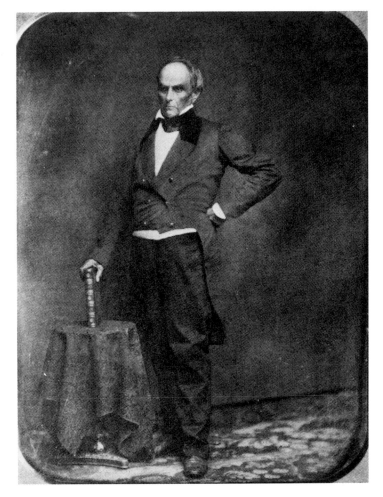

JOSIAH HAWES: Daniel Webster.

ded to truth of style in its mellow sheen. The short duration of its sway will steadily increase its esthetic importance. Although after its suppression it lingered on for a decade or more in various versions, it was in fashion only in the forties and fifties, and it will continue to represent this period to us. Impressions that impress art lovers generally have the flavor of rarity. This quality among *objets d'art* is granted only to a chosen few. The daguer-reotype speaks a language of its own that touches the common chords of life. The daguerreotype possesses the pictorial magic and historic power to fascinate the many as well as expert minds; for it conjures up to contemporary view and truthfully portrays forms and faces long passed away, things that are dead and lost to living eyes because it was, as James[9] would put it, "the real right thing" in its own peculiar time.

—1912

18

What Remains

THE PHOTOGRAPHIC exhibition at the Albright Art Gallery is a thing of the past.[1] There are many rooms in that white marble mansion, and they will be devoted as heretofore to the display of art in all its varied aspects. But its hospitable doors may never swing open again for a similar array of photographic prints. It was not an ordinary exhibition, this November show at Buffalo. It was a conquest, the realization of an ideal. Its triumph will rarely be repeated and even if repeated will assume a different aspect. It is not my intention to dwell upon any official reports of this successful venture. It is not a question of favorable comments or the number of visitors that availed themselves of the intellectual treat. They fail to tell the story. May it suffice to say that the general consensus of opinion agreed that pictorial photography had never been presented to the public in so effective, comprehensive, and beautiful a manner. I endorse this estimate with absolute sincerity. I have seen numerous exhibitions, photographic and otherwise, but I do not remember any which excelled this one in clarity and precision of presentation. This is now a matter of history and its harmony of lines, the charm of its individual exhibits, and the artistic excitement which was evident in assembling them, are merely a memory.

After hearing a symphony the score remains. After seeing a play the text remains. An exhibition, as soon as it is dispersed, leaves nothing but the general impression and a few cherished recollections, that we may realize again only according to their general sensitiveness and strength.

What is it that remains of the exhibition? Of what significance is photography artistically in these days of eclectic art expressions? This, I maintain, is what interests the true lover of photography most of all. Questions like these have nothing to do with the style of presentation, of mounting, hanging, and the exquisite proportions of the exhibition halls. It is the print itself, stripped of all embellishment, and the eye, brain, and hand behind it which must tell the story.

I believe the old cry "art for art" has become meaningless. That some pictorialists have fashioned for themselves a personal mode of expression is an established fact. The victory over the photographic bureaucracy has been won long ago. It needs no further argument. We have learnt that a photographic print can be a thing of beauty aside from reference to any subject it portrays. The high average of excellence thoughout the exhibit was astounding as it was exquisite.

Now, as heretofore, the pictorial army is divided in two camps, the Demachy-Eugene-Steichen camp who favor painter-like subjects and treatment, and the Stieglitz-White-Craig-Annan class who flock around the standard of true *photographic themes and texture*. The camp of the former, true evidently, becomes more and more deserted, the old flag hangs limp and the fires burn low—only the dense and indifferent public, which is always behind the time, begins to patronize what was popular ten years ago. But in the rank and file the old feuds are forgotten. The artist who rose at dawn and measured swords with his critics has acquiesced. Each man went his way, made his own audience, and challenged it for his own specific purposes.

The contention has become a much subtler one. What we would like to fathom is what photography can do better than any other monochrome medium, not what it may do eventually, but what it has done. This is strictly a matter of technical consideration, as the aesthetic satisfaction derived from an art is in exact proportion to the public's knowledge of that art's technique. We know more about photography, and consequently are more deeply interested in the intricacies of the process. Photographic draftsmanship commands three technical preferences which are always evident when photography is at its best.

1. The image is actually drawn by light, and no other black and white medium can compete with this conveyance of the actual flow and shimmer of light, as it flits from object to object to the deepest shadows, still capable of preserving a degree of delicacy in the most solid black. Prints like White's "Portrait of Mrs. White," Laura Armer's "Mother and Child" and Käsebier's "The Manger," to mention but a few, brought this out distinctly. As soon as the light is manipulated, it loses its greatest charm, and often becomes dull and chalky.

2. Line is invariably suggested by the gradation

GERTRUDE KÄSEBIER: The Manger. IMP-GEH.

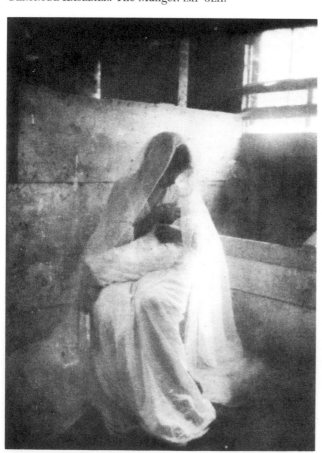

CLARENCE H. WHITE: Portrait of Mrs. C. H. White. IMP-GEH.

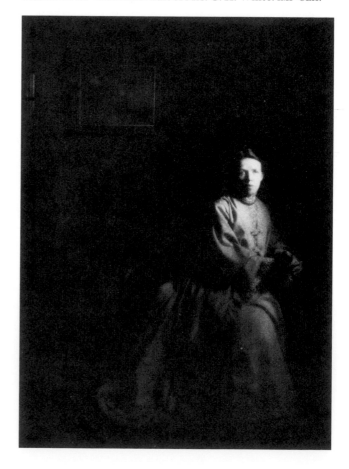

of tonal planes. Precise, or blurred, it is drawn entirely by the differentiation of values. This absence of actual line is possible also in other mediums but achieved only with great difficulty, while it is natural to photography and consequently one of its powerful characteristics. All prints excepting those of the extreme tonalists express this quality.

3. As it is impossible to emphasize line except by juxtaposition of values, that tone (a subtle variation of hues within one tint) is one of the most favorable formulae of photographic picture-making (viz., Craig Annan[2] and De Meyer[3] still-lifes). Tone in this sense has never been produced with equal perfection except by American wood engraving.

In subject matter the studio print and landscape photography have advanced but few new themes, if any have been brought out. They are borrowed largely from the other arts. It is the men who have preferred the city streets, the impressionism of life, and the unconventional aspects of nature to costuming and posing, who have occasionally enriched our wealth of pictorial impressions. In many instances they have discovered and subdued new and unusual motifs and improvised upon the laws of composition with the skill of true virtuosos. I refer in particular to Stieglitz's skyscrapers and dock scenes, and some of Coburn's interpretations of city views.

One can hardly say that photographic picture-making up to this day has revealed much of spiritual gravity. It is mobile and complete, but not splendidly audacious conceptionally. Only in rare instances does it reflect actual mentality, as in the work of Steichen and the Viennese.[4] Perhaps this is a limitation of the pictorial print of portfolio size. Its masterpieces may be defined as perfect beauty of visional appreciation joined to perfect beauty of technical expression. Elaborate figure compositions belong rather to the domain of snapshot photography. It is the single image, the attitude of a figure, the tonal fragment, a glass among shadows, a fleeting expression or some atmospheric condition, which adds something to our consciousness of beauty.

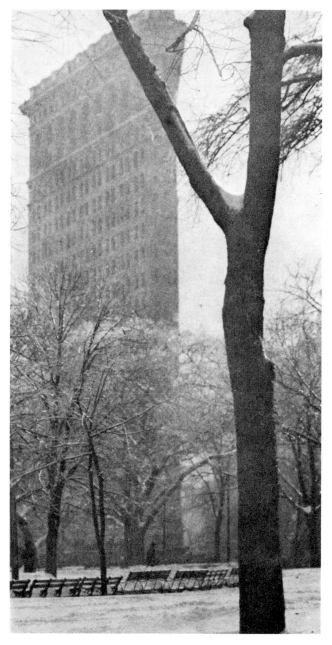

ALFRED STIEGLITZ: The Flatiron Building, New York, 1903. IMP-GEH.

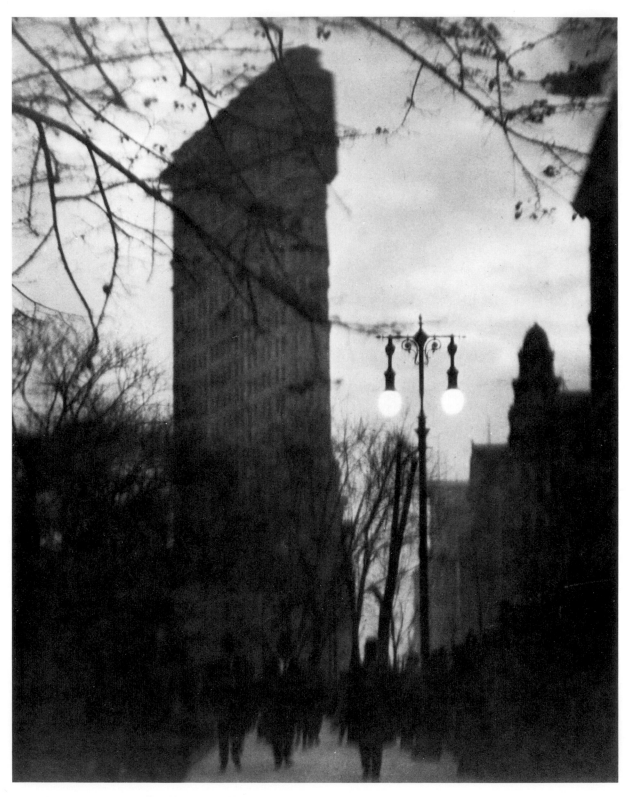

ALVIN LANGDON COBURN: The Flatiron Building, New York. IMP-GEH.

These reflections in a way are the result of my visit to the Albright Art Gallery. No doubt, any student of photography bent upon analysis of its aesthetic significance, has arrived at similar conclusions, but it was never brought out more clearly, more convincingly than at Buffalo. The photographer had a chance to realize the possibilities and limitations of his medium.

But there was something else which could not be seen, but only felt, which emanated as it were from the walls, and which pervaded the entire exhibit. It is difficult to express it in words. An ensemble so exceptional, aside of all actualities, teaches a lesson of deeper significance. It was combined in the spirit which provoked it. I sit at my desk and wonder how such a refined sensation of visional joy mingled with an appreciation of the mind so deep and true, as I experienced walking through these large peaceful galleries, could have ever been conjured up in this diffident commerce-sodden community. It can only be the result, I mused, of the natural exaltation of a mind free from prejudices (except it were directed against insincerity), solely as the pursuit of some lofty ideal. And I must confess that I have never met a group of men who have taken their vocation more seriously and disinterestedly than these pictorialists.

Art today in many instances is so mechanical and imitative, so time-pleasing and coin-of-fact that one greets these workers with exceptional feelings of sympathy and appreciation. Not that they are necessarily visionary and fanatic. No, they are practical enough, for it demands a peculiar temperament to be a successful pictorialist. There enters into his make-up a certain amount of patience and scientific calculation which is foreign to the average artist's nature. But they possess the vital spark. Their art expression is germinal, not mimetic. They have put themselves at the service of a new medium, and they endeavor to conquer it. No matter how eclectic they may be, they at least freshly comprehend, reassimilate, readopt accepted principles of beauty to a new virile condition. And thanks to these finer artistic faculties and sensibilities, to their subjective process of taste and ideality the success of the exhibition was due. These workers realize that their art instincts must blossom forth into wholesome consciousness as natural expansion before their medium of expression can take its proper and its fullest meaning. And it was this spirit which made the Albright Exhibit of November, 1910, memorable in the annals of photography and art.

Like the delicious odor in some mirrored cabinet that lingers indefinitely for years, this spirit will not fade. It will be remembered long after individual efforts have lost their immediate usefulness. The few masterpieces will remain, the rest will be forgotten, but the spirit will continue to remain an active force, and produce fresh impressions of light and tone, of form and grace.

—1911

19

The Esthetic Significance of the Motion Picture

No OTHER FORM of popular amusement to-day enjoys as steady and general a patronage as the moving picture shows receive.

The people in the larger cities can hardly imagine what this entertainment means to town and village populations. It is cheap and within the reach of all. And it is in many communities the one regular amusement that is offered. A town of six thousand inhabitants will easily support three to four houses with continuous performances of three reels each. Larger towns, of sixty thousand residents, where concerts, lectures and theatrical performances occur more frequently, furnish sufficient patronage for eighteen to twenty of these amusement halls. This shows a decided decrease in the percentage of attendance. In the larger cities where the motion picture is taken less seriously, the percentage is still smaller. It takes the place of the theatre only among the lower strata of society.

But its popularity is undeniable. It contains some element that appeals to the masses; and whenever I see one of these auditoriums packed to standing room only, I become conscious that I am in the presence of something that touches the pulse-beat of time, something that interests a large number of people and in a way reflects their crude esthetic taste. And is it not curious, with the popularity of this kind of pictorialism, regular art exhibits should be deprived of a similar appreciation. Generally no admission is charged and yet the public does not take advantage of these opportunities with any sort of enthusiasm.

The public is fond as ever of illustrations, stationary art, and cheap reproductions, perhaps more so than formerly, but it does not feel at home in art galleries. The fine arts seem to evade popularity. Works of art are generally so high-priced that they are beyond the means of the middle class. And merely to study them is too much of an intellectual exertion. People understand a Tschaikowsky symphony as little as an impressionist exhibit; nevertheless ninety-nine out of a hundred will prefer to hear the concert—while one solitary individual will derive a similar pleasure and satisfaction from the paintings—for the simple reason that music is easier to enjoy. One pays a comparatively small admission, sits down and listens, and the music drifts without any personal effort into one's consciousness.

Paintings are seen to the best advantage in daylight, when most people are busy in the more material things. They have to be enjoyed standing and walking about. One is forced to make one's own selections. Rather a laborious task, even for connoisseurs and critics.

No, there is something wrong in the present distribution of art products. Exhibitions are naught but battlefields for the survival of the fittest, and museums the morgues for pictures that are unsuitable or too unwieldy for private possession. Pictures and books should be owned by the people. Museums and circulating libraries are the products of a trust civilization. They are abnormal. Historical collections and reference libraries, like those of the Louvre and the Vatican, are not included in this statement.

Of course, there are many solitary works of art that can claim a certain popularity. Botticelli's "Spring" shares this distinction with "The Doctor's Visit" by Lucas Fildes.[1] Madame Le Brun's[2] portrait of herself and daughter is popular and so is Gibson's[3] latest drawing. It is largely the problem of quality—of the work, versus quantity—of the appreciation. An explanation is difficult. My contention is that every masterpiece must possess some of the "buckeye" element; or in other words, no matter how elaborate, fascinating and exquisite in finish a painting may be, it must offer some tangible, ordinary interest that the average mind can seize in order to be truly popular. And it is this element which modern painting lacks, and which the motion picture possesses to an almost alarming degree, for it contains all the pictorialism the average person wants, plus motion.

Readers may ask whether I take these pictures seriously and whether I see any trace of art in them. Yes, honestly, I do. I know that most cultivated people feel a trifle ashamed of acknowledging that they occasionally attend moving picture shows. This is due to caste prejudice, as the largest percentage of the attendance belongs to the illiterate class (at least as far as art esthetics are concerned). To my mind there is not the slightest doubt that these performances show much that is vivid, instructive, and picturesque, and also occasionally a fleeting vision of something that is truly artistic.

Judging from the ideal standpoint that a moving picture reel should reveal action in a series of perfect pictures, of course the majority are still very imperfect and unsatisfactory. There is too much bad acting and stage scenery in most of them. And many are absolutely tawdry and foolish in execu-

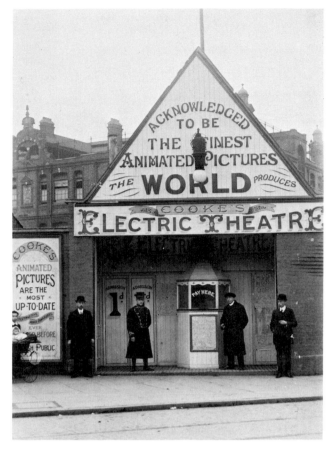

PHOTOGRAPHER UNKNOWN: Early motion picture theatre. Courtesy of Daniel Lawton.

tion and sentiment. My arguments in favor refer necessarily to the more practical ones.

The French film makers are in every way our superiors. They succeed in making excursions even into purely imaginary realms. I saw a Pathé reel in color representing Poe's "The Masque of the Red Death" which was done in a masterly way. There was more real art in the composition and arrangements of these groups and natural backgrounds than can be found in the majority of paintings of our annual exhibitions. The French command better talent and more picturesque scenery. They know how to handle costume and scenes of dramatic interest. The Americans excel only when they put aside cheap studio interiors, go into the open and handle realistic episodes of modern life.

Of course, it is generally not the story which interests me but the representation of mere incidents, a rider galloping along a mountain path, a handsome woman with hair and skirts fluttering in the wind, the rushing water of a stream, the struggle of two desperate men in some twilight atmosphere. These fragmentary bits of life, or merely of scenery, with the animating spirit of motion as main attraction, contain all the elements of pure esthetic pleasure, although we still hesitate to acknowledge it. But the motion picture will steadily gain in recognition, for it has come to stay.[4] No doubt it will undergo many transformations. It will be in color and accompanied by phonographic speech. It may become like the piano-player, a home amusement, and also enter the domain of home portraiture. And the reels will be free of all blemishes that will obscure the image on the screen. All this, however, will not make it more artistic.

More artistic it will become solely by more artistic handling, and there is no reason why some genius like Henry Irving,[5] Gordon Craig,[6] or Steichen should not invade the realm of motion picture making and more fully reveal its esthetic possibilities. As long as dramatic action, story telling or records of events will constitute the principal aim, it will remain imitative of the stage. Only when poetic and pictorial expression become the main object will it develop in esthetic lines. Some literary theme will always be necessary to support the action, but it could be the theme of a painter that is stage-managed by a poet or vice versa.

Imagine Böcklin's[7] "Villa at the Sea" as a motion picture: Old Roman architecture with waving pinions, and the approach of a coming storm. The waves would caress the shore, the leaves would be carried away by the wind, and into this scene of melancholy and solitude would enter a dark draped figure who in a few superb gestures would express the essence of grief. Many paintings of Leighton[8] could be rendered in such a poetic fashion. And also themes of more realistic painters, like Breton,[9] Cottet,[10] and Liebermann,[11] would be available. Short episodes in which all the laws of composition, color and chiaroscuro are obeyed, just as in a painting, only with the difference that there would come to our vision, like a series of paintings, one perfect picture after the other, linked together by action.

Would this not be an art equally as beautiful as the painting of to-day—while more intricate, and more in harmony with our present life's philosophy!

—1912

PROFILES OF PHOTOGRAPHIC PIONEERS

20
ALFRED STIEGLITZ

An Art Critic's Estimate

Leave routine to the timid, clear with one bound the common track, and when thou shalt have created a path where none can follow thee; when thou shalt have given life to a free work, loosened from the fetters of ordinary rule, thy place will be fixed and thou wilt see, coming towards thee with an even step, both glory and fortune.

—FROM "HOFFMAN'S TALES"

WHENEVER I HAVE spoken of the possibilities of photography becoming so independent and artistic that it can claim to be ranked as one of the expressions of pictorial art, the work of men like Robert Demachy[1] and Alfred Stieglitz has formed the basis and starting point for my speculations.

Alfred Stieglitz is to me indisputably the foremost artistic photographer of America—and I say this with due consideration of Eickemeyer's scientific realism and F. H. Day's decorative portraiture—a man whose personality and accomplishments are worthy of being treated by the critic with the same consideration as the life and work of a master artist. What differentiates the genius from the ordinary being and lifts him above the multitude? To me it is the mastery of three gifts, which also others possess, only not to the same degree and not united, namely, first, the power of selection in which technical accomplishments find their expression; second, the depth of emotion, which formulates the conception of the idea to be por-

trayed; and thirdly, perseverance largely dependent on temperament and constitution.

In his selection of his subject, the photographer is as much an artist as a painter, only forced to limit himself, like the *plein air* painter, voluntarily to the reproduction of realities. He must have mastered the science of composition, the laws of perspective, the effects of empty space and linear beauty, the massing of light and shade, and the art of values (rendered particularly difficult by the unreliability of photographing color values); in short be a connoisseur to such an extent that he knows at what moment to realize a certain sentiment and express it on the plate. The ability to select, after the setting of the picture has been satisfactorily chosen and composed, the moment when atmospheres and figures passing by make a perfect harmony with the premeditated conception, surpasses all other ways of expressing an artistic idea. In this moment, the photographer can show genius. To wait for days at the same hours for a certain effect, to wait for years

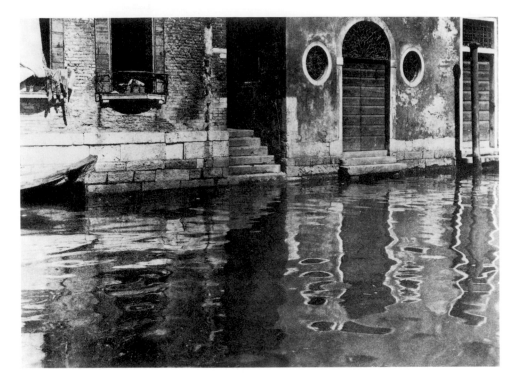

ALFRED STIEGLITZ:
Reflections of Venice,
1894. UNM.

for a certain atmospheric expression, and, later on, the developing of the plate, the process of printing, and not quite legitimate procedure of retouching, demand principally the practice of perseverance, with knowledge, judgment, and chance as guidance.

This is merely to prove that genius is possible in photography.

How far Alfred Stieglitz realizes these conditions I will leave to the judgment of the readers. The domain of criticism is to analyze the actual results of an artist's work.

Although the recipient of scores of medals at international exhibitions, in correspondence with the leading artistic photographers of Europe and recognized by them as their equal, continually sought by the American profession for advice and criticism, his position is a solitary one, as it necessarily must be, of a man who is a pathfinder and pioneer in a new direction of art.

His work, fairly well known to the profession of amateur photographers, has remained compara-

tively unknown, not only to the larger public—easily enough explained by the general indifference in art matters—but also to the artists, who on the average do not disdain photography as a mechanical helpmate for a sort of plagiarism from nature, yet do not condescend to recognize it as a possible rival to their productions. It would be in their own interest to surmount this prejudice, as an artist should not be only conscious of the scope but also the limitations of his art, both of which are dependent on the intellectual drift of the time.

Alfred Stieglitz has recently for the first time given the general public an opportunity to estimate his work by letting the publishing firm of R. H. Russell reproduce twelve of his original photographs in photogravure (*Picturesque Bits of New York, and Other Studies*).[2]

We have seen so many paintings and illustrations that look like photographs that it is refreshing to see once photographs that look somewhat like paintings.

Although I am aware that I cannot do perfect

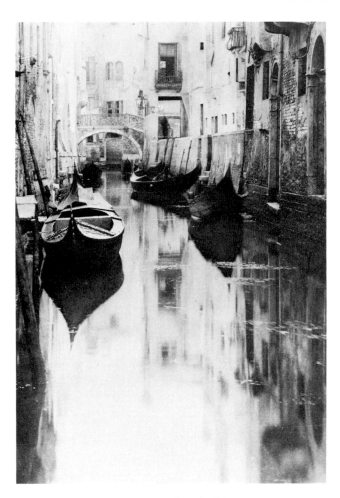

ALFRED STIEGLITZ: A Venetian Canal, 1894. UNM.

delicacy and vibratory force. Reproductions of works of art are always most dignified in black, or at least one dark tonal color.

"The Old Mill," a picturesque nook somewhere in the Black Forest, is one of those bits of realism that become romantic not so much by the handling of the artist, but by the reminiscences that such old landmarks awaken in us. It shows competent composition and exquisite gradation of light and shade—strong and powerful in the foreground, and fragile in the remoter parts.

Also, "The Letter Box," two little barefoot peasant girls in their neat *Badenser* costume, depositing a letter, with the diagonal wall of a house as background is merely a genre study, an attempt at story telling that arouses no special interest. Other men could do it, and I am only interested in that part of a man's work which the majority would find rather difficult to perform.

Of the two studies of Venice the reflections in the canal of the one termed "Reflections" are entirely too harsh in outline and values to allow a satisfactory enjoyment. The water is too opaque and has lost in parts all power to convey fluidity. It seems to be one of the most difficult tasks to photograph reflections in a sheet of water, as nearly all attempts at it seem exaggerated and untrue to me. That the difficulties, however, can be overcome, Stieglitz shows in his "Bit of Venice." A stretch of water of a canal as a foreground, losing its perspective in its gondola-lined embankments of quaint weather-stained house walls with a bridge and the suggestion of another cross-thoroughfare as background. The texture of the reflection is superb, mellow, blurred, and of manifold variation; only where the sky is mirrored in the foreground a delicate tint is lost which lends a special charm to the original. The composition of the upper part is perfect. It gives a better idea of Venice than many a painting. It conveys the true spirit of Venice, that poetical city of "broken fragments and washed out colors" that reflects in its quaint melancholy the history of a sumptuous past.

justice to Mr. Stieglitz by criticizing the contents of this map—realizing fully how much is lost by the process of reproduction—it will after all be more advisable than to criticize the originals themselves, of which only two or three perfect copies are in existence and which but few will have an opportunity to study.

The map contains two complete failures: "The Incoming Boat," which is in every respect commonplace; and "The Glow of Night," Fifth Avenue with a full view of the Savoy with its long rows of lighted candelabra reflected on the wet pavement, which is utterly spoiled by the attempt of lending it a color effect, a cheap yellow monotony which has robbed the otherwise excellent picture of all its

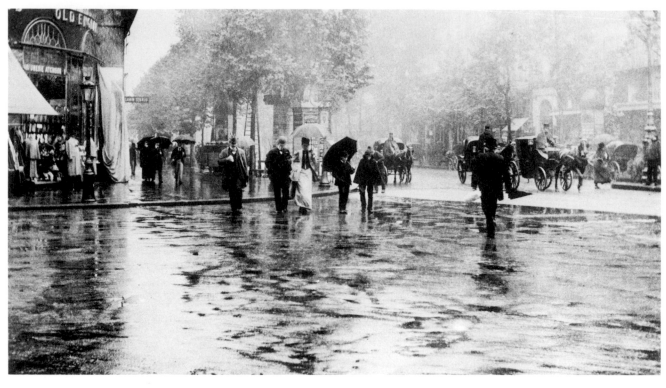

ALFRED STIEGLITZ: Wet Day on the Boulevard, Paris, 1895. UNM.

In his "Wet Day on the Boulevard" the photographer has attempted figure composition on a large scale. Although not quite satisfactory from a painter's viewpoint, it has many excellent qualities. The empty foreground, the store in the left hand corner, and, in particular, the hazy vista of the boulevard with its cabs is worthy of a de Nittis.[3] The only potent criticism I have to make is that the pedestrians coming toward us crossing the street lift their feet in a way that does not seem natural, although instantaneous photography has proven beyond dispute the correctness of such fugitive movements. The problem is whether we are not accustomed enough to the representation of such instantaneous reality to discover any beauty in it, or whether there is no beauty in the scientific analysis of movements, the details of which our eyes are not capable of reporting. More characteristic pedestrians, a grisette daintily lifting her skirts, or some other more typical type of the boulevards would have probably improved the picture.

The rotunda at Fifth Avenue and Fifty-ninth Street, with the Savoy and New Netherlands Hotels as backgrounds, is a bold attempt at night photography.[4] The effect is very beautiful, but at closer scrutiny one finds the blacks rather monotonous, in particular the defoliated branches of the trees which form a confused network that disturbs.

A special compliment has to be paid, however, to the photographer for discovering for art one of the most picturesque spots of nocturnal New York. I do not know a single painting in recent exhibitions that attempts a similar subject with equal grasp of pictorial beauty. It is a lesson to our painters that cannot be undervalued.

A "Winter Sky," a solitary fir tree on a snow-covered hill with the sun struggling through a cloudy veil and glistening on the ice-crusted branches. Stieglitz has tried himself as a virtuoso. The effect is remarkable, but is too near the border line of sensationalism to be considered a work of art.

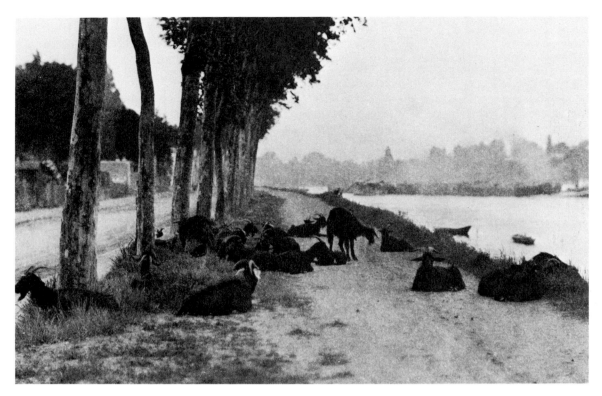

ALFRED STIEGLITZ: On the Seine—Near Paris, 1897. UNM.

Now we come to the three last pictures—"On the Seine," "Scurrying Home," and a "Winter Day." They are, with his "Net Mender," (not in this collection) a young girl sitting on the dunes mending her nets, a simple poem of nature like a canvas of Liebermann[5]—the masterpieces of his career. Before them criticism necessarily grows silent or becomes largely descriptive, as it always does when art approaches perfection.

"On the Seine," a double road on the embankment of the river with a row of trees in the middle, loses itself in an obtuse angle in the distance. A flock of goats has grouped itself in the road nearest to the river. To the right a vista on the Seine, a tug boat with a line of barges, and a silhouette of the housetops of Paris in the distance. It is a decorative panel filled with the musical cadence of a waning day, and that peculiar atmosphere which roads where city and country blend together always have for me. What patience the artist must have exercised before the goats grouped themselves so ade-

quately! In fact Mr. Stieglitz told me that for more than a week he stood every afternoon with his camera at the same spot, until at last he saw before him what he considered essential for a picture. The cluster of dark foliage, the border of grass along the edge of the water, and the distance have lost in values through the reproduction, but otherwise it is a picture which any modern master could be proud of. It is a well balanced artistic composition of rare decorative suggestiveness which shows that the artist understands the charm and power of linear and *spacial* beauty. "On the Seine" is a tribute to the undeniable truth that the future of art lies largely in decoration.

"Scurrying Home" could teach many an artist what composition means. It is more simple and direct than the previous picture. Two Dutch women crossing an open waste of sand, with the Katwyk Church, made famous by modern painters, in the distance. How interesting the texture of the foreground! How well its oblique lines cut those of

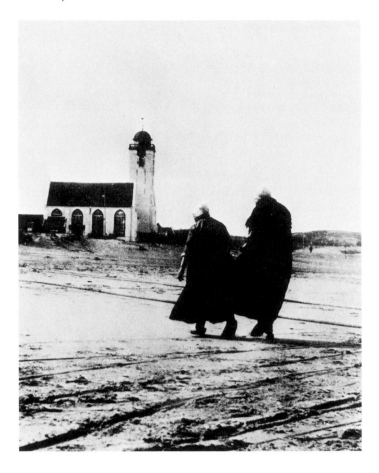

Above. ALFRED STIEGLITZ: Scurrying Home, 1897. UNM.

Opposite page. ALFRED STIEGLITZ: Winter on Fifth Avenue, 1893. IMP-GEH.

the middle distance! How well the distance is managed! And how marvelously the figures are placed, considering that if they had been photographed one second sooner or later the picture would have been spoiled. Their movement is as natural as it can be; it suggests the breeziness of the weather; only the feet of the larger one are somewhat indistinct, and the skirts of both are too opaque. It seems almost impossible in photography to attain Whistleresque subtleties of tone in a dark object.

"Scurrying Home" is a landmark in the domain of camera art and worth alone a trip to Europe. Many an artist after a three years' sojourn abroad returns without being able to show half as much. "Scurrying Home" shows better than any other American photograph I know the possibilities of artistic photography.

A "Winter Day," a Fifth Avenue stage coach ploughing through chaotic masses of snow, is perhaps less pictorial from a painter's point of view, but for that very reason more original and individual than the others because it reminds one of nothing else, while most of the others suggest in some way or another faint reminiscences of some school of art. It is a realistic expression of an everyday occurrence of metropolitan life under special atmospheric conditions, rendered faithfully and yet with consummate art. I, as a literary man, would feel proud if I could express a "Winter Day" in words with the same vigor, correctness, and individual note as Mr. Stieglitz in his photographic plate. His achievements in this picture are not merely finger posts for amateur photographers but for our American art world in general.

Let us scrutinize a little closer the personality of this man. Like so many other more or less prominent amateur photographers, he is so situated in life as to allow himself a constant devotion to his art, which is fortunate not so much because it lifts him beyond the dangers of mercenariness (since artistic photography is still in that idyllic stage where a market value of its productions is an unheard of thing), but because it enables him to indulge freely

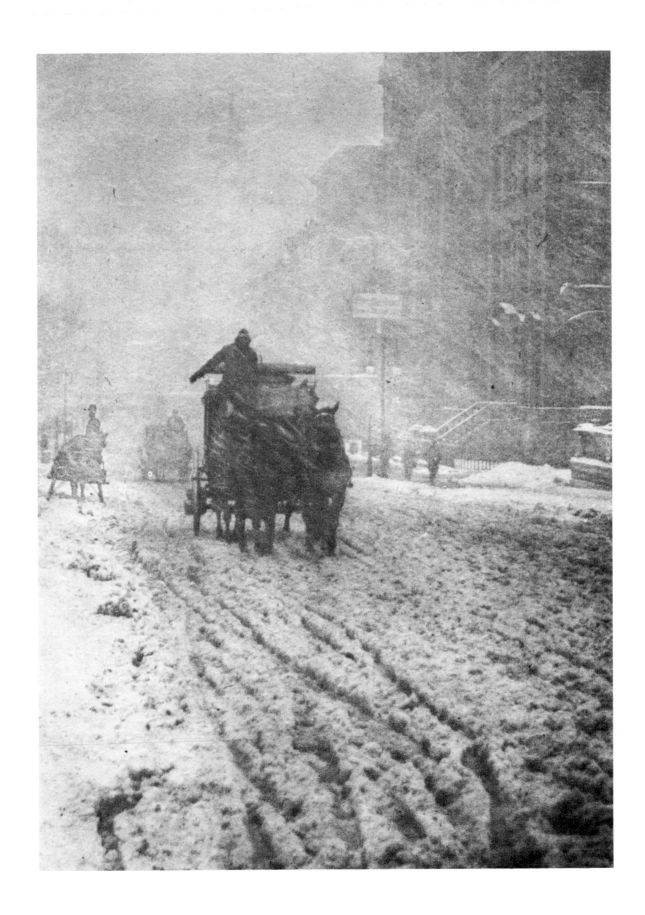

PROFILES OF PHOTOGRAPHIC PIONEERS

in costly experiments that are quite beyond the purse of ordinary mortals.

Stieglitz is a university man; he has taken a three years' course of chemistry and photochemistry at the Berlin University under Vogel[6] and Hoffman.[7] He is a thorough master of his technique, although he has never tried to improve the technical mediums by inventions of his own; he has been satisfied with doing his utmost in artistic expression.

He has traveled much, has been in touch with all the various phases of modern art and artistic thought, and associated with quite a number of European painters. In my first conversation with him, he told me that his favorite painters were Thaulow[8] and Besnard,[9] and that he went to see Duse[10] every night, and that he was also a great admirer of Yvette Guilbert.[11] This I mention simply to show that the trend of his intellectual life is strictly modern.

Simplicity is the keynote of his work. He recognizes that "art is hidden in nature," as Dürer so aptly said, "and that he who can tear her out of it, owns her." He does not try to idealize nature—look at his vigorous Bonnat-like portraits,[12] that are likenesses and not like so many other decorative whims or individual commmentaries—he merely represents picturesque ideas that suggest themselves in a simple natural manner. He endeavors to represent space and atmosphere, and groups his figures according to laws which nature offers itself. This seems simple enough and yet is rarely met with even in modern art. In Mr. Stieglitz was

necessarily from the very beginning the material for an artist, but by taking up camera and chemicals instead of brush and paint, he has succeeded in finding a new expression of pictorial art and in lifting it by incessant experiments to such heights that it can no longer remain unrecognized by the artists. He has revealed principles that apply to all arts.

The principal merit of Mr. Stieglitz' works, however, lies in his bold independence which enabled him to resist all temptations to overstep the limits of photography. He never applied anything but photography "pure and simple" and disdained the assistance of retouching by which Demachy has attained some of his most marvelous results. He realizes that artistic photography, to become powerful and self-subsistent, must rely upon its own resources and not ornament itself with foreign plumes in order to resemble an etching, a charcoal or wash drawing, or the reproduction of an old master.

I am confident that Mr. Stieglitz works in the right direction, and if he will also free himself absolutely in regard to conception and composition from all existing schools of art, trust his judgment and experience alone, and discover for us in a score of pictures the picturesqueness of New York City, as he intends to do, he will gain himself a place in our art life which the future art historian cannot overlook. At any rate, the last word about Alfred Stieglitz has not yet been said.

—1898

21
ZAIDA BEN-YÚSUF

A Purist

Whenever lately the subject of photography was broached in artistic circles I had an opportunity to frequent, invariably the name of Miss Zaida Ben-Yúsuf was mentioned as one of the most gifted exponents of the branch of portraiture.[1] I often overheard exclamations like "that only Miss Ben-Yúsuf could do!" or admonitions like "you should try that lady photographer with the peculiar name," given to people who had been repeatedly disappointed in getting a satisfactory likeness.

It would be interesting to investigate if, or how far, this lady's work deserves the high opinion which people seem to entertain about it, and to that purpose I today sit down at my writing desk, covered with prints from her workshop, and seize my pen.

The getting of a likeness, which everybody who sits for a photograph demands, and with perfect right, is not so easily infused with something of artistic merit as a bystander might imagine; hence any worthy result is specially welcome, as in this field the capable workers are distinctly limited so far. We all have observed what a contrast there is at times between the individuality of the personage the photographers portray and the whimsical results they obtain.

In looking through a pile of mounted prints—albums, I believe, have gone entirely out of fashion, except in flat and tenement houses, and in the country—one is confronted for the most part with very inartistic attempts; the likeness may be there, but the art is to seek. By this I do not mean that slovenly execution or inexact presentation of fact makes them conspicuously uninteresting, but they lack distinction. It is a palpable and instructive fact that if we were to take the representative works of half a dozen of the leading professional photographers, there would be but little difference in their productions. Their work is equally mechanical, equally the result of a stereotyped system of posing, lighting, and subsequent retouching.

Miss Ben-Yúsuf, on the contrary, endeavors to produce impressions more individual to the artist, and yet manages to get a likeness, and what is still more difficult, to please her customers. Each of her prints is easily recognizable as her work; they are, so to speak, infused with her personality, even in cases when they are more commonplace than they ought to be from a person who craves new fields to conquer. For she pretends to be a sworn foe to the fashion of popular photography and intends her prints to represent a sort of artistic revolt against the minutiae of detail, the glossy surfaces, and the mathematical precision still displayed in the show cases of Daguerre's successors.

Although she apparently does not always live up to her ideals, she has some, at least, and that alone is much to her credit. To eulogize the artist as some

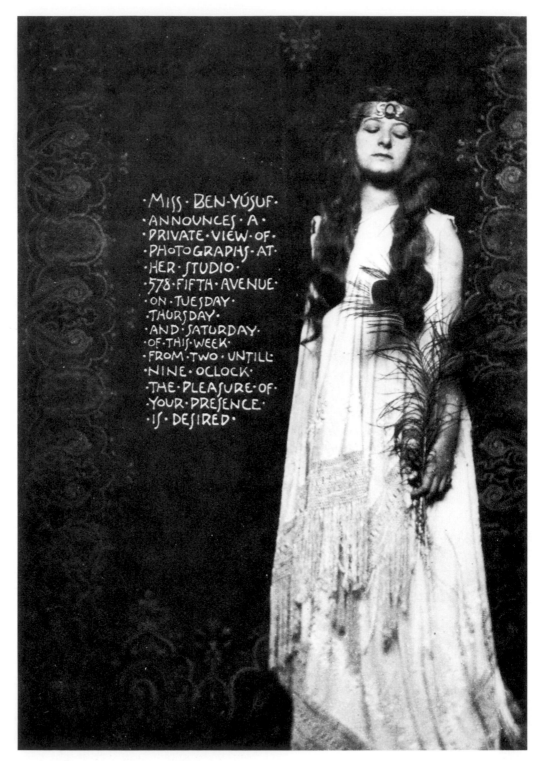

Zaida Ben-Yúsuf (Zeda Ben-Yúsuf): Exhibition Announcement: Self Portrait with Feathers. Gift of Mrs. Guy Bullock. MOMA.

writers have done is too easy to be of any value; to speak of her in a patronizing manner or to take a superior tone, would be impertinent, for it is doubtful if there is in the entire United States a more interesting exponent of portrait photography than she is; certainly it would take no little search to bring together half a dozen such individuals. One has simply to analyze her work, consider it calmly from all sides, point out its various defects and merits and, if possible, trace the origin of the various aspects of her art.

First of all, I would like to settle the question whether Miss Ben-Yúsuf is an "artistic" or a "professional" photographer. Of course, I consider Miss Ben-Yúsuf a professional photographer. A person who keeps a studio for the purpose of photographing people for a monetary remuneration is *professional,* no matter whether she avoids the ordinary hackneyed ways of advertising her business, or whether she has a show case standing before her door or not. Her methods of securing customers are simply different from others, and for that very reason, perhaps, more shrewd. There exists in New York a clan of Bohemians who pretend they do not care a rap for money, and who only accept it for their more or less artistic services because they have to live after all. This is merely a pose in most cases. When the manager of Julia Marlowe introduced her to the public without the customary bill posters and press agents' notices, he was perfectly aware that, once for a change, the best way of advertising his star was not to advertise her at all. And because Miss Ben-Yúsuf and Miss Käsebier have found such a new way of getting customers, they do not wish to be called professionals. Besides, they claim to be superior craftsmen of their trade; they fancy limited editions of prints and exhibits in photographic salons and understand how to surround themselves with a certain air of exclusiveness. It almost seems as if they wish to convey that they confer a special favor in photographing a person for twenty-five dollars per dozen. This is absurd, and the sooner they abolish it the better, as they will find out that they have only harmed themselves, for as soon as other professionals discover the trick, we will have artistic photographers galore all over the city.

In my opinion only men like Messrs. Stieglitz, Day, and Keiley[2] are artistic photographers; like the true artist, they only depict what pleases them, and not everybody who offers them twenty-five dollars in return. That is the line which divides artistic and professional photography, as it does art and potboiling. Money has nothing to do with it. Mr. Stieglitz has received for a single print as much as eighty dollars, I believe, and surely he was after that transaction an artistic photographer as much as ever, for it was a picture at the making of which its possible market value never entered his head. It would be different if encouraged by such a success he would set out to make a dozen or two of other photographs that would also sell for eighty dollars or more; then his art would necessarily deteriorate. Miss Ben-Yúsuf and Miss Käsebier, however, only on rare occasions produce something to suit themselves, as, for instance, Miss Ben-Yúsuf in her panels "Spring" and "The Book;" they adapt themselves to what their business offers them and are, for that reason—even if they were really indifferent to financial success—strictly professional.

The next point which I would like to dwell upon is the nature of Miss Ben-Yúsuf's aims. During a conversation the lady told me that her ambition was to become the "Mrs. Cameron of America,"[3] i.e., to photograph all celebrities she could get hold of, and thus go down to posterity with them as a depicter of geniuses.

How far will she succeed in this? We can only judge the past, and looking over her work of the last few years we must come to the conclusion that until now she has not accomplished her ambition. She has taken quite a number of men and women whose names are known and who might get an obituary notice when they die, like Anthony Hope, Le Gallienne,[4] Admiral Sampson, Emmeline Rives, Governor Roosevelt, Julia Marlowe, Ada Rehan,

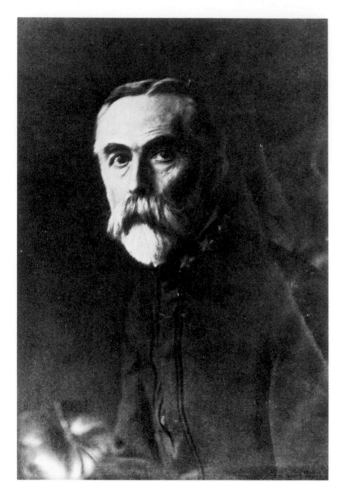

ZAIDA BEN-YÚSUF: Admiral Sampson.

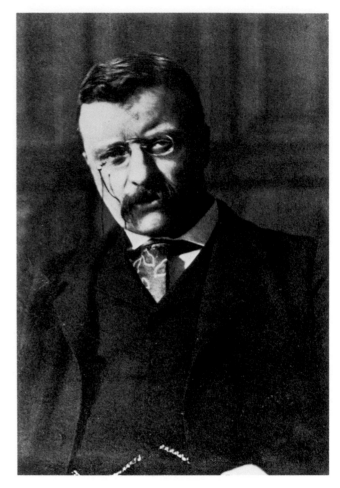

ZAIDA BEN-YÚSUF: Governor Roosevelt.

etc., but all of them are only celebrities of the hour. The only man she has portrayed who has some claim to after fame is W. D. Howells. In depicting celebrities she competes in no way with Hollinger and several other photographic studios, although she, possessing a special gift of summing up a person's individuality at the first glance, seems better equipped for such a task. She has failed to use her opportunity. So many great men have passed through New York in recent years, only to mention Nansen,[5] Boldini, Raffaelli,[6] Cazin, Duran, Prince Kropotkin,[7] Bourget, Holger Drachmann, the Danish poet of the sea, Kipling, Yvette Guilbert, Bernhardt, Sonnenthal, the opera singers, famous

orchestra leaders and soloists, not to speak of what New York itself offers in this respect, personalities like St. Gaudens, Ingersoll, Edison, Tesla, etc. For a woman it may be extremely difficult to approach all these different personalities with success, and in particular for one as independent as Miss Ben-Yúsuf seems to be. But why select then such a difficult path!

Perhaps we find an explanation in her artistic temperament. She is supersensitive; she has perhaps the desire to grow famous in the momentary association with geniuses, and yet is too self-centered to stoop in any way to reach her aim. Personally she is very fastidious in her taste, one of

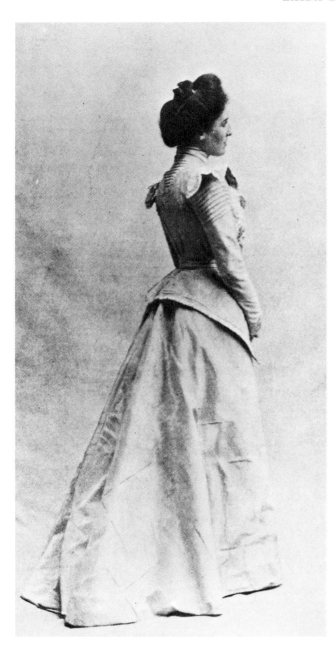

Zaida Ben-Yúsuf: Portrait of a Lady.

those peculiar persons who can only live in a room with wall paper of a most violent blue. In her dresses she is a second Mrs. Hovey,[8] although not quite as eccentric. She attends Ibsen performances, and everything else that mildly stirs up the Bohemian circles, reads decadent literature, and fancies high-keyed pictures such as outshout each other in color, best.

And yet, strange to say, in her photography she almost escapes her environment. There is no suggestion of it; everything is sober, intelligent, and refined. She perfectly understands the limitations of photography, and in producing pictorial results relies more on the mechanical assistance of the soulless camera than on her own creative power. There is no affectation in her art. And although the majority of her pictures have noticeable qualities that mark them as peculiarly noteworthy and interesting to an observer, the effects are all obtained legitimately.

When compared with the versatility and scientific composition of an Eickemeyer, the epigrammatic Japanism of a Keiley, or the decorative lyricism of a Day, Miss Ben-Yúsuf's work looks rather monotonous. It lacks depth and concentration, which is unavoidable in commercial pursuits, and besides, consisting entirely of portraits, is in itself not very interesting.

Her artistic training is defective, her code of aesthetics not very voluminous, her imagination not out of the ordinary, but she is somewhat of a psychologist, ever on the alert, ever seeking to grasp and to express in material form the characteristics of her subjects.

She understands posing, and yet relies for her poses mostly on her sitters. The charm of the *nonchalant* pose of Anthony Hope, perhaps, is due more to Mr. Hope than to Miss Ben-Yúsuf. It was undoubtedly an accidental pose, but it was her merit that she at once noted and appreciated it. In subordinating her knowledge of composition to that which the momentary situation in gestures and attitudes affords, she is a truer artist than if she would try, like Miss Käsebier, to introduce her own personality at every occasion. Perhaps she relies too much on unforeseen happy incidents, but as they happen rather frequently, the critic has no special reason to find fault with her method.

Nor does she depend much on accessories, although her backgrounds, if perhaps too frugal at times, generally show sensitive treatment. Particularly successful is she in the reproduction of hands; they become almost as eloquent a medium of recording the character of the sitter as the face. The garments, except when they are in some way interesting, she suppresses and modifies to masses of light and shade.

Of her technical shortcomings I will mention only one, which seems to be the most serious. She takes everybody under a top-light. True enough, top-light accentuates and emphasizes all the characteristic traits and features in a face. It is excellent for reproducing plaster casts. Look what wonderful work the Carbon Studio[9] has achieved for instance with Mr. St. Gaudens' relief of Stevenson, but it is not true to life. Human beings, except artists, are never seen under top-light, and their family and circles of friends and acquaintances are not used to seeing them in that particular light. It is a fault that nearly all professionals have in common, and Miss Ben-Yúsuf is no innovator in technical methods, only in style.

In her work we find the influence of London, where she has been active in photography, strongly marked. She is a so-called "purist," that is, she leaves her work largely to the camera, the chemicals, and the sun, and only retouches to a certain extent—what Mr. Stieglitz calls "dodging."

All these characteristics make out her individuality. She is no copyist. Each of her pictures shows her predilection, her personal bent, her own peculiar conception of life—however, only as far as the laws she herself has made for her art allow—even if it is only expressed in the quality and shape of her printing paper and mounting boards. She thoroughly succeeds in carrying out the object she has in view in justice to herself and what she considers legitimate in photography. Setting aside the delight that her consummate technique affords, which may or may not be entirely satisfying in a majority of her prints, there can be little doubt that in their reliable likeness, in the spontaneity of their poses, and the decorative disposition of the masses, they make up a pleasing total. The accompanying reproductions need not be taken as a final test; they were selected by herself because they show partly the average of the artist's work. One feels that her pictures represent a faction which must exercise some influence on American portrait photography sooner or later.

I shall look forward to Miss Ben-Yúsuf's work with interest and curiosity, and if I have induced my readers to share my feelings as far as interest and curiosity for her work are concerned, I shall have realized my expectations to the full.

—1899

22
FRANK EUGENE

Painter-Photographer

In FRANK EUGENE, a New York portrait painter who has devoted much study to the peculiar branch of art in which he is known, we find an able and versatile wielder of the brush suddenly deviating from the trodden paths of his art and producing a number of photographs which, both in conception and execution, show a distinct departure from the average artistic photograph.[1]

A visit to his studio affords great pleasure. He is, one might say, the painter of theatrical celebrities. He has painted Joe Jefferson more than a dozen times in all his parts—Rip Van Winkel, Bob Acres, and old Caleb Plummer. One of them is owned by Henry Irving. His portrait of Irving as Becket hangs in the Players' Club.[2] He has also portrayed Irving as King Arthur, Mrs. James Brown Potter as Marie Antoinette, Mrs. Corinne Jackson as Tillie Slowboy, Mme. Calve as Carmen (owned by Jefferson), and Anton Seidl—quite an interesting collection. The principal merit of his work is a certain richness of color that is subdued to a harmony of tone, rarely met with in pictures, suggesting all colors of the solar spectrum. Another characteristic of his portraits is that they look—particularly those of Jefferson—more like genre pictures than ordinary portraits, which is rather refreshing in a time when everybody has his portrait painted.

But the visitor who strays into the studio at present sees but little of these accomplishments; the painter has turned photographer, and wants everybody to share his enthusiasm and hopes about the artistic possibilities of photography.

Mr. Eugene has practiced photography for quite a number of years, and the number of his prints amounts to several hundred. Looking them over carefully, as I have done, one by one, I have been impressed by two facts: that nearly all his prints contain technical imperfections, such as could be easily pointed out by any moderately accomplished critic; and that—despite these glaring, almost unpardonable mistakes—they have, in almost every instance, pictorial qualities which the majority of artistic photographs lack.

Look at his "Henry Irving." Surely a remarkable bit of portraiture, in many respects the best I have ever seen, and yet the left leg is all out of proportion. Then again his "Madonna." What a marvelous contrast of light and shade; the first impression is that of a perfect composition, but how disappointed one feels when one discovers that the plate has been scratched all over, and that the hand of the mother is almost twice as large as it should be. The same mistake we find in his otherwise so beautifully composed picture, "The Misses H." The accessories are handled with remarkable cleverness; only the two large light spots in the background, overlooked by mere carelessness I suppose, disturb.

This strange combination of shortcomings and

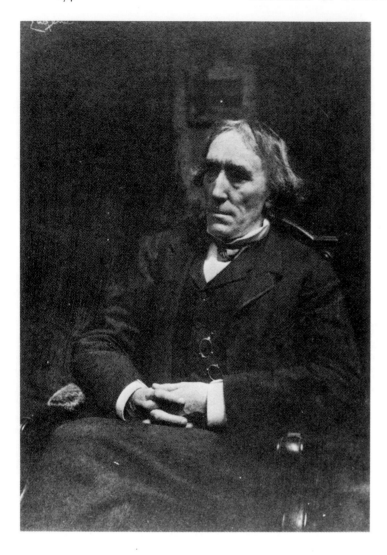

Above. FRANK EUGENE: Sir Henry Irving.

Opposite page. FRANK EUGENE: Frau von Holwein. IMP-GEH.

meritorious traits can be only explained by taking into consideration that Mr. Eugene, whose versatility has led him to exploit nearly every graphic art, (like etching, pencil, pen and ink, and charcoal drawing, etc.), looks at photography merely as a new medium to express his artistic temperament, overlooking entirely that photography, as soon as it rises above mechanical picture-making, is a science which can only be mastered by long years of apprenticeship and experimentation.

The ambition to get painter's results is nothing new. All photographers of high standing and ability have striven for it, and a few in this country, principally Messrs. Stieglitz, Day, and Miss Käsebier, have achieved it. With few exceptions, their knowledge of drawing, light and shade, composition, however, is simply theoretical, acquired by the study of galleries, reproductions, and books, and not by practical application in some other art. They endeavor to reflect the principles of painting, and to imitate its effects as to tonality and chiaroscura. Mr. Eugene, on the contrary, being a wielder of the pencil, etching needle and brush, strives to introduce the technical characteristics of other arts into his prints. They look like reproductions of paintings and etchings. He imitates linear expression and brush work in the same way as Mr. Keiley does Japanese wash drawings.

Let us investigate his method of working. It is most peculiar. His routine as a portrait painter gives him the advantage of posing his subjects at once in adequate surroundings that are in themselves artistic. Like most studios, his contains all sorts of paraphernalia, the use of which no ordinary mortal can solve, but which lend the place that atmosphere, apparently indispensable, to the production of a work of art. It is interesting to watch Mr. Eugene manipulate these odds and ends. He places, for instance, a lady sitter against a most unconventional background, formed of a gobelin or painting, throws an old piece of drapery over her lap and surrounds her with plaster casts, fans, large faded flowers, picture frames, books—in short, whatever falls into his hands or impresses his fancy

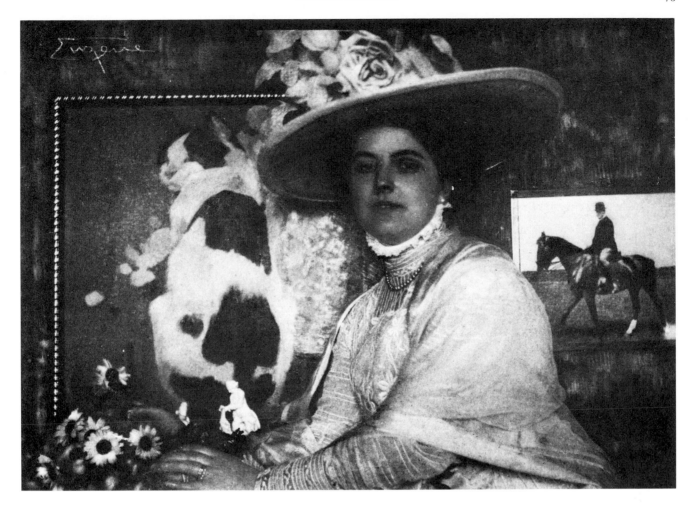

for the moment. While doing so he keeps up a most entertaining conversation, in order to make his fair sitter feel in no way embarrassed at finding herself suddenly in such an artistic curiosity shop; he continually adds one thing or another to his pictorial arrangement, and patiently watches for the moment when the lady, by accident, assumes a pose that pleases him. Thereupon he lets somebody hold a mirror at a certain angle, so as to throw a reflex of light on the shadowy side of the face, and then relies upon the camera to do the rest.

But the camera refuses to obey him. He has arranged his subject nearly as a portrait painter might do, who can rectify any shortcoming of the composition while painting. He has paid no particular attention to the foreshortening (very likely the fault of his lens), he has overlooked the fact that the action of light accentuates and often exaggerates every detail, and that the colors always turn out differently from what the layman expects. The result is a plate abundant with obtrusive details, meaningless dark and light spots, and, worst of all, with a false perspective. There is hardly any excuse for such oversight, not to say ignorance. A man like Eickemeyer knows exactly what he will get when he presses the rubber ball, while with Mr. Eugene a perfect plate, in which no retouching is required (like his portrait of Miss Jones, remarkable in its suggestion of color, and his large head of Kyrle Bellew as Cardinal de Rohan), is simply a lucky incident.

Any other photographer would despair at such

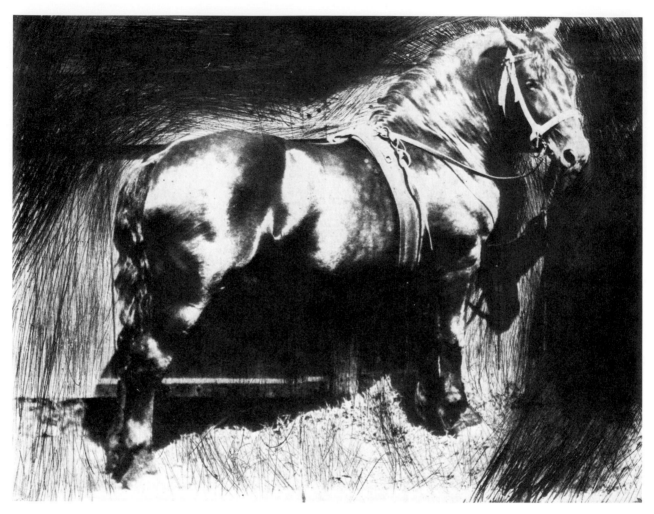

FRANK EUGENE: The Horse, 1895. IMP-GEH.

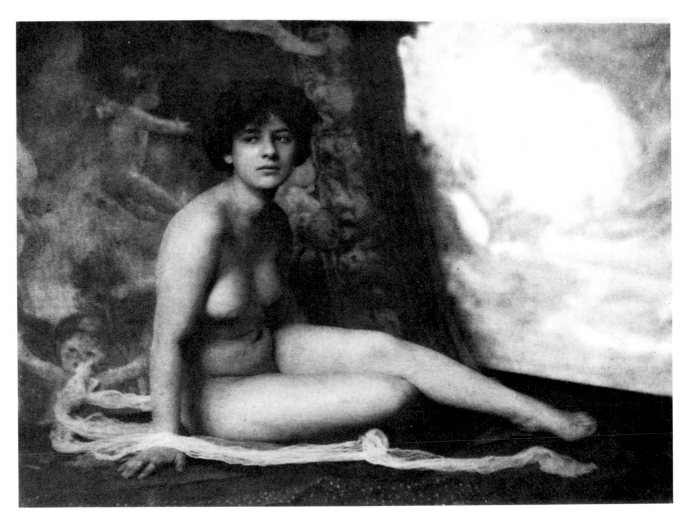

FRANK EUGENE: Nude—A Study. IMP-GEH.

dire results; to Mr. Eugene, on the contrary, they suggest all sorts of pictorial possibilities; they call his artistic temperament into play, and not only by the most extraordinary methods of suppression and modification, but also by actually adding absolutely new matter, he succeeds in producing something whose artistic merit can not be denied. He alters entirely the aspect of the subject depicted as seen by the eyes of the camera; for instance, he is capable of changing a gobelin background into a forest interior, as one can witness in his Madonna composition. The left part of the background of the portrait of Mrs. H. is produced by oil color, manipulated on the negative by means of thumb and index.[3] The same you can observe in his portraits of Miss M. W., and many others. Another of his retouching methods is a peculiar application of lines. The tonality which the camera refuses to repeat for him, he strives to attain by covering up and hiding all defects with cross-hatching. I have seen a portrait of the sculptor D. C. French by Mr. Eugene in which only the face was pure photography; all the remainder was the work of an etcher. Traces of these etched lines you can find in nearly every one of his prints.

The merit of his work lies distinctly outside the domain of photography; and although I do not undervalue his peculiar gift of imbuing a technically most hopeless subject with artistic feeling, I fail to see how the art of Daguerre can particularly benefit by such proceedings.

Every art has its limitations, and only he can claim to master it who accomplishes something within these very limitations. For that one must have its entire mechanism at one's fingers' ends. Nobody would dare to compose a symphony unless he were thoroughly acquainted with musical rhythm and form, the laws of harmony, and the construction of counterpoint. Why should it be different with photography?

Mr. Eugene defends his method by saying: "I do not see how my way of retouching is more illegitimate than the gum process," and with some right.[4] To make a photograph look like a sepia wash

drawing is really as unsatisfactory as to make it resemble an etching, the more so as the men who apply the gum process are generally no draughtsmen, and have no experience in handling a water color brush. Mr. Eugene at least can draw; but for his photographic career it would be more essential if he knew the difference of long and short focus lenses, and had given a little study to the chemical principles brought into action.

It is a great pity that the majority of artistic photographers are as deficient in artistic temperament as Mr. Eugene is in the technique of photography. The artistic photographers with their great stores of knowledge have, with few exceptions, but little to express, while Mr. Eugene has too much to express for his insufficient mastery of technical agencies. And for that reason Mr. Eugene's work is worth careful study. It represents an interesting phase in the development of artistic photography in America. It contains at times wonderful passages, almost as astonishing as the feats of an Ole Bull on the violin.[5]

The student of photography can therefore go to his works as proofs of what could be done in the art, if feeling and technique would go hand in hand, and derive from them the lesson that whenever a print fails to express something worth expressing, the fault lies in unskillfulness and not in any defect of the process. On the other hand, it would not be desirable to rival Mr. Eugene on his own ground, which would anyhow be impossible unless the photographer were himself an uncommonly clever artist to begin with. Even Mr. Day, with his rare decorative talent, could not approach it on its own ground.

His work also shows that artistic photography is capable of performing a good deal more than it has accomplished hitherto. And although I look at Mr. Eugene's achievements merely as an experimentation in a direction not quite desirable, it enables us to estimate all the nonsense said to the effect that photography cannot do this thing and cannot do that at its true value.

Artistic photography is still in its infancy, and it

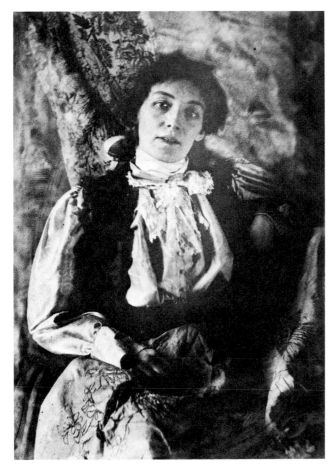

FRANK EUGENE: Elizabeth Blanche Walsh (Hartmann's first wife. This may be the photograph referred to as "Mrs. H."), 1896. WHL-UCR.

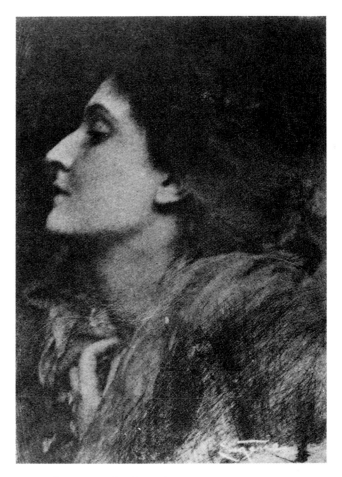

FRANK EUGENE: Lady of Charlotte.

will not reach maturity before it has freed itself from the influence of painting; for nearly all prize pictures of the Photographic Salons, with few exceptions (for instance the "Winter on Fifth Avenue" by Alfred Stieglitz) remind us of pictures that we have seen before. This is also the most grievous fault I have to find with Mr. Eugene's work; it is reflective, not original. In quite a number of his productions I can distinctly trace the first cause of their inspiration—his "Lady of Charlotte," one of his most graceful and delicate compositions, to a pastel drawing of Fernand Khnopff,[6] the profile of a pre-Raphaelite lady kissing the air; the portrait of "Miss Lillian" to the Glasgow school, etc. He has

the ability to re-create. Instead of exploring new realms for photography, he has been satisfied with endowing it with a certain pictorial beauty. It matters not from what source, as long as it pleases his artistic fancy.

We must be grateful to him even for that. In a decade or so his work may attract but little attention, but, at present despite the fierce opposition it will meet with on account of its technical shortcomings, it may command a position and perhaps even have followers, as it is the first time that a truly artistic temperament, a painter of generally recognized accomplishments and ability, asserts itself in American photography.

—1899

23

CLARENCE H. WHITE

A Meteor Through Space

Clarence h. white of Newark, Ohio sprang into being as an artist with the rapidity of a meteor rushing through space. I do not speak of the fashionable vogue which may suddenly illuminate the efforts of a man, long watched by friends and fellow-practitioners. This he could only gain if he would come to New York, and it would in no way concern the true merit of his work. Mr. White matured very quickly, if you look at the many years it took to ripen Demachy[1] or Craig Annan,[2] for instance. It is only three or four years ago that Mr. White asserted himself in the photographic world, and now, thanks to a peculiar rapidity of growth, he suddenly finds himself at the top to share the honors with men who have labored twice and three times as long and have yet remained comparatively incomplete.

Mr. White is as strong an individuality as I have met among American photographers. True enough his powers are more limited than those of others; he lacks versatility and is only a specialist, if you like; but nevertheless he is a well-rounded individuality. What he does is consistent, often beautiful, and entirely independent of other photographic work, for even if he takes his matter at secondhand from those he venerates, he understands how to imbue it with a spirit of his own.

The range of his subjects is very limited—satisfied largely with one female model, who, although not beautiful, has a remarkable talent for posing; he has succeeded in making a series of genre studies which, despite their similarity and uniformity of method, claim our attention at the first glance. At the beginning one merely notes a solemn, low-toned key of relative values, a certain weird fancifulness of subject, and a breadth of handling, at times delicious; but one is still uncertain as to what produces the general sense of unity and singleness of their impression. By studying what they mean to represent, one gradually begins to understand that this man's art is a product of the environment in which he lives. I have never been in Newark, Ohio, but I presume that it is one of those provincial little towns of the West with about 16,000 or 18,000 inhabitants, who probably live quite comfortably—perhaps even more so than the average New Yorker—but who know but little of the attractions and luxuries of a great city. Now imagine a man of artistic instincts placed in such surroundings. There are no opportunities for studying; all the ordinary thoroughfares for pursuing art are out of his reach; he cannot devote himself to it in spare hours, as he has to follow a mercenary profession and consequently lead a routine life. All he sees of the world's art is in stray magazines—and surely not always of the best—which come to the little town. A man in such a position has to rely largely upon himself and the observation of that which surrounds him in daily life. He will trust to the report of his own eyes and pick out from his surroundings that which seems to him practical and worthy of artistic treatment. This is exactly what Mr. White has done.

In his prints one can read as in an open book. Those old-fashioned interiors taken against the light of big windows, those old staircases, doors, and porches, the quaintly patterned gowns of the women who people these scenes, all tell their story. There is something so idyllic in his pictures, something so simple and subtle that the impression they make upon one is not unlike the peculiar fascination which Miss Wilkins' New England stories have for one.[3] It is a poetry which comes naturally, and yet at times can be romantic, (as in his Chest studies), or mystical, (as in his "Spring" panel or the delightful composition entitled "The Bubble"). As long as he is true to himself he succeeds, but as soon as he attempts to set forth his ideas with the eloquence of other masters, he fails. He has no skill in compilation, as Mr. Eugene has, for instance, and is unable to cloak his sentiments in the nervous elegance of Boldini. He is even incapable of depicting ladies of fashion in magnificent robes or dazzling evening toilette, which is astonishing, as he succeeds marvelously well as long as his sitters wear ordinary tailor-made gowns, as, for instance, his "Mrs. H." and his "Lady in Black," which I consider among his best work. He seems to have no eye for decorative magnificence or the management of gorgeous accessories, which take a completer training than was his share to enjoy. His strength lies rather in a vital love of reality, subdued only as far as the imagination of a simple-minded man can accomplish it. Simple subjects, like "The Readers," he can handle to perfection.

Technically, Mr. White's work belongs to the most perfect we have seen in recent years; it is satisfactory in all details; even the mounting and framing, done by himself, shows good taste and judgment. The ensemble of his exhibition[4] was very harmonious; there was nothing to offend the eye,

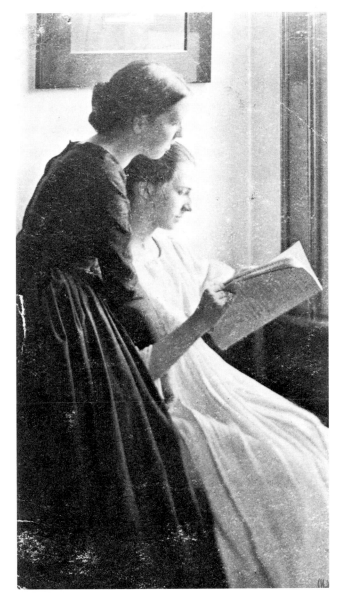

CLARENCE H. WHITE: The Readers. IMP-GEH.

which is more than I can say of most exhibitions; everything was so quiet and subdued that one almost overlooked a certain monotony of appearance, which, with inferior work, would have been simply intolerable.

This shortcoming is very easily explained, for as masterly as he is in the observation and expression of relative value, so deficient he is in the suggestion of color. That is his weak spot. The filmy, sugges-

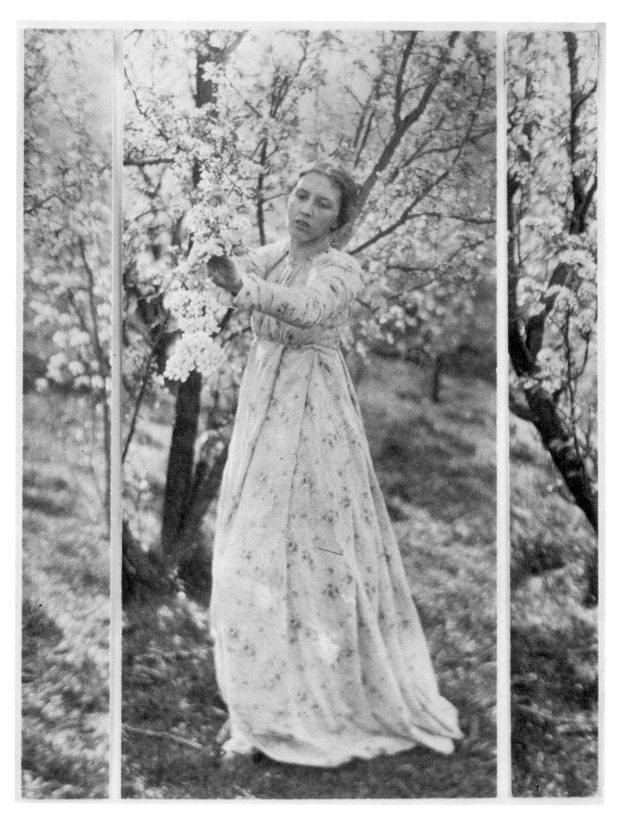

CLARENCE H. WHITE: Triptych, Spring, 1898. Gift of Mrs. Mervyn Palmer. MOMA.

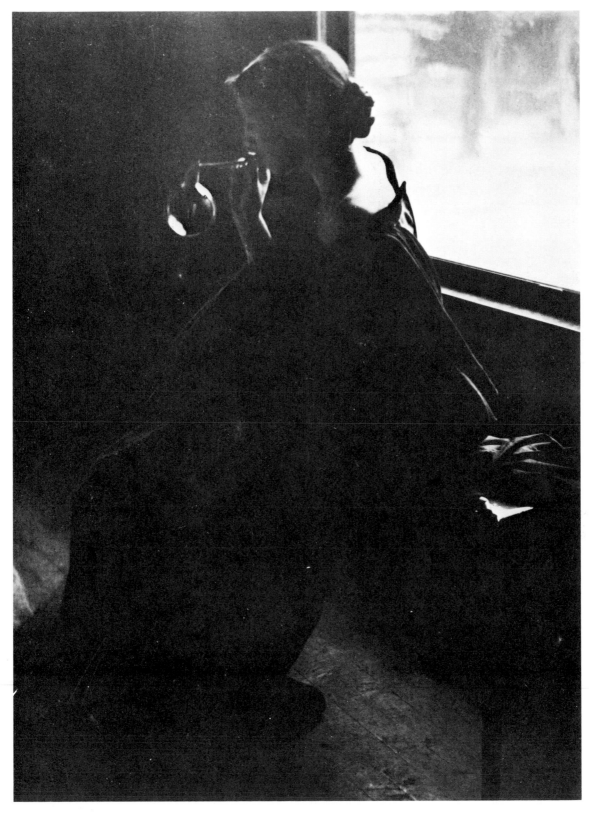

CLARENCE H. WHITE: The Bubble, 1898. Gift of Mr. and Mrs. Clarence H. White, Jr., MOMA.

tive, and mysterious manner in which he handles his interiors allows of no strong contrasts—the general tone would be spoiled, and with it the sentiment. He regards colors as relating to the prevailing note of the whole field of vision rather than to each other, and thus he invariably obtains an effective scale of relative importance in tone. He has learned to reveal things with the mystery of a true chiaroscura, but he only masters her in her most modest moods, and wisely avoids all violent effects. He probably knows that he would fail in attempting atmospheric effects of a more joyous nature than those which he likes to depict over and over again. Superb at times is the way in which he subordinates all unnecessary details to a mass of black. His blacks, however, are not as rich and deep as Mr. Day's, which, although they never seem mere willful emptiness, fail to express depth of space.

A certain frugality is the keynote of Mr. White's work. He is not brimful of ideas like some men; he has only a few and his resources for expressing them are very limited, but what he can give, he gives whole-souled, in a sincere and conscientious manner. And these two qualities should not be undervalued if they are combined with genuine inborn talent. They have made a great sculptor of Mr. St. Gaudens,[5] and although Mr. White's abilities can in no way be compared to those of our greatest sculptor, they might in time ripen Mr. White's individuality so that it will bear still more beautiful fruit.

As we know him at present he is one of the very best exponents of figure-photography we have, a man who always aims at completeness, at an extremely high finish, at beauty of sentiment handled so reverently that it becomes part of the imagination, an accomplishment still very rare in modern photography.

The mild, melancholy mood which we can trace in all his prints, and which is achieved with such frugal means, is to me the most interesting note of his work. I always believed that the most individual

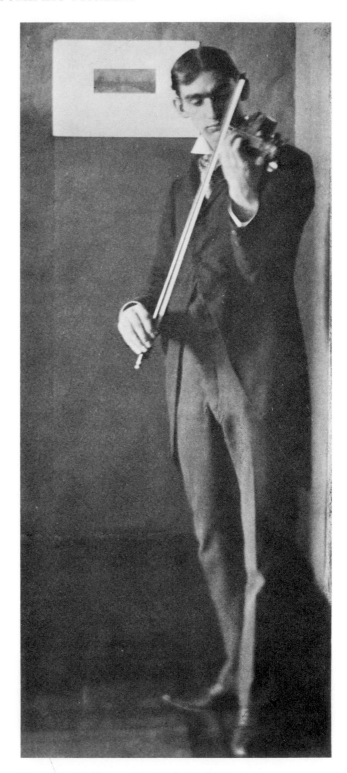

CLARENCE H. WHITE: The Violinist, 1897. MOMA.

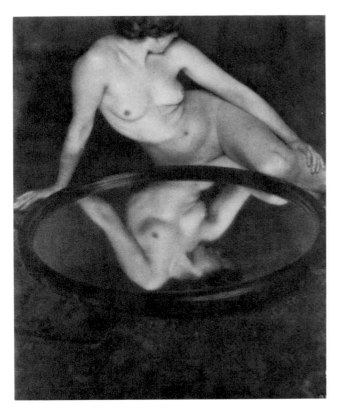

CLARENCE H. WHITE: Nude. The Mirror, 1909. MOMA.

My final test of an artist's work is to consider what of it I would care to hang up on the walls of my own home; the larger the number is, the more favorable becomes my estimate of the artist; for a man who has seen as much as I have, can only *live* with pictures that possess intrinsic value. Let me apply this test to Mr. White's photographic prints.

His "Spring" I consider one of the masterpieces of American photography; it belongs to my framed collection of photographic prints, in which every man is only represented by two or three prints. Also "The Bubble," "The Lady in Black," and several of his interiors and standing figures like "The Violinist" would do honor to any wall. I am doubtful about his "Old Chest Studies." They have been accused of being theatrical. I do not agree there; they have sprung from genuine feeling, and show how far Mr. White's imagination may venture successfully. They are like scenes illustrating some strange story of people of bygone days moved by some heart-rending sorrow or feverish desire. A lurid light hovers over these quaintly draped women who bend over an old chest and clasp in their pale hands some relic, a sword or a chain, with the ardor of some deep emotion called up from the graves of the past. They have a great fascination for me, and yet I do not believe they would remain longer than two weeks on my wall. A story has to be marvelously well told to be permissible in pictorial art, and the "Old Chest Studies" do not reach, despite their merits, that state of perfection; they are, after all, only studies. But they, like two-thirds of his exhibited prints, should find a place in the portfolio of every collector of artistic photographs.

—1900

representatives of American art would come from the West. In the Eastern large cities we are too much influenced by European art to develop strong self-reliant individualities who, after once having entered upon a path, pursue it to the end. We Easterners are apt to shift from one ideal to another; we know too much and yet scarcely know our own trend of mind; suggestions come too easily to us, and we find it difficult to concentrate upon one aim.

24

F. HOLLAND DAY

A Decorative Photographer

M<small>R. F. H. DAY'S</small> photographic art is an art full of delicacy, refinement, and subtlety, an art full of deep thought and charm, full of dreamy fascinations. This is as much as to say that it is not the kind of work to please everybody. It appeals rather to the intellectual and the refined; to those, in a word, who can understand and can feel—such as those who love and appreciate Mr. Day's work; their support is enough to establish an artist's reputation, and that in a manner far preferable to the notoriety achieved by much of the transient, garish work of the day.

First and foremost, Mr. F. H. Day is a figure-photographer, intentionally and passionately decorative. As I stated recently in *Camera Notes,*[1] I know of no photographer who can drape a figure more pictorially or adorn a man's or a woman's hair with flowers in a more picturesque manner. He has proved in a rapid succession of admirable pictures what possibilities lie in decoration. His decorative feeling, however, is not complete in itself or affected by nothing beyond itself. It is dependent on many external incongruities, as dramatic effect, poetical sentimentalism, aesthetic emotion, and at times even complete story-telling.

He strives to render our modern life more harmonious. No easy task, truly, in this age of ours, when everything tends toward the effacement of character, when uniformity of dress is almost universal, when the leveling of the classes is every day causing our personality to disappear more and more. A risky task, too, and one requiring a rare gift of perception for its thorough accomplishment; for it is really a fine and fertile subject of study for an artist conscious of his mission—an age like our own, full of elegancies and refinements of every kind and instilled with a feverish activity, throbbing perpetually throughout the civilized world with its thirst for the joys of the moment, its love of pleasure and luxury, its craving for a life crowded with the greatest possible variety of sensations.

Mere talent for arrangement does not suffice, and neither does it suffice Mr. Day. He is a psychologist, ever on the alert, ever seeking for this—to grasp and to express in material form the individual characteristics of his subject. What do I care for the blood flowing beneath the skin, for the network of swelling and throbbing veins? What matters the sight of the straining muscles full of life, if the invisible part, the mystery of this living being, be absent from the picture, if I cannot enter into communication with its spirit? I care not how rightly, how truly, the eyes may shine, if I know nothing of the thought, the fancy, animating them. Even a flatness, or the projection of a bone, or the irregularity of a line, a deformity even, gives evidence of some

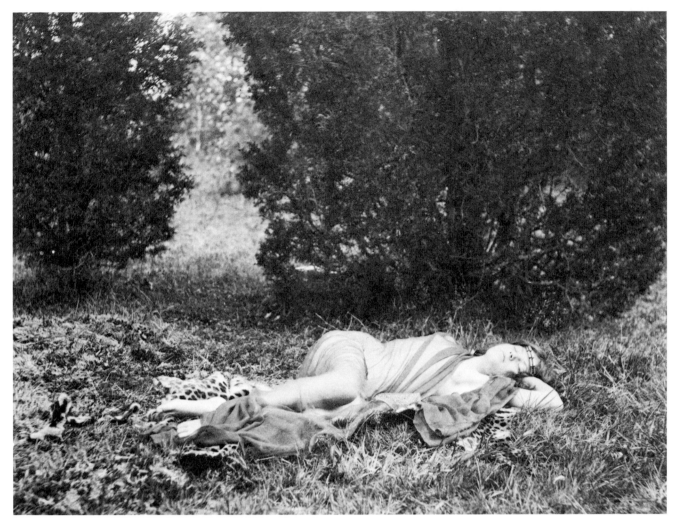

F. Holland Day: Fragment of Armageddon. LC.

habitual trait which, if at times contradictory, is nevertheless always full of interest.

As I said before, Mr. Day's art is one of delicacy and subtle refinement. To prove this, examine carefully the figures he so delights in. His subjects are intensely alike with the inner he; they seem heedless of all that might bar them from their own secret dreamings. They make no attempt at futile agitation, but are content with the thoughtful gestures of repose, the special poses and attitudes of pensive grace, in which the artist has fixed them. Look, for instance, at his portrait of Miss Ben-Yúsuf. How well he has caught her habit, her ordinary way of being, "all her little ways." One feels at once that the artist has photographed her with his heart, if such a thing can be said. The portrait thus conceived becomes a plastic psychological synthesis of the person represented.[2] He is not always equally successful with his portraits. He is too full of decorative effect to consider the getting of a likeness the most important quality. But his series of women's portraits, including Ethel Reed, Mrs. James Brown Potter, Julia Arthur, Miss Devens, and Mrs. Käsebier, are conspicuous illustrations of the harmonious concentration of vision peculiar to him. Full of grace and investing the true likeness of their

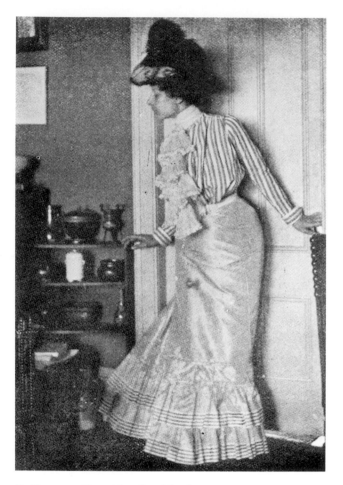

F. HOLLAND DAY: Miss Ben-Yúsuf.

subjects with an exquisite fascination, they have a certain something about them (which very likely could be traced to the arrangement of the backgrounds, the objects around, and the costumes) that seems to suggest the very spirit of decorative lyricism.

We find that all his scrupulously studied figure compositions have a setting of their own and a special atmosphere. Mr. Day will have none of that strict exactitude, the importance of which is so greatly exaggerated by most photographers. Imagination has too strong a hold on him for that; hence the air of harmony pervading his pictures—a skillful harmony, perhaps somewhat pedantic and affected at times, but generally deep and concen-

trated, substantial and mellow, expressing exactly what he wishes to express, adding merely emough to transfigure, magnify, and generalize reality.

The decorative side of Mr. Day's work can, in my estimation, be hardly overvalued. It is this which impels him to those subtle effects of light and shade and those surprising arrangements of costumes and accessories, giving to each of his figures just those surroundings which are proper to that particular subject, which give such an irresistible charm.

Mr. Day is fond of strange and wayward fancies. He likes to strike rich chords, but muffled, as it were, by the mist of his dreams. What delicate poems can be found among his studies after the nude—those graceful, youthful forms showing in calm repose on a background of some idyllic landscape! They appear in the twilight air, in which he likes to envelop them, like lovely figures of the past, telling of glories that have faded long ago. They are nearly always broad in treatment, without a trace of coarseness.

One feels that in all his works he is master of himself, master of gifts, laboriously developed in a most conscientious study and observation. Only in his "Christ Studies" he failed (with the exception of a few plates); the simplicity of "Open Air" effects proved too strong for him, but we have hardly the right to criticize, as he himself is not satisfied and willing to tackle the subject again and again until he finally succeeds. I, personally, wish him every success, for it is the boldest and most ambitious venture ever undertaken by a photographer, but at the same time I doubt very much if he will ever accomplish something perfect in that particular line of pictorial photography.

His peculiar *tournure d'esprit*, recognizable in his whole behavior, is decidedly against him; he has always lived the life of an aesthete, who appears to all at the first glance as an extraordinary, extravagant personality, one that excites immediate curiosity. Strange stories, both astonishing and ridiculous, are told about him, and he in no way objects to them. In serious dignity, he applies more

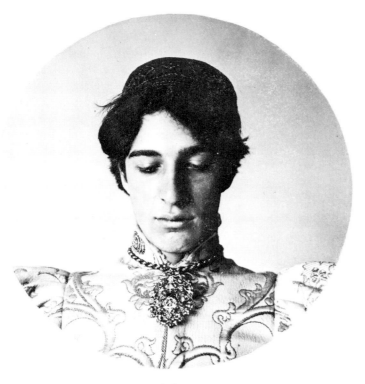

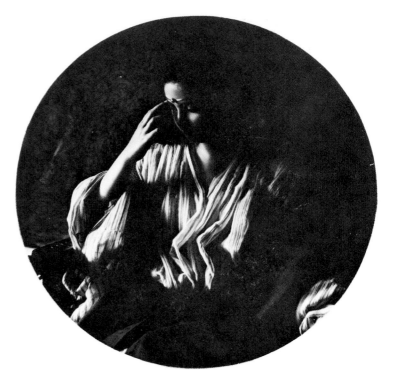

F. HOLLAND DAY: Untitled. LC.

F. HOLLAND DAY: Study of Drapery. LC.

of his imagination, for instance, to his mounting of prints than to his artistic productions themselves. To pose is a necessity to him, as it is only when he believes himself something out of the ordinary that he can accomplish good work, which is always an endeavor to realize something out of the ordinary.

Many anecdotes are circulated about him.[3] Once a stranger visited him and knocking at the door heard a most cheerful "come in," but entering found to his great astonishment nobody present. He looked around everywhere, but could find no trace of Mr. Day; then suddenly he heard a clucking sound, he looked up and saw Mr. Day sitting on a shelf right under the ceiling, wrapped in an oriental costume, smoking a water pipe! There exist also dozens of variations of the curious theme of how he made his "Christ Studies." He left Boston with a whole troop of male and female models, accompanied by a wagon load of costumes, a wooden cross and other paraphernalia, for some secluded country

spot in the vicinity of the modern Athens. Out there he went at once to work, had the cross erected on the top of a hill, built a sepulchre and prepared for a long stay. Then began the rehearsing of his company and the sacred tragedy was played more than a hundred times on the top of that hill, while curious farmers on their wagons with their entire families came from far and near to gaze at the strange spectacle. There is still some doubt in the profession whether he posed himself for the Saviour or not. I can hardly associate the appearance of this man, carrying always a portfolio with prints under his arm almost as large as himself, with the idea of his impersonating such an august personality, and yet his Christ in the sepulchre looks very much like him.

But it is time to come to an end; these general remarks are not, I think, out of place, inasmuch as they have a special bearing upon his individuality and the place occupied by him among those few

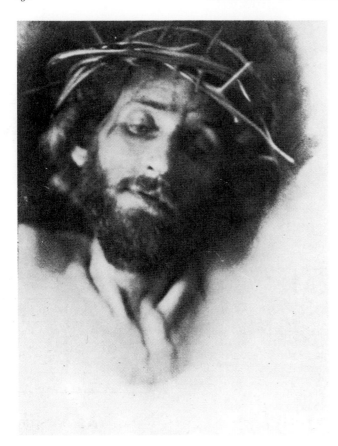

F. HOLLAND DAY: "I Thirst."

artists, of whom it may be said that they will in the future be considered the representatives of American artistic photography. If Mr. Day is not yet acknowledged as a leader he will be surely some day; he is winning his way slowly but surely, with admirable patience, by dint of honest work, backed up by gifts of the highest order, to the first rank in the near future.

Imitators he has in abundance, equals—in his own peculiar line of work—he has none, and he has probably done more for the creating of the "new school" than any other individual photographer.

—1900

25
RUDOLF EICKEMEYER, JR.

Master of the Foreground

IN SPEAKING OF Rudolf Eickemeyer, I do not introduce a new subject to the photographic public; he is well known as a professional, as well as an amateur, so I am neither tempted, on the one hand, to treat him as a whale among minnows, nor, on the other hand, induced by a certain timidity to underestimate the artist's talent.

The business of assigning a place to a living artist, however fascinating as a pastime, is a dangerous affair for the critic. In the case of an artistic photographer, it would be mere foolhardiness to attempt it, as even the vocation he follows has not yet been recognized as an art. And yet it seems to me that without indiscretion one may be sure of some things in regard to him. There are some artistic photographers whose art is less strikingly the outcome of what has gone before; others, again, have perhaps made a more gracious use of the art of the past. On the other hand, there are very few who have worked on old methods and preserved more of the truly pictorial element in their prints. And moreover, there are not very many whose work, if much of it be seen at the same time, is more interesting. It appears to me that nothing about Eickemeyer's work is more welcome and surprising than the variety and freshness of his choice of subjects.

The examples which illustrate this article give some hint of his variety. His well-composed *genre*

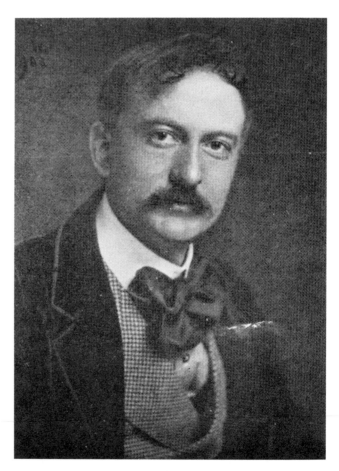

CAMPBELL ART COMPANY: Portrait of Rudolf Eickemeyer, Jr.

191

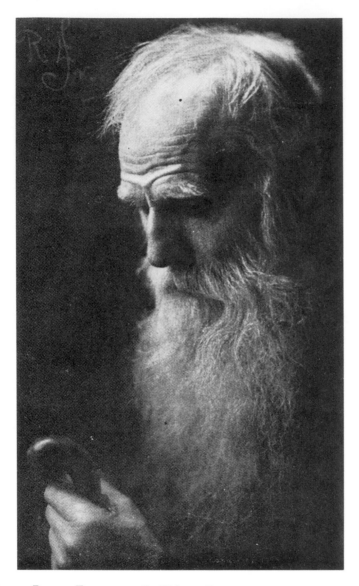

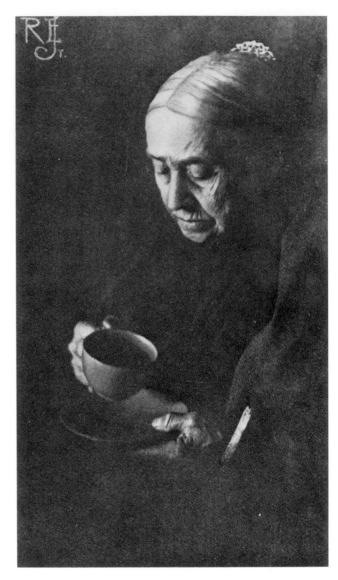

RUDOLF EICKEMEYER, Jr.: Halcyon Days.

RUDOLF EICKEMEYER, Jr.: When Age Comes Stealing On.

pictures like "The Dancing Lesson," his pictur-esque winter landscapes, his charming foreground studies, his draped figures, like his straight forward portraiture (viz., the "Ranchman" and "Halcyon Days"), show widely different aspects of Eicke-meyer's talent. He has entered every branch of pictorial photography with more or less success, and that is more than can be said of most of his colleagues who limit themselves largely to studio pictures. This versatility is the keynote of Eick-emeyer's work; he is in that respect like Craig Annan, which alone, with the immense amount of his output, entitles him to a high position among our artistic photographers.

The technical processes by which his pictures are produced are straightforward enough, and differ only in details from the usual methods of the purists. There is in his technique a directness and simplicity which are in a sense reflections from his personality, and which give to his execution a significance and exact meaning that are not to be ignored. These qualities, which were evident years ago in his earliest works, have never deserted him—not even in his latest triumph, the simple rendering of a block-house, behind which the sun has just set, radiating the sky with a last dazzling glow. It is the most pictorial photograph I have ever seen.

There are but a few technicalities which Eick-emeyer does not master, but he has limited his technique to purely scientific devices, and it is this simplicity which makes the adequate presentation and successful realization of his thoughtful fancies possible, and that his pictures afford to the profes-sion at large. Without the power to give shape to one's own convictions and to present them to the passerby in their most persuasive guise, the efforts of the most gifted person would remain ineffectual. The mastery of technical difficulties is an indis-pensable aid to fluent art-expression.

Each of his prints (of course I do not refer to his commercial work) convinces by an absolute sincer-ity of thought and expression. The only serious fault

(although one that he cannot help) I find in all his work, is the lack of temperament. One cannot look at forty or fifty of his prints without feeling, despite their diversity of subject, a sort of monotony. He incessantly strives for the expression of poetical sentiment, as in his "The Day is Done," "A Faun," "After the Haul," and yet, with a very few excep-tions, he always falls short of creating something positively beautiful. His conception is always greater than his actual realization. Eickemeyer is constantly handicapped by his lack of tempera-ment, but he employs the little he has to the best advantage, and at times even with amazing elasticity.

He is a man who has made earnest investigations into the theories of art. He inquired the reasons why the great painters did certain things before he had learned to do these things himself, and he had so much respect for custom that he preferred to train his intelligence even more highly than in the mechanical rudiments demanded by photography, declining to depend merely upon manual dexterity to get him through the difficult phases in the path of art.

His principle is still today preeminently an intellectual one, making demands upon his sense of observation, analysis, and upon his power to create on lines individual to him. It is one which guided him first in the collection of mental material and afterwards in the assimilation of the items of knowledge so gathered.

His genre-pictures, although exceedingly care-fully composed (viz., how in his "Dancing Lesson," the toys around the boy are placed, how the folds of the woman's dress are arranged, how the music sheet is turned down, and how the monotony of the mantlepiece and wall is broken by the vase) never pleased me. I am not over-fond of pictorial story-telling, at least not of this kind. There must be a deeper meaning to it than a mere superficial incident of life can afford. The "Vesper Bell" is by far his best effort in this direction.

His studies of the Southern Negroes are interest-

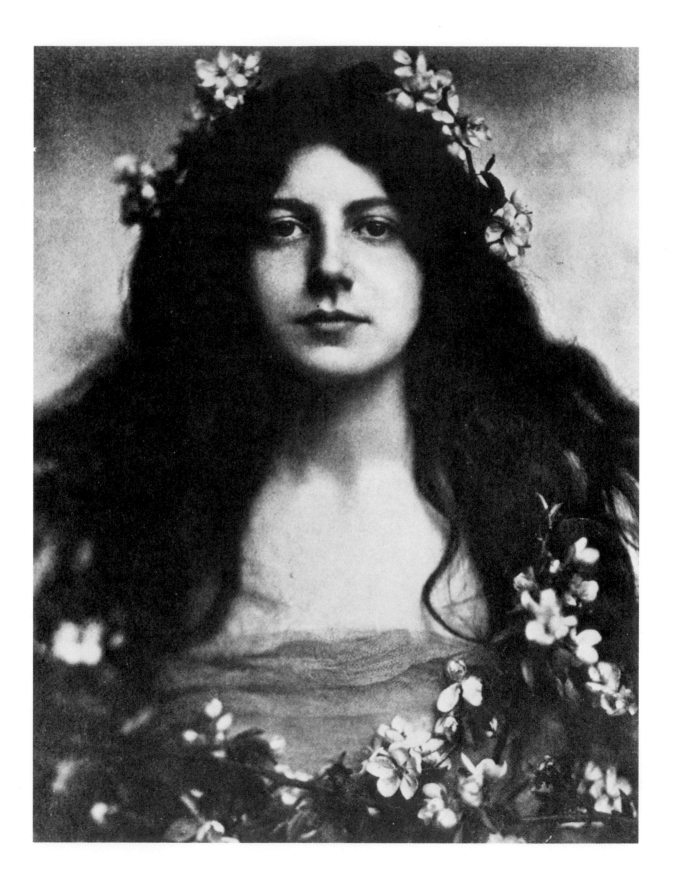

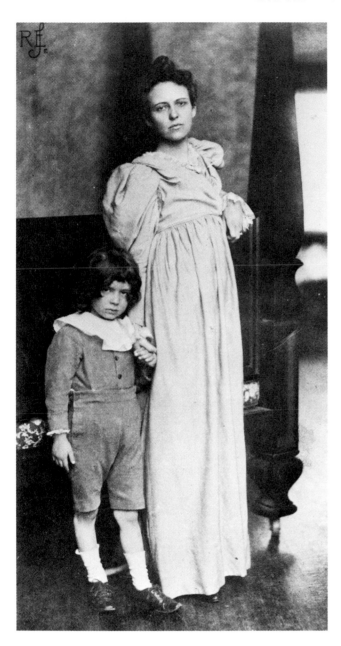

Above. RUDOLF EICKEMEYER, JR.: Portrait of Mrs. R. and Son.

Opposite page. RUDOLF EICKEMEYER, JR.: An Idyll of Spring.

ing from an ethnological viewpoint, but have but little pictorial value, with the exception of his "Peanut Field," which possesses the qualities of a good picture of the realistic school. He told me one afternoon, in his logwood study in Yonkers, that he made them with the intention to do something similar for the Southern Negro as Millet did for the French peasant. That was very ambitious, but he did not accomplish his ambition. They fall short in every respect of such a high aim. He undertook too much; his intellect continually runs away with him; his artistic abilities cannot keep pace with it.

Also his costume studies, in my estimation, do not reach very high. There is too much pose and premeditation in them. His portraits, on the contrary—that is, those in whom he is really interested—belong to the very best that are made. There is something so simple, direct, and yet virile about them, which is delightful. I would almost take it upon myself to proclaim him as the best portrait photographer I am acquainted with. I believe him capable of making a satisfactory likeness which at the same time would have decided pictorial qualities. It is no small thing to do either of these, but to do both is indeed a considerable thing.

His landscapes, with or without figure work, are at times full of suggestion, and appeal strongly to one's emotions and imaginations.

I am very fond of his winter studies, when everything sleeps beneath the glimmering mantle of snow, and only the light penetrates deeper than ever into the woods with their interlacing branches and many-textured barks.[1]

But it is, I venture to think, in his foreground studies that Eickemeyer gives the most convincing and most interesting proofs of his talent. There he shows himself a true lover of nature. Three out of four of his foreground studies would pass the scrutiny of the most exacting critic. They point out how little material is really required to make a successful picture. Two or three fern fronds, a stretch of bramble and a cluster of flowers are amply sufficient. The pictorial value of a fore-

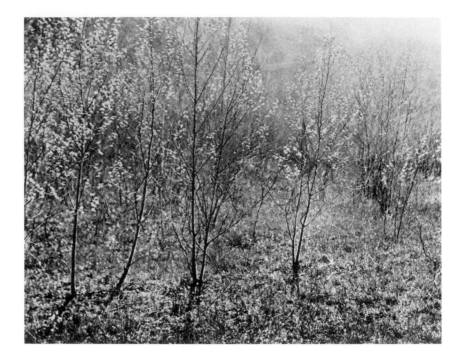

RUDOLF EICKEMEYER, Jr.: Spring.

ground study depends nearly entirely on selection of the right spot, and this gift Eickemeyer possesses to a rare degree; and his love of nature makes him at times unconsciously, despite the wise lore he has stored in his mind, a poet, as, for instance, in those magnificent "Fleur de Lys." In my opinion it is one of the best photographs ever produced in America, and only second to Stieglitz's "Winter on Fifth Avenue."

Eickemeyer should stick to these foreground sketches, make a specialty of it, or devote at least most of his time to them, for he owns the key to this fairyland where Oberon and Titania hold their moonlight revels. A few branches of foliage through whose tracery the sunlight filters, a handful of nodding grass whispering to the wind, a group of nettles, spreading burdocks or tangled bracken on the roadside, or a field of flowers in which we like to pause and rest, these are the subjects which he has perfectly at his command. In these he is unexcelled.

What will be the future developments of Eickemeyer's art it is impossible now to say. He has passed from one step to another, and has, in apparent obedience to the aesthetic instincts which control him, varied his performances to suit each phase. There are worlds full of variety which he may yet conquer. He has more than most artistic photographers, the chance of securing consideration and acceptance for any new departures that he may be moved to make, for he has already gained for himself a place which he shares with no one else. He has the reputation of being an innovator of judicious and well-balanced views; he is, with justice, given by the popular voice a position amongst the most capable of his profession, and well established in regard to medal and honorary mentions upon the ladder of fame.

He has enough of the true artist in him to desire to do justice to himself, and in leisure hours he may be trusted to waste nothing of his energies in trivialities and to make no mistakes that are not sincere. Indeed, we may look to Eickemeyer as one of the most representative types of the artistic photographer, one who, having had a past, has still left a future.

—1900

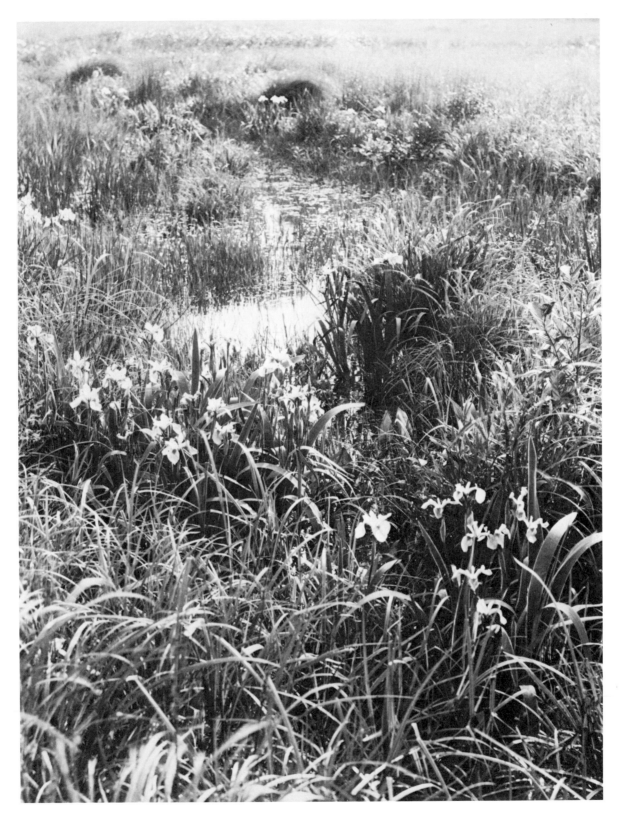

RUDOLF EICKEMEYER, Jr.: Fleur-de-lys. SI.

26
GERTRUDE KÄSEBIER

A Sense of the Pictorial

*F*EW ARTISTIC photographers there are who of late have so much attraction for the public as Gertrude Käsebier. Many of her colleagues praise and admire her; she apparently claims the attention of all eyes in the photographic world, and boasts powers of fascination which none can resist. Käsebier's individuality is of a very special order.

It consists of a highly developed sense for the pictorial, a gift which belongs rather to the *expression* than the *technique*. The technical means, which she controls, consist largely of a knowledge to obtain chiaroscural and tonal effects. In lines she is deficient, her values are often painfully faulty, her space composition with few exceptions is nothing above the ordinary. Clever distribution of light and shade and harmony of tone, however, can be found in nearly all her pictures. And the pictorial element is always predominant.

This gift of Mrs. Käsebier is incontestably a great gift; and her merit is the more remarkable in that, to obtain her effects, she makes no vulgar sacrifice, such as would degrade her work artistically.

But I cannot agree with Mr. Stieglitz who once declared in his *Camera Notes*[1] that she was the leading artistic portrait photographer in America, thus indirectly making the statement that he considered her in no way inferior in point of originality to such an artist as F. H. Day. Of course this is a matter of opinions. But Day strikes me as being far

more original than Käsebier by his exquisite imagination, his delightful caprices, his grace, and his fancifulness. Käsebier may be his equal in some respects, but her individuality, although very apparent, almost obtrusive, is rather a superficial one, one which can be analyzed and traced to various origins.

She has an ardent love of the picturesque, but her art is not based on observation. Nothing that is going on around her in this great city seems to interest and excite her. Her sympathies are entirely restricted to a certain artistic atmosphere which she has created in her studio, and into which every sitter, no matter how eager for actual, immediate reality he may be, is forced when he wants a picture.

They are not allowed to reveal the secrets of their existence or to lead the lives they live outside, they are simply transformed into pictorial visions, such as Mrs. Käsebier sees fit to conjure up from her store of knowledge. She knows the old masters so well that she can imitate them to perfection. Of course I do not wish to convey the idea that she is nothing but a plagiarizer. She is a dreamer, and if you like a poet—but the old master and other phrases and formula of art are so deeply ingrained in her whole system that she cannot help herself. The visions of the past will invariably rise, and as "the combination of subtle faculties" constituting

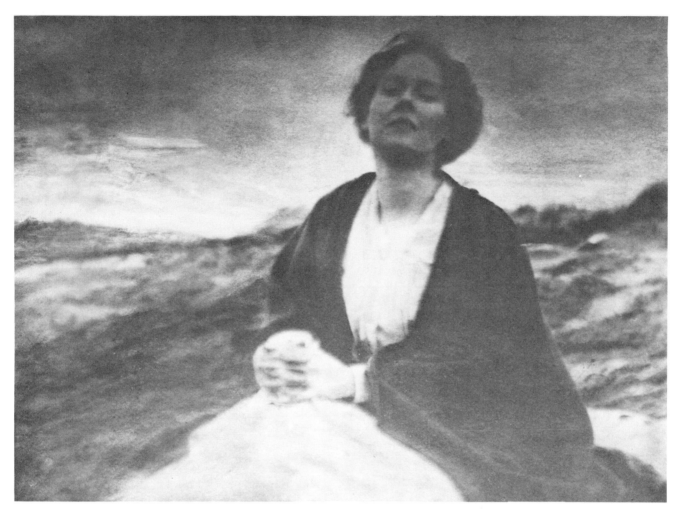

GERTRUDE KÄSEBIER: The Heritage of Motherhood. Gift of Mrs. Hermine M. Turner. UNM.

her power of expression only obey her at times, she does everything—posing the sitter, arranging her camera, developing and printing—more or less by chance.

If I go to her studio today, she may make a Holbein of me, tomorrow it would be a Rembrandt, or a Mary Cassatt. Thus, her vision of things will satisfy largely those temperaments who, without deep culture and true appreciation, long for something bizarre and out of the ordinary, and demand of art that it shall principally amuse them, and titillate their nerves. Of course, they do not acknowledge this; they consider themselves the true connoisseurs, and anybody who does not share their views is not trained sufficiently to do so. For they hold that art should ever remain a mystery reserved for the elect, an appendage of the fit and few—that is to say, themselves!

Nevertheless, there are few who have done as much as Mrs. Käsebier towards making commercial portraiture more refined and *recherché*. From this point of view, her experiments deserve the fullest encouragement, and they have been amply justified in many cases. It is only in bringing artistic photography to bear directly upon ordinary production that any aesthetic growth can be effected in the public taste.

On the other hand, without wishing to ascribe to a dominant artistic influence the credit due to Mrs. Käsebier, I may safely say that her work affords one

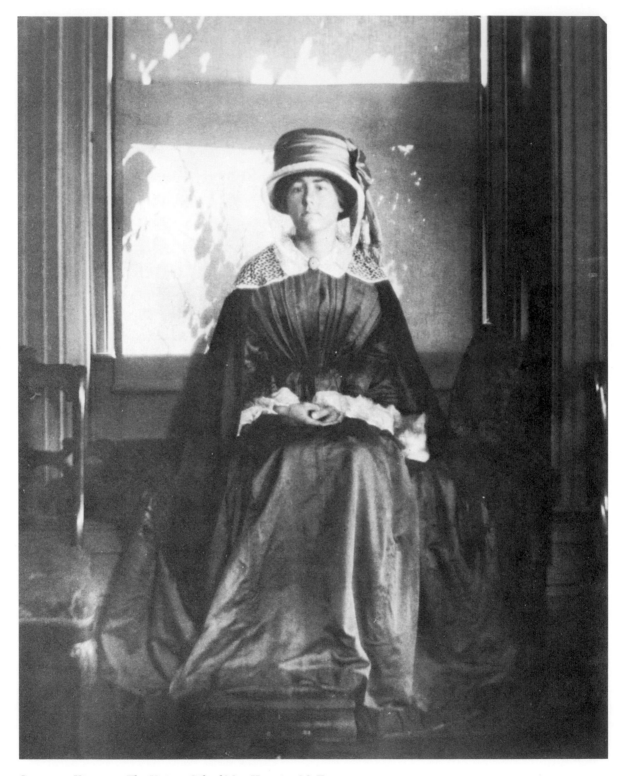

GERTRUDE KÄSEBIER: The Visitor. Gift of Mrs. Hermine M. Turner. UNM.

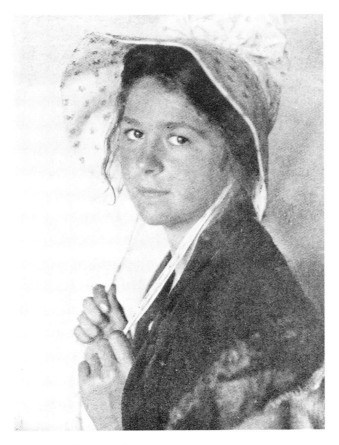

GERTRUDE KÄSEBIER: Portrait.

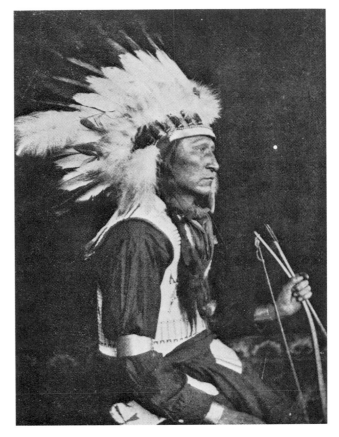

GERTRUDE KÄSEBIER: Lone Bear.

of the examples of the influence of a certain movement in modern art upon photography. In painting, this movement is represented in our country by men like H. W. Ranger,[2] A. B. Davies,[3] and Pamela Smith,[4] etc., all of whom are remarkably clever, but lack concentration. They feed upon the past and are influenced by every suggestion they receive within the limited sphere of their environment. They may possess a certain style of their own, but one which invariably reflects others, more or less in familiar use.

An artist, however, with the keen sensitiveness and the intensity of vision possessed by Käsebier, has no need to borrow the manner of other artists, be they who they may. When one is impressed so powerfully, so melodramatically, and at times so delicately, by the pictorial and ever varying spectacle of light and shade and tone harmonies, why use any language but one's own to express one's feelings and one's fancies? As well address a fellow countryman in some foreign tongue. The artist who has anything worth saying must say it in an original manner—that is, unlike anyone else; for if in the course of his expression he should allow himself to employ methods that are not original with him, but merely adopted and adapted, it will mean that what he had to say was really not worth the trouble saying.

These are the reasons why I have attacked Mrs. Käsebier in my criticisms.[5]

—1900

27

EDWARD STEICHEN

A Visit to Steichen's Studio

A DARK, CHILLY December afternoon. The rain falls in thin, straight lines on the streets of New York, and the lighted shop windows are reflected, like some blurred and golden dream, on the slushy pavement.

You mount the slippery iron stairs of a humble and reticent office-building on Fifth Avenue. To the Negro, who comes to your ring, you say: "Mr. Steichen." He takes you up to the top floor, and carelessly, indifferently, as one points to a door, he points to the right. "Right in there, sir," he says.

You knock at the door. It is Mr. Steichen who admits you. It is a plain little room, without skylight, but with an artistic atmosphere of its own. The first impression is one of cool grays and pale terra-cotta, a studio void of furniture, but full of artistic accessories—a vagrom place, where a sort of orderly disorder, a sort of gypsy fashion prevails. The light of the waning day seems to rest in the center of the walls, while the corners are filled with twilight shadows, whose monotony is only here and there relieved by the color-notes of a Japanese lantern, a large glass vessel, or some other quaint accessory. A little plaster fragment of one of Rodin's statues hangs in proud isolation over the mantelpiece.

Mr. Steichen looms tall among his canvases, his arms crossed. With his square shoulders, his pallid, angular face, his dark, disheveled hair, his steady eyes, he reminds one of some old statue carved of wood, a quaint personality which has at times the air of some classical visionary, "a modern citizen of Calais," and at other times the deportment of some gallant figure of Sir Reynold's time.

He showed me his paintings, sketches, and photographs in rapid succession, which is one of the ordeals the art critic has to go through if he wants to become acquainted with a new man. I have probably passed through this severe experience oftener than any other man. I remember having visited at least four hundred and fifty American studios for a similar purpose—as I have convinced myself that it is the only way to get at a man's individuality. And art criticism is to me nothing but a peculiar mania for searching in every expression of art, and life as well, for its most individual, perhaps innermost, essence.

Biographical data do not interest me. What is the difference where a man is born, how old he is, where he studied, and where he was medaled? His art must speak—that is all I care for.

The first picture that attracted my attention in Steichen's studio was his Beethoven. It is all black and gray, huge and grim (though no canvass of colossal size) almost Doric in its severity. Everything is sacrificed to the idea, a study in the somber supremacy of genius and the martyrdom of the artist. It is Beethoven of the Fifth, not of the Ninth

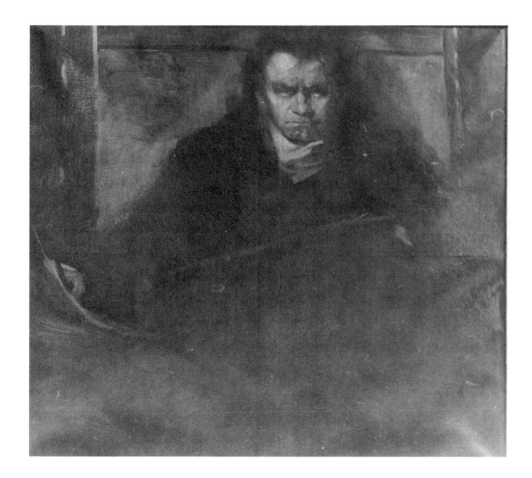

Edward Steichen:
Beethoven. Courtesy
Seminary of the Immaculate
Conception, New York.

Symphony. It contains more strength and power than beauty. The simplicity of its composition is remarkable. This dark pyramidal shape of a seated figure, harsh and angular, as if cast in iron, crowned by a pale, apocalyptic face, is seen against a slab of grayish stone, whose monotony is scarcely broken by a vista of dark, twisted tree-trunks in the upper corners. The face, haggard as a ghost of Dante's Inferno, makes one think of stormy tortuous nights, of sinister shadows trailing obstinately along the ground. It is a picture barbaric as the clangor of iron chains against each other, the only attempt of the young painter in the epic field. It presents Steichen at the height of his ambition; but being a solitary effort, it is difficult to judge the artist's individuality solely from this exalted point of view. One cannot

fully grasp his intentions, and it is very likely that he is not conscious of them himself.

In his landscapes, he reveals himself much more clearly. He has created a world of his own, but one based on actual things, translated into dreams. The rain still falls in thin, straight lines upon the blurred symphony of black and gold that glistens and glimmers on the wet pavements of Fifth Avenue, and there seems to be something analogous in the vertical lines of Steichen's landscapes and the gray lines of the rain outside. Nobody has carried the composition of lines further than Mr. Steichen. All his pictures are composed in vertical, diagonal, and outer-twisting line-work, but the lines are not as distinct and scientific as in Chavannes'[1] or Tryon's[2] pictures. They are not outlines, they only serve as

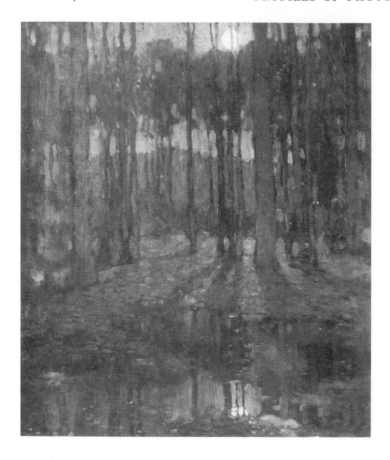
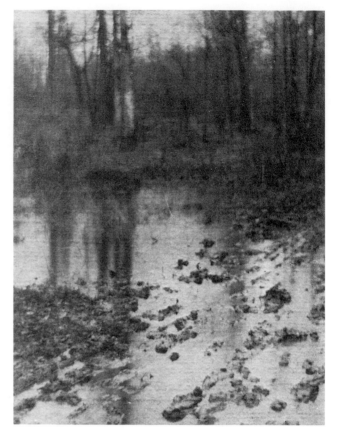

accentuation. He endows each line with a mystic quality, and they run like some strange rune through his tonal composition. French critics have compared his pictures with musical compositions, but I beg to differ. To me all his tree-trunks, whether ethereally thin, repeating their wavering lines in some moon-hazed water, or crudely massive, towering into some dismal twilight atmosphere, are purely decorative. In order to be musical, the line composition has to serve as outlines for the color-patches which should in turn repeat or accentuate the motive of the spacing. In Steichen's pictures color is always subordinate to one tonal value, and the dominating idea is rather the expression of a single sentiment than the varying subtleties of a musical theme.

To me Steichen is a poet of rare depth and significance, who expresses his dreams, as does Maeterlinck,[3] by surface decoration, and with the simplest of images—for instance, a vague vista of some nocturnal landscape seen through various clusters of branches, or a group of beech- and birch-trees, whose bark forms a quaint mosaic of horizontal color suggestions—can add something to our consciousness of life. His lines, blurred and indistinct as they generally are, are surprisingly eloquent and rhythmical. They become with him as suggestive as the dividing-line of some sad woman's lips, as fragile as some tremulous flower-branch writing strange hieroglyphics on the pale-blue sky, or as mystic as the visionary forms which rise in our mind's eye, as we peer through the prison-bars of modern life into some nocturnal landscape or twilight atmosphere. The only fault that I find with his landscapes, as with the majority of his pictures, is that they are not finished pictures. They are sketches. A mere suggestion suffices him. It is left to the imagination of the spectator to carry them out to their full mental realization.

There are many other pictures of interest, mixtures of fantasy and reality clearly characteristic of the gifts and methods of Steichen. I mention some at random. A violent color-study of a sailor, reclining, with a red bowl in his hand; the heads of four Parisian types; an old man; an artist with his model supposed to be crossing one of the Seine bridges, with the silhouette of another bridge, and a vague suggestion of the Louvre in the background; the sphinx-like profile of some phantom woman; portraits of F. H. Day and Mrs. Käsebier; and color-schemes of various types of womanhood, one of a young girl and another of a woman of the world. The manner in which he used flowers to tell the characters of his sitters (in the two latter portraits) shows how deeply he can read into the human soul. The young girl folds her hands listlessly around a large round flower with a straight stem, the other flowers resting in a long and narrow vase; while the woman of fashion throws a weary glance at the few pink blossoms which loom from some large, round vase and which repeat the color-note of her face.

To look immediately at monotypes after you have looked at a lot of paintings would prove in most cases very disastrous to the former. But, strange to say, Steichen's photographs hold their own. It proved to me once more that in art the method of expression matters naught; that every effort, no matter in what medium, may become a work of art provided it manifests with utmost sincerity and intensity the emotions of a man face to face with nature and life.

The artistic photograph answers better than any other graphic art to the special necessities of a democratic and leveling age like ours. I believe this, besides some technical charms like the solidity of dark tones and the facility with which forms can be lost in shadows, is the principal reason why Steichen has chosen it as one of his mediums of expression.

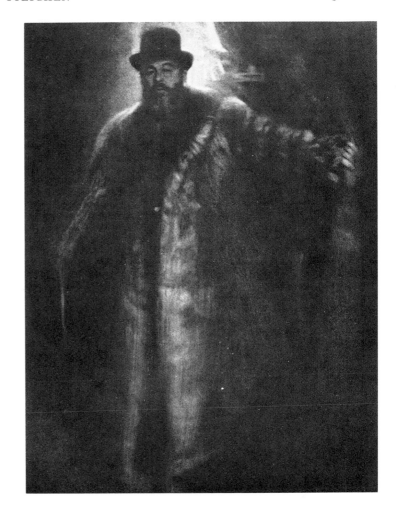

Above. EDWARD STEICHEN: Besnard. IMP-GEH.

Opposite page left. EDWARD STEICHEN: Night Landscape, 1905. Oil on canvas. Whitney Museum of American Art, New York. Gift of Mr. and Mrs. Ira Spanierman.

Opposite page right. EDWARD STEICHEN: The Pool. IMP-GEH.

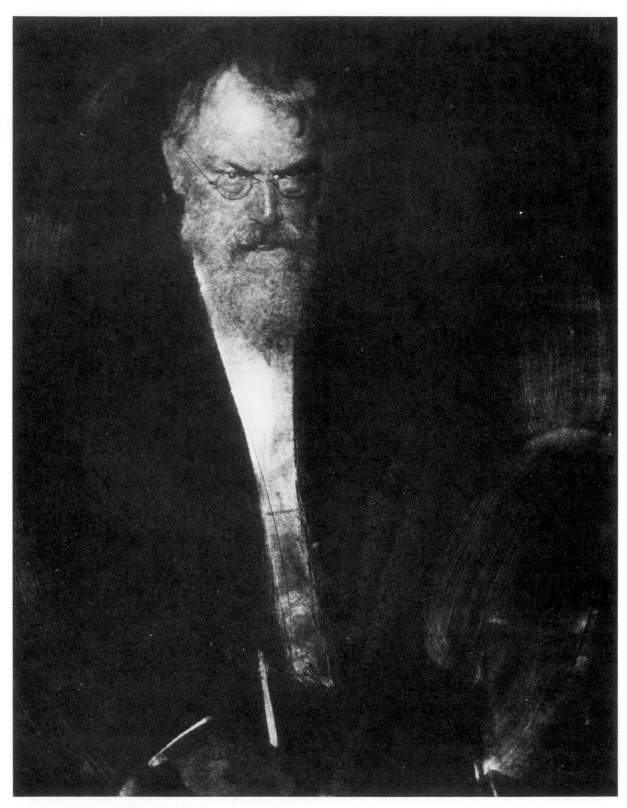

EDWARD STEICHEN: Lenbach. IMP-GEH.

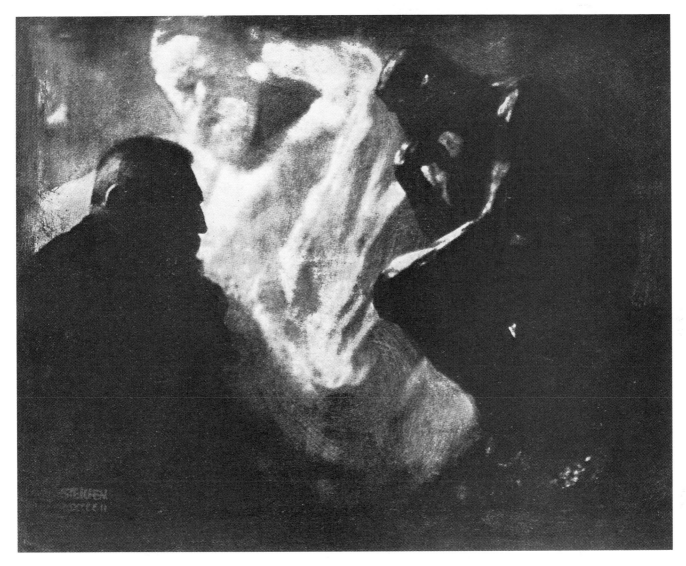

EDWARD STEICHEN: Rodin—Le Penseur, 1902. IMP-GEH.

He never relies upon accidents; he employs in his photographic portraits the same creative faculty which he employs in his paintings. That is the secret of his success. Look at his portraits of Lenbach, Stuck, Watts, Maeterlinck, Besnard, Bartholomé, and Rodin. In each, with the exception of Maeterlinck—and Maeterlinck's face seems to be one of those which do not lend themselves to pictorial representation, being too subtle, perhaps—he has fully grasped the sitter's personality. Lenbach he has treated like a "Lenbach," with the light-effects of an old master and with copious detail bristling with intellectuality, such as the Munich master is apt to use in all his important portraits. The Stuck portrait is full of a riotous technique, with a *bravado* touch in the white glare in the corner of the eyes. This is a man often vulgar and crude, but with healthy blood in his veins—an artist personifying the *storm and stress* element in genre art. How calm and dignified in comparison is Steichen's handling of Watts! And then, again, his Besnard, direct and realistic, and yet unforeseen in

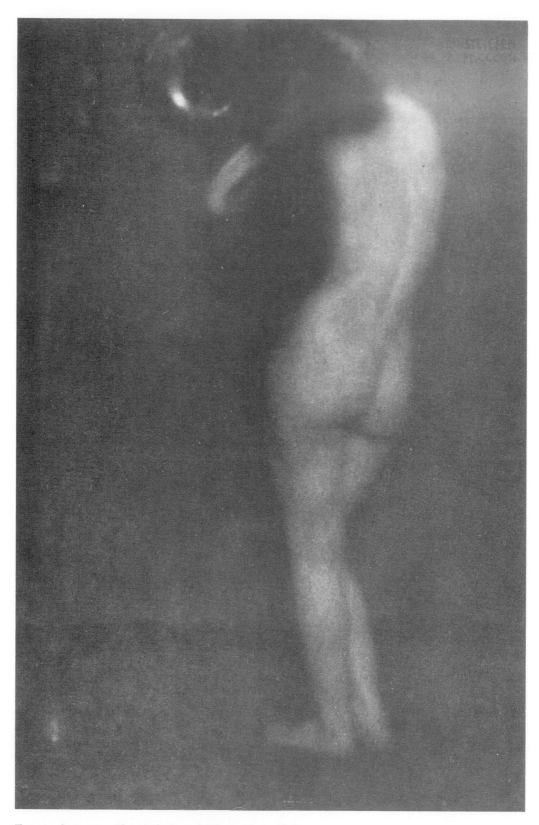

Edward Steichen: The Little Round Mirror, Paris, 1902. moma.

its effect. The treatment of the big fur mantle, with which the bulky form of the painter is clad, is symbolical of his tumultuous technique, and the burst of light behind the curtains suggestive of Besnard color-orgies in violent yellows, blues, and reds. The Bartholomé is deficient in composition, the Greek column against which the sculptor is leaning and the huge caryatid, which he is contemplating and which fills the rest of the picture, are too obtrusive, and yet they intimate the dreams of this poet of form, with their mixed savor of the modern and archaic.

But the masterpiece of this collection is the Rodin. It can not be improved upon. It is a portrait of Rodin, of the man as well as his art, and to me by far more satisfactory than Alexander's portrait of the French sculptor, excellent as it is. It is a whole man's life condensed into a simple silhouette, but a silhouette of somber splendor, powerful and personal, against a vast background, where black and white seem to struggle for supremacy. This print should, once and for all, end all dispute whether artistic photography is a process indicative of decadence, an impression under which so many people and most artists will seem to labor. A medium, so rich and so complete, one in which such a masterpiece can be achieved, the world can no longer ignore. The battle is won!

But it is getting late. Only a few more words, about Mr. Steichen's nudes.

"These nudes nobody seems to understand," Mr. Steichen remarks. "Do they mean anything to you?" It has grown dark and the rain is still tapping, curiously and faintly, at the window panes.

My answer is a smile. He does not know that my whole life has been a fight for the nude, for liberty of thought in literature and art, and how I silently rejoice when I meet a man with convictions similar to mine.

Steichen's photographic nudes are not as perfect as the majority of his portraits, but they contain perhaps the best and noblest aspirations of his artistic nature. They are absolutely incomprehensible to the crowd.

To him the naked body, as to any true lover of the nude, contains the ideals, both of mysticism and beauty. Their bodies are no paeans of the flesh nor do they proclaim absolutely the purity of nudity. Steichen's nudes are a strange procession of female forms, naive, non-moral, almost sexless, with shy, furtive movements, groping with their arms mysteriously in the air or assuming attitudes commonplace enough, but imbued with some mystic meaning, with the light concentrated on their thighs, their arms, or the back, while the rest of the body is drowned in darkness.

What does this all mean? Futile question. Can you explain the melancholy beauty of the falling rain, or tell why the slushy pavements, reflecting the glaring lights of Fifth Avenue stores, reminds us of the golden dreams the poets dream?

I seize my umbrella and say "Good night" indifferently as I might say it to any stranger, and he answers absent-mindedly "Come again!" He is thinking of his soul, and I am thinking of mine. What a foolish occupation is this busy, practical world of ours!

—1903

28
H. H. PIERCE
A Traveling Photographer

I MET H. H. PIERCE for the first time under rather trying circumstances for a critic. It was at the Washington Convention.[1] I was strolling through the exhibition gallery—one of the darkest places for such a purpose I have ever encountered, which made all prints two or three shades darker than they really were—when I was called over to a group of men who discussed the merits of a certain print.

"I want you to look at this print," exclaimed the jovial rotund president, who now and then makes a good thing himself, "Tell us what you think about it."

I looked at it. It hung all by itself in a little corner away from the other exhibits. One of those dismally dark tonalities that I designate as "mock-turtle soup!" A bust portrait of a woman with the smallest possible quantity of light on her face and shoulders. Everything else was hopelessly weird and brown— no composition to speak of and scarcely any feeling for flesh quality—and yet there was a peculiar fascination about the print, produced either by the peculiar facial expression or by the relation of certain values to each other.

"That's a nightmare, a freak picture," I smiled in my blunt fashion, "and yet I find it mighty interesting. It has some individuality to it."

The men who had discussed the print continued to shake their heads and gradually dispersed with a laugh or shoulder shrug. One man remained. He had attracted my attention from the first. A strapping young fellow in a big slouch hat, cape-coat and flowing tie, with a grim expression in his eyes as if he were in charge of a battery.

It was H. H. Pierce, the perpetrator of that pictorial fancy. He had been present when I made the remark, but he did not seem to mind its harshness. On the contrary he seemed rather anxious to enter into a discussion about the criticism. People still open to improvement are never offended at any frank and honest statement about their work.

Pierce had an excellent exhibit at Washington, and I soon found out that his nightmare print was only an exception with him. The average of his work was of a very high percentage, photographically as well as pictorially, in no way freakish, but astonishingly sane despite all its beauty and inventive force.

Pierce is to me the most "pictorial" of professional photographers, and I say this with due consideration of Garo, whose portrait of A. T. Proctor[2] is as wonderful a bit of chiaroscura as I have seen in a photographic portrait. Pierce has, perhaps, made less serious studies in composition than the majority of our leading men, but he has the gift of finding something picturesque in anything he "takes." His perception of the pictorial may be even keener because of being less studied. Every photographer who lays special stress on composition is naturally influenced by the art of painting and generally by the old masters, but there is comparatively little trace of it in Pierce. It is not necessarily the vocation of a critic "to clinch the photographer" and whenever he has made a new exhibition print to enumerate several paintings or painters which it closely resembles. All serviceable criticism, however (and I hope mine is), traces the filiation of pictorial idea, sorts and labels them, and cultivates a keen eye for family likenesses. Keeping this keen eye wide open, it observes the same motif persistently reappearing under varying forms.

Very little of conventional arrangements and old masters in composition appear in Pierce's work. It is novel and delightfully unconventional.

There is more of the true temperament of the artist in this man than in most photographers. He does not proceed as scientifically, but is nevertheless equally sure of his result.

"What are your methods and theories?" I queried.

He answered that he didn't have any to speak of; that it was different each time (it is naturally more so with home-portraiture then any other branch of portrait photography); that his sole aim and purpose was to get a beautiful result, "you know what I mean."

And when I had the opportunity to see him make an exposure or rather a dozen of them, I understood what he "meant." I never saw a man behind the camera more enthusiastic than he was. He peered into the sitter's face from all sides and in all possible attitudes, getting up into a chair and down on the floor to do it; in restless activity he moved about the furniture, arranged the hands of the sitter, or the edges of his coat, and lit up the shadows of the "living composition" before him by the artificial reflections from a newspaper, which he held every second in a different position. The thing he seemed to be particularly susceptible to was the play of delicate light and shade values, the gradations of shifting tints, the shimmering notations of the

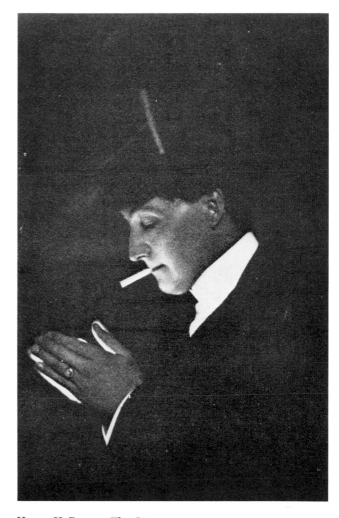

HENRY H. PIERCE: The Cigarette.

high-lights. A perfect control of light is the ideal of every true photographer. To reproduce its vibratory quality seems well nigh impossible in photography. It has been approached in rare cases (as in Garo's prints) but it seems to be accidental, a more or less uncontrollable chemical effect. For this reason several of our leading men, for instance Garo and Pirie MacDonald, have reduced the control of light to a kind of a system. Garo concentrates his principal light plane on the face, and divides it into three lights of different value and size, with one predominating the other two; while Pirie Mac-Donald subordinates everything to one large commanding light plane that emphasizes the foreheads and eyes of his portraits.

Pierce has no such rule. He scatters his lights promiscuously all over his figures. He does not care if the largest part of a face remains in shadow (as for instance in the mother's face in "Love"); but each of his light-spots tells, they invariably combine to a brilliant and accomplished picture. He is never purely and simply a portraitist; he always tries to introduce some pictorial element into his composition. He wants a "picture" rather than strictly a portrait. This is his strength and at the same time his weakness.

If he could draw I fear Pierce would turn Secessionist, unlike Pirie MacDonald, who used his *academic* training to become more efficient in the rendering of photographic texture. Pierce professed to me an ardent admiration for Steichen's work. I can readily understand this. There is something so intellectually vivacious about Steichen's portraits, despite their utter pictures as likenesses, that a man with pictorial instincts must take a liking to them. But Steichen always wants to assert himself. He gives us a commentary on the sitter. He is not satisfied with showing us how a person looks, but how he thinks the person should look.

Pierce is remarkably free of this quality of arrogance; he is at all times truly photographic in texture, and I believe it is his ignorance of the

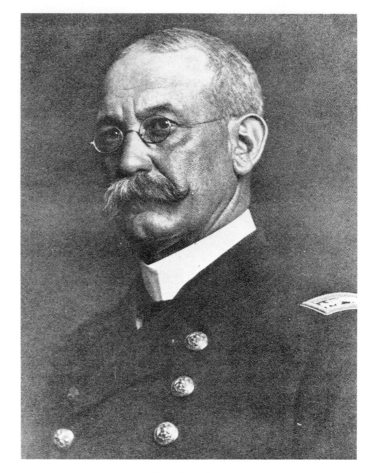

HENRY H. PIERCE: Rear Admiral Sigsbee, U.S.N.

painter's technique which has saved him. Let us be thankful for that, for it is just men like him that we need most in the profession—men who have an artistic temperament and perhaps even the artist's ability, but who have never exerted the latter and therefore can use their gifts exclusively for the idealization of the photographic processes.

In keeping with his temperament is also the way in which he follows his profession. He is a true Bohemian, a nomad by disposition. At the time he entered photography the clamor for art was at its highest, so he came under its influence; but he was more than an accomplished technician, more than a clever manipulator of values, and was not one to

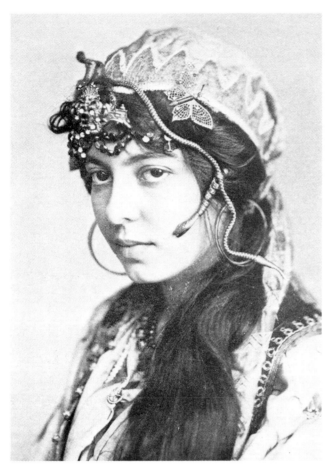

Henry H. Pierce: A Dancing Girl.

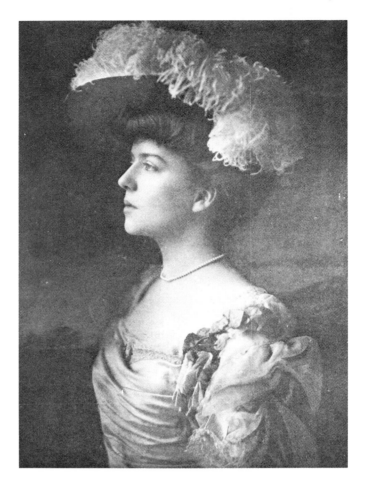

Henry H. Pierce: Mrs. N. Longworth, 1905.

sit steadily in one studio. He went his own way, independent, audacious. He became a traveling photographer.

Like so many of our earlier painters he travels from place to place, executing portrait orders wherever there is a demand. Only he does not stop at the villages, but, like our fashionable portrait painters of today, makes straight for those places where the best of society congregates. Last summer he was in Newport, this season he is in Narragansett Pier, and next year for all we know may be in Marienbad or Biarritz. And during the rest of the year he wanders from one city to the other, never staying more than a month or so in any place.

Rather an interesting vocation this, to see the world, to meet interesting people everywhere, and to make one's living at the same time.

"But is such a method really conducive to good work, and is it a paying proposition," some of my readers may ask.

I believe I can answer the first question in the affirmative. Pierce does good work, and the continual change is surely more conducive to inspiration and new arrangements than one particular place. Of course, he has to work under great difficulties. Although he has a permanent studio at Boston, and executes or has most of his orders executed there or at some other convenient workshop, he is often obliged to use a closet in his hotel room or a steamer cabin as a dark room and do some proof-printing under the most trying conditions. But his finished work does not seem to lose thereby.

The second question only concerns him. I believe that the only man who has a right to talk about such matters is the man himself. His peculiar method, however, sets one thinking, and as business methods are open to criticism, it might be interesting to discuss Pierce's.

There is a great danger about continually changing one's domicile, of being an eternal wanderer, and changing one's life into an Odyssey. If one stays in one town one grows prosperous with the growth of the population, one gets known for a certain kind of work that one can do better than any one else, one has made friends amongst one's customers upon whom one can depend, and as the years roll on things begin to run more smoothly as by themselves. The transient photographer is really nowhere at home; he quickly makes friends and is as quickly forgotten. He has no clientele except the one of which he is dealing with at present, and which is created by the necessity of the moment.

Of course, it is a free and easy life from the artist's viewpoint, and a man who has a frank and genuine passion for his profession may find it very enjoyable. But does it not after all smack a little bit—pardon me, I mean just a trifle—of the peddler who goes from house to house? A successful photographer should not solicit his business; it should come to him. And a man who comes to a city that is strange to him must necessarily drum up his business even with the best of introductions.

Of course, I perfectly understand what is in Mr. Pierce's mind. Nearly all the foremost portrait painters have turned globe trotters. They shift hither and thither from one metropolis to the other, holding exhibitions, painting portraits and filling their coffers with gold. Why could not a photographer do likewise?

Possibly—although the conditions are not quite the same—at all events it could only be accomplished by a photographer of international reputation. But I will say so much, that if it ever were accomplished it would do more to raise the standard of the profession in the eye of the public than anything I can imagine.

Follow your natural inclinations, do your chosen work as well as you can, fashion your happiness of the hours as they come, and at all events make some good photographs. This, I take it, is the philosophy of Pierce's life and work. Is he a great photographer? He is more: He is alive, impulsive, courageous, and ambitious, and may yet startle the world, not only the photographic one. He is traveling at a fast pace. I should not be surprised to meet him on the road to Windsor or the Berliner Schloss.

—1905

29
ELIAS GOLDENSKY

In the Proletarian Interest

$\mathcal{N}$OBODY WHO HAS ever heard Goldensky take part in a convention debate will deny that his mental attitude is a peculiar one. He is always ready to deny and to revolt. He preaches individualism and at all times is willing to indulge in that rare and dangerous luxury of—telling the truth. He is a serious student of social economics and, at the same time a mystic who dreams of Utopias, of absolute freedom, of a society in which all men shall be intelligent and naturally good.

Fond of expounding his theories, he is always on the stump for his ideas—in his reception room as well as on the convention platform. He is a victim of his vocabulary; he utters his socialistic paeans, inspired by the altruism which one finds on the East Side of New York, in blunt and vehement words.

A strange personality, this Russian Hebrew with a studio at the outskirts of the Philadelphia slums, making photographs of such taste and refinement that the most fashionable society people do not consider it beneath their dignity to look him up and sit for him.

The craftsmanship of his portraits and the subtlety of characterization is singularly fine and accomplished. They do not, however, reflect his mental agitation. They apparently have undergone a clarifying process, for the ideas back of them are of a turbulent, riotous order.

He is one of the few photographers who has

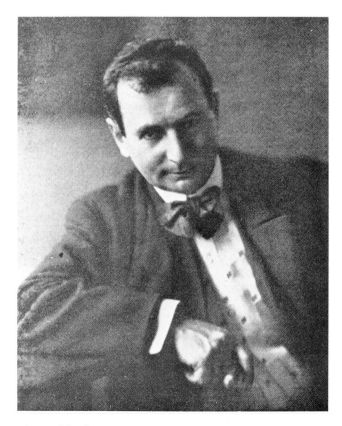

Elias Goldensky.

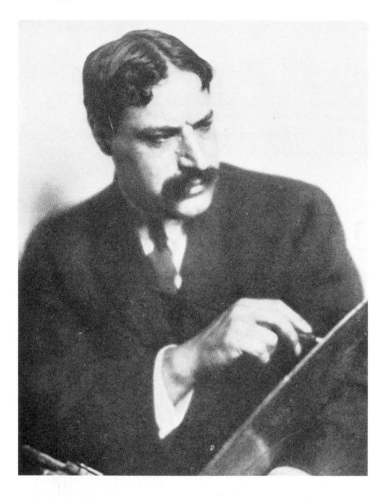

Above. ELIAS GOLDENSKY: The Artist.

Opposite page right. ELIAS GOLDENSKY: Portrait.

Opposite page left. ELIAS GOLDENSKY: Gum Print.

thought deeply about all the details of his craft. He has a theory for everything, and at least a half-dozen different ideals. His arguments are wonderfully lucid, though often disconnected and contradictory to previous statements. There is some classic standard he is searching for, some formidable expression that would solve the various problems of portraiture, and in the meanwhile he is doing work of excellent quality.

His present method under the light is a very interesting one. He explained it to me in his colorful, vivacious language.

Contrary to Pirie MacDonald, Strauss, and Pierce, who believe that the photographer must *influence* the facial expression of the sitter, Goldensky holds the opinion that the sitter alone can control the expression. "How do they know when a man looks most like himself? Those photographers who say they know a man as soon as they see him are not telling the truth. Nobody can do that. And facial expression is surely not helped by intimidation or by a deliberate effort to force the features into a certain characteristic expression. That's all wrong about hypnotizing people. Let them be themselves."

From Goldensky's viewpoint the application of the photographer's personal magnetism is no improvement on the old "Now please look pleasant" method. In both the real expression is perturbed and disturbed. The Hollinger method of dragging his sitter on a pushcart platform all over the studio until he discovers what seems the most typical expression is not bad in principle; but it is difficult to feel at one's ease—the situation is rather a ridiculous one—one feels as if one is pushed about on some tumbril awaiting one's photographic execution.

How can the problem be solved? Is there a way in which the photographer can receive his customers and make them feel perfectly natural? I hardly think so. People are too self-conscious, and the majority of studios are, after all, queer places, hardly conducive towards making one feel *en son aise*.

It has to be remedied in some way. The creating of a mood or of a composite likeness (by a longer exposure), however successful it may be at times, is necessarily guess work unless one is an unerring character reader, as Pirie MacDonald claims to be. If one can afford the time to study each sitter at one's leisure, one's talent for discerning character—which I consider the most essential faculty in a portrait photographer—may be shown to good advantage. But how about six or eight sittings in an hour? For this reason men like Charles H. Davis[1] taboo the idea of creating a mood. They treat the human face like still life and produce likenesses, perhaps not of a high order as some of the other more or less accidental ones, but after all they are likenesses such as the average intelligent public wants.

The problem is a very intricate one; it is really inexhaustible. Now, how does Goldensky get around it?

His policy is to let people stroll into the studio, and do very much as they like. He may point out a chair, or suggest a pose, but he has made it a rule to interfere as little as possible. At the start he makes several snapshots (which are rarely ordered) merely to get the sitter "used to his new experience," and thereupon follows it up with a "continuous sitting," often to twelve prolonged exposures, which is largely due, first, to the fact that the low-keyed pictures temporarily in fashion need more time, and, secondly, that "with most sitters an expression requires time to grow."

Goldensky does not believe in the growth of expression. He talks to his sitters, but not in order to keep their interest alive. He does not want any particular expression. Like everybody else, he

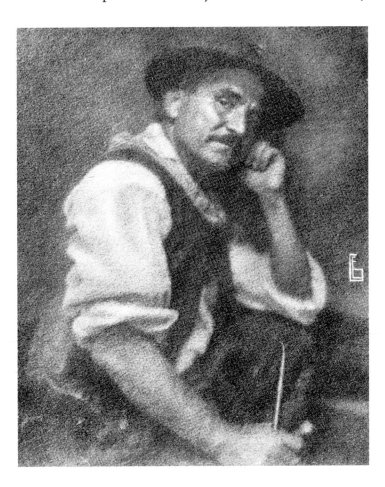

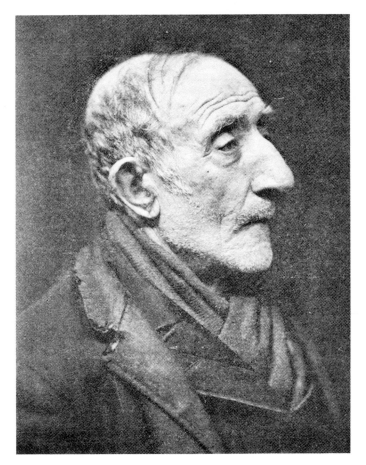

begins with positions and lightings which are not quite satisfactory, striving continually for better lighting and a better pose, but it must come naturally and not through any conversation or psychological explorations.

The Goldensky idea of leaving the sitter undisturbed impresses me as being not much better or worse than any of the other ones. I don't consider it tenable. Looking over some of his albums of proofs containing up to twenty different poses, I came to the conclusions that either his sitters must have been remarkably clever in posing themselves or—that he after all had more to do with the varied attitudes than he is willing to admit.

Of course, Goldensky, philosophizing photographer that he is, has all sorts of curious ideas to back up his theory. He claims that the less one knows a sitter, the better are the conditions for making a good portrait. "If one knows people too well, one can't photograph them!" he exclaimed. "I can't photograph my wife or my boy. I know them from too many different viewpoints. One picture cannot express it."

This may be true enough. But it is dangerous ground to enter upon. What he says of members of his own family is just as true of yours or mine. Likeness is always evasive, only the majority has not such a high standard and is easier to satisfy. If this were not the case the profession of portrait making might come to an abrupt end. To tell people that it is an impossibility to make a satisfactory portrait of them may be more honest than to assure them "they will get the very best they ever had," but it is hardly good business. It has the flavor of revolt about it; a revolt that is abstract and largely sentimental.

And so it is with everything Goldensky advocates. He continually gropes for the stars. He has the Griffith[2] idea of studios; of long spacious rooms, furnished like the interior of houses, containing fragments of libraries, boudoirs, parlors, music rooms, etc.—with a complete absence of ordinary photographic paraphernalia—so that his sitters may proceed from one natural environment to another. A capital idea that is carried out in a way by Core,[3] whose operating room resembles a nursery; and by Stein,[4] whose studio has all the sombre luxury of some aristocratic family of Teutonic origin. Goldensky would like to go them one better. He would like to have special studios for ladies, men, and children. He would like—even as Garo would—to make large, three-quarter, life-size portraits single-handed, only one of each; just suit his own fancy; leave it to the customer whether they would care to purchase it, and only in case they like it, ask his own exorbitant price for it.

And thus Goldensky dreams his bold, esthetic dreams, while he continues to lead his good industrious life at the borders of the slums, photographing some Armenian peddlar, or some newly-married Hebrew couple.

We talked of Pirie MacDonald and his scientific method. There is a mental affinity between the two men. They are both thinkers of far more than ordinary acumen; they are innovators and have the analytical turn of mind, but with the one difference; Pirie MacDonald knows how to catalogue and classify his multitudinous photographic speculations. He has erected a distinct style of his own; he has found an archetype without neglecting the individual. Whenever he reaches perfection (or anything near it), he is quite sure of it. Goldensky, on the other hand, is never satisfied with his results; he is merely experimenting, trying to do his best, and like so many of us, unable to judge his work until some time has elapsed. "There can be no system!" he proclaims. "With each case conditions change. One person has to be lighted in such a way, another one in an entirely different way."

Goldensky at all times remains the ideal opportunist; he continues to experiment, and each day fights for a new conviction.

This appreciation—and it is an appreciation, as I find very much to admire in this man, and the strange mixture of proletarianism and aristocratic artistry which he represents—may seem rather

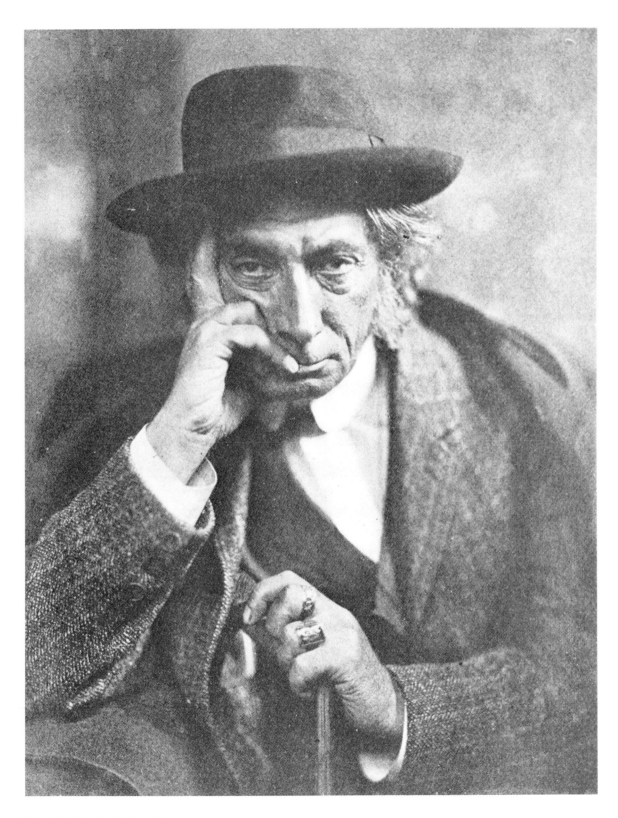

Elias Goldensky: Imber, Esq.

vague and unsettled to the reader. I wish it to be so. I change my method of writing with each man. I want to reflect the character of that man.

He is the most turbulent spirit in photographic circles today. He is instructive, rather than interesting. He looks out at the vehement play of causes with the dull hatred of a Jewish phylactery. He sees in photography, as everywhere else, a war of the many against the few, of the weak against the strong, of the individual against the material and despotic power. Goldensky is inspired by a true love of his profession, of the minor talents, of the owners of smaller galleries in provincial towns, and some day he may have a message to deliver; but the crude violence of words, which is the chief defect of reformers, stands at present in the way of any clear understanding of the fierce crusade for the ideal he

is fighting. Even serene and thoughtful men like Stein and Richard[5] have a tendency to scream when you touch them on their theories.

I admire the man for his ardor, but I do not feel like applauding him too loudly. I do not take things quite as seriously as he; I look rather skeptically and shrewdly through my eyeglasses upon this generation and have no particular sympathy for a man who turns from a dark and troubled present to a future all rose.

But Goldensky is sincere, and as long as he can turn out of all the turmoil and tumult so many beautiful and characteristic portraits as he has shown in recent years, we can not help admiring his candour and analytical spirit of revolt. It is the development of the conditions of the day, and had to come in photography as well as everywhere else.

—1905

30

J. H. GARO

Wanderer on New Roads

WHEN I FIRST met J. H. Garo I hardly trusted my eyes. Surely that man can be no adherent of old pictorial formulae and a T-square art—no ordinary photographer! Why, with his hat tipped over his eyebrows, and a hand shaped like that of a painter's, caressing a mustache that is defiantly twisted up—he has the air of some bobadil of Tripolis, of a pirate of the Algerian coast.

Nevertheless, he is a photographer, but one who can draw and who does not hesitate to make use of these qualities and paint like an artist in his portraiture. His aim is to attain the maximum of personal intensity in his photographic work.

The *Garograph,* as he has termed his photographic production, does not necessarily decry conventional photography. There is a place for the clear, sharp, over-retouched portrait. There are times when the old ways are aptest and best. But Garo himself wanders on new roads. He has a personal mode of feeling and thinking, and searches for an adequate and personal fashion of expressing himself. If he had only conventional things to say, the old style would suit him well enough, but as he has—like Pierce and others—something special to say, he must find for himself a special and unique mode of expression.

He is an Armenian by birth; he came to America when he was sixteen. Slowly he has made his way. Ten years ago he entered the photographic field.

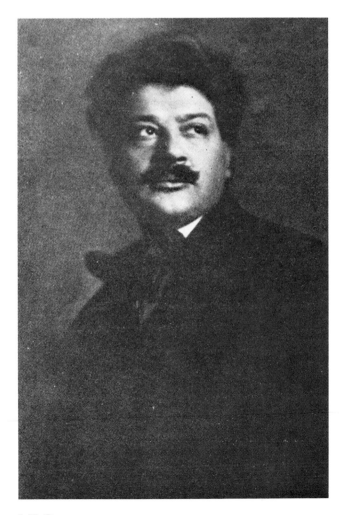

J. H. GARO.

221

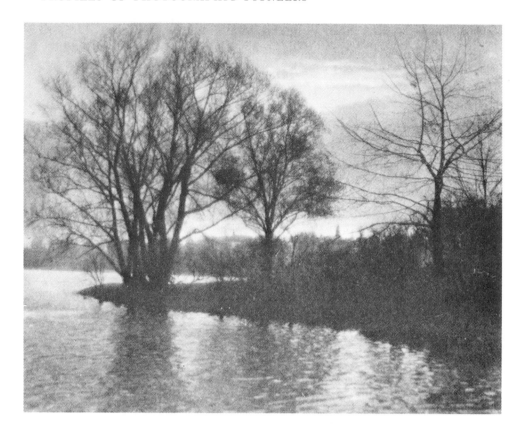

JOHN H. GARO:
Early Morning.

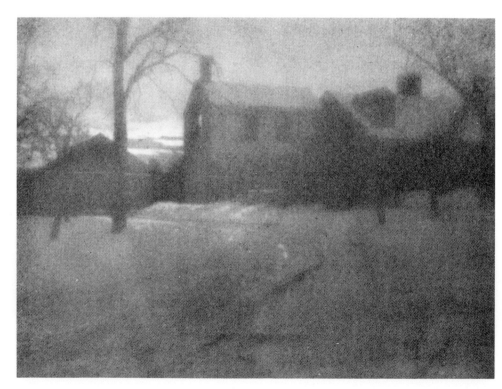

JOHN H. GARO:
Winter Evening.

Four years ago he opened his studio, the most beautiful studio in Boston, unlike any one I have ever seen. Since then he has rowed lustily against the stream. He does not wish to make any concessions to popularity. He does not want any pictorial expression learned by rote, or garrotted by a thousand rules which others have invented—but that personal touch which is inveterately the artist's own.

In simple words, Garo's ambition is to produce in photographic monotone pictorial qualities such as we admire in painting. It is surely a tribute to Garo's ability that his work accomplishes this in a more pronounced degree than we are used to encounter, even in the most advanced professional realms, and that he is able to run a studio on these artistic lines.

Little by little his work has become known to those whom it was once the mode to call *cognoscenti*. He gained admirers and disciples. Last year he received a splendid recognition at the national convention. He sent one single print to the Exhibition, and it attracted more attention than all the other exhibits together.[1]

Chiaroscura should be to the photographer what color is to the painter. Few have realized this as fully as Garo. To him light creates space and roundness, and he distributes his light planes scientifically by emphasizing them on the face and "using less light" on the body. In his standing figures both head and body are seen under common daylight, but the light values in the figure grow more and more subdued the farther they recede from the predominating light. Sometimes his strongest light accents shimmer like pearls set in a deep rich tone to which the rest of his composition is subordinate. Reserve and fidelity go hand in hand in his work, and although I am not quite prepared to become an adherent of his peculiar style, of composing solely in two principal tones—a light and dark one (six or eight tones would be more to the point)—I admire the characteristic breadth of his treatment joined as it is to an extreme delicacy of execution.

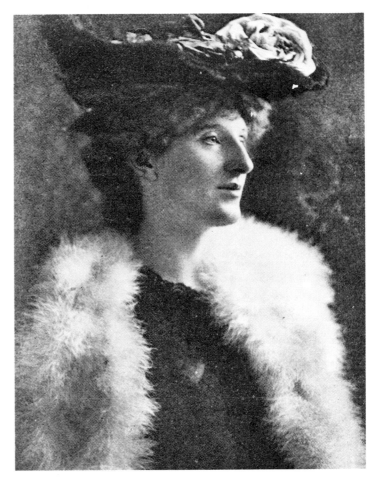

JOHN H. GARO: Bertha Cushing Child—Contralto.

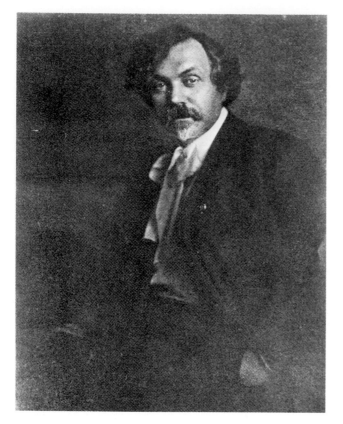

John H. Garo: H. H. Kitson, Sculptor.

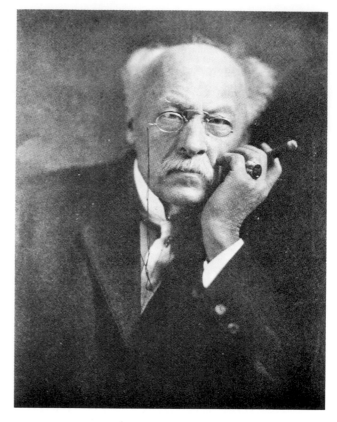

John H. Garo: Portrait of Mr. B.

His technique is rather an elaborate one, and would hardly bear the endorsement of the advocates of straight photography. Garo is a painter, water colorist, monotypist almost as much as he is photographer, and consequently a very clever and industrious manipulator of the negative. Involuntarily a comparison with E. J. Steichen suggests itself. Both men understand the value of the subordination of parts of the main subject, of right emphasis, of more careful definition at the chief points of interest, and of that general harmony of line, mass, tone, light and shade which we look for among the fundamentals of an ordinary picture. Both men are deficient in producing likenesses, and too much given to "esthetic subtlety," "decorative harmony," and "soulful composition" and that sort of thing. They claim too much interest for the artistic quality of their portraits and become

utterly oblivious to the fact that too much "poetic atmosphere" may offend the fundamental laws of depiction.

There is no doubt that Steichen is by far the more fluent and versatile of the two in artistic expression, but he is absolutely deficient of photographic texture. He is just like the man who in a race of sailing yachts would have no scruples in using a propeller in addition to his sails. Garo, although not half as clever, is hardly ever *unphotographic*, technically as little as in the choice of his subject. He is never guilty of producing figures that have no faces, hands that look like flappers, or pictures that are entirely clouded over by a granular veil. Nor do his faces stare at us as familiarly as out of well-known masterpieces of painting. Also Garo's work contains certain of the ideals and characteristics, together with the same general conception of things, that

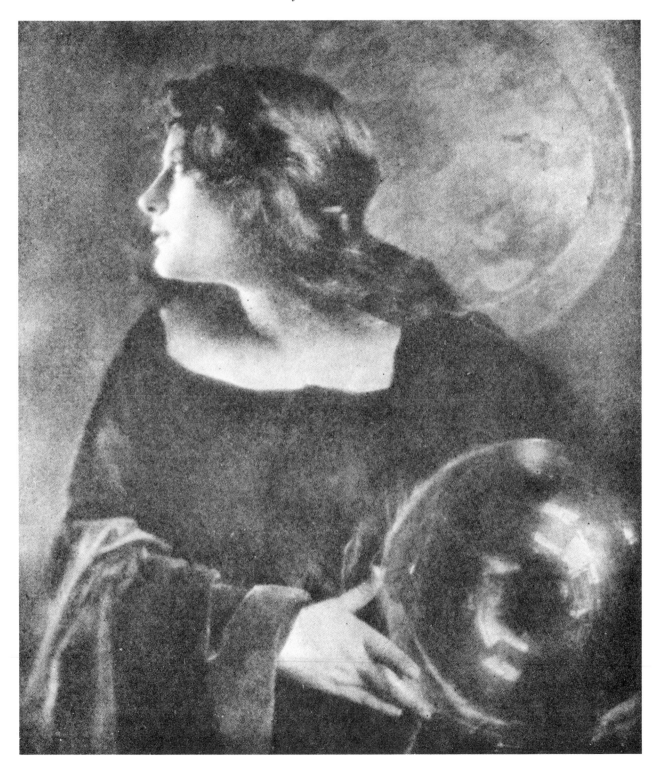

JOHN H. GARO: Portrait.

one finds in the work of a Watteau, for instance, but his pictorial conception does not necessarily copy from the past; it carries on the tradition, yet is different, transformed as it were, because more truly photographic.

Garo's men's portraits are often beautiful. His photographic drawing, although soft and blurred, is always nervous, full of accent and virility. What could be more forceful than the drawing of the nose and mouth in the portrait of Mr. F. E. Aiken, and yet what more sensitive! Look, too, at the rendering of the wrinkles and the firmness in the otherwise so smoothly washed contour. And behind all this is that sense of something being passionate and alive which so few portraitists give us. Also his Joe Jefferson is a fine piece of work. There is much power in the face, an infinite delicacy in the modeling of the high cheek bones, thin temples, and faintly humorous mouth, while the necessary accent is obtained by the depth of the eyes. And then his improvisation of Proctor.[2] (One can scarcely call it a portrait.) Where did he acquire that wonderful control of light? The eye lingers lovingly over the exceptional richness of the execution, the superb chiaroscural display, which is of the very first order, while faithfully playing at the same time its proper part in the ensemble—it is a notable portrait, indeed.

Among his women's portraits I was particularly attracted by the one photograph which hangs in his "waiting" or "getting into the right mood" room (Garo has a special one for this purpose) among a lot of oil paintings, and yet holds its own. It is a full length portrait of a young lady, and especially attracts our attention by the manner in which she has been surprised in her most characteristic attitude, quietly poised, looking straight ahead, and yet carrying out the nervous accent and all the instinctive grace of the American woman. It shows him to be as enthusiastic an observer of character as a passionate admirer of tone.

And why is such a man not a wielder of the brush? Not to be able to be oneself is indeed a sad affair; or does he really believe that he is the photographer who "will bring mighty things to pass"?

At thirty-three a man stands only at the threshold of his life, and one, therefore, may be warranted in prophecying without fear of contradiction that Garo's peculiar line of work will gain a widespread and deserved approbation. His energetic, far-seeing and vigorous development of "a method for the few" that he has consistently believed in and labored for is worthy of the success he has already achieved, and of the encouragement of all those who like to see themselves portrayed as another personality views them. His ideal would be to make only one (or a very limited number of copies) of each person, to carry it out in large size, to make it absolutely a personal creation, as Boldini[3] has painted Whistler and Whistler the violinist Sarasate. Some golden day in the future (he does not necessarily need to wait until Goldensky brings about the new era) his studio will be open solely to those who desire original work, thus preserving his style of expression from the degradation which it would certainly suffer from ordinary routine portraiture, so that each pictorial masterpiece issued from his studio will possess the additional value of being the only one of its kind in existence. It is difficult, indeed, not to become enthusiastic over the idea of the gorgeous aspect of such a portrait gallery. Each one of his own choice, representing a unique specimen of character or beauty, and embellished with the most varied and brilliant effects.

The motto which has always expressed Garo's artistic aspiration is, "The utmost for the highest." And he has always lived up to it. In a day when the only form of portrait photography which is financially successful is the pleasing likeness, he has preferred to devote himself to the dictates of his fancy, and only to take portraits of people who interest him personally. His object has always been to produce pictures which came to him in his own way, and to satisfy his inner vision before anything else. May he flourish in the land of his adoption.

—1906

31

B. J. FALK

An Exquisite Temperament

Strange that I should have never run across this man before now. Only when my editor suggested his name did I recall that there was such a photographer in existence.

Although the name "Falk" is as popular as any in the photographic world, the man himself has understood to keep away from the glare of the limelight. He does not know the value of the pompous phrase, he has no pet theories to exploit, and has never tried to make himself a mode of the day. Not that he would not take his firm stand whenever there is a stir and bustle of thought—as, for instance, now in the copyright question—but he does it with an amiable and unassuming grace, keeping his own personality in the background. He prefers to let the products of his studio do the talking. The operating room is his field of action, and he is satisfied if the results reach the highest standard of excellence that his ability is capable of.

A new acquaintance is very much like a new book. It is only with old friends and old books that we may chat the hours away. A new friend, like a new book, may come into your life, and you may find both winsome. But it is not until the book is dog-eared and the man is worn down into a certain intimacy that you take a real pleasure in them. It is the familiar book—with its friendly savor of a favorite dish—that give the greatest satisfaction; in equal measure you cannot really like a man until you know what to expect of him.

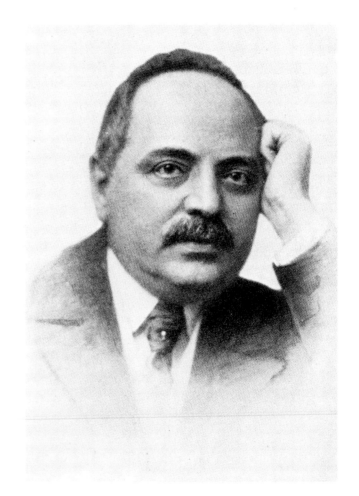

B. J. Falk.

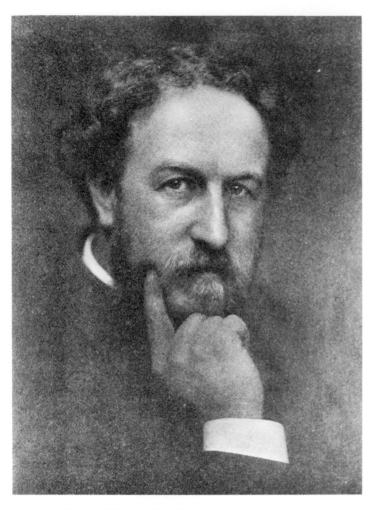

B. J. FALK: H. Snowden Ward.

But there are exceptions, men that give themselves so naturally that even at the first meeting you feel perfectly at ease, as if you knew them for a long time. Such a personality is B. J. Falk.

He impressed me by the gentleness of his manners, the sincerity of his opinions, and the loyalty to his profession.

Falk belongs to the old guard—having established himself as early as 1877—but to the old guard that never surrendered; on the contrary, shrewd man of affairs that he was, he kept apace with the technical innovations and the fads and fancies of each decade, and is today as successful as any of the younger men. He began in the old collodion days, was one of the first to adopt the dry plates, and after years of so-called "professional work" branched out as a society photographer. Who else would have had the courage and insight to open a fashionable studio in the Waldorf-Astoria? And after all these experiences of a long career of twenty-eight years—he is now situated in West 33d Street opposite the Waldorf-Astoria—he is as alert and progressive as at the start. The best proof for this is that he is the only *portrait photographer* who went seriously into color photography. He clearly sees, even as I had occasion to state at various times, that portraiture in color will be the most important development in the evolution of photography, and he only regrets that his present business does not allow him to take it up as a specialty.

The advent of portraiture in color is to him inevitable. It has been coming all this time. Already, fifteen years ago—one and a half years before Prof. Vogel[1] in Germany—E. Bierstadt,[2] in Reid Street (N.Y.), tried to solve the problem. More recently Kurtz[3] experimented with still lifes on three plates.

Becqueral,[4] Poitevin,[5] Lippmann,[6] Joly,[7] Clerk-Maxwell[8] have since endeavored in various ways to mirror the colors of nature. New cameras, filters and printing papers for that purpose are continually invented. It has become merely a question of time. In the meanwhile a studio has been opened in

Berlin that devotes itself entirely to color portrait photography. Falk, in turn, sent over for one of those experts. The experiments which he made in his studio were quite successful, but he found that the difficulty of successive or simultaneous exposures, of registration, of keeping the apparatus in order, etc., were still too elaborate and expensive to be handled as "a side issue" in any photographic establishment.

"One had to devote all one's time to it, and I can't afford that," he modestly remarked, "so I have shelved it for the present; but it is one of my dearest wishes to see it effective, in good working order, before I make my departure from this earth."

The way he said it showed me the man in a clear light. He does not seem to care a snap for any personal glory; of course, he would not object to it, he would even feel proud of it, but the principal concern is after all the welfare of photography. I have met few men in my life with such an impersonal attitude toward their own accomplishments.

Glancing over the work on his walls, I was surprised at the unevenness of the display. There were a few as perfect as photographic craftsmanship can make them, others merely represented a fair average, while some were disappointing to say the least. I do not remember ever having seen the work of one studio cover such a wide range in character and quality, from the commonplace to the most exquisite specimen of portraiture. Why, some of his portraits, particularly one of the profile of a young girl rather curiously spaced, were even "secessionist" in tendency.

"It is rather easy to make that sort of a thing, if one wants to make it," he remarked. "To put good, strong qualities into the average run of your work is by far more difficult. You see every man is subject to moods. Did you never notice, looking at the different show cases, that the expressions on the faces of one photographer are all serious, while those of another are all gay and cheerful? The temperament of a photographer always gets into his work. There is no escape from it. And the temperament itself is

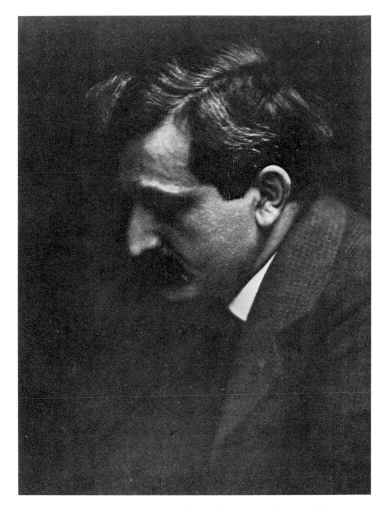

B. J. Falk: Dr. Emanuel Lasker, Chess champion of the world.

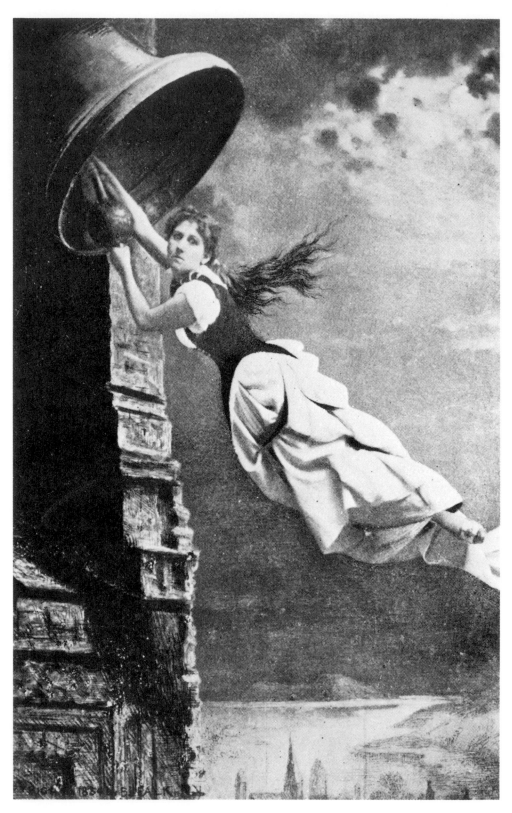

B. J. Falk: "Curfew Shall Not Ring Tonight."

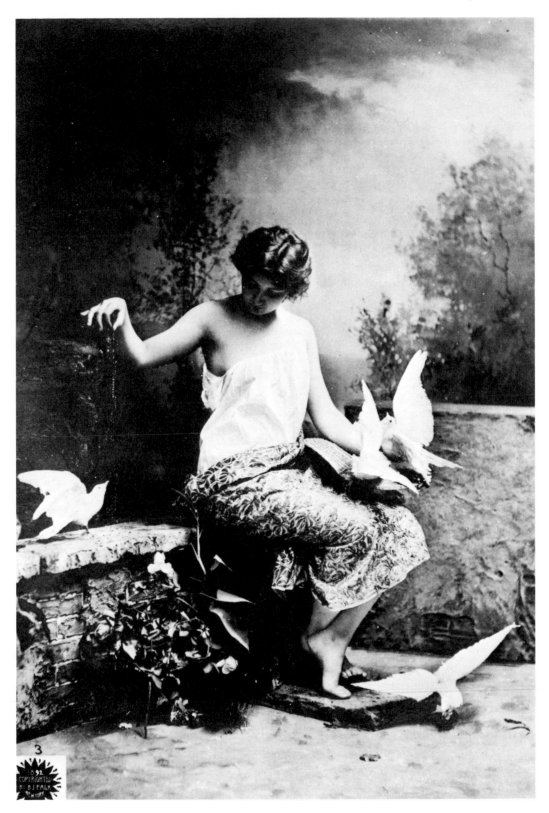

B. J. FALK: Untitled.

due to changes. Some mornings when I am in bad humor, no matter what I may do, all my sitters will have a sour expression in their faces. On the other hand, when I feel particularly happy or elevated over some good news, my feeling is sure to impact itself to the countenance of my sitters."

This sounded very plausible, and in a way explained to me the unevenness of his work. Yet, after all it seems to me only possible with a man who possesses a temperament generally so exquisite in tune that even its slightest discords will influence those who come in contact with it.

"For that reason," Falk continues, "I try to work as quick as possible. Already in 1881 I was in favor of rapid exposure. I divided the usual time of exposure: ten or twenty seconds by ten, which gave me one to two seconds. I worked under the strongest light I could get. My idea was the photographer has to do it all; if he does not succeed in getting a straightforward, life-like expression, he alone is to blame for it. And for that quick work is absolutely essential. At that time, when nearly all my time was taken up by theatrical work, I was also fond of making all sorts of stunts—for instance, a clown jumping through a hoop" (and he showed me the negative). "I wanted to give the impression of instantaneousness."

"And do you still work in the same fashion?"

"The light in this studio is not good enough for very rapid work. You see, my skylight is of blind glass, and in summer I have to screen off the light by two sets of curtains, as the reflections of the red walls opposite interfere considerably."

Falk seems to me to be one of those men who do not fret much about possible disadvantages and that sort of a thing, but who readily adapt themselves to conditions and always do the best they can under the prevailing circumstances.

Talking of lighting he spoke of Sarony,[9] who really had an ideal arrangement for lighting. "No fancy light, the light was more direct—a matter of angles—very strong and always of the same quality. He merely had to pose a person there and was sure

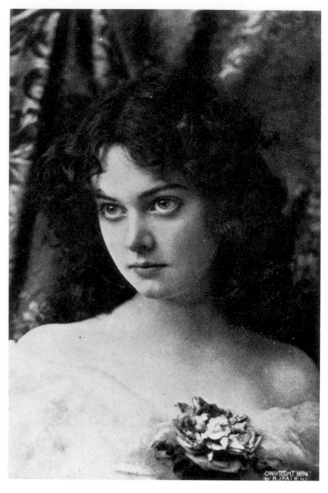

B. J. FALK: Minnie Ashley.

of a result. Of course he differentiated the light values. I do not agree at all with those photographers who light all persons in the same way."

"You are of the opinion that different types of character should be differently lighted?"

"Decidedly so. One has to find for each character the light which is best suited to the complexion, the color of the hair, the expression of the face, or any physical characteristic. For instance, if a girl has a peculiar interesting curve in her shoulder or arm one wants to emphasize it, as long as it is beautiful."

Glancing at his collection of "theatrical" backgrounds,[10] which are of a most astounding variety, I asked him whether he had not found it necessary to simplify his general studio outfit as so many of his contemporaries have done.

"No, I have always worked very much the same way," he replied.

"You seem to be peculiarly free of any theory or pose," I interrogated.

"Yes, I don't go in for that sort of thing. I haven't the gift of talking as some other men have. All I try for is a good, satisfactory likeness, a pleasing effect, well posed and well lighted."

After inspecting the reception room and the studio, Mr. Falk invited me to his private den, a large and curious room crammed full with books, pictures, statuary and souvenirs of every description. Also the growlery—so familiar in western studios but sadly absent in New York establishments—was not missing. One could not help feeling at home.

And there we sat in the twilight and talked of conventions and exhibitions, of color and "freak photography," of the Metropolitan Section of the New York State Society and the copyright law. Noticing a few of the charming photographic crayons of Sarony on the wall, the latter became for awhile the topic of our animated conversation. We both agreed that he was a wonderful man, a true genius in his way. Unphotographic? Why, of course, in that particular kind of work, even as Steichen is to-day. Steichen and Sarony, an inadequate comparison! Not at all. Each man represents a different phase of art, and one as good as the other, I suppose, in the long run of time. Sarony will always occupy a little niche in the estimation of photographers. Let us be just and hope that Steichen will do the same.

Falk told me how he had admired Sarony, how much he had learned from him; that he really owed "an awful lot" to him. Be that as it may, I cannot quite agree with it. In my humble opinion Falk owes all that has made him dear to his friends and valuable to the profession solely to himself, to his modesty, his sincerity, his adaptability and rare craftsmanship, his loyalty and unselfishness in all that pertains to the welfare and progress of photography, and above all else to his exquisite temperament—that has won me over to his side the first time I had occasion to feel the firm grasp of his hand in mine.

—1906

32

J. C. STRAUSS

The Man Behind the Gun

IT IS WELL-NIGH impossible to talk ten minutes about photography without mentioning the name of J. C. Strauss. No other—neither Pirie MacDonald's nor the cryptic Steichen's—suggests itself so readily to our mind, comes so easily tripping on our tongue, though we may have never enjoyed the hospitality of the Growlery[1] nor idled away a gray afternoon amidst the roseate pleasures of the tower room. Strauss, more than any other of his brother craftsmen, has realized the necessity of making concessions to popularity, and he has made them in a broad and brilliant Western fashion. His "shop," with the air of a French castle, with its elegant and yet matter-of-fact equipments and it insolent waste of space, boldly proclaims the advance the profession has made in recent decades, and proves beyond doubt that also a portrait photographer may possess a striking and even pompous personality.

Tall and brusque, with hair that curls and eyes that twinkle ironically and continually—the sort of man at whom women look regardfully—he lives in St. Louis and has made his studio one of the sights of that lightest and most coquettish of Western towns. He has made the city photographically his own by right of personal conquest.

Twenty-seven years ago he opened there a little shabby gallery, and did the ordinary down-town trade. His work was probably not much worse nor much better than the average encountered in such premises. They represented the attempts through which every young ambitious photographer passes on his way to a knowledge of his own thought and his own style. But he was shrewd; he sized up his competitors; he studied the wants of his time with all its conventions and limitations (over which man has no control); sought how best to turn to account the material he had on hand, and slowly but steadily made his way into public favor, until he completely mastered the trick of pleasing the public. His cleverness in that respect is, in these days, amazing, almost diabolical.

As a portraitist Strauss is what I would call a "brutalist." He does not merely endeavor to control, but actually tries to force the countenance of a sitter into its most favorable expressions. He makes his sitter assume an attitude, a gesture, a twist of the body that he considers characteristic, and then, with bulb in hand, lies in wait for some fugitive expression that will yield a significant and impressive representation of the subject, and lend life and suggestive force to the objective record of the camera. Like a bandit ready to seize upon a victim and rob it of all the beauty it calls its own, he crawls around his sitter, restless as a panther, peering into his face and rearranging the light effect at every moment (his sidelights are frequently the best part of the performance), and when the reflection of a congenial mood flits across the features before

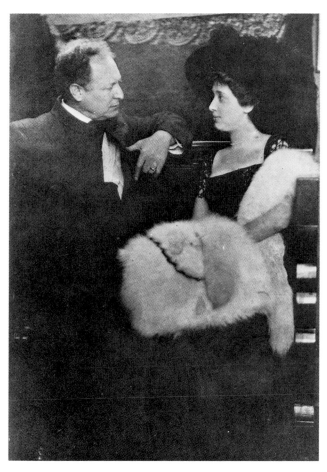

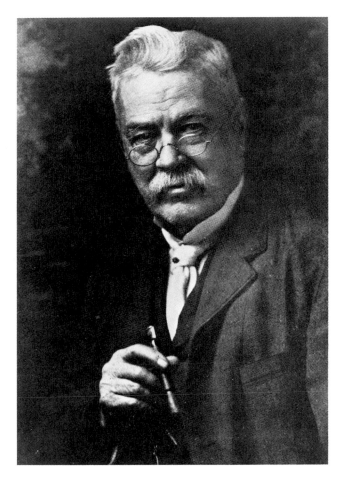

J. C. STRAUSS: Miss Maude Hellman and J. C. Strauss.

J. C. STRAUSS: Portrait.

him—presto! Before the sitter is aware of it, the thing is accomplished, and you only have the familiar remark of Strauss to his assistant, "Boy, did you get that?"

And the "boy" is so wonderfully trained that he invariably realizes Strauss's intentions. Strauss's operating tactics are really marvels of rapidity. Four to six exposures a minute are mere play to him. He works his camera like a breech-loading gun. It is very much like target practice at high sea, he aims at a certain facial expression, and whenever any indication of it appears, he fires away in rapid succession, operating his bulb with amazing alacrity. Also Falk and Pierce deserve the title of "men behind the gun," but there is a difference. Falk,

learned as he is in photographic ballistics, is not quite nimble enough to fire away in volleys; and Pierce (really a disciple of Strauss), although courageous enough to sail over torpedoes or any house portraiture obstruction, somehow, does not aim quite as accurately. And this is, after all, the secret of success of all portraiture of this kind.

Strauss seems to be more versed in the knowledge of human nature, seems to be a more efficient character reader. He has the changes of physiognomy, the range of external appearances at his beck and call. Using a rubber tube of extraordinary length—I have never seen a longer one—his movements are in no way handicapped; he can stand twenty feet away from his sitter and still practice

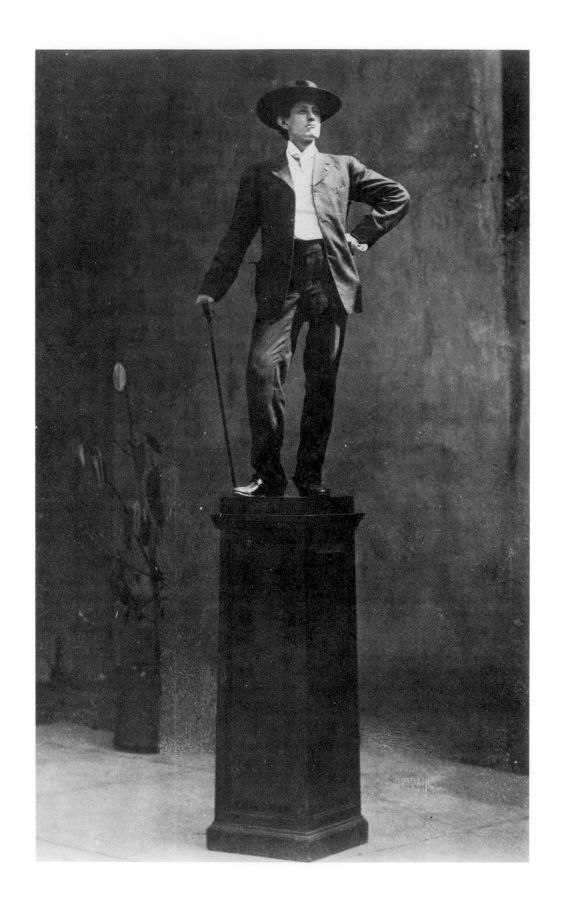

his hypnotic coaxing and invigorating methods. And he juggles so expertly with rubber bulb and tube that he almost persuaded me that photography was all slight of hand.

The natural fugitive expression is Strauss's strength and weakness. Portraiture of this kind is surprisingly interesting, but a trifle impersonal, not so much as far as the photographer is concerned—this particular method gives as much scope to the display of individuality as any other—but from the sitter's standpoint. A snap-shot portrait—and what else is it!—rarely becomes typical, the exposure is too short to enable one to seize upon the essential characteristics of a face. An idealization is purely accidental. And yet—after many a sleepless night—I have come to the conclusion that it is, after all, the most logical method, and the one which I most heartily endorse.

What the public wants first of all is a natural likeness. Coburns are no photographic commodity. A momentary expression may look at times very queer, notwithstanding that it may be perfectly accurate. No matter how intimately we may be acquainted with a person, it is impossible to compete with the camera and discover all the subtle variations of his or her (as it may be) facial expressions. It is at this point where the genius of the portrait photographer comes in, his ability to read character, to reflect through external appearances the disposition of the sitter. A long exposure, the composite of several fugitive expressions, on the other hand, may be more typical, but it has the disadvantage of being less subtle, more stereotype and less natural. And for that reason, mark my word, the "brutalist" will win out in the long run.

And this brutal interpenetration into a person's character is really what interests me most in Strauss's work. His workmanship is as elegant and elaborate as that of a dozen other men—not more so and not less. He has, of course, also been influenced, but not to his undoing, by the tonal movement, and indulges in the harmless pastime of painting meaningless pictorial backgrounds into his pictures. But

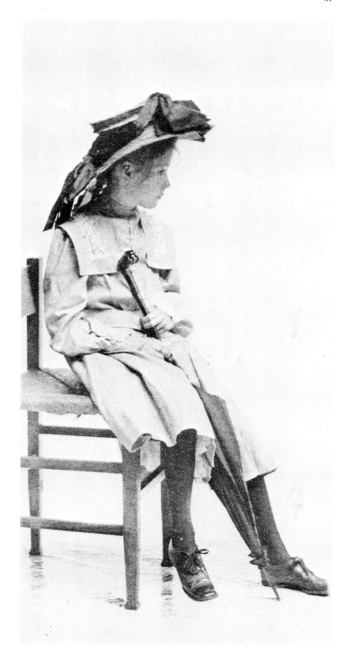

Above. J. C. STRAUSS: Portrait.

Opposite page. J. C. STRAUSS: Sadakichi on Pedestal, ca. 1898.

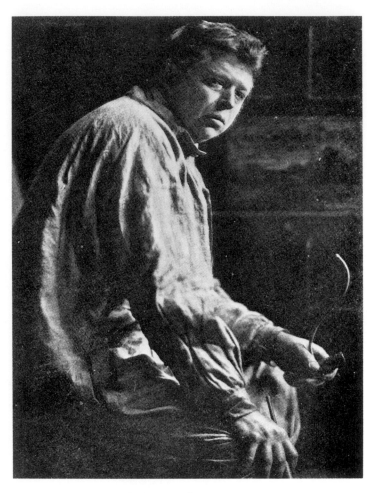

J. C. Strauss: Convention Picture.

these are merely mannerisms that do not count in the final summing up of his abilities.

What I admire in Strauss is that he works with the true intensity of an artist. His work is visible. He has faith in himself, and is in love with the work he does. His special faculty as a reader of physiognomies is self-centered; it revolves on its own pivot. He has not enriched the world with morbid pictorial fragments like Steichen, but poured forth a rich and vivid stream of average excellence. He is a natural man, who loves all that tends to expand his emotions, and his portraits (mediocre as at least 10 per cent of them are) are merely the expression of his joy in expansive life. And for that reason I like best to think of Strauss, sitting in his tower room when the strain of work is over, giving his friends the benefit of his wholesome, spendthrift nature, his wit, his heart, his intelligence. He is as whole-souled and magnetic a personality as I have ever known, and he is always triumphantly himself.

But what does it really matter what I or anybody else think of him! He is one of the men who has made good in his profession, as well as in his life, and that is, after all, the principal thing in all nooks and byways of our earthly existence.

Strauss is not merely playing a very important role—if not the most important—in American portrait photography of the last ten years; but has also created a mode of doing things in a gallant and lavish way that has attracted and influenced all the photographers of his generation. In his profession he is the most accomplished man of affairs living—master of all the artifices and secrets of pleasing the public and yet, withal an excellent craftsman, an expert portrait photographer, full of originality, insight and selection, whom I admire and whom all, I presume, respect.

—1906

33

JOSEPH BYRON

"The Stage Is My Studio"

IN THIS AGE, specialism is the order of the day. It is generally accompanied by success. The man who is wise enough to concentrate his faculties and restrict his field of action to what he can do best has a better chance than his more versatile competitor. Of course the start is difficult for the specialist. He has to assert himself; he has to create his own specialty and convince his prospective customer of its necessity and his superiority in the particular line he has chosen to exploit. But as soon as he has made good, provided he has the necessary business foresight, patience and perseverance, he will have a comparatively easy time of it. Orders will drift to him of their own accord; one customer will recommend another, and his trade will steadily increase the more he insists upon his specialty—that he is the one man who can do a certain thing better than anybody else.

Byron is such a specialist. He is known as the photographer of the stage; the theatrical flashlight man. He prefers to call it *artificial* light, but of that anon. In the theatrical world, as well as in the profession, he has gained the reputation of being the leading "flashlight" photographer, and the epithet "will he nil he" will stick to him as long as he lives.[1]

He can be justly proud of it. He has been one of the first to apply flashlight photography—some forty-three years ago or more; he has mastered all of its intricate technicalities and brought it to a higher grade of perfection, pictorially as well as practically, than anybody else.

One wintry morning last November I sat at his office—for he has no reception room—"the stage being his studio" and he told me of his varied experiences. Byron is as candid, jovial, and whole-souled a Britisher as I have ever met, and he still drops his h's with the same alacrity as if he had just crossed the big pond, instead of being with us for more than eighteen years.

Byron made his first flashlight, using magnesium wire, on March 10, 1863, at the occasion of some festivity at which the Prince of Wales (the present King) furnished the central figure of attraction. The result was not a very startling one. He only succeeded in getting silhouettes with the slightest indication of detail. Slowly he conquered the difficulties of the process and when he came to this country in 1887[2] I believe he was an expert in the game with considerable experience behind him.

Yet at that time nobody wanted flashlights. The theatrical managers had no use for them. Byron went from one office to the other explaining the advantage of flashlight pictures, its merits as an advertising medium, as actual pictorial reports and records showing at a glance the character of a production, its scenery, costumes, and placing of accessories, but they would have none of it. They

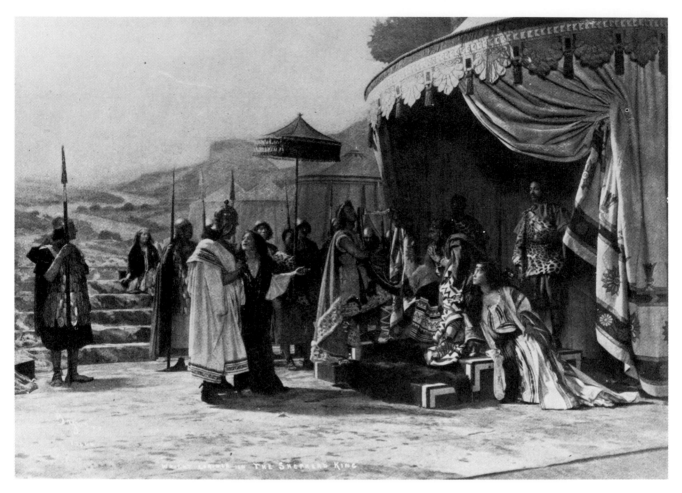

Joseph Byron: Scene from "The Shepherd King."

were of the opinion that the customary way of sending out diagrams served their purpose better than any new method. So Byron got connected with a newspaper. Flashlights as illustrations were a decided novelty and Byron made a hit with them; the managers, however, continued to shrug their shoulders at the innovation and only reluctantly gave permission to have some of their performances photographed. They considered it a great nuisance.

But there came a time when the public had grown so used to this kind of illustrations that it would have been very unwise to discontinue them. For a while there was a decided danger that this would happen. The editors did not see any reason why they should pay for illustrations that adver-

tised the theaters, and the managers did not yet fully realize the value of this pictorial réclame. Byron, a true pioneer, was equal to the emergency. He knew his time had come. Again he approached the managers, and this time with some success. They began to consider it. First one came around— Lederer[3] I believe—then others followed suit. They paid Byron for his work and furnished the photographs gratuitously to the papers. And suddenly Byron found himself the possessor of a lucrative trade created by himself.

That was about twelve years ago. Today, it is difficult to believe that there was even a time when theatrical flashlight photography was not an established fact. No manager would think of sending out a production on the road without having secured a full set of all the principal scenes in the play. It has really become his helpmate in booking engagements and advertising his plays, and seems to do its work more effectually than press clippings or any other method of recommendation. Of course Byron has many competitors now, but he still holds his own, and as far as workmanship and pictorial treatment is concerned, he is still king of them all.

The secret is that he has steadily improved. He did not rest on his laurels and energetic worker that he is—the number of his negatives reached the 23,000 mark some time ago—did not allow his work to become stereotype. It is now better than ever.

I had the opportunity to look at some of his work of fourteen or fifteen years ago. It looked very much like some of the work his competitors are doing now. His photographs of that early period are good flashlights, well-posed, well-lighted, and clear in detail, but there is no discrimination in values. A white gown is simply rendered white. There is no gradation, no subtlety, no finer pictorial effect. The pictures look blank and bald like so many we see standing in the theatre entrances.

The Byron of today is made of entirely different mettle. His pictures are no longer mere records, they are studies in light and shade. The lightest spot of the picture is skillfully reserved for the principal character of each scene, and the rest of the figures and accessories are subdued without loosing their distinctness. Everybody familiar with the garishness of stage scenery will realize how difficult it must be at times to eliminate its objectionable elements, for instance the netting and sharp outlines of drops and wings, and to give to mere daubs of paint something like depth and natural appearance.

Besides, good lighting is very scarce. It is generally done without real understanding in a kind of slipshod manner. Irving[4] and Duse[5] were notable exceptions. Their scenes could be taken very much as they were represented to the audience.

But the majority of productions need re-composition, and Byron has learnt to overcome, to a large extent, the difficulties caused by inadequate lighting. He conceives his pictures like a painter and prints his compositions and light effects with his flashlights, of which he uses frequently as many as eight. They are really not flashlights, but continual artificial lights which he has under perfect control as he prepares his own magnesium powder. Contrary to the general custom and belief, he does not take his pictures by a single flash but by one to two second exposures. He allows himself time to wait for the most opportune moment, and yet he works with lightning rapidity, making sometimes as many as thirty exposures in an hour and a half. One of his peculiarities in operating is that he never shuts out any source of light, but on the contrary, that he uses every illuminative available, may it be the footlights or a streak of daylight, to heighten his effects. A twelve foot stand enables him to get a full view of the stage and his pictures all show a stretch of foreground that help the naturalness of the scene depicted.

With his lights he plays like a magician. He orders his men about all over the stage and auditorium, places one man in the flies, another in a proscenium box, a third quite near the principal actor and so on until he has finished the composition in his mind's eye. It is wonderful how he manages to concentrate a streak of light on one person. This is, no doubt, done with some special device which controls the expansion of light, perhaps by a funnel-like shade attached to the stand; but we do not know, we can only guess at it. He admits that there are some tricks in his trade, but he is not willing to disclose them, or even use them when the coast is not entirely clear. "Not that I object so much to letting them know, and to profit by my experience," he remarked to me, "but I object to their claiming it as their own invention, which they have done in more instances than one."

The great fault of flashlight photography lies in the falsity of its lighting. There are interiors where the light is supposed to come from the window, while the shadows of the furniture indicate that it comes from the opposite direction. In some of his

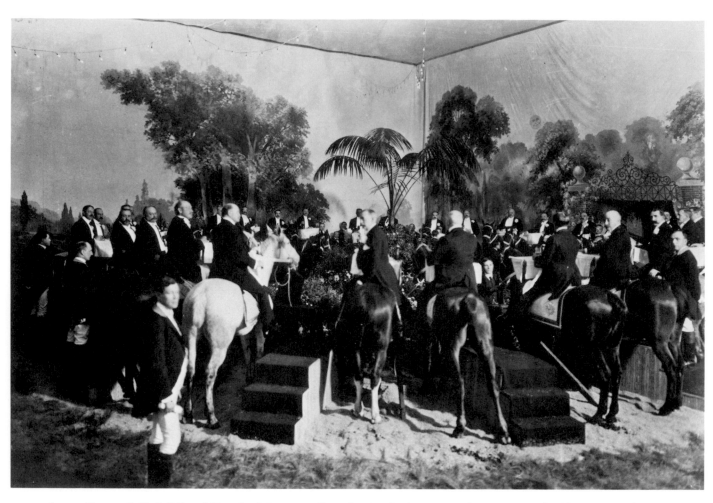

JOSEPH BYRON: C. K. G. Billings' Horseback Dinner at Sherry's, March 28, 1903. Southwest corner of Fifth Avenue and Forty-Fourth Street. MCNY.

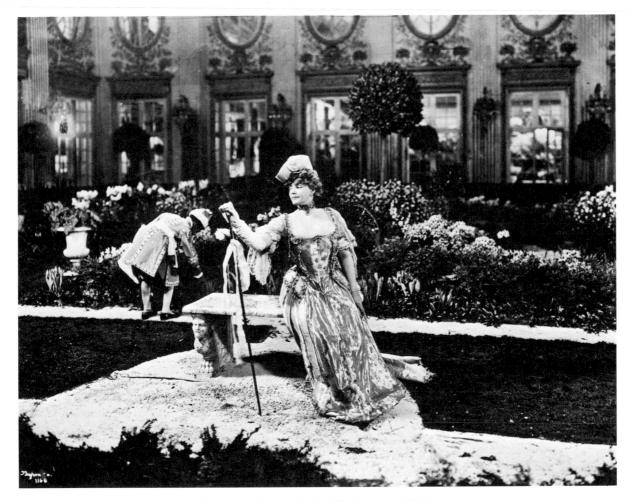

JOSEPH BYRON: Madame Réjane at the James Hazen Hyde Ball, January, 1905. MCNY.

pictures I discovered so many sources of light that the chiaroscural scheme was reduced to a battle of lights against each other. They, however, perfectly balanced each other and eliminated all darkness in the shadows.

"You do not strive for any accurate lighting?" I asked the photographer.

"No, that is out of the question," he replied, "just as plain truth wouldn't do in a story, accurate lighting would not make a good picture. Something has to be added."

I was not quite satisfied with his answer. To go contrary to all laws of lighting can hardly be right. And yet in a stage representation everything is artificial; the whole aim is to produce an illusion, and as long as pictures of it produce a similar effect I suppose one has to excuse the chaos of conflicting lights. The principal thing is, after all, to make a good effective picture that plainly tells its story, and this Byron invariably does, adding to it a certain artistic refinement that enhances its value to the more critical and fastidious mind.

The life of a theatrical flashlight photographer seems to be rather a strenuous one. He has to keep up with all the new productions, familiarize him-self with the dramatic situations and be ready to be called away at any moment to photograph a play during a dress rehearsal or perhaps late at night after a first night production. The latter are generally in out-of-town places, and at short notice, he and his assistants with all the necessary implements have to journey to New Haven, New London, Boston, Baltimore, or Washington (sometimes even as far as Pittsburgh or Chicago) and as soon as they arrive look up the theatre and get ready at once for action.

The number of engagements Byron has covered in the last ten years is an astounding one. The majority of all leading productions, with their original cast, scenery, and costumes, during that period have been duly recorded by him and there is hardly an actor or actress of prominence who has remained unrepresented. Irving, Duse, Réjane,[6] Bernhardt, and all our native favorites, are there. It is an interesting assembly that will increase in interest with every year. It is a pictorial history of our stage, and it is Byron's merit that he has told it in an expressive and artistic manner far beyond the average of photographic records.

—1907

34

BURR MCINTOSH

Photographer of Fads and Fancies

How to classify him! A photographer who is no specialist (in the ordinary sense of the word) and yet who can give most specialists a beating at their own game must be a remarkable sort of camera craftsman.

I, who am not easily abashed, stand perplexed before this virile and versatile personality. The usual terms do not apply to him. He occupies a unique position in the photographic field, and I find it difficult to make up my mind from what side I might best approach him.

He is generally called a society photographer. This is true to a certain extent. Burr McIntosh is, at all times, at the service of polite society, but in a somewhat different fashion than the rest. The average "society" photographer sits in his studio, sends out a general invitation to fashionable people, and waits until they come or do not come to him. Burr McIntosh, on the other hand, actually goes into society; he has the entrée into political and military circles and various coteries of our fashionable world, and while enjoying himself in their very midst plies his tools of trade nonchalantly like a gentleman-amateur. Only the results, photographically as well as financially, are strictly professional in character.

To understand more clearly his peculiar vocation, it may be interesting to dwell, for a few moments, upon his earlier life before he became a photographer. As a college student he was greatly interested in athletics and, I believe, made quite a hit as a baseball player. After leaving college he followed the theatrical profession for fifteen years, and not earlier than ten or twelve years ago did he take up photography as a profession.

And how well he understood to adapt his new vocation to the wants of his own personality! It furnishes an object lesson to every man in the profession. The temperament of the strolling player, something lusty, restless, and unabashed, was still in him and it has never entirely left him to this very day. He is a nomad by nature. Change is absolutely necessary to him. He can not occupy himself with anything for any length of time. He went his own way, always splendidly and aggressively himself; one of the few men who have fashioned out of photography a resonant instrument capable of expressing the virile and individual emotions of his own life. This is to me Burr McIntosh's chief distinction.

But what of his workmanship? It is OK of course; I have said so at the very start. Should one wish to be critical one might say that his prints are generally a trifle too hard or too light. Well, these faults are not of a very serious nature.

By choice, he is largely a recorder of facts, and distinctness and clearness are not always possible without hardness in the outlines and the transition

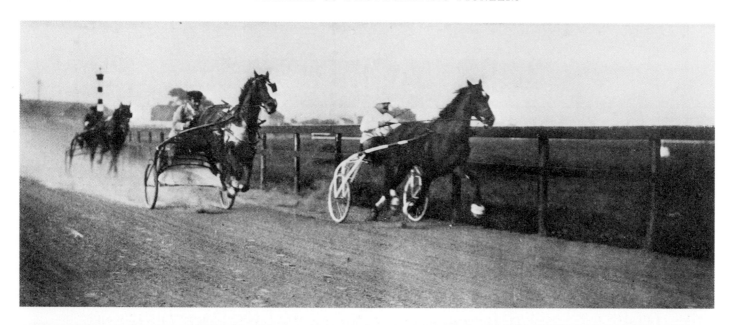

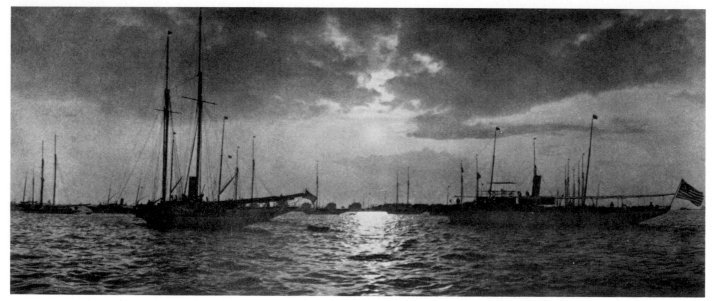

Top. BURR MCINTOSH: Lou Dillon, World's Champion Trotter (Two Minute), 1903.

Above. BURR MCINTOSH: At Rest (The New York Yacht Club Cruise, Newport, Friday Evening), 1903.

of light to shadows. Whether a print is too light or not is really a matter of taste; some people like it, and his portraits on that order had, for a time, quite a vogue. His prints, however, do not interest me as specimens of workmanship. Workmanship I study at Strauss' studio, or at Falk's, or at Steffens'[1] or Stein's.[2] The subject matter attracts all my attention. It is poured forth in an endless stream. It is like a society encyclopaedia in pictures. The range of subjects is simply astounding. I believe Burr McIntosh has photographed everything under the sun.

Rummage about in his studio and you will get a vague idea of this man's prodigality. There is Ethel Barrymore in her prime, a vaguely colored enlargement, as handsome a "professional" picture as I have ever seen. Right near it stands a picture of the Sultan of Sulu on horseback accompanied by two runners. Nor far away from it I espy a camp scene of the Spanish-American War, with Colonel Roosevelt, General Wheeler, and several other military notables as leading figures; and with the grasp of my hand, for a change, lies the portrait of the pet dog of some languid lady of fashion. Everywhere prints galore: of children in smart frocks and coats; of frequenters of clubs; of society débutantes in delicate fluffy gowns; of tally-ho parties; of picnic and garden scenes; of an equestrienne taking a hurdle on her favorite hunter; of yachts and automobiles, etc. There seem to be no end to his energy.

But this kind of photography is really only a side issue with him. It occupies very little of his time, for he is generally away on some trip, on some photographic exploitation. Some lumber king of the West wants to give the world an impression of the vastness of his possessions, of his yards and forest land. Burr McIntosh is at his disposal. A railroad company desires the beauty of some mountain scenery depicted for advertising purposes. Burr McIntosh will start to-night for the spot. As panoramic views are most suitable for this kind of work, McIntosh has made quite a study of this sort of kodaking. I have seen several of these views, some of them forming a complete circle; a lumber yard

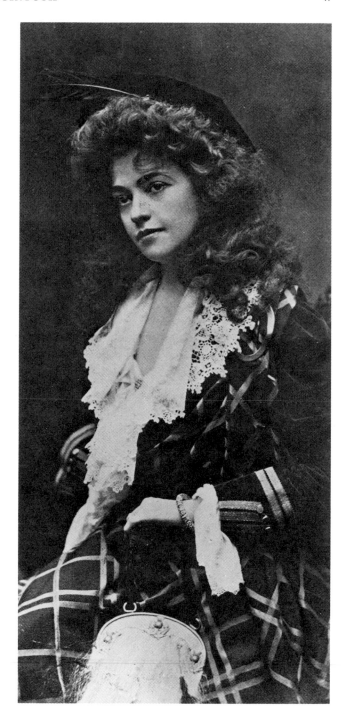

BURR McINTOSH: Louise Gunning.

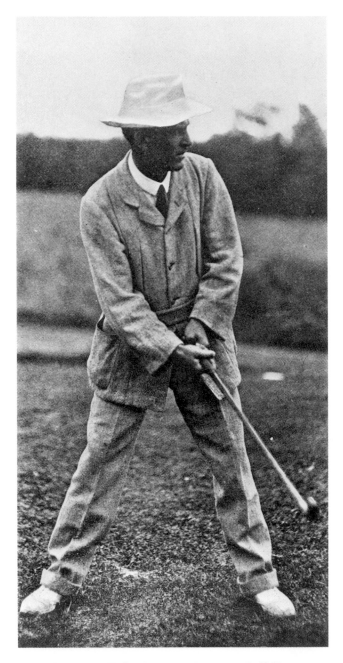

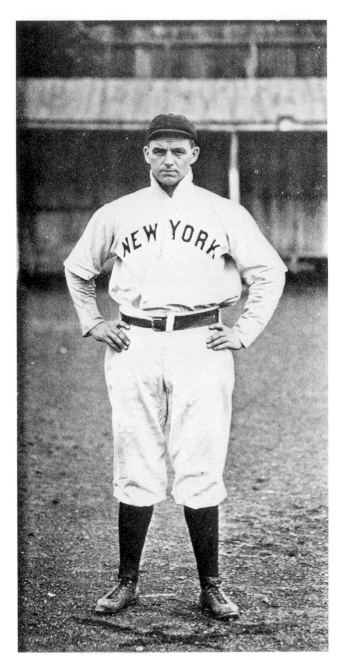

BURR McINTOSH: Walter J. Travis, American Golf Champion.   BURR McINTOSH: "Iron Man" Joe McGinnity, 1903.

and a baseball field (taken from the centre) which were exceedingly well handled, without a blur or break, clear in every part and perfect as regard to detail. Of course a man like McIntosh has no distinct method. I asked him whether he had one. He answered in a vague way: "One has to reckon with the conditions, the light, the weather, and atmosphere."

But before I forget, I must point out to you McIntosh's principal claim to photographic honors. He is in a way the special photographer to his Excellency, the President of the United States, Theodore Roosevelt. It is not an official position, he would be the last to take one, but he simply has leave of way whenever something of importance happens in the solemn affairs of state. Thus he accompanied the Rough Riders as war photographer on their Cuba campaign, and was the only member of his clan who succeeded in snapshotting several phases of the famous charge on San Juan Hill. And thus he went with the Taft party to the Orient, chronicling the scenes and incidents of that memorable semi-diplomatic journey. The number of pictures he made during this trip goes into the thousands, and to the initiated they are very much like illustrations to some "Alice in Wonderland." We see her slender girlish form, *en famille* so to speak, in attitudes and poses unknown to the public with the beauties of the Orient. Perchance, the Temple of Shiba or some Chinese gateway as a fitting background.

Yes, Burr McIntosh knows how to get some enjoyment out of his profession. I never wished that I were a photographer, but if I had to be one I would rather change places with him than with anyone else. He is alive, masculine, vital, and in his work he has made his own personality live; and that is more than art, it is the art of life which few of us manage to introduce in our every-day business life.

The life of most photographers is hodden-gray. Always the same thing, going to the shop in the morning and going home in the evening. The same wearisome promenades from the reception-room to the operating-room and back again; the same experiences under the skylight. This man knows how at least to give his life an interesting twist. He goes to the big athletic games and takes part in the Meadow Brook hunt. But does this diversified occupation really add to the prosperity of his business? Well, this is not for me to answer. That is every man's own affair. I only know that he is "a hale fellow well met," who understands the art of spending money.

He has great capacity for work. He has always several "irons in the fire."

He is afraid of nothing, and we can expect everything from him. Attending to the ordinary routine of his business, and furnishing all the material for the Burr McIntosh magazine every month,[3] he still finds time to lecture on his trip to the Orient, and to work on the libretto of a musical comedy entitled "The Photographer," which will be produced by some New York manager early in spring. In the meanwhile he will proceed to Los Angeles, where he dreams of opening a gorgeous studio in the Mission style of vast dimensions—the largest and most beautiful studio in America, surrounded by acres of ground. In the winter, for a few months, he will conduct his business in New York as heretofore; but, the remainder of the year he will live in some summer clime, among the fairy-like surroundings of his own creation, which can not fail to give to his personality the proper setting which it should have enjoyed long ago. Let us hope, for his sake, that this dream will come true.

Burr McIntosh has travelled on many highways, but he has always remained master of himself. He has exploited the fads and fancies of society, but in a way that has lifted the profession one peg higher in the esteem of the world. Photography is to him a sport, useful, pleasing, and lucrative at times, specially made for a man of roving disposition as he is, and the least we can do is admire his versatility. He may have never produced a single photograph that is perfect, artistically speaking—who does? But I am sure that he has produced more photographs that will live than the majority of photographers I know.

—1907

35

GUIDO REY

A Master of Detail Composition

*T*HE MORE I look at pictorial prints, the more I come to the conclusion that the majority of "successful" photographs are the result of accident rather than of any distinct evidence of artistic feeling and execution, or in other words that they are chance pictures. If a camera worker shows me several dozen pictures and only a few—as is often the case—reach a reasonable standard of excellence, probability points to those two or three pictures as a result of mere chance, as a mere happening that proves absolutely nothing as to the ability of the maker.

This became particularly clear to me when I sat for my portrait at the studio of one of our best known amateur portraitists, a man who can boast of an international reputation. He made twenty-nine exposures in order to produce one satisfactory result. Would it not be quite logical to argue that said picture was the product of experiment rather than of a masterly application of art laws. In photography, number is the supreme test of skill. If a man exhibits ten pictures, nine of which are merely matter of fact records and the remaining one fairly artistic, it is reasonable to suppose that the one is a chance picture. If, on the other hand, another man exhibits twenty pictures that all show artistic composition, it is equally reasonable to suppose them to be the work of an artist.

On my desk before me lies at this moment a small collection of prints by Guido Rey,—an Italian worker (semi-professional I suppose)—which records this uniformity of excellence. I have lived with them for a few days, and I have found in them considerable knowledge of composition, skill in artistic treatment, and a rare appreciation for the details of life—faculties that can be due only to a mind which, after hard fought struggles, slow artistic growth, and long years of observation, has finally gained the power to materialize his imagination.

From the tonal point of view—the accepted standard in recent years—the prints of Guido Rey show but little merit, but as he has said himself in a letter to the editor, he strives for different ideals. He considers detail and transparency the most important features of art photography, and a man with such convictions can naturally not enter the field of tonal competition with any sort of success. The tonalists strive for blurred effects, and the elimination of detail. Guido Rey sacrifices breadth of expression for subtler effects of lights and lines.

One of the principal merits of his work seems to me to be in his choice of subjects. Our American amateurs are favorably known for their excellent workmanship, but there is an appalling dearth of interesting subjects in most exhibitions. I have a vague recollection of a recent exhibition that contained at least twelve figure compositions, in which showing brass vessels and crystal balls played the most conspicuous parts. Surely this world does not consist entirely of brass vessel collectors and crystal ball gazers. The latter may be a very aesthetic occupation, but is it not a rather whimsical excuse for the making of a pictorial masterpiece? This lack of appreciation may be entirely my fault, but I cannot help myself. I prefer a man who has something to say or convey and I find it refreshing, to say the least, to come into contact now and then with a photographer who has ideas like Guido Rey.

This man of Turin composes his pictures like a genre painter. All his prints reveal a thorough knowledge and study of that popular branch of painting. Some are slightly imitation, as for instance: "The Encyclopedist" which reminds of Meissonnier;[1] and "Feeding the Pigeons" which looks like a reproduction of an Alma-Tadema[2] or a Coomans;[3] while others like the "Ciociara" and the "Morning Prayer" show true originality of pictorial conception. Yet no matter whether they are the products of skillful adaptation or careful invention, they invariably have a charm of their own, a certain poetical suavity which roots in personal feeling and ability.

Let us now take up each print separately and dwell upon the principal merits and short comings in each case. The "Morning Prayer" is exceedingly delicate in treatment. A man who can drape a figure in such an exquisite fashion and yet at the same time be historically accurate, avoiding all theatricality of effect, must have a strong poetical vein in him. With the conception and the placing, no fault can be found. Also the light (I suppose artificial light) is well concentrated; the only objection I have is that the outlines of the figure and the drooping veil should not be so abruptly lost in the darkness of the right hand corner. A faint indication of the form would in my opinion help the composition. A pity that he did not use real flowers instead of artificial ones. This is an infinitesimal detail, but a photographer who prides himself on

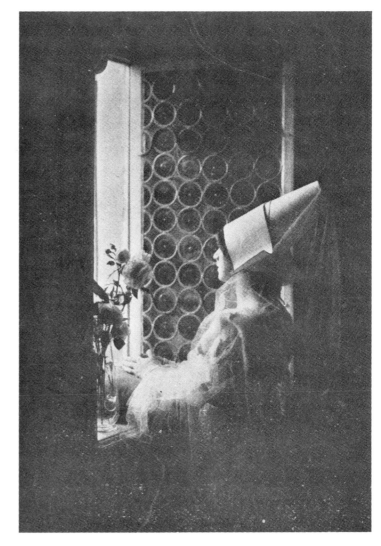

GUIDO REY: Morning Prayer.

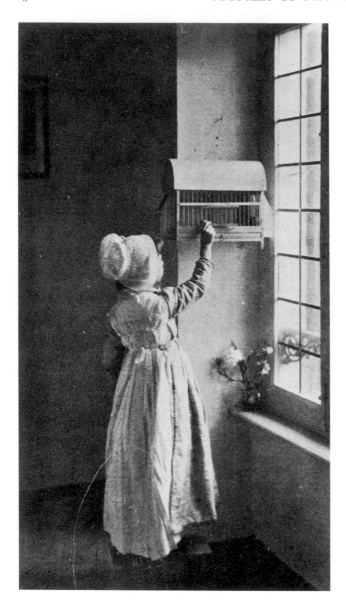

Above. GUIDO REY: The Cage of the Blackbird.

Opposite page top. GUIDO REY: Lady Tying her Bonnet.

Opposite page bottom. GUIDO REY: Little Girl Reading.

his handling of detail, should consider everything that might make his picture more perfect.

The next picture that we have to consider is "The Cage of the Blackbird." It is one of the very best. Its simplicity alone is convincing. The feeling for straight lines, in particular of the vertical ones, are unusually pronounced in this composition, but the little hooded and aproned figure is so well placed, that it destroys every trace of awkwardness and angularity. This is further helped by the distribution of light. The dark floor and the semi-darkness of the big stretch of wall with the black lines of the frame perfectly balance the light that comes pouring in through the window. In this case, however, the highest light merely strikes the lower part of the figure; the principal part of interest, the hand opening the door of the cage, is emphasized by the greatest accumulation of detail, the linear arrangement of the cage; and the manner in which the tiny pot of flowers is utilized to hide the angle formed by wall and window sill is a master touch of which only a man with an artistic knowledge is capable of.

The "Lady Tying her Bonnet" is not half as carefully composed as the preceding print, it is beautiful only in parts, notably in the way the model is costumed and posed. The principal fault of the picture is that its vertical and horizontal lines are all out of perspective. The left side of the picture holds its place, its vagueness helps the figure, but the arrangement of objects on the table and window sill is not up to his usual standard. It is too confused.

Excellent in every detail is his "Little Girl Reading." I consider it the masterpiece of this little collection. Notice how well the space is divided in regard to light and shade, how the flowers break the monotony of the curtain, how beautifully the hand rests on the highly illumined pages of the book. The little girl is poring over some picture book. This is the subject of the picture, the reason why it was made, and the eye of the beholder is lead straight to the main object of interest, the book, from there to

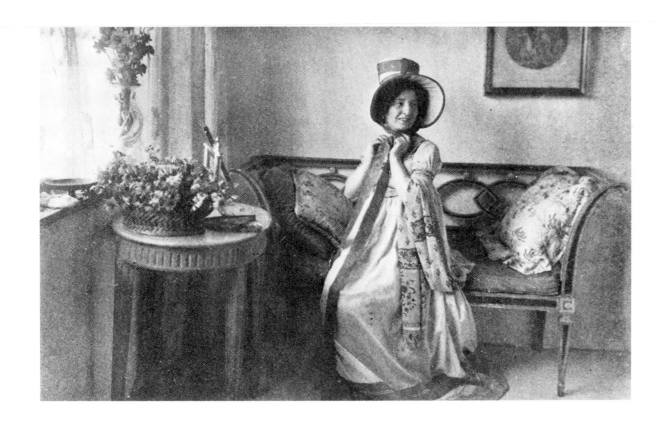

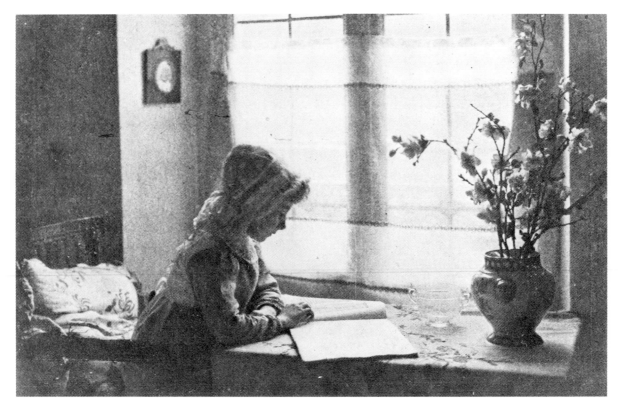

the exquisitely posed hands and the silhouette of the little girl's face. Then the eye is caught by the over-hanging flower, and in a circle taking in the other flowers, the vase, and the crystal bowl, returns to the book. Only gradually one discovers all the charming details, the elaborate costume of the girl, the arrangement of the cushion, the little picture which hangs just at the right spot, and the peculiar line arrangement and diffused light effect of the window. This picture is a triumph in the mastery of detail, without spoiling the general effect of the picture.

Rather trite in subject is his "The Encyclopedist." We have seen that kind of picture so often that most of us will pass it with a shoulder shrug no matter how well it is done, and yet this picture, as far as composition is concerned, is one of the best Guido Rey has produced. Only to mention one instance, observe how well the empty space on the left side of the picture is filled by the reclining back of the chair. A decided shortcoming in the treatment, however, is the lack of transparency in the blacks of the man's coat; furthermore, the line formed by the map and the canvas behind the table should be more subdued.

"Feeding the Pigeons" is equally successful in the handling of detail, but the composition is not quite as satisfactory. The interest is too divided. The little Greek child, the pair of pigeons, the table with the still life in the background, all absorb an equal share of attention. The picture is spotty, and the eye errs restlessly from one object to another. The large light space in the upper part of the picture may possibly help to convey the impression of sunlight but does not balance well with the rest of the picture. Some tall object, where the bottle stands, would have helped the composition. Not too much in praise, however, can be said of the loving way in which all the minor objects are treated. There are few photographers who could pose and drape a figure more simply and artistically than Guido Rey in this little Greek child study.

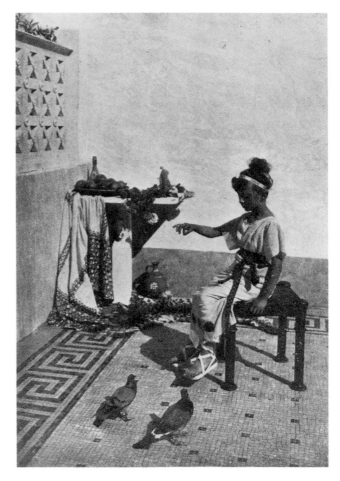

GUIDO REY: Feeding the Pigeons.

Truly Italian in character is his "Ciociara." The true meaning of the picture, perhaps one of local interest, is difficult to discern. All that concerns us is its pictorial quality and significance. The pose of the peasant woman, holding so picturesquely her huge basket while her eyes sweep over the distant valley, is superb. It conveys to us a feeling of outdoor life among the hills of Piedmont, the native country of the artist photographer. Too bad that the sky is so empty and meaningless. How easily a sky could have been faked in that it would have enhanced the beauty of the scene. But Guido Rey never *retouches*, and it is perhaps well that he sticks to the rule that he has laid down for himself. With a flat poster-like effect, the lineal arrangement should have been more strongly accentuated.

"Reading the Bible" is a good example of the so-called "full-face" composition. The subject demands concentration, and there was no other way but to make the arrangement a symmetrical one. This was done not merely by placing the figures in the centre and by balancing the tulips with the hour glass, but by giving the shape of the picture an archlike effect. The concentration of light towards the side of the little girl, and the vagueness of objects in the background are handled with the true understanding for pictorial effect.

I believe I have amply proven that the work of Guido Rey is exempt from the element of chance. When he sets out to make a picture, it is all ready in his mind; he may not always succeed in realizing it, but even his weakest effort is not accidental, but the product of a trained and sensitive mind; and if we agree on the point that the final test of a photographer's ability is the production of a *number* of artistic pictures, then Guido Rey is entitled to the highest honors, as he has shown by numerous and varied examples that he is a master in the application of art laws.

—1907

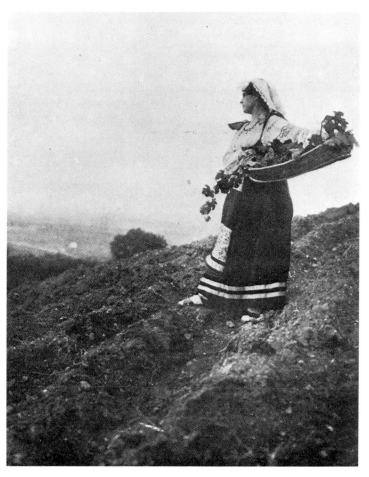

GUIDO REY: Ciociara.

him everything depends on premeditation and pre-arrangement; he strives to get the final result in the exposure without further manipulation. One can only respect him for this determination, and I who have always advocated straight photography welcome his as a true exponent of my theory.[4]

A pretty conceit is also his "Bowl of Milk," and it might belong to the very best of his pictures, if there was more differentiation of values, and the floor, mantelpiece and wall not of the same uniform tint. As it is, figure and accessories are seen almost as silhouettes, and the feeling of space which every interior should convey is spoiled thereby. On the other hand, if the photographer wished to produce

36

ALVIN LANGDON COBURN

Secession Portraiture

AT THE RECENT One-Print Exhibition of the Professional Photographers' Society of New York,[1] I was greatly astonished to find several prints, notably those of Strauss, Pirie MacDonald, and Partridge[2] that reminded me—there was no getting away from it—of Coburn's peculiar method of portraying celebrities.

Were those pictures accidents, or did the photographers wish to convey the idea that they also could do that sort of a thing? Hardly. I believe it was done on their part more or less unconsciously. They are all three men who are well posted and keep apace with new achievements. They may have made experiments in that direction years ago, and only now dare to come out with them because there is a general tendency all over the country for softer and more blurred effects. This, of course, is the influence of the Secession, but it is not imitation. Such things are in the air. I have seen forced highlights, such as Steichen used at times with more bravado than discrimination, in pictures of one-horse-town photographers who had never enjoyed the aesthetic pleasure of gazing at a Steichen print.

Of course, Coburn is an extreme. His delicate and poetical pictorial fancies are not for the public at large; nor can his portraiture be applied to common humanity. He is preëminently a depictor of picturesque personalities.

He shows us forms and faces as we may see them in a dream immaterialized as it were, and yet in a strongly decorative manner. He is in photography what Carrière[3] with his nebulous portraits is in painting. Portraits of this sort have no utilitarian but only an esthetic importance. If you get attached to them at all, you get attached to them deeply.

I have not yet arrived at that point. To be transformed into a pictorial phantasm may grant an acute sensation to the fastidiously inclined, but I prefer line and clear modeling to vagueness.

I asked Mr. Coburn the naive question, how he came to see everything in such an abnormal way. He responded with the equally naive answer, that there was nothing abnormal about it; that he considered the way other photographers represented life abnormal.

Well, that is merely an attitude of mind, as I do not believe that any man can actually see things that way, just as little as the impressionist painters see nature actually in color dots. Impressionism is a style of expression, and so is Coburn's method of diffusion.

There is really nothing new in this way of treating subjects, although it impresses me as unfamiliar and in a way unique. Tom Harris[4] made a portrait of me in 1901 (displayed at various Secession exhibits) which was done very much in the same manner; of course, it was a solitary example. It is Coburn's merit to have developed

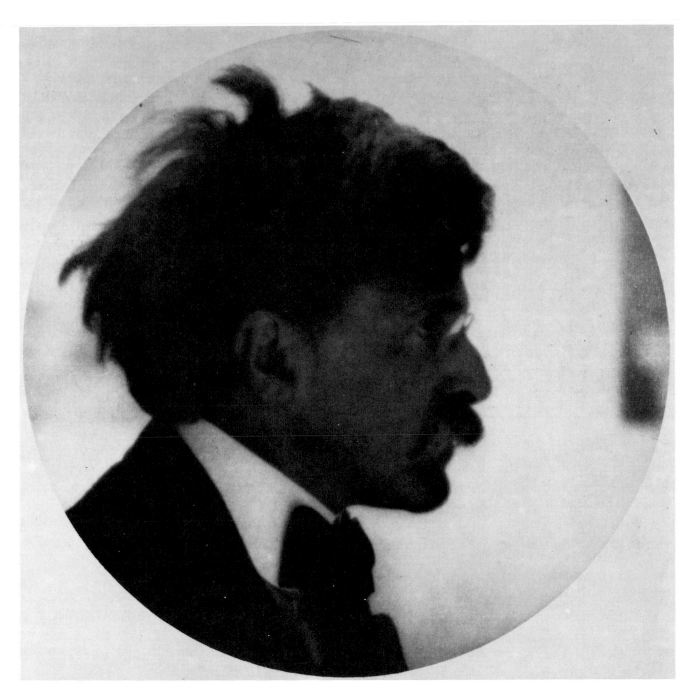

ALVIN LANGDON COBURN: Alfred Stieglitz. IMP-GEH.

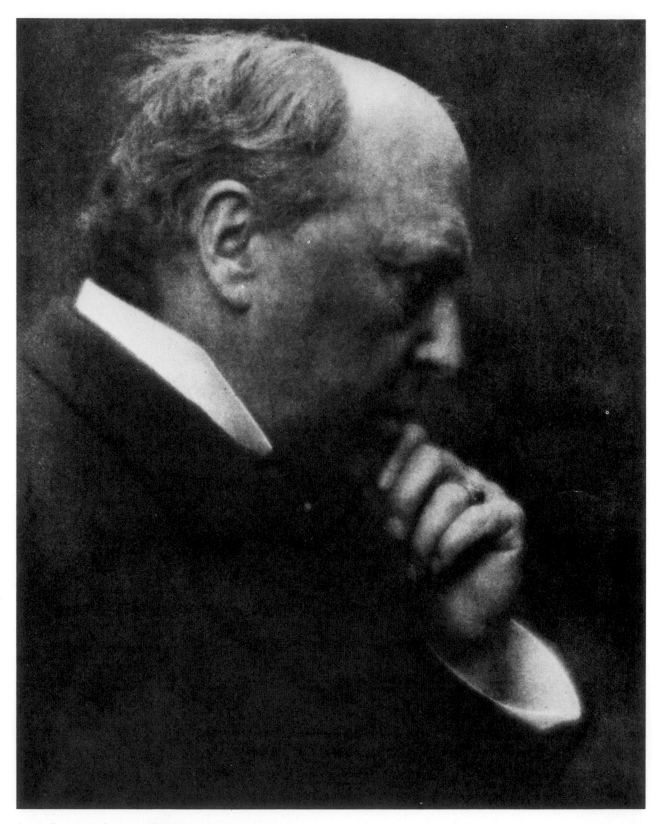

ALVIN LANGDON COBURN: Henry James. IMP-GEH.

this vagueness of effect into a style of his own. He has mastered it completely, and after once accepting his viewpoint (as a critic should) one will find much of interest in his work.

As may be easily understood, there is in this sort of pictorialism not much scope for character interpretation, at least as we generally understand it, yet there is something in it that is perhaps equally eloquent. As I looked at his Rodin in scull cap with flowing beard; at his Arthur Symons, very thoughtful-looking with one hand at his chin; and his Chesterton, all washy and blurred, it seemed to me that I did not merely see the faces of three distinct personalities, but something beyond; something of their life, their occupation, etc,; a vague impres-

sion, such as we may get of the personality of an author perusing one of his books. Is it merely because I am familiar with the work of these men, and does my imagination add this intangible something? Very likely; but is it not rather curious that a photograph can set your imagination going in such a direction? It seems so to me. Steichen never accomplished it. His portraits of celebrities were always self-explanatory, even melodramatic. Coburn is subtler, more poetic and elegant. One only has to look at the two men. Steichen was proud, eccentric, intolerant. Coburn is genial, cheerful, more temperamental. And just as his personality vaguely reminds me of some quaint character that we have seen in daguerreotypes, a young esthete of

ALVIN LANGDON COBURN: Chesterton. IMP-GEH.

ALVIN LANGDON COBURN: Rodin in Skull Cap. IMP-GEH.

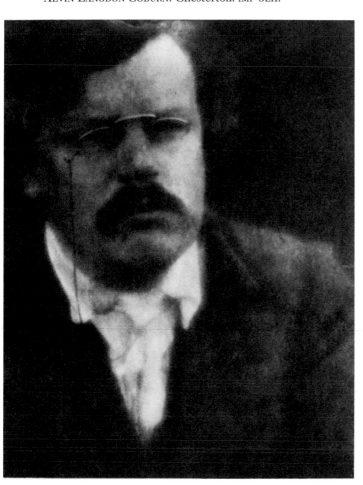

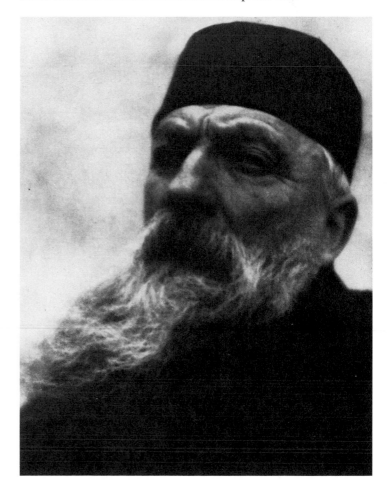

some Anglicized "Bohemia" (note: stove pipe, finger rings, and aureole of beard), his prints, grave and all, have a certain old-fashioned breadth and charm about them. His Shannon, Carpenter, James, Soloman Soloman, Shaw, Meredith, Sargent, etc., have what the critic calls soul quality. They give us more than we see at the first glance, yet we feel that all has not been said.

Technically this is easy enough to explain. Of course, I do not refer now to photographic technique, but that higher technique of conception. Every painter who thinks (sorry to say there are many who do not, just as there are such photographers), knows that mystery is produced by vagueness. Form ordinarily is something tangible, but as soon as its outlines are blurred and its texture diffused, it will begin to mystify us. This is—if not the aim—at least the final result of Coburn's work.

Whether these ghostlike apparitions have any permanent place in portraiture, I do not dare to decide. There is rarely an excuse for their existence, and I have never heard it better explained than by a young amateur at the Metropolitan School of Photography. We discussed Coburn, and he asked: "Is that, after all, not the right way, as we have never anything but a rather vague idea about great men?"

Coburn is not so much an impressionist as a symbolist. He knows that the character of a great man cannot be conveyed fully in one portrait; he therefore creates before our eyes an elegant and graceful vision, suggestive by its very formlessness of something subtly intellectual, and lets us add with the help of our imagination what the picture lacks in actual facts.

Although I do not endorse his method, not even for great men, I admire the energy with which he seeks out his subject and the exquisite taste with which he handles them. His management of silhouette and middle tints (never approaching pure white or the deepest black) is masterly. He is today by far the most progressive member of the Secession. Despite its ardent estheticism, his art is sane and healthy. He has heightened the key of tone composition, and it is largely due to him that—to talk with an English critic—"the gloomy glimmering and Aubrey Beardsley-like straining after effect of American pictorial photography" is changing into something brighter, more beautiful, and less painful to contemplate.

Yet the most remarkable thing, after all, is that one can write about a photographer as I have done, just as if he—well, dear reader, you will come to your own conclusion. It is my old argument, well nigh threadbare by this time, but just as true as ever. In my opinion Coburn is an artist, but the term portrait photography cannot be applied to such delicate fantasies as he has chosen to do.

—1907

37

RUDOLF DÜHRKOOP

A German Pictorialist

THE WORK OF Rudolf Dührkoop is fairly well known in this country. He is one of the few German professionals who can claim this distinction. During his visit to America in 1904 as commissioner to the St. Louis Exposition, he made many friends, and ever since has been exceedingly generous in sending specimens of his average studio work across the ocean. During my recent trip in the West I came across several portfolios filled with examples from his Hamburg workshop.

Dührkoop occupies in Germany a similar position to Garo, Pierce, Goldensky, and Strauss here, men who carry the artistic element in their prints as far as their customers allow them to do it. The German pictorialists—of whom Rudolf Dührkoop and Fritz Greiner[1] of Munich are typical—are perhaps a trifle more ambitious than their American colleagues. They tackle more difficult problems, in particular more elaborate interior compositions, and in consequence often lack the naturalness and simplicity of our work.

I do not believe that an American professional would ever produce a composition like "The Lovers." It is even beyond the grasp of the Secessionists. Its sentimentality is strictly Teutonic. I do not know the particular *raison d'etre* of this picture, whether there are really people in aristocratic, purse-proud Hamburg who fancy such effusions and accept them as portraiture, or whether it is merely a study, a flight of Herr Dührkoop's muse into the pictorial-emotional domain of life. As a composition, it is excellent. The management of light, putting the strongest highlights in the man's forehead, leaving the rest of the face in shadow, and distributing a shimmer of subdued light on the lower part of the girl's face is worthy of an illustrator. Even A. E. Sterner[2] who excells in such depictions could not do it any better. The placing of the folded hands is a difficult proposition. They are a trifle large and could be better in line feeling, but they help to carry out the sentiment and perfectly balance the higher planes in the upper part of the picture. The arm of the girl is rather carelessly draped, but hardly enough in praise can be said as to how the rest of the garments have been subdued and kept back. Also the natural treatment of the girl's hair deserves favorable comment.

The "Young Man in the Panama Hat" is a good study of subdued flesh-tints. Despite the whiteness of the tie and coat, the face has remained the principal point of attraction. I believe this has been accomplished by the dark accent of the hair and by producing, with the help of the hat (almost of the same tone value as the face), a large uniform plane of middle tints. The background, although subjected to manual manipulation, is restful and effective. The ear and the jaw line seem to be a trifle out of drawing.

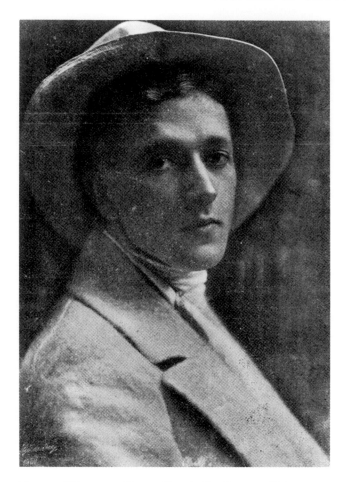

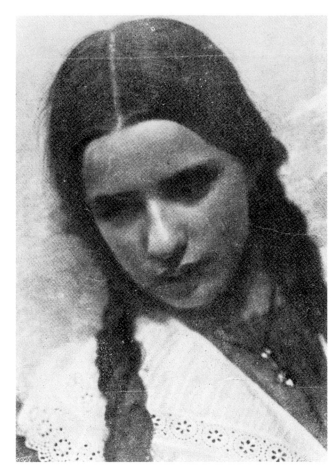

RUDOLF DÜHRKOOP: Young Man in the Panama Hat.

RUDOLF DÜHRKOOP: Head of a Girl.

The "Head of a Girl" is an interesting study in oblique lines. Again the face is lower in key than the dress. The darkness of the hair, accentuated by the light background, helps the complexion of the face. It does not impress one as being too dark. Dührkoop seems to lay special stress upon a clearly defined light and shade distribution, a quality which is apt to lend strength to the modeling and which is generally neglected in this country. Few of our men would dare to apply such pronounced shadows as these under the nose, lower lip, and chin. Even a Pierce seems to be afraid of such decided contrasts.

The "Lady in Riding Habit" reminds one of the work of Rose Clark[3] and Eli abeth Flint Wade.[4] The subtlety of the black and dark gray tones is exceedingly fine. The lower hand is too dark, and one is also left in doubt as to what she holds in her hands. In a good picture everything should explain itself. The modeling of the face is treated with charming breadth. The features have undergone a flattening process and yet suggest roundness. The fragment of the frame in the right upper corner is well placed and helps the composition considerably. On the whole this is a most satisfactory print. It seems, however, to show American influence and it is not quite as original as most of Dührkoop's work.

The group of the three children is too full of detail to suit me. There is a decided lack of composition in this picture. It is overcrowded and too diversified in interest. The poses of the children, each taken separately, are natural enough but the

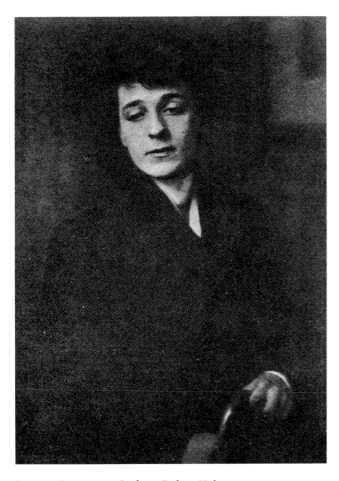

RUDOLF DÜHRKOOP: Lady in Riding Habit.

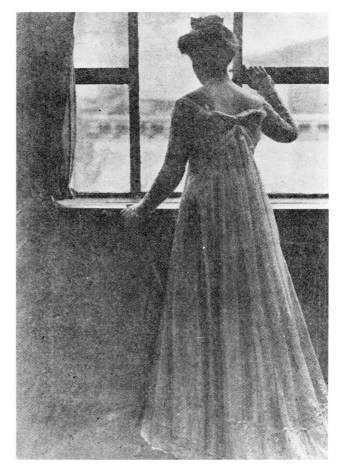

RUDOLF DÜHRKOOP: Study.

figures do not pull together. If the smallest girl had been left out entirely and the background treated in a more sketchy manner, the composition would be greatly improved. As it is, this picture falls short of Dührkoop's best efforts. Eickemeyer could easily beat him in this kind of work.

In the "Study," a lady in evening dress standing at a sort of studio window, we have a poster-like effect. It is produced principally by the straight lines of the window-frame, the silhouette-like treatment of the figure and the train of the dress disappearing in the lower right corner. Particularly note-worthy is the handling of the upper part of the figure. It is full of charming details, kept in such a low tone, however, that they are hardly noticed at the first glance. The Hamburg pictorialist seems to

be specially fond of such low-toned effects, and I would find it difficult to mention anybody who could compete with him in this specialty. If the picture were changed into an upright by trimming it about an inch and a quarter at the left hand side (eliminating the suggestion of the side wall), the pictorial quality of the composition would be greatly enhanced. The length of the figure seems to call for it.

We now come to the three most beautiful prints of this collection. The portraits of an Old Lady, of the poet Froensen, and of a young girl are specimens of such excellent workmanship that every studio could well afford to be proud of them. They are exceedingly simple and unaffected as all good portraiture should be. The photographer tried for

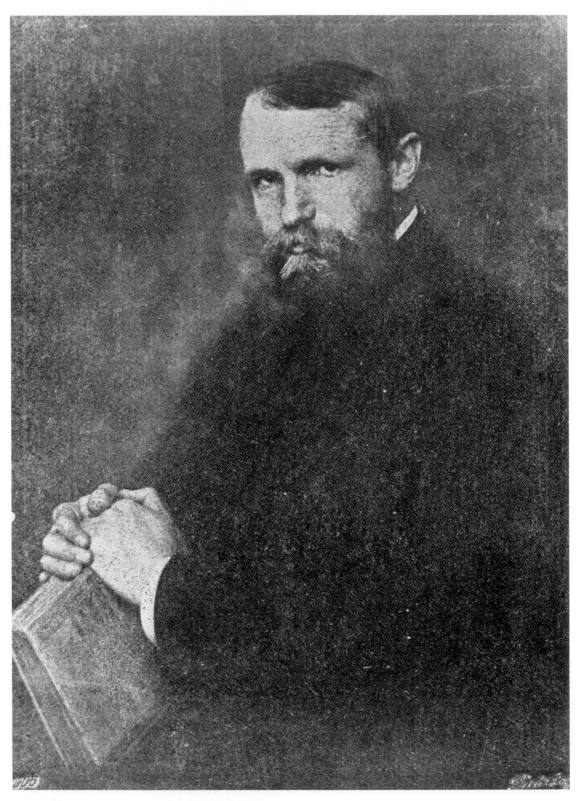

Rudolf Dührkoop: Portrait of the Poet Froensen.

nothing but the salient characteristics of each sitter, and he succeeded in recording them. It would be difficult to say which of the three is the best one. They seem to be powerfully and rapidly improvised direct from nature.

How naturally the thoughtful old lady wrapped in meditation is seated. She truly conveys the idea that she was not posing. This is frank and sane portraiture without a trace of arrogance and striving for queer and quaint effects. It is inspired only by the spectacle of life as visible to his own eyes. It seems almost cruel to pick out minor faults in such an excellent print, and yet this is the critic's duty. I wish the photographer had not considered it necessary to accentuate the highlights of the hand on which the old woman's face is resting. The face does not need this contrast, and the form of the hand is not beautiful enough to warrant accentuation. The highlights in the lace cap would have proved sufficient to throw the face into relief. Otherwise, the picture is perfect, unless somebody should find fault with the three perpendicular folds in the background.

The portrait of the poet is equally successful, perhaps even more so. However hard I might try, I would find it difficult to criticize anything in this print. There is nothing to criticize. The simple arrangement, the pose of the thoughtful face, the masterly treatment of the hands resting so naturally on the book, the elimination of all unnecessary details, the quality of the background, are all above fault finding; and it is really a critic's greatest pleasure to find something where argument becomes unnecessary. A pity that it occurs so seldom.

There is something, however, in this print that demands special consideration. You will notice that the strongest highlight, the tone nearest to white (as in the majority of Dührkoop's pictures) is not in the face but on the collar and cuff. It proves the fallacy of the general opinion (Poore's,[5] Bement's,[6] Beck's[7] and Dundas Todd's[8] included) that the highest light effects must be concentrated on the face, in order to make it stand out. Garo's and Pirie MacDonald's

theories are well enough—for them, but they are only one solution of the problem of lighting a face. The Dührkoop method is a much subtler one and well worth analysis and experiments under the skylight. The expression of a face handled in a gradation of middle tints is much finer than one produced by big chalky splotches on forehead and nose.

In the "Portrait of a Young Girl" we have a peculiar top light effect which strikes neither forehead nor chin, but only a part of the eyebrow, the cheek bone, and one side of the nose, and of the upper and lower lip. Dührkoop apparently searches continually for new light effects. They give variety to his prints and in this instance give a

RUDOLF DÜHRKOOP: Portrait of a Young Girl.

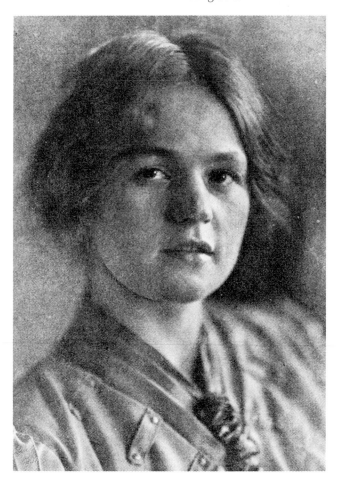

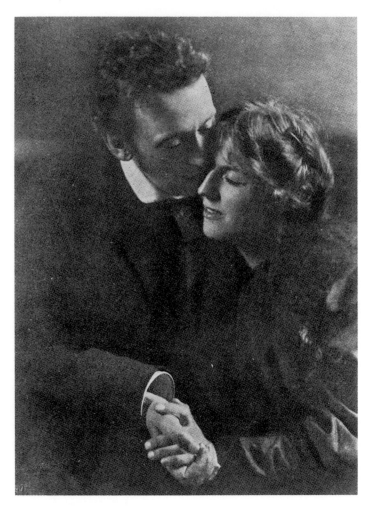

RUDOLF DÜHRKOOP: The Lovers.

special impression of vivacity to the typically German face of the young girl. In this picture, as in the "Lady in Riding Habit" and "The Lovers," the strongest highlights are to be found in the face, but in each instance they are treated in an unconventional, novel sort of a manner. He does not believe in any stereotyped method of picture construction. The prevailing tone of mushiness invented by gloom-imbued souls whose artistic feeling can find no other outlet than in the portrayal of dark vagaries and misty agonies, has also found its way to Germany. But no person of superior judgment like Dührkoop would apply this preponding note of gloom to the depiction of a happy laughing child. Käsebier would. That is the difference.

In summing up the manifold merits of Rudolph Dührkoop as a portraitist, it seems that special stress should be laid upon his unconventionality of expression. Also following at times to some extent the tonal compositions of American pictorialists, he invariably produces work which is strongly marked by personal sentiment. He recognizes the great truth that the charm of a face does not necessarily lie in the accurate rendering of its features, but in the expression of those deeper and more subtle beauties by which nature appeals to the imagination. To him a portrait is not merely a record, not merely actuality, but the means by which he can give utterance to poetic sentiments and aspirations. He revels in the mysteries of light and shade—one of the greatest problems portraiture has to offer— and makes his prints sparkle with that delightful freshness which is one of the great charms of all good pictures.

—1907

38

E. S. CURTIS

Photo-Historian

ALTHOUGH IT IS difficult to tell the whereabouts of E. S. Curtis at this moment, there is no doubt that he is just now the most talked-of person in photographic circles.

His publisher or manager, whoever that may be, seems to be engaged in a huge advertising campaign. Wild rumors are afloat that Pierpont Morgan is backing Curtis with immense sums. There is much talk about the forthcoming edition de luxe of *The North American Indian* in ten to twelve volumes, at three thousand dollars per copy; and President Roosevelt who, like the German Emperor, likes to have his say about everything has endorsed the work with a foreword.[1]

The publication of such a work which will contain 2200 photogravure illustrations (a third of which will be twelve by sixteen inches) is, of course, a stupendous undertaking. Some noise has to be made, in order to avoid too great a loss of invested money. But it is not particularly dignified. One would prefer to see less glamour and lime-light flare connected with a serious scientific publication, as this pretends to be.

I never had the pleasure of meeting Mr. Curtis personally, but I have heard a good deal about him indirectly. A friend of mine, Albert L. Groll[2] the painter of "Arizona," has met him while photographing the Hopi Indians, and told me all about the photographer's field outfit and his curious way of working. There is no doubt that this man is sincere. His fifteen years of camplife devoted to the task prove it. He probably knows about the Indians as much as any other man alive, and seems to possess the faculties necessary for making valuable records of his knowledge and observations.

As the Indian Commissioner Francis E. Leupp says in the introduction: "*The North American Indian* will give a complete written description of every detail of the lives, customs, and folklore of every Indian tribe in the United States. All phases are pictured—the Indians in their environment, the types of the old and young, their primitive home structure, their handicrafts, their ceremonies, games, customs—with an object first to truth, then to art composition."

Truly a gigantic task. And I believe it is safe to say that the work will satisfy all expectations as far as truth is concerned. It will give a truthful record of the Indian race, and as an ethnological document will be invaluable.

Walt Whitman, in his prose writings, expressed more than once his regret at the ultimate fate and extinction of this wild and beautiful race. And although some authorities claim that "the Indian race is not dying out, and that some tribes are steadily increasing (as, for instance, the Cherokees, who adopt all who marry into their tribe)," one can hardly be very sanguine on that subject. I perfectly

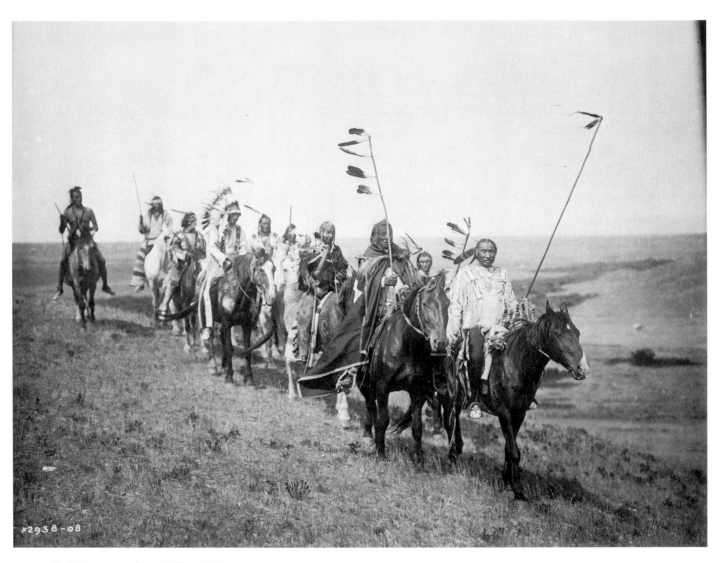

E. S. Curtis: Indians Riding, 1908. lc.

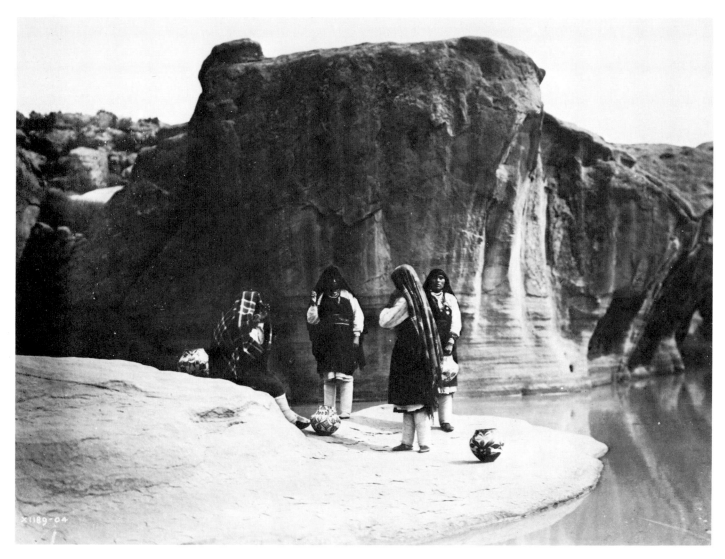

E. S. Curtis: A Morning Chat, Acoma, 1904. LC.

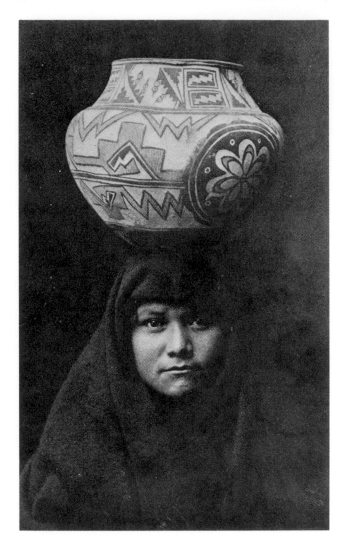

Above. E. S. Curtis: Pueblo Zuni Girl.

Opposite page. E. S. Curtis: A Desert Cahuilla Woman (Rose-belle Nombre of Torres-Martinez Reservation).

agree that Mr. Curtis' undertaking is one that can not easily be repeated. The red savage Indian is fast changing into a mere ordinary, uninteresting copy of the white race. And although opportunities for similar records may continue to exist for some years to come, there will probably be no other Curtis to do it. He is an enthusiast and has made it his life's work, and none of his occasional competitors will succeed in gathering a more valuable and complete accumulation of material.

Curtis is the pictorial historian of the Red Man, and he has done more in that respect than any painter has been able to do. And it was the camera that won out for him. A painter is apt to let his imagination run away with him. He is never to be relied upon for accuracy, and accuracy is what makes Curtis' records valuable to posterity. There is no making of pictures for pictures' sake; a Sioux must be a Sioux, an Apache an Apache. In fact every picture must be primarily an ethnographic record. Being photographs from life they show what exists and not what one in the artist's studio presumes might exist.

Of course, black and white reproduction has its drawbacks. "An Indian is only half an Indian without the blue-black hair and the brilliant eyes shining out of the wonderful dusky ochre and rose complexion." Also his paraphernalia, feathers and paint, etc., suffer greatly by monochrome depiction. Another serious objection is the photographic process itself. It cannot grasp ideal traits. It necessarily falls short in the highest characteristic representation, that which the painter can add by his thought. A photograph will never go beyond the record, and the more faithful the photograph is the truer this will be.

Pictures as George de Forrest Brush[3] has painted, notably his Indian plucking a water lily and his Indian in a canoe gazing at the flight of a wild swan overhead, will convey to posterity a finer conception of the aboriginal American than any photograph can ever do. And yet there is a question whether the Indian is really such a wonderfully

inspiring subject for an artist. Despite their characteristic make-up, their primitive way of living, and
their peculiar ceremonious rites they can hardly
claim to be as picturesque as, for instance, the
Arabian horsemen that Schreyer[4] paints. Their
circlet of eagle feathers, necklaces of bear claws,
headdresses of colored braid, blankets and drab
buckskin leggings, hideous wooden masks and moc-
casins embroidered with glass beads are too gaudy,
too loud to be truly pictorial. Everything has to be
subdued, reduced in value, idealized, made more
poetical, but also less real. All the painters who
have tackled this subject, Wimar,[5] Shirlaw,[6] Gaul,[7]
Cary,[8] Farny,[9] Deming,[10] Hamilton,[11] Latoix,[12] De
Cost Smith,[13] Mosler,[14] etc., have had the same
experience. The material was too uncouth for
them; they either produced pictures that were a
trifle awkward and prosaic, or idealizations that do
not ring quite true.

In a black and white delineation harmony is
much easier obtained. It is only necessary to
transfer the record into a low tone; and it is this
toned quality which Curtis applies in the majority
of his pictures—and I fear artistically almost to his
undoing. The majority of his pictures I have seen
were all a trifle muddy. That of course is a fault of
the handling and not of the process. The workmanship of the Curtis print could be improved upon and
I do not agree with some of his lay critics that "he
has created the most beautiful and artistic series of
photographs that the world has ever known."

Not even as far as photographs of Indians are
concerned. Some of the Käsebier and even Goldensky's Indian pictures are way ahead artistically.[15]
But they are merely isolated examples. They do not
count when one considers the aim and intrinsic
value of Curtis's work. He has done what no other
photographer has done. He is *the* photographer of
Indians, and will live as such.

Much could be said, I suppose, about his methods
as a photographer, and the adventures of his various
canvas wagon journeys when he is "gunning with
his camera," but as I am not familiar with either it

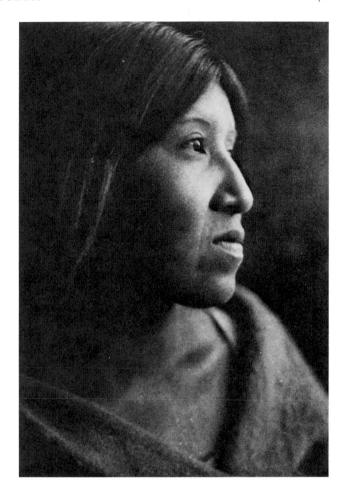

is best to leave it to others. He himself would
probably prove the best narrator of his manifold
experiences. The majority of his prints seem to be
snapshot enlargements, no doubt the safest way to
arrive at results.

The scope of his book is absolutely exhausting.
The first volume treats of the Apaches, Jicarillas,
and Navahoes. Volume two will cover the many
tribes in Southwestern Arizona and in the Colorado, Gila, and Salt River valleys. The different
Sioux tribes of North and South Dakota will come
next in order, in volume three; and volume four will
treat of the tribes of Eastern Montana. The fifth
volume will depict the tribes of Western Montana
and Idaho and the sixth the tribes of Eastern
Washington.

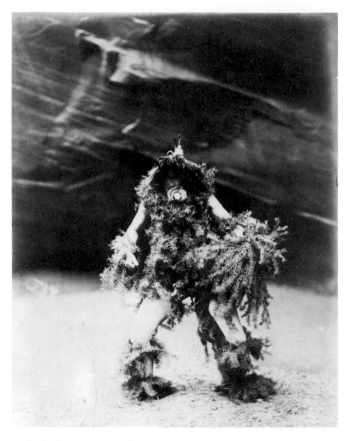

E. S. Curtis: Tonenli ("Water Sprinkler"), Navaho Rain God, 1904. LC.

Other volumes will take up the Mission Indians of Southern California, the aborigines of Northern California and Oregon, those on the Northern Pacific coast and Puget Sound, and the coast Indians of Alaska and the Pacific coast. One will be devoted to the Hopis and one to the other different Pueblo tribes. There probably will be a volume on the Seminoles of Florida, and Canada will have, without doubt, one volume which will practically be what might be called a treatise on the "Woods Indians." The final volumes will take up the tribes in the Oklahoma and Indian territory.

We will become acquainted with the tribes of the mountains and the plains. We will learn to know them as they hunt, as they travel, as they go about their various avocations on the march and in the camp. We will be introduced to their medicine men, sorcerers, and story tellers, their chiefs and warriors, their young men, squaws, and children. And we will not only see their vigorous outward existence, but catch glimpses of that strange spiritual life of theirs, their mythology, folklore, and religious ceremonies—whose innermost recesses were never fathomed by white men.

—1907

39

PIRIE MACDONALD

Psychology in Portraiture

PORTRAITURE, AS IT is practised to-day, even when at its very best, is nothing but an aesthetic enjoyment for the few who like to see a personality delineated as another personality sees it. The pride and surprise of performance has become the predominant quality, and the note of psychology—the record of the inner life of man in contrast to outward appearance—is lacking.

The painter is too much absorbed in the individuality of brush-work, in the color-scheme and composition, in the effect, perchance, of some passing light, to give due attention to the delineation of character. Of course there are exceptions like Watts,[1] Lenbach[2] and Bastien-LePage,[3] who, all three in their own way, undertook to blend character with artistic qualities. But the technique of the painter is inseparable from the conception of his mind, and the stronger his personality is, the more active will his imagination be in the presence of an interesting sitter. He unconsciously will give his own interpretation to the features and forms before him, and the result will be a commentary on them rather than an accurate representation of the same.

Their medium of expression is a too elaborate one, the action of the hand too closely connected with activity of the brain that it could grasp objective phenomena; and the likeness they render

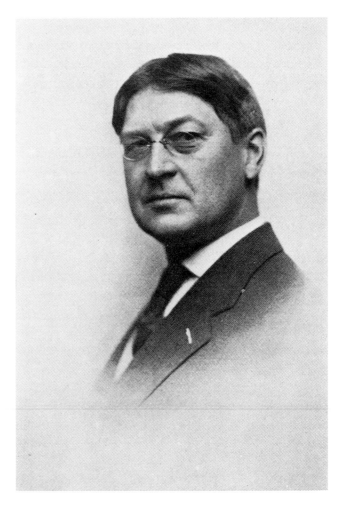

PIRIE MacDONALD.

273

is not likeness *per se*, but likeness as seen through a temperament. Many of the leading portrait-painters have realized this deficiency and tried to substitute for it a mechanical registration of facts. They have welcomed the camera as an obliging assistant to overcome the difficulties of actual structure.

Photography is the one medium of pictorial expression which records independently; only the selection of its subjects is under control, but what it is asked to represent, it represents mechanically. And it is one of those inexplicable cases of human shortsightedness that the artists of the camera have not recognized the fact that the originality of camera expression is dependent, no, stands or falls, with this one quality of independent registration. Instead of blindly imitating the formula of other arts, they should have recognized that their technical means were capable of a new style of expression.

For who can say what a portrait-painter might not accomplish, if he could devote his entire knowledge and all those qualities which constitute genius in a painter to the arrangement, investigation and full comprehension of his subject, leaving the labor of actual representation to a mechanical process of reproduction.

"But a photograph is so matter-of-fact, so bald in appearance!" will be the argument. True, it is matter-of-fact, and this is the sole reason why so many photographers lose themselves in imitative eclecticism, in the endeavor to substitute what their process is lacking. I am not so certain, however, about the baldness of effect. The technique of photography is becoming more fluent and flexible every day, and, barring color, it has a peculiar solidity of dark tints, a richness of tonal gradations, and a faculty to lose form in its background and environment which compares favorably with other graphic arts. If one approves an etched portrait, one has no ground to find fault with a photographic portrait.

The great difficulty at present is that so few men enter the profession who have the necessary faculty for its proper and successful manipulation. Not every man is an appreciator of character and facial expression and at the same time endowed with good taste, pictorial insight, and that peculiar patience which the scientific practice of photography demands. Pirie MacDonald is such an exception. He is a man of great intellectual resources, naturally endowed with good taste and a peculiar gift for his profession. He underwent a thorough academic training in order to become more conversant with the technical methods of art and the laws of composition. Few have carried the photographic art to such a pitch as MacDonald. He was a masterly technician from the start. From the time of his first successes at photographic expositions he was hailed, I believe, as a recruit of high value to the camp of artistic photography. He was already in possession of a style. Slowly his style gained in delicacy and assurance, in the faculty to render character in a straightforward, sympathetic manner. Then he became a master of light and shade, and added the poetry of atmosphere to his character delineation. Finally, he carried his style to the highest point by expressing those subtle emotions which might be called the psychological element in art.

His portraits, glanced over *en masse*, have all a certain virility and robustness in common; although at first glance there is a deceptive smoothness, resulting from a perfect technique, about them. His subjects are, of course, such as thousands might have to interpret; but how they reflect each human expression! He gives the exact translation of his thought about a person, without changing the actual resemblance. With him photography has become pure tact of vision.

Two of Pirie MacDonald's recent portraits, which it must have been a delight to interpret—I allude to those of General Chaffee and Russell Sage—show his conception of character. It is evident in the massive and erect head of the one and the arrangement of light which forms the setting of the slim, long face of the other. He enables us to see in the shrewd, wrinkled countenance of Russell

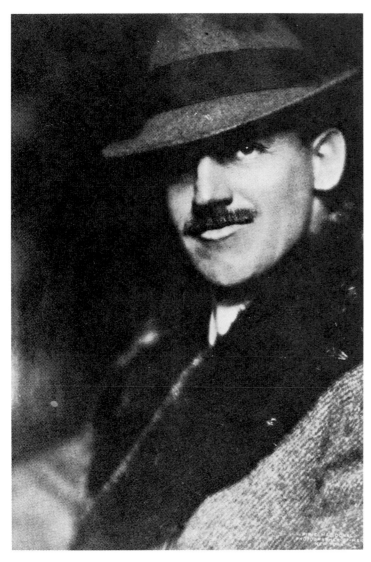

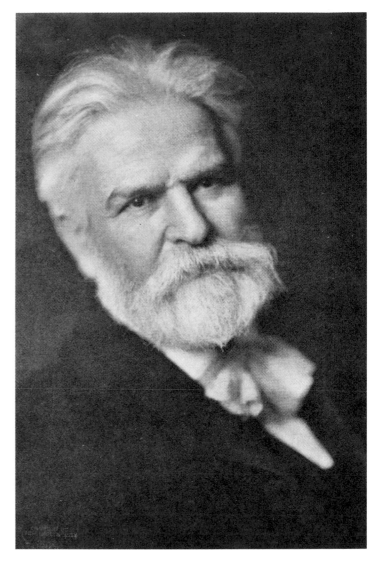

Pirie MacDonald: Portrait.

Pirie MacDonald: Edwin Markham.

Sage all the power of concentrated thought and patient labor that is valuable in the man; and in the face of General Chaffee, he suggests squareness of form, indicative of firmness and manly vigor, by features and form that are perfectly round.

Another brilliant production is the portrait of Rev. Parkhurst. The well-known preacher and reformer is quite a picturesque character, and the photographer expressed it by a more pictorial arrangement. It is shown in the energetic twist of the head and in the usually strong contrasts between the light and shadowy parts. His keen and thoughtful and his absorbed and concentrated gaze gains a deeper significance by this treatment.

MacDonald's power of interpretation is also much in evidence in his portrait of Jacob Riis.[4] The sympathetic nature of Roosevelt's "best citizen," his faculty for observation and his frankness in expressing it, are apparent in the simple and genial facial expression.

And with what breadth of sympathy and keenness of insight has the photographer depicted the face of Marshall Field, a man of calculation, restless energy and rare organizing-power. The first impression MacDonald received when Mr. Field entered his studio was that of an officer who, with perfect ease of manner, is used to command large masses of people. "Why, he is the merchant-militant," suggested itself to the photographer's mind, and out of this idea he created the portrait which carries out the most familiar phase in Mr. Field's outward appearance.

MacDonald's activity has been confined almost exclusively to portraiture and, as he was attracted most by character, he has devoted himself in recent years exclusively to the portrayal of men. Laying particular stress upon the beauty of features and those parts of the face that express intellectuality and rare mental gifts, he concentrates all his light upon the eyes and forehead, while the failings and weaknesses of humanity are absorbed in the shadows. For the same reason he seldom attempts standing figures, but prefers the simplicity and

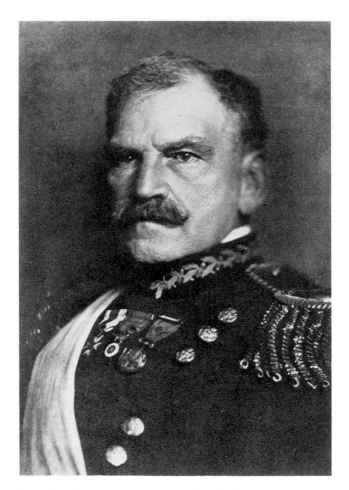

PIRIE MacDONALD: General Adna R. Chaffee.

directness of the bust portrait without any embellishments and accessories. MacDonald simplifies, but simplifies with taste and unerring precision. What big, sweeping masses of light and shade, and what a shimmer of light upon the faces! He is not imitating the chiaroscuro scheme of any painter or school, but has invented his own method.

My admiration for this distinguished work is such that I am perhaps in danger of overstating its merits; but it is worth taking into account that to-day, after several years of acquaintance with it, its merits seem more and more to justify enthusiasm. His photographs have the sign of portraits of the first order, and their style alone—I can't call it

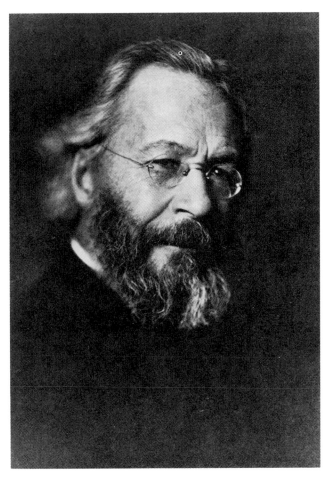

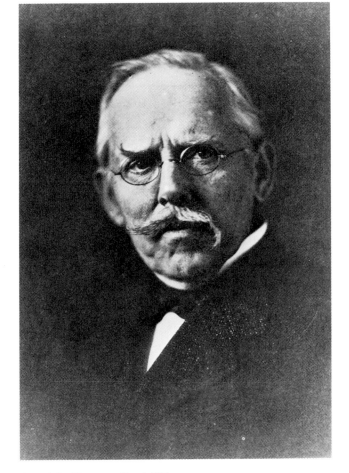

PIRIE MacDONALD: Rev. Charles H. Parkhurst.

PIRIE MacDONALD: Jacob Riis.

otherwise—would save them if everything else should change: our measure of the value of resemblance, their expression of character, and the particular association they evoke.

The gift that he possesses he possesses completely—the immediate perception of the final result and the means he can employ. Putting aside the question of the subject (and to a great portrait a common sitter will doubtless not always conduce),

the highest result is achieved when to the element of quick perception a certain faculty of lingering reflection is added. I use this term for lack of a better; I mean the quality which enables the artist to see deep into a subject, to absorb it, to discover in it new things that are not on the surface of expression, and to become patient and almost reverent with it—thus elevating and humanizing the pictorial problem.

—1907

40
BESSIE BUEHRMANN

Under the Influence of the Secession

$\mathcal{I}$ HAD GONE to East Aurora for a vacation. I thought I would indulge for a change in Elbert Hubbard's[1] philosophy of sunshine, get interested in flowers, trees and Roycroft products, and forget for a while all about art and photography. But somehow one can't escape one's destiny. There was a whole congregation of photographers assembled on the porch when I arrived. I had to face the artillery of their cameras more than half a dozen times during the next days and was inveigled into dissertations on art in photography at all hours of the day and night.

Among these enthusiastic craftsmen of the camera was a young lady, Miss Bessie Buehrmann of Chicago, whose work attracted my attention. I had never heard of her, but there was something about her prints which fascinated me. The liberal size, the quality of the material, the way of mounting, the blurred effect, the pictorial notes and tonal arrangement in the composition of the portraits—all betrayed the Secession influence. There is something in the way in which she poses people, or rather in the way in which she lets her sitters pose themselves, which reminds of Eva Watson Schütze,[2] and the general effect particularly of the bust portraits shows all the ear marks of Coburn's masterly technique. And true enough Miss Buehrmann told me that she had worked with Eva Watson Schütze, that she knew Stieglitz, and ad-

mired Coburn's style of portraiture above all others. She had only recently returned from a trip to Europe, and was familiar with the pictorial work on both continents.

A good basis to start work upon. Of course one can hardly expect that Miss Buehrmann at the age of twenty-one is a full-fledged artistic personality. But there is no gainsaying that her work has distinction, and that it is particularly interesting to the critic as it represents in a way a further development of the Secessionist movement. Until now, when we came across a "Secession" print, it was one by the regular workers who had grown up in the rank and file of the Secessionists. The movement in itself is only a few years old, and there was no time as yet to bring to light a younger generation of Secessionists. There were followers and sympathisers and imitators galore, but no younger photographers who developed directly under the influence of the movement.

Miss Buehrmann is no Secessionist, and as far as I know no candidate at present, yet it is well nigh impossible to classify her work in any other way than I have done. Her work is at present exceedingly uneven. At times it is perfectly satisfactory, at others, decidedly open to criticism. There is as yet no mathematical precision about it. I heard somebody criticize her work to the effect that it was strictly accidental. I beg to differ. Her portraiture may be bad in instances, but is never mediocre and, for that reason, possesses some notes of individuality which she alone can lend to it.

There are three kinds of pictorial photographers. The first class consists of those who have a premeditated conception of the subject they are going to take, and who master the medium of photography so perfectly that they are capable of translating the color and light values of life and nature with as much truth as is possible into monochrome. In other words, they know beforehand the result of the exposure, and they really need under favorable conditions not more than a single plate to produce a satisfactory picture. This is Stieglitz's ideal, but pictorialists who work in that manner can be counted on the fingers of one hand. The second class has numerous exponents. They still have the premeditated conception, but not enough of the technical ability to carry out their original plan to the letter, and so they expose half a dozen plates or more until they get something that resembles their first idea. The members of the third class have no premeditated conception, merely a vague idea of what they want. They rely on the inspiration of the moment, and as it is impossible for any person to be technically so well-equipped as to master all the various conditions of light, atmosphere, etc. (particularly so in home portraiture), the results, at least the larger percentage of them, are strictly experimental.

The majority of the better amateurs—and, sorry to state, also many of the Secessionists—work in that fashion. No wonder that a young photographer like Miss Buehrmann has not yet risen beyond the experimental stage, and yet she would not fare so badly in comparison with others.

When she took my portrait for the first time, she made five exposures. They were all failures. Even in the two better ones, the likeness was snapshotty and in no way typical. Then I told her what I wanted, a portrait that would go with a book, gotten up somewhat in Japanese fashion with margin, illustrations, etc. She made four more exposures in the open, against a background of shrubbery; three of them I never saw, but the fourth one was entirely satisfactory for the special purpose it was intended for. This I thought was doing fairly well, considering that Steichen made twenty-nine exposures of me to produce the portrait which appeared in "Camera Work" two or three years ago.[3]

Let us take a look at Miss Buehrman's portfolio and critically examine some of her best prints. The print entitled "An Artist" is solely taken for pictorial purposes. Why it is called "An Artist" I do not know, but the composition is quite original. The entire interest of the picture is concentrated in the upper left corner. The highlight on the shoulder,

BESSIE BUEHRMANN: An Artist.

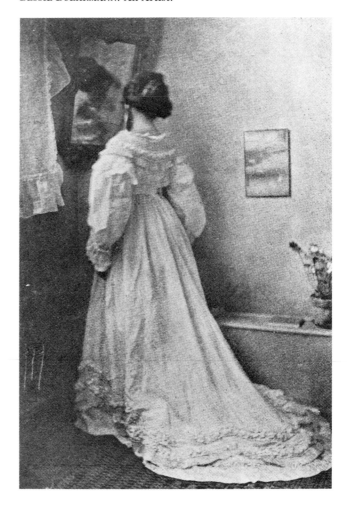

the dim reflection in the mirror with its oblique lines balanced by another slanting line of the curtain, are well managed. The values of the white gown (a trifle ill-fitting I fear) are soft and harmonious and fill the rest of the picture in a satisfactory manner. The lower left corner is perhaps a trifle too dark, but after all furnished a good note of contrast. Exceedingly clever is the management of the background to the right. Notice how the empty space is broken by the Japanese print on the wall and the line of the seat, with book and flower pot. There is nothing forced in the arrangement, everything is simple, and yet every object tells and helps towards the general harmony of the picture.

I also have very little fault to find with the portrait of Donald Robertson. The pose is unconventional, though natural, and it seems to be a good likeness. Even if one is unacquainted with the sitter,

one can generally tell from the expression of the face whether there is any resemblance or not. The foreshortening of the right arm is a trifle careless; it looks too small in comparison with the other. The background is well handled, the dark mass on the left gives solidity to the picture, but I object to the spotty manipulation behind the head. It is the one false note in the composition. There could be of course stronger highlights in the face, but as the modeling of the feature is satisfactory, perhaps little could be gained by it. The Coburn style avoids strong accents, and although the print has very few Coburn characteristics, it after all strives for the softness of effect which he has introduced into portraiture.

The study head "Erna" is more ordinary. It is merely a pretty face taken in a conventional way. The hand is rather bad; it is awkwardly placed, and

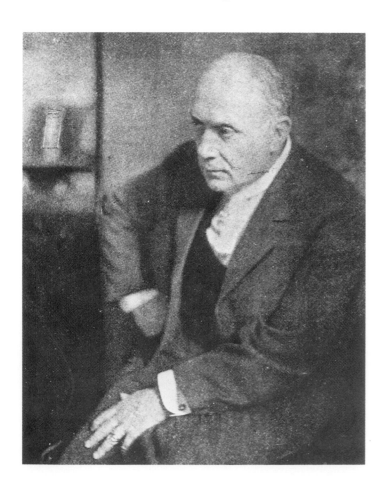

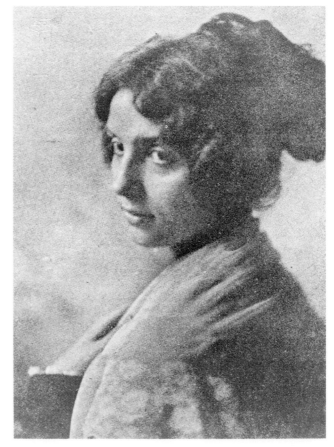

has lost all resemblance to human shape. The background is too monotonous. The best part is the silhouette of the head. The flesh tints are a trifle muddy, and the hair entirely too opaque. These however are minor shortcomings; on the whole it is a pleasing picture of the popular kind.

The "Portrait of Mme. Modjeska" comes very near being a masterpiece. I told Miss Buehrmann that her fame would be assured if she could make a dozen portraits as good as that. There is something in the management of the lines, in the distribution of light and shade, and in the sympathetic attitude of the aged actress (once the ideal "Rosalind" and "Viola" of the American stage) which gives this portrait a superior quality to the others. I do not know how much this may have to do with the sentiment that the beholder involuntarily adds to the pictorial qualities of the portrait. I only know that if a picture is capable of arousing even a particle of emotion which makes one forget or at least look less critically at the composition, it is superior portraiture. What we want is character, as artistically rendered as possible, and here we have both. Anybody who has ever seen Modjeska in the heydays of her triumphs must like this portrait. It tells its story.

One can hardly believe that the *decolletée* fur-beruffled lady in profile is meant for a portrait. It looks more like a whimsical fancy, a study in eccentricity. It is a space arrangement, cleverly handled. The dark mass of the hair (cut off at the top in the impressionistic manner) is well balanced by the flesh-tints of the shoulders and back. By making these a trifle lighter than the face, the eye, strange to say, is lead directly to the soft yet distinct outlines of the face. From the point of composition (although I do not approve of the heavy lines on the neck), this is the most interesting head I have yet seen by Miss Buehrmann. It shows that she is guided at all times by an exquisite taste. Whenever she fails it is lack of experience, and she could easily cover up that deficiency by merely showing her successful prints. One can also show good taste in the discrim-ination of one's own work.

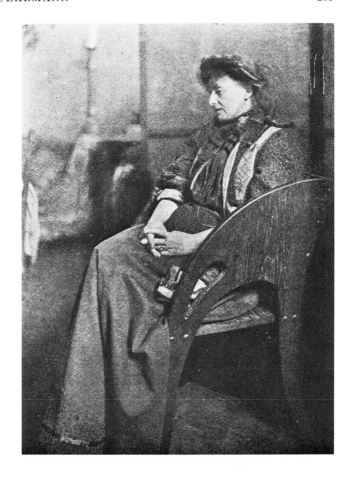

Above. BESSIE BUEHRMANN: Portrait of Mme. Modjeska.

Opposite page right. BESSIE BUEHRMANN: Erna.

Opposite page left. BESSIE BUEHRMANN: Portrait of Donald Robertson.

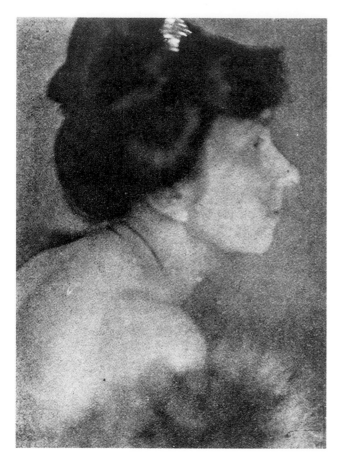

BESSIE BUEHRMANN: Portrait.

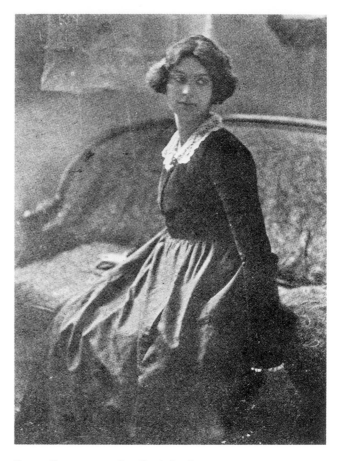

BESSIE BUEHRMANN: In a Paris Studio.

The last picture of our series, "In a Paris Studio," is another delightful composition. Apparently Miss Buehrmann favors arrangements in slanting lines. They break up the space better than horizontal and vertical ones, and adapt themselves more readily to picturesqueness of effect. The pose of the girl is a graceful one. She is slightly out of proportion, and the left arm looks entirely too long, but one hardly notices these shortcomings. The tonal arrangement as in most of her pictures envelops all details in an atmosphere of harmony, and the light coming from some unknown source (one of the greatest charms of home portraiture) accentuates the figure just enough to make it the principal object of interest.

The accompanying reproductions need not be taken as a final test; they were selected because they show a fair average of a photographer's work, portraits far superior in conception and quality than she has produced hitherto. I shall look forward to her work with interest and curiosity, and if I have induced my readers to share my feelings, I shall have realized my expectations to the full.

—1907

41

MEREDITH JANVIER

With a Rush

HERE WE HAVE a man who is neither to hold nor to bind. He is the most energetic, "go-ahead" man in the business. He has made up his mind to get to the top and he will get there by sheer nerve and pluck. He is almost there now, and yet a few years ago he was absolutely unknown to the profession. He was an amateur who exhibited at the Philadelphia Salon, the Pennsylvania Academy of Fine Arts, and at the Linked Ring, London.[1]

And now look at his record. He himself has furnished the data:

1900	Began as amateur.
1900–1902	Amateur work—all classes.
1903 (July)	Began a one-man's studio.
1904	Began home and studio portraiture. Hired one woman assistant.
1905	Hired one man assistant.
1906	Hired one more man and one more woman assistant.
1907	Hired one more man assistant. Rebuilt studio (entire four-story house). Made trip to Europe on money made after the first four years.

This is doing fairly well. Plugging away, building up his business steadily, step by step; from a one-man plant with one room for studio and work-room, to nine rooms and five selected assistants within four years. Very few men could repeat this feat; to take up a profession in that short span of time, own a place to work in, and top the fourth year's close by a trip to Europe, having made the money out of his business in competition with the best men in America. It seems to become the fashion for successful photographers to summer in Europe. It is meant to convey to the outsider a certain air of prosperity, but as going abroad is (or at least comparatively) cheaper than staying here, I do not attach so very much importance to it.

The Janvier studio is a quaint and old building—built, some say, as early as 1812. Its decorations were, many of them, made by Mr. Janvier's own hands. Thus, in some cases, if the artist could not secure in the shops just the right sort of an Indian mask or the totem pole he wanted, he carved them himself. He also made many of the frames in which his portraits are shown, and he always asks his sitters to allow him to select the frames for their portraits, so that a good print may not be ruined by its surroundings.

The studio proper is quite different from the ordinary gallery. It has no skylight and there are no painted backgrounds, no iron headrests, and none of the regulation accessories in sight. Large, single slanting side-light (facing north) with top skylight connected (à la Notman[2] of 1879), side windows

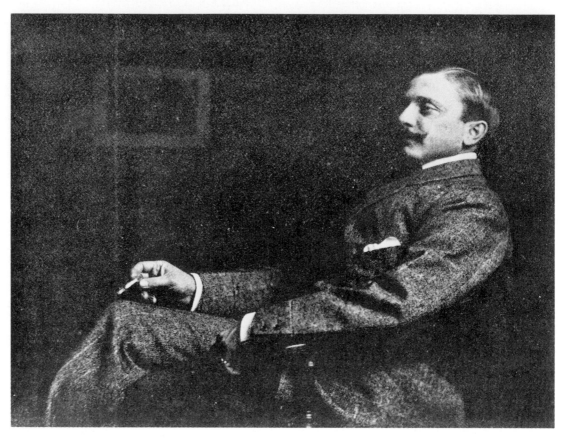

MEREDITH JANVIER: Portrait Study.

eight feet up from the floor at each end, and green burlap in place of wall paper. On entering the room it seems to be almost empty. There are two of the King light controllers—a rotary dais, and, of course, a camera. There is a movable frame, too, with which he can utilize dark, gray, or white backgrounds. The new studio opens where a section of wall was removed into the old room, a part of the house proper. A cozy fire is burning in the open grate. The walls are covered with old arms, paintings, and engravings; and some bits of unique furniture make the room attractive.

Personally, the photographer is quite interesting. He has a fine, sensitive face allied to a stalwart person. He is a short man, possibly not more than five feet eight inches tall. In his studio he wears a gray Norfolk jacket, but it is not of velvet, and his hair is not long, for which his admirers praise the saints. His manners are easy and very cordial; he says he is a man without nerves and he looks it. It might be added that he was eight years a lawyer; his butting up against all kinds of people has made him a good "mixer." He is never off his guard and handles conversation "like a Jap juggling tennis balls" (these are his own words). And really the best way to get an idea of the man and his method is to let him explain things.

"The average man," he may tell you, "comes into the studio and throws himself down in a chair and says: 'Take my photograph as soon as you can, please. I don't want it, but my wife does, and I suppose I will have to humor her.' He is a good subject. He will walk away forgetting all about himself, and I will snap him for one of his best

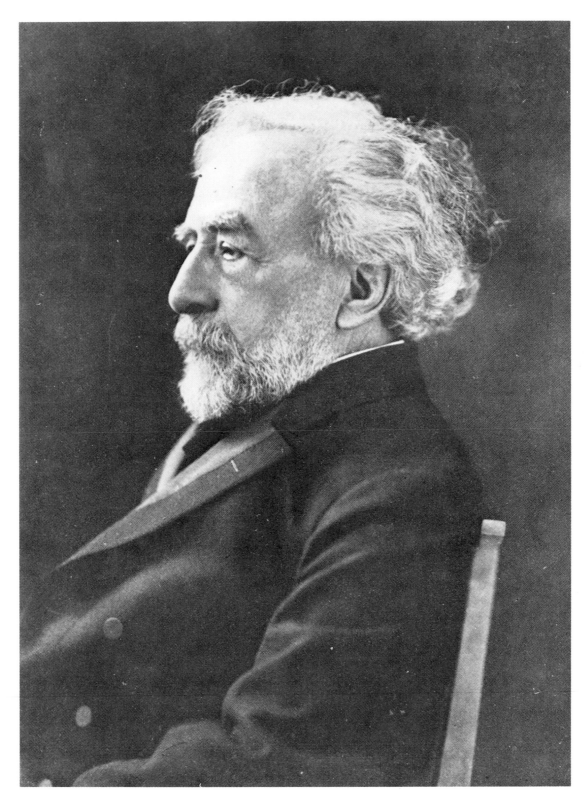

MEREDITH JANVIER: Dr. Jacobi, New York.

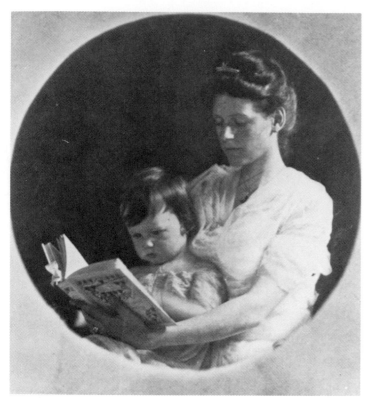

MEREDITH JANVIER: Mother and Child.

expressions, and the picture will be a great success, and so pronounced by his friends. This is the average man. There is another class which is as particular about the folds of its coats and the sets of its cravats as a woman could possibly be about her gown. I leave it to you to determine whether it is above or below the average. A third class is much more fastidious than women and is very troublesome. There is only one rule to observe in taking the portrait of a woman, and that is one of the English school of artists—to flatter, flatter, and flatter. As a rule, pretty women take ugly photographs and homely women usually take pretty ones."

"My object in taking a photograph is to catch my subject while he is in repose, of course, but with as alert and forceful an expression on his face as possible. In order that I may do this I bring him into the studio, if he is going to have his likeness taken here, and ask him to sit down. I have the camera here in the only dark corner of the room, as you see. Then I begin to talk with my sitter, having first ascertained that his chair is properly focused. When he is interested I say suddenly, 'When did you say you were going to Washington?' or something of the sort. Of course, he hasn't said he was going to Washington, and so when he looks up, surprised, and eager to correct my false impression, I snap him. During the course of our conversation I ask something else which calls forth another good expression, and I snap that. Thus I have two negatives, one of which, at least, will probably be good. After this I pose my subject and try to get one or more of him as he sits more artistically posed."

Like Mr. Stieglitz in New York, Mr. Janvier in Baltimore enjoys the reputation of being a splendid lunch entertainer and of dining his sitters first before he snaps them.

"Come about lunch time," he will say, "and take the whole course—lunch, a talk, and be photographed. Thus will you learn much more about my methods than I can possibly tell you. You know," he will furthermore explain to you, "it was a rule of Sir Joshua Reynolds never to paint a subject until he had dined with him, and I do like to have a long talk with my people and a chance to study them before I place them in front of the camera. I am not an artist. I could not in a hundred years sit down here and paint a portrait of anyone, and I have not the patience to paint it if I could; but I hope I am artistic. One reason I like the camera is because it gives quick results. You can see what you have done before you have time to cool off. You have results before discouragement comes. There are lots of discouragements in the work you know. It is a discouragement in a way to find that you got as good a picture the first week you began this work as you can the fourth year after you have been in the profession. And yet an accident of this sort often happens, and it brings a shade of discouragement with it. In this, as in everything else, one likes to feel that he has progressed. But there is so much that is delightful about photographic portraiture that it is idle and foolish to dwell on the occasional bad moments one has."

I have not yet said anything about his work. I have seen portraits by him of all kinds—low key, high key, and a conversative of lines. His tones and gradations are at times very soft and delicate. For a time he made a specialty of carbons transferred on porcelain and canvas, and of enlarged negative work, head studies of children half life-size, along artistic lines. I will refrain from further criticism. I do not know whether I would patronize him; I might and I might not. Certain it is that he charges as much for his work as anybody in the business. It is not his work I am particularly interested in. In this instance it is the man.

I admire him for his determination, for his ambition, and for his ability to deliver such goods as to make him successful. He ferrets things out for himself; he does not need conventions, he teaches himself; he is ever on the alert, picks up things here and there, and experiments until he has put into practice what he wants and is in need of.

Every photographer in business could learn a lot from Meredith Janvier.

—1907

42

F. BENEDICT HERZOG

A Master of Decorative Composition

THE NAME OF F. Benedict Herzog—absolutely unknown four years ago—has of late become fairly well known in photographic circles. He has received an unusual amount of publicity, and publicity that can not be sniffed at—an article in the *Century Magazine* being after all the highest literary appreciation a photographer, and for that matter also an artist, can get in this country.[1] Although his method, or rather his photographic technique, has been subject to severe criticism, the general trend of these articles is by far more laudatory than otherwise.

The "art gentlemen" who penned these appreciations seemed to realize that Herzog attempted something new, and that "story telling" in photography had never before been treated in such an ambitious and elaborate manner as, for instance, in his "Tale of Isolde," "Banks of Lethe," etc. They were not far from the truth, although their estimates on the whole lacked definiteness; they arrived at no conclusions, they failed to tell us in what particular phase of artistic endeavor Herzog excels, and why he, perhaps more than anybody else, has the right to call himself an exponent of "the higher photography."

I believe I was one of the first art writers who became acquainted with his work, and I was attracted by it from the very start, but somehow I had no opportunity until today to express my opinion about his work in print. I met Herzog for the first time about four years ago in the New York Camera Club. It was a chance meeting. I was introduced to him as a man who "was trying to do some new stunts," and soon after Herzog produced a wallet containing some hundred photographs of draped figures and nudes. I was astonished at the apparent ease with which he posed and draped figures. I did not remember of ever having encountered in painting, as well as in photography, a more decided talent for the handling of drapery as was revealed to me in those tattered proofs. And this criticism still holds good today.

As a photographic critic, with straight photography as an ideal, I of course am not in the position to fully endorse Herzog's departure. Even as Bernard Shaw did with Demachy[2] I have to do with Herzog and call him a traitor in the photographic camp. My objection is not so much to his method of arranging and bringing together various photographs, and by some intelligent means or other to build up a pictorial mosaic, but rather to his neglect of certain technical qualities which to me constitute the greatest charm of photography. The natural gradation of values, the principal characteristic of photographic texture, cannot be brought into perfect harmony with such "control and embellishment," no matter how cleverly it may be imparted. The means cannot be entirely concealed, and as

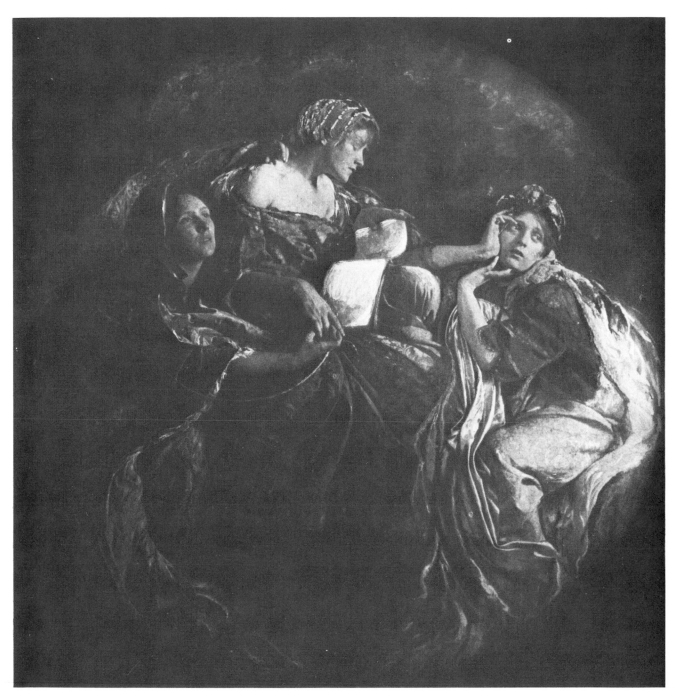

F. Benedict Herzog: The Tale of Isolde. imp-geh.

long as they are not concealed the photographic texture will suffer thereby. But this is an old story, and although there is no getting around it, it should not influence one's judgment of other accomplishments.

Herzog has probably realized as well as I have certain technical shortcomings in his work. But they seem small and unimportant to him, as he tries for other and perhaps bigger things. He conceives his pictorial visions as a master painter would, on a grand scale, in decorative friezes and panel compositions of several feet in length, built up of several groups. There are twenty to thirty or even more figures in some of his compositions. This is the new note he has added to pictorial photography. He has lifted it out of the ruck of one-figure composition, and proved beyond doubt that it lends itself to the display of higher constructive and creative qualities. This was Herzog's aim, and he could not accomplish it in any other way. Already Salomon,[3] in the seventies of the last century, and the ingenious Rejlander,[4] who combined thirty different negatives in his "Two Ways of Life" (1887), realized this, and Herzog is a true descendant of these two men. Only he reaches farther and attempts subject-matter from the fields of poetic romance and allegory which were far beyond the pale of combination printing.

Herzog, if I understand him rightly, does not so much wish to be ranked as a pictorial photographer (in the sense of Stieglitz and Steichen), but rather as an artist who uses photography solely as a medium for the expression of art problems and emotions. If that is his standpoint, of course he should be judged accordingly. A critic's business is largely to find out what a man is driving at and to convey his observations in a logical manner to the public. It may be difficult to classify Herzog for some time; but what of that? Innovations, no matter in what field of activity, are always difficult to classify. They arouse our curiosity, and we are apt to regard them as strange phenomena whose ultimate value we are unable to determine; time alone can do that. And so it will be with Herzog's work.

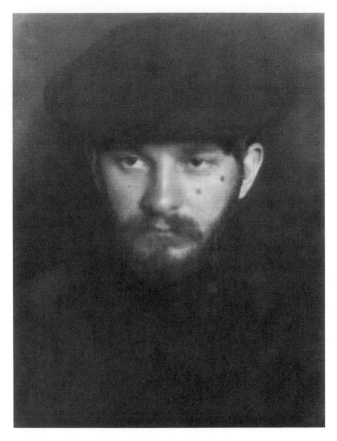

F. Benedict Herzog: Portrait of Alvin Langdon Coburn. imp-geh.

In the meanwhile let us admire what there is to admire, and there is much. First of all, I admire how he goes about his work. He does not believe in portfolio photography. Nearly all his finished prints are enlargements, some fourteen by twenty inches or more, and they are made with an idea of that size. They are story-telling pictures, but conceived for no other purpose than decorative embellishments. They are *objets d'art*, pure and simple.

Having looked at hundreds of them, again and again, during the last four years of our acquaintance, I must confess that they impress me as something very apart and praiseworthy. I have met many artists in my day, but I do not remember of ever having met an artist (and I refer to artists of high standing and superior skill) who had such a wide and intimate knowledge of drapery. Considering that Herzog sometimes makes forty to fifty

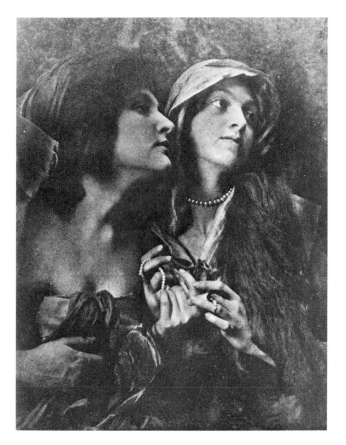

F. BENEDICT HERZOG: Two Maids of St. Ives.

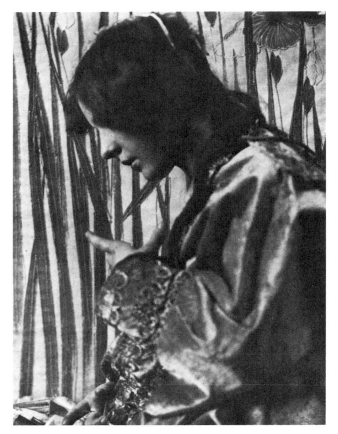

F. BENEDICT HERZOG: Angela. IMP-GEH.

exposures in an afternoon—compositions of a never-ending variety and all of a fair average excellence—one can not help pronouncing this gift an extraordinary one. He is at home in all styles. No matter whether it is the crushed and crumpled drapery of the Pre-Raphaelites, the pompous style of the Venetians with its broad planes of shining velvet, or the pliable, soft, stunning effects of a Reynolds or a Gainsborough, he masters them all; and, although his imagination is haunted with the souvenirs of former, more-picturesque periods in the history of costume, he is invariably the interpreter of his own moods. His feeling for line is exceedingly fine, in detail as well as in the rhythm of long, sweeping curves, and is perhaps nowhere better expressed than in his management of hands and the twist he knows how to give to the neck and shoulders of his figures. In his big compositions he is

at times a true poet; he has in his mind some vague idea, suggestive of some poetical sentiment, as, for instance, in his "Men Kiss and Ride Away," and he carries it out with rare sympathy and grace, and a perfect balance as far as lines and masses are concerned.

To be able to do this in photography is indeed a rare accomplishment, as all photographers who have entered upon the pictorial field well know from experience, and they will no doubt agree with Herzog's own words on these "photographic difficulties":

"To costume, pose, light, and arrange the bodies, draperies, hands, and faces of a group of even only two or three of the most adaptable and willing models; to watch until the end of the exposure every fold of the drapery, every changing shadow which may be cast at some undesired point as the models are moved tentatively; to study every movement of the head or expressive feature of the face or the nervous and often unconscious change in the fingers or hands of the nerve-strained models— all this furnishes an exercise in patience, invention, and concentration of faculties which I find about as good a test of what engineers call 'the maximum efficiency' as any task I have ever performed."

Herzog is by profession a civil engineer and inventor, and was also for some time engaged in art work, I believe as a poster painter, previous to his photographic exploitations; and I believe his success is largely due to this combination of scientific precision and artistic aspiration.

His decorative schemes are no productions of chance—he is too much a constructionist for that— they are carefully planned and patiently carried out, and he has at all times enough of the temperament and enthusiasm of an artist to lend grace and beauty to his original ideas.

Herzog has said a new word. He has widened the scope of pictorial photography and fashioned for himself an individual and personal mode of expression—and if that be not genius, it is at least a serviceable substitute, and we cannot but admire it.

—1907

43

FREDERICK I. MONSEN

The Stamp of Reality

"AMERICAN INDIANS are undoubtedly pictorial and perhaps semi-picturesque," was Walter Shirlaw's[1] verdict about the possibilities of the American Indians as artistic material. This was after a western trip which he and Gilbert Gaul,[2] the battle painter, had made in the interest of the Indian Department. The verdict, over-exacting as it may seem, comes nearer to the truth than one may imagine at the first glance. The native tribes with their characteristic make-up, their wild way of living, and their peculiar ceremonial rites, contain for the artist all the elements of the pictorial; but even to the layman, they do not seem as picturesque as, for instance, the Arabian horsemen that Schreyer[3] paints.

The majority of our American painters, if they have given the subject any thought at all, apparently share Walter Shirlaw's opinion, as the number of those who have made the Indians their special genre is very limited. Among them we find the well-known names of C. Wimar,[4] W. Cary,[5] Farny,[6] E. W. Deming,[7] Gaspard Latoix,[8] Schreyvogel,[9] Frederick Remington,[10] De Cost Smith,[11] de Forrest Brush[12] (the last the most successful artistically of all, though not always archaeologically correct), and the latest recruit to this rank of artists, Louis Akin.[13] Of those painters who have handled the subject occasionally, Henry Mosler,[14] Shirlaw, Gaul, and Dodge[15] should be mentioned.

Among the sculptors Bush-Brown[16] has made some busts of different Indian types and Cyrus Dallin[17] and Hermon MacNeil[18] several statues which are quite effective.

In photography the real Indian has been a less popular subject than one might expect and suppose. Of course any amount of amateurs have photographed an Indian, but there are few who have produced any notable achievements like Mrs. Käsebier, or Goldensky.

The trouble is that the subject is rather difficult to get at. The ordinary art school model will hardly do, except for artistic studies. Pictures of ethnological value, of the true Indian as he really is, leading a wild open-air life with all its curious customs and manners and strange spectacular ceremonies, are only accessible at the spot. To get satisfactory and comprehensive results, one must live years and years among the various tribes, just as Monsen has done.

Monsen is a serious photographer who photographs with a purpose. He has made the southwest his specialty. His observation has been long and thorough. He has studied attentively every phase and detail of America's Wonderland, during eighteen years of extensive travels and long sojourns in Mexico, New Mexico, and Hopi Land, the Land of the Navaho, and the mountains of California. He has followed the trail of the Spanish pioneers that

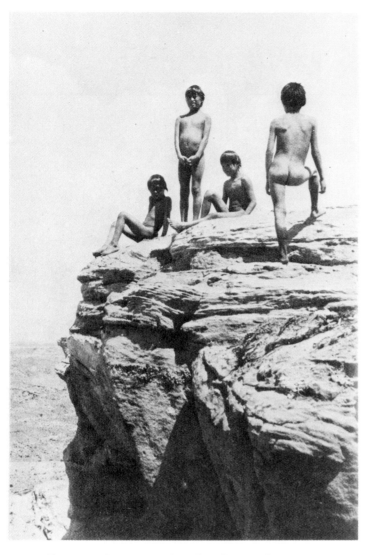

FREDERICK I. MONSEN: The Edge of the Cliff.

leads from the city of Mexico to the villages of Pueblo Indians; he has lingered among the picturesque old churches of Mexico, and camped out in the ancient habitations of the Cliff Dwellers. He has tramped through Death Valley and explored the Colorado River and the Grand Canyon of Arizona.

A collection of more than three thousand photographs; numerous note books filled with valuable observations; a dozen lectures or more, illustrated by colored transparencies, panoramic motion and transition pictures; and animated pictures of aboriginal sports and dances are the splendid results of Monsen's extraordinary gift of exploration and pictorial representation. Each part of this country, and each tribe has its peculiarities, and this photographer succeeds in showing us their characteristic features, and manages to tell us in pictorial representations how little these people of the desert have been changed by the influences of the world around. Being as successful in landscape as in figure subjects, his work has a double interest.

The Kodak always gets nearer to this sort of subject than the painter's brush. Of course a painting has its own beautiful value, as a fragment of nature, but it does not really make us acquainted with the characteristics of the depicted scene, which may exist more in the imagination of the painter than in reality. If we get interested in far away countries of such vastness and beauty as the southwest, we want to become acquainted with its topographical peculiarities, the structure of the barren plateaus and gorges, the scant vegetation of the desert, and the life of the strange people in the reservations. Paintings rarely give us this information. Look for instance at the paintings of Arizona, by A. L. Groll[19] and F. Lungren.[20] The former draws the sky lines so very low that the depicted scene occupies one-fourth of the canvas, while the rest is all sky and rolling clouds. The other draws the sky line so high that three-quarters of the picture is devoted to the depiction of the desert with a mere strip of sky at the far horizon. Both try to express the immensity and desolation of the country, but at the same time sacrifice the actual material to their individual conception of the esthetic possibilities of the subject.

Monsen is proud to give us facts; true enough facts that are rendered as artistically as possible—but they are after all pre-eminently records that give us the desired information in a pleasant and interesting manner. Some of his photographs are strikingly pictorial, as for instance the young Mexican girl stooping down to fill a water jug, or "The Edge of the Cliff," a group of Hopi children looking down from some sunburnt rock to the plain below. But he never forgets that instruction is their principal aim and object. Though an enthusiast, he never allows his enthusiasm to mar his judgment. His pictures are excellent specimens of clear straight photography. His sympathies are not with the Secession method which sacrifices everything to clever decorative use and arrangement. He is as a matter of course a realist and likes to take his subjects with their natural incident and interests. The distribution of light is particularly fine. They are always to the point, *i.e.*, they tell their story in a simple straightforward manner.

Not unlike most photographers who wish to obtain descriptive result, Monsen has had the experience that a large camera and plates of the same size as the finished picture seldom produce atmosphere, perspective, or unconventionality of pose. Monsen began to work in the early days of the dry plate when every subject had to be posed and focused. The pictures somehow lacked naturalness and convincing local color, but gradually as Kodak and films reached their present state of perfection, Monsen was able to realize his long cherished ambition—to reproduce the unconscious expression of pose and character, results that were impossible by the old method of using plates.[21]

Monsen's particular method of working is to carry three Kodaks of small size which fit in cases without covers that are slung to a belt around his waist, so they are ready for use by a single turn of his hand; long practice in focusing has made it possible for him to get the unobtrusive desired snapshots

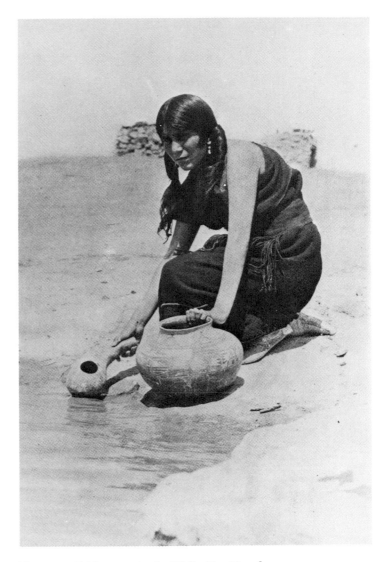

FREDERICK I. MONSEN: At the Well—Hopi Land.

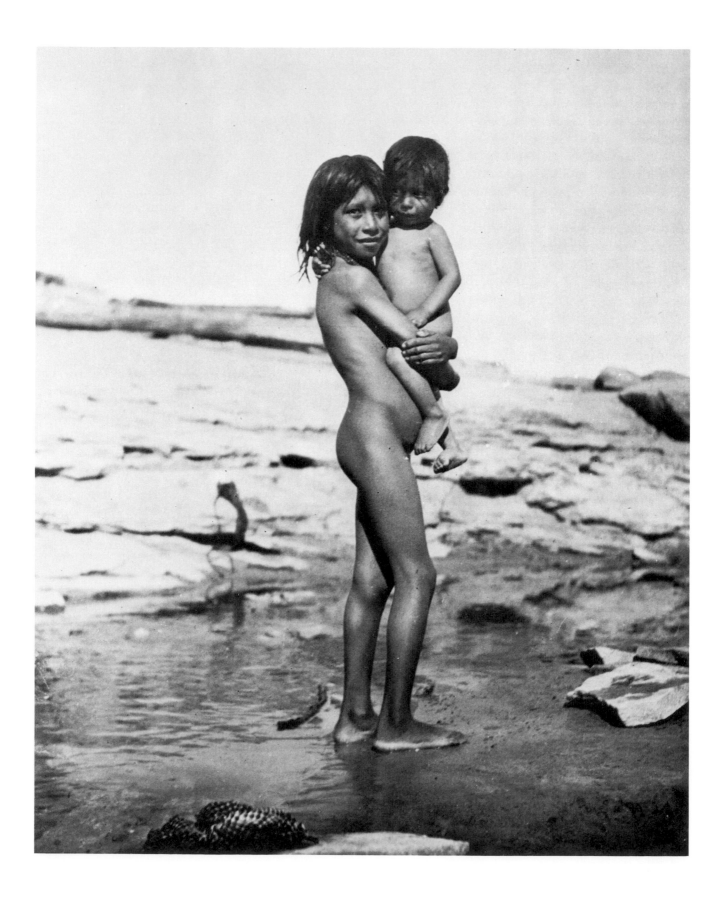

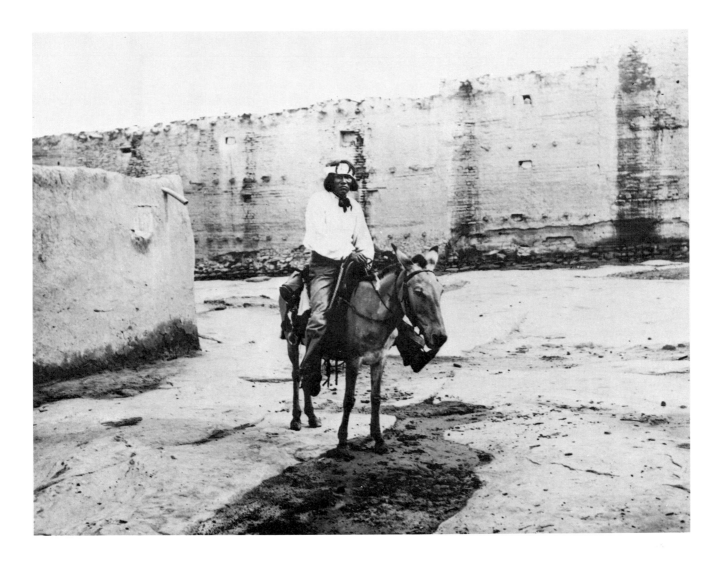

Above. FREDERICK I. MONSEN: Untitled. Courtesy of the Museum of Photography, University of California, Riverside.

Opposite page. FREDERICK I. MONSEN: Untitled Portrait of Indian Children. Courtesy of the Museum of Photography, University of California, Riverside.

almost by instinct, "as an expert rifleman will hit the target when firing from the hip." His subjects seldom knew when they are photographed. They are not on dress parade or posing for costume picture, but are presented just as they are with all their individual characteristics. Some of the figure compositions look a trifle overcrowded, but as they were taken for the special purpose of being thrown upon the canvas, this is a virtue not a shortcoming. A cartridge film picture must be sharp and full of interesting details. The enlargement will mellow the effect, soften the outlines, diffuse the light and deepen the shadows, and convey to the print as well as the slide the feeling of distance and sunshine, of atmosphere and color.

Visiting an exhibition of Frederick Monsen's photographs, one realizes that he has accomplished his task of producing "the most complete ethnographic series of pictures of Indian life and manners of Southwestern United States." He has dealt effectively with the vast subject, so suggestive and so full of the deepest interest. His work bears the unmistakable imprint of sincerity and practical utility. His collection appeals not only to the traveler and student of foreign parts of the world, but also to the general public whose interest in the American Indians with their ancestral manners and ceremonies has been greatly on the increase in recent years.

Every print of this collection bears the stamp of reality, and long after the tribal communities will have passed from their native conditions, these pictures will serve to call back to every true lover of the human race, the noble figure of the American Indian.

In Frederick Monsen we possess an indefatigable draftsman of the camera who has not been spoiled by successes already achieved, and who continues to devote infinite patience and a rare fund of knowledge to the laudable employment of registering for future generations the aspects of a vanishing race.

—1909

44
ARNOLD GENTHE

A Photographer of Japan

$\mathcal{T}$HAT JAPAN IS a land of poetry is evident to all who, seeking below the outward appearance of things Japanese as stray to this country, probe into the heart of them. The simple designs of flowers and birds that decorate our screens or porcelain ware, or illuminate with a few flashing touches the dainty folding fan, are oftentimes reminiscent of some vague poetical thought, of some pleasant emotion or happy inspiration.

But the real Japan, its temples and bridges, its cherry trees and ancient statuary, its mountains and picturesque population, is to most people but a sealed book; the student of sights and scenes longs in vain for a magic key to unlock the treasures, the soft contours, and subtler suggestions of her scenic beauty. The solitary instances of adequate artistic depiction—beyond examples of ordinary view photography, exquisite as they are at times—have only whetted our appetite for more, and the work of Dr. Arnold Genthe of San Francisco, which we have now under view, is therefore especially welcome.

Direct products of snapshot photography, with a rare command of pictorial possibilities, Genthe has presented us with a number of original prints, all of which are of interest and some of great beauty. One thing that is very evident in these pictures is the manner in which the photographer has given free rein to his imagination in selecting his subject. For this type of photography there are rules prescribed

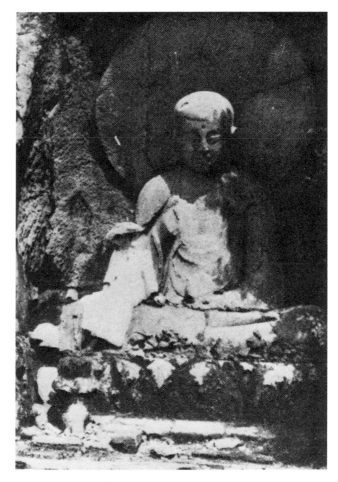

ARNOLD GENTHE: Statue—Hakone Road.

299

by custom and long usage, fixed conventions which are held to be good enough to guide the camera worker, simply because they have served his predecessors for many years. He is supposed to confine himself to recognized formalities, and in a large number of instances he is not, it must be admitted, any too anxious to put himself to the trouble of seeking out new forms of expression.

For one thing, those people which may put his interpretations to practical usage are quite disposed to be satisfied with the sort of work to which they are accustomed, and ask only that the work he gives them should be executed with sufficient skill. For another, the repetition of old ideas with, perhaps, some slight modifications which will pass as new readings of the unfamiliar stories, is easier to

manage and imposes no task upon his inventive capacities. Only the conscientious artist who finds pleasure in thinking out things for himself and rebels against stereotype modes of expression would exert himself to do for his own satisfaction what the general public does not specially demand of him.

Dr. Genthe undertook the trip as a recreation; he tramped and "jinrickisha'd" all over the islands. Many a mechanical or technical problem—caused partly by the climatic conditions and partly by unforeseen difficulties of travel in a foreign land—had to be overcome. But nowhere can he be said to have failed to show himself equal to the task which was calculated to test him severely, and his success is all the greater because it has been attained under

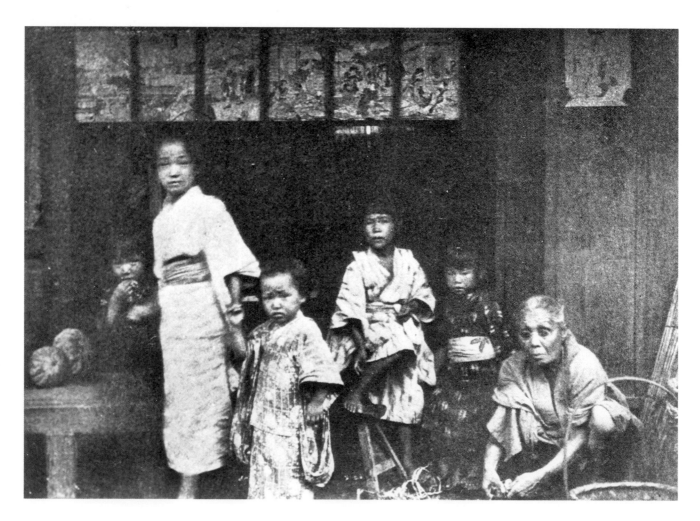

conditions which might well have excused many deficiencies.

What is most remarkable in these pictures is that the most interesting qualities emanate from Genthe himself.

He is first of all a master of composition who seeks and finds in scenes, landscapes, of figure groups, special opportunities for carrying to completion a logical design. About the pattern of each of his pictures he greatly concerns himself; he adjusts lines and harmonizes forms by selecting the most favorable viewpoint, and he plans his light and dark grays with the closest consideration for its balance, not only of area but of degree. As a consequence his work has definitely the charm and suavity and repose; it bears the stamp of scholarly consideration and matured judgment, and there is in its restraint evidence that he has mastered the most perplexing of artistic problems, how to use his material to the best advantage.

A motive, which pictorially may be without any special significance, can become valuable by emphasizing certain natural subtleties of local values or illumination which are in themselves worthy of being studied and recorded. And Genthe's intention is always to visualize a mood or sentiment, to present a scene which has impressed him in its entirety as being beautiful and photographable.

We recognize this characteristic particularly in his pictures of Japan. Here, one feels, is not only a faithful rendering of the scenes depicted, but an insight into the more subtle charms of their peculiar beauty. The series of Japan is, perhaps, the more interesting partly because the artist was exploiting a country which has not hitherto been much interpreted by American amateurs, but principally because the softer and more subdued tones were more in harmony with his natural leaning towards "atmospheric" composition and he could be more entirely himself.

One of the best pictures of the series is the one reproduced here, "Fuji from Hakone," a strong and simple composition, showing delightful freedom in the handling of forms, combined with rich and

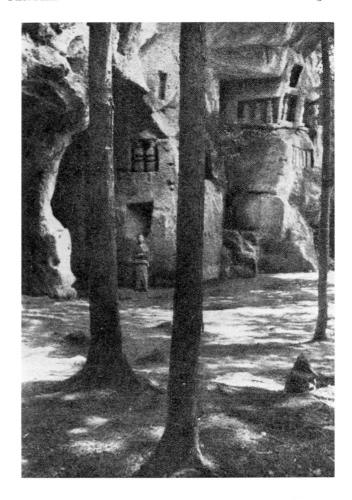

Above. ARNOLD GENTHE: Cave Temple—Northern Japan.

Opposite page. ARNOLD GENTHE: Japanese Shop Front.

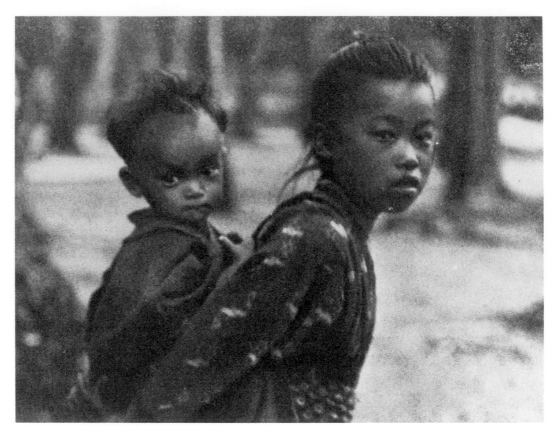

ARNOLD GENTHE: Little Nursemaid.

sober tones. Hardly less successful are his "Japanese Shop Front,"—a delightful study of Eastern physiognomies—and his Jigo statue, which well display the artist's facility of adding a human or sentimental interest to inanimate objects.

In most instances, however, he takes more pains to arrive at unity of effect than to tell a story or to illustrate an episode in which the people he photographs might be supposed to be concerned. His love of picturesqueness is the dominant factor in his art, and it influences him as much in his treatment as in his choice of subjects. He aims at recording the life he sees about him, but he aims also at recording it with its right sentiment, its right atmosphere, and above all with its true balance of essentials.

The pictorialism in which he believes is neither half-hearted nor one-sided; it influences every stage of his practice as nearly as it determines his point of view and controls the manner of his observation. Indeed not many photographers who depict figures in combination with landscapes strive so consistently to keep all parts in their pictures in strictly correct relation, and not many attain to such thorough mastery over subtleties of representation.

Genthe is as free from conventions of observation as he is from tricks of handling, and he allows no mannerism to cramp the freedom or to sap the vitality of his representation. Breadth and reticence are among the chief characteristics of his work, but they come from perfect adjustment of complex details, and from singularly skillful use of the material which nature makes available. He sees things in a big way, in a few large and impressive facts, but he is fully conscious of the small matters as well, and quite ready to give them the place that is due to them.

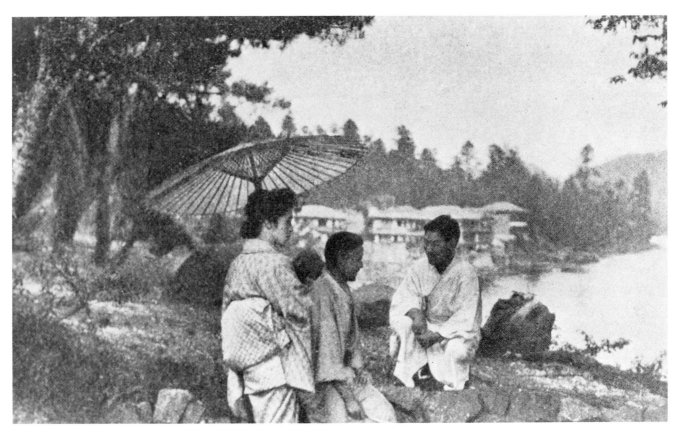

ARNOLD GENTHE: A Japanese Family.

Concerning his powers as an executant there is this to be said, that he has a thorough command over the mechanism of his machine, that he is an expert in the process of bromide enlargement, and that he possesses a sense of values and tones that is quite unusual. His use of materials is always skillful and always free from trickery; he affects neither painter-like freedom nor minute precision of handling; his prints lack finish but they are executed in a simple, broad and direct fashion, with a touch that is flexible and full of meaning. His technique is that of the ideal recorder, the photographic illustrator *par excellence* who knows what he wants to do and how it should be done, and who is so far sure of himself that he has no desire to imitate the executive devices of anyone else. He photographs, in a word, with an individuality that is much to be commended in the present day, when pictorialists

are far too apt to follow fashions and to work in the manner introduced by this or that school.

As an instance of the sensitiveness of his line and space composition, his "Fuji from Hakone" and "Cave Temple, Northern Japan" are well worth studying; and as an illustration of the sincere appreciation of form and graceful contours his "Japanese Family" and "Little Nursemaid" are not less deserving of consideration.

Some of the prints of his "Japanese Series" have made their appearance in public from time to time in magazines and at various exhibitions in London, Dresden, and the Secession, but the number of works thus exhibited are few compared with the entire number he executed. The examples now reproduced have been selected from a large accumulation with the idea of showing his versatility and various styles of interpretation.

—1910

45

MAUDE WILSON

Poet of Sunshine and Mist

SOFT GRAY DAYS along the coast, lone tracts of duneland basking in shimmering sunlight, scant vegetation straggling its way through the dry soil, mission-buildings with the play of light and shadow on the white walls, the surf among quaint rock-formations, the mist from the ocean rolling in among the hills, bare foregrounds with a few decorative weed-stalks, sunshine and mist, mist and moonlight—such is California, at least the California which Maude Wilson depicts.

Maude Wilson is a new name in the world of pictorialism. Her prints, hitherto, have escaped exploitation in the magazines. She is an alien to the Annual Salon, competitions and camera-club exhibitions; in fact, she had never exhibited. She has worked quietly for several years in a studio at Carmel-by-the-sea, doing professional portraiture for the transient tourists, and indulging in her leisure hours in view-photography. She endeavored to record the beauty of her native State in the way she saw it, what it meant to her; and there vague atmospheric versions and misty scenes gained so much recognition that the proceeds of a few years' work enabled her to make a study-trip to Europe.

On her return she may settle in the East and devote herself entirely to pictorial photography. This is about all there is to say about her biographically. She has developed under the influence of Genthe, and is like him an adherent of the snap-shot-and-enlargement school, but she went her way quite independently, and her work—however we may value it—shows strange subtleties of workmanship and a clean artistic aim.

Is it not strange that a talent like hers can grow up, unnoticed and unappreciated, right in our midst? Her indifference to ordinary photographic ways and honors may be the cause of it. Or is it the difficulty of reproducing and popularizing her poetic visions that reject all detail, and are as faint as "fleeting dreams"?

She is an extremist in elimination. She does not care for any subject-matter. She focuses upon the lyrical vein of things. A shiver of light in the eager morning air, a moon rising behind dew-drenched trees, a whitewashed wall where wavering lights and shadows come and go—impressions like these furnish the inspiration for her prints. And she succeeds in recording these impressions in such a manner that they produce in the beholder very much the same emotion as the author received from the original. She invented a technique of her own to produce these effects. She underexposes, the image is vague from the start, and from these thin negatives she enlarges up to portfolio size. The result is generally an extremely light (or middle-tint) tonality, an annihilation of all detail, contour and modeling, a process of reducing to two or three tones in which form is expressed in blurred shapes

MAUDE WILSON: Mist From the Ocean.

and silhouettes. Her range of values is frequently limited to five per cent of what is possible in the medium. She frees her art-ideas from all the trammels of material flaws, but does not succeed in making her technique equally bold and free. Although her black and white palette possesses both tint and tone, it represents merely a limited phase of photographic expression.

Most of her *motifs* are uninteresting as far as grace of landscape is concerned. The lines are ineffective in themselves; there is no mastery of composition, no selection of a favorable view-point, no picturesqueness, even, merely an atmospheric mood; and with this mood of shimmering light-mist or spume, she clothes, like a magician, each scene of her selection with a touch of beauty. She sacrifices everything else—line, form, space-

arrangement spotting, chiaroscuro, relief, highlights, contrast, suggestion of color. It is all obliterated. There is rarely a trace of it. She avoids all stronger accents. In her seashore-delineations she does not give broad generous sunlight, a sudden glow of pleasure, but rather a mystical veil of radiance that hovers calmly over the sandhills. Her "Surf at Point Lobos" reduced the frolicsome seas to dark indistinct shapes and large sweeps of foam in which all wave and rock structures are lost.

Pictorially her prints create no *illusion;* they are naught but haphazard fragments of nature that *suggest the feeling,* the inner law of beauty of the object shown. They are whimsical, like Whistler's lithographs; they have their shy suggestion, but naturally lack the seductive ease, the mental flavor which lend a special fascination to the painter's

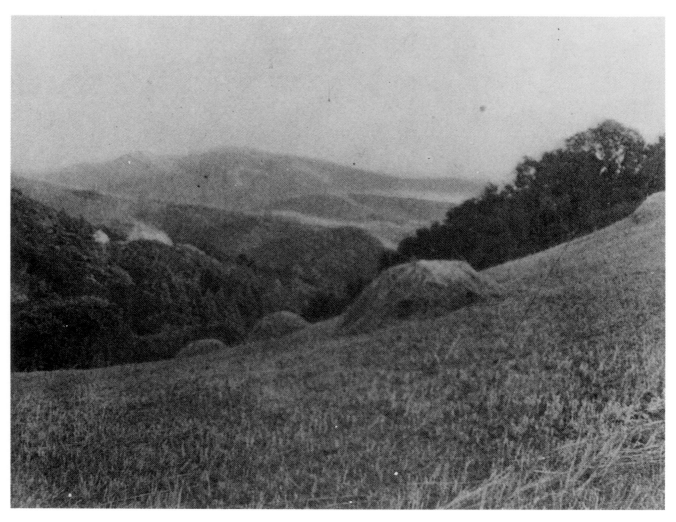

MAUDE WILSON: Among the Hills.

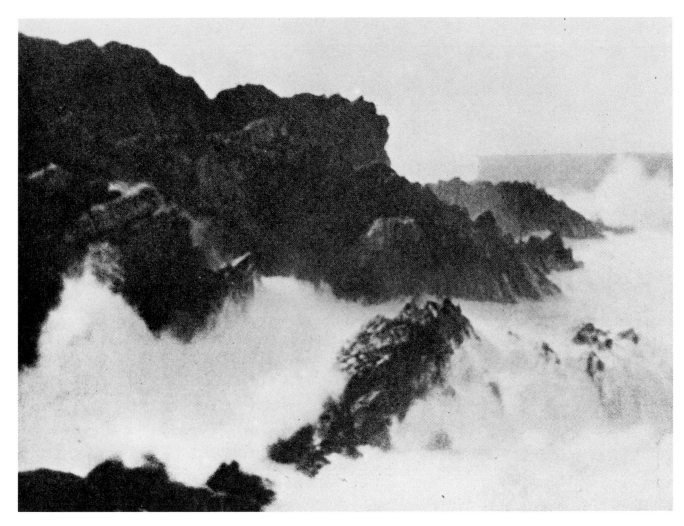

Maude Wilson: Surf at Point Lobos.

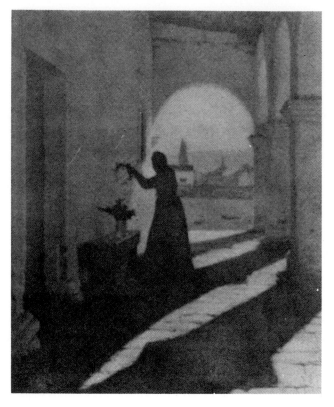

Maude Wilson: An Altar-Dresser—San Juan Capistrano.

work. A bromide enlargement cannot compete in textural qualities with a crayon lithograph, and a few gray touches do not prove sufficient to enliven a large area of white.

Elimination in photography is one of the qualities which may reflect the range and limit of the craftsman's thought, but there is also a limit to this elimination and it is easier reached than in the other graphic arts. Our nocturne painters, Dabo,[1] Wuerpel,[2] Lucas,[3] in their vague fashion of repre-

senting twilight and night—although they deal with juxtaposition of colors—never go as far as Maude Wilson. They still cling to a decided division of space. As soon as all line and suggestion of detail are lost, the planes lose their translucency, they become monotonous and not even the vibration of atmosphere (which is the saving grace in all of Maude Wilson's pictures) will prevent the texture from becoming flat, cold and motionless.

Even Maude Wilson is best in those pictures where she is least vague. Of course, there are differentiations. In one of her masterpieces, "Silence," there is actual palpitation, the tones melt into each other; while in her "Moonlight," a more popular rendition (and one which she does not herself fancy), we have the ordinary mellow sheen of a shining sea. No subtlety, no elusive changes, merely vividness of effect.

In "Silence" we feel the stillness of evening, the muffled pulsing vibration of light conquering darkness, and yet there is still a distinct suggestion of form, contrast, and the repetition of shapes in the branches which by their very parallelism of indistinctness produce the optical effect of tremor and wavering masses. I do not believe mood-representation can go any farther.

Maude Wilson, as we see her to-day, is not a versatile performer. She merely sings one song, but that one well. In her little way she has a new message to deliver, she has a style of her own—a rare thing to say!—a tempered technique and a convincing grace that will please amateurs and experts alike.

—1911

46

J. E. MOCK

A Study in Backgrounds

ONE EVENING IN Kodak town, I strayed to that old tavern—the Lafe Heidell Café, known for generations to all travelers as one of the gay landmarks of Rochester—and was astonished to be confronted not with the marble seat rotunda that has sheltered so many illustrious spirits, but with a few large genre-pictures of a monk that brought me straight back to the very beginning of pictorialism, when Dumont[1] shared the enviable reputation of an advanced amateur with Stieglitz, Eickemeyer and Bullard[2] of Philadelphia.

Dumont's story-telling pictures were perfection in a way. His "Clarinet-Player" has never been surpassed. But there were three factors in his success: first, the presence of an excellent actor-model in the person of the tavern-keeper, jovial Lafe; second, his own artistic appreciation combined with a genial enthusiasm for photography; and, third, the technical craftsmanship of J. Ernest Mock, who at that time had only an unpretentious gallery.

Mock was a serious student from the start. He was not only a good reliable technician, sensitive to all changes and improvements, but a lover of art with sufficient skill to make a vivid and interesting crayon-sketch. He had only one ambition—to get to the top of the ladder, to make portrait-photography as beautiful an expression of interpretation of character as possible, and so he studied composition

as thoroughly, I believe, as any man in the profession. He has told me himself that he has re-read Beck's and Poore's books on composition,[3] as well as my humble efforts in that direction, three or four times. Mock was also a level-headed business-man, so the ladder-climbing after all came not so very difficult to him.

Mock's work has been familiar to me for nearly twenty years. He represented to me for many years the photographer's straining for "dramatic expression," as all I ever saw of him were strange concoctions of draped women, of tragic deportment, endeavoring to represent passion by the help of dagger and sinister facial expression. They were clever "stunts" at the best—exhibition pictures. And yet I recall one head of a woman (reproduced in *Photo-Era* years ago), dramatic in expression, with chin thrust upwards, treated in regard to drapery and background with the utmost simplicity which showed that it was in Mock to do a truly artistic thing.

Since then many years have passed and Mock to-day is known to the profession as a successful portraitist who has his own artistic notions—or principles if you prefer the term—and who pursues his path unabashed and with more genuine enthusiasm than most of his contemporaries are able to muster.

He has become known as a master of back-

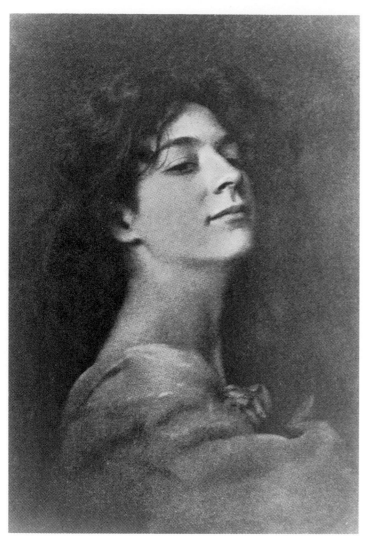

J. E. Mock: Lady Vere de Vere.

grounds.* He is the professed champion of back-grounds. It is his hobby (unless it were his beautiful country-home in Irondequoit) and he can talk background for hours at a stretch. Of course his Van Dyck-Gainsborough column and park-vista back-grounds are a trifle old-fashioned. But can anything that has ever made good in art in a big way really become old-fashioned? Does not my attitude arise either from my status of taste or my desire of novelty, as I have been too long in criticism and am tired of things that I am too well acquainted with?

Sir Joshua Reynolds said that the most difficult thing in a portrait was the background, and no doubt he meant the selection as well as treatment of it. What kind of a background can the modern portraitist select? It is either the plain background, the home-portraiture background, or the back-ground suggested by the old masters. The plain background is rarely artistic, particularly so in photography, as it is too monotonous in texture and incapable of suggesting atmosphere except in some cases (when handled by a Carrière or a Whistler, for instance). The background of modern accessories is always too accidental, and it is difficult to make the interiors of most homes conform to esthetic and fundamental laws of background-composition. The background of the English portrait-school has made good. It may look a little out of place in this material world of ours, but it is, after all, reliable. If handled with skill, it always produces an effect, and the peculiar setting of the scene adds a certain poetic sentiment and charm that can be attained in no other manner.

Mock is versatile. He can express himself in many ways. The big head proves that. It is an excellent up-to-date space-composition. But is there a demand for this kind of work? Only a very limited one. The public clings tenaciously to the conventional and traditional. It may be induced

*The editors were unable to secure satisfactory copies of the photographs discussed as representative of Mock's best work in backgrounds.

to patronize a—shall we call it—"photographic sketch," as of the boy. Although this is neither photography nor drawing, it may appeal as a novelty and something special. But in the ordinary portrait the public wants something that it understands, and it understands only such things as have become familiar through long usage.

Mock, knowing this, has endeavored to attain perfection within the very limitations of his medium of expression. He has experimented for many years. In the two full-length portraits the backgrounds are too elaborate. The one is a modern interior background, the other of the Gainsborough order. In the latter there are too many lines, and yet they display a rare knowledge of composition. The principal lines of the background radiate from the figure and balance each other. All the picture lacks is simplicity. The simpler a background is (one that suggests distance, space, perspective or atmosphere), the more difficult the test becomes.

Mock has made wonderful strides towards this frugality of expression. The two women holding roses—the seated bride and the full-face view of the woman with the necklace—are masterful in treatment. They are surpassed, however, by the portrait of the young girl leaning against a column. This is not far from being a masterpiece, and surely it is a masterpiece of Mock's career as a photographer.

Mock's backgrounds are all painted and specially composed. One may object to this method as a method; but no one can deny Mock's rare artistic discrimination. His figures all stand in space (outdoor-space at that), and they are correctly lighted—the rarest accomplishment in portrait-photography. Most photographers who apply this method introduce the background in a haphazard manner, merely for pictorial effect, and thereby commit the unpardonable blunder of having lighted the figure from one side and the accessories from another, or of having a strong light come from some "exit" in the background without influencing the outlines of the figures. Mock's pictures are all judiciously lighted; it is one source of light that is

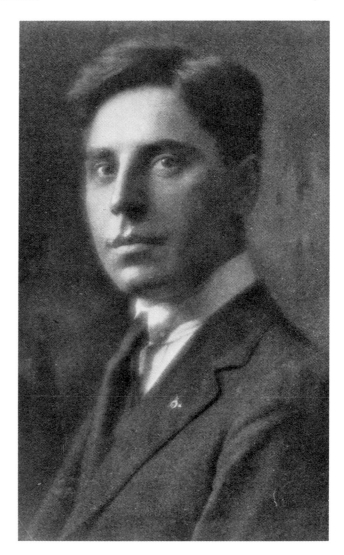

J. E. MOCK: H. Oliver Bodine.

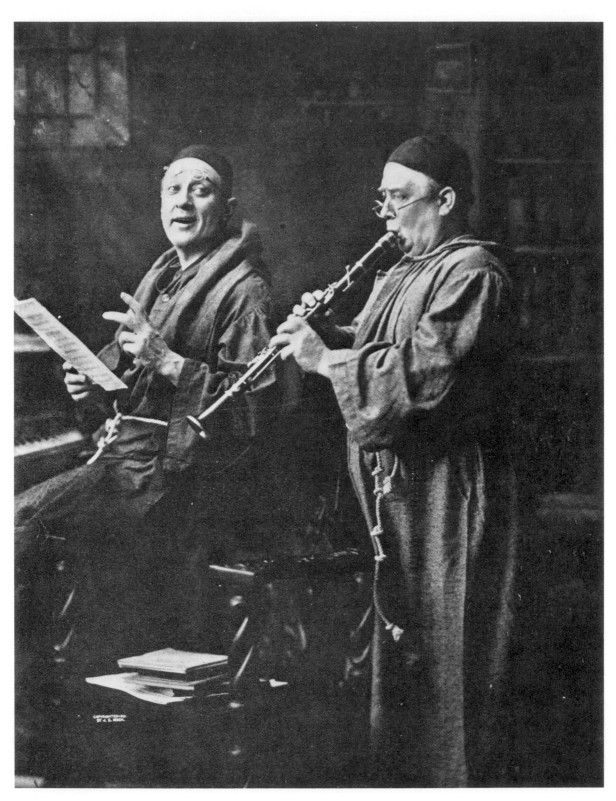

J. E. Mock: The Duet.

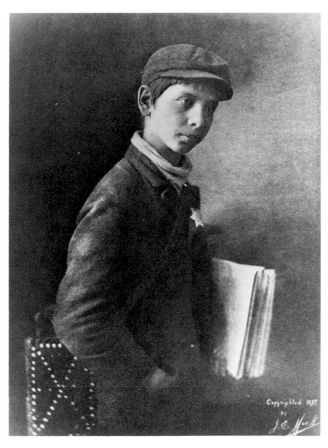

J. E. Mock: A Convention Prize Winner, 1897.

carried triumphantly throughout the whole composition and which pervades the entire picture. Study the accompanying pictures and you will see that the light throughout is logical and masterful. There is the proper entrance and exit, combination of highlights just at the right place and a suggestion of receding distance.

Mock's art has many other distinguishing traits. I mention only his manipulation of drapery, and the ability to bring out a pleasing facial expression. He discovers in every face a beauty which the casual observer fails to see. But it is in the realm of backgrounds that Mock reigns preëminent, and where he soars far above even the most accomplished efforts of contemporary portraiture.

It has always been a characteristic of my criticisms to bring out the one quality in which a man excels—as an object-lesson to others, and that is what I have endeavored to do in this brief analysis. Mock has solved one of the most serious and difficult problems of portraiture in a popular yet superior manner; this should command the respect and admiration of every practitioner in the profession. The public is with him, and if his contemporaries appreciated his point of view and accomplishments and would themselves adopt his principles, they might have less reason for the everlasting complaints of slack seasons and non-patronage.

—1913

NOTES

FOREWORD

1. For additional discourse on the criticism of photography and Hartmann's aesthetics see: Kay Tucker, *The Educated Innocent Eye: Some Criteria for the Criticism of Photography* (Berkeley: The Image Circle, Inc., 1972).

2. *Camera Notes* 4 (Dec, 1903):183. The essay is published under Hartmann's pseudonym of Sidney Allan.

3. "A Few Reflections on Amateur and Artistic Photography," *Camera Notes* 2 (Oct. 1898):41.

4. Ibid.

5. Tucker, *The Educated Innocent Eye*, p. 7.

6. Representative of his least successful work is the piece signed Sidney Allan on "Scherril Schell, Portrait-Pictorialist," *Photo Era* 28 (Apr. 1912):141–145.

7. Hartmann's connections within the Stieglitz circle come to mind, but more indicative of his wide range of investigations are the several hundred essays written for the German language newspaper *New Yorker Staats-Zeitung* between 1898 and 1902. A number of these pieces were translated by Hans-Peter Breuer of the University of Delaware for the *Sadakichi Hartmann Newsletter*.

EDITORS' INTRODUCTION

1. Thomas F. Barrow, "A Letter With Some Thoughts on Photography's Future," *Album* 6 (July 1970):3.

2. See Alexander S. Horr, "Sadakichi Hartmann as a Photographic Writer," *Photo-Beacon* 16 (Oct. 1904):308. The article incorrectly quotes "E. W. Stimson" rather than J. W. Stimson. Stimson was a contributor to Hartmann's magazine, *The Art Critic* (1893–94).

3. Benjamin De Casseres, "Five Portraits on Galvanized Iron," *American Mercury* 9 (Dec. 1926):398.

4. Ibid., pp. 397–98. To his disciple, De Casseres, Hartmann was a "Dionysiac wobbly," who was "Half God, half Hooligan, all artist." De Casseres describes one of Hartmann's drunken sprees: "Or Sadakichi doing his dervish dances at Joel's at 5 A.M., passing around the hat among the boozers, one of whom kicks the hat full of cash in the air, Sadakichi throwing a tableful of glasses in our faces. Unforgettable rough-house."

5. *Des Moines Register and Leader*, Oct. 5, 1906. Clipping in Hartmann scrapbook titled "Revelations" (Wistaria Hartmann Linton Collection, Library of the University of California, Riverside).

6. Jerome F. Mellquist, *The Emergence of an American Art* (New York: Charles Scribner's Sons, 1942), p. 232.

7. Ibid.

8. Barbara Rose, ed., *Readings in American Art Since 1900* (New York: Frederick A. Praeger, 1967), p. 50.

9. James Gibbons Huneker claimed to have been the first American writer to mention Gauguin, apparently in an American newspaper sometime after 1900, according to Oliver W. Larkin, *Art and Life in America* (New York: Rinehart & Co., Inc., 1940), p. 325. Hartmann, a naturalized American, appears to have precedence. He mentions Gauguin in passing among a group of French impressionist painters in his unsigned article, "Modern French Painting: An Art Historical Study (Unfinished)," *The Art Critic* 1 (Jan. 1894):29.

10. See Hartmann's attack on "sur-realists [sic], abstractionists, and whatnots" in his *Strands and Ravelings of the Art Fabric* (Hollywood: Author's Edition, 1940), pp. 5–8.

11. James Gibbons Huneker, "Younger American Painters," *Camera Work*, No. 31 (July 1910), pp. 43–44; Sadakichi Hartmann, review in Huneker, "Younger American Painters," pp. 47–49.

12. Sadakichi Hartmann, "Structural Units," *Camera Work*, No. 36 (Oct. 1911), pp. 18–20.

13. Hartmann, review in Huneker, "Younger American Painters," p. 48.

14. Sadakichi Hartmann, "Through Semi-Japanese Eyes," *Camera Notes* 4 (July 1900):47.

15. W. M. Chase, "Foreword," in Sidney Allan, *Composition in Portraiture* (New York: Edward L. Wilson, 1909), p. 5.

16. Horr, "Sadakichi Hartmann as a Photographic Writer," p. 307.

17. Roland Rood, "The Three Factors in American Pictorial Photography," *The American Amateur Photographer* 16 (Aug. 1904):348. Rood repudiated the article *in toto* after publication, charging that the magazine's editor and Hartmann had made unwarranted alterations and additions without his permission (see "Letters to the Editor," *The American Amateur Photographer* 16 [Oct, 1904]:421). J. P. Chalmers, assistant editor of the magazine, replying in the same letters' column (pp. 421–22), assailed Rood's writing ability, denied Hartmann had any hand in the editing, and insisted numerous corrections were necessary to render the article in "readable English." He said the only addition was twenty lines at the end of the article about Curtis Bell and the newly-formed American Federation of Camera Clubs, designed to bring the essay up to date. Hartmann jumped into the dispute with a letter to *The Camera* 8 (Oct. 1904):403–404. He defended the editing of the article (which Chalmers had shown him in manuscript), charged Rood was an amateurish writer who needed blue penciling, and said he had been embarrassed by Rood's "puerile and sycophantic appreciation of my efforts in the photographic field." He admitted instigating the article, which suggests he was on friendly terms with Rood prior to publication. The ramifications of the quarrel are complex and an outgrowth of squabbles occurring at the time between partisans and opponents of Curtis Bell and his American Photographic Salon. Hartmann had joined the Bell faction, whereas Rood appears to have favored the Photo-Secession group. It seems doubtful if the section of the manuscript dealing with Hartmann was altered in any significant way by editing, since this would have then been the probable focus of Rood's attack.

18. Hartmann's claim that he discovered Frank Eugene is reinforced in a letter to Stieglitz, Sept. 2, 1904, Alfred Stieglitz Archive, Collection of American Literature, Yale University. Berating Stieglitz for having been "abusive" to him after a Hartmann reading at Steichen's studio, Hartmann says: "It was a similar case as once with Eugene whom you call 'the sloppy fellow with the black finger nails, I don't want him to come to my house' until he revealed himself as a fairly good photographer."

19. Roland Rood, "The Three Factors in American Pictorial Photography," pp. 348–49.

20. Dennis Longwell, assistant curator of photography, Museum of Modern Art, is of the opinion that the amount of hatred generated between Hartmann and the younger critic was founded upon a genuine sense of betrayal, presupposing a "prior period of friendship and trust" (ltr. to Michael Elderman, Jan. 24, 1972). He notes that Rood in a 1906 letter to Stieglitz speaks of having been assisted by Hartmann in selling articles to the photographic press.

21. See the editorial tribute, "J. Wells Champney," *Camera Notes* 6 (Dec. 1903):196–97. The writer observes that Champney served for many years as Club Critic of the Camera Club, finally resigning "simply from the dread of hurting 'some one's' feelings."

22. Horr, "Sadakichi Hartmann as a Photographic Writer," p. 308.

23. The reference is to Paragot, Bohemian hero of William J. Locke's *The Belovéd Vagabond* (London: John Lane Company, 1900). There is no basis to claims made repeatedly by Hartmann's friends that the popular best-seller was modeled on his life and character. Probably Hartmann encouraged this apocryphal story.

24. Edward Weston in Nancy Newhall, ed., *The Daybooks of Edward Weston: California* (New York: Horizon Press & George Eastman House, 1966), II, p. 60.

25. Tape-recorded interview by Harry Lawton of Mr. and Mrs. Peter Krasnow, Los Angeles, June 6, 1970.

26. Weston, *The Daybooks* p. 61.

27. Sadakichi Hartmann, "Black Butterflies," *Forum* 51 (Feb. 1914):299–304.

28. C. Sadakichi Hartmann, "My Autobiography," *The Theatre* 6 (July 1890):248.

29. Sadakichi Hartmann, "Uncle Ernst," Chap. 6, pp. 20–21 of the unfinished manuscript titled "Autobiography." Hartmann's copy is in the Wistaria Hartmann Linton Collection, Library of the University of California, Riverside. A

second copy, formerly owned by Gene Fowler with marginal annotations in his own hand, is in the Special Collections, Library of the University of California, Riverside.

30. Sadakichi Hartmann, "Learning the Language of Sense Perception," Chap. 5, p. 10 of an unpublished manuscript, "Esthetic Verities." The original is in the Ridgeway Branch of the Library Company of Philadelphia. A copy is in the Wistaria Hartmann Linton Collection, Library of the University of California, Riverside.

31. Sadakichi Hartmann, *Conversations with Walt Whitman* (New York: E. P. Coby, 1895). See also George Knox and Harry Lawton (eds.), *The Whitman-Hartmann Controversy: Including Conversations with Walt Whitman and Other Essays* (Frankfurt: Lang, 1976).

32. Hartmann, "Learning the Language of Sense Perception," pp. 11–12.

33. Ibid., p. 12.

34. [Unsigned, untitled.] *The Weekly Review* 3 (18 March 1893):336.

35. "List of Artist Subscribers," *The Art Critic* 1 (Jan. 1894):42.

36. Sadakichi Hartmann, *Christ: A Dramatic Poem in Three Acts* (Boston: Privately Printed, 1893). (Reprinted in Sadakichi Hartmann, *Buddha, Confucius, Christ: Three Prophetic Plays*, ed. Harry Lawton and George Knox [New York: Herder and Herder, 1971].)

37. For an account of the short-lived life of the *Daily Tatler* see Carolyn Wells, *The Rest of My Life* (Philadelphia: J. B. Lippincott Company, 1937), pp. 174–175. See also her "Post-Mortem Statement," *The Chap-Book* 6 (1 Feb. 1897):251–52.

38. [Unsigned.] "The Death of Napoleon Sarony," *The Daily Tatler* 1 (11 Nov. 1896):4.

39. Sadakichi Hartmann, "The New York Camera Club," *Photographic Times* 32 (Feb. 1900):59.

40. See account of the merger in Robert Doty, *Photo-Secession: Photography as a Fine Art* (Rochester: The George Eastman House, 1960), pp. 17, 19. For an excellent early history of the Society of Amateur Photographers see F. C. Beach, "The Society of Amateur Photographers of New York," *American Amateur Photographer* 6 (Apr. 1895):157–69.

41. Sadatichi [sic] Hartmann, "Die Kunst-Photographie in ihrer Beziehung zur Malerei," *Sonntags-blatt der N.Y. Staats-Zeitung*, 30 Jan., 1898, p. 17, cols, 1–6.

42. Ibid.

43. *Camera Notes* 2 (April 1899):162.

44. Ibid., p. 178.

45. Hartmann, "The New York Camera Club," p. 60.

46. Ibid., p. 60.

47. Gorham Munson, "The Limbo of American Literature," *Broom* 2 (June 1922):252. Munson also writes on the same page; "Harte and Monahan and Sadakichi Hartmann will probably always remain in the limbo and be discovered only by the curious from time to time. Their talents lack momentum, but let us honor them for their level heads and true eyes and gallant spirits which, in a time of most confused provincialism, chose and fought on the intelligent side."

48. S. H., "Puritanism, Its Grandeur and Shame," *Camera Work*, No. 32 (Oct. 1910), p. 17. For a much earlier attack by Hartmann on Puritanism in America, see the unsigned column, "As You Like It," *The Weekly Review* 3 (15 April 1893):472–73.

49. Roger P. Hull, "The Stieglitz-Hartmann Letters: The Toy Balloonist and the Great Aerialist," *Sadakichi Hartmann Newsletter* 2 (Fall 1971):1–2, 4–7.

50. When Hartmann's prose poem, "White Chrysanthemums," originally published in *Camera Work* (Jan. 1904) reappeared in Hubbard's magazine, *The Fra* (April 1909), Stieglitz wrote to Hubbard providing a detailed explanation of the essay's history, stating that he felt "inclined to believe that Mr. Hartmann has probably sold you something which does not belong to him. . . " Ltr., Stieglitz to Hubbard, May 3, 1909, Alfred Stieglitz Archive, Collection of American Literature, Yale University Library.

51. See Robert Eugene Haines, "Image and Idea: The Literary Relationships of Alfred Stieglitz," Diss. Stanford University, 1967, pp. 65–66.

52. Ltr., Stieglitz to Hartmann, May 25, 1915, Alfred Stieglitz Archive, Collection of American Literature, Yale University.

53. Sadakichi Hartmann, "An Art Critic's Estimate of Alfred Stieglitz," *Photographic Times* 30 (June 1898):259.

54. Sadakichi Hartmann, "A Walk Through the Exhibition of the Photographic Section of the American Institute," *Camera Notes* 2 (Jan. 1899):86–89.

55. Ibid., p. 88.

56. J. T. Keiley, "The Philadelphia Salon: Its Origin and Influence," *Camera Notes* 2 (Jan, 1899):125. Keiley specifically mentions a Hartmann pastel, "Poe's Cottage." A list kept by Hartmann of pastels sold or given away records Keiley

purchasing this pastel for $15 in 1896 (Wistaria Hartmann Linton Collection, Library of the University of California, Riverside). Hartmann also gave pastels to Zaida Ben-Yúsuf, Rudolf Eickemeyer, Jr., and Paul B. Haviland.

57. Ltr., Hartmann to Stieglitz, undated, Alfred Stieglitz Archive, Collection of American Literature, Yale University.

58. Sadakichi Hartmann, "The Broken Plates," *Camera Work*, No. 6 (April 1904), pp. 35–39.

59. Following Harris' death, Stieglitz selected the Hartmann portrait as an entry in the International Art Exhibition of 1901 in Glasgow. See "The American Pictorial Photographs for the International Art Exhibition in Glasgow," *Camera Notes* 4 (April 1901):275. This was possibly the earliest portrait of Hartmann by a prominent art photographer, and appears to have been taken in 1898. Cliff Wesselmann was a photographer for the *Los Angeles Examiner*.

60. Sadakichi Hartmann, "In Search of My Likeness," p. 1, unpublished essay. The typed original draft is in the Wistaria Hartmann Linton Collection, University of California, Riverside. Hartmann in this essay satirizes the many "pictorial transfigurations" of his face by photographers.

61. Ltr., Hartmann to Stieglitz, July 26, 1899, Alfred Stieglitz Archive, Collection of American Literature, Yale University.

62. The address was reprinted in *Wilson's Photographic Magazine* 42 (Sept. 1905):422–26; *Saint Louis and Canadian Photographer* 29 (Oct. 1905):452–58; and *The American Amateur Photographer* 17 (March 1905):469–75.

63. Sadakichi Hartmann, "Random Thoughts on Criticism," *Camera Notes* 3 (Jan. 1900):103.

64. A fuller account of Day's exhibition may be found in Doty, *Photo-Secession*, pp. 24–25. See also Beaumont Newhall, *The History of Photography From 1839 to the Present Day* (New York: The Museum of Modern Art & George Eastman House, 1964), p. 104.

65. Sadakichi Hartmann, "A Few Reflections on American Amateur and Artistic Photography," *British Journal of Photography* 45 (7 Oct. 1898):650–51.

66. [Unsigned.] "Plastic Psychological Syntheses at Russell Square," *British Journal of Photography* 47 (26 Oct. 1900):677–78.

67. Ibid.

68. Ibid., p. 678.

69. Frederick H. Evans, "To The Editors," in "The Exhibition of American Photography at Russell Square," *British Journal of Photography* 48 (2 Sept. 1900):702.

70. Sadakichi Hartmann, "The Photo-Secession Exhibition at the Carnegie Art Galleries, Pittsburgh, Pa., *Camera Work*, No. 6 (April 1905), p. 48.

71. Sadakichi Hartmann, "A Photographic Enquête," *Camera Notes* 5 (April 1902):233–38.

72. "An Apology," *Camera Work*, No. 1 (Jan. 1903), p. 15.

73. See Roger Hull, "Hartmann in Camera Work: A Bibliography," *Sadakichi Hartmann Newsletter* 1 (Fall 1970):1–3.

74. Roger Hull, "The Stieglitz-Hartmann Letters: The Toy Balloonist and the Great Aerialist," *Sadakichi Hartmann Newsletter* 2 (Fall 1971):5.

75. Sidney Allan, "The Value of the Apparently Meaningless and Inaccurate," *Camera Work*, No. 3 (July 1903), p. 17.

76. Sadakichi Hartmann, "Structural Units," *Camera Work*, No. 36 (Oct. 1911), pp. 18–20.

77. Hartmann, "The Esthetic Significance of the Motion Picture." *Camera Work*, No. 38 (April 1912), pp. 19–21.

78. Sidney Allan, "The 'Flat-Iron' Building—An Esthetical Dissertation," *Camera Work*, No. 4 (Oct, 1903), pp. 36–40.

79. Hartmann, "The Photo-Secession Exhibition at the Carnegie Art Galleries, Pittsburg, Pa.," p. 47.

80. Klingsor the Magician, "A Pilgrimage to the Secession Shrine at Pittsburgh," *Camera Work*, No. 6 (April 1904), pp. 54–56.

81. Sadakichi Hartmann, "The Salon Club and the First American Photographic Salon at New York," *American Amateur Photographer* 16 (July 1904):305.

82. Ltr., Hartmann to Stieglitz, undated (received Sept. 2, 1904), Alfred Stieglitz Archive, Collection of American Literature, Yale University.

83. Walter Zimmermann, "Another Letter to the Editor," *Camera Craft* 10 (April 1905):246–48. After the First American Salon, a controversy occurred in the photographic press over whether European exhibitors were promised that their work would be shown *hors de concours*. One of Hartmann's letters was published by *Camera Craft* on page 247, substantiating that such a promise was made. Zimmerman, first vice-president of the American Federation of Photographic Societies, stated in his letter that he and officers of the Salon could not read German and therefore were ignorant of any offer which Hartmann might have made in the invitations.

84. Ltr., Keiley to Stieglitz, undated, Alfred Stieglitz Archive, Collection of American Literature, Yale University. Quoted at greater length in Doty, *Photo-Secession*, pp. 36–37.

85. Juvenal, "Little Tin Gods on Wheels," *Photo-Beacon* 16 (Sept. 1904):282–86.

86. Alfred Stieglitz, "The 'First American Salon at New York'," *Camera Work*, No. 9 (Jan. 1905), pp. 50–52.

87. Newspaper clippings in Hartmann's scrapbook "Revelations" (Wistaria Hartmann Linton Collection, Library of the University of California, Riverside).

88. In a ltr. to Stieglitz, July 19, 1918, Hartmann writes from Homestead, San Mateo County: "Bruguière is coming to New York. Doing real good stuff at times. Otherwise photography out here (with the exception of a gum printer in Santa Barbara [Maude Wilson?]) is as dead as the true spirit of democracy." Alfred Stieglitz Archive, Collection of American Literature, Yale University. Hartmann's relationship with Bruguière is explored by James Enyeart, director of the Friends of Photography, Carmel, California, in a forthcoming monograph titled *Francis J. Bruguière* to be published by Alfred Knopf.

89. [Juan C. Abel] "National Convention Notes: Foremost Art Critic of Country Engaged to Give Public and Private Criticisms of Pictures at the National Convention." *Abel's Photographic Weekly* 10 (13 July 1912):32–34.

90. Ltr., Hartmann to Stieglitz, Aug. 22, 1908, Alfred Stieglitz Archive, Collection of American Literature, Yale University.

91. Ltr., Hartmann to Stieglitz, Nov. 3, 1912, Alfred Stieglitz Archive, Collection of American Literature, Yale University.

92. Ltr., Stieglitz to Hartmann, Dec. 22, 1911, Alfred Stieglitz Archive, Collection of American Literature, Yale University. The first two sentences of this passage and two later sentences are quoted in Doty, *Photo-Secession*, p. 58.

93. Ltr., Hartmann to Stieglitz, Oct. 21, 1912, Alfred Stieglitz Archive, Collection of American Literature, Yale University.

94. Hartmann, originally given the leading supporting role of the Chinese prince in Fairbank's film, suffered a severe asthmatic attack after three weeks of shooting, which he partly attributed to a costume weighing forty pounds. Fairbanks was forced to shoot around his role, reputedly at a cost of thousands of dollars. Letters between Fairbanks and Hartmann (Wistaria Hartmann Linton Collection, Library of the University of California, Riverside) support Sadakichi's illness, contrary to apocryphal accounts that he walked out to inconvenience Fairbanks. See Sadakichi Hartmann, "My Experience at the Fairbanks Studio," *Camera!* 6 (Feb. 2 1924):16–18.

95. Ltr., Stieglitz to Hartmann, April 27, 1919, Alfred Stieglitz Archive, Collection of American Literature, Yale University.

96. Ltr., Stieglitz to Hartmann, Nov. 22, 1930, Alfred Stieglitz Archive, Collection of American Literature, Yale University.

97. Hull, "The Stieglitz-Hartmann Letters: The Toy Balloonist and the Great Aerialist," p. 6.

98. Ltr., Hartmann to Stieglitz, Dec. 16, 1930, Alfred Stieglitz Archive, Collection of American Literature, Yale University.

99. The unpublished "Autobiography" (314 pp.) ends with Hartmann's meeting his first wife, Elizabeth Blanche Walsh, in 1891. An outline for other volumes indicates one chapter would have dealt with Stieglitz (Wistaria Hartmann Linton Collection, Library of the University of California, Riverside, California).

100. See "Sadakichi's Autobiography," in Hartmann, *White Chrysanthemums: Literary Fragments and Pronouncements,* edited by George Knox and Harry W. Lawton (New York: Herder & Herder, 1971), pp. 23–29. Hartmann writes: "1898. Wrote first article on pictorial photography. This has become a regular habit with the author. It would be easy to wallpaper a palace with his contributions to photographic literature. His pseudonym 'Sidney Allan' became as well known as Sadakichi. . . ."

101. See Foreword, Note 3; also *Wilson's Photographic Magazine* 42 (Sept. 1905):422–26.

102. See *Camera Work*, No. 3 (Apr. 1910), pp. 21–23.

103. See *Camera Work*, No. 4 (Oct. 1903), pp. 36–40.

104. Sidney Allan, "A Visit to Steichen's Studio," *Camera Work*, No. 3 (Apr. 1903), p. 25. See Chap. 28, p. 202.

105. Sidney Allan, "John H. Garo—An Appreciation," *The Camera* 19 (Apr. 1915):195–99.

106. See Kay Tucker, "Sadakichi's Impact on Photography," *Sadakichi Hartmann Newsletter* 1 (Summer 1974):1–3.

107. See Vance Thompson, "Sadakichi Hartmann, Art Critic," in George Knox and Harry W. Lawton (eds.), *The Life and Times of Sadakichi Hartmann,* 1867–1944, (Riverside: University Library and The Riverside Press-Enterprise Co., 1970), p. 11. Catalog of an exhibition of paintings and photographs on the life of Sadakichi Hartmann held from May 1-30, 1970, University of California, Riverside.

108. See Henry Holmes Smith, "Models for Critics," in Van Deren Coke (ed.), *One Hundred Years of Photographic History: Essays in Honor of Beaumont Newhall* (Albuquerque: University of New Mexico Press, 1975), pp. 139–43.

109. See Peter Plagens, "The Critics: Hartmann, Huneker, De Casseres," *Art in America* 61 (July-Aug. 1973):66–71.

1. PORTRAIT PAINTING AND PORTRAIT PHOTOGRAPHY

1. Prince Peter Kropotkin (Piotr Alekseyevich Kropotkin, 1842–1921), Russian social philosopher and anarchist, who wrote *Memoirs of a Revolutionist* (1899). Hartmann, a friend of Emma Goldman, Alexander Berkman, and many of the other anarchists of his period and a contributor to Goldman's magazine, *Mother Earth,* claimed to have briefly served as a voluntary attache to Kropotkin during the latter's American visit in 1900. Hartmann and Goldman are central characters in the anarchist milieu of J. F. Burke's novel, *Noah* (New York: Bantam Books, 1969).

2. Gotthold Ephraim Lessing (1729–1781), German dramatist and critic, and one of the most influential literary figures of the eighteenth century. Hartmann discusses Lessing's impact on his own aesthetic and critical ideas in several unpublished manuscripts (Wistaria Hartmann Linton Collection, Library of the University of California, Riverside).

3. León-Joseph-Florentin Bonnat (1833–1922), French religious, historical, and portrait painter, known for his portraits of many famous contemporaries.

4. Giovanni Boldini (also cited as Giordigino Boldini, 1845–1931), Italian portrait painter. Boldini's portrait of Whistler appears on the cover of Hartmann's *The Whistler Book* (Boston: L. C. Page & Co., 1910).

5. Franz von Lenbach (1836–1904), Bavarian portrait painter, noted as a brilliant colorist and technician. See Sidney Allan, "Masters in Portraiture—Franz von Lenbach," *Wilson's Photographic Magazine* 46 (Oct. 1909):454–59.

6. Jean François Raffaeli (1850–1924), French painter, etcher, and lithographer known for genre scenes of the poor. See Hartmann's unsigned essay, "*A Conversation with Jean François Raffaelli About American Art,*" Hartmann's *Art News* 1 (April 1897):3–4; also "Should an Artist be National or Cosmopolitan? A Conversation with Jean François Raffaeli," *Greenwich Village* 2 (June 23, 1915):7–9.

7. Henri Gervex (1852–1929), French painter and member of the impressionist school.

8. Jacques Émile Blanche (1861–1942), French still-life painter and portraitist, strongly influenced by English masters of the seventeenth century.

9. Jan van Beers (1852–1927), Belgian painter of historical subjects, later of genre portraits, especially of women, and finally landscapes.

10. Pierre Puvis de Chavannes (1824–1898), French painter known for his symbolical and allegorical decorations and murals, particularly in America for a mural commissioned in 1900 by the Boston Public Library. See Hartmann's essay, "Puvis de Chavannes," *The Art Critic* 1 (Jan. 1894):30–31; also Hartmann's column "Art and Artists," *Musical America* 1 (Nov. 12, 1898):39.

11. Edouard Manet (1832–1883), French painter credited with originating impressionism, who was a victim of critical hostility throughout his life, dying before recognition of his genius had become general. See Hartmann's essay on Manet, "The Fight for Recognition," *Camera Work,* No. 30 (April 1910) pp. 21–23.

12. Claude Monet (1840–1926), French painter, one of the founders of impressionism and a great landscape painter.

13. George Frederich Watts (1817–1904), English painter known for his portraits of notable contemporaries. See Hartmann's essay, "Masters in Portraiture—George Frederich Watts," *Wilson's Photog. Mag.* 46 (Nov. 1909):506–511.

14. Eleonora Duse (1859–1924), famous Italian actress, who interpreted Sardou, Ibsen, D'Annunzio, Maeterlinck, etc. See Hartmann's unsigned essay, "Eleonora Duse," *The Weekly Review* 3 (Jan. 28, 1893):32.

15. F. P. Vinton (1846–1911), Boston painter, who studied in Munich and Paris, and is best known for his portraits.

16. Thomas Wilmer Dewing (1851–1938), American painter who studied in Paris under Lefebre and was a member of the Society of the Ten American painters (organized in Jan. 1898). See Hartmann's essays, "The Tarbellites," *Art News* 1 (March 1897):3–4; and "Thomas W. Dewing," *The Art Critic* 1 (Jan. 1894):34–36. Hartmann's essay "On the Elongation of Form," *Camera Work,* No. 3 (April 1905) is illustrated with Dewing's painting "In the Garden," a popular painting even today under the title of "In the Moonlight" at the National Gallery of the Smithsonian Institution, Washington, D.C. In Hartmann's unpublished biography, he describes Dewing's model for three Graces—identified only as "Ruth"—as his first girl friend in 1888 in Boston (Wistaria Hartmann Linton Collection, Library of the University of California, Riverside). He writes: "She embodied the American pre-Raphaelite type to me, and I composed a sort of rhapsodical description of her in my essay on Thomas W. Dewing, which was dragged all over the country, printed innumerable times, and finally embedded in my *History of American Art* [Boston: L. C. Page & Co., 1901, Vol. 1, pp. 302–04]."

17. Alfred Stevens (1828–1906), Belgian genre painter and impressionist, whose chief subjects were society women and fashionable interiors.

18. Jules Bastien-LePage (1848–1884), French painter and disciple of Courbet and Manet. See C. Sadakitshe [sic]

Hartmann, "A Picture of Bastien-LePage," *Boston Evening Transcript*, Oct. 15, 1887, p. 6. In about 1890, Hartmann began dispensing with the Germanic transcription of *Sadakitshe* and started writing under the name of C. Sadakichi Hartmann, later dropping the first initial.

19. Gustave Courbet (1819–1877), French realist who painted scenes of everyday life and autobiographical events.

20. Anders Leonhard Zorn (1860–1920), Swedish etcher, impressionistic landscape painter, and portraitist who achieved fame as an etcher with studies of Verlaine, Proust, Rodin, etc., and a series of nude studies. His paintings deal mainly with Swedish peasant life.

21. Théobald Chartran (1849–1907), French painter, whose works are chiefly portraits and religious subjects. In 1885, 1886, and 1887, Hartmann made summer trips to visit relatives in Germany with many side excursions to see painters and theatrical personalities whom he admired. He may have seen Chartran on one of these excursions or in 1892 during his honeymoon in Paris with Elizabeth Blanche Walsh.

22. Joseph T. Keiley (1869–1914), associate editor of *Camera Work* and pictorial photographer. See Hartmann's review of Keiley's work, "Through Semi-Japanese Eyes," *Camera Notes* 4 (July 1900):46–47.

23. Lafcadio Hearne (1850–1904), American journalist, novelist, and travel writer, who became a naturalized Japanese citizen in 1893 and wrote many works centered on Japan. Although Hartmann frequently mentioned Hearne in his writings, he appears not to have met him.

24. The physiognomists listed by Hartmann appear to be Giambattista della Porta (1540–1615), Italian natural philosopher and alchemist, who published the first account of the *camera obscura* in his *Natural Magic* (1558); John Kaspar Lavater (1741–1801), Swiss poet and theologian, who was founder of the so-called science of physiognomy; Theodor Piderit, a nineteenth century writer on physiognomy; and Klaus Harms (1778–1855), a German protestant theologian. The editors were unable to identify Shyler. Hartmann's interest in physiognomy dates back to the 1880s in Boston when he taught Delsarte and was fascinated by what some psychologists today call "body language."

25. W. M. Hollinger, New York portrait photographer. See Hartmann's review of Hollinger's work, "The Man With A System—W. M. Hollinger." *Wilson's Photog. Mag.* 43 (May 1906):201–04.

26. Emmeline Rives (Princess Troubetzkoy Amélie Rives, 1863–1945), American novelist, playwright, and poet, whose first book, *The Quick, or the Dead?*, was a sensational best-seller in 1889.

27. Anthony Hope (pseudonym of Sir Anthony Hope Hawkins, 1863–1933), English novelist, best known for *The Prisoner of Zenda* (1894).

28. Moritz Rosenthal (1862–1946), Polish piano virtuoso, pupil of Franz Liszt, noted for his brilliant technique.

29. Saxe-Meiningen: a former duchy of central Germany, now in East Germany. In the second half of the nineteenth century the ducal theater of Meiningen acquired an international reputation and set the style for German dramatic performances.

30. Sir Henry Irving (1838–1905), English actor and stage manager, who took over the Lyceum Theatre in New York in 1878. See the review of Irving and Ellen Terry in "The Merchant of Venice" by C. Sadakichi Hartmann, "Recent New York Productions," *The Theatre Magazine* 6 (Feb. 15, 1890):264–66. See also Hartmann's essay, "Where Are the Gestures of Yesterday," *The Curtain* 9 (January 1930):3–4.

31. Fritz-Karl von Uhde (1848–1911), German genre painter, best known for pictures of scriptural subjects in modern costumes and setting.

32. Albert Gustav Edelfelt (1854–1905), Finnish artist who worked in many different media in a naturalistic style. Hartmann may be alluding to one of his best known paintings, *Christ and the Magdalene.*

33. Cécile Louise Stéphanie Chaminade (1861–1944), French composer, best known for her piano pieces.

34. Robert Demachy (1859–1937), Parisian banker and leading French photographer, who perfected the bichromate printing process and in 1911 introduced the oil transfer process for prints. See Hartmann's essay, "Constructive Criticism—No. 10. A Weekly Pictorial Review," *Bull. of Photog. and the Photographer* 5 (Aug. 11, 1909):81, 84.

35. Georg Einbeck, German photographer, gifted amateur in the *art noveau* movement in Hamburg.

36. George C. Cox (?–1902), American photographer, particularly known for his portrait of Walt Whitman, seated facing camera, wearing a large hat, right hand in coat pocket, left hand on the head of a cane. See Ida M. Tarbell, "A Great Photographer," *McClure's Magazine* 9 (May 1897):558–64. See Sadakichi Hartmann's booklet, *A Note on the Portraits of Walt Whitman* (New York: At the Sign of the Sparrow, 1921). See also Knox and Lawton, *The Whitman-Hartmann Controversy,* pp. 115–22.

37. John White Alexander (1856–1915), American painter influenced by Whistler, who specialized in portraits. Alexander's oil painting of Whitman is in the Metropolitan Museum of Art. Hartmann mentions the portrait in *A Note on the Portraits of Whitman,* p. 115. See Hartmann's essay on Alexander, "A Painter of Women," *The Stylus* 1 (Jan. 1910):1–4.

38. James L. Breese, professional New York photographer. From 1895 to 1900 he was a partner with Rudolf Eickemeyer, Jr., operating the Carbon Studio in New York.

39. Yvette Guilbert (1869–1944), French comedienne and songstress, who achieved fame in the 1890s with a revival of the old French ballads. Hartmann wrote about Guilbert prior to her American tour of 1896 in an unsigned essay, "Notes on the Fin de Siécle Movement in Parisian Art and Literature," *The Art Critic* 1 (Nov. 1893):4–9.

40. See Note 37 above.

2. A PLEA FOR THE PICTURESQUENESS OF NEW YORK

1. Théophile Alexandre Steinlen (1859–1923), French painter, etcher, lithographer, and illustrator, particularly known as a chronicler of Montmartre life.

2. *Gil Blas,* a French newspaper. The illustrated supplement ran from June 1891 to Aug. 1903.

3. Emile Zola (1840–1902), French writer, critic, and leader of the naturalist movement. While a correspondent for the McClure Syndicate in 1892, Hartmann wrote an interview with Zola. See Hartmann's "A Chat With Emile Zola," *The Louisville Courier-Journal,* Nov. 13, 1892, p. 15. See also Hartmann's unpublished essay "Confessions of an Ex-Journalist" (Wistaria Hartmann Linton Collection, Library of the University of California, Riverside). In this essay, Hartmann describes journalistic practices of the nineteenth century and competitive pressures that led newspaper reporters to heavily embroider or fabricate news stories and interviews. According to Hartmann, he succeeded in interviewing Zola, his editor found his story dull, and he rewrote it with embellishments gathered from library research. His account of common reporting methods during the period should make any scholar wary of celebrity interviews in the press of that era.

4. The Sezession (*Sécession*) emerged first in Munich in 1892 after the furor caused by an Edvard Munch exhibit, then it appeared in Berlin. The Viennese *Sezession* was apparently organized in the 1890s under the leadership of Gustav Klimt and associated with *Jugendstil* (Art Nouveau). These movements were part of a larger European and Russian turn to new standards and an escape from Academism. See Hartmann's essay "Notes on the Fin de Siécle Movement in Parisian Art and Literature," *The Art Critic* (Nov. 1893):4–9.

5. John George Brown (1831–1913), American genre painter, best known for his humorous studies of street urchins. See Hartmann's review of Brown in his Column "Art and Artists," *Musical America* 1 (November 26, 1898):31.

6. Vance Thompson (1863–1925), biographer, essayist, critic, and poet, best known for his book on the French symbolist movement, *French Portraits* (1900), and as co-editor with James Gibbons Huneker of the magazine, *M'lle New York*. Hartmann first met Thompson at the New York debut of Yvette Guilbert and later frequently in the company of Huneker. He described the man's whimsical personality and Beau Brummel tastes in "Reminiscences of Vance Thompson," *The Literary Digest International Book Review* 3 (Sept. 1925):688. Thompson's reputation suffered a severe blow with the publication of Bruce A. Morrissette's "Vance Thompson's Plagiarism of Teodor de Wyzewa's Articles on Mallarmé," *Modern Language Notes* 68 (1952):175–78. Morrissette showed that Thompson's exposition of Mallarmé's theories in *French Portraits* was plagiarized from Wyzewa's *Nos maîtres*. This fact appears to have been known to some of Thompson's contemporaries, however, who did not take such cut-and-paste "cribbing" as seriously as modern scholars. In his own piece on Thompson, Hartmann first called attention to his friend's book as a "clever assembly of borrowed materials" constructed with "skill and sympathy" through a "judicious use of the scissor" from *Figaro, Gil Blas,* and other literary magazines of the period. Hartmann's article has been overlooked by Morrissette, Haskell Block, and other modern scholars of the symbolist movement. Our own research on Hartmann has convinced us that such cribbing was relatively common in the nineteenth century. For example, many paragraphs from Hartmann's earliest published essays on art may be found spliced into S. C. de Soisson's book, *Boston Artists: A Parisian Critic's Notes* (Boston: Privately Printed, 1894).

7. Claude Lorrain (1600–1682), French landscape painter of idyllic scenes known for their golden light.

8. Dudley Hardy (1866?–1922), English painter and illustrator for many magazines.

9. Gaston Latouche (1854–1913), French painter and etcher, influenced by Manet and the naturalistic motifs of Zola.

10. See Chap. 1, Note 6.

11. Vasili Vereschagin (1842–1904), Russian painter of battles and executions and author of a book of travel sketches.

3. ON PLAGIARISM AND IMITATION

1. Joost Van den Vondel (1587–1679), Dutch poet and dramatist. Hartmann is referring to *Lucifer* (1654), a powerful dramatic poem, thought by some to be an allegorical account of the rise of the Netherlands against Philip II of Spain.

Miltonists with whom the editors have consulted discount the possibility that Milton was influenced by the poem, although there are certain parallels with *Paradise Lost.*

2. John Addington Symonds (1840–1893), English literary critic, historian, and scholar, author of *History of the Renaissance in Italy* (1875–1886).

3. Victorien Sardou (1831–1908), popular French dramatist and leading innovator of the "well-made play."

4. See Chap. 1, Note 4.

5. Clifford Prevost Grayson (1857–1951), American painter of landscapes, street scenes, and genre pieces.

6. Frederick Leighton (1830–1896), English historical and portrait painter.

7. Edwin Howland Blashfield (1838–1936), American painter known for his monumental decorations including one in the central dome of the Congressional Library, Washington, D.C. See Hartmann's review of Blashfield's work in his column, "Art and Artists," *Musical America* 10 (Dec. 10, 1898):39.

8. Max Liebermann (1847–1935), German genre painter, portraitist, and etcher.

4. RANDOM THOUGHTS ON CRITICISM

1. August Emile Bergerat (pseudonym, "Caliban" 1845–1923, French journalist and dramatic writer.

2. *Le Figaro*, satirical Parisian journal, founded in 1826, discontinued in 1833, and refounded by Villemessant in 1854.

3. Gilbert Hamerton (1834–1894), English artist and essayist. Hartmann is referring to his masterwork, *Etching and Etchers* (1866).

4. See Chap. 1, Note 2.

5. Nicholas Boileau[-Despréaux] (1637–1711), French critic and poet, whose chief work is *Ars Poétique* (1674).

6. Hippolyte Taine (1828–1893), French philosopher, historian, and critic. Hartmann is alluding to his *La Philosophie de l'Art* (1865–69).

7. See Chap. 1, Note 34.

5. ON COMPOSITION

1. Jean Léon Gérôme (1824–1904), French painter, especially of historical subjects and romantic eastern scenes.

2. Anton Mauve (1838–1888), Dutch painter and one of the greatest landscapists of his time, influenced by Corot and Millet.

3. Jean Baptiste Camille Corot (1796–1875), French landscape painter, who sacrificed unity of detail to harmony of effect.

4. See Chap. 1, Note 22.

5. A. Wesley Dow (1857–1922), painter and art theorist, author of *Composition* (Boston: Bowles, 1899).

6. Unidentified. Possibly Elizabeth Mill Reid (1858–1931), owner of the *New York Tribune* and wife of Whitelaw Reid, Ambassador to the Court of St. James.

7. Mrs. James Brown-Potter (*née* Cora Urquhart, 1859–1936), American actress and author of a number of books of essays and poetry.

6. ON GENRE

1. Mariano y Carbo Fortuny (1839–1874), Spanish genre painter and aquafortist, known for his rococo pictures.

2. Ludwig Knaus (1829–1910), German genre painter.

3. Franz von Defregger (1835–1921), Austrian genre and historical painter, noted for popular pictures of Tyrolean life.

4. Very likely Pierre Vauthier (1845–1916), French landscape painter.

5. Henry Mosler (1841–1920), American genre painter.

6. Josef Israëls (1824–1911), Dutch genre painter.

7. See Chap. 3, Note 8.

8. Jean Louis Ernest Meissonier (1825–1891), French painter, noted for small, meticulous genre pictures, frequently of military subjects.

9. Eduardo Zamaçois (1842–1871), Spanish figure painter.

10. See Chap. 1, Note 17.

11. See Chap. 5, Note 1.

12. John E. Dumont of Rochester, New York, who in 1898 exhibited his work with Stieglitz and Eickemeyer, Jr. at the exhibition of the Royal Photographic Society, London. See Hartmann's review, "The John E. Dumont Exhibition," *Camera Notes* 3 (July 1899):38.

13. Edmund Stirling, Philadelphia photographer, and one of the twelve founders with Stieglitz of the Photo-Secession on Feb. 17, 1902.

14. Probably Frederick Dielman (1847–1935), German-

born genre painter, whose chief subjects were society women and fashionable interiors.

7. A PHOTOGRAPHIC ENQUÊTE

1. Daniel Chester French (1850–1931), American sculptor, known for character studies and decorative, idealized motifs.

2. George C. Barnard (1863–1938), American sculptor, strongly influenced by Rodin.

3. William Merritt Chase (1849–1916), American painter, academic in tradition, who established a school of landscape painting in the Shinnecock Hills, Long Island. See Hartmann's review of a Chase exhibition, "A Special and Unique Event," *The Stylus* 1 (Feb. 1910):200–31.

4. Frederick Stuart Church (1842–1923), American painter, illustrator, and etcher.

5. Albert Pinkham Ryder (1847–1917), American painter of glowing compositions, particularly moonlit seas and night scenes. See the following Hartmann essays: "A visit to A. P. Ryder," *Art News* 1 (March 1897):1–3; "Eremites of the Brush," *American Mercury* 11 (June 1927):192–96; "Albert Pinkham Ryder," *Magazine of Art* 31 (Sept. 1938):500–03, 550. Hartmann visited Ryder frequently over a twenty-three-year period, beginning in 1893, and a number of addresses for the painter may be found in Hartmann's address books (Atma Dorothea Gilliland Collection, Library of the University of Oregon). One of the fullest accounts of Ryder's life as a painter is Hartmann's unpublished 17,000-word manuscript, titled *The Story of an American Painter* (Wistaria Hartmann Linton Collection, Library of the University of California, Riverside).

6. Childe Hassam (1859–1935), American painter and etcher, known for his impressionistic landscapes. See Hartmann's discussion of Hassam's work in the column "Studio Talk," *International Studio* 29 (1907):267–70.

7. George de Forest Brush (1855–1941), American painter, best known for his poetical renderings of American Indian scenes.

8. Dwight Williams Tryon (1849–1941), American landscape painter. See Hartmann's essay, "W. D. [sic] Tryon: A Painting in Prose," *Art News* 1 (April 1897):1–3.

8. THE INFLUENCE OF PHOTOGRAPHY ON INTERIOR DECORATION

1. See Chap. 7, Note 8.

2. See Chap. 1, Note 16.

3. Horatio Walker (1858–1938), Canadian painter, known for his scenes of simple life on the Ile d'Orleans in the St. Lawrence River.

4. Stanford White (1853–1906), leading American architect, responsible for designing such structures as the old Madison Square Garden, the Washington Arch in Washington Square, New York, and Trinity Church, Boston. White was shot to death by Harry Thaw in one of the most sensational scandals of the period as a result of his pursuit of Thaw's wife, Evelyn Nesbit. In 1896, Hartmann worked briefly as a librarian for the architectural firm of McKim, Mead, and White. Later, he appears to have encountered White regularly at New York social events, including those hosted by "Miss Kuehme Beveridge, that remarkable hetaera who entertained at her *petits levees,* in a studio atmosphere sick with sex, such remarkable personalities as Stanford White, Richard Harding Davis, Buffalo Bill, Blaine, and sculptor Noble." (See Sadakichi Hartmann's *White Chrysanthemums* [New York: Herder and Herder, 1971], pp. 153–54.

5. A wall picture composed of an oblong piece of silk, framed in strips of brocade, and mounted on a long narrow strip of canvas with wooden rollers.

6. John Rogers (1829–1904), American sculptor, best known for his statuettes illustrating literary and dramatic figures and scenes from American country life.

7. George Romney (1734–1802), English portrait painter.

8. William Morris (1834–1896), English artist and poet, whose manufacturing and decorating firm of Morris & Co. created new standards of taste in furniture, stained glass, and textiles.

9. REPETITION WITH SLIGHT VARIATION

1. See Chap. 2, Note 4.

2. See Chap. 1, Note 10.

3. See Chap. 7, Note 8.

4. Maurice Maeterlinck (1862–1949), Belgian dramatist, poet, and essayist, whose symbolic dramas such as *Pelléas et Melisande* (1892) were clearly an influence on Hartmann's own symbolist plays of the 1890s: *Christ: A Dramatic Poem in Three Acts* (Boston: Privately Printed, 1893), and *Buddha: A Drama in Twelve Scenes* (New York: Author's Edition, 1897). Hartmann may have corresponded with Maeterlinck, and he served as translator of the short essay "Message from Maurice Maeterlinck," which arrived too late for inclusion in *Camera Work*, No. 2 as planned by Stieglitz and therefore was circulated with *Camera Work*, No. 3 for insertion in No. 2.

5. A vaudeville troupe of the 1890s.

6. See Chap. 7, Note 7.

7. Abbott H. Thayer (1849–1921), American painter, whose figure paintings were characterized by an unaffectedness and healthy vitality. See Hartmann's discussion of Thayer, "Eremites of the Brush," *American Mercury* 11 (June 1927):192–96.

8. F. H. Tompkins, Boston figure painter of genre scenes. See Hartmann's essay, "A Boston Artist: F. H. Tompkins," *The Art Critic* 1 (Nov. 1893):17–18. A copy of a sketch of Hartmann drawn in 1896 by Tompkins may be found in the Wistaria Hartmann Linton Collection, Library of the University of California, Riverside.

9. Mary Cassatt (1845–1926), American figure painter and etcher, who spent most of her life in France. A friend of Manet and Degas, her paintings were influenced by the French impressionists. In a letter written in 1894 from Paris to Hartmann in Boston, the American artist Frederick Dana Marsh reported encountering Cassatt at Degas' studio. Marsh's letter also asked Hartmann about the progress of Robert Henri, indicating that Sadakichi was familiar with that painter's work as early as 1894 in Philadelphia, which was prior to Henri's establishing himself in New York and joining other artists in laying the foundations for the famous "Ash Can School" of American painting (Wistaria Hartmann Linton Collection, Library of the University of California, Riverside).

10. THE PHOTO-SECESSION EXHIBITION AT THE CARNEGIE ART GALLERIES, PITTSBURGH, PA.

1. The exhibition at the Corcoran Art Galleries, held in January, 1904, was arranged by the Secession under the auspices of the Capitol Camera Club. The Carnegie Institute exhibition opened on February 6, 1904 and attracted 11,000 visitors in three weeks.

2. Lee has not been identified by the editors.

3. Oscar Maurer, San Francisco photographer and member of the Photo-Secession.

4. Augustus Saint-Gaudens (1849–1907), famous American sculptor, who worked on numerous commemorative monuments. Saint-Gaudens was a subscriber to Hartmann's magazine, *The Art Critic* (1893–1894). In a publication announcement for Hartmann's first collection of short stories, *Schopenhauer in the Air* (New York: Privately Printed, 1899), Saint-Gaudens is quoted as having written Hartmann in Oct. 1896, saying: "What you think in matters of art, I think of high value." The editors have been unable to locate this ltr. or a

second ltr. to Hartmann from Saint-Gaudens, dated Sept. 5, 1896, comprising three pages. The latter ltr. was sold together with a photograph of Saint-Gaudens mounted in the same frame on Oct. 17, 1913, at an auction of the library of Mary M. Ward by Merwin Sales Company, New York. An early Hartmann essay on Saint-Gaudens appeared in his column "Art and Artists," *Musical America* 1 (Oct. 29, 1898):31.

5. Emmanuel Signoret (1870–1900), founder of the symbolist magazine *Le Saint-Graal* (1892–1899) and author of *Daphne* (1894). Hartmann met many of the French symbolists on his excursion to Europe in 1892, and later corresponded with Mallarmé and quite possibly several other members of the movement. He described meeting Mallarmé, Henri de Régnier, and Stuart Merrill in his essay, "A Tuesday Evening at Stéphane Mallarmé's," *The Art Critic* 1 (Nov. 1893):9–11. See also Thomas B. Brumbaugh, "Odilon Redon and Sadakichi Hartmann," *Sadakichi Hartmann Newsletter* 2 (Fall 1972):6–7; Elizabeth Stanton Blake, "Un Correspondent Américain de Mallarmé Avec Deux Lettres et un Document Inédits," *Revue d'Histoire Littéraire de la France* 68 (Jan.-Feb. 1968):26–35; and Hans-Peter Breuer's translation of an article written by Hartmann in German for the *New Yorker Staats-Zeitung* of March 4, 1899, "An Essay on Henri de Régnier and the Symbolists," *Sadakichi Hartmann Newsletter* 1 (Winter 1970): 10–12.

6. See Chap. 5, Note 5.

7. *Eben Holden* (1900), a popular novel by Irving Bacheller (1859–1950).

8. A short story by Clara Morris, illustrated by White photographs, which appeared in *McClure's Magazine* 22 (Feb. 1904):429–34.

9. See Chap. 6, Note 13.

10. W. F. James, Chicago photographer and a member of the Photo-Secession.

11. John G. Bullock, Philadelphia photographer and a member of the Photo-Secession.

12. William B. Post, photographer from Fryeburg, Maine, and a member of the Photo-Secession.

13. Rose Clark, pictorialist photographer from Buffalo, New York. See Hartmann's review of her work in Sidney Allan, "The Recent Exhibition of the Photo-Secession Society," *Camera Craft* 8 (May 1904):243–48. Rose Clark often collaborated with Elizabeth Flint Wade, another Buffalo pictorialist.

14. Mary Devens, Boston photographer and a member of the Photo-Secession.

15. C. Yarnall Abbott, Philadelphia photographer, who served as president of the Photographic Society of Philadel-

phia and was a prolific contributor of articles to the photographic journals of the 1890s, particularly *Photo-Era*.

16. William B. Dyer, Chicago photographer and a founding member of the *Photo-Secession*.

17. S. L. Willard, Chicago photographer and a member of the Photo-Secession.

18. Herbert G. French, Cincinnati photographer and a member of the Photo-Secession.

19. Ernest Walter Histed (1860–1947), Anglo-American photographer who was usually referred to in the photographic press only as "Histed." He had a studio at 569 Fifth Avenue, New York City, and was a summer resort photographer in Newport, Rhode Island. See Hartmann's essay, "Histed—Photographer of Celebrities," *Wilson's Photographic Magazine* 44 (Oct. 1907):457–59. See also Harry H. Brodine's essay, "Up and Down Fifth Avenue," *Wilson's Photographic Magazine* 50 (Oct. 1913):418–22.

11. A PLEA FOR STRAIGHT PHOTOGRAPHY

1. See Chap. 10, Note 15.

2. See Chap. 10, Note 14.

3. Charles Emile Jacque (1813–1894), French painter and etcher, who excelled in etchings of rural life.

4. Adolphe Appian (1819–1898), French etcher.

5. Jules Jacques Veyrassat (1828–1893), French painter, engraver, and etcher.

6. Charles Meryon (1821–1868), French etcher, best known for a series of etchings on the old sections of Paris, *Eaux-Fortes sur Paris* (1850–1854).

7. See Chap. 6, Note 12.

8. See also Hartmann's essay, "The Gum Process and Its Proper Application," *Photo-Era* 19 (July 1907):3–4. Here again Hartmann argues for moderation in the application of the gum-bichromate process to preserve the photographic texture of the finished print.

9. See Chap. 1, Note 33.

10. See Chap. 10, Note 11.

11. See Chap, 10, Note 13.

12. See Chap. 10, Note 16.

13. See Chap. 10, Note 18.

14. Russel has not been identified by the editors.

15. Eva Watson Schütze (1867–1935), Chicago photographer and a founding member of the Photo-Secession.

16. See Chap. 10, Note 9.

17. See Chap. 10, Note 17.

12. THE BROKEN PLATES [A Short Story]

1. Hartmann experimented periodically with photography, and this short story probably reflects his abandonment of the idea of becoming an artistic photographer even though he is on record as disclaiming ever having had such an ambition. A few examples of Hartmann's photographic work may be found in the Wistaria Hartmann Linton Collection, Library of the University of California, Riverside.

13. THE SALON CLUB AND THE FIRST AMERICAN PHOTOGRAPHIC SALON IN NEW YORK

1. See Hartmann's essay, "A Note on Louis Fleckenstein and His Work," *The Photographic Times-Bulletin* 36 (Oct. 1904):433–37.

2. Jeanne E. Bennett, Baltimore photographer.

3. Curtis Bell, New York photographer and chairman of the Salon Club. For a description of his New York studio see the anonymous article, "The Photographer's Metropolis," *Abel's Photographic Weekly* 3 (Jan. 16, 1909):74–75.

4. Adolph Petzold, Philadelphia photographer.

5. See Hartmann essay, "The Landscape Work of the Salon Club," *American Annual of Photography and Photographic Times Almanac* 19 (1905):139–42.

6. See Chap. 1, Note 4.

7. Baron Wilhelm von Gloeden (1856–1931), German count and photographer, who settled in the Sicilian village of Taormina, selling to magazines and connoisseurs photographs of local male youth in the nude or draped in togas and wreathed with laurel crowns.

8. Albert L. Groll (1866–1952), American painter and etcher. See Sidney Allan, "An Appreciation of Albert L. Groll—Landscape Painter," *Brush and Pencil* 11 (Oct. 1902):36–41.

14. RECENT CONQUESTS IN NIGHT PHOTOGRAPHY

1. Aart Van der Neer (1603–1677), Dutch painter.

2. Godfried Schalcken (1643–1706), Dutch portraitist.

3. W. M. Van der Weyde (1871?–1929), New York photographer.

16. UNPHOTOGRAPHIC PAINT: THE TEXTURE OF IMPRESSIONISM

1. Marsden Hartley (1878–1943), American landscape and still-life painter, who, influenced by the Italian impressionist Segantini and other European modern painters, adopted an impressionist technique based on form and color.

2. In 1905 Edward Steichen suggested that Stieglitz take over two rooms adjoining his own quarters at 291 Fifth Avenue and run it as a gallery for the Photo-Secession. The "Little Galleries of the Photo-Secession" opened formally on Nov. 24, 1905.

3. Giovanni Segantini (1858–1899), Italian impressionistic genre painter.

4. Adolphe Joseph Thomas Monticelli (1824–1886), French painter, whose work was characterized by masses of color and almost invisible figures in an impressionistic style.

5. Antonio Mancini (1852–1930), Italian genre portrait and landscape painter.

6. Guido Reni (1575–1642), Italian painter.

7. Andrea del Sarto (1486–1531), Florentine painter, noted for his draftsmanship and harmonious use of color.

8. Beato Angelico, also Fra Angelico, real name Guido di Pietri (1387–1455), Italian painter, beatified after his death, whose ethereal treatment of angels gave him his name.

9. Camille Pissarro (1830–1903), French impressionistic painter whose landscapes were characterized by the use of fine small strokes and subtle tonal shading.

10. Alfred Sisley (1839–1899), French impressionist painter.

17. THE DAGUERREOTYPE

1. Gilbert Stuart (1755–1828), American portrait painter, known for his portraits of Washington, Jefferson, Madison, and other notable men and women of his time.

2. Thomas Sully (1783–1872), American portrait painter, born in England, best known for his painting, "Washington Crossing the Delaware."

3. Hartmann is incorrect in asserting that the daguerreotype never became popular in America. The first successful daguerreotype in the United States, a view of St. Paul's Church, New York, was taken in 1839 by D. W Seager, an English resident of New York. Within two years almost every major town in the United States had a daguerreotype studio, and by 1853 there were approximately 10,000 people earning their living as daguerreotypists. Hartmann is right about the short-lived reign of the daguerreotype, although its popularity continued on into the 1860s, longer than in Europe and elsewhere. See Helmut and Aline Gernsheim, *L. J. M. Daguerre: The History of the Diorama and the Daguerreotype* (New York: Dover Publications, Inc., 1968), pp. 129–42.

4. John W. Draper (1811–1882), chemist, physiologist, and historian, who helped found the medical school of New York University and was renowned for his research into photochemistry and spectrum analysis.

5. Dorothy Catherine Draper. The portrait was taken during the summer of 1840.

6. Louis Jacques Mandé Daguerre (1789–1851), Parisian scene painter who, beginning in 1826 after correspondence with Niépce, set out on the path that led to development of the daguerreotype.

7. Joseph Nicéphore Niépce (1765–1833), French chemist, lithographer, and inventor of heliography, whose attempts at true photography began in 1816, when he discovered how to briefly fix the images of pictures taken by the *camera obscura*. Hartmann unknowingly—in the light of recent research—minimizes Niépce's achievements. See Helmut Gernsheim, "The 150th Anniversary of Photography," *History of Photography* 1 (Jan. 1977):3–8.

8. Alexander S. Wolcott (1804–1844), a New York manufacturer of dental supplies who, with his partner John Johnson, began experimenting with photographic portraiture in the 1830s. The camera apparatus he designed was patented on May 8, 1840, becoming the first invention in the United States to receive a patent relating to photography. See Gernsheim, *L. J. M. Daguerre: The History of the Diorama and the Daguerreotype*, pp. 132–34.

9. Henry James, Jr. (1843–1916), American novelist. Hartmann is alluding to James' short story, "The Real Thing" (1892).

18. WHAT REMAINS

1. The Albright Gallery exhibition, which opened on Nov. 4, 1910 and ran through Dec. 1, has been credited with vindicating the belief that photography had a right to recognition as a fine art. The show, organized by Stieglitz with the encouragement of Cornelia B. Sage, acting director of the gallery, was under the control of the Photo-Secession, although Stieglitz planned to include the Photo-Pictorialists of

Buffalo as well as an open section. The Buffalo group refused to participate and the show was attacked bitterly by many of the photographic journals. See Robert Doty, *Photo-Secession: Photography as a Fine Art* (New York: George Eastman House, 1960), pp. 56–57.

2. James Craig Annan (1846–1946), leading English art photographer.

3. Baron Adolph De Meyer (?–1946), founder of the elegant style of fashion photography, beginning with the reproduction of his work in *Vogue* in 1913.

4. The Vienna Camera Club, whose members included Heinrich Kühn, Dr. Hugo Henneberg, and Dr. Frederick Spitzer, was one of the world's most illustrious pictorialist groups, having been affiliated with the Linked Ring in England as early as 1895. See Helmut and Alison Gernsheim, *The History of Photography from the Camera Obscura to the Beginning of the Modern Era* [1685–1914] (New York, St. Louis, San Francisco: McGraw-Hill Book Company, 1969), p. 465.

19. THE ESTHETIC SIGNIFICANCE OF THE MOTION PICTURE

1. Lucas Fildes (1844–1927), English genre and portrait painter.

2. Elizabeth Vigeé-Lebrun (1755–1842), French portrait painter.

3. Charles Dana Gibson (1867–1944), American illustrator, creator of the "Gibson Girl," whose work appeared in many magazines, including *Life, Harper's, Century,* and *Scribner's.*

4. Hartmann first referred to some of the possibilities of cinematography in his 1898 essay on portrait painting and portrait photography (see Chap. 1, p. 35). He accurately prophesized the future of home cinematography in "The Chances of Moving Picture Portraiture," *Wilson's Photographic Magazine* 51 (Sept. 1914):408–10. See also Howard A. Burton, "A Gift for Film Theory: The Film Criticism of Sadakichi Hartmann," *Sadakichi Hartmann Newsletter* (Winter 1972):1–3. Burton commenting on the essay presented here states: "The remarkable thing about Hartmann's 'The Esthetic Significance of the Motion Picture,' published in *Camera Work,* No. 38 (April, 1912), pp. 19–21, is that he wrote it at all. In 1912 the art of the film was still almost as primitive as it had been in the 1890's when the films were first shown in public . . . Hartmann's looking beyond the flimsy sets, the over-acting, the complete artificiality, the awkwardness of silence in vehicles whose point lay in their dialogue is really an important bit of prophesy . . . Hartmann's predicting sound, color, and home movies deserves recognition . . ."

5. See Chap. 1, Note 30.

6. Edward Gordon Craig (1872–1966), English actor, stage designer, and producer. Craig carried on a correspondence with Hartmann in the 1930s and some of his letters to Sadakichi may be found in the Wistaria Hartmann Linton Collection, Library of the University of California, Riverside.

7. Arnold Böcklin (1871–1901), Swiss painter, mostly of mythological subjects.

8. See Chap. 3, Note 6.

9. Jules Adolphe Aimé Breton (1827–1906), French painter of rustic scenes and peasant life.

10. Charles Cottet (1863–1925), French landscape and genre painter.

11. See Chap. 3, Note 8.

20. ALFRED STIEGLITZ: AN ART CRITIC'S ESTIMATE

1. See Chap. 1, Note 34.

2. Alfred Stieglitz, *Picturesque Bits of New York and Other Studies* (New York: R. H. Russell, 1897).

3. Guiseppe de Nittis (1845–1884), Italian genre painter known for his Parisian and London street scenes.

4. See Hartmann's discussion of night photography, Chap. 14.

5. See Chap. 3, Note 8.

6. Hermann Wilhelm Vogel (1834–1898), professor of photography, Technische Hochschule, Berlin.

7. August Wilhelm von Hoffmann (1818–1892), great German chemist whose students included famous persons in many fields.

8. Fritz Thaulow (1847–1906), Scandanavian impressionist painter.

9. Albert Besnard (1849–1934), French impressionist painter.

10. See Chap. 1, Note 14.

11. See Chap. 1, Note 39.

12. See Chap. 1, Note 3.

21. ZAIDA BEN-YÚSUF: A PURIST

1. Hartmann probably first viewed Miss Ben-Yúsuf's work at her exhibition in 1898. See William M. Murray, "Miss Zaida Ben-Yúsuf's Exhibition (Nov 24 to 26)," *Camera Notes* 2 (April

1899):168–72. See also Richard Hines, Jr., "Women in Photography," *Wilson's Photographic Magazine* 36 (March 1899):137–41. Hines described Miss Ben-Yúsuf as "an English girl, transplanted to America," who conducted a studio on Fifth Avenue, and had already exhibited at the Vienna Camera Club and had two pictures represented at a Kodak loan exhibition.

2. See Chap. 1, Note 22.

3. Julia Margaret Cameron (1815–1879), noted English photographer of eminent persons, who won many gold medals in Europe and America.

4. Richard Le Gallienne (1866–1947), English poet and essayist, first visited America in 1898 and resided in New York for many years. Hartmann and Le Gallienne were drinking companions and moved in the same Bohemian circles. The two writers parted company when Hartmann punched Le Gallienne in the nose during a drinking bout.

5. Fridtjof Nansen (1861–1930), Norwegian explorer. Hartmann speaks of interviewing Nansen in New York Harbor after his North Pole attempt of 1896 (unpubl. ms., "Confessions of an Ex-Journalist," Wistaria Hartmann Linton Collection, Library of the University of California, Riverside). Hartmann was then working as a feature writer for the German language newspaper, the *New Yorker Staats-Zeitung*.

6. See Chap. 1, Note 6.

7. See Chap. 1, Note 1.

8. Henriette Hovey, a student of Delsarte and wife of the American poet Richard Hovey, was noted for her eccentric dress. In 1896, Hartmann served as art columnist for the Hovey's short-lived magazine, *The Daily Tatler*.

9. See Chap. 1, Note 38.

22. FRANK EUGENE: PAINTER-PHOTOGRAPHER

1. Hartmann first wrote about Eugene as a painter in his column "Art and Artists," *Musical America* 1 (Oct. 22, 1899):27.

2. An essay by Hartmann on the Player's Club of New York appeared in the *New Yorker Staats-Zeitung* on Oct. 15, 1899. See Hans-Peter Breuer's transl. "The Player's Club of New York," *Sadakichi Hartmann Newsletter* 2 (Spring 1971):7–10.

3. The reference appears to be to a portrait of Elizabeth Blanche Walsh, Hartmann's first wife. An original Eugene portrait of her manipulated in the manner described is in the Wistaria Hartmann Linton Collection, Library of the University of California, Riverside. See portrait on p. 13.

4. See Chap. 11, Note 8.

5. Ole Bull Bornemann (1810–1889), Norwegian violinist who after a triumphal tour of America in 1848 established a Norwegian settlement, Oleana, in Pennsylvania.

6. Fernand Khnopff (1858–1928), Belgian painter and sculptor and one of the founders of the *Cercle des Vingt*.

23. CLARENCE H. WHITE: A METEOR THROUGH SPACE

1. See Chap. 1, Note 34.

2. See Chap. 18, Note 2.

3. Mary Wilkins Freeman (1852–1930), New England novelist and short story writer, married in 1902 to Dr. Charles Freeman.

4. Hartmann is referring to the exhibition of White's work at the New York Camera Club, Oct. 10 to 31, 1899. See the review by Joseph T. Keiley, "Exhibition of the Pictures of Clarence H. White of Newark, Ohio (Oct. 10 to 31, 1899)," *Camera Notes* 3 (Jan. 1900), 123–24.

5. See Chap. 10, Note 4.

24. F. HOLLAND DAY: A DECORATIVE PHOTOGRAPHER

1. See Chap. 1, p. 46 (*Camera Notes* 3 [July 1899], p. 15).

2. British photographic journals and critics seized with great glee upon the term "plastic psychological synthesis" in debunking American photographic criticism and American photographers. See discussion in Editors' Introduction, p. 19.

3. According to Elbert Hubbard, Day's eccentricities also included affecting a fez and turned-up Turkish slippers, worshipping a squat number ten joss, and writing only by the light of thirteen candles. See Herbert White Taylor's essay, "F. Holland Day: an Estimate," *Photo-Era* 4 (March 1900), p. 77.

25. RUDOLF EICKEMEYER, JR.: MASTER OF THE FOREGROUND

1. Eickemeyer's winter studies were the subject of his book, *Winter, Pictured by Rudolf Eickemeyer, Jr.* (New York: R. H. Russell, 1903) to which Hartmann contributed an introduction. According to critic Roland Rood ("A Retrospect," *The Burr McIntosh Monthly* 18 [Dec, 1908]:6 pp. [unnumbered]) credit for first introducing photographs as illustrations in the big literary magazines of America belonged to Eickemeyer. Hartmann collaborated for several years with Eickemeyer on a series of nature studies in the tradition of

Thoreau and John Burroughs, which were published as "illustrated essays" or as Sadakichi termed them "photo-essays." See, e.g., "A Winter Ramble," *Harper's Monthly Magazine* 103 (Nov. 1901):989–96. Since Hartmann had published nature essays prior to becoming acquainted with Eickemeyer, he may have been the collaborator who first perceived the possibility of illustrating such articles with photographs.

26. GERTRUDE KÄSEBIER: A SENSE OF THE PICTORIAL

1. See Stieglitz's note, "Our Illustrations," *Camera Notes* 3 (July 1899):24.

2. Henry Ward Ranger (1858–1916), American landscape painter.

3. Arthur Bowen Davies (1862–1920), American romantic painter and key figure in the New York Armory Show of 1913, the first major exhibition of modern art in America. Hartmann was an early supporter of Davies in his magazine *The Art Critic* 1 (Jan. 1894):40. Subsequently, Hartmann attacked Davies as having become an imitator rather than an innovator in his essay, "The Echo," *Art News* 1 (June 1897):4–5. Yet Hartmann stood ready to revise his critical opinions in the face of later work by any artist or photographer he wrote about. In *A History of American Art* (New York: L. C. Page & Company, 1902), Vol. 2, p. 267–69, Hartmann described Davies as "the most intellectual painter we possess" and said that if Davies develops into a great painter, his deep culture will have made him one."

4. Pamela Colman Smith's drawings were displayed by Stieglitz in Jan. 1907 at the first non-photographic exhibition of the "Little Galleries of the Photo-Secession."

5. Mrs. Käsebier's generosity of spirit was reflected in the fact that the editor of *The Photographic Times* showed the manuscript of this article to her and offered to blue-pencil some passages he considered unduly harsh. Mrs. Käsebier insisted the article be published as written by Hartmann. See "Editorial Notes," *The Photographic Times* 32 (May 1900):237. For another studio interview with Mrs. Käsebier see R. Child Bayley, "A Visit to Mrs. Käsebier's Studio," *Wilson's Photographic Magazine* 40 (Feb. 1903):73–74.

27. EDWARD STEICHEN: A VISIT TO STEICHEN'S STUDIO

1. See Chap. 1, Note 10.

2. See Chap. 7. Note 8.

3. See Chap. 9, Note 4.

28. H. H. PIERCE: A TRAVELING PHOTOGRAPHER

1. The reference is to the 1905 convention of the Photographer's Association of Pennsylvania, Maryland, and the District of Columbia. At one of the afternoon sessions, Hartmann took the delegates on a tour of the Smithsonian Institution and the Corcoran Art Gallery in Washington, D.C.

2. A. T. Proctor of Huntington, West Virginia, whose photographic work was exhibited in many smaller galleries. See Sadakichi Hartmann, "A. T. Proctor—A Maker of Exhibition Prints," *Wilson's Photographic Magazine* 44 (April 1907):169–71.

29. ELIAS GOLDENSKY: IN THE PROLETARIAN INTEREST

1. Charles H. Davis of Davis & Sanford, New York City. Hartmann used Davis frequently in his essays as an example of the "ideal average" of craftsmanship to which every professional photographer should aspire. See Sidney Allan, "The Ideal Average—Charles H. Davis," *Wilson's Photographic Magazine* 43 (Jan. 1906):7–10.

2. Possibly A. H. Griffith, director of the Detroit Art Museum. Hartmann and Griffith delivered the major address before the Ohio-Michigan Photographer's Convention in 1905.

3. E. B. Core, New York specialist in children's portraits.

4. S. L. Stein, Milwaukee professional photographer. See Sidney Allan, "The Man Without a Pose—S. L. Stein," *Wilson's Photographic Magazine* 43 (Dec. 1906):557–59.

5. Richard was unidentified by the editors.

30. J. H. GARO: WANDERER ON NEW ROADS

1. The reference is to the twenty-fifth convention of the Photographer's Association of America, Aug. 8–11, 1905, in Boston.

2. See Chap. 28, Note 2.

3. See Chap. 1, Note 4.

31. B. J. FALK: AN EXQUISITE TEMPERAMENT

1. Vogel (see Chap. 20, Note 6) was the first to discover

that by dyeing photographic emulsion could be made sensitive to light waves. This made possible color photography.

2. The editors have no information on Bierstadt's experiments. Born in Solingen, Germany, Bierstadt was an art photographer and a brother of the American painter, Albert Bierstadt. He was in charge of the Photo-Mechanical Section of the American Photographic Exhibition held Sept. 6 to Oct. 8, 1898 in the National Academy of Design, New York City. Color work was one of the three classes featured in this section of the exhibition. Further information on Edward Bierstadt may be found in Robert Taft's *Photography and the American Scene* (New York: The Macmillan Company, 1938), pp. 432, 515.

3. William Kurtz of New York, collaborating with Ernst Vogel, made the first satisfactory three-color prints in 1892, employing azaline plates. See Josef Maria Eder, *History of Photography*, transl. by Edward Epstead (New York: Columbia University Press, 1945), pp. 653–654. See note on Kurtz attributed to Hartmann, *The Weekly Review* 3 (March 11, 1893):366.

4. Edmond Becquerel of France, who between 1847 and 1855 made several major contributions to photochromy.

5. Alphonse Louis Poiteven (1819–1882) of France, inventor of callotype (1855) and pigment printing.

6. Gabriel Lippmann (1845–1921), professor at Sorbonne and Nobel prizewinner in physics (1908), produced direct color photographs in 1891 by the phenomena of interference of light waves.

7. John Joly (1857–1933), credited with producing the first mosaic-screen color photographs in 1897.

8. James Clerk-Maxwell (1831–1897), Scottish physician and first person to conceive of color reproduction by means of three-color light filters.

9. Napoleon Sarony (1821–1896), pioneer photographer in Europe and New York. See anonymous editorial obituary attributed to Hartmann, "The Death of Napoleon Sarony," *The Daily Tatler* 1 (Nov. 11, 1896):4.

10. Many of Falk's photographs of theatrical personalities and the world of the stage may be found throughout the 1890s in *The New York Dramatic Mirror*. The magazine is a rich, unmined source for photo-historians.

32. J. C. STRAUSS: THE MAN WITH A SYSTEM

1. The "Growlery" was a huge tile room in the basement of Strauss' St. Louis tower studio, where photographers, writers, painters, and other friends of the photographer met for convivial drinking sessions.

33. JOSEPH BYRON: THE STAGE IS MY STUDIO

1. More commonly "willy-nilly," which is to say Byron could not escape the label of being the "theatrical flashlight man."

2. Grace M. Mayer in *Once Upon a City* (New York: The Macmillan Company, 1958), p. xi, gives 1888 as the year in which Mr. and Mrs. Joseph Byron arrived in America. The Byron photographic collection, presented in 1942 to the Museum of the City of New York by Byron's son, Percy, contains over 10,000 prints and negatives of every aspect of the city.

3. George W. Lederer (1861–1939), American theatrical producer and originator of the word "vaudeville."

4. See Chap. 1, Note 30.

5. See Chap. 1, Note 14.

6. Gabrielle Réjane (1856–1920), French actress, equally gifted in comic and tragic roles, enjoyed considerable popularity in both England and America. See Byron's photograph of Madame Réjane, p. 243.

34. BURR McINTOSH: PHOTOGRAPHER OF FADS AND FANCIES

1. M. J. Steffens, Chicago photographer specializing in social celebrities. See Sidney Allan, "The Well-Made Print—Steffens," *Wilson's Photographic Magazine* (Nov. 1906):43: 498–500.

2. See Chap. 29, Note 4.

3. McIntosh was publisher of the *Burr McIntosh Monthly* (1903–1910), a journal reflecting his interest in society, sports, and mass culture.

35. GUIDO REY: A MASTER OF DETAIL COMPOSITION

1. See Chap. 6, Note 8.

2. Sir Lawrence Alma-Tadema (1863–1912), Dutch-English painter of classical subjects.

3. Pierre Oliver Joseph Coomans (1816–1889), Belgian painter of genre and historical subjects.

4. See Sidney Allan, "A Plea for Straight Photography," *American Amateur Photographer* 16 (March 1904):101–09. See also Chap. 11.

36. ALVIN LANGDON COBURN: SECESSION PORTRAITURE

1. See Sidney Allan, "The One-Print Exhibition," *Wilson's Photographic Magazine* 44 (May 1907):217–19.

2. W. H. Partridge, a member of the Lens and Brush Club of Boston (see *Photo-Era* 14 [April 1904]:217–19).

3. Eugene Carrière (1859–1906), French painter with misty, monochromatic style, known for melancholic atmosphere and maternal subject matter.

4. The Harris portrait appeared as the frontispiece for Sidney Allan, "A Plea for Straight Photography," p. 101.

37. RUDOLF DÜHRKOOP: A GERMAN PICTORIALIST

1. Probably a typographical error for Franz Grainer. Hartmann discussed the work of the German photographer Franz Grainer (1871–1948) in Sidney Allan, "Composition in Portraiture—On the Arrangement of Groups," *Wilson's Photographic Magazine* 45 (Oct. 1908):453–59.

2. Albert Edward Sterner (1863–1946), American portrait painter and book and magazine illustrator. See Hartmann's essay on Sterner in his column, "Art and Artists," *Musical America* 1 (Nov. 1898):31.

3. See Chap. 10, Note 13.

4. See Chap. 10, Note 13.

5. Henry Rankin Poore (1859–1940), author of *Pictorial Composition and Critical Judgment of Pictures.*

6. Alon Bement (1878–1954), painter, educator, and author of *Figure Composition* (New York, Chicago: The Gregg Publishing Co., 1921).

7. Otto Walter Beck (1864–1938), art and photographic critic. Author of *Art Principles in Portrait Photography* (Chicago: The Photo-Beacon Co., 1897–1899).

8. F. Dundas Todd (1858–1926), editor of *The Photo-Beacon* and author of *A Reference Book in Practical Photography* (Chicago: The Photo-Beacon Co., 1897–99).

38. E. S. CURTIS: PHOTO-HISTORIAN

1. Edward S. Curtis, *The North American Indian* (Seattle: E. S. Curtis; Cambridge: The University Press, 1907–1930), 20 vol.

2. See Chap. 13, Note 8.

3. See Chap. 7, Note 7.

4. Adolf Schreyer (1826–1899), German painter, primarily of military scenes, mostly involving cavalry, and of North African scenes, featuring Arabian horses.

5. Carl [Karl] Ferdinand Wimar (1829–1863), German-born American painter, who worked in St. Louis, and sketched various frontier scenes along the Missouri River.

6. Walter Shirlaw (1838–1932), American painter, muralist, and illustrator, who painted the Crow and Northern Cheyenne, while serving as a special agent on the U.S. Census of 1890 of the Indians.

7. Gilbert Gaul (1855–1932), American painter and illustrator, known for his battle scenes. In September, 1890, while serving as a special agent on the U.S. Census of Indians, Gaul painted a portrait of Sitting Bull a few months before the chieftain's death.

8. William de la Montagne Cary (1840–1922), prominent western illustrator of the 1850s and 1860s, who captured many phases of frontier life. His work appeared in *Harper's Weekly, Leslie's Weekly, Scribner's,* and other magazines.

9. Henry T. Farny (1847–1916), American painter and illustrator, who had studios in Cincinnati, and made a specialty of Indian portraits and drawings.

10. Edwin Willard Deming (1860–1942), American painter, whose first training as a professional artist occurred in 1887 when he visited the Apaches and the Pueblos in the Southwest and the Umatillas in Oregon. De Cost Smith and Deming traveled together in the 1890s, sketching the Sioux and Crow Indians.

11. E. W. D. Hamilton (1862–?), Boston painter, best known for his painting titled "Canal, Venice" in the Boston Museum of Fine Arts.

12. Not identified by the editors.

13. De Cost Smith (1864–1939), American painter, who lived among various Indian tribes, including the Sioux, Crow, Omaha, and Winnebago, studying their customs and languages and painting and sketching them.

14. See Chap. 6, Note 5. Although living most of his life in France and best known for his genre scenes of Brittany, Mosler visited Santa Fe in 1886 with two commissions for Indian paintings.

15. Both Gertrude Käsebier and Elias Goldensky made a number of portraits of Indians. Käsebier's best known Indian portrait is titled "Lone Bear."

39. PIRIE MacDONALD: PSYCHOLOGY IN PORTRAITURE

1. See Chap. 1, Note 13.

2. See Chap. 1, Note 5.

3. See Chap. 1, Note 18.

4. Jacob Riis (1849–1914), noted journalist and reformer, who in waging battle against conditions in New York tenements first enlisted photography as a weapon in reform. His *How the Other Half Lives* (1890) resulted in child labor laws, elimination of New York's worst slum, and other reforms.

40. BESSIE BEUHRMANN: UNDER THE INFLUENCE OF THE SECESSION

1. Hartmann's first extended visit to Elbert Hubbard's semi-communal Roycroft colony at East Aurora, New York, occurred in the summer of 1907. He participated in a socialist symposium on the night of July 13, which featured Hartmann and Carl Sandburg as guest speakers. Between 1911 and 1916 Hartmann lived intermittently at East Aurora, where he undertook ghost-writing assignments for Hubbard. It was there he met his second wife, Lillian Bonham. See Charles Hamilton, "The Roycroft Period: Hartmann, Hubbard, and East Aurora," *Sadakichi Hartmann Newsletter* 2 (Spring 1907):1–5.

2. See Chap. 11, Note 15.

3. See "Sadakichi Hartmann," a portrait by Edward J. Steichen, *Camera Work*, No. 7 (July 1904), [4].

41. MEREDITH JANVIER: WITH A RUSH

1. In 1872 George Davison and other artistic photographers seceded from the Royal Photographic Society of Great Britain and founded the Linked Ring Brotherhood, whose international exhibitions were the most important events in the photographic world up to 1914.

2. William Notman (1826–1891), Canada's first internationally known photographer; his studio, William Notman and Son, was based in Montreal and had branches in several cities, including New York and Boston.

42. F. BENEDICT HERZOG: A MASTER OF DECORATIVE COMPOSITION

1. See Christian Brinton, "Herzog's Decorative Photographs," *The Century Magazine* 44 (May 1907):81–87.

2. See Chap. 1, Note 34.

3. Anthony Adam-Salomon (1818–1881), Parisian photographer who contributed outstanding portraits of contemporary celebrities to the *Galerie Contemporaine*.

4. Oscar G. Rejlander (1813–1875), great Swedish photographer, noted for his allegorical compositions.

43. FREDERICK L. MONSEN: THE STAMP OF REALITY

1. See Chap. 38, Note 6.

2. See Chap. 38, Note 7. Hartmann is alluding to their role as special agents in the U.S. Census of 1890 of Indians.

3. See Chap. 38, Note 4.

4. See Chap. 38, Note 5.

5. See Chap. 38, Note 8.

6. See Chap. 38, Note 9.

7. See Chap. 38, Note 10.

8. See Chap. 38, Note 12.

9. Charles Schreyvogel (1861–1912), American painter, most of whose canvasses dealt with cavalry soldiers on the frontier. He was catapulted into sudden popularity at the turn of the century for his painting "My Bunkie" (1899).

10. Frederick Remington (1861–1902), the best known and greatest of all American painters and illustrators of the Old West.

11. See Chap. 38, Note 13.

12. See Chap. 7, Note 7.

13. Louis B. Akin (1868–1913), American painter who specialized in Indians and decorated the Southwestern Room at the American Museum of Natural History in New York City.

14. See Chap. 38, Note 14.

15. William de Leftwich Dodge (1867–1935), American mural painter, known for his classic themes and ornate decorative compositions. See Hartmann's discussion of Dodge in his column, "Art and Artists," *Musical America* 1 (December 10, 1898):39.

16. Henry Kirke Bush-Brown (1857–1935), sculptor, best known for his "Indian Buffalo Hunt," exhibited at the Chicago Exposition of 1893.

17. Cyrus Edwin Dallin (1861–1944), American sculptor,

particularly of Indian subjects. His works include two equestrian statues, "The Medicine Man" and "A Signal for Peace," and the life-size nude "The Indian Hunter." See Hartmann's *Modern American Sculpture* (New York: The Architectural Book Company, 1918).

18. Hermon Atkins MacNeil (1907–?), American sculptor, who executed many monuments and assisted in the decoration of buildings for the World's Columbian Exposition in Chicago in 1893.

19. See Chap. 13, Note 8.

20. Ferdinand Harvey Lungren (1872–1932), American magazine illustrator.

21. See Monsen's own essay, "Picturing Indians with the Camera," *Photo-Era* 25 (Oct. 1910):165–72. See also Monsen's "The Colorado Desert and the Colorado Delta," *Camera Craft* 5 (May 1902):1–8.

45. MAUDE WILSON: POET OF SUNSHINE AND MIST

1. Leon Dabo (1868–1960), American landscape and mural painter.

2. Edmund Henry Wuerpel (1866–?), American painter.

3. Albert Pike Lucas (1862?–1945), American painter and sculptor.

46. J. E. MOCK: A STUDY IN BACKGROUNDS

1. See Chap. 6, Note 12.

2. Bullard is probably a typographical error for Bullock. See Chap. 10, Note 11.

3. See Chap. 37, Notes 5 and 7.

SADAKICHI HARTMANN: A PHOTOGRAPHIC BIBLIOGRAPHY

Extensive as this bibliography of Sadakichi Hartmann's photographic writings may appear, there are still areas which might profitably yield further citations. Several foreign and American periodicals were not available to us for consultation or were seen only in broken runs. In addition, no thorough search was made of newspapers. Scrapbooks in the Wistaria Hartmann Linton Collection at the University of California, Riverside, indicate that Hartmann wrote about the arts for newspapers in many major American cities. Undoubtedly, some of these newspapers contain articles by Hartmann on photography.

Although many articles on arts other than photography are included here, such entries are confined to those appearing in photographic periodicals, such as *Camera Notes* and *Camera Work*, where Hartmann was writing for an essentially photographic audience. Although ostensibly about other arts, such essays are often concerned with the relationship between art and photography—a relationship which Hartmann particularly explored in *The Whistler Book* (1910). The wisest course in selection, therefore, appeared to be to include all publications by Hartmann from the photographic press.

The first section of the bibliography contains all articles written by Hartmann under his own name or pseudonyms; all unsigned articles attributed to Hartmann are presented in the second section. Publications by other authors in which Hartmann is mentioned and those of an associational nature are presented in the third section. Often a brief annotation in brackets follows an entry to clarify a source of possible confusion or to provide additional information. Essays appearing in the text of this volume are noted with an asterisk preceding the entry, which is then followed by a bracketed reference to the chapter number.

The bibliography would not have been possible without the aid and encouragement of many people. I particularly wish to thank the General Reference and Humanities Staff of the New York Public Library for two years of continuous assistance in compiling bibliographic data. I also want to express appreciation to the reference staffs of the San Francisco Public Library, the Los Angeles Public Library, the University of California Library at Berkeley, the University of Texas Library at Austin, the Boston Public Library, the Library of the Philadelphia Museum of Art, the Library Company of Philadelphia, the Pennsylvania Historical Society, the St. Louis Public Library, the University of Southern California Library, and the Riverside Public Library.

My special gratitude goes to Miss Gladys Finley of the California State Library at Sacramento, who worked hard and long to expedite interlibrary loans of literally hundreds of volumes from which came much of this bibliography. Assisting in a similarly arduous capacity were Mrs. Hazel Schupbach and the Interlibrary Loan Staff at the University of California, Riverside, and Diane Bennett, Gail Dameworth, Bernita Ginsburg, and Jim Robison of the Bio-Agricultural Library of the College of Natural and Agricultural Sciences, University of California, Riverside. Other important assistance came from Mrs. Hilda Bohem, Special Collections, University of California at Los Angeles; Mr. Richard Dillon of the Sutro Library, San Francisco; Miss Aileen Pringle and Mr. F. W. Howton, both of New York City; Mr. Robert Lang, associate university librarian, and Mrs. Betty Lang, English Department bibliographer, both at the University of California, Riverside; and Roger P. Hull, associate professor of art, Willamette University.

I should also like to express my appreciation for numerous favors to the International Museum of Photography, George Eastman House, Rochester, New York, and specific indebtedness to Mr. Dennis Longwell, assistant curator of photography at the Museum of Modern Art. Finally, I want to thank George Knox and Harry Lawton for their innumerable suggestions and contributions.

—MICHAEL J. ELDERMAN

I. BIBLIOGRAPHY OF THE PHOTOGRAPHIC PUBLICATIONS OF SADAKICHI HARTMANN

ALLAN, SIDNEY. [Pseud.] "A. T. Proctor—A Maker of Exhibition Prints." *Wilson's Photog. Mag.* 44 (April 1907):169–71.

———. "Academic Portraiture: Pirie MacDonald." *Wilson's Photog. Mag.* 43 (Oct. 1906):440–42.

———. "Advance in Artistic Photography." *Leslie's Weekly* 98 (28 April 1904):388–89.

———. Advertisement. Endorsement for the Ansco Company, Binghamton, New York. *Abel's Photog. Weekly* 9 (15 Feb. 1913):145.

———. "After a Snowstorm." *The Photog. Times* 35 (March 1903):97–104. [Illustrated by Rudolf Eickemeyer, Jr.]

°———. "Alvin Langdon Coburn—Secession Portraiture." *Wilson's Photog. Mag.* 44 (June 1907):251–52. [See Chap. 36.]

———. "The Annual Exhibition of the Wilkes-Barre Camera Club." *The Photog. Times* 42 (June 1910):216–21.

———. "An Appreciation of C. H. Davis." *The Camera* 13 (Oct. 1909):347–50.

———. "Appreciation Overdone." *Wilson's Photog. Mag.* 45 (Nov. 1908):482.

———. "Art in Child-Portraiture." *Smith's Mag.* (1907), pp. 472–75. [Part of a "Special Art Insert in this number."]

———. "Art Principles in Portrait Photography, By Otto Walter Beck. Review by Sidney Allan." *Wilson's Photog. Mag.* 44 (July 1907):313–15.

°———. "Bessie Buehrmann—Under the Influence of the Secession." *The Photog. Times* 39 (Nov. 1907):435–41. [See Chap. 40.]

———. "The Book as a Point of Interest." *Bull. of Photog.* 10 (7 Feb. 1912):164–66.

———. "The Boss of the Family." *Bull. of Photog.* 10 (28 Feb. 1912):262–64.

———. "Bread and Butter Talks. Give Your Customers What They Want." *Bull. of Photog. and the Photographer* 5 (8 Sept. 1909):155.

———. "Bread and Butter Talks. On Amateurs." *Bull. of Photog. and the Photographer* 5 (15 Sept. 1909):167.

———. "Bread and Butter Talks. On Management." *Bull. of Photog. and the Photographer* 5 (8 Sept. 1909):155.

———. "Bread and Butter Talks. On Prices." *Bull. of Photog. and the Photographer* 5 (15 Sept. 1909):167. [Byline omitted.]

———. "Bread and Butter Talks. On Success." *Bull. of Photog. and the Photographer* 5 (22 Sept. 1909):186.

———. "Bread and Butter Talks. What to Study." *Bull. of Photog. and the Photographer* 5 (22 Sept. 1909):186.

°———. "Burr McIntosh, Photographer of Fads and Fancies." *Wilson's Photog. Mag.* 44 (March 1907):99–101. [See Chap. 34.]

°———. "Byron—'The Stage is My Studio,'" *Wilson's Photog. Mag.* 44 (Jan. 1907):25–28. [See Chap. 33.]

———. "Camera Impressionism. Dr. Arnold Genthe." *The Camera* 14 (Dec. 1910):503–09.

———. "The Camera in a Country Lane." *Scribner's Mag.* 31 (June 1902):679–88. [Illustrated by Rudolf Eickemeyer, Jr.]

———. "Children at Play." *Bull. of Photog.* 10 (17 Jan. 1912):68–71.

———. "Clearness of Interpretation." *Bull. of Photog.* 16 (14 April 1915):456–59.

———. "Color Photography at the New York State Association." *Bull. of Photog.* 10 (6 March 1912):298–99.

———. "Comparative Portraiture." *Wilson's Photog. Mag.* 44 (March 1907):129–32. [Originally "An Address given before the students of the Milton Waide School of Photography, New York."]

———. "Composition by Repetition of Shapes." *Bull. of Photog.* 10 (12 June 1912):792–94.

———. "Composition and the Functions of the Eye. The Laws of Vision as Applied to Portraiture. I. The Mechanism of Vision." *Portrait* 8 (Jan. 1917):6–11.

———. "Composition and the Functions of the Eye. II. The Laws of Vision as Applied to Portraiture. II. The Pyramid Form." *Portrait* 8 (Feb. 1917):7–13.

———. "Composition and the Functions of the Eye. III. Triangular Vision." *Portrait* 8 (March 1917):6–12.

———. "Composition and the Functions of the Eye. IV. Circular and Oval Forms." *Portrait* 8 (April 1917):6–12.

———. "Composition and the Functions of the Eye. V. Preferred Shapes." *Portrait* 9 (May 1917):6–12.

———. "Composition and the Functions of the Eye. VI. Elements of Space Arrangement." *Portrait* 9 (June 1917):9–14.

———. "Composition and the Functions of the Eye. VII. Rectangular Arrangements." *Portrait* 9 (July 1917):5–10.

———. "Composition and the Functions of the Eye. VIII. Irregular Arrangements." *Portrait* 9 (Aug. 1917):4–9.

———. "Composition and the Functions of the Eye. IX. Likeness, Facial Expression, and Character Interpretation." *Portrait* 9 (Sept. 1917):611.

———. "Composition and the Functions of the Eye. X. The Perception of Light and Shade." *Portrait* 9 (Oct. 1917):6–11.

———. "Composition and the Functions of the Eye. XI. Contrast, Diffusion, and Detail." *Portrait* 9 (Nov. 1917):7–13.

———. "Composition and the Functions of the Eye. XII. The Balance of Parts and Motions." *Portrait* 9 (Dec. 1917):8–13.

°The asterisk precedes entries for all essays appearing in this volume.

————. "Composition in Child Photography." *Wilson's Photog. Mag.* 46 (Jan. 1909):22–27.

————. *Composition in Portraiture.* New York: Edward L. Wilson, 1909.

————. "Composition in Portraiture. Introduction to a Series of Articles on the Law of Composition." *Wilson's Photog. Mag.* 45 (Jan. 1908):25–28. [The series was reprinted in the book cited above.]

————. "Composition in Portraiture—The Placing of the Head." *Wilson's Photog. Mag.* 45 (Feb. 1908):70–76.

————. "Composition in Portraiture—The Profile View." *Wilson's Photog. Mag.* 45 (March 1908):117–23.

————. "Composition in Portraiture—The Full Face and Three Quarter View. Part I." *Wilson's Photog. Mag.* 45 (April 1908):166–71.

————. "Composition in Portraiture—The Full Face and Three Quarter View. Part II." *Wilson's Photog. Mag.* 45 (May 1908):214–19.

————. "Composition in Portraiture. Chapter IV. The Management of Hands." *Wilson's Photog. Mag.* 45 (June 1908):260–71.

————. "Composition in Portraiture. Chapter V. Standing Positions." *Wilson's Photog. Mag.* 45 (July 1908):310–15.

————. "Composition in Portraiture—On Sitting Positions." *Wilson's Photog. Mag.* 45 (Aug. 1908):358–63.

————. "Composition in Portraiture—On Backgrounds." *Wilson's Photog. Mag.* 45 (Sept. 1908):405–11.

————. "Composition in Portraiture—On the Arrangement of Groups." *Wilson's Photog. Mag.* 45 (Oct. 1908):454–59.

————. "Composition in Portraiture—On Tone and Values." *Wilson's Photog. Mag.* 45 (Nov. 1908):502–06.

————. "Composition in Portraiture—On Light Effects." *Wilson's Photog. Mag.* 45 (Dec. 1908):558–63.

————. "Constructive Criticism—No. 1. A Weekly Pictorial Review." *Bull. of Photog. and the Photographer* 4 (16 June 1909):376–77. [On the work of Rudolf Dührkoop.]

————. "Constructive Criticism—No. 2. A Weekly Pictorial Review." *Bull. of Photog. and the Photographer* 4 (23 June 1909):392–93. [On the work of Hugo Erfurt and Jacob Hilsdorf.]

————. "Constructive Criticism—No. 3. A Weekly Pictorial Review." *Bull. of Photog. and the Photographer* 4 (30 June 1909):408–09. [On the work of H. J. Springer and Rudolf Dührkoop.]

————. "Constructive Criticism—No. 4. A Weekly Pictorial Review." *Bull. of Photog. and the Photographer* 5 (7 July 1909):4–5. [On the work of Herman Link and Rudolf Dührkoop.]

————. "Constructive Criticism—No. 5. A Weekly Pictorial Review." *Bull. of Photog. and the Photographer* 5 (14 July 1909):17–18, 26. [On the work of Paul Fournier and H. H. Pierce.]

————. "Constructive Criticism—No. 6. A Weekly Pictorial Review." *Bull. of Photog. and the Photographer* 5 (21 July 1909):33–34, 36. [On the work of Elizabeth Flint Wade & Rose Clark and W. M. Van der Weyde.]

————. "Constructive Criticism—No. 7. A Weekly Pictorial Review." *Bull. of Photog. and the Photographer* 5 (28 July 1909):49, 52. [On the work of W. M. Van der Weyde and Rudolf Dührkoop.]

————. "Constructive Criticism—No. 8. A Weekly Pictorial Review." *Bull. of Photog. and the Photographer* 5 (4 Aug. 1909):65, 69. [On the work of Morris Burke Parkinson and Paul Fournier.]

————. "Constructive Criticism—No. 9. A Weekly Pictorial Review." *Bull. of Photog. and the Photographer* 5 (11 Aug. 1909):81, 84. [On the work of Otto Scharf and Robert Demachy.]

————. "Constructive Criticism—No. 10. A Weekly Pictorial Review." *Bull. of Photog. and the Photographer* 5 (18 Aug. 1909):97–98, 100. [On the work of Davis & Eickemeyer and Pirie MacDonald.]

————. "Constructive Criticism—No. 11. A Weekly Pictorial Review." *Bull. of Photog. and the Photographer* 5 (25 Aug. 1909):113, 116. [On the work of Paul Fournier and Rudolf Dührkoop.]

————. "Constructive Criticism—No. 12. A Weekly Pictorial Review." *Bull. of Photog. and the Photographer* 5 (1 Sept. 1909):130, 135. [On the work of S. H. Lifshey and Gustave Lorey.]

————. "Constructive Criticism—No. 13. A Weekly Pictorial Review." *Bull. of Photog. and the Photographer* 5 (8 Sept. 1909):146, 152–53. [On the work of S. H. Lifshey and Curtis Bell.]

————. "Constructive Criticism—No. 14. A Weekly Pictorial Review." *Bull. of Photog. and the Photographer* 5 (15 Sept. 1909):164–65. [On the work of W. M. Van der Weyde and Wm. Shewell Ellis.]

————. "Constructive Criticism—No. 15. A Weekly Pictorial Review." *Bull. of Photog. and the Photographer* 5 (22 Sept. 1909):181–82. [On the work of Curtis Bell and Pirie MacDonald.]

————. "Constructive Criticism—No. 16. A Weekly Pictorial Review." *Bull. of Photog. and the Photographer* 5 (29 Sept. 1909):193, 196. [On the work of B. J. Falk and Curtis Bell.]

————. "Constructive Criticism—No. 17. A Weekly Pictorial Review." *Bull. of Photog. and the Photographer* 5 (6 Oct. 1909):214–15. [On the work of Mishkin and W. M. Van der Weyde.]

————. "Constructive Criticism—No. 18. A Weekly Pictorial Review." *Bull. of Photog. and the Photographer* 5 (13 Oct. 1909):230–31. [On the work of J. C. Strauss and W. M. Van der Weyde.]

————. "Constructive Criticism—No. 19. A Weekly Pictorial Review." *Bull. of Photog. and the Photographer* 5 (20 Oct. 1909):248–49. [On the work of H. H. Pierce and William Orpen.]

———. "Constructive Criticism—No. 20. A Weekly Pictorial Review." *Bull. of Photog. and the Photographer* 5 (27 Oct. 1909):266–67. [On the work of Pirie MacDonald and Eastman Johnson.]

———. "Constructive Criticism—No. 21. A Weekly Pictorial Review." *Bull. of Photog. and the Photographer* 5 (3 Nov. 1909):278–79. [On the work of Leopold Horowitz and C. Puyo.]

———. "Constructive Criticism—No. 22. A Weekly Pictorial Review." *Bull. of Photog. and the Photographer* 5 (10 Nov. 1909):290–95. [On the work of H. J. Springer and Carl Frederiksen.]

———. "Constructive Criticism—No. 23. A Weekly Pictorial Review." *Bull. of Photog. and the Photographer* 5 (17 Nov. 1909):310–11. [On the work of Curtis Bell and Alfred Krauth.]

———. "Constructive Criticism—No. 24. A Weekly Pictorial Review." *Bull. of Photog. and the Photographer* 5 (8 Dec. 1909):358–59. [On the work of S. H. Lifshey.]

———. "Constructive Criticism—No. 25. A Weekly Pictorial Review." *Bull. of Photog. and the Photographer* 5 (15 Dec. 1909):374–75. [On paintings by W. M. Chase and Dawson Watson.]

———. "Constructive Criticism—No. 25 [sic: No. 26]. A Weekly Pictorial Review." *Bull. of Photog. and the Photographer* 5 (22 Dec. 1909):390–92. [On a painting of Franz von Lenbach, and the work of Clarence H. White and Bessie Buehrmann.]

———. "Constructive Criticism—No. 26 [sic: No. 27]. A Weekly Pictorial Review." *Bull. of Photog. and the Photographer* 6 (5 Jan. 1910):4. [On the work of S. H. Lifshey and Davis & Eickemeyer.]

———. "Constructive Criticism—No. 27 [sic: No. 28]. A Weekly Pictorial Review." *Bull. of Photog. and the Photographer* 6 (12 Jan. 1910):26. [On the work of S. H. Lifshey and Mrs. Jeanne E. Bennett.]

———. "Constructive Criticism—No. 28 [sic: No. 29]. A Weekly Pictorial Review." *Bull. of Photog. and the Photographer* 6 (26 Jan. 1910): 59. [On the work of Curtis Bell and Rose Clark & Elizabeth Flint Wade.]

———. "Constructive Criticism—No. 29 [sic: No. 30]. A Weekly Pictorial Review." *Bull. of Photog. and the Photographer* 6 (2 Feb. 1910): 76–77. [On the work of B. J. Falk and S. H. Lifshey.]

———. "Constructive Criticism—No. 30 [sic: No. 31]. A Weekly Pictorial Review." *Bull. of Photog. and the Photographer* 6 (9 Feb. 1910):91. [On the work of H. H. Pierce and W. M. Van der Weyde.]

———. "Constructive Criticism—No. 31 [sic: No. 32]. A Weekly Pictorial Review." *Bull. of Photog. and the Photographer* 6 (16 Feb. 1910):frontis., 105. [On the work of Davis & Eickemeyer and Leachy.]

———. "Constructive Criticism—No. 32 [sic: No. 33]. A Weekly Pictorial Review." *Bull. of Photog. and the Photographer* 6 (23 Feb. 1910):frontis., 122. [On the work of A. Marshall and Mishkin.]

———. "Constructive Criticism—No. 33 [sic: No. 34]. A Weekly Pictorial Review." *Bull. of Photog. and the Photographer* 6 (2 March 1910):frontis., 140. [On a painting of F. H. Tompkins and the work of Franz Grainer.]

———. "Constructive Criticism—No. 34 [sic: No. 35]. A Weekly Pictorial Review." *Bull. of Photog. and the Photographer* 6 (9 March 1910):frontis., 154. [On the work of Davis & Eickemeyer and Franz von Lenbach.]

———. "Constructive Criticism—No. 35 [sic: No. 36]. A Weekly Pictorial Review." *Bull. of Photog. and the Photographer* 6 (16 March 1910):172. [On the work of E. Gaiduschek.]

———. "Constructive Criticism—No. 36 [sic: No. 37]. A Weekly Pictorial Review." *Bull. of Photog. and the Photographer* 6 (23 March 1910):frontis., 186. [On the paintings of A. P. Lucas and Wm. M. Chase.]

———. "Constructive Criticism—No. 37 [sic: No. 38]. A Weekly Pictorial Review." *Bull. of Photog. and the Photographer* 6 (30 March 1910):202. [On the paintings of Max Koner and Franz von Lenbach.]

———. "Constructive Criticism—No. 38 [sic: No. 39]. A Weekly Pictorial Review." *Bull. of Photog. and the Photographer* 6 (6 April 1910):220. [On the work of Coubillier and Anonymous.]

———. "Constructive Criticism—No. 36 [sic: No. 40]. A Weekly Pictorial Review." *Bull. of Photog. and the Photographer* 6 (11 May 1910):298–99. [On the work of Renée Le Bègue and Hugo Erfurth.]

———. "Constructive Criticism—No. 37 [sic: No. 41]. A Weekly Pictorial Review." *Bull. of Photog. and the Photographer* 6 (18 May 1910): 316–17. [On the work of Rudolf Dührkoop and E. Gaiduschek.]

———. "Constructive Criticism—No. 38 [sic: No. 42]. [A] Weekly Pictorial Review." *Bull. of Photog. and the Photographer* 7 (20 July 1910):34, 42. [On the work of Davis & Eickemeyer.]

———. "Constructive Criticism—No. 39 [sic: No. 43]. [A] Weekly Pictorial Review." *Bull. of Photog. and the Photographer* 7 (31 Aug. 1910):134–135. [On the work of E. Gaiduschek.]

———. "Constructive Criticism—No. 39 [sic: No. 44]. [A] Weekly Pictorial Review." *Bull. of Photog. and the Photographer* 7 (7 Sept. 1910):146, 154. [On the work of W. McLean and Guido Rey.]

———. "Constructive Criticism—No. 41 [sic: No. 45]. [A] Weekly Pictorial Review." *Bull. of Photog. and the Photographer* 7 (14 Sept. 1910):166–67. [On the work of Rudolf Dührkoop and S. H. Lifshey.]

———. "Constructive Criticism—No. 42 [sic: No. 46]. [A] Weekly Pictorial Review." *Bull. of Photog. and the Photographer* 7 (21 Sept. 1910):187. [On a painting of Frans Hals and the work of Peter Orr.]

———. "Constructive Criticism—No. 43 [sic: No. 47]. [A] Weekly Pictorial Review." *Bull. of Photog. and the Photographer* 7 (28 Sept. 1910):frontis., 203. [On the work of Nicola Perscheid and Guido Rey.]

———. "Constructive Criticism—No. 43 [sic: No. 48]. [A] Weekly Pictorial Review." *Bull. of Photog. and the Photographer* 7 (5 Oct. 1910):218. [On the work of the Munich School.]

———. "Constructive Criticism—No. 44 [sic: No. 49]. [A] Weekly Pictorial Review." *Bull. of Photog. and the Photographer* 7 (12 Oct. 1910):234–35. [On the work of Anonymous and Rudolf Dührkoop.]

———. "Constructive Criticism—No. 45 [sic: No. 50]. [A] Weekly Pictorial Review." *Bull. of Photog. and the Photographer* 7 (26 Oct. 1910):294–95. [On the work of Guido Rey and E. T. Holding.]

———. "Constructive Criticism—No. 46 [sic: No. 51]. [A] Weekly Pictorial Review." *Bull. of Photog. and the Photographer* 7 (2 Nov. 1910):310–11. [On the work of Carine Cadby and D'Ora.]

———. "The Control of Expression and Attitude. How to Guide the Sitter Toward a Natural Expression. Introduction." *Portrait* 7 (Dec. 1915):6–9.

———. "The Control of Expression and Attitude. How to Guide the Sitter Toward a Natural Expression. I. The Look of Interest." *Portrait* 7 (Jan. 1916):6–11.

———. "The Control of Expression and Attitude. II. The Control of Facial Expression." *Portrait* 7 (Feb. 1916):3–8.

———. "The Control of Expression and Attitude. How to Guide the Sitter Toward a Natural Expression. III. The Mechanism of Movement in Standing Positions." *Portrait* 7 (March 1916):1–7.

———. "The Control of Expression and Attitude. How to Guide the Sitter Toward a Natural Expression. IV. How to Seat a Person Naturally." *Portrait* 7 (April 1916):4–12.

———. "The Control of Expression and Attitude. How to Guide the Sitter Toward a Natural Expression. V. On the Arrangement of Hands." *Portrait* 8 (May 1916):5–10.

———. "The Control of Expression and Attitude. How to Guide the Sitter Toward a Natural Expression. VI. How to Suggest Figure Poses to Women." *Portrait* 8 (June 1916):7–11.

———. "The Control of Expression and Attitude. How to Guide the Sitter Toward a Natural Expression. VII. How to Pose Young Women for Bust Portraits." *Portrait* 8 (July 1916):7–11.

———. "The Control of Expression and Attitude. How to Guide the Sitter Toward a Natural Expression. VIII. How to Manage Men for Figure Compositions." *Portrait* 8 (Aug. 1916):5–9.

———. "The Control of Expression and Attitude. How to Guide the Sitter Toward a Natural Expression. IX. How to Gain the Confidence of Children." *Portrait* 8 (Sept. 1916):4–9.

———. "The Control of Expression and Attitude. How to Guide the Sitter Toward a Natural Expression. X. How to Represent Brides' Dresses." *Portrait* 8 (Oct. 1916):6–10.

———. "The Control of Expression and Attitude. How to Guide the Sitter Toward a Natural Expression. XI. Mother and Child Pictures." *Portrait* 8 (Nov. 1916):9–13.

———. "The Control of Expression and Attitude. How to Guide the Sitter Toward a Natural Expression. XII. How to Direct Artistic Grouping." *Portrait* 8 (Dec. 1916):6–11.

———. "Correspondence." *The Photographer* 6 (16 April 1907):396. [Hartmann claims authorship of the article "Art Terms Explained," and denies that J. P. Chalmers wrote it. Also see Chalmers, J. P., below.]

———. "Criticism of Our Cover Design." *The Camera* 20 (April 1916):214.

———. "The Difficulty of Photographing Sculpture." *The Photog. Jour. of America* 60 (May 1923):163–72.

———. "Drapery in Portraiture." *Wilson's Photog. Mag.* 46 (May 1909):217–19.

°———. "E. S. Curtis, Photo Historian." *Wilson's Photog. Mag.* 44 (Aug. 1907):361–63. [See Chap. 38.]

———. "Eduard J. Steichen, Painter-Photographer." *Camera Notes* 6 (July 1902):15–16.

———. "Elaborate Figure Composition." *Bull. of Photog.* 10 (21 Feb. 1912):230–32.

———. "Elias Goldensky, Maker of Gum Prints." *Wilson's Photog. Mag.* 49 (June 1912):frontis., 257–67.

———. "Exhibition of Photographs by Members of the Camera Club of New York, April 13–30, 1904." *American Amateur Photog.* 16 (May 1904):207–09.

°———. "An Exquisite Temperament—B. J. Falk." *Wilson's Photog. Mag.* 43 (April 1906):146–49. [See Chap. 31.]

°———. "F. Benedict Herzog—A Master of Decorative Composition." *Wilson's Photog. Mag.* 44 (Dec. 1907):553–55. [See Chap. 42.]

———. "The Features of the Human Face. Introduction." *Portrait* 6 (Nov. 1914):5–6.

———. "The Features of the Human Face. I. The Forehead." *Portrait* 6 (Nov. 1914):7–11.

———. "The Features of the Human Face. II. The Eyebrows." *Portrait* 6 (Dec. 1914):6–8.

———. "The Features of the Human Face. III. The Eye." *Portrait* 6 (Jan. 1915):5–8.

———. "The Features of the Human Face. IV. The Eye in Profile." *Portrait* 6 (Feb. 1915):4–6.

———. "The Features of the Human Face. V. The Nose." *Portrait* (6 March 1915):10–12.

———. "The Features of the Human Face. VI. The Mouth." *Portrait* 6 (April 1915):9–12.

———. "The Features of the Human Face. VII. Wrinkles and the Cheek." *Portrait* 7 (May 1915):8–11.

———. "The Features of the Human Face. VIII. The Chin and the Ear." *Portrait* 7 (June 1915):10–13.

————. "The Features of the Human Face. IX. The Hair and the Beard." *Portrait* 7 (July 1915):10–13.

————. "The Features of the Human Face. X. The Neck." *Portrait* 7 (Aug. 1915):3–5.

————. "The Features of the Human Face. XI. Expressions of Pleasure." *Portrait* 7 (Sept. 1915):7–10.

————. "The Features of the Human Face. XII. Intellectual Expressions." *Portrait* 7 (Oct. 1915):10–13.

————. "The Feldman Studio, El Paso, Texas." *Bull. of Photog.* 18 (2 Feb. 1916):133–40.

————. "A Few American Portraits." *Wilson's Photog. Mag.* 49 (Oct. 1912):454–59.

————. "A Few Genre Subjects." *The Camera* 16 (May 1912):202–05.

————. "A Few Notes on Drapery." *Bull. of Photog.* 10 (27 March 1912):390–93.

————. "Five Minute Talks to Photographers—First Talk." *Bull. of Photog.* 13 (3 Dec. 1913):718.

————. "Five Minute Talks to Photographers—Second Talk." *Bull. of Photog.* 13 (10 Dec. 1913):755.

————. "Five Minute Talks to Photographers—Third Talk." *Bull. of Photog.* 13 (17 Dec. 1913):780.

————. "Five Minute Talks to Photographers—Fourth Talk." *Bull. of Photog.* 13 (24 Dec. 1913):814.

————. "Five Minute Talks to Photographers—Fifth Talk." *Bull. of Photog.* 13 (31 Dec. 1913):845.

————. "The 'Flat Iron' Building—An Esthetical Dissertation." *Camera Work*, No. 4 (Oct. 1903), pp. 36–40.

————. "Foreign Types." *Bull. of Photog.* 10 (1 May 1912):581–82.

°————. "Frederick I. Monsen." *The Photog. Times* 41 (Jan. 1909):79–82. [See Chap. 43.]

°————. "A German Pictorialist—Rudolph [sic] Dührkoop." *The Photog. Times* 39 (June 1907):243–51. [See Chap. 37.]

————. "A German Practitioner: A. Gottheil of Danzig." *Photo-Era* 34 (Feb. 1915):54–59.

°————. "Guido-Rey—A Master of Detail Composition." *The Photog. Times* 39 (March 1907):98–107. [See Chap. 35.]

————. "The Gum Process and its Proper Application." *Photo-Era* 19 (July 1907):3–4.

————. "Hats in Portraiture." *Wilson's Photog. Mag.* 46 (March 1909):118–22.

————. "The Head in Portraiture." *Wilson's Photog. Mag.* 46 (May 1909):207–16.

————. "Histed—Photographer of Celebrities." *Wilson's Photog. Mag.* 44 (Oct. 1907):457–59.

————. "The Hoffman Studio, Philadelphia, Pa." *Wilson's Photog. Mag.* 49 (Sept. 1912):frontis. (facing p. 385): 401–11.

————. "How to Make Large Heads: A New Phase of Photographic Portraiture." *Wilson's Photog. Mag.* 50 (March 1913):111–22.

————. "How Photographers May be Helped by the Study of Paintings: In Two Parts—Part I." *The Photog. Times* 40 (Oct. 1908):290–97.

————. "How Photographers May be Helped by the Study of Paintings: In Two Parts—Part II." *The Photog. Times* 40 (Nov. 1908):323–38.

————. "The Ideal Average—Charles H. Davis." *Wilson's Photog. Mag.* 43 (Jan. 1906):7–10.

°————. "In the Proletarian Interest: Elias Goldensky." *Wilson's Photog. Mag.* 42 (Dec. 1905):541–44. [See Chap. 29.]

————. "In Quest of Pictorial Incidents—River Scenes." *The Camera* 20 (June 1916):325–26.

————. "In Quest of Pictorial Incidents—A Few Words on Line Interest." *The Camera* 20 (July 1916):381–83.

————. "In Quest of Pictorial Incidents—Silhouette Effects in Landscape Work." *The Camera* 20 (Aug. 1916):431–33.

————. "In Quest of Pictorial Incidents—Various Methods of Figure Delineation." *The Camera* 20 (Sept. 1916):503–04.

————. "In Quest of Pictorial Incidents—How to Add a Special Interest to a Landscape." *The Camera* 20 (Oct. 1916):562–63.

————. "In Quest of Pictorial Incidents—The Picturesque Value of Tree-Trunks." *The Camera* 20 (Nov. 1916):616–19.

————. "In Quest of Pictorial Incidents—Have Pictorial Incidents an Artistic Significance?" *The Camera* 20 (Dec. 1916):675–77.

————. "In Quest of Pictorial Incidents—The Tang of the Sea." *The Camera* 21 (Jan. 1917):30–31.

————. "In Quest of Pictorial Incidents—Domestic Pets." *The Camera* 21 (Feb. 1917):96–98.

————. "In Quest of Pictorial Incidents—Snow as a Picture Maker." *The Camera* 21 (June 1917):293–94.

————. "In Quest of Pictorial Incidents—About a College Town." *The Camera* 21 (July 1917):331–33.

————. "In Quest of Pictorial Incidents—On Portraiture." *The Camera* 21 (Aug. 1917):389–92.

°————. "The Influence of Artistic Photography on Interior Decoration." *Camera Work*, No. 2 (April 1903):31–33. [See Chap. 8.]

————. "The Influence of Visual Perception on Conception and Technique." *Camera Work*, No. 3 (July 1903):23–26.

————. "John H. Garo—An Appreciation." *The Camera* 19 (April 1915):195–99.

————. "The Landscape Work of the Salon Club." *American Annual of Photog. and Photog. Times Almanac* 19 (1905):139–42.

————. "Letter to the Editor." *Wilson's Photog. Mag.* 44 (May 1907):240. [Claims the authorship of "Art Terms Explained": see Chalmers, J. P.]

————. "Local Subjects." *Bull. of Photog.* 10 (17 April 1912):504–07.

———. "Looking for the Good Points." *Bull. of Photog.* 17 (8 Sept. 1915):303–04. [On treatment of pictorial incidents, using the work of Frank S. Clark as illustration.]

———. "Looking for the Good Points. 'Child Portrait.' May L. Smith, Binghamton, N.Y." *Bull. of Photog.* 18 (22 March 1916):364–65.

———. "Looking for the Good Points. 'A Family Group.' Jane Reece, Dayton, O." *Bull. of Photog.* 18 (10 May 1916):588–89.

———. "Looking for the Good Points. 'Hortense.' Frederick Pohle, Buffalo, N.Y." *Bull. of Photog.* 18 (15 March 1916):330–31.

———. "Looking for the Good Points. 'An Idyllic Pastime.' Toloff, Evanston, Ill." *Bull. of Photog.* 17 (27 Oct. 1915):522–24.

———. "Looking for the Good Points. 'In the Library.' Elizabeth Schliepmann, St. Louis, Mo." *Bull. of Photog.* 18 (5 April 1916):430–31.

———. "Looking for the Good Points. 'Lou Tellegen.' Gledhill, Santa Barbara, Calif." *Bull. of Photog.* 18 (1 March 1916):270–71.

———. "Looking for the Good Points. 'Mother and Child.' May L. Smith, Binghamton, N.Y." *Bull. of Photog.* 17 (13 Oct. 1915):453–54.

———. "Looking for the Good Points. 'Mother and Infant.' W. E. Burnell, Buffalo, N.Y." *Bull. of Photog.* 18 (24 May 1916):654–55.

———. "Looking for the Good Points. 'Out of Door Group.' J. C. Strauss, St. Louis, Mo." *Bull. of Photog.* 17 (17 Nov. 1915):617–19.

———. "Looking for the Good Points. Portrait by R. C. Nelson, Hastings, Neb." *Bull. of Photog.* 17 (22 Sept. 1915):362–63, 365.

———. "Looking for the Good Points. 'Portrait.' Frank Scott Clark, Detroit, Mich." *Bull. of Photog.* 18 (3 May 1916):556–57, 559.

———. "Looking for the Good Points. 'Portrait.' Fred J. Feldman, El Paso, Tex." *Bull. of Photog.* 18 (14 June 1916):748–49.

———. "Looking for the Good Points. 'Portrait.' Helmar Lerski, Milwaukee, Wis." *Bull. of Photog.* 17 (10 Nov. 1915):585–86.

———. "Looking for the Good Points. 'Portrait.' L. J. Buckley, Binghamton, N.Y." *Bull. of Photog.* 17 (20 Oct. 1915):489–91.

———. "Looking for the Good Points. 'Portrait.' W. E. Burnell, Buffalo, N.Y." *Bull. of Photog.* 18 (12 April 1916):458, 460–61.

———. "Looking for the Good Points. 'Portrait of William J. Connors.' Frederick W. Pohle, Buffalo, N.Y." *Bull. of Photog.* 17 (3 Nov. 1915):550–51.

———. "Looking for the Good Points. 'Rockabye Baby.' Knaffl Bros., Knoxville, Tenn." *Bull. of Photog.* 18 (17 May 1916):620–21.

———. "Looking for the Good Points. 'Ruth St. Denis.' J. D. Toloff, Evanston, Ill." *Bull. of Photog.* 18 (8 March 1916):298–99.

———. "Looking for the Good Points. 'Sisters.' Elizabeth Schliepmann, St. Louis, Mo." *Bull. of Photog.* 17 (29 Sept. 1915):388–90.

———. "Looking for the Good Points. 'Youngsters.' G. J. Sipprell, Buffalo, N.Y." *Bull. of Photog.* 18 (29 March 1916):396–97.

*———. "The Man Behind the Gun—J. C. Strauss." *Wilson's Photog. Mag.* 43 (July 1906):290–92. [See Chap. 32.]

———. "The Man With a System—W. M. Hollinger." *Wilson's Photog. Mag.* 43 (May 1906):201–04.

———. "The Man Without a Pose: S. L. Stein." *Wilson's Photog. Mag.* 43 (Dec. 1906):557–59.

———. "The Management of Hands." *The Photog. Jour. of America* 56 (Nov. 1919):548–53.

———. "Masterly Unfinish." *Bull. of Photog.* 10 (10 April 1912):473–75.

———. "Masterpieces of American Portraiture." *Bull. of Photog.* 16 (2 June 1915):684–86. [On the work of Richard E. Miller.]

———. "Masterpieces of American Portraiture." *Bull. of Photog.* 16 (9 June 1915):722–23. [On the work of Alden Weir.]

———. "Masterpieces of American Portraiture." *Bull. of Photog.* 16 (16 June 1915):747–48. [On the work of Gari Melchers.]

———. "Masterpieces of American Portraiture." *Bull. of Photog.* 16 (23 June 1915):780–81. [On the work of James J. Shannon.]

———. "Masterpieces of American Portraiture." *Bull. of Photog.* 16 (30 June 1915):810–11. [On the work of George B. Butler.]

———. "Masterpieces of American Portraiture." *Bull. of Photog.* 17 (7 July 1915):13–14. [On Whistler.]

———. "Masterpieces of American Portraiture." *Bull. of Photog.* 17 (14 July 1915):46–47. [On Sargent.]

———. "Masterpieces of American Portraiture." *Bull. of Photog.* 17 (21 July 1915):73–74. [On Robert McCameron.]

———. "Masterpieces of American Portraiture." *Bull. of Photog.* 17 (4 Aug. 1915):141–43. [On Thomas Eakins.]

———. "Masterpieces of American Portraiture." *Bull. of Photog.* 17 (11 Aug. 1915):175–78. [On William M. Chase.]

———. "Masterpieces of American Portraiture." *Bull. of Photog.* 17 (25 Aug. 1915):238–39. [On Louis Betts.]

———. "Masters in Portraiture—Edouard Manet." *Wilson's Photog. Mag.* 46 (Aug. 1909):358–63.

———. "Masters in Portraiture—Auguste Renoir." *Wilson's Photog. Mag.* 46 (Sept. 1909):406–11.

———. "Masters in Portraiture—Franz von Lenbach." *Wilson's Photog. Mag.* 46 (Oct. 1909):454–59.

———. "Masters in Portraiture—George Frederick Watts." *Wilson's Photog. Mag.* 46 (Nov. 1909):506–11.

———. "Masters in Portraiture—Hubert Herkomer." *Wilson's Photog. Mag.* 46 (Dec. 1909):550–55.

———. "Masters in Portraiture—Max Koner." *Wilson's Photog. Mag.* 47 (Jan. 1910):22–27.

———. "Masters in Portraiture—Friedrich August von Kaulbach." *Wilson's Photog. Mag.* 47 (Feb. 1910):70–74.

———. "Masters in Portraiture—Dante Gabriel Rossetti." *Wilson's Photog. Mag.* 47 (March 1910):118–23.

———. "Masters in Portraiture—James McNeil Whistler." *Wilson's Photog. Mag.* 47 (April 1910):166–71.

———. "Masters in Portraiture—John W. Alexander." *Wilson's Photog. Mag.* 47 (May 1910):214–18.

———. "Masters in Portraiture—Lucien Simon." *Wilson's Photog. Mag.* 47 (July 1910):310–15.

———. "Masters in Portraiture—Caro Delvaille." *Wilson's Photog. Mag.* 47 (Aug. 1910):358–63.

———. "Masters in Portraiture—W. Q. Orchardson." *Wilson's Photog. Mag.* 47 (Sept. 1910):407–11.

———. "Masters in Portraiture—Francisco Goya." *Wilson's Photog. Mag.* 47 (Oct. 1910):454–59.

———. "Masters in Portraiture—Thomas Gainsborough." *Wilson's Photog. Mag.* 47 (Nov. 1910):502–07.

———. "Masters in Portraiture—Wilhelm Leibl." *Wilson's Photog. Mag.* 47 (Dec. 1910):550–55.

———. "Masters in Portraiture—Joshua Reynolds." *Wilson's Photog. Mag.* 48 (Feb. 1911):70–75.

———. "Masters in Portraiture—Joshua Reynolds." *The Photog. Jour. of America* 54 (Feb. 1917):65–69. [Reprint of preceding article. Byline omitted.]

———. "Masters in Portraiture—Anton Van Dyck." *Wilson's Photog. Mag.* 48 (March 1911):166–70.

———. "Masters in Portraiture—Albrecht Durer." *Wilson's Photog. Mag.* 48 (June 1911):262–66.

———. "Masters in Portraiture—Jean Baptiste Greuze." *Wilson's Photog. Mag.* 48 (July 1911):310–14.

———. "Masters in Portraiture—Jean Baptiste Greuze." *The Photog. Jour. of America* 54 (March 1917):110–13. [Reprint of preceding article. Byline omitted.]

———. "Masters in Portraiture—Diego Velasquez." *Wilson's Photog. Mag.* 48 (Aug. 1911):358–63.

———. "Masters in Portraiture—Rembrandt." *Wilson's Photog. Mag.* 48 (Nov. 1911):502–07.

———. "Masters in Portraiture—Rembrandt." *The Photog. Jour. of America* 55 (Jan. 1917):18–22. [Reprint of preceding article. Byline omitted.]

———. "Masters in Portraiture—Gilbert Stuart." *Wilson's Photog. Mag.* 49 (Jan. 1912):19–27.

———. "Masters in Portraiture—De La Tour." *Wilson's Photog. Mag.* 49 (March 1912):118–22.

———. "Masters in Portraiture—Hans Holbein." *Wilson's Photog. Mag.* 49 (Aug. 1912):358–63.

———. "Masters in Portraiture—Hans Holbein." *The Photog. Jour. of America* 55 (Feb. 1918):64–67. [Reprint of preceding article. Byline omitted.]

———. "Masters in Portraiture—Peter Paul Rubens." *Wilson's Photog. Mag.* 49 (Nov. 1912):502–07.

———. "Masters in Portraiture—Titian." *Wilson's Photog. Mag.* 49 (Dec. 1912):550–54.

———. "Masters in Portraiture—Raphael." *Wilson's Photog. Mag.* 50 (Feb. 1913):70–74.

———. "Meredith Janvier—With a Rush." *Wilson's Photog. Mag.* 44 (Nov. 1907):494–500. [See Chap. 41.]

———. "Methods of Character Interpretation. Paper I. By Straightforward Realism." *Bull. of Photog.* 15 (21 Oct. 1914):518.

———. "Methods of Character Interpretation. Paper II. By Emphasis of Physiognomy." *Bull. of Photog.* 15 (11 Nov. 1914):614–16.

———. "Methods of Character Interpretation. Paper III. By Emphasis of Personality." *Bull. of Photog.* 15 (25 Nov. 1914):679.

———. "Methods of Character Interpretation. Paper IV. By Idealization." *Bull. of Photog.* 15 (9 Dec. 1914):741–42.

———. "Methods of Character Interpretation. Paper V. By Symbolization." *Bull. of Photog.* 15 (23 Dec. 1914):807–08.

———. "Methods of Character Interpretation. Part VI. By Manipulation." *Bull. of Photog.* 16 (6 Jan. 1915):7–8, 10.

———. "Methods of Character Interpretation. Part VII. By One Indirect Source of Light." *Bull. of Photog.* 16 (20 Jan. 1915):71–72, 74.

———. "Methods of Character Interpretation. Part VIII. By Diffused Light." *Bull. of Photog.* 16 (3 Feb. 1915):135–36, 138.

———. "Methods of Character Interpretation. Part IX. By Pictorial Treatment." *Bull. of Photog.* 16 (17 Feb. 1915):212–14.

———. "Methods of Character Interpretation. Part X. By Dress and Accessories." *Bull. of Photog.* 16 (3 March 1915):264–66.

———. "Methods of Character Interpretation. Part XI. By Decorative Treatment." *Bull. of Photog.* 16 (24 March 1915):360–63. ·

———. "Methods of Character Interpretation. Part XII. By Flat Treatment and Pattern Device." *Bull. of Photog.* 16 (7 April 1915):426–28.

———. "Milton Waide: One Man Method of Photography." *Wilson's Photog. Mag.* 44 (Feb. 1907):73–75.

———. "Modern Portraits." *Portrait* 9 (Jan. 1918):8–10. [On the work of Eduardo Chicharro.]

———. "A More Rapid Perception of Pictorial Possibilities." *Bull. of Photog.* 10 (19 June 1912):827–29.

———. "The Mother and Child Picture in Portraiture." *Wilson's Photog. Mag.* 46 (April 1909):166–70.

———. "Motion and Atmosphere." *Bull. of Photog.* 11 (2 Oct. 1912):494–97.

———. "Natural Picture Makers." *Bull. of Photog.* 15 (22 July 1914):102–06.

———. "A New Departure in Photography." *The Lamp* 28

(Feb. 1904):19–25. [On the work of Alvin Langdon Coburn.]

———. "A New European Departure." *The Photog. Jour. of America* 52 (Jan. 1915):33–35. [On the work of Charles Gerschel and the Dührkoops.]

———. "The New Kodachrome Process of Color Photography." *Bull. of Photog.* 16 (26 May 1915):654–55.

———. "A New Phase of Activity." *The Photog. Times* 36 (Oct. 1904):442–44. [On Curtis Bell and the First American Photographic Salon.]

———. "A New Power of Artistic Expression. The Pictorial Movement in Photography." *Smith's Mag.* (Jan. 1908), pp. 567–78.

———. "A Note on Louis Fleckenstein and His Work." *The Photog. Times-Bull.* 36 (Oct. 1904):433–37.

———. "The Old Man as Subject." *Bull. of Photog.* 10 (14 Feb. 1912):196–99.

———. "An Old Topic Once More. Discussion of Tonal Qualities." *The Photog. Times* 45 (Jan. 1913):8–15.

———. "On the Arrangement of Groups." *The Photog. Jour. of America* 57 (Jan. 1920):52–56.

———. "On the Arrangement of the Skirt in Portraiture." *Wilson's Photog. Mag.* 46 (Feb. 1909):70–74.

———. "On the Composition of Two-Figure Portraits." *Wilson's Photog. Mag.* 46 (July 1909):309–15.

———. "The One-Print Exhibition." *Wilson's Photog. Mag.* 44 (May 1907):217–19.

———. "On Exhibitions, Juries and Awards." *The Photographer* 7 (14 May 1907):36.

*———. "On Genre." *Camera Notes* 6 (July 1902):10–11. [See Chap. 6.]

———. "On Impressionism." *The Camera* 9 (July 1905): 254–58.

———. "On Pictorial and Illustrative Qualities." *Camera Notes* 6 (Dec. 1902):181–83.

———. "On Portraits of Actors in Parts." *Bull. of Photog.* 10 (20 March 1912):359–61.

———. "On Sitting Positions." *The Photog. Jour. of America* 57 (March 1920):98–102. [Essentially a reprint of article published under the same title by Sadakichi Hartmann with one additional paragraph.]

———. "On Strictly Commercial Lines. Theo. Marceau." *Wilson's Photog. Mag.* 43 (June 1906):269–71.

———. "On Tree Forms." *Bull. of Photog.* 10 (22 May 1912):681–84.

———. "On the Use of Furniture in Portraiture." *Wilson's Photog. Mag.* 46 (June 1909):262–67.

———. "On Vignetting." *Bull. of Photog.* 10 (24 Jan. 1912):103–06.

———. "An Open Letter." *In:* "An Answer to an Open Letter." *The Photographer* 7 (11 June 1907):100–02. [Allan's ltr. is on p. 100, the editor's response on pp. 100–02.]

———. "An Open Letter." *The Camera* 11 (June 1907):236–38. [An attack on the management of photographic conventions, the ltr. resulted in a long controversy.]

———. "An Open Letter From Sidney Allan." *Wilson's Photog. Mag.* 44 (June 1907):243–45.

*———. "A Painter Photographer—J. H. Garo." *Wilson's Photog. Mag.* 43 (March 1906):99–102. [See Chap. 30.]

———. "Perspective as a Means of Expression." *Bull. of Photog.* 10 (31 Jan. 1912):132–34.

———. "The Photographer in a Small Town." *Wilson's Photog. Mag.* 48 (Dec. 1911):550–55.

*———. "A Photographer of Japan—Arnold Genthe." *The Photog. Times* 42 (Dec. 1910):458–64. [See Chap. 44.]

———. "A Photographer of New York Society—A. F. Bradley." *Wilson's Photog. Mag.* 43 (Feb. 1906):57–59.

———. "The Photographer with an Artist's Temperament." *The Amer. Annual of Photog., 1914* 28 (1913):168–73. [On the work of Robert R. McGeorge.]

———. "Photography vs. Old Masters. Series I—A Few Madonna Pictures." *The Camera* 14 (March 1910):95–99.

———. "Photography vs. Old Masters. Series I—A Few Madonna Pictures." *Bull. of Photog.* 7 (9 Nov. 1910):323–25. [Reprinted (acknowledged) from *The Camera*.]

———. "Photography vs. Old Masters. Series II—The Choice of Subject." *The Camera* 14 (April 1910):127–33.

———. "Photography vs. Old Masters. Series II—The Choice of Subject." *Bull. of Photog.* 7 (23 Nov. 1910):353–54. [Reprinted (acknowledged) from *The Camera*.]

———. "Photography vs. Old Masters. Series III—The Principles of Portraiture." *The Camera* 14 (May 1910): 176–81.

———. "Photography vs. Old Masters. Series III—The Principles of Portraiture." *Bull. of Photog.* 7 (30 Nov. 1910):372–74. [Reprinted (acknowledged) from *The Camera*.]

———. "Photography vs. Old Masters. Series IV—The Conventions of Drapery." *The Camera* 14 (June 1910): 219–24.

———. "Photography vs. Old Masters. Series IV—The Conventions of Drapery." *Bull. of Photog.* 7 (7 Dec. 1910):385–87. [Reprinted (acknowledged) from *The Camera*.]

———. "Photography vs. Old Masters. Series V—A Few Remarks on the Nude." *The Camera* 14 (July 1910):269–74.

———. "Photography vs. Old Masters. Series V—A Few Remarks on the Nude." *Bull. of Photog.* 7 (14 Dec. 1910):406–08. [Reprinted (acknowledged) from *The Camera*.]

———. "Photography vs. Old Masters. Series VI—Fancy and Study Heads." *The Camera* 14 (August 1910):317–21.

———. "Photography vs. Old Masters. Series VI—Fancy and Study Heads." *Bull. of Photog.* 7 (21 Dec. 1910):418–

20. [Reprinted (acknowledged) from *The Camera*.]

————. "Picturesque New York, in Four Papers. The Esthetic Side of Jewtown." *Camera Notes* 6 (Feb. 1903):143–48. [The remaining three papers in this series were not published after *Camera Notes* ceased publication with this volume.]

————. "A Plea for Good Taste and Common Sense." *Wilson's Photog. Mag.* 42 (Sept. 1905):422–26. [Read before the National Convention of the Photographers' Association of America, in Boston, 10 August 1905.]

————. "A Plea for Good Taste and Common Sense." *Saint Louis and Canadian Photog.* 29 (Oct. 1905):452–58. [See above.]

————. "A Plea for Good Taste and Common Sense." *American Amateur Photog.* 17 (Oct. 1905):469–75. [See preceding.]

————. "A Plea for Localism." *The Camera* 9 (Dec. 1905):449–53.

————. "Pleasing Expressions: An Appreciation of the Working Methods of A. O. Titus, of Titus & Burnell, Buffalo, N.Y." *Bull. of Photog.* 17 (6 Oct. 1915):420–24.

°————. "A Poet of Sunshine and Mist—A Recorder of Atmosphere: Maude Wilson." *Photo-Era* 27 (Dec. 1911): 283–85. [See Chap. 45.]

————. "Pointers on Composition From Sidney Allan." *Wilson's Photog. Mag.* 47 (Feb. 1910):85.

————. "Pointers on Composition From Sidney Allan." *Abel's Photog. Weekly* 5 (25 June 1910):1–2. [Reprint of the preceding article.]

————. "The Popular Element in Pictures." *The Photog. Times* 40 (June 1908):162–69.

————. "The Popularity of the Dutch School." *Bull. of Photog.* 11 (31 July 1912):154–56.

————. "Popular Landscape Photography." *The Photog. Times* 47 (Sept. 1914):354–59.

————. "A Popular Woman Portraitist—Vigée-Le Brun." *Bull. of Photog.* 10 (3 April 1912):431–34.

————. "Portraits at the Paris Salon, 1910." *Wilson's Photog. Mag.* 47 (June 1910):262–67.

————. "Portraiture at the Buffalo Exhibition." *Wilson's Photog. Mag.* 47 (Dec. 1910):530–32.

————. "Portraiture and Picture Making." *Wilson's Photog. Mag.* 50 (May 1913):201–10.

————. "Possibilities—Figure Composition." *The Camera* 16 (Feb. 1912):59–64.

————. "'The Prince of Photographers,' Morris Burke Parkinson." *Wilson's Photog. Mag.* 42 (Nov. 1905):498–501.

————. "Print-in-Ground." *The Camera* 13 (Oct. 1909): 359–60.

————. "Print-in-Ground Backgrounds." *Bull. of Photog.* 5 (1 Sept. 1909):139.

————. "The Problem of Double Lighting." *Bull. of Photog.* 14 (20 May 1914):614–16.

————. "The Problem of Grouping." *Bull. of Photog.* 15 (12 Aug. 1914):198–200.

————. "The Problem of Perfect Illusion." *The Camera* 16 (April 1912):161–65.

————. "Professional Photography in Japan." *Bull. of Photog.* 11 (3 July 1912):13–20.

————. "A Professional Pictorialist—S. H. Lifshey." *The Camera* 9 (Oct. 1905):382–88.

————. "Professional Pictorialism. Illustrated by May L. Smith." *Wilson's Photog. Mag.* 50 (Nov. 1913):frontis., 449–51, 473–80.

°————. "Psychology in Portraiture." *Photo-Era* 19 (Aug. 1907):57–62. [On Pirie MacDonald; see Chap. 39.]

————. "The Recent Exhibition of the Photo-Secession Society." *Camera Craft* 8 (May 1904):243–48.

————. "Review of the Exhibition." *Bull. of Photog. and the Photographer* 4 (14 April 1909):235–36. [The Exhibition of the Professional Photographer's Society of N.Y., April 7, 8, 9, 1909.]

————. "Roaming in Thought (After Reading Maeterlinck's Letter)." *Camera Work*, No. 4 (Oct. 1903), pp. 21–24.

°————. "Rudolf Eickemeyer, Jr. An Appreciation." *Photo-Era* 15 (Sept. 1905):78–83. [See Chap. 25.]

————. "Sherril Schell, Portrait-Pictorialist." *Photo-Era* 28 (April 1912):141–45.

————. "Sidney Allan on Criticism." *Wilson's Photog. Mag.* 45 (Aug. 1908):339.

————. "The Silhouette Idea in Landscape Photography." *The Photog. Times* 47 (April 1915):139–47.

————. "Simple Separate Persons. Illustrated by the Lerski Studio." *Wilson's Photog. Mag.* 50 (Jan. 1913):17–26.

————. "Sir Thomas Lawrence, Portraitist." *Bull. of Photog.* 10 (13 March 1912):329–32.

————. "Some New Ideas in Picture Frames." *The Photog. Times* (Oct. 1913):21–29.

————. "Some New Ideas in Portrait Photography. A Visit to the Studio of Howard D. Beach, Buffalo." *Wilson's Photog. Mag.* 48 (Oct. 1911):449–59.

————. "Some Problems in Home Portraiture." *Photo-Miniature*, No. 12 (Sept. 1915), pp. 413–50.

————. "Some Whistler Etchings." *The Camera* 16 (June 1912):255–59.

————. "Standing Positions." *The Photog. Jour. of America* 57 (April 1920):139–42.

————. "Story Telling Photography. An Appreciation of H. B. Conyer's Work." *The Photog. Times* 40 (April 1908):98–105.

————. "Studio Bonaventura, Rome, Italy." *The Photog. Jour. of America* 52 (Sept. 1915):415–17, 419, 421, 423, 427, and facing p. 415.

————. "Studios of Sweet—An Appreciation." *The Camera* 19 (Aug. 1915):461–65.

°———. "A Study in Backgrounds." *Photo-Era* 31 (Nov. 1913):225–30. [On J. E. Mock. See Chap. 46.]

———. "A Summer Revery in the Woods." *The Photog. Times* 34 (Oct. 1902):432–41. [Illustrated by Rudolf Eickemeyer, Jr.]

———. "Talks on Composition. I—Training the Pictorial Sense." *Kodakery* 2 (April 1915):16–18.

———. "Talks on Composition. II—Emphasizing the Point of Central Interest." *Kodakery* 2 (May 1915):5–7.

———. "Talks on Composition. III—Controlling Shapes." *Kodakery* 2 (June 1915):12–14.

———. "Talks on Composition. IV—Reliable Formulae in Landscape Work." *Kodakery* 2 (July 1915):6–7.

———. "Talks on Composition. V—Avoid Unnecessary Detail." *Kodakery* 2 (Aug. 1915):12–14.

———. "Talks on Composition. VI—How to Obtain a Decorative Effect." *Kodakery* 3 (Sept. 1915):12–14.

———. "Talks on Composition. VII—Significance of Geometrical Shapes." *Kodakery* 3 (Oct. 1915):10–11.

———. "Talks on Composition. VIII—Foreground, Distance, and Middle Distance." *Kodakery* 3 (Nov. 1915):10–12.

———. "Talks on Composition. IX—On the Division of Light and Dark Planes." *Kodakery* 3 (Dec. 1915):18–20.

———. "Talks on Composition. X—The Pictorial Value of Shadows." *Kodakery* 3 (Jan. 1916):11–14.

———. "Talks on Composition. XI—Place Your Figures in Space." *Kodakery* 3 (Feb. 1916):13–14.

———. "Talks on Composition. XII—Have Your Values Correct." *Kodakery* 3 (March 1916):14–15.

———. "The Technique of Mystery and Blurred Effects." *Camera Work*, No. 7 (July 1904), pp. 24–26.

———. "Texture in Photography." *American Annual of Photog. and Photog. Times Almanac*, ed. Walter E. Woodberry 14 (1900):105–09.

———. "Three Self Portraits." *Bull. of Photog.* 10 (24 April 1912):539–41.

———. "The Towles Studio." *Wilson's Photog. Mag.* 45 (Nov. 1908):495–501.

°———. "A Travelling Photographer: H. H. Pierce." *Wilson's Photog. Mag.* 42 (Oct. 1905):450–53. [See Chap. 28.]

———. "Twenty-five Years of Photographic Activity." *Wilson's Photog. Mag.* 46 (Jan. 1909):2–3.

———. "The Unconventional in Portrait Photography." *Photo-Era* 13 (Aug. 1904):129–32.

———. "Unusual Portraiture." *Bull. of Photog.* 10 (29 May 1912):718–21.

———. "The Value of the Apparently Meaningless and Inaccurate." *Camera Work*, No. 3 (July 1903), pp. 17–18, 21.

°———. "A Visit to Steichen's Studio." *Camera Work*, No. 2 (April 1903), pp. 25–28. [See Chap. 27.]

———. "The Well-Made Print. Steffens." *Wilson's Photog. Mag.* 43 (Nov. 1906):498–500.

———. "What Is the Best Way to Take a Wedding Gown?" *Bull. of Photog.* 15 (1 July 1914):6–10.

———. "What Is a Camera Club?" *The Camera* 16 (March 1912):122–23.

———. "What Is the Commercial Value of Pictorial Prints?" *The Photog. Times-Bull.* 36 (Dec. 1904):539–41.

———. "What Photographers May Learn From the Old and New Masters. Paper I. On the Choice of Subjects." *The Photog. Times* 42 (Sept. 1910):332–41.

———. "What Photographers May Learn From the Old and New Masters. Paper II. On Interiors." *The Photog. Times* 42 (Oct. 1910):383–90.

———. "What Photographers May Learn From the Old and New Masters. Paper III. On the Nude." *The Photog. Times* 42 (Nov. 1910):420–26.

———. "What Photographers May Learn From the Old and New Masters. Paper IV. On Drapery." *The Photog. Times* 42 (Dec. 1910):471–78.

———. "White Backgrounds." *American Annual of Photog.* 29 (1915):218–20.

———. "Why Was Rembrandt?" *American Annual of Photog.* 30 (1916):144–47.

———. "Wilkes-Barre Camera Club Exhibition." *The Camera* 19 (May 1915):295–97.

ALLEN [sic], SIDNEY. "The Chances of Moving-Picture Portraiture." *Wilson's Photog. Mag.* 46 (Sept. 1909):408–10.

———. "How Leading Photographers Mount Their Prints." *Wilson's Photog. Mag.* 51 (June 1914):272–77.

———. "The Younger Generation." *Wilson's Photog. Mag.* 51 (Aug. 1914):frontis., 347–50, 357–63. [Illustrated by Elizabeth Schliepmann.]

A. CHAMELEON. [Pseud.] "Modern Chiaroscural Deficiencies and Their Influence on Pictorial Art." *Camera Work*, No. 26 (April 1900), pp. 19–21.

CALIBAN. [Pseud.] "The Inquisitorial System." *Photo-Beacon* 16 (Nov. 1904):346–49. [Hartmann attacks Stieglitz and the Photo-Secession as dictatorial.]

———. "Gessler's Hat." *The Camera* 8 (Nov. 1904):431–34. [Another attack on the Photo-Secession, concentrated particularly on Stieglitz.]

"THE CHIEL." [Pseud.] "Supplement to *Camera Work*—Notes and Comments." *Camera Work*, No. 33 (Jan. 1911), pp. 71–72.

°———. "The Salon Club and the first American Photographic Salon at New York." *American Amateur Photog.* 16 (July 1904):296–305. [See Chap. 13.]

HARTMANN, SADAKICHE [sic]. "My Experiences at the Fairbank's [sic] Studio." *The Curtain* 4 (Feb. 1925):26–28. [The second of two articles; the first appears under Hartmann, Sadakichi.]

HARTMANN, SADAKICHI. "Aesthetic Activity in Photography." *Brush and Pencil* 14 (April 1904):24–41.

———. "American Photography at Russell-Square. [Ltr.]

To The Editors." *Brit. Jour. Photog.* 47 (30 Nov. 1900): 767–68.

———. "Amerikanische Kunstphotographen. Eine zeitgenossiche Studie." *Dekorative Kunst* 8 (8 May 1905):330–36.

———. "An Analysis of Facial Expression: With Special Reference to Photographic Portraiture and Pictorial Representation. Introduction." *Abel's Photog. Weekly* 9 (24 Feb. 1912):598–99.

———. "An Analysis of Facial Expression: With Special Reference to Photographic Portraiture and Pictorial Representation. Chapter 1. The Study of a Face." *Abel's Photog. Weekly* 9 (9 Mar. 1912):646–48.

———. "An Analysis of Facial Expression: With Special Reference to Photographic Portraiture and Pictorial Representation. Chapter II. The Elementals of Facial Expression." *Abel's Photog. Weekly* 9 (23 Mar. 1912):694–96.

———. "An Analysis of Facial Expression: With Special Reference to Photographic Portraiture and Pictorial Representation. Chapter III. Methods of Rectification." *Abel's Photog. Weekly* 9 (6 Apr. 1912):742–44.

———. "An Analysis of Facial Expression: With Special Reference to Photographic Portraiture and Pictorial Representation. Chapter IV. Methods of Rectification." *Abel's Photog. Weekly* 9 (20 Apr. 1912):790–92.

———. "An Analysis of Facial Expression: With Special Reference to Photographic Portraiture and Pictorial Representation. Chapter V. On the Shape of the Head." *Abel's Photog. Weekly* 9 (4 May 1912):838–40.

———. "An Analysis of Facial Expression: With Special Reference to Photographic Portraiture and Pictorial Representation. Chapter VI. The Proportions of the Face." *Abel's Photog. Weekly* 9 (18 May 1912):887–88.

———. "An Analysis of Facial Expression: With Special Reference to Photographic Portraiture and Pictorial Representation. Chapter VII. The Minor Expressions." *Abel's Photog. Weekly* 9 (1 June 1912):934–36.

———. "An Analysis of Facial Expression: With Special Reference to Photographic Portraiture and Pictorial Representation. Chapter VIII. On The Forehead." *Abel's Photog. Weekly* 9 (15 June 1912):981–83.

———. "An Analysis of Facial Expression: With Special Reference to Photographic Portraiture and Pictorial Representation. Chapter IX. On the Expression of the Human Eye." *Abel's Photog. Weekly* 9 (29 June 1912):1029–31.

———. "An Analysis of Facial Expression: With Special Reference to Photographic Portraiture and Pictorial Representation. Chapter X. On the Expression of the Human Eye." *Abel's Photog. Weekly* 10 (20 July 1912):30–32.

———. "An Analysis of Facial Expression: With Special Reference to Photographic Portraiture and Pictorial Representation. Chapter XI. On the Expression of the Human Eye." *Abel's Photog. Weekly* 10 (27 July 1912):78–80.

———. "An Analysis of Facial Expression: With Special Reference to Photographic Portraiture and Pictorial Rep-

resentation. Chapter XII. The Nose." *Abel's Photog. Weekly* 10 (10 Aug. 1912):125–26.

———. "An Analysis of Facial Expression: With Special Reference to Photographic Portraiture and Pictorial Representation. Chapter XIII. The Lips." *Abel's Photog. Weekly* 10 (3 Aug. 1912):197–98.

°———. "An Art Critic's Estimate of Alfred Stieglitz." *The Photog. Times* 30 (June 1898):257–62. [See Chap. 20.]

———. "The Art of Coercion." *The Curtain* 7 (July 1928):83.

———. "Art and Artists." *Musical America* 1 (22 Oct. 1898):27–28. [On the paintings of Frank Eugene.]

———. "Artistic Photography and Interior Decoration." *The House Beautiful* 17 (Dec. 1904):44–45.

———. "Ausstellung der Amerikanischen Photo Secession in dem Carnegie-Institut zu Pittsburg." *Photographische Rundschau und Photographisches Centralblatt* 18 (1 Mai 1904):111–16.

———. "The Autonomy of Pantomime." *The Curtain* 9 (Oct. 1930):125.

———. "Broken Melodies." *Camera Work*, No. 38 (Apr. 1912), pp. 33–35.

°———. "The Broken Plates." *Camera Work*, No. 6 (Apr. 1904), pp. 35–39. [See Chap. 12.]

———. "The Carnegie Art Institute at Pittsburg." *The Burr McIntosh Monthly* 17 (Oct. 1908):[8 pp.].

———. "Charles Rohlfs: A Worker in Wood." *Wilson's Photog. Mag.* 49 (Feb. 1912):67–70, 73–76.

———. "Chaplin's City Lights." *The Curtain* 10 (Mar. 1931):38.

———. "Children As They Are Pictured." *Cosmopolitan* 43 (July 1907):235–47.

°———. "Clarence F. [sic] White." *The Photog. Times* 32 (Jan. 1900):18–23. [See Chap. 23.]

———. "Color and Texture in Photography." *Camera Notes* 4 (July 1900):9–14.

———. "Composition in Child Photography." *The Photog. Jour. of America* 53 (Apr. 1916):153–58.

———. *Composition in Portraiture. In:* The Literature of Photography Series, Peter C. Bunnell and Robert A. Sobieszek, eds. New York: Arno Press, 1975. [Reprint of the original 1909 edition published under the pseudonym of Sidney Allan.]

———. "The Conquest of Light." *Photog. Progress* 4 (Sept. 1909):111–14.

°———. "The Daguerreotype." *Photo-Era* 29 (Sept. 1912): 100–05. [See Chap. 17.]

———. "A Day in the Salt Meadows." *Harper's Monthly Mag.* 106 (May 1903):957–63.

°———. "A Decorative Photographer. F. H. Day." *The Photog. Times* 32 (Mar. 1900):102–06. [See Chap. 24.]

———. "Drapery and Accessories." *The Photo Miniature* 10 (June 1910):3–37.

———. "En Passant." *The Stylus* 1 (Dec. 1909):29. [A short appreciation of *Wilson's Photog. Mag.* Hartmann was editor of *The Stylus.*]

————. "Essentials in Portraiture." *The Photo Miniature* 8 (Nov. 1908):471–516.

°————. "The Esthetic Significance of the Motion Picture." *Camera Work*, No. 38 (Apr. 1912), pp. 19–21. [See Chap. 19.]

————. "Eugene R. Hutchinson—Professional Pictorialist." *Photo-Era* 32 (June 1914):266–73.

————. "The Exhibition of Children's Drawings." *Camera Work*, No. 39 (July 1912), pp. 45–46.

————. "Exhibition of Photographs by Elias Goldensky at the New York Camera Club, Feb. 10–27, 1904." *American Amateur Photographer* 16 (Apr. 1904):150–56.

————. "Exhibition of Photographs by Rudolph [sic] Eickemeyer, Jr." *Camera Notes* 3 (Apr. 1900):216–17.

————. "Exhibition of Prints by Virginia M. Prall (Nov. 14–26, 1900)." *Camera Notes* 4 (Apr. 1901):276–77.

————. "Exhibition of Prints by Wm. B. Post (December 1–10, 1900)." *Camera Notes* 4 (Apr. 1901):277–78.

————. "Feminine Beauty the World Around. Illustrated from Photo-Studies by Rudolf Eickemeyer, Jr." *The Metropolitan Mag.* 21 (Oct. 1904):119–28.

————. "A Few Reflections on Amateur and Artistic Photography." *Camera Notes* 2 (Oct. 1898):41–45.

————. "A Few Reflections on American Amateur and Artistic Photography." *Brit. Jour. of Photog.* 45 (7 Oct. 1898):650–51.

°————. "Frank Eugene. Painter-Photographer." *The Photog. Times* 31 (Dec. 1899):555–61. [See Chap. 22.]

————. "Frank Scott Clark—The Man and His Work." *The Photog. Jour. of America* 52 (March 1915):115–22.

————. "From a Hollywood Studio. Charlie Chaplin—His Methods—His Imitators—'The Most Lonesome Man in Hollywood.' " *The Curtain* 5 (Feb. 1926):19.

————. "From a Hollywood Studio." *The Curtain* 6 (Nov. 1927):132–33.

————. "From a Hollywood Studio. Chaplin's Personality." *The Curtain* 5 (June 1926):82.

————. "From a Hollywood Studio. Chapter I.—Chaplin the Conceited—His Luck—and his Genius." *The Curtain* 4 (Nov. 1925):146.

————. "From a Hollywood Studio. VIII. Film Critics—Some Advice to Fairbanks—Art and Money-making." *The Curtain* 5 (Dec. 1926):160.

————. "From a Hollywood Studio. Hollywood in Fiction and Fact." *The Curtain* 5 (July 1926):92.

————. "From a Hollywood Studio. The Meteoric Career of Aileen Pringle—Screen Technique—Pictorial Values." *The Curtain* 5 (Jan. 1926):4.

————. "From a Hollywood Studio. Patrons of the Pictures—The Amateurs and The Aspirants—'Fame in a Month.' " *The Curtain* 4 (Dec. 1925):158.

————. "From a Hollywood Studio. The Future of the Films—Chaplin and Immortality." *The Curtain* 6 (Sept. 1927):108.

————. "The Full-Face and Three Quarter View. Part I." *The Photog. Jour. of America* 53 (Oct. 1916):424–27. [From Sidney Allan's *Composition in Portraiture*.]

————. "The Full-Face and Three-Quarter View. Part II." *The Photog. Jour. of America* 53 (Nov. 1916):462–66. [From Sidney Allan's *Composition in Portraiture*.]

°————. "Gertrude Käsebier." *The Photog. Times* 32 (May 1900):195–99. [See Chap. 26.]

————. "Hats in Portraiture." *The Photog. Jour. of America* 53 (Aug. 1916):342–48.

————. "Henry Havelock Pierce. An Appreciation." *The Photog. Jour. of America* 52 (Apr. 1915):185–89.

————. *A History of American Art.* Boston: L. C. Page & Co., 1902. 2 vols.

————. *A History of American Art.* New York: Tudor Publishing Co. New Revised Edition. 1932. pp. 150–59, 303–04, 337. [Includes "An Art Wrangler's Aftermath," a new chapter in which Hartmann discusses photography.]

————. "Home Portraiture." *The Photo-Miniature* 12 (Sept. 1915):413–50.

————. "How a Talkie Dialogue Is Written." *The Curtain* 10 (Nov. 1931):143–44.

————. "How to Win a Competition." *Camera and Dark-Room* 8 (Oct. 1905):330–32.

————. "International Exhibition of Pictorial Photography—Albright Art Gallery. The Most Comprehensive Review of the Buffalo Exhibition." *Wilson's Photog. Mag.* 48 (Jan. 1911):2–4.

————. "In Search of My Likeness." 3 pp. unpubl. [Ms. in the Wistaria Hartmann Linton Collection, University of California, Riverside. A satire on Hartmann's experiences in being photographed.]

————. "Introduction." *Winter, Pictured by Rudolf Eickemeyer, Jr.* Rudolf Eickemeyer, Jr. New York: R. H. Russell, 1903.

————. "The Invisible Drama." *The Curtain* 11 (Jan. 1932):3.

————. "A Japanese Practitioner: Oki Seizo." *Wilson's Photog. Mag.* 51 (Dec. 1914):507–13.

————. "John Donoghue." *Camera Work*, No. 21 (Jan. 1908), pp. 23–26.

————. *Landscape and Figure Composition.* New York: The Baker & Taylor Company, 1910, 121 pp. [Illustrated.]

————. *Landscape and Figure Composition. In:* The Literature of Photography Series, Peter C. Bunnell and Robert A. Sobieszek (eds.) New York: Arno Press, 1975. [Reprint of original 1910 edition.]

————. Letter [in German]. *Camera Craft* 10 (Apr. 1905):247. [Ltr. from Hartmann as a representative for Curtis Bell's First American Photographic Salon to German and Austrian salons inviting exhibitors to participate.]

————. "Briefkasten." *Photographische Rundschau und Photographisches Centralblatt* 19 (15 Juni 1905):168. [The ltr., signed "Sadakichi Hartmann, Sidney Allan," is a German printing of the preceding citation.]

———. "[Letter to the] Editor of *The Camera.*" *The Camera* 8 (Oct. 1904):403–04. [On the Chalmers-Hartmann-Rood controversy.]

———. "Looking for the Good Points—." *The Camera* 21 (Oct. 1917):490–93. [On the work of W. E. Burnell and L. L. Higgason.]

———. "Looking for the Good Points—." *The Camera* 21 (Nov. 1917):558–60. [On the work of Jane Reece.]

———. "Looking for the Good Points—." *The Camera* 21 (Dec. 1917):610–12. [On the work of Gledhill.]

———. "Looking for the Good Points—." *The Camera* 22 (Jan. 1918):22–25. [On the work of Percy Newman and James Cooper.]

———. "Looking for the Good Points—." *The Camera* 22 (Mar. 1918):138–40. [On the work of Miss Reineke.]

———. "Looking for the Good Points—." *The Camera* 22 (July 1918):344–47. [On the work of George French, Belle Johnson, and Frank Scott Clark.]

———. "Looking for the Good Points—." *The Camera* 22 (Sept. 1918):460–62.[On the work of Edward H. Weston.]

———. "Looking for the Good Points—." *The Camera* 22 (Oct. 1918):514–17. [On the work of May L. Smith.]

———. "Looking for the Good Points—. Portrait—May L. Smith." *The Camera* 22 (Oct. 1918):517–18.

———. "Looking for the Good Points—." *The Camera* 22 (Nov. 1918):573–75. [On the work of L. D. Sweet.]

———. "Lumiere's 'Autochrome.' " *The Stylus* 1 (Jan. 1910):13–18.

———. "The Man Behind the Gun—J. C. Strauss." *In: An Appreciation of J. C. Strauss as a Photographer.* [A pamphlet, n.d., n.p.], pp. 2–5.

———. "A Master in Child Portraiture." *Photo-Era* 29 (Jan. 1912):8–9.

———. "A Midsummer Night's Dream." *The Lantern* (Aug. 1913):111–19.

———. "Mob Psychology." *The Curtain* 8 (June 1929):77.

———. "Modern Portraits." *Bull. of Photog.* 16 (21 Apr. 1915):486–88. [On a painting of Lucien Simon.]

———. "Modern Portraits." *Bull. of Photog.* 16 (28 Apr. 1915):527–28. [On a painting of Charles W. Hawthorne.]

———. "Modern Portraits." *Bull. of Photog.* 16 (31 Mar. 1915):400–01. [On a painting of Jean Jacques Henner.]

———. "Modern Portraits." *Bull. of Photog.* 16 (12 May 1915):581–82. [On a painting of William M. Chase.]

———. "Modern Portraits." *Bull. of Photog.* 16 (19 May 1915):623–24. [On a painting of Jean van Beers.]

———. "Modern Portraits." *Bull. of Photog.* 16 (26 May 1915):652–53. [On a painting of Robert Henri.]

———. "Modern Portraits." *Portrait* 7 (Nov. 1915):6–8. [On a painting of Albert Rosenthal.]

———. "A Monologue." *Camera Work,* No. 6 (Apr. 1904), p. 25. [Poetry on photography.]

———. "The Mother and Child Picture in Portraiture." *The Photog. Jour. of America* 53 (July 1916):303–06.

———. "My Experience at the Fairbanks Studio." *Camera!* 6 (2 Feb. 1924):16–18.

———. "My Experiences at the Fairbank's [sic] Studio." *The Curtain* 4 (Jan. 1925):11–13. [Reprint of preceding article. This was the first of two articles. The second is cited under Hartmann, Sadakiche (sic).]

———. "A New Departure in Light and Shade Arrangement." *Photo-Era* 29 (Nov. 1912):226–28.

———. "New Studies of the Mechanism of Composition. I. Local Values." *Portrait* 10 (Jan. 1919):4–8.

———. "New Studies of the Mechanism of Composition. II. Contrast." *Portrait* 10 (Feb. 1919):8–12.

———. "New Studies of the Mechanism of Composition. III. Tone." *Portrait* 10 (March 1919):7–12.

———. "New Studies of the Mechanism of Composition. IV. The Pose." *Portrait* 10 (Apr. 1919):4–9.

———. "The New York Camera Club." *The Photog. Times* 32 (Feb. 1900):59–61.

———. *A Note on the Portraits of Walt Whitman.* New York: At the Sign of the Sparrow, 1921. [Contains a discussion of the photographers of Walt Whitman.]

———. "A Note on the Portraits of Walt Whitman." *In:* Knox, George and Harry Lawton (eds.) *The Whitman-Hartmann Controversy, Including Conversations with Walt Whitman and Other Essays.* Frankfurt and Munich: Herbert Lang Bern/Peter Lang, 1976. pp. 115–16.

———. "Once More Matisse." *Camera Work,* No. 39 (July 1912), pp. 22, 33.

———. "On Backgrounds." *The Photog. Jour. of America* 54 (Jan. 1917):10–15. [From Sidney Allan's *Composition in Portraiture.*]

°———. "On Composition." *Camera Notes* 4 (Apr. 1901): 257–62. [See Chap. 5.]

———. "On the Composition of Two-Figure Portraits." *The Photog. Jour. of America* 53 (May 1916):208–12.

———. "On Exhibitions." *Camera Notes* 5 (Oct. 1901):105–10.

———. "On the Lack of Culture." *Camera Work,* No. 6 (Apr. 1904), pp. 19–22.

———. "On Light Effects." *The Photog. Jour. of America* 54 (Mar. 1917):103–07. [From *Composition in Portraiture.*]

———. "On Originality." *Camera Work,* No. 37 (Jan. 1912), pp. 19–21.

°———. "On Plagiarism and Imitation." *Camera Notes* 3 (Jan. 1900):105–08. [See Chap. 3.]

°———. "On the Possibility of New Laws of Composition." *Camera Work,* No. 30 (Apr. 1910), pp. 23–26. [See Chap. 15.]

———. "On Sitting Positions." *The Photog. Jour. of America* 53 (Dec. 1916):510–13. [From Sidney Allan's *Composition in Portraiture.*]

———. "On Tone and Values." *The Photog. Jour. of America*

54 (Feb. 1917):57–60. [From Sidney Allan's *Composition in Portraiture*.]

———. "On the Use of Furniture in Portraiture." *The Photog. Jour. of America* 53 (June 1916):252–59.

———. "On the Vanity of Appreciation." *Camera Work*, No. 5 (Jan. 1904), pp. 21–23.

———. "Phono-Film Infection." *The Curtain* 8 (Apr. 1929):47–48.

°———. "A Photographic Enquête." *Camera Notes* 5 (Apr. 1902):233–38. [See Chap. 7.]

———. "The Photographing of Types." *The Photog. Jour. of America* 59 (May 1922):175–82.

°———. "The Photo-Secession Exhibition at the Carnegie Art Galleries. Pittsburg, Pa." *Camera Work*, No. 6 (Apr. 1905), pp. 47–51. [See Chap. 10.]

———. "Pictorial Progress." *Wilson's Photog. Mag.* 50 (Dec. 1913):501–03.

———. "Picturesque Features of the Ghetto: The Esthetic Side of Jewtown." *Mother Earth* 5 (Aug. 1910):200–05. [Reprinted from *Camera Notes* 6 (Feb. 1903):143–48.]

———. "Placing of the Head." *The Photog. Jour. of America* 53 (Feb. 1916):65–70. [From Sidney Allan's *Composition in Portraiture*.]

———. "A Plea for the Amateur." *Burr McIntosh Monthly* 14 (Nov. 1907):Unpaginated.

°———. "A Plea for the Picturesqueness of New York." *Camera Notes* 4 (Oct. 1900):91–97. [See Chap. 2.]

°———. "A Plea for Straight Photography." *American Amateur Photog.* 16 (Mar. 1904):101–09. [See Chap. 11.]

———. "Pictorial Aims of Modern Portraiture. I. Whistler's Lesson of Simplicity." *Portrait* 9 (Jan. 1918):3–6.

———. "Pictorial Aims of Modern Portraiture. II. Definition of Composition." *Portrait* 9 (Feb. 1918):8–11.

———. "Pictorial Aims of Modern Portraiture. III. The Importance of Character Delineation." *Portrait* 9 (Mar. 1918):8–12.

———. "Pictorial Aims of Modern Portraiture. IV. The Problem of Space in Standing Figures." *Portrait* 9 (Apr. 1918):7–11.

———. "Pictorial Aims of Modern Portraiture. V. The 'Interior' Device." *Portrait* 10 (May 1918):7–10.

———. "Pictorial Aims of Modern Portraiture. VI. A Realistic Group." *Portrait* 10 (June 1918):7–9.

———. "Pictorial Aims of Modern Portraiture. VII. On Foreshortening." *Portrait* 10 (July 1918):7–9.

———. "Pictorial Aims of Modern Portraiture. VIII. The So-Called 'Painter-Like' Technique." *Portrait* 10 (Aug. 1918):7–11.

———. "Pictorial Aims of Modern Portraiture. IX. Unusual Arrangements." *Portrait* 10 (Sept. 1918):4–7.

———. "Pictorial Aims of Modern Portraiture. X. Theatrical Effects." *Portrait* 10 (Oct. 1918):10–13.

———. "Pictorial Aims of Modern Portraiture. XI. The Graceful Pose, its Mechanism and Pictorial Value." *Portrait* 10 (Nov. 1918):3–7.

———. "Pictorial Aims of Modern Portraiture. XII. Decorative Inventions." *Portrait* 10 (Dec. 1918):4–7.

———. "Portrait." *Photo-Era* 29 (Sept. 1912):110.

°———. "Portrait Painting and Portrait Photography." *Camera Notes* 3 (July 1899):1–20. [See Chap. 1.]

———. "The Portrait Print—Its Significance in Interior Decoration." *Wilson's Photog. Mag.* 46 (Aug. 1909): 367–69.

———. "The Pretty Woman in Photography." *Cosmopolitan Mag.* 43 (May 1907):3–16.

———. "The Profile View." *The Photog. Jour. of America* 53 (Mar., 1916):111–16. [From Sidney Allan's *Composition in Portraiture*.]

°———. "A Purist." *The Photog. Times* 31 (Oct. 1899):449–55. [On Zaida Ben-Yúsuf; see Chap. 21.]

———. "Quite in the Gentlemanly Interest." *The Photog. Times-Bull.* 36 (Sept. 1904):385–88. [On the work of W. G. Corthell.]

°———. "Random Thoughts on Criticism." *Camera Notes* 3 (Jan. 1900):101–04. [See Chap. 4.]

°———. "Recent Conquests in Night Photography." *The Photog. Times* 41 (Nov. 1909):441–50. [See Chap. 14.]

———. "Recent Work by J. C. Strauss." *Wilson's Photog. Mag.* 51 (Oct. 1914):frontis., 431–34, 445–50.

———. "A Reverie at the Seashore." *Harper's Monthly Mag.* 105 (Sept. 1902):561–68. [A photo-essay illustrated by Rudolf Eickemeyer, Jr.]

———. "Reviews of the Exhibition of Photographic Studies by Charles I. Berg (Feb. 14-Mar. 13, 1900)." *Camera Notes* 4 (July 1900):37–38.

———. "Rudolph [sic] Eickemeyer, Jr." *The Photog. Times* 32 (Apr. 1900):161–66.

———. "The St. Louis World's Fair Photographer's Impressions." *The Photog. Times-Bull.* 26 (Nov. 1904):480–89.

———. "The Solitary Horseman." *Camera Work*, No. 7 (July 1904), pp. 17–18.

———. "Structural Units." *Camera Work*, No. 36 (Oct. 1911), pp. 18–20. [On the paintings of Max Weber.]

———. "Subject and Treatment." *Camera Notes* 5 (Jan. 1902):177–87.

———. "Talks on Composition—Some Individual Forms of Landscape Composition." *The Camera* 20 (June 1916): 338–40.

———. "Talks on Composition—Second Paper. Legitimate Imitation." *The Camera* 20 (July 1916):390–92.

———. "Talks on Composition—Third Paper. Divided Points of Interest." *The Camera* 20 (Aug. 1916):437–39.

———. "Talks on Composition—Fourth Paper. The Repetition of Shapes." *The Camera* 20 (Sept. 1916):509–11.

———. "Talks on Composition—Fifth Paper. The Diagonal Foreground Line." *The Camera* 20 (Oct. 1916):566–67.

———. "Talks on Composition—Sixth Paper. Line Feeling in Figures." *The Camera* 20 (Nov. 1916):620–21.

———. "Talks on Composition—Seventh Paper. The Vanishing Point in Out-Of-Door Work." *The Camera* 20 (Dec. 1916):666–67.

———. "Talks on Composition—Eighth Paper. The Picturesqueness of Odd Forms." *The Camera* 21 (Jan. 1917): 32–34.

———. "Talks on Composition—Ninth Paper. On Pattern Design." *The Camera* 21 (Feb. 1917):94–96.

———. "Talks on Composition—Tenth Paper. The Japanese Foreground Idea." *The Camera* 21 (Mar. 1917): 145–47.

———. "Talks on Composition—Eleventh Paper. Color Values in Monochrome Representation." *The Camera* 21 (Apr. 1917):199–201.

———. "Talks on Composition—Twelfth Paper. The Pictorial Importance of Rhythm." *The Camera* 21 (May 1917):250–52.

———. "The Ten Leading Styles of Portraiture. I: The Old Master Idea." *Portrait* 5 (Nov. 1913):8–11.

———. "The Ten Leading Styles of Portraiture. II: The Dutch School." *Portrait* 5 (Dec. 1913):10–13.

———. "The Ten Leading Styles of Portraiture. III: The German Method. Exploitation of Detail." *Portrait* 5 (Feb. 1914):2–5.

———. "The Ten Leading Styles of Portraiture. IV: The Rembrandt Style. Light and Shade Composition." *Portrait* 5 (Mar. 1914):4–7.

———. "The Ten Leading Styles of Portraiture. V: The Allegorical Form." *Portrait* 5 (Apr. 1914):4–7.

———. "The Ten Leading Styles of Portraiture. VI: The French Spirit. Vivacity and Brilliancy." *Portrait* 6 (May 1914):4–7.

———. "The Ten Leading Styles of Portraiture. VII: The Gainsborough Style." *Portrait* 6 (June 1914):4–8.

———. "The Ten Leading Styles of Portraiture. VIII: The Decorative Manner." *Portrait* 6 (Aug. 1914):4–7.

———. "The Ten Leading Styles of Portraiture. IX: The Whistler Mode." *Portrait* 6 (Sept. 1914):4–7.

———. "The Ten Leading Styles of Portraiture. X: The Impressionistic Way." *Portrait* 6 (Oct. 1914):6–9.

———. "Texture in Photography." *American Annual of Photog. and Photographic Times Almanac* 1 (1900):105–09.

———. "Through Semi-Japanese Eyes." *Camera Notes* 4 (July 1900):46–47.

———. "A Visit to the Chicago Art Institute." *Wilson's Photog. Mag.* 48 (Mar. 1911):118–23.

———. "A Walk Through the Exhibition of the Photographic Section of the American Institute." *Camera Notes* 2 (Jan. 1899):86–89.

———. "Walter Zimmerman's Travel Pictures." *American Amateur Photog.* 16 (Sept. 1904):390–94.

———. "What Is the Matter with Eisenstein?" *The Curtain* 9 (Dec. 1930):159.

°———. "What Remains." *Camera Work*, No. 33 (Jan. 1911), pp. 30–32. [See Chap. 18.]

———. "Where Are the Gestures of Yesterday?" *The Curtain* 9 (Jan. 1930):3–4.

———. *The Whistler Book*. Boston: L. C. Page & Co., 1910. Pp. 164–65.

———. "White Chrysanthemums." *Camera Work*, No. 5 (Jan. 1904), pp. 19–20. [On James McNeil Whistler.]

———. "White Chrysanthemums." *The Fra* 3 (Apr. 1909):20–21. [Stieglitz protested Hartmann's selling this article to Elbert Hubbard's *The Fra* after it had already appeared in *Camera Work*. See preceding.]

———. "A Winter Ramble." *Harper's Monthly Mag.* 103 (Nov. 1901):989–96.

———. "The Works of Rudolf Eickemeyer, Jr." *The Photo American* 15 (July 1904):195–99.

———. "Younger American Painters." *Camera Work*, No. 31 (July 1910), pp. 47–49. [Exhibition, Little Galleries of the Photo-Secession, 291 Fifth Avenue, New York.]

HARTMANN, SADAKITCHI [sic]. "The Photo-Secession: A New Pictorial Movement." *The Craftsman* 6 (Apr. 1904):30–37.

HARTMANN, SADATICHI [sic]. "Die Kunst-Photographie in ihrer Beziehung zur Malerei." *Sonntags-blatt der N.Y. Staats-Zeitung*, Jan. 30, 1898, p. 17, cols. 1–6. [Hartmann's earliest known article on photography as a fine art. See Breuer, Hans-Peter (below).]

JUVENAL. [Pseud.] "Little Tin Gods on Wheels." *Photo-Beacon* 16 (Sept. 1904):282–86.

KLINGSOR, THE MAGICIAN. [Pseud.] "Our Second Pilgrimage." *Camera Work*, No. 33 (Jan. 1911), p. 72. [On the Photo-Secession Exhibition at Buffalo.]

———. "A Pilgrimage to the Secession Shrine at Pittsburg." *Camera Work*, No. 6 (Apr. 1904), pp. 54–56.

S. H. [Initials only.] "Dawn Flowers." *Camera Work*, No. 2 (Apr. 1903), p. 29. [A poem dedicated to Maurice Maeterlinck, suggested by Steichen's photograph of the same title.]

———. "De Zayas." *Camera Work*, No. 2 (Apr. 1903), pp. 31–33.

———. "Dolor." *Camera Work*, No. 2 (Apr. 1903), p. 35. [A poem suggested by Steichen's photograph of the same title.]

———. "The John E. Dumont Exhibition. (Apr. 11–25)." *Camera Notes* 3 (July 1899):38.

———. "A Photographer of Pretty Women. Will Armstrong." *American Amateur Photog.* (Feb. 1906):58–65.

———. "Puritanism, Its Grandeur and Shame." *Camera Work*, No. 32 (Oct. 1910), pp. 17–19.

———. "Rodin's Balzac." *Camera Work*, No. 34–35 (Apr.-July 1911), pp. 19–21.

————. "That Toulouse-Lautrec Print!" *Camera Work*, No. 29 (Jan. 1910), pp. 36–38.

————. "To the 'Flat-Iron.'" *Camera Work*, No. 4 (Oct. 1903), p. 40. [Poem.]

————. "Visions of the Nude." *Camera Work*, No. 31 (July 1910), pp. 29–31.

UNSIGNED. "A Branch of Cherry Blossoms." *Camera Work*, No. 29 (Jan. 1910), pp. 21–22. [Firmly attributed to Hartmann on the basis of a list prepared by him ca. 1940 of articles which he identified as his own work.]

————. "The Death of Napoleon Sarony." *The Daily Tatler* 1 (11 Nov. 1896):4. [As art critic for Richard Hovey's literary magazine, Hartmann in all likelihood wrote this editorial obituary.]

————. "The Fight for Recognition." *Camera Work*, No. 30 (Apr. 1910), pp. 21–23. [Initialed by Hartmann as his work in a scrapbook of *Camera Work* material which he gave to the actress Aileen Pringle.]

————. "Old Colonial Rooms." *Camera Work*, No. 32 (Oct. 1910), pp. 24–25. [Included by Hartmann in a list of 33 essays which he planned to publish in an anthology of his work.]

————. "The Elements of Pictorial Composition." *American Amateur Photog.* 17 (July 1905):318–24. [Attributed to Hartmann on the basis of internal textual evidence. Cf., "On Composition," *Camera Notes* 4 (Apr. 1901):257–62.]

————. "On the Elongation of Form." *Camera Work*, No. 10 (Apr. 1905), pp. 27–34. [Attributed to Hartmann with a high degree of confidence on the basis of an analysis of style and content.]

°————. "Unphotographic Paint:—The Texture of Impressionism." *Camera Work*, No. 28 (Oct. 1909), pp. 20–23. [Initialed by Hartmann as his work in the Aileen Pringle scrapbook. See Chap. 16.]

————. [Untitled.] News item on the development of the three-color halftone process in the plant of William Kurtz, New York. *The Weekly Review* 3 (18 Mar. 1893):336. [Attributed to Hartmann who was serving as the primary editorial staff member of this small Boston periodical. Prior to his joining the staff, the magazine contained no articles; its content was solely a weekly compilation listing major articles in magazines and newspapers, probably assembled by clerical help.]

III. PUBLICATIONS CONTAINING MATERIAL RELATING TO SADAKICHI HARTMANN

[ABEL, JUAN C.] "A Boil-Down of the Current Photographic Magazines. You Can't Read Them All. This Is a Page of This Week's Good Stuff. Composition in Portraiture." *Abel's Photog. Weekly* 1 (18 Jan. 1908):65.

————. "Editorial: A Brief Review of the Picture Show at the P.P.S.N.Y. Convention." *Abel's Photog. Weekly* 3 (27 Mar. 1909):185–86.

————. "Editorial: A Valuable Book." *Abel's Photog. Weekly* 3 (23 Jan. 1909):81.

————. "Editorial Comment: Hartmann Again." *Abel's Photog. Weekly* 1 (22 Feb. 1908):115.

————. "Editorial Comment: Hartmann's New Attack on MacDonald." *Abel's Photog. Weekly* 2 (8 Aug. 1908):339.

————. "Editorial Comment: Prizes or No Prizes." *The Photographer* 7 (21 May 1907):51.

————. "In Passing By." *Abel's Photog. Weekly* 9 (17 Feb. 1912):571. [Announcement of Hartmann's series "An Analysis of Facial Expression."]

————. "In Passing By." *Abel's Photog. Weekly* 10 (26 Oct. 1912):387.

————. "National Convention Notes. Foremost Art Critic of Country Engaged to Give Public and Private Criticisms of Pictures at the National Convention." *Abel's Photog. Weekly* 10 (13 July 1912):32–34.

————. "The Photographer's Metropolis." *Abel's Photog. Weekly* 3 (16 Jan. 1909):75.

————. "Program of the W.Va. Convention to be Held in Wheeling, Oct. 9-10-11, 1912. *Abel's Photog. Weekly* 10 (28 Sept. 1912):293–94.

————. "The Week in Review." *Abel's Photog. Weekly* 7 (21 Jan. 1911):47–48.

ANON. Untitled article on Wistaria Hartmann Linton collection at the University of California, Riverside. *At UCR*, 1, No. 6 (Sept.-Oct. 1976), 8–9. [Includes photographs of Hartmann by J. C. Strauss, Cliff Wesselman, one sculpture by Leon Saulter, one pastel by Leslie Cauldwell, one photograph of Hartmann as the Magician in "The Thief of Bagdad," and one photograph of Hartmann with John Barrymore.]

BARROW, THOMAS F. "A Letter With Some Thoughts on Photography's Future." *Album*, No. 6 (July 1970), p. 23.

BEACH, HOWARD D. "Portrait of Sadakichi Hartmann." *Photo-Era* 29 (July, 1912):3. [Photograph.]

BEN-YÚSUF, ZAIDA. "Portrait of Sadakichi Hartmann," *Camera Notes* 3 (July 1899):8. [Photograph.]

————. "Portrait of Sadakichi Hartmann." *Sadakichi Hartmann Newsletter* 3 (Winter, 1972):8.

————. "Sadakichi Hartmann," *Brush and Pencil* 14 (Apr. 1904):51. [Photograph.]

BLOISS, HARRY A. "The 'Open Letter.'" *The Photographer* 8 (9 July 1907):174. [Response to Sidney Allan ltr. in June 11 issue.]

BRADLEY, A. F. "Reply to Sidney Allan's Open Letter." *Wilson's Photog. Mag.* 44 (June 1907):245. [Allan's ltr. appears in the same issue.]

BREUER, HANS-PETER (Transl.) "Sadakichi's First Photography Essay." *Sadakichi Hartmann Newsletter* 5 (Summer, 1974):3–6. [A reprint of Hartmann's "Art Photography in Its Relationship to Painting." See above, Hartmann, Sadakitchi (sic).]

BURTON, HOWARD A. "A Gift for Film Theory: The Film Criticism of Sadakichi Hartmann." *Sadakichi Hartmann Newsletter* 3 (Winter, 1972):1–3.

CHALMERS, J. P. "Art Terms Explained. Definitions of Words and Phrases Used by Picture Critics and Writers on Art Subjects." *American Amateur Photog.* 19 (Jan. 1907): 11–14. [Authorship of this article was claimed by Sidney Allan.]
———. "Correspondence." *The Photographer* 7 (14 May 1907):43. [Ltr. dated 13 May 1907. Chalmers says he was "fully justified in signing" "Art Terms Explained." Says Hartmann furnished "at my request" some notes. But "fully three-fourths of the article" was Chalmers' own work.]
———. "The Facts in a Personal Matter." *American Amateur Photog. and Camera and Dark Room* 19 (May 1907):268–69.
———. "An Open Letter." *American Amateur Photog.* 15 (Oct. 1904):421–22. [Reply to Rood's letter repudiating "The Three Factors" article. See Rood, Roland.]
CLATTENBURG, ELLEN FRITZ. *The Photographic Work of F. Holland Day.* Introduction and Catalogue by Ellen Fritz Clattenburg. Wellesley, Mass: Wellesley College Museum, 1975, pp. 17, 22, 23, 29, 33, 36, 63. [Catalogue of an exhibition held Feb. 21–Mar. 24, 1975.]
COBURN, ALVIN LANGDON. *A Portfolio of Sixteen Photographs.* Introduction by Nancy Newhall. Rochester, N.Y.: George Eastman House, 1962, p. 5. [Hartmann quoted twice.]
COKE, VAN DEREN. *The Painter and the Photograph.* Albuquerque: Univ. of New Mexico Press, 1964, pp. 15, 306.
———. *The Painter and the Photograph.* Albuquerque: Univ. of New Mexico Press, 1972. Revised and enlarged edition. Pp. 15, 306.
"Composition in Portraiture." *The Camera* 14 (Feb. 1910):following p. 82. [Advertisement.]
CORE, E. B. "Reply to Sidney Allan's Open Letter." *Wilson's Photog. Mag.* 14 (June 1907):246–47. [Allan's ltr. appears in the same issue.]
CORN, WANDA M. "The New New York." *Art in America* 61 (July-August 1973):59–65. [Hartmann (Sidney Allan) cited twice and quoted once (p. 59) from "The 'Flat-Iron' Building—An Esthetical Dissertation." The article appeared originally in *Camera Work*, No. 4 (Oct. 1903), pp. 36–40.]
CROUGHTON, G. HANMER. "Criticism of Illustrations." *Saint Louis and Canadian Photog.* 29 (Oct. 1905):479. [On a photograph of Hartmann by W. M. Hollinger. The photograph faces p. 447. See Hollinger, William M.]
———. "Echoes." *Saint Louis and Canadian Photog.* 29 (Oct. 1905):449–50.
———. "Echoes." *Saint Louis and Canadian Photog.* 29 (Nov. 1905):497–98.
———. "Echoes. Concentration—Art Students in Photographic Studies." *Abel's Photog. Weekly* 9 (23 Mar. 1912): 693.
———. "Echoes. Impressions of the Convention." *Abel's Photog. Weekly* 10 (24 Aug. 1912):173–74.

DOTY, ROBERT. *Photo-Secession: Photography as a Fine Art.* Foreword by Beaumont Newhall. Rochester: The George Eastman House, 1960. George Eastman House Monograph Number 1, pp. 33, 34, 36, 58.
"Doug Discovers New Types for 'Bagdad.'" *Camera!* 6 (23 June 1923):13. [On the casting of Hartmann as the Chinese prince in "The Thief of Bagdad."]
DRINNON, ROBERT. *Rebels in Paradise: A Biography of Emma Goldman.* New York: Harper/Colophon Books, 1976, pp. 62, 99.

EDENS, STEPHANIE T. "The Silent Decade[:] 1900–1910. Chronology." *Art in America* 61 (July-August 1973):32–33. [Hartmann is mentioned as having written *The History of American Art.*]
[EDITOR] "American Photographic Criticism." *British Jour. of Photog.* 47 (23 Mar. 1900):182–83.
———. "Among the Camera Clubs." *The Photog. Times* 41 (July 1909):273. [Short item concerning Hartmann's judging an exhibition of the Wyoming Valley Camera Club in Wilkes Barre, Pa. on June 18, 1909.]
———. Announcement of Sidney Allan's reading of "A Plea for Good Taste and Common Sense." *Wilson's Photog. Mag.* 42 (July 1905):292.
———. "Camera Work, No. 1." [Review.] *American Amateur Photog.* 15 (Feb. 1903):90–91.
———. "Camera Work, No. 6." [Review.] *American Amateur Photog.* 16 (Apr. 1904):186.
———. "Camera Work, No. 21." [Review.] *British Jour. of Photog.* 55 (31 Jan. 1908):89.
———. "Copying Daguerreotypes." *Photo-Era* 29 (Dec. 1912):316. [Commentary on Hartmann's article in the September issue of *Photo-Era:* "The Daguerreotype," *Photo-Era* 29 (Sept. 1912):101–05.]
———. "Conventions and Their Methods." *Wilson's Photog. Mag.* 44 (June 1907):241–42.
———. "Criticism Department." *Bull. of Photog. and the Photographer* 4 (16 June 1909):375. [Introducing Hartmann's series, "Constructive Criticism."]
———. "Editorial Notes." *American Amateur Photog.* 18 (July 1906):307–08. [An attack on "that discredited critic" Sidney Allan.]
———. "Editorial Notes." *The Photog. Times* 32 (Jan. 1900):40.
———. "Editorial Notes." *The Photog. Times* 32 (May 1900):237.

———. "Editor's Table." *Wilson's Photog. Mag.* 43 (Aug. 1906):384.

———. "Editor's Table." *Wilson's Photog. Mag.* 44 (Dec. 1907):576.

———. "Editor's Table." *Wilson's Photog. Mag.* 45 (Nov. 1908):528.

———. "Editor's Table." *Wilson's Photog. Mag.* 45 (Dec. 1908):576.

———. "Editor's Table." *Wilson's Photog. Mag.* 46 (Mar. 1909):144.

———. "Editor's Table." *Wilson's Photog. Mag.* 46 (Apr. 1909):192.

———. "Editor's Table." *Wilson's Photog. Mag.* 47 (Feb. 1910):96.

———. "Editor's Table." *Wilson's Photog. Mag.* 47 (Mar. 1910):144.

———. "Editor's Table." *Wilson's Photog. Mag.* 47 (Oct. 1910):480.

———. "Editor's Table." *Wilson's Photog. Mag.* 47 (Nov. 1910):528.

———. "Editor's Table." *Wilson's Photog. Mag.* 47 (Dec. 1910):568.

———. "Ex Cathedra." *British Jour. of Photog.* 47 (30 Nov. 1900):754.

———. Excerpt from Hartmann's "Letter to the Wyoming Valley Camera Club." *The Camera* 13 (Aug. 1909):280.

———. *"Landscape and Figure Composition."* [Review.] *The Nation* 91 (Nov. 1910):482.

———. "The Last Year of the Century." *The Photog. Times* 32 (Jan. 1900):37.

———. "New Books." *British Jour. of Photog.* 51 (15 Jan. 1904):55. [Review of *Winter Pictured by Rudolf Eickemeyer, Jr.*]

———. "New Books." *British Jour. of Photog.* 51 (18 Nov. 1904):993. [Review of *Photograms of the Year, 1904* in which Hartmann's essay "A New Departure in American Pictorialism" appeared.]

———. "New Books." *British Jour. of Photog.* 57 (12 Aug. 1910):617. [Review of Hartmann's essay "Drapery and Accessories."]

———. "New Books." *Wilson's Photog. Mag.* 47 (Dec. 1910):566. [Review of Hartmann's *The Whistler Book.*]

———. "News and Notes." *Wilson's Photog. Mag.* 46 (Apr. 1909):190.

———. "Notes and News." *Photo-Era* 14 (Apr. 1905):151.

———. "Our Book Shelves." *Camera Craft* 17 (Oct. 1910):378. [Review of Hartmann's *Landscape and Figure Composition.*]

———. "Our Monthly Digest." *The Photog. Times* 32 (Feb. 1900):83.

———. "Our Table." *American Amateur Photog.* 10 (Oct. 1898):471. [Review of *Camera Notes* for October.]

———. "Our Table." *American Amateur Photog.* 11 (July 1899):312. [Review of *Camera Notes* for July.]

———. "Our Table." *American Amateur Photog.* 12 (May 1900):234. [Review of *Camera Notes* for April.]

———. "Our Table." *American Amateur Photog.* 12 (July 1900):331. [Review of *Camera Notes* for July.]

———. "Our Table." *American Amateur Photog.* 12 (Nov. 1900):524. [Review of *Camera Notes* for October.]

———. "Our Table." *American Amateur Photog.* 15 (Feb. 1903):90–91. [Review of *Camera Work*, No. 1.]

———. "Our Table." *American Amateur Photog.* 15 (May 1903):232. [Review of *Camera Work*, No. 2.]

———. "Our Table," *American Amateur Photog.* 15 (Nov. 1903):521–23. [Review of *Camera Work*, Nos. 1–4.]

———. "Our Table." *American Amateur Photog.* 16 (Feb. 1904):92. [Review of *Camera Work*, No. 5 (Jan. 1904).]

———. "Our Table." *American Amateur Photog.* 16 (Mar. 1904):138. [Review of the Catalogue of the Exhibition of the Work of the Photo-Secession.]

———. "Our Table." *American Amateur Photog.* 16 (Apr. 1904):186. [Review of *Camera Work*, No. 6.]

———. "Our Table." *American Amateur Photog.* 16 (June 1904):281–82. [Review of *Camera Work*, No. 8.]

———. "Our Table." *American Amateur Photog.* 22 (Dec. 1910):724. [Review of Hartmann's *Landscape and Figure Composition.*]

———. "Our Table." *American Amateur Photog.* 17 (Mar. 1905):132. [Review of *Photograms of the Year, 1904.*]

———. "Our Table." *American Amateur Photog.* 18 (May 1906):242–43. [Review of *Camera Work* and the Steichen Supplement; April, 1906, No. 14.]

———. "Photographers' Association of America. Quarter Centennial Convention, Boston, Mass., August 8th to 11th, 1905." *Camera Craft* 11 (Jan. 1905):31–32.

———. "Photographic Reviews." *The Photog. Times* 41 (Feb. 1909):66. [Review of *Composition in Portraiture.*]

———. "Plastic Psychological Syntheses at Russell Square." *British Jour. of Photog.* 47 (Oct. 1900):677–78. [Attack on Hartmann's criticism and the F. Holland Day exhibition sponsored by the Royal Photographic Society.]

———. "The Quarter Centennial Convention of the P.A. of A." *Photo-Era* 15 (Sept. 1905):110.

———. "Sadakichi Hartmann Here." *Camera Craft* 23 (Dec. 1916):504. [Brief announcement of Hartmann's move to San Francisco.]

———. "That Hartmann Letter in Our Last Issue." *Camera Craft* 10 (May 1905):310.

———. "What the Editors Are Saying of 'Composition in Portraiture.' " *Wilson's Photog. Mag.* 46 (June 1909): 273–76.

ELLIS, WILLIAM SHEWELL. "Portrait of Sidney Allan (Sadakichi Hartmann." *In:* Taylor, Charles Stillman. "Winter Work." *American Annual of Photog.* 27 (1913): 267.

ENYEART, JAMES. *Francis J. Bruguière.* New York: Alfred A. Knopf, 1977. (In press.) [Contains considerable material on the Hartmann-Bruguière relationship.]

EUGENE, FRANK. "Nirvana." *Camera Notes* 3 (Apr. 1900):197. [According to Hartmann, the last act of his play *Buddha* (1897) inspired Eugene's taking this photograph.]

———. "Portrait of Mrs. Hartmann." *Camera Craft* 7 (May 1903):261. [A portrait of Hartmann's first wife, Elizabeth Blanche Walsh. The original photograph is in the Wistaria Harmann Linton collection at the University of California, Riverside.]

———. "Sadakichi Hartmann." *Camera Notes* 3 (Apr. 1900):193. [A portrait.]

EVANS, FREDERICK H. "American Photography at Russell Square. [Letter] To the Editors." *British Jour. of Photog.* 47 (16 Nov. 1900):736.

———. "The Exhibition of American Photography at Russell Square. [Letter] to the Editors." *British Jour. of Photog.* 47 (2 Nov. 1900):702. [Editor's response, pp. 702–03.]

FAGIN, C. F. "A Reply to Sidney Allan's Criticism." *Wilson's Photog. Mag.* 44 (Nov. 1907):525–26.

FALK, B. J. "A Portrait by B. J. Falk, 'Made at the demonstration before members of the Professional Photographers' Society of New York, April 2, 1907.' " *Wilson's Photog. Mag.* 44 (June 1907):264. [Photograph of Hartmann.]

———. "Reply to Sidney Allan's Open Letter." *Wilson's Photog. Mag.* 44 (June 1907):245–46. [Allan's ltr. appears in the same issue.]

FOURNIER, PAUL. "Sidney Allen [sic]." *Photo-Era* 20 (Feb. 1908):71. [Winning Photograph in the "Professional Portrait Class" of *Photo-Era's* Fifth Annual Photographic Contest of 1907.]

FLECKENSTEIN, LOUIS. "Sadakichi Hartman [sic], Pittsburgh Salon, 1909." *American Photog.* 13 (June 1919):321. [A photograph.]

FRANK, WALDO, et al., (eds.). *America and Alfred Stieglitz.* New York: The Literary Guild, 1934, p. 83.

From 1839: Revolution in a Box. Catalogue of Exhibition. An Historical Survey of Photographica in two parts, Presented by the Art Departments at Pomona College, and the University of California, Riverside, 1973, [6.] [J. C. Strauss' portrait of Hartmann on a pedestal is included in the photographs reproduced in the catalogue.]

"From a Hollywood Studio." *The Curtain* 4 (Oct. 1925):143. [Announcement of Hartmann's series of the same title, to begin Nov. 1925.]

GREEN, JONATHAN (ed.) *Camera Work: A Critical Anthology.* Millerton, New York: Aperture, 1973, pp. 11, 12–13, 14, 15, 16, 21, 28–33, 37–39, 43–47, 89, 183–86, 190–92, 196–202, 204–07, 220–23, 337.

GREENOUGH, SARAH E. *The Published Writings of Alfred Stieglitz.* Unpublished MFA Thesis in Art History, Graduate School of the University of New Mexico, Albuquerque, New Mexico, 1976, pp. 106, 108, 121, 133, 182.

GOULD, JEAN. *Winslow Homer.* New York: Dodd, Mead & Co., 1962, p. 260. [Gould states that Winslow Homer's picture "The Lookout," which he had priced at $850 "was hailed as a 'great painting' by the most discerning of critics, Sadakichi Hartmann, and (Thomas B.) Clarke bought it soon afterward."]

GRIFFIN, G. TAYLOR. "Reply to Sidney Allan's Open Letter." *Wilson's Photog. Mag.* 44 (June 1907):248. [Allan's ltr. appears in the same issue.]

HAGELL, EDGAR. "Reply to Sidney Allan's Open Letter." *Wilson's Photog. Mag.* 44 (July 1907):336. [Allan's ltr. appears in the same issue.]

HARRIS, TOM. "Portrait of Sadakichi Hartmann." Also listed in "The American Pictorial Photographs for the International Art Exhibition at Glasgow." *Camera Notes* 4 (Apr. 1901):275. [Photograph.]

HARTMANN, NURVA. "How I Made My First Pictures." *The Camera* 14 (June 1910):247–50. [Hartmann undoubtedly gave his twelve-year-old daughter help in writing this article.]

"Hartmann's *Composition in Portraiture.*" *Bull. of Photog. and the Photographer* 5 (17 Nov. 1909):317. [Advertisement.]

HILEY, MICHAEL. "The Photographer as Artist." *Studio International* 190 (July-August 1975):10–11.

HOLLINGER, WILLIAM M. "Portrait of Sidney Allan." *Saint Louis and Canadian Photog.* 19 (Oct. 1905):facing p. 447. [Photograph only.]

———. "Portrait of Sidney Allan." *Wilson's Photog. Mag.* 42 (Dec. 1905):facing p. 537. [Photograph only.]

———. "Portrait of Sidney Allan." *Sadakichi Hartmann Newsletter* 4 (Spring 1973):1. [Photograph.]

HOMER, WILLIAM INNES. Alfred *Stieglitz* and the American Avant-Garde, Boston: New York Graphic Society, 1977, pp. 26, 37, 48, 67, 68, 78, 282.

HORR, ALEXANDER S. "Sadakichi Hartmann as a Photographic Writer." *Photo-Beacon* 16 (Oct. 1904):307–09.

HULL, ROGER P. "Hartmann in *Camera Work:* A Bibliography." *Sadakichi Hartmann Newsletter* 1 (Fall 1970):1–3.

———. "Nature Writings of Sadakichi Hartmann." *Sadakichi Hartmann Newsletter* 5 (Spring 1975):1–4.

———. "The Stieglitz-Hartmann Letters: The Toy Balloonist and the Great Aerialist." *Sadakichi Hartmann Newsletter* 2 (Fall 1971):1–6.

———. *Poetry and Politics in American Photography: The Forgotten Story of Rudolf Eickemeyer, Jr.* [Unpublished ms. in the author's possession, Department of Art, Willamette University.]

———. "Rudolph Eickemeyer, Jr. and the Politics of the

Photo Secession. *New Mexico Studies in the Fine Arts.* [In press.]

JUHL, ERNST. "The Jubilee Exhibition at the Hamburg Art Galleries," transl. by Mrs. S. H., *Camera Work*, No. 5 (Jan. 1905):46–49. [The translator of this German review was Hartmann's first wife, Elizabeth Blanche Walsh.]

KÄSEBIER, GERTRUDE. Photograph of Sadakichi Hartmann. *In: The Woman's Eye.* Ed., with an introd. by Anne Tucker. New York: Alfred A. Knopf, 1973, p. 27.

KEILEY, J. T. "The Philadelphia Salon. Its Origin and Influence." *Camera Notes* 2 (Jan. 1899):125.

KLINTWORTH, C. VERNE. "A Florida Photographer Recalls Sadakichi." *Sadakichi Hartmann Newsletter* 1 (Fall 1970):4.

KNOX, GEORGE, and HARRY W. LAWTON (eds.). "Introduction." *Buddha, Confucius, Christ: Three Prophetic Plays.* By Sadakichi Hartmann. New York: Herder and Herder, 1971. [On photography see specifically pp. xi-xii, xiv.]

———. (eds.) *The Life and Times of Sadakichi Hartmann, 1867–1944.* Riverside: University of California Library, 1970. [On photography see pp. 2–17 passim.]

LAWTON, HARRY, and GEORGE KNOX (eds.). "Introduction." *White Chrysanthemums: Literary Fragments and Pronouncements.* By Sadakichi Hartmann. Foreword by Kenneth Rexroth. New York: Herder and Herder, 1971. [On photography see pp. ix, xx-xxi.]

LYONS, NATHAN, (ed.). *Photographers on Photography.* Englewood Cliffs, New Jersey: Prentice-Hall, 1966, p. 13. In Collaboration with the George Eastman House, Rochester, New York.

MacDONALD, PIRIE. "Criticism." *Wilson's Photog. Mag.* 45 (Aug. 1908):338.

MADDOX, JERALD C. "Photography in the First Decade." *Art in America* 61 (July-August 1973):72–79. [See especially pp. 77–78, in which Hartmann's review of the exhibition in 1910 at Buffalo's Albright Museum is quoted.]

MADIGAN, MARY JEAN. "Rudolf Eickemeyer, Jr.—A Biographical Appreciation." *Photography of Rudolf Eickemeyer, Jr. Hudson River Museum. March 12-April 30, 1972.* [Catalogue of the Exhibition.] Yonkers, New York: The Hudson River Museum, 1972, pp. 1, 7, 9, 19, 30. [Hartmann is quoted and cited in the catalogue's bibliography.]

MAETERLINCK, MAURICE. "Maurice Maeterlinck on Photography." *American Amateur Photog.* 15 (Nov. 1903):510. [Hartmann's translation of "Message from

Maurice Maeterlinck," which appeared in *Camera Work*, No. 2 (Apr. 1903).]

———. "Message from Maurice Maeterlinck" *Camera Work*, No. 2 (Apr. 1903). [Unpaginated.] [Transl. by Sadakichi Hartmann. This letter from Maeterlinck arrived too late to be incorporated in *Camera Work*, No. 2 and was circulated in *Camera Work*, No. 3 for insertion in *Camera Work*, No. 2.]

———. "Message from Maurice Maeterlinck." *Camera Work*, No. 14 (Apr. 1906). [Unpaginated.] [Transl. by Sadakichi Hartmann.]

———. "Message from Maurice Maeterlinck." *Camera Work*, No. 37 (Jan. 1912), pp. 41–42. [Transl. by Sadakichi Hartmann.]

MITCHELL, J. D. "Correspondence. 'The Open Letter.' " *The Photographer* 7 (25 June 1907):140. [Response to Sidney Allan's ltr. in June 11 issue.]

NEWHALL, BEAUMONT. *The History of Photography.* New York: The Museum of Modern Art in Collaboration with the George Eastman House, 1949, p. 138.

———. *The History of Photography From 1839 to the Present Day.* New York: The Museum of Modern Art in Collaboration with the George Eastman House, 1964. Revised and enlarged edition, p. 109.

NEWHALL, NANCY, (ed.). *The Daybooks of Edward Weston. Vol. I: Mexico.* Rochester: George Eastman House, 1962, p. 142.

———. (ed.). *The Daybooks of Edward Weston. Vol. II: California.* New York: Horizon Press, 1961, pp. 60, 61. In Collaboration with the George Eastman House.

NICOL, JOHN. "Personal." *American Amateur Photog.* 16 (Oct. 1904):427–28. [The editor of the magazine apologizes to readers for the handling of Roland Rood's "Three Factors" article. See Rood, Roland.]

NUSSBAUMER, J. GEO. "Correspondence [.] 'The Open Letter.' " *The Photographer* 7 (25 June 1907):140–41. [Response to Sidney Allan's ltr. in the June 11 issue.]

OTA, SABURO. "Sadakichi Hartmann: A Colorful Eccentric With Talent." *Gakuen*, No. 384 (Dec. 1971), pp. 2–16. [In Japanese.]

"Painters and the Public." The New York *Evening Sun.* Vol. 20, No. 259 (14 Jan. 1907):8, cols. 2–3. [Editorial in which Hartmann is mentioned.]

"Painters and the Public." *Wilson's Photog. Mag.* 44 (Feb. 1907):51–52. [Reprint of preceding citation.]

PECK, CHARLES L. Portrait of Lillian Bonham [Hartmann's second wife] by photographer Charles L. Peck, Buffalo, New York. "Special Supplement to *Abel's Photographic*

Weekly." *Abel's Photog. Weekly* 9 (17 Feb. 1912):593. [Miss Bonham poses satirically as "Whistler's Mother."]

PHILLIPS, RYLAND W. "Reply to Sidney Allan's Open Letter." *Wilson's Photog. Mag.* 44 (June 1907):248. [Allan's ltr. appears in the same issue.]

PLAGENS, PETER. "The Critics: Hartmann, Huneker, De Casseres." *Art in America* 61 (July-August 1973):66–71. [Hartmann is called "the most compelling and tragic figure. . . . "]

POLLACK, PETER. *The Picture History of Photography.* Revised and enlarged edition. New York: Harry N. Abrams, 1969, pp. 263, 273.

"Program of the W.Va. Convention to be Held in Wheeling, Oct. 9-10-11, 1912." *Abel's Photog. Weekly* 10 (28 Sept. 1912):293–94.

REEDY, W. M. "J. C. Strauss—A Kindly Caricature." *Camera Craft* 11 (Aug. 1905):74–75. [Reprinted from Reedy's *St. Louis Mirror.*]

———. "Kindly Caricatures—J. C. Strauss." *In: 'Appreciation of J. C. Strauss as a Photographer.* [A pamphlet, n.d., n.p.; also contains Hartmann's essay "The Man Behind the Gun—J. C. Strauss," pp. 6–8].

ROCKWOOD, GEO. G. "Correspondence." *Bull. of Photog. and the Photographer* 5 (10 Nov. 1909):295.

ROOD, ROLAND. "A Retrospect." *The Burr McIntosh Monthly* 18 (Dec. 1908):6 pp.

———. "Letter to the Editor." *American Amateur Photog.* 16 (Oct. 1904):421. [Rood repudiates the authorship of his article "The Three Factors in American Pictorial Photography."]

———. "The Three Factors in American Pictorial Photography." *American Amateur Photog.* 15 (Aug. 1904):346–49. [The three "factors" are Stieglitz, Eickemeyer, and Hartmann. Rood repudiated the article in the ltr. above.]

ROSE, BARBARA (ed.). *Readings in American Art Since 1900.* New York: Frederick A. Praeger, 1967, pp. 4, 50–53. [Includes excerpts from Hartmann's essays "Puritanism, Its Grandeur and Shame" and "The American Picture World, Its Shows and Shams."]

RUBINCAM, HARRY C. "Caliban." *The Photographer* 2 (19 Nov. 1904):52–53.

———. "A Letter to the Editor of *Camera Craft.*" *Camera Craft* 10 (Mar. 1905):184–85.

———. "Pointed Paragraphs." *Camera Craft* 10 (Mar. 1905):153–55.

———. "The Photo-Secession and the First American Salon." *American Amateur Photog.* 17 (Mar. 1905):149–50. [Letter to the editor.]

SCHARF, AARON. *Art and Photography.* Allen Lane: The Penguin Press, 1968, p. 277.

SMITH, CLARENCE H. "Reply to Sidney Allan's Open Letter." *Wilson's Photog. Mag.* 44 (June 1907):247–48. [Allan's ltr. appears in the same issue.]

STEICHEN, EDUARD J. "Photo: 'Sadakichi Hartmann.'" *Camera Work,* No. 7 (July 1904), p. 49.

"Portrait of Sadakichi Hartmann." *In: A Collection of American Pictorial Photographs by the Photo-Secession and Exhibited under the Auspices of the Capital [sic] Camera Club at the Corcoran Art Galleries at Washington January MDCCCCIV.* [Catalogue of the exhibition. The Hartmann photograph is number 125 of the exhibition. For materials related to the exhibition, see *Camera Work,* No. 6 (Apr. 1904), pp. 39–40 and pp. 45–46.]

STIEGLITZ, ALFRED. "A New Journal." *Camera Craft* 5 (Sept. 1902):204.

[TENNANT, JOHN.] "Books and Prints." *Photo-Miniature* 9 (Feb. 1909):94. [Reviews *Composition in Portraiture.*]

———. "Books and Prints." *Photo-Miniature* 10 (Sept. 1910):199. [Review of Hartmann's *Landscape and Figure Composition.*]

———. "Notes." *Photo-Miniature* 1 (July 1899):203. [Review of *Camera Notes,* Vol. 3, No. 1.]

———. "Notes and Comment." *Photo-Miniature* 10 (Feb. 1912):536.

———. "Notes and Comment." *Photo-Miniature* 6 (July 1904):232–33. [Review of September *Metropolitan Magazine,* including a Sidney Allan article.]

———. "Notes and Comment." *Photo-Miniature* 12 (Nov. 1915):563–64.

———. "Posing the Figure in Portraiture." *Photo-Miniature* 12 (Jan. 1915):179–80.

THE OFFICE BOY. "'Camera Work' for October—An Appreciation." *Photo-Era* 11 (Dec. 1903):360, 371–72.

———. "'Camera Work' for October—An Appreciation." *Image* 15 (July 1972):25–28. [Reprint of the preceding.]

THOREK, MAX. *Creative Camera Art.* Canton, Ohio: Fomo Publishing Company, 1937, p. 110. [In the chapter "Purism Versus Control in Photography," Thorek cites Hartmann as a dogmatist. "There are many victims of dogmatism. To cite: Sadakichi Hartmann believes that portraits *must* be made in only one way and that backgrounds must have only certain characteristics and that composition must be limited."]

TUCKER, KAY. *The Educated Innocent Eye: Some Criteria for the Criticism of Photography.* Berkeley, Calif.: The Image Circle, Inc., 1972.

———. "Sadakichi's Impact on Photography." *Sadakichi Hartmann Newsletter* 5 (Summer 1974):1–3.

VANCE, ADRIAN. "West Coast." *Popular Photog.* 77 (Nov. 1975):42, 76. [Hartmann collection at University of California, Riverside, mentioned in connection with UCR's growing collection of cameras and photographic equipment.]

WALSH, ELIZABETH BLANCHE. "Letter to the Editor of the [New York] *Sun*." *Photo-Miniature* 7 (Oct. 1905):43. [A ltr. by Hartmann's first wife.]
———. See JUHL, ERNST.
WARD, W. E. "The Cult of the Godlings." *Wilson's Photog. Mag.* 37 (July 1900):292–99. [A hostile attack on Hartmann's criticism and the new American photography.]
———. "The Cult of the Godlings." *British Jour. of Photog.* 47 (3 Aug. 1900):487–90. [Reprinted from *Wilson's Photog. Mag.* of July 1900.]
WESTON, EDWARD. "Photograph of Sadakichi Hartmann." *In:* "Weston to Hagemeyer: New York Notes." Center for Creative Photography, No. 3 (Nov. 1976):15.
WILSON, E. L. "American Photography." *Wilson's Photog. Mag.* 37 (July 1900):289.
———. "American Photography." *British Jour. of Photog.* 47 (3 Aug. 1900):48. [Reprint of the preceding.]

ZIMMERMAN, WALTER. "Another Letter to the Editor." *Camera Craft* 10 (Apr. 1905):246–48.

INDEX OF NAMES